The Oxford Handbook of Cognitive
and Behavioral Therapies

OXFORD LIBRARY OF PSYCHOLOGY

OXFORD LIBRARY OF PSYCHOLOGY

Editor in Chief **PETER E. NATHAN**

The Oxford Handbook of Cognitive and Behavioral Therapies

Edited by

Christine Maguth Nezu

Arthur M. Nezu

OXFORD
UNIVERSITY PRESS

OXFORD
UNIVERSITY PRESS

Oxford University Press is a department of the University of
Oxford. It furthers the University's objective of excellence in research,
scholarship, and education by publishing worldwide.

Oxford   New York
Auckland   Cape Town   Dar es Salaam   Hong Kong   Karachi
Kuala Lumpur   Madrid   Melbourne   Mexico City   Nairobi
New Delhi   Shanghai   Taipei   Toronto

With offices in
Argentina   Austria   Brazil   Chile   Czech Republic   France   Greece
Guatemala   Hungary   Italy   Japan   Poland   Portugal   Singapore
South Korea   Switzerland   Thailand   Turkey   Ukraine   Vietnam

Oxford is a registered trademark of Oxford University Press
in the UK and certain other countries.

Published in the United States of America by
Oxford University Press
198 Madison Avenue, New York, NY 10016

Library of Congress Cataloging-in-Publication Data
The Oxford handbook of cognitive and behavioral therapies / edited by Christine Maguth Nezu, Arthur M. Nezu.
    pages cm. — (Oxford library of psychology)
Includes bibliographical references and index.
ISBN 978–0–19–973325–5 (alk. paper)
1. Cognitive therapy.   I. Nezu, Christine M., editor.   II. Nezu, Arthur M., editor.
RC489.C63O96 2015
616.89′1425—dc23
2015019572

9 8 7 6 5 4 3 2 1
Printed in the United States of America
on acid-free paper

We dedicate this book to our grandchildren, Alex, Jacob, Maxwell, and Elle. May you learn, grow, and flourish in your life dreams.

SHORT CONTENTS

The *Oxford Library of Psychology*, a landmark series of handbooks, is published by Oxford University Press, one of the world's oldest and most highly respected publishers, with a tradition of publishing significant books in psychology. The ambitious goal of the *Oxford Library of Psychology* is nothing less than to span a vibrant, wide-ranging field and, in so doing, to fill a clear market need.

Encompassing a comprehensive set of handbooks, organized hierarchically, the *Library* incorporates volumes at different levels, each designed to meet a distinct need. At one level are a set of handbooks designed broadly to survey the major subfields of psychology; at another are numerous handbooks that cover important current focal research and scholarly areas of psychology in depth and detail. Planned as a reflection of the dynamism of psychology, the *Library* will grow and expand as psychology itself develops, thereby highlighting significant new research that will impact on the field. Adding to its accessibility and ease of use, the *Library* will be published in print and, later on, electronically.

The *Library* surveys psychology's principal subfields with a set of handbooks that capture the current status and future prospects of those major subdisciplines. This initial set includes handbooks of social and personality psychology, clinical psychology, counseling psychology, school psychology, educational psychology, industrial and organizational psychology, cognitive psychology, cognitive neuroscience, methods and measurements, history, neuropsychology, personality assessment, developmental psychology, and more. Each handbook undertakes to review one of psychology's major subdisciplines with breadth, comprehensiveness, and exemplary scholarship. In addition to these broadly conceived volumes, the *Library* also includes a large number of handbooks designed to explore in depth more specialized areas of scholarship and research, such as stress, health and coping, anxiety and related disorders, cognitive development, or child and adolescent assessment. In contrast to the broad coverage of the subfield handbooks, each of these latter volumes focuses on an especially productive, more highly focused line of scholarship and research. Whether at the broadest or most specific level, however, all of the *Library* handbooks offer synthetic coverage that reviews and evaluates the relevant past and present research and anticipates research in the future. Each handbook in the *Library* includes introductory and concluding chapters written by its editor to provide a roadmap to the handbook's table of contents and to offer informed anticipations of significant future developments in that field.

An undertaking of this scope calls for handbook editors and chapter authors who are established scholars in the areas about which they write. Many of the nation's and world's most productive and best-respected psychologists have agreed to edit *Library* handbooks or write authoritative chapters in their areas of expertise.

For whom has the *Oxford Library of Psychology* been written? Because of its breadth, depth, and accessibility, the *Library* serves a diverse audience, including graduate students in psychology and their faculty mentors, scholars, researchers, and practitioners in psychology and related fields. All will find in the *Library* the information they seek on the subfield or focal area of psychology in which they work or are interested.

Befitting its commitment to accessibility, each handbook includes a comprehensive index, as well as extensive references to help guide research. And because the *Library* was designed from its inception as an online as well as a print resource, its structure and contents will be readily and rationally searchable online. Further, once the *Library* is released online, the handbooks will be regularly and thoroughly updated.

In summary, the *Oxford Library of Psychology* will grow organically to provide a thoroughly informed perspective on the field of psychology, one that reflects both psychology's dynamism and its increasing interdisciplinarity. Once published electronically, the *Library* is also destined to become a uniquely valuable interactive tool, with extended search and browsing capabilities. As you begin to consult this handbook, we sincerely hope you will share our enthusiasm for the more than 500-year tradition of Oxford University Press for excellence, innovation, and quality, as exemplified by the *Oxford Library of Psychology.*

Peter E. Nathan
Editor-in-Chief
Oxford Library of Psychology

Christine Maguth Nezu

Christine Maguth Nezu, PhD, ABPP, is professor of psychology in the College of Arts and Sciences and professor of medicine in the School of Medicine at Drexel University. She has maintained a private practice as a licensed psychologist for over 25 years and is board-certified by the American Board of Professional Psychology (ABPP) in clinical as well as in cognitive and behavioral psychology. She is also a program consultant to the Department of Veterans Affairs in Washington, DC, as well as a program consultant for the Joint Programs of the Departments of Veterans Affairs and Defense, and a past president of the ABPP. She is a fellow of the American Academy of Cognitive and Behavioral Psychology, the Academy of Clinical Psychology, and the Academy of Cognitive Therapy, and she is the recipient of the 2014 ABPP Award for Distinguished Contributions.

Dr. Maguth Nezu has authored or coauthored over 125 scholarly publications, including 18 books, and is the coeditor of several distinguished book series. Her publications cover a wide range of topics in mental health and behavioral medicine, many of which have been translated into a variety of foreign languages. She is considered an international expert regarding cognitive-behavioral assessment and treatment, and embraces an evidence-based approach to clinical intervention, advocating the use of an individual case formulation as a bridge between science and practice.

Dr. Maguth Nezu was also a member of the board of directors for the Association for Behavioral and Cognitive Therapies and a representative for that organization to the World Congress Committee for Cognitive and Behavioral Therapies. She was a board member and representative to ABPP for the Academy of Cognitive & Behavioral Psychology and received the 2011 ABPP Award for Outstanding Contributions to the Specialty of Cognitive and Behavioral Psychology, which was jointly sponsored by the Cognitive & Behavioral Board and Academy.

Although her contributions cover many areas of clinical psychology, it is her collective work as the codeveloper of contemporary problem-solving therapy and its current application as a transdiagnostic and evidence-based intervention, as well as to programs for both active service members and veterans, that has brought her national and international recognition.

With regard to this level of recognition, Dr. Nezu has served as a distinguished visiting professor, consultant, and trainer for the US Air Force, the FBI, and for universities around the world and served on the editorial board of several professional journals in the United States and abroad.

Arthur M. Nezu

Arthur M. Nezu, PhD, DHL (Hon.), ABPP, is distinguished university professor of psychology, professor of medicine, and professor of community health and prevention at Drexel University in Philadelphia. He is the current editor of the *Journal of Consulting and Clinical Psychology*, a current associate editor for the *Archives of Scientific Psychology*, and past editor of *The Behavior Therapist*. Dr. Nezu previously was president of the Association for the Advancement of Behavior Therapy (ABCT; now known as the Association of Behavioral and Cognitive Therapies), the American Board of Cognitive and Behavioral Psychology (ABCBP), and the Behavioral Psychology Specialty Council. He also served as chair of the board of directors of the World Congress of Behavioural and Cognitive Therapies (WCBCT) and trustee and secretary of the American Board of Professional Psychology (ABPP). Dr. Nezu is board certified by ABPP in cognitive and behavioral psychology, clinical psychology, and clinical health psychology. He is a fellow of multiple professional organizations, including the American Psychological Association (APA), the American Psychological Society, the Society of Behavior Medicine, and the Academy of Cognitive Therapy.

Dr. Nezu has received awards from the WCBCT, ABCBP, ABCT, and the American Academy of Cognitive and Behavioral Psychology. An annual award for an outstanding doctoral dissertation in diversity was named in his honor by the ABPP. Dr. Nezu received an honorary doctoral degree from the Philadelphia College of Osteopathic Medicine and recently received the Florence Halpern Award for Distinguished Professional Contributions to Clinical Psychology by the Society of Clinical Psychology (Division 12 of the American Psychological Association). He is the codeveloper of contemporary problem-solving therapy, which is considered an evidenced-based intervention by numerous professional and government organizations. His research has been sponsored by the Veterans Administration, the National Cancer Institute, and the National Institute of Mental Health. Dr. Nezu has also served as a research and clinical consultant to numerous national and international academic institutions, as well as US government agencies, including the Department of Veterans Affairs and the Department of Defense. He has published over 200 research and professional journals articles and book chapters, as well as 22 books on a wide variety of topics.

CONTRIBUTORS

Michelle M. Braun, PhD, ABPP
Department of Neurology and
  Neurosurgery
Wheaton Franciscan Healthcare—All Saint's

Jacqueline R. Bullis, MA
Center for Anxiety and Related Disorders
Boston University

James J. Collard, DPsych, GradDipPsych
Cognitive Behaviour Therapy Australia
Cairnmillar Institute

Richard J. Contrada, PhD
Department of Psychology
Rutgers, The State University of New Jersey

Mike J. Crawford, MD
Centre for Mental Health
Imperial College London, UK

Sara B. Danitz, MA
Psychology Department
Suffolk University

Lee J. Dixon, PhD
Department of Psychology
University of Dayton

Gareth R. Dutton, PhD
Department of Medicine
Division of Preventive Medicine
University of Alabama at Birmingham

Kyle E. Ferguson, PhD
St. Peter Family Medicine and University
  of Washington

Audrey File, MA
University of Tennessee

Edna B. Foa, PhD
Center for the Treatment and Study
  of Anxiety
University of Pennsylvania

Seth J. Gillihan, PhD
Department of Psychology
Haverford College

Kristina Coop Gordon, PhD
Department of Psychology
University of Tennessee–Knoxville

Alexandra P. Greenfield, BS
Department of Psychology
Drexel University

Gordon C. Nagayama Hall
Department of Psychology
Center on Diversity and Community
University of Oregon

Stephen N. Haynes, PhD
Department of Psychology
University of Hawaii at Manoa

Bridget A. Hearon, PhD
Department of Psychology
McLean Hospital and Harvard
  Medical School

Stefan G. Hofmann, PhD
Department of Psychological and Brain
  Sciences
Boston University

Derek R. Hopko, PhD
Department of Psychology
The University of Tennessee

Alicia Yee Ibaraki
Department of Psychology
University of Oregon

Suzanne Jolley, PhD
Department of Psychology
Institute of Psychiatry, Psychology and
  Neuroscience
King's College London

Joseph Keawe'aimoku Kaholokula, PhD
Department of Native Hawaiian Health
John A. Burns School of Medicine
University of Hawaii at Manoa

Bradley E. Karlin, PhD, ABPP
Education Development Center, Inc.
Department of Mental Health, Bloomberg
  School of Public Health
Johns Hopkins University
School of Nursing, Bouvé College of
  Health Sciences
Northeastern University

Philip C. Kendall, PhD, ABPP
Child and Adolescent Anxiety
  Disorders Clinic
Department of Psychology
Temple University

Megan Kirouac, MS
Department of Psychology
Center on Alcoholism, Substance Abuse,
  and Addictions
University of New Mexico

Elizabeth Kuipers, PhD
Department of Psychology
Institute of Psychiatry, Psychology and
  Neuroscience
King's College London

Marsha M. Linehan, PhD, ABPP
Department of Psychology
Department of Psychiatry
University of Washington
Behavioral Research and Therapy Clinics

James K. Luiselli, Ed.D., ABPP, BCBA-D,
Department of Applied Research, Clinical
  Training, and Peer Review
May Institute

Anita Lungu, PhD
Behavioral Research and Therapy Clinics
University of Washington

Sarah L. Mann, MS
Department of Psychology
Rutgers, The State University of New Jersey

Crystal McIndoo, PhD
Department of Psychology
The University of Tennessee

Mary McMurran, PhD
Institute of Mental Health
University of Nottingham, UK

Bryon G. Miller, MA, BCBA
Department of Child and Family Studies
University of South Florida

Raymond G. Miltenberger, PhD, BCBA-D
Department of Child and Family Studies
University of South Florida

Matthew Mychailyszyn, PhD
Department of Psychology
Towson University
Division of Psychology and
  Neuropsychology
Mt. Washington Pediatric Hospital

Cory F. Newman, PhD, ABPP
Center for Cognitive Therapy
University of Pennsylvania, Perelman
  School of Medicine

Arthur M. Nezu, PhD, (Hon.) DHL, ABPP
Departments of Psychology, Medicine, and
  Community Health and Prevention
Drexel University

Christine Maguth Nezu, PhD, ABPP
Departments of Psychology
  and Medicine
Drexel University

William H. O'Brien, PhD
Department of Psychology
Bowling Green State University

William T. O'Donohue, PhD
Department of Psychology
University of Nevada, Reno

**Monica E. O'Kelly, Dip Ed, MBSc,
PhD, FAPS**
Cognitive Behaviour Therapy Australia
Monash University

Kelly A. O'Neil Rodriguez, PhD
Child and Adolescent Anxiety
  Disorders Clinic
Department of Psychology
Temple University

Juliana Onwumere, DClinPsy, PhD
Department of Psychology, Institute of
  Psychiatry, Psychology and
  Neuroscience
King's College London, UK
The National Psychosis Unit, South
  London and Maudsley NHS
  Foundation Trust, London, UK

Susan M. Orsillo, PhD
Psychology Department
Suffolk University
Michael W. Otto, PhD
Center for Anxiety and Related Disorders
Boston University
Michael G. Perri, PhD, ABPP
Department of Clinical and Health
Psychology
College of Public Health and Health
Professions
University of Florida
Jeremy S. Peterman, MA
Child and Adolescent Anxiety
Disorders Clinic
Department of Psychology
Temple University
Sarah Ricelli, MS
Department of Psychology
Drexel University
C. Steven Richards, PhD
Department of Psychological Sciences
Texas Tech University
Lizabeth Roemer, PhD
Psychology Department
University of Massachusetts Boston

Marlena M. Ryba, PhD
The University of Tennessee
Jessica B. Stern, MS
Department of Psychology
Drexel University
Marianne A. Villabø, PhD
Center for Child and Adolescent
Mental Health
Oslo, Norway
Katie Wischkaemper, PhD
Department of Psychology
University of Tennessee-Knoxville
Katie Witkiewitz, PhD
Department of Psychology
Center on Alcoholism, Substance Abuse,
and Addictions
University of New Mexico
Antonette Zeiss, PhD
Office Mental Health Services
Department of Veterans Affairs
Central Office
(Retired)
Heather M. Zerger, MA
Department of Child and Family Studies
University of South Florida

CONTENTS

The Oxford Handbook of Cognitive
and Behavioral Therapies

Introduction

Christine Maguth Nezu *and* Arthur M. Nezu

Abstract

This introductory chapter presents an overview of *The Oxford Handbook of Cognitive and Behavioral Therapies.* We delineate a definition of this specialty area of psychology as well as describe the purpose of this particular volume of the Oxford Library of Psychology series. We provide a description of the Handbook including its 26 chapters and present them under the following section headings: Conceptual Foundations, Major Cognitive and Behavioral Therapy Approaches, Major Psychological Problems and Populations, and Special Topics. The contributors of the chapters in each section of the volume represent the most prominent names in the field regarding cognitive and behavioral theory and research and evidence-based clinical treatment in the specialty area.

Key Words: cognitive and behavioral therapies, behavior therapy, cognitive therapy, clinical psychology, psychotherapy, intervention

It is important at the outset, especially to those only somewhat familiar with this particular area of psychology, to distinguish between cognitive-behavioral therapy (CBT) and cognitive and behavioral therapies (C&BT). The acronym *CBT*, which is often used as the shorthand term to identify this group of clinical interventions, should not be viewed as a single therapeutic strategy. Instead, it is the umbrella term for an expanding cadre of treatment approaches that share a common history and worldview (Nezu, Nezu, & Lombardo, 2004). For instance, in their "CBT" encyclopedic compendium, O'Donohue, Fisher, and Hayes (2003) include descriptions of over 65 differing cognitive and behavioral techniques (see also Freeman, Felgoise, Nezu, Nezu, & Reinecke, 2005). As such, we use the nomenclature of cognitive and behavioral therapies (C&BT) in this handbook's title to more accurately describe this area of applied psychology.

This important distinction is apparent by simply viewing the actual names of the various major professional organizations that focus on this theoretical orientation. For example, the major international organization is called the World Congress of Behavioural and Cognitive Therapies. The name of the largest North American association is the Association of Behavioral and Cognitive Therapies. The United States national credentialing organization that awards the diplomate (i.e., board certification) in this area of psychological specialization is named the American Board of Cognitive and Behavioral Psychology. The major European organization is named the European Association of Behavioural and Cognitive Therapies, and so forth. As such, the acronym *C&BT* used in this chapter refers to the myriad of various cognitive and behavioral treatment strategies as compared to a singular intervention. Note that the order C&BT, rather than B&CT, is used purely for convention purposes, rather than suggesting the primacy or importance of one type or set of strategies over the other.

What Is C&BT?

We define C&BT as a worldview that emphasizes an empirical approach to assessment, case conceptualization, intervention, and evaluation regarding human problems (Nezu et al., 2004). It is a conceptual framework to help us understand, based on the scientific literature, both "normal" and "abnormal" aspects of human behavior, as well as to articulate a set of empirically based guidelines by which such behavior can be changed. It can be said that an overall C&BT approach easily falls within an experimental clinical framework that incorporates a broad definition of human (and, where relevant, animal) functioning that focuses on the role of overt actions, internal cognitive phenomena, the experience of affect, underlying neurobiological activities, and social interactions. These components can range in complexity from molecular events, such as smoking a cigarette, hyperventilation, or a critical comment made by a spouse, to more molar and multidimensional constructs, such as complex social skills or attempts to manage relationships or cope with traumatic stressors.

During its birth and adolescence, the field of behavior therapy was defined as the application of "modern laws of learning" (e.g., Hersen, Eisler, & Miller, 1975) and included clinical interventions that were based on operant (e.g., token economies) and classical (e.g., systematic desensitization) conditioning paradigms. It initially emerged from the philosophical framework of behaviorism, which traditionally focused exclusively on events and behaviors that were observable and objectively quantifiable. A major hallmark of this approach was its insistence on the empirical verification of its various interventions, which continues as a fundamental precept in C&BT.

However, during the early 1970s, behavior therapy, along with psychology in general, underwent a partial paradigm shift, whereby a "cognitive revolution," in part, influenced traditional behavioral researchers and clinicians to underscore the mediational role that cognitive processes could play regarding behavior (Miller, 2003). This shift suggested that cognitive mechanisms of action in their own right should serve as meaningful targets for change. These cognitive processes included self-control mechanisms, self-efficacy beliefs, social problem solving, negative self-schemas, and irrational beliefs. As such, during the past 20–40 years, the domain, concepts, and methods of this overarching approach have continued to expand greatly to incorporate a myriad of both behavioral and cognitive therapy

strategies (Nezu et al., 2004). Since its nascent stages as based in experimental bases of behavior and conditioning theories, C&BT has been a dynamic and evolving approach to treatment and, more recently, has incorporated perspectives of early emotional learning experiences, contextual change, theories of evolution, and neurobiology. Some people in the field have referred to this as the emergence of "third wave" of treatment strategies. For example, Hayes has characterized this recent evolution in the field as involving an "openness to older clinical traditions, a focus on second order and contextual change, an emphasis of function over form, and the combination of flexible and effective repertoires" (Hayes, 2004, p. 639).[1] We endeavor to include descriptions of many of the full breadth of various cognitive and behavioral interventions in this handbook.

Why Focus on C&BT?

Not only is there increasing evidence that multiple C&BT approaches are considered evidenced based or empirically supported, as demonstrated throughout this handbook, but psychotherapy experts continue to predict that many strategies subsumed under the C&BT umbrella will increase in usage by health and mental health professional in the future (Norcross, Pfund, & Prochaska, 2013). As such, it seems reasonable to suggest that a handbook focused on this approach is relevant and useful.

Structure of This Handbook

This volume is organized into four major sections containing a total of 26 chapters. Part I consists of four chapters that address various conceptual foundations underlying C&BT broadly defined. In Chapter 2, O'Donohue and Ferguson provide a general overview of the theoretical and philosophical underpinnings of C&BT and begin by echoing the idea set forth earlier that "contemporary cognitive-behavioral therapy is not monolithic." In line with the competency movement in professional psychology, we define the specialty of cognitive and behavioral psychology in Chapter 3. Moreover, we describe the various functional and foundational core competencies that comprise this area of specialization in psychology. An integral partner to C&BT interventions is behavioral assessment. In Chapter 4, O'Brien and colleagues describe the conceptual foundations of this form of assessment, which features the functional analysis. In Chapter 5, we advocate and describe a problem-solving-based model of case conceptualization that clinicians can use as a "roadmap" when attempting to integrate the available scientific literature in order to design a C&BT ideographic intervention for a given client.

Part II focuses on describing the various major C&BT interventions and treatment approaches. Historically tied more to a behavioral approach that initially was based on an operant conditioning paradigm, Miltenberger and colleagues provide an overview of the field of applied behavior analysis in Chapter 6. In Chapter 7, Gillihan and Foa describe the principles that underlie exposure-based interventions for anxiety disorders among adults. Newman describes cognitive restructuring techniques that are central to the practice of cognitive therapy in Chapter 8. In Chapter 9, O'Kelly and Collard offer an overview of rational-emotive behavior therapy, an approach that focuses on disputing irrational demands and evaluations. We describe the conceptual underpinnings and clinical guidelines of contemporary problem-solving therapy in Chapter 10, an approach that teaches individuals a set of adaptive emotional regulation and problem-solving activities geared to foster their ability to cope effectively with stressful life events. Orsillo and colleagues, in Chapter 11, focus on the use of mindfulness and acceptance-based practices across certain C&BT interventions. Dialectical behavior therapy, as described by Lungu and Linehan in Chapter 12, was originally developed as a treatment for individuals with borderline personality disorders. Over the past few decades, it has emerged as an effective C&BT intervention to treat individuals with severe mental disorders. Chapter 13 focuses on relapse prevention strategies. Witkiewitz and Kirouac address such efforts that are geared to either prevent an initial lapse or to provide management tools if a lapse does occur. Hopko and colleagues describe behavioral activation, an approach that emphasizes structured attempts to increase overt behaviors in order to help bring individuals more into contact with reinforcing environmental contingencies in Chapter 14. The last chapter in this section on C&BT intervention approaches by Mann and Contrada addresses strategies geared to help reduce stress.

C&BT interventions have been successfully applied to a wide range of disorders, clinical problems, and patient populations. Part III contains chapters that address a particular problem or population and describes how various C&BT interventions have been applied as treatment approaches.

For example, in Chapter 16, Bullis and Hofmann describe how certain C&BT strategies have been used as treatments for a variety of adult anxiety disorders, including generalized anxiety disorder, obsessive-compulsive disorder, social anxiety disorder, panic disorder, specific phobias, and post-traumatic stress disorder. Richards, in Chapter 17, addresses how various C&BT interventions have been applied to treat major depressive disorder. Kuipers and colleagues focus on the treatment of psychosis in Chapter 18, whereas Braun and colleagues describe various treatments for older adults in Chapter 19. Kendall and his coauthors describe C&BT interventions for treating a variety of childhood and adolescent disorders in Chapter 20. In Chapter 21, Gordon and colleagues address how C&BT interventions have been applied for couples treatment. In Chapter 22, Luiselli provides an overview of how C&BT strategies have been used in the treatment of children and adults with developmental disabilities. Dutton and Perri, in Chapter 23, focus on the treatment of obesity, whereas McMurran and Crawford, in Chapter 24, describe the application of various C&BT interventions to help individuals diagnosed with various personality disorders.

The last section, Part IV, contains two chapters that have a specific focus. Hall and Ibaraki, in Chapter 25, provide a conceptual model for assessing an individual's goodness of fit with his or her sociocultural and cultural environments and for determining implications for C&BT interventions. In Chapter 26, Otto and Hearon address the issues, advantages, and liabilities involved in combining C&BT interventions with various forms of pharmacotherapy for the treatment of affective disorders.

Whereas the scope, relevance, importance, and breadth of the material contained in this handbook suggest that it could easily be expanded into a multivolume large encyclopedia, we attempted to provide concise overviews of the most important and timely information regarding C&BT. If we achieved this goal, it is truly because of the quality of the expertly written chapters themselves. As such, we wish to extend our deep gratitude to these contributors.

Note

1. It should be noted that multiple authors have criticized the use of the term "third wave," highlighting the idea that more similarities than differences exist between "traditional C&BT" interventions and those termed "third wave" approaches (e.g., Hofmann, 2008). See also Chapter 2 of this volume for a more detailed discussion of these issues.

References

Freeman, A., Felgoise, S. H., Nezu, A. M., Nezu, C. M., & Reinecke, M. A. (Eds.) (2005). *Encyclopedia of cognitive behavior therapy.* New York: Springer Publishing.

Hayes, S. C. (2004). Acceptance and commitment therapy, relational frame theory, and the third wave of behavioral and cognitive therapies. *Behavior Therapy, 35,* 639–665.

Hofmann, S. G. (2008). Acceptance and commitment therapy: New wave or Morita therapy? *Clinical Psychology: Science and Practice, 15,* 280–285.

Miller, G. A. (2003). The cognitive revolution: A historical perspective. *Trends in Cognitive Science, 7,* 141–144.

Nezu, A. M., Nezu, C. M., & Lombardo, E. R. (2004). *Cognitive-behavioral case formulation and treatment design: A problem-solving approach.* New York: Springer.

Norcross, J. C., Pfund, R. A., & Prochaska, J. O. (2013). Psychotherapy in 2022: A Delphi poll on its future. *Professional Psychology: Research and Practice, 44,* 363–370.

O'Donohue, W., Fisher, J. E., & Hayes, S. C. (Eds.). (2003). *Cognitive behavior therapy: Applying empirically supported techniques in your practice.* New York: Wiley.

PART 1

Conceptual Foundations

Historical and Philosophical Dimensions of Contemporary Cognitive-Behavioral Therapy

William T. O'Donohue *and* Kyle E. Ferguson

Abstract

Behavior therapy is heterogeneous and parallels what Wittgenstein called "family resemblances," as it is impossible to delineate necessary or sufficient definitional criteria for what constitutes behavior therapy or cognitive-behavioral therapy. Since its infancy, behavior therapy has been sometimes associated with one or more forms of behaviorism, the basic learning and/or cognitive principles, and a grab bag of practical ideas, as well as the varieties of problems it endeavors to solve, among many other complex relations. Behavior therapy has become increasingly intricate as it matures and, to some extent, has developed into what Kuhn (2001) termed "micro-communities." Subcommunities within behavior therapy employ different concepts, point to various influences, utilize different research methodologies, prioritize different problems, and incorporate diverse clinical strategies into routine practice. This chapter provides a general overview of the theoretical and philosophical underpinnings of behavior therapy.

Key Words: classical conditioning, operant conditioning, behavior therapy, cognitive therapy, cognitive-behavioral therapy, philosophy of science, scientific revolution, logical positivism, falsificationism, methodological anarchism

Contemporary cognitive-behavioral therapy is not monolithic. In this it shares a property with behavior therapy when it first emerged in the 1950s and 1960s: It, too, was heterogeneous in its infancy (Kazdin, 1978; O'Donohue et al., 2001). Currently, behavior therapy resides in the activities of tens of thousands of individuals who have (1) a diverse set of professional identities (although most are clinical psychologists); (2) a diverse set of interests that includes, but is not limited to, broad theoretical allegiances that can include applied behavior analysis, experimental analysis of behavior, radical behaviorism, cognitive therapy, experimental cognitive psychology, and neuroscience; (3) broad interests in certain kinds of systems of psychotherapy such as dialectical behavior therapy, behavioral activation, contemporary problem-solving therapy,

acceptance and commitment therapy, and mindfulness; (4) applied to a wide variety of problems and populations, including developmental delays, enuresis, oppositional defiant disorder, attention-deficit/hyperactivity disorder, depression, anxiety disorders, schizophrenia, obesity, chronic pain, dementia, marital problems, sexual deviance, sexual dysfunction, behavioral medicine, integrated care, psychotropic medications, children, adolescents, adults, the elderly, various cultural groups; and (5) a more difficult to classify but substantive set of additional interests that may include learning and conditioning, radical critics of psychiatry, prevention, social policy, management, single-subject experimental designs, statistics, behavioral genetics, personality, training and education, research methodologies, behavioral assessment, and functional analyses, among many others. Interested readers should consult the following archival sources for more complete definitions of cognitive, cognitive-behavioral, and behavioral psychology—developed by numerous consensus panels, representing many experts in cognitive, experimental, behavioral, and cognitive-behavioral psychology (American Board of Behavioral Psychology [ABBP]; American Board of Professional Psychology [ABPP]; Council of Specialties in Professional Psychology [CSPP]).

One can see that there are many permutations of these interests—so much so that it is really impossible to delineate any necessary or sufficient definitional criteria for what constitutes "behavior therapy" or "cognitive-behavioral therapy." Rather, it appears that this complexity is best captured by Wittgenstein's (2009) notion of "family resemblance." Wittgenstein famously argued that all words do not have simple definitional properties. Although the concept "brother" may be simply explicated as a male sibling, Wittgenstein argued that other terms—and there are many of these—cannot be defined in this manner. For example, more complex concepts such as "games" elude simple and straightforward definitions. Wittgenstein (2009) stated:

Consider for example the proceedings that we call "games." I mean board-games, card-games, ball-games, Olympic games, and so on. What is common to them all?

—Don't say: "There must be something common, or they would not be called 'games'"—but look and see whether there is anything common to all.

—For if you look at them you will not see something that is common to all, but similarities, relationships, and a whole series of them at that. To repeat: don't think, but look!

Look for example at board-games, with their multifarious relationships. Now pass to card-games; here you find many correspondences with the first group, but many common features drop out, and others appear. When we pass next to ball-games, much that is common is retained, but much is lost.

—Are they all "amusing"? Compare chess with noughts and crosses. Or is there always winning and losing, or competition between players? Think of patience. In ball games there is winning and losing; but when a child throws his ball at the wall and catches it again, this feature has disappeared. Look at the parts played by skill and luck; and at the difference between skill in chess and skill in tennis.

Think now of games like ring-a-ring-a-roses; here is the element of amusement, but how many other characteristic features have disappeared! And we can go through the many, many other groups of games in the same way; we can see how similarities crop up and disappear.

And the result of this examination is: we see a complicated network of similarities overlapping and criss-crossing: sometimes overall similarities.

I can think of no better expression to characterize these similarities than "family resemblances"; for the various resemblances between members of a family: build, features, colour of eyes, gait, temperament, etc. etc. overlap and criss-cross in the same way.—And I shall say: "games" form a family (pp. 66–67).

Thus, it may be the case that our conceptual analysis of "behavior therapy" reveals a similar complexity that Wittgenstein called "family resemblances." We must not have the simple model that we will always find simple necessary and sufficient properties. We can see these commonalities emerging and disappearing. Some good candidates for these commonalities can be found in the conceptual origins of cognitive-behavioral therapy. What might be seen as the key traits in the family? According to Goldberg, there are nine underlying assumptions or properties of behavioral therapy (Goldberg & Goldberg, 1996, p. 254):

1. All behavior, normal or abnormal, is acquired and maintained in identical ways (that is, according to the same principles of learning).

2. Behavior disorders represent learned maladaptive patterns that need not presume some inferred underlying cause or unseen motive.

3. Maladaptive behavior, such as symptoms, is itself the disorder, rather than it being a manifestation of a more basic underlying disorder or disease process.

4. It is not essential to discover the exact situation or set of circumstances in which the disorder was learned; these circumstances are usually irretrievable anyway. Rather, the focus should be on assessing the current determinants that support and maintain the undesired behavior.

5. Maladaptive behavior, having been learned, can be extinguished (that is, unlearned) and replaced by new learned behavior patterns.

6. Treatment involves the application of the experimental findings of scientific psychology, with an emphasis on developing a methodology that is precisely specified, objectively evaluated, and easily replicated.

7. Assessment is an ongoing part of treatment, as the effectiveness of treatment is continuously evaluated and specific intervention techniques are individually tailored to specific problems.

8. Behavioral therapy concentrates on "here-and-now" problems, rather than uncovering or attempting to reconstruct the past. The therapist is interested in helping the client identify and change current environmental stimuli that reinforce the undesired behavior, in order to alter the client's behavior.

9. Treatment outcomes are evaluated in terms of measurable changes. Research on specific therapeutic techniques is continuously carried out by behavioral therapists.

Missing from the aforementioned assumptions are the skills-building aspects of behavior therapy. When individuals lack the requisite skills required to successfully function in a given environment, the appropriate response class (i.e., different topographical behaviors producing comparable outcomes) must be shaped by contingencies carefully arranged by other people (e.g., the behavior therapist)—the contingencies must be programmed (Skinner, 1966). Shaping, technically speaking, is the differential reinforcement of successive approximations toward effective performance (Holland & Skinner, 1961; Martin & Pear, 1978; Miltenberger, 2001; Skinner, 1953). The following list includes various client behaviors that may be targeted for shaping or differential reinforcement: learning new social skills, assertiveness training, rational problem-solving skills training, relaxation training (e.g., autonomic, progressive muscle relaxation, diaphragmatic breathing), and distress tolerance, among countless other behaviors.

It has been argued that cognitive-behavioral therapy developed out of three waves—with the first wave being (1) behavior therapy, the second wave being (2) cognitive-behavioral therapy, and the (3) third wave being largely mindfulness-based psychotherapies (see Hayes, 2004; Hayes et al., 2006). Behavior therapy developed, in part, out of dissatisfaction with psychoanalysis—due to the lack of outcome data meeting minimal scientific standards as well as numerous conceptual problems; because clinical outcomes did not produce large treatment effects; and on account of problems with psychoanalytic theory's vague constructs, unclear measurement operations, and unclear predictions (Eysenck, 1952). Behavior therapy, although highly effective with a number of clinical conditions, also realized its limits—especially with higher functioning patients—which gave rise to the second wave of behavior therapy, cognitive-behavioral therapy. The third wave developed out of dissatisfaction with second-wave cognitive approaches. The third wave introduced a number of new concepts and terms to the behavioral canon, including metacognition, cognitive fusion, emotional regulation, emotional avoidance, acceptance, mindfulness, dialectics, and commitment to meaning, among other constructs (Kahl, Winter, & Schweiger, 2012).

Not included in the notion of "waves," of course, are the recent contributions of evolutionary and emotional theories developed out of basic neuroscience. Evolutionary concepts emphasize how functional systems are selected to bolster inclusive fitness (i.e., reproductive success; see Confer et al., 2010 for a recent discussion). That is to say, evolution works toward selecting humans based on reproductive advantage, not on the basis of whether an individual possesses "psychological wellness" or is free from "psychiatric illness." From this vantage point, therefore, there is no "disorder" in the usual sense of the term if symptoms and behaviors are unrelated to reproductive success. Nature simply does not "care" whether someone has what might be called schizophrenia, obsessive-compulsive disorder, or depression, only whether individuals are able to contribute their genetic information to the next generation of our species. Moreover, evolutionary psychology does not constitute a new kind of therapy, nor does it compete with extant approaches. Rather, its aim is to inform or augment other therapeutic approaches. Namely, "every kind of therapy should make use of evolutionary principles...by defining phenotypes and identifying evolved behavior regulation mechanisms" (Nesse, 2005, p. 920). Interested readers are directed to Buss's (2008) textbook titled *Evolutionary Psychology: The New Science of the Mind* (3rd ed.). Moreover, it should be noted that Skinner's radical behaviorism is at its essence an evolutionary account (see O'Donohue & Ferguson, 2001; O'Donohue, 2013).

Advances in neuroimaging (e.g., functional magnetic resonance imaging [fMRI]; positron emission tomography [PET]; and magnetoencephalography [MEG]) have revolutionized our basic understanding of brain function, which eluded neuroscientists until recent decades. These technological innovations have enabled scientists to study the metabolic activity of living brains (e.g., cerebral blood flow) as research participants perform various mental functions while lying in scanners. Interestingly, researchers have also investigated brain activity during down time (or when the brain is presumably idle) revealing so-called default networks. Much of this work has informed our basic understanding of broad classes of psychiatric conditions involving anxiety and fear (e.g., panic disorder, posttraumatic stress disorder, generalized anxiety disorder, and obsessive-compulsive disorder; Damasio & Carvalho, 2013). Moving beyond simple stimulus-response interpretations of classical ("Pavlovian") conditioning processes, for example, LeDoux and colleagues identified neural circuits that mediate fear conditioning; particularly, the convergence of neural inputs from conditioned stimulus (CS) and unconditioned stimulus (US) pathways onto the lateral nucleus of the amygdala (LeDoux et al., 1988, 1990; Rodrigues, Schafe, & LeDoux, 2004). Interested readers should consult the excellent book by Charney and Nestler (2008), *Neurobiology of Mental Illness*. Popular books include Damasio's (1999) *The Feeling of What Happens: Body and Emotion in the Making of Consciousness* and Ledoux's (1998) *The Emotional Brain: The Mysterious Underpinnings of Emotional Life.*

Readers should note that the notion of waves is not analogous to scientific revolutions as shown in physical sciences, although one can see how it could be misinterpreted as such (cf., biology, physics, or chemistry; Kuhn, 1962, 1974; Lakatos, 1970, 1978; Popper, 1959, 1962, 1972). An older paradigm is not supplanted by a new paradigm that better accounts for anomalous data. A new paradigm is not replacing an older paradigm because of its deficiencies, pragmatically speaking, or otherwise. Rather, waves appear to be additive. Namely, first-generation behavioral therapists still exist and may even be said to be flourishing. Collectively, they would now call themselves applied behavior analysts. Cognitive-behavioral therapy still has a strong presence in treating countless clinical problems, from panic disorder and posttraumatic stress disorder, to bipolar disorder and chronic pain. The third-wave or third-generation therapies simply now "share" in some of the work. With that as background, let us turn to the historical roots of cognitive-behavioral therapy. Given space limitations, this chapter can neither be exhaustive of the historical antecedents of cognitive-behavioral therapy nor sufficiently detailed enough to expound on recent influences, including evolutionary psychology, cognitive neuroscience, and epigenetics. Rather, the chapter authors focus on what they feel to be the most influential historical factors that affected the development of cognitive-behavioral therapy, broadly speaking.

Historical Background

The earliest influences of cognitive-behavioral therapy can be found in the experimental learning laboratory (O'Donohue, 2009). The first generation of behavior therapy was influenced, namely, by basic classical (or Pavlovian) conditioning and operant research involving nonhuman subjects. The first generation of behavior therapists included Joseph Wolpe, Hans Eysenck, and Ogden Lindsely, among others. Their work began appearing in the behavioral science literature between the 1940s and 1950s. The first-generation behavior therapists provided highly effective interventions for such clinical conditions as simple and complex phobias, chronic anxiety, schizophrenia, and neurodevelopmental disorders like autism and severe intellectual impairments.

Arguably, the two most influential figures during the first wave were the conditioning researchers Ivan P. Pavlov and B. F. Skinner. Let us now turn to the contribution of Pavlov as his work served as the cornerstone for Skinner's work and, later, for the work of other behavioral scientists. Although volumes can be and have been written about such highly influential intellectuals as Pavlov, Wolpe, Eysenck, and Lindsely, among others, we chose to focus on the work of Skinner because we believe that he has had the greatest impact on the field of behavior therapy and cognitive-behavioral therapy, either directly or in response to his writings.

The Russian physiologist Pavlov identified several basic learning mechanisms in the early twentieth century: habituation/sensitization and classical conditioning processes (Pavlov, 1927, 1928). These learning mechanisms entailed two-term and four-term relations between stimulus/stimuli and response/responses (S-R).

Habituation and sensitization are the most fundamental types of behavioral processes (nonassociative or perceptual learning). These involve a two-term relation between stimulus and response. In the case of habituation, repeated presentations of an eliciting stimulus (i.e., S) result in a decrease in response (R) magnitude. White coat hypertension, for example, can diminish with sufficient exposure to a doctor's office (Chrysant, 2000). Sensitization, in contrast, results in an increase in response (R) magnitude with repeated presentations of an eliciting stimulus. A learning history involving repeated trauma, for example, can produce hypervigilance and an exaggerated startle response when introduced to certain types of novel environments (American Psychiatric Association, 2013).

In the four-term relation in classical conditioning (CS-US-UR-CR), a neutral stimulus, CS (e.g., an auditory or visual stimulus), is paired with a US (e.g., food or shock). Through repeated pairings of the US/CS, the CS will eventually elicit topographically similar responses to the UR (unconditioned response). In Pavlov's classic studies involving dogs, his research subjects began salivating (CR) in response to hearing the bell (CS). The dogs, of course, would only salivate after there had been a sufficient amount of pairings of the bell (CS) with the food powder (US). That is to say, the dog began to salivate to the bell after transfer of stimulus functions had occurred.

The CS can also serve an *excitatory* or *inhibitory* function, signaling the presence or absence of the US, respectively. This process is called stimulus discrimination, because certain respondent behaviors are elicited under specific contextual circumstances but not under others (Pierce & Epling, 1999). As we shall see later, the CS can also serve as a discriminative stimulus, which evokes a characteristic operant response associated with a given reinforcement history. In operant conditioning, the CS in the former case might simultaneously serve as a prompting or discriminative stimulus. After operant conditioning, for example, the discriminative stimulus or SD signals to the organism that the reinforcer is likely available in the environment (e.g., the Wi-Fi bars signal when the Internet is likely available). In the latter case, the CS stimulus might also serve as an S-delta (S^Δ). An S-delta, in contrast, signals that the reinforcer will likely be withheld regardless of behavior (e.g., no Wi-Fi bars on one's smartphone or tablet).

Pavlov's work on classical conditioning mechanisms provided the foundations for Mowrer's (1947, 1951, 1956) important two-factor theory of emotion, which has been the most influential theory of fear and avoidance to this day. Wolpe—a contemporary of Mowrer—based his treatment, systematic desensitization, and theory of reciprocal inhibition on the work of Pavlov as well (Wolpe, 1958). Systematic desensitization is a counterconditioning strategy designed to treat "neurotic-anxiety response habits" (Wolpe, 1990, p. 150). Systematic desensitization employs the use of progressive muscle relaxation, which is thought to reciprocally inhibit an anxiety response (Wolpe, 1976).

Pavlov's work on classical conditioning mechanisms had a profound influence on the work of B. F. Skinner. And Skinner's influence on applied behavior analysis, in turn, is vast and uncontroversial. He is also one of the most influential figures on the formation of behavior therapy in the 1950s and 1960s; although Joseph Wolpe, as indicated earlier, and Albert Ellis also played considerable roles in the development of behavior therapy (see O'Donohue et al., 2001, for treatments of their relative influences). Wolpe, particularly, established a sustainable program of research that had a noteworthy impact on how clinicians practiced during his time and even now, for that matter (O'Donohue, 2009).

B. F. Skinner

Given that Skinner retired in the 1970s, it is perhaps the case that younger generations of behavioral scientists might not fully appreciate the breadth of his work or the extent of his influence on the field of psychology and allied professions (the reader is referred to O'Donohue & Ferguson, 2001, for a book-length treatment of Skinner's psychology). Skinner was a polymath and prolific writer who wrote technical papers for scientific audiences, and articles and books for the lay public. He was an important philosopher in psychology and education, and he was highly influential with his work in animal and human learning. Generations of basic and applied behavioral scientists, inspired by the basic tenets of Skinner's work, went on to develop more sophisticated analyses of behavioral phenomena, including matching, behavioral momentum, and response deprivation, among many other examples (Pierce & Epling, 1999). Skinner's theoretical work in verbal behavior stimulated many empirical efforts in human language and cognition, including, though not limited to, stimulus equivalence and, most recently, relational-frame theory, which, in turn, have been influential in the formation of acceptance and commitment therapy. Skinner even devised a plan for a utopian society, which was solidly based on his science of behavior. Of course, his views on bettering society never fully materialized beyond a few fringe experimental communities—nor did his work on education, which, to this day, remains subject to the latest fads. It goes without saying that, were he still alive, Skinner would be greatly disappointed by what has become of modern-day society, its impact on the natural environment, and what has become of education.

Skinner's Radical Behaviorism

Skinner called his philosophy of science *radical behaviorism*. His first use of the term in a publication appeared in his oft-cited paper, "The Operational Analysis of Psychological Terms" (Skinner, 1945a, p. 294). Unlike methodological behaviorism's eschewal of "all reference to consciousness" and introspective methods, and insistence on intersubjective verifiability, among other positivistic sentiments, Skinner's radical behaviorism considered "events taking place in the private world within the skin" as admissible in a scientific analysis (Skinner, 1957, p. 15). That is to say, although he questioned "the objects observed and the reliability of the observations," Skinner believed cognitions played a legitimate role in science—which, in one sense, made his brand of behaviorism "radical" (Skinner, 1957, p. 15). Skinner (1953) went on to write,

> We need not suppose that events which take place within an organism's skin have special properties for that reason. A private event may be distinguished by its limited accessibility but not, and so far as we know, by any special structure or nature. We have no reason to suppose that the stimulating effect of an inflamed tooth is essentially different from that of, say, a hot stove. The stove, however, is capable of affecting more than one person in approximately the same way. (Skinner, 1953, pp. 257–258)

As will be taken up shortly, the notion that private/public behavior is fundamentally one and the same is the foundation of Skinner's (1957) work, *Verbal Behavior*. The only distinction Skinner (1957) made between nonverbal and verbal behavior is the way in which behavior influences the environment—verbal behavior is behavior that alters the environment "through the mediation of other persons," whereas nonverbal behavior "alters the environment through mechanical action" (pp. 1–2). Regardless of behavioral topography (e.g., vocal, written, or use of skeletal muscles), therefore, both verbal and nonverbal responding are subjected to the same contingencies of reinforcement (i.e., reinforcement, extinction, and punishment).

Skinner's Experimental Analysis of Behavior

Skinner pioneered the science of behavior analysis or the experimental analysis of behavior. Skinner (1981) considered the experimental analysis of behavior a branch of biology and argued that all human behavior results from three levels of variation and selection: "(i) contingencies of survival responsible for natural selection and (ii) contingencies of reinforcement responsible for the repertoires of individuals, including (iii) the special contingencies maintained by an evolved social environment" (p. 501).

Natural selection accounts for why "we have a body and a brain at all" (Skinner, 1990, p. 1206). The contingencies of natural selection determine what physical attributes or "behavior makes it more probable that individuals will survive and breed . . . over long periods of time" (Skinner, 1974, p. 37). The sympathetic branch of the autonomic nervous system (ANS), for example, facilitates rapid responding to threats in the environment by dilating pupils and bronchi, channeling blood flow from unnecessary muscles (like those used in digestion), and supplying oxygenated, nutrient-rich blood for energy metabolism to skeletal muscles. These complex biological events enabled our ancestors to step out of harm's way when predators were dangerously close or defend themselves in the event of an attack (Skinner, 1974, p. 38ff.). In contrast, those humans with an inadequate ANS were presumably selected out by nature before passing their genes on to the next generation, becoming another animal's meal.

Natural selection operates in the order of hundreds of thousands, perhaps millions of years, as genetic variation occurs via two very slow, gradual processes: (1) meiosis (sexual recombination) and (2) mitosis (mutation of genes or chromosomes). Accordingly, natural selection has certain faults that hinder organisms' ability to rapidly adapt to ever-changing environments. According to Skinner (1990),

> Classical conditioning prepares a species only for a future that resembles the selecting past. Species behavior is only effective in a world that fairly closely resembles the world in which the species evolved. If we were to wait for natural selection to fashion a relatively simple behavioral repertoire, this would take millions of years spanning countless generations, as selection is contingent on genetic variation. That fault was corrected by the evolution of a second type of variation and selection, operant conditioning, through which variations in the behavior of the individuals are selected by features of the environment that are not stable enough to play any part in evolution. (p. 1206)

Moreover, as it turns out, only the second level of variation and selection, "operant conditioning, occurs at a speed at which it can be observed from moment to moment" (Skinner, 1984, p. 478). Among the three levels of variation, therefore, operant conditioning is the only level that lends itself well to work in the research laboratory or in the clinic.

Before proceeding, it is important to note that the field of epigenetics did not emerge until after Skinner's death (August 18, 1990); in fact, not until quite recently. Epigenetics is knowledge about how a gene's function or expression can be changed without altering a gene's basic structure. Epigenetics might have, therefore, tempered Skinner's view in the earlier quotation. This is speculative, of course.

Regarding levels of analysis, natural selection involves species, whereas selection by consequences pertains to individuals and their unique conditioning histories. Conditioning histories that shape behavioral repertoires enable individual organisms to adapt more efficiently to similar environments and, in the case of more generalizable repertoires, to adapt more effectively to novel ones. An operant is behavior that "operates" on—changes—the immediate environment to produce certain consequences (Skinner, 1953, p. 65). The environment ultimately "selects" which responses effectively "operate" on it to produce events that function as reinforcers for the individual's behavior. Through this differential reinforcement or shaping process, the environment also selects which behavioral variants go unreinforced (i.e., operant extinction) or eventuate in punishment. Readers should note that a stimulus "does not elicit the response in the sense of forcing it to occur . . . It is simply an essential aspect of the occasion upon which responses are made and reinforced" (Skinner, 1969, p. 7). In other words, stimuli as used here are probabilistically based—that is, either more of less likely to occur in the presence of other stimuli, related or otherwise.

In mathematical terms, the probability (P) of these events (E) or any event for that matter would be expressed as follows: The $P(E)$ must be greater than or equal to 0 and less than or equal to 1.0. Namely, $0 \leq P(E) \leq 1.0$. A probability of 0, therefore, would reflect no contingency or relation between a given stimulus and response. The two events would thus be truly random. Any value above zero, conversely, would reflect degrees of association and, therefore, suggest a contingent relation of variable strength between the stimulus and response; the closer to 1.0, the stronger the association. Conversely, the closer the probability is to 0, the weaker the association or contingent relation.

Behavior always varies topographically—that is, no two responses are exactly the same. Responses vary along certain dimensional parameters and thus reflect "average performance" (Baum, 1994, pp. 64–65). The distribution of dimensional parameters might fall along a normal distribution (i.e., Gaussian distribution) or, perhaps, appear positively or negatively skewed were the data depicted graphically. For example, a native living in the Galapagos might strike a coconut with comparable (not identical) force every time. Of course, the force would likely vary with fatigue levels, time of day (midday versus middle of the night), whether someone experiencing a migraine headache is around, ripeness of the coconut, type of coconut, and so on. Perhaps, if one were to graph responding, the force of impact might look similar to a normal distribution—with most responses distributing around the mean and fewer responses distributing along the tails of the distribution.

The fundamental behavioral process responsible for such variability in performance is extinction (Galbicka, 1994). Failing to meet the environment's reinforcement criterion (in an adequately motivated individual, say, at 90% of ad libitum body weight) will likely result in extinction-induced behavior or a so-called extinction burst. An extinction burst includes a temporary increase in response frequency, a resurgence of behavior that was perhaps effective in the past, and/or emotional responding or aggressive behavior (Pierce & Epling, 1999). Soda machines are chained to walls because of extinction-induced behavior. Individuals have been known to crush themselves emitting extinction-induced behavioral variability, which involves rocking the machine until it succumbs to the force of gravity with the person under it!

The interplay between reinforcement and responding is ongoing. This interplay or certain contingency configurations are called schedules of reinforcement (Skinner, 1953). Skinner discovered the effects of schedules of reinforcement serendipitously. Skinner was an avid tinkerer and would often fashion apparatus out of old scraps lying around his shop. Out of scraps, he built teaching machines (Skinner, 1960), baby tenders (Skinner, 1945b, October), and cumulative recorders (Skinner, 1956). Cumulative recorders, particularly, yielded data of critical importance for Skinner's scientific analysis of behavior. In the following passage, Skinner recounts of his discovery of schedules of reinforcement:

> The disc of wood from which I had fashioned the food magazine was taken from a storeroom of discarded apparatus. It happened to have a central spindle, which fortunately I had not bothered to cut off. One day it occurred to me if I wound a string around the spindle and allowed it to unwind as the magazine was emptied . . . I would get a different kind

of record. Instead of getting a mere report of the up-and-down movement of the runway, as a series of pips as in the polygraph, I would get a *curve*. And I knew that science made great use of curves … as it turned out the curve revealed things in the rate of responding, and changes in that rate, which would certainly otherwise have been missed. (Skinner, 1982, pp. 81–82)

In collaboration with his student Charles Ferster, Skinner almost exhausted every permutation of reinforcement schedule using his cumulative recorder, which culminated in their magnum opus, *Schedules of Reinforcement* (Ferster & Skinner, 1957). Reinforcement schedules are either (1) continuous or (2) intermittent. Continuous schedules of reinforcement deliver the reinforcer after every operant response. Intermittent reinforcement schedules dispense the reinforcer after a certain number of responses or after a certain time has elapsed.

The former refers to ratio schedules. These are either *fixed* or *variable*. For example, the reinforcer might be delivered after every fifth response (fixed-ratio schedule 5 [FR5]) or, on average (i.e., based on a mean value), after every fifth response (variable-ratio schedule 5 [VR5]). Interval schedules of reinforcement are temporally based. As with ratio schedules, they, too, are either *fixed* or *variable*. A fixed interval schedule might dispense the reinforcer following a response after 5 seconds have elapsed (fixed-interval 5 seconds [FI5 sec.]). A variable interval schedule might deliver the reinforcer following a response after an average of 5 seconds has elapsed (variable-interval 5 seconds [VI5 sec.]). Because reinforcer delivery is based on a mean value, the response interval ranges from, say, 3, 4, 5, 6, and so on, seconds for any given response.

Interestingly, different schedules of reinforcement produce different patterns of responding (see Ferster & Skinner, 1957, for countless cumulative records depicting these behavioral phenomena). With fixed-ratio schedules, for example, a high rate of responding occurs, followed by a long postreinforcement pause after delivery of the reinforcer (i.e., a characteristic break-and-run pattern; Pierce & Epling, 1999). Similarly, with fixed-interval schedules there is also a long postreinforcement pause; however, responding generally occurs at a lower rate than ratio schedules throughout much of the interval (i.e., until the end of the interval, producing a characteristic scalloped pattern on a cumulative record; Ferster & Skinner, 1957).

On variable-ratio schedules, organisms respond at the highest rate of any schedule. Moreover, there often is little or no pause after reinforcement occurs. As an aside, VR schedules are essential for the success of the gambling industry. In fact, this industry has to be carefully monitored to prevent patrons from exhausting their savings on certain VR schedules. Variable-interval schedules also produce little or no postreinforcement pause; however, rate of responding is generally low, relatively speaking.

Another interesting empirical regularity discovered with schedules of reinforcement concerns resistance to extinction—the so-called partial reinforcement effect (which is synonymous with the term "resistance to extinction"; Pierce & Epling, 1999). Intermittent reinforcement schedules result in more responding during extinction than continuous reinforcement schedules. This might occur because it takes more responses, initially, to contact the prevailing contingencies with variable schedules.

Skinner's Verbal Behavior

Skinner applied his experimental analysis of behavior to the investigation of language—an intellectual pursuit, which commenced in 1934 after a chance encounter with the eminent philosopher Alfred North Whitehead. Skinner (1957) answered Professor Whitehead's challenge that the science of behavior was ill equipped to tackle human language with his tome titled *Verbal Behavior*—a work, incidentally, which Skinner regarded as his greatest intellectual achievement. Unfortunately, Chomsky's (1959) scathing review was received by a much wider audience, despite the fact that it had been based on bad exegesis.

Skinner was critical of linguists who regarded language "as a system of rules which relate sound sequences to meanings" (Hayes, Orstein, & Gage, 1988, p. 2)—seeing the referential nature of those approaches as problematic with respect to "words like *atom* or *gene* or *minus one* or *the spirit of the times* where corresponding nonverbal entities are not easily discovered" (Skinner, 1957, p. 8). Skinner (1957), in contrast, viewed language from a wholly different vantage point, within the purview of behavior analysis:

> The "LANGUAGES" studied by the linguist are the reinforcing practices of verbal communities. When we say that *also* means *in addition* or *besides* "in English," we are not referring to the verbal behavior of any one speaker of English or the average performance of many speakers, but to the conditions

under which a response is characteristically reinforced by a verbal community. (p. 461)

Verbal communities are thus broadly defined. They may include members of a given geographic area, virtual communities online (like message boards and social media), or the verbal community of one's profession, to name only a few. Verbal communities either explicitly or implicitly state the prevailing contingencies. Message boards and social media, for example, explicitly state the contingencies in their "terms of use." Implicit rules might be understood by observing subtle social behavior like averting eye contact, sighing to oneself, looking at one's watch, and so on.

Although verbal behavior bears similarities with nonverbal behavior (e.g., it can be reinforced, punished, or extinguished), it differs in how it operates on the environment. Verbal behavior indirectly influences the environment. It requires a listener to have an impact on the environment.[1] Uttering "water" is ineffective in obtaining a glass of water without a listener within earshot to get it. Of course, there is a presumption that both speaker and listener have similar verbal conditioning histories. Saying *voda* (Czech), *maji* (Swahili), or *vesi* (Finnish), for example—all of which mean "water" in their respective languages—would not likely evoke the correct response on the part of the listener who, say, speaks English as her first and only language. In this case, rather, the speaker would have to engage in nonvocal verbal behavior to evoke effective action on the part of the listener (e.g., pantomiming someone drinking water, pointing to an empty glass that recently contained water, or sketching a glass of water on an iPad).

Skinner (1957) defined functional relations between controlling variables and verbal responding. Skinner's unit of analysis of speech was the *total verbal episode*. A total verbal episode can be understood using the three-term contingency, which applies to both speaker and listener.[2] In our example, the verbal operant "water" belongs to the response class, *mand*, presuming that our speaker has gone without water for some time (whose behavior has been reinforced with water in the recent past; Skinner, 1957). A mand is defined as a verbal operant in which the response is reinforced by a characteristic outcome and, as such, is under the momentary influence of conditions of deprivation or aversive stimulation (Michael, 1993). The verbal behavior emitted by the earlier speaker is more likely to be reinforced by the receipt of water

the longer she has gone without it (or any revitalizing fluids for that matter). Should the listener echo back the response, "water," Skinner would call this *echoic behavior*. Had the speaker written the word, "water," or drawn a picture of it on a napkin—and the listener uttered "water"—Skinner would call this *textual behavior* (i.e., the vocal response is controlled by a verbal stimulus, which is not heard).

A *tact* is a verbal response of a particular form that is evoked by a characteristic nonverbal stimulus (Skinner, 1957, pp. 81–82). Perhaps, our speaker uttered the response, "water," while working on a puzzle of an ocean scene. Had our listener written down the response in lieu of a vocal response, Skinner would call this *transcription*. With transcription, "all the characteristics of echoic behavior follow, except they are now expressed in visual rather than auditory terms" (Skinner, 1957, p. 70). Presumably, the logic would also extend to American Sign Language as well, despite it being nonvocal or an inherently inaudible form of communication (i.e., the echoed response from, say, lip-reading, is now expressed visually).

Autoclitics are said to "lean on" or otherwise depend on other verbal behavior. They essentially serve grammatical functions in language. A listener, for example, might respond very differently to "Burrhus *is* at home" versus "Burrhus *was* at home" if she were trying to drop off a time-sensitive, registered letter addressed only to him. While the autoclitics *is* and *was* are meaningless in and of themselves, they "lean" on the nouns and prepositions in the aforementioned sentences, which attribute contextual "meaning." Let us briefly turn to Skinner's analysis of meaning and understanding as these concepts are both important with any discussion on language.

According to Skinner (1974), "meaning" is not found in words, rather:

> The meaning of a response … is to be found in its antecedent history … In other words, meaning is not properly regarded as a property either of a response or situation but rather of the contingencies responsible for both the topography of behavior and the control exerted by stimuli. To take a primitive example, if one rat presses a lever to obtain food when hungry while another does so to obtain water when thirsty, the topographies of their behavior may be indistinguishable, but they may be said to differ in meaning: to one rat pressing the lever "means" food; to the other it "means" water. Both of these are aspects of the contingencies which have brought

behavior under the control of the current occasion. (pp. 93–94)

Accordingly, "when someone says that he can see the meaning of a response, he means that he can infer some of the variables of which the response is usually a function" (Skinner, 1957, p. 14). Meaning is thus found in the context, in the interaction between behavior and environment—it is an extrapolation of sorts.

Verbal behavior cannot arise in the absence of an audience. According to Skinner (1957), an audience serves as a discriminative and reinforcing stimulus in whose presence verbal behavior is typically strong (i.e., more probable). Of course, when individuals are alone, they may talk to themselves (e.g., " 'I' before 'E' except after 'C' "; "turn left on Horsehead Bay Drive"; "Easy now, she's your boss")—serving as both speaker and listener simultaneously.

Any discussion of audiences or listeners involves the notion of *understanding*. Skinner maintained that understanding, as conceived in a scientific analysis of behavior, entails several levels of comprehension. "In a simple sense of the word, I have understood what a person says if I can repeat it correctly" (Skinner, 1974, p. 146). This definition would reflect Skinner's (1957) notion of echoic or textual behavior. "In a somewhat more complex sense, I understand it if I respond appropriately" (Skinner, 1974, p. 146). Lastly, the deepest level of understanding would entail specifying the contingencies of which behavior is a function. Behavior under the control of *contingency-specifying stimuli* is called rule-governed behavior (Pierce & Epling, 1999). In what follows, Skinner (1974) describes this level of understanding:

Understanding sometimes means knowing reasons. If I throw a switch to put a piece of apparatus into operation and nothing happens, I may try the switch again, but my behavior quickly undergoes extinction, and I may then look to see whether the apparatus is connected with the power source, or whether a fuse is blown, or whether the starting switch is broken. In doing so, I may come to understand why it has not worked in the sense of discovering reasons. I have acquired understanding by analyzing the prevailing contingencies. (pp. 146–147)

Skinner's Views on Bettering Society

In the third level of selection, cultural selection, Skinner maintained that this was only possible after nature selected certain physical features in humans, their vocal apparatus (e.g., larynx and pharynx), which enabled the production of speech sounds. Skinner (1986) wrote,

The human species took a crucial step forward when its vocal musculature came under operant control in the production of speech sounds. Indeed, it is possible that all the distinctive achievements of the species can be traced to that genetic change. (p. 170)

Made possible by verbal behavior, rules were formulated. Rules including, but not limited to, customs, government legislation, and religious and secular law enabled cultures to influence the behavior of their members (Skinner, 1953). Rules permitted leaders to influence members of society even when those members were not under direct observation. Take the Decalogue, for example. These so-called sacred laws likely lowered the probability of stealing, killing one another (within one's own religion, at least), or engaging in adulterous acts (which could incite violence) in devote Christians, Jews, and Muslims.

Over the millennia, of course, rule-governed behavior continues to evolve in sophistication and complexity in keeping with technological advances, as industrial societies continue to grow exponentially. Antipiracy and antispying Internet laws, and the inordinately complex bureaucratic rules and regulations of a constantly changing health care system, are a few such examples.

Skinner's major contribution to bettering society was his writings on freedom and control. Skinner's views incited a major backlash from critical audiences and the lay public alike, who maligned Skinner as a proponent of despotism and other tyrannical governments. Carl Rogers, one of Skinner's contemporary intellectual adversaries, deemed his book, *Walden Two*, and George Orwell's nightmarish dystopian society, *1984*, as one and the same (Skinner, 1972). The irony in this, of course, is that Skinner was vehemently opposed to the use of punishment, as he found most of the benefits to be only temporary, and the behavioral and emotional byproducts of punishment as highly undesirable.

Skinner, among other behavior analysts, viewed all behavior as determined and, thus, controlled. Skinner (1971), in fact, went further to state that believing in *autonomous man* only harms society in the end, for all of society's ills are behaviorally based—from pollution, domestic violence, starvation, obesity, sexual assaults, homelessness, stockpiling nuclear weapons, drug abuse, crime, and so on. Polluting the environment, striking others, withholding food from those in need, overeating, sexually assaulting others, evicting vulnerable individuals, accumulating weapons of mass destruction, using excessive amounts of illicit substances at the expense of a comfortable and sustainable quality of life, and robbing others entail some form of behavior. Concern for autonomous man or free will, in Skinner's view, only leads to developing techniques, which are largely ineffectual; the "just-say-no-to-drugs" campaign of the 1980s and, more contemporarily, "good girls only kneel for Jesus" illustrate this point nicely, as neither campaign has had an appreciable influence on drug-related or sexual behavior.

Because all behavior is controlled all the time, "we cannot choose a way of life in which there is no control…We can only change the controlling conditions" (Skinner, 1974, p. 195). As mentioned, Skinner, particularly, urged members of society to promote positive behavioral contingencies as opposed to using coercive methods because those kinds of contingencies had a tendency to engender undesirable behavioral byproducts like anger, aggression, and countercontrol.

Skinner believed that those positive societal practices should be shaped experimentally, "in piecemeal fashion" (Skinner, 1971, p. 156). Practices, for example, might be developed on a smaller scale at first—after which, those successful practices might be adopted and further refined by larger groups of individuals (see Skinner, 1948). Ineffective practices, and those characterized by unintended negative consequences, might therefore be discarded before investing further resources.

Of course, in the spirit of Skinnerian pragmatism, those deemed as successful theories and practices would only be provisionally held until something more efficacious or effective is discovered that might one day supplant it. With this in mind Skinner, for example, presaged that his own science of behavior would eventually be supplanted by neuroscience in the future, with the advancement of structural and functional neuroimaging technologies ("An answer will probably come from neurology, but only in the distant future" [Skinner, 1988, p. 65]).

In what follows is Skinner's "Decalogue" to building a better world:

(1) No way of life is inevitable. Examine your own closely. (2) If you do not like it, change it. (3) But do not try to change it through political action. Even if you succeed in gaining power, you will not be able to use it any more wisely than your predecessors.

(4) Ask only to be left alone to solve problems in your own way. (5) Simplify your needs. Learn how to be happy with fewer possessions … (6) Build a way of life in which people live together without quarreling, in a social climate of trust rather than suspicion, of love rather than jealousy, of cooperation rather than competition. (7) Maintain that world with gentle but pervasive ethical sanctions rather than a police or military force. (8) Transmit the culture effectively to new members through expert childcare and a powerful educational technology. (9) Reduce compulsive labor to a minimum by arranging the kinds of incentives under which people enjoy working. (10) Regard no practice as immutable. Change and be ready to change again. Accept no eternal verity. Experiment. (Skinner, 1948, pp. vii–viii)

The Emergence of Cognitive and Cognitive-Behavioral Therapy

There was a breaking point in the history of psychology during the late 1940s and 1950s. On the one hand, there were those psychologists who remained faithful to the behavioral tradition and continued on this path. Those behavioral psychologists have, in fact, departed little from the Skinnerian tradition in the fields of basic and applied behavior analysis. They use the same technical language proffered by Skinner and the same direct observation methods and single-case methodology. On the other hand, there were those psychologists, dissatisfied with the applied technologies and theoretical work of the first generation, who broke ties with that tradition. Those psychologists led the way for cognitive psychology (Baars, 1986; Hergenhahn, 1997).

Two important dates that were attributed to this watershed event were 1948 and 1956 (Leahey, 1992). The year 1948 marked the Hixon Symposium on Cerebral Mechanisms in Behavior (Gardner, 1985). The year 1956 marked the Symposium on Information Theory at the Massachusetts Institute of Technology (Baars, 1986). Basic research in cognitive psychology provided the fundamental concepts and terms for cognitive therapy. Among other things, cognitive therapy adopted the notion that behavior results from information processing, and how knowledge and experience are organized around various schemas.

It is unclear who initiated cognitive therapy, if any individual could lay claim to this. Judith Beck (1995) stated that "cognitive therapy was developed by Aaron T. Beck at the University of Pennsylvania in the early 1960s as a structured, short-term, present-oriented psychotherapy for depression, directed toward solving current problems and modifying dysfunctional thinking and behavior" (p. 1). Albert Ellis (2009), however, explicitly stated that he began work in cognitive therapy somewhat earlier: "In 1955…I started to do rational emotive behavior therapy (REBT) and to forcefully favor cognitive restructuring and the disputing of irrational client beliefs" (p. 189). He added: "I was not the first therapist to use what became known as cognitive behavior therapy (CBT), since a few practitioners—such as Herzberg (1945) and Salter (1949)—had employed aspects of it previously" (Ellis, 2009, p. 189). Surely other pioneers of cognitive therapy would acknowledge other theoreticians and practitioners as major players in the cognitive therapy movement (e.g., George Kelly's, construct theory; or clinical theorists such as Michael Mahoney and Arnold Lazarus).

Readers should note that Ellis and Beck were not especially influenced by the literature on basic cognitive psychology. Rather, they relied heavily on folk notions of rationality (e.g., don't catastrophize or "make mountains out of molehills") and informal notions of what constitutes pernicious irrational beliefs (e.g., "I have to be perfect at everything I do"). Ellis and Beck, however, have been criticized for this. Hollon (Dimidjian & Hollon, 2010; Hollon, Shelton, & Davis, 1993) and McFall (1991, 1996), for example, have regarded their overreliance on folk wisdom as a poor basis for clinical theories. These authors, in contrast, argue that cognitive therapy ought to be based on experimental cognitive science, insofar as behavior therapy is based on the empirical regularities discovered in the basic learning laboratory.

The key cognitive and cognitive-behavioral approaches of the second generation of behavior therapists are Beck's (1976) cognitive therapy, Ellis's rational-emotive therapy (1962; though he has since renamed it rational-emotive behavior therapy), Meichenbaum's (1977) self-instructional training, and metacognitive therapy (Wells & Matthews, 1994). As in the case of first-generation behavior therapy, second-generation approaches elude simple and straightforward definitions. Invoking Wittgenstein's (2009) notion of family resemblance, there are several assumptions underlying most cognitive-behavioral therapy interventions. First, thoughts or beliefs, emotions, and behavior exert bidirectional influence. Thoughts, for example, affect how one feels. Feelings might, in turn, affect how one behaves (of course, as used here, emotions would serve a secondary function). Consider the behavior of someone who is severely depressed: She moves more slowly, talks more slowly, and there are notable changes in prosody. Of course, behaving in certain ways (e.g., incongruent with one's values) might eventuate in negative cognitive appraisals of one's actions, which, in turn, elicit the emotions of guilt, shame, and/or embarrassment. Guilt, shame, and embarrassment always involve some form of behavior—imagined (i.e., covert behavior) or overt behavior. A second assumption concerns the notion of directly modifying one's "automatic thoughts," core beliefs, and or behavior in an effort at influencing one's mood status. Negative or dysfunctional beliefs, therefore, would be identified and acted upon accordingly. Third, most cognitive-behavioral therapy interventions are centered on one core strategy, cognitive restructuring, to which we turn (Edmondson & Conger, 1996).

Cognitive restructuring is the core strategy in cognitive therapy and cognitive-behavioral therapies (Mahoney, 1977). Cognitive restructuring is designed to directly modify specific thought patterns or beliefs that purportedly mediate maladaptive behavioral and emotional responding (Foa & Rothbaum, 1998; Last, 1985). When working with suicidal teens, for example, the therapist might assist the client in developing an awareness of how her negative self-talk reinforces feelings of hopelessness and helplessness. The client may be encouraged to replace her negative cognitive messages with more positive ways of thinking about her current life situation, as a means of overcoming her sense of hopelessness and empowering her so that she feels less helpless.

A number of behaviorally based psychotherapies emerged out of dissatisfaction with second-wave cognitive approaches. Proponents of one of the most influential approaches, called acceptance and commitment therapy (ACT), maintain that ACT and related therapies represent a "third wave" (Hayes, 2004). The third wave is comprised largely of ACT, dialectical behavior therapy (DBT), functional analytic psychotherapy (FAP), and behavioral activation (BA), among others (Hayes et al., 2006). Readers should note that Marsha Linehan—the founder of DBT—stated that DBT is not a third-wave therapy. Rather, she identifies DBT with "classic CBT that includes acceptance strategies" (David & Hofmann, 2013, p. 116).

Although not explicitly stated as such, asserting that one's approach is part of a third wave might imply that there has been a scientific revolution of sorts. However, the notion of a "generation" or "wave" is not the same as the concept of scientific revolution as seen in basic science (cf. physics, biology, or chemistry; Kuhn, 1962, 1974; Lakatos, 1970, 1978; Popper, 1959, 1962, 1972). Older paradigms have not been supplanted by newer ones. First- and second-generation therapies still flourish in applied behavior analysis and cognitive-behavioral therapy, respectively. Accordingly, if newer therapies indeed represent a "wave," these approaches add to extant approaches—nothing has been superseded. Moreover, it is important to note that these so-called waves also produce heterogeneity in how behavior therapy is practiced as individual behavior therapists pursue various interests and maintain allegiances more or less to particular therapeutic orientations.

The third generation introduced new concepts and terms such as metacognition, cognitive fusion, emotional regulation, acceptance, mindfulness, dialectics, and committed actions (Kahl, Winter, & Schweiger, 2012). Moreover, a third-wave perspective on cognitive phenomena as found in ACT places a premium on how verbal behavior interacts with nonverbal behavior in a bidirectional manner (Hayes & Gifford, 1998). Through this interaction, functions of stimuli are transferred or otherwise transformed (Hayes, 2004). For example, a client might develop a shoe fetish after repeated pairings with sexual stimuli (i.e., certain types of shoes might become associated with the positive sensations associated with sex). Accordingly, shoes would then elicit sexual arousal in their presence alone.

ACT is a principles-driven therapy designed to evoke behavior and thinking patterns that are more flexible and adaptive for the client (Wilson, & Roberts, 2002). ACT modifies psychological functioning and behavior by altering the social and verbal contexts that are said to link thoughts and feelings to overt behavior. Dialectical behavior therapy (DBT) utilizes behavior analytic strategies (e.g., behavioral chain analyses and basic case conceptualization; Linehan, 1993, pp. 258–264). It also employs dialectical strategies. Dialectical strategies bear much resemblance to cognitive restructuring or cognitive reframing as found in cognitive therapy and cognitive-behavioral therapy. Functional analytic psychotherapy (FAP)—purportedly based on the principles of radical behaviorism—explores clinical factors related to the psychoanalytic concepts of transference and countertransference (Kohlenberg & Tsai, 1991). FAP, rather, refers to these as clinically relevant behaviors (CRBs), which are said to emerge in session within the context of the therapist–client relationship. A CRB1 is the behavior that is problematic for the person (e.g., fear of intimacy). More adaptive behavior is also evoked and shaped by the therapist in session (CRB2). Clients are eventually taught how to tact (or describe) the contingencies that are believed to evoke CB1s and CB2s (so-called CRB3s).

Jacobson and colleagues developed a new treatment approach called behavioral activation therapy (BA; Jacobson, Martell, & Dimidjian, 2001). Behavioral activation was designed for individuals with depression, though there is no reason why the principles and therapeutic strategies could not be extended to other clinical conditions as well. Behavioral activation focuses on increasing access to reinforcement and developing more active behavioral coping strategies. At the same time, it targets problematic avoidance behavior (i.e., passive coping strategies) because problematic passive coping behaviors serve as a major barrier to accessing reinforcement. For example, an individual who would like to date spends weekend nights with her three cats lest she run the risk of asking someone out in her building only to get turned down.

Contemporary problem-solving therapy (PST) is another transdiagnostic intervention that incorporates cognitive strategies, psychoeducation (targeting problem-solving skills), and mindfulness strategies to increase awareness of how thoughts and feelings impact an individual (Nezu, Nezu, D'Zurilla, 2013; Nezu & Nezu, 1989; Nezu, Nezu, & Perri, 1989). Similar to therapeutic approaches like ACT and DBT, PST also employs experiential emotional regulation strategies in order to assist clients in pursuit of valued goals.

Cognitive-Behavioral Therapy and the Philosophy of Science

If there is one property that would appear to be central to cognitive and behavior therapies, it would be a commitment to scientific reasoning. The general idea is that negative automatic thoughts and distorted negative core schemas, treated as hypotheses/predictions, would be tested alongside reality-based alternative hypotheses—at which point, negative core schemas might be falsified in the face of contradictory evidence uncovered by behavioral experiments. For example, the core belief, "I'm too scared to go out in public" might be tested by walking one's dog in a nearby dog park—in which case, although scared, the notion that the individual is too scared to engage in the behavior would be refuted, especially when the outcome is replicated multiple times without incident.

Similarly, from the standpoint of the cognitive-behavioral therapist, her own beliefs about behavioral phenomena might be "put to the test of science" before they are practiced or—even better—become products of basic scientific research. A case in point would be a behavior therapist who is teaching contingency management to parents to decrease their child's defiant behavior. The cognitive-behavioral therapist could readily defend this practice by arguing along the lines of multiple basic research studies corroborating reinforcement principles as well as multiple treatment outcome studies on the efficacy of contingency management. This would be in stark contrast to therapies that could do neither of these—that is, could neither support the basic principles through basic scientific research nor show outcomes studies revealing the beneficial effects of the treatment.

This raises the question of exactly "What is science?" as well as "What exactly is the conceptualization of science that is associated with cognitive and behavior therapies?" These sorts of questions can be important because (1) at times behavior therapists have argued along the lines of "we are scientific—other disciples like psychoanalysis are not"; (2) at times some cognitive-behavioral therapists have argued that certain practices (e.g., eye movement or vibrations or tapping movements in eye movement desensitization and reprocessing [EMDR]) ought not to be part of cognitive-behavioral therapy because the scientific credentials of the candidate are suspect—consider the controversies about the scientific status of EMDR, for example (Lohr et al, 2003); and finally (3) some cognitive therapists have argued that if the epitome of rational belief formation is science, perhaps cognitive therapy ought to teach the client who is having difficulty with irrational beliefs how to "think like a scientist" (e.g., Ellis, 1981; Mahoney, 1987). However, the problem in all of this is that the answers to the two questions initially posed in this paragraph have yet to be resolved. We turn now to this controversy by examining some of the major accounts of science found in the philosophy of science.

Cognitive-Behavioral Therapy and Logical Positivism

The logical positivists were quite influential in both philosophy and the philosophy of science

in the first half of the twentieth century. The logical positivists were initially concentrated in Vienna and Berlin and were forced to scatter to the English-speaking world with the rise of Nazi Germany. The logical positivists were influenced by the Scottish philosopher David Hume (1887) when he stated:

> If we take in our hand any volume; of divinity or school metaphysics, for instance; let us ask, Does it contain any abstract reasoning concerning quantity or number? No. Does it contain any experimental reasoning concerning matter of fact and existence? No. Commit it then to the flames: for it can contain nothing but sophistry and illusion. (p. 86)

Identifying and eliminating metaphysics was thus the central concern of the logical positivists. They argued that metaphysical statements were meaningless—not false—but literally, nonsense. Metaphysical claims may fool speakers and listeners (in their terms "the bewitchment of intelligence by language") because metaphysical statements might appear syntactically well constructed though, in actuality, are nonsensical, semantically. For example, "Green ideas sleep furiously" is syntactically sound, though clearly meaningless, semantically.

Logical positivists constructed and used the *verifiability criterion of meaning* to demarcate scientifically meaningful from meaningless statements; although because of many problems with the verifiability criterion, this criterion went through several versions. A widely accepted version appears as follows:

> A statement is verifiable if it is analytic (e.g., "Squares have four sides") or if there is some finite set of observation statements that entails the statement.

Smith (1986) has done an excellent historical analysis that clearly shows that the early behaviorists did not import logical positivism to formulate their views on science or language but instead developed their own indigenous epistemologies. Thus, Smith argues the behaviorists and the logical positivists do share "linked fates." The same can be said for cognitive-behavioral therapy. There is no clear historical record that shows either the first-generation behavior therapists or subsequent behavior therapists were importing the views of the logical positivists.

The concerns of the two were quite distinct: cognitive and behavior therapists were not concerned with eliminating metaphysics; they were not using any form of the verifiability criterion; and they generally were not concerned with semantics. The first-generation behavior therapists did want to make their movement scientific and did have various notions for understanding what "science" is, which will be taken up shortly. However, it is fair to say that logical positivism had little influence on cognitive and behavior therapies either through behaviorism (per Smith, 1986) or more directly.

This might not be wholly advantageous to cognitive and behavior therapies. The strength of logical positivism was its central interest in understanding language and using it carefully and precisely. Some of this linguistic metaconcern can be seen in early twentieth-century behaviorism, particularly with Skinner (1957), and this might be the reason why some scholars have made the mistake of conflating the two or claiming they had a much closer relationship than they did in actuality (e.g., see Mahoney, 1988).

There is a proliferation of terms in contemporary cognitive and behavior therapies —from classic terms such as "contingencies" or "automatic thoughts" as well as terms that are imported from other influential sources such as the *DSM* (e.g., "mental disorder" or "major depressive episode") but also new terms such as "experiential avoidance" and "mindfulness." The field has a good methodology for clarifying the meaning of these terms, which, if left unchecked, can result in substantial confusion and limitation in research quality.

Cognitive and Behavior Therapies, and Popperian Falsification

Karl Popper is one of the most influential philosophers of science. A number of Nobel laureates, for example, attribute their scientific success to utilizing his views on what constitutes good science. In fact, although Albert Ellis (1980) originally attributed the Stoics as providing the greatest philosophical influence on his cognitive therapy, in his later years, he claimed that one of Popper's students, W. W. Bartley and his pan-critical rationalism had the most influence on rational emotive therapy.

Popper claimed that the goal of science is error elimination and to do this the scientist must attempt to falsify his or her theories. The essence of science is, therefore, not induction and confirmation but rather falsification. Falsification is implemented by determining what states of affairs a theory or belief rules out—states that cannot occur—and then experiments are designed and conducted to see if these states of affairs occur. For example, if my theory is "Ministers never swear," I would then attempt to delineate what states of affairs this rules

out—for example, a minister saying "God damn" or using the F-word, and so on. Ideally, then I would do what Popper calls a "severe (falsificatory) test" by conducting an experiment that has the most likelihood of observing the states of affairs that the theory rules out. For example, it is a more severe test to examine ministers after they hit their thumbs with a hammer or hit a poor golf stroke than to examine them when they are giving a sermon or at a child's birthday party.

Popper had a complex and rich philosophy of science. He wrote on the links between evolution and science; on what he calls "objective knowledge" and even political philosophy. A full treatment of this richness is beyond the scope of this chapter (see O'Donohue, 2013, for a more extended treatment). However, part of the complexity of his views is that he thought a different principle was necessary for explaining human behavior, what he called the rationality principle—which somewhat surprisingly he thought was never falsifiable. The rationality principle is roughly "Agents always act rationally to their views of their problem situation." This is coming quite close to some of the views of cognitive therapy, but again it is beyond the scope of this chapter to investigate the interrelationships.

It is not at all clear exactly what influence Popper has had on cognitive-behavioral therapy. Beyond Ellis, few cognitive behaviorists have explicitly stated a debt to Popper. For example, it is not at all clear that cognitive-behavioral therapists when conducting their research are using severe tests to attempt to falsify their theories or therapy beliefs. To the contrary, it may be the case that the explicit strategy is to show that the therapy works. This can be due both to the reward systems of science (i.e., "positive" results are valued more than "negative" results) and due to practical influences (i.e., any verisimilitude of a therapy can be used to benefit clients). Moreover, it is not clear that at the level of therapy that cognitive therapists teach their clients the importance of falsification as opposed to confirmation. However, it is fair to say that the richness of Popper's views on eliminating error, evolutionary epistemology, and rationality have not been mined either at the level of improving cognitive therapies or the metalevel of better understanding of what good science might be.

Cognitive and Behavior Therapies, and Kuhnian Paradigms

Kuhn's (1962) *Structure of Scientific Revolutions* is often shown to be the most highly influential book on both the philosophy of science as well as upon psychology. However, the quality of the exegesis of Kuhn can be questioned (O'Donohue, 2013); for example, his central notion of "paradigm" has been shown to have over 20 distinct meanings in his writings.

Kuhn claims through his study of selective episodes in biology and physics that there are three kinds of science: (1) preparadigmatic science, (2) normal science, and (3) revolutionary science. Preparadigmatic science occurs before a general problem-solving exemplar has emerged: In this phase there is little agreement in a field regarding fundamentals but instead there are numerous debates about what are proper objects of study, methods of study, and definitions of terms.

According to Kuhn, therefore, some scientists solve an important problem, which becomes the paradigm (roughly, the "exemplar" in Kuhn's terms) for other scientists to try to solve other problems in their domain. When scientists are using a paradigm to try to solve other problems, Kuhn calls this "normal science." However, during this period of normal science, all problems are not solved—scientists experience what Kuhn calls "anomalies" in that their attempts at problem solving are thwarted. These anomalies are the basis for what Kuhn calls a "scientific revolution," which occurs when someone solves one of these anomalies with a new strategy/problem-solving exemplar/paradigm. This new strategy becomes the new paradigm defining a new period of normal science. This alternation between normal and revolutionary science is perpetual, according to Kuhn.

Several aspects of Kuhn's account of science have been problematic for many. For example, Kuhn questions whether science actually shows progress—for him the new paradigms involved in scientific revolutions are so novel compared to the old paradigm that they involve what he calls a "Gestalt switch." The old and new paradigms are simply incommensurable, according to Kuhn, and because they cannot be compared one cannot say that the newer one represents progress.

O'Donohue (2013) has criticized the rather sloppy and informal use of the notion of Kuhnian paradigm among psychologists and behavior therapists. First, a paradigm by definition involves a problem solution—one can only say X is a paradigm—at least in the Kuhnian sense—after X has solved a problem. This term is not synonymous with "theory" or "hypothesis." It is only correct,

for example, to use the phrase "the psychoanalytic paradigm" or the "Rogerian paradigm" if these can be shown to solve some clinical problem. Thus, it can be validly said that there are cognitive and behavioral paradigms because, for example, problem solutions can be found in the Chambliss list. However, other usages are simply exegetically incorrect.

Cognitive and Behavior Therapies and Feyerabendian Anarchism

The views of Paul Feyerabend—a student of Popper's—are particularly challenging for both philosophers of science and cognitive-behavioral therapists—but perhaps the way in which the challenge is framed can be instructive. Feyerabend argued that a proper examination of the history of science as well as best fulfilling the Popperian question of maximizing criticism in order to root out error requires what he calls *methodological anarchism*—anything goes. Any other rule inhibits progress, according to Feyerabend.

Here are a few key quotes to get a better idea of Feyerabend's views. One should also examine Feyerabend's (1975) rhetorical style—he is quite the provocateur:

> Everywhere science is enriched by unscientific methods and unscientific results … the separation of science and non-science is not only artificial but also detrimental to the advancement of knowledge. If we want to understand nature, if we want to master our physical surroundings, then we must use all ideas, all methods, and not just a small selection of them. (pp. 305–306)

> Given any rule, however "fundamental" or "necessary" for science, there are always circumstances when it is advisable not only to ignore the rule, but to adopt its opposite. For example, there are circumstances when it is advisable to introduce, elaborate and defend *ad hoc* hypotheses, or hypotheses which contradict well-established and generally accepted experimental results, or hypotheses whose content is smaller than the content of the existing and empirically adequate alternative, or self-inconsistent hypotheses, and so on. (pp. 23–24)

> Unanimity of opinion may be fitting for a church, for the frightened or greedy victims of some (ancient, or modern) myth, or for the weak and willing followers of some tyrant. Variety of opinion is necessary for objective knowledge. And a method that encourages variety is also the only method that

is comparable with a humanitarian outlook. (p. 8, emphasis in original)

Feyerabend's methodological anarchism has had little influence upon cognitive therapy. In some way it is antithetical to a metaview held by many cognitive-behavioral therapists—that science is special and it does have special rules and what distinguishes cognitive and behavior therapies from many other approaches to therapy is that cognitive-behavioral therapy follows these rules better or more often. However, Feyerabend is useful to at least raise the question of whether our notion of scientific method is too restrictive. The view that Skinner greatly modified this view by introducing single-subject methodologies and the view that soft psychology has made "slow progress" to use Meehl's (1978) term suggests that we ought to be perpetually examining our metanotions of valid scientific methods.

Cognitive and Behavior Therapies, and Laudan's Problem Solving

Larry Laudan stressed that science is essentially a problem-solving enterprise—an emphasis, for example, shared in Nezu and Nezu's problem-solving therapy in cognitive and behavior therapies. Laudan states:

The rationale for accepting or rejecting any theory is thus fundamentally based on the idea of problem-solving progress. If one research tradition has solved more important problems than its rivals, then accepting that tradition is rational precisely to the degree that we are aiming to "progress," i.e., to maximize the scope of solved problems. In other words, the choice of one tradition over its rivals is a progressive (and thus a rational) choice precisely to the extent that the chosen tradition is a better problem solver than its rivals. (p. 109)

Laudan also said that science has two distinct types of problems: (1) empirical problems, such as "What causes depression?" but also (2) conceptual problems, such as "But what actually is meant by 'depression'?" Laudan stated a theory must be appraised by evaluating its effectiveness in solving both kinds of problems. Laudan's problem-solving model "argues that the elimination of conceptual difficulties is as much constitutive of progress as increasing empirical support" (p. 147). Laudan even stated: "it is possible that a change from an empirically well-supported theory to a less well-supported one could be

progressive, provided that the latter resolved significant conceptual difficulties confronting the former (p. 147)." The better theory solves more conceptual problems while minimizing empirical anomalies.

It has been the case that cognitive-behavioral therapists have placed too little value in identifying and attempting to solve conceptual problems. Wittgenstein (2009) famously said about psychology,

The confusion and barrenness of psychology is not to be explained by calling it a "young science"; its state is not comparable with that of physics, for instance, in its beginnings. For in psychology there are experimental methods and conceptual confusion. The existence of the experimental method makes us think we have the means of solving the problems that trouble us; though problem and method pass one another by. (p. 232)

It might be very valuable in the future of cognitive-behaviorists to begin to identify and make progress on their conceptual problems. There are many examples of this kind of confusion, but O'Donohue and Casselles (1993) have written about the conceptual problems of the term "homophobia" and O'Donohue and Benuto (2011) have written about the conceptual issues in the notion of "cultural sensitivity."

Cognitive and Behavior Therapies, and Grossian Rhetorical Analyses

Alan Gross in his *Rhetoric of Science* claimed that the practice of science is fundamentally a rhetorical activity—an activity meant to persuade. Gross states, "Rhetorically, the creation of knowledge is a task beginning with self-persuasion and ending with the persuasion of others" (Gross, 1990, p. 3). The rhetorical analysis of science becomes "the application of the machinery of rhetoric to the texts of sciences" (p. ix). Traditionally, one of the purposes of language—texts or talks—is persuasion (Quine & Ullian, 1970). However, in this strong view, rhetoric does not just influence beliefs; rhetoric becomes constitutive of knowledge. Bazerman (1988) stated:

Persuasion is at the heart of science, not at the unrespectable fringe. An intelligent rhetoric practiced within a serious knowledgeable committed research community is a serious method of truth seeking. The most serious scientific communication is not that which disowns persuasion, but which persuades in the deepest, most compelling manner, thereby sweeping aside more superficial arguments. Science has developed tools and tricks that make nature the strongest ally of persuasive argument, even while casting aside some of the more familiar and ancient tools and tricks of rhetoric as being only superficial and temporarily persuasive. (p. 321)

It is beyond the scope of this chapter to critically analyze this account in much detail. However, it has become very influential in recent decades. The reader is referred to O'Donohue (2013) for a more extended treatment. It is fair to say that a rhetorical analysis of cognitive-behavioral therapy might be long overdue. Therapy—as well as science—can be seen as a fundamentally rhetorical activity—clients are attempting to persuade their therapists ("My smoking is really not a problem") and therapists are attempting to persuade clients ("Therapy X can help you, but only if you do your homework"). The field probably has been a bit naïve in assuming a Joe-Friday-just-the-facts-ma'm is sufficiently persuasive. It is probably the case that Bill Miller's motivational interviewing is the intervention that both explicitly recognizes the rhetorical burden of the therapist as well as having processing that may enhance the therapist's rhetorical effectiveness.

Cognitive and Behavior Therapies, and Postmodernism

If the reader is to be conversant in twenty-first-century metascience, he or she must have a basic understanding of the major dimensions of these views and the controversies that they have spawned. Koertge (1998) provided a nice summary of the relevance of postmodernist and social constructionist views to science:

• Every aspect of that complex set of enterprises that we call science, including, above all, its content and results, is shaped by and can be understood only in its local historical and cultural context.

• In particular, the products of scientific inquiry, the so-called laws of nature must always be viewed as social constructions. Their validity depends on the consensus of "experts" in just the same way as the legitimacy of a pope depends on a council of cardinals.

• Although scientists typically succeed in arrogating special epistemic authority to themselves, scientific knowledge is just "one story among many." The more epistemological authority that science has in a given society, the more important it is to unmask its pretensions to be an enterprise dedicated to the pursuit of objective knowledge. Science must be "humbled."

• Because the quest for objective knowledge is a quixotic one, the best way to appraise scientific claims is through a process of *political* evaluation. Because the "evidence" for a scientific claim is never conclusive and is always open to negotiation, the best way to evaluate scientific results is to ask who stands to benefit if the claim is taken to be true. Thus, for the citizen the key question about a scientific result should not be how well tested the claim is but, rather, *Cui bono?*

• "Science is politics by other means"; the results of scientific inquiry are profoundly and importantly shaped by the ideological agendas of powerful elites.

• There is no univocal sense in which the science of one society is better than that of another. In particular, Euroscience is not objectively superior to the various ethnosciences and shamanisms described by anthropologists or invented by Afrocentrists.

• Neither is there any clear sense in which we can talk about scientific progress within the European tradition. On the contrary, science is characterized chiefly by its complicity in all the most negative and oppressive aspects of modern history: increasingly destructive warfare, environmental disasters, racism, sexism, eugenics, exploitation, alienation, and imperialism.

• Given the impossibility of scientific objectivity, it is futile to exhort scientists and policymakers to try harder to remove ideological bias from the practice of science. Instead, what we need to do is deliberately introduce "corrective biases" and "progressive political values" into science. There is a call for "emancipatory science" and "advocacy research" (pp. 3–4).

As was stated in the beginning of the chapter, there are diverse streams inside cognitive-behavioral therapy. The streams most influenced by postmodernism appear to be feminist approaches to cognitive and behavior therapies—with their emphasis on the importance of political analysis and emancipatory goals; as well as, more generally, the interests of many cognitive behaviorists in cultural sensitivity, as there are political and advocacy interests within this stream. However, it is fair to say that this postmodernist influence within cognitive and behavior therapies is rather restrained—not too many are radically critiquing science or advocating native indigenous epistemologies to replace the narrative of science.

Conclusions

Behavior therapy was never a monolithic enterprise. From its beginning it had complex relationships to behaviorisms (radical, methodological, and others); it had complex relationships with learning theories (operant, Hullian, classical, observational); it had complex relationships to theoretical accounts of behavior (reciprocal inhibition vs. two-factor theory or vs. operant accounts); it had complex relationships with critiques of the medical model; it had complex relationships to what kind of problems it was attempting to solve (children's defiance, nocturnal enuresis, or elective mutism), and so on. As it matured, these complexities increased. Kuhn (2001) has suggested that as sciences mature it often morphs into what he calls "micro-communities," which roughly are small groups of scientists who share a number of beliefs—agree on what problems ought to be worked on—what methodologies are best for this, and so on, and these can be quite distinct from other micro-communities. It appears that there is some truth in this analysis when looking into contemporary behavior therapy.

It would be advantageous, however, for behavior therapy to understand its conceptual, theoretical, and empirical roots. It is worrisome that the new generation of behavior therapists may not realize the worth of some of these initial values—for example, the sound grounding in the basic learning laboratory—or the willingness to address the conceptual underpinnings of the power structure. It is also timely for behavior therapists to have a better understanding of their understanding of science because this is a complex and important question given its centrality to cognitive-behavioral therapists.

Notes

1. Of course, a speaker can serve as one's own listener in which case she herself serves as a "mediator" of sorts ("Julie, get up and get yourself a glass of water.").
2. A detailed description of a total verbal episode is beyond the scope of the present chapter. For readers interested in this topic, please see the following for examples (Skinner, 1957, pp. 38–39, 57, 84–85).

References

American Board of Behavioral Psychology. (n.d.). *Archival description of behavioral psychology*. Retrieved January 2015, from http://www.personal.kent.edu/~edowd/ABPP/definition.htm

American Board of Professional Psychology. (n.d.). *Cognitive and behavioral psychology*. Retrieved January 2015, from http://www.abpp.org/i4a/pages/index.cfm?pageid=3358

American Psychiatric Association. (2013). *Diagnostic and statistical manual of mental disorders* (5th ed.). Washington, DC: Author.

Baars, B. (1986). *The cognitive revolution in psychology*. New York: Guilford.

Baum, W. M. (1994). *Understanding behaviorism*. New York: Harper Collins College Publishers.

Bazerman, C. (1988). Shaping written knowledge: The genre and activity of the experimental article in science. University of Wisconsin Press, Madison.

Beck, J. S. (1995). *Cognitive therapy: Basics and beyond*. New York: Guilford.

Buss, D. M. (2008). *Evolutionary psychology: The new science of the mind* (3rd ed). Boston: Allyn & Bacon.

Charney, D. S., & Nestler, E. J. (2008). *Neurobiology of mental illness* (3rd ed). Oxford, UK: Oxford University Press.

Chomsky, N. (1959). Review of Skinner's Verbal Behavior. *Language*, 35, 26–58.

Chrysant, S. G. (2000). Treatment of white coat hypertension. *Current Hypertenions Reports*, 2(4), 412–417.

Confer, J. C., Easton, J. A., Fleischman, D. S., Goetz, C. D., Lewis, D. M. G., Perilloux, C., & Buss, D. M. (2010). Evolutionary psychology: Controversies, questions, prospects, and limitations. *American Psychologist*, 65(2), 110–126.

Council of Specialties in Professional Psychology. (n.d.). *Behavioral and cognitive psychology*. Retrieved January 2015, from http://cospp.org/specialties/behavioral-and-cognitive-psychology

Damasio, A. R. (1999). *The feeling of what happens: Body and emotion in the making of consciousness*. New York: Harcourt Brace.

Damasio, A., & Carvalho, G. B. (2013). The nature of feelings: Evolutionary and neurobiological origins. *Nature Reviews Neuroscience*, 14, 143–152.

Dimidjian, S., & Hollon, S. D. (2010). How would you know if psychotherapy was harmful? *American Psychologist*, 65, 21–33.

Edmondson, C. B., & Conger, J. C. (1996). A review of treatment efficacy for individuals with anger problems: Conceptual, assessment, and methodological issues. *Clinical Psychology Review*, 16, 251–275.

Ellis, A. (1980). *Growth through reason*. Chatsworth CA: Wilshire Book Company.

Ellis, A. (1981). *Rational-emotive therapy and cognitive behavior therapy*. New York: Springer.

Ellis, A. (2009). Cognitive restructuring of the disputing of irrational beliefs. In W. O'Donohue & J.E. Fisher (Eds.), *General principles and empirically supported techniques of cognitive behavior therapy* (pp. 189–193). Hoboken, NJ: John Wiley & Sons, Inc.

Eysenck, H. J. (1952). The effects of psychotherapy: An evaluation. *Journal of Consulting Psychology*, 16, 319–324.

Ferster, C. B., & Skinner, B. F. (1957). *Schedules of reinforcement*. New York: Appleton-Century-Crofts.

Feyerabend, P. (1975). Against method: Outline of an anarchistic theory of knowledge. London: Verso.

Foa, E., B., & Rothbaum, B. O. (1998). *Treating the trauma of rape: Cognitive-behavioral therapy for PTSD*. New York: The Guilford Press.

Galbicka, G. (1994). Shaping in the 21st Century: Moving percentile schedules into applied settings. *Journal of Applied Behavior Analysis, 27*, 739–760.

Gardner, H. (1985). *The mind's new science: A history of the cognitive revolution*. New York: Basic Books.

Goldberg, H., & Goldberg, Irene. (1996). *Family therapy, an overview* (4th ed.). Pacific Grove: Brooks/Cole Publishing Company.

Gross, A. G. (1990). *The rhetoric of science*. Cambridge, MA: Harvard University Press.

Hayes, S. C. (2004). Acceptance and Commitment Therapy, Relational Frame Theory, and the Third Wave of Behavioral and Cognitive Therapies. *Behavior Therapy, 35*, 639–665.

Hayes, S. C., Luoma, J. B., Bond, F. W., Masuda, A., & Lillis, J. (2006). Acceptance and Commitment Therapy: Model, processes and outcomes. *Behaviour Research and Therapy, 44*, 1–25.

Hayes, C. W., Orstein, J., & Gage, W. W. (1988). *The ABC's of languages and linguistics: A basic introduction to language science*. Lincolnwood, IL: National Textbook Company.

Hergenhahn, B. R. (1997). *An introduction to the history of psychology* (3rd ed.). Brooks/Cole.

Holland, J. G., & Skinner, B. F. (1961). *The analysis of behavior: A program for self-instruction*. New York: McGraw-Hill.

Hollon, S. D., Shelton, R. C., & Davis, D. D. (1993). Cognitive therapy for depression: Conceptual issues and clinical efficacy. *Journal of Consulting and Clinical Psychology, 61*, 270–275.

Jacobson, N. S., Martell, C. R., & Dimidjian, S. (2001). Behavioral activation treatment for depression: Returning to contextual roots. *Clinical Psychology: Science and Practice, 8*, 255–270.

Kahl, K. G., Winter, L., & Schweiger, U. (2012). The third wave of cognitive behavioral therapies. *Current Opinion in Psychiatry, 25*(6), 522–528.

Kazdin, A. E. (1978). History of behavior modification: Experimental foundations of contemporary research. Baltimore, MD: Univ. Park Press.

Koertge, N. (1998). Postmodernisms and the problem of scientific literacy. In N. Koertge (Ed.), *A house built on sand: Exposing postmodernist myths about science*. New York: Oxford University Press.

Kuhn, T. S. (1962). *The structure of scientific revolutions*. Chicago: University of Chicago Press.

Kuhn, T. S. (1974). Second thoughts on paradigms. In F. Suppe (Ed.), *The structure of scientific theories* (pp. 459–482). Urbana: University of Illinois Press.

Kuhn, T. S. (2001). *The road since structure* (J. Conant & J. Haugeland, Eds.). Chicago: University of Chicago Press.

Lakatos, I. (1970). Falsification and the methodology of scientific research programs. In I. Lakatos & A. Musgrave (Eds.), *Criticism and the growth of knowledge* (pp. 91–195). New York: Cambridge University Press.

Lakatos, I. (1978). Falsification and the methodology of scientific research programs. In J. Worrall & G. Currie (Eds.), *The methodology of scientific research programmes* (pp. 8–101). Cambridge, UK: Cambridge University Press.

Last, C. G. (1985). Cognitive restructuring. In A. S. Bellack & M. Hersen (Eds.), *Dictionary of behavior therapy techniques* (pp. 59–60). New York: Pergamon.

LeDoux, J. E. (1998). *The emotional brain: The mysterious underpinnings of emotional life*. New York: Simon & Schuster.

LeDoux, J. E., Cicchetti, P., Xagoraris, A., & Romanski, L. M. (1990). The lateral amygdaloid nucleus: Sensory interface of the amygdala in fear conditioning. *Journal of Neuroscience, 10*, 1062–1069.

LeDoux, J. E., Iwata, J., Cicchetti, P., & Reis, D. J. (1988). Different projections of the central amygdaloid nucleus mediate autonomic and behavioral correlates of conditioned fear. *Journal of Neuroscience, 8*, 2517–2529.

Leahey, T. H. (1992). The mythical revolutions of American psychology. *American Psychologist, 47*, 308–318.

Lohr, J. M., Hooke, W., Gist, R. & Tolin, D. F. (2003). Novel and controversial treatments for trauma-related stress disorders. In S. O. Lilienfeld, S. J. Lynn & J. M. Lohr (Eds.), *Science and pseudoscience in clinical psychology* (pp. 243–272). New York: Guilford Press.

McFall, R. M. (1991). Manifesto for a science of clinical psychology. *Clinical Psychologist, 44*, 75–88.

McFall, R. M. (1996). Elaborate reflections on a simple manifesto. *Applied and Preventive Psychology, 9*, 5–21.

Mahoney, M. J. (1977). Reflections on the cognitive learning trend in psychotherapy. *American Psychologist, 32*, 5–13.

Mahoney, M. J. (1987). The cognitive sciences and psychotherapy. In K. S. Dobson (Ed.), *Handbook of cognitive-behavioral therapies* (pp. 357–386). New York: Guilford.

Mahoney, M. J. (1988). The cognitive sciences and psychotherapy: Patterns in a developing relationship. In K. S. Dobson (Ed.), *Handbook of cognitive-behavioral therapies* (pp. 357–386). New York: Guilford Press.

Martin, G., & Pear, J. (1978). *Behavior modification: What it is and how to do it*. Englewood Cliffs, NJ: Prentice Hall.

Meehl, P. E. (1978). Theoretical risks and tabular asterisks: Sir Karl, Sir Ronald, and the slow progress of soft psychology. *Journal of Consulting and Clinical Psychology, 46*(4), 806–834.

Michael, J. (1993). *Concepts and principles of behavior analysis*. Kalamazoo, MI: Association for Behavior Analysis.

Miltenberger, R. G. (2001). *Behavior modification: Principles and procedures* (2nd ed.). Belmont, CA: Wadsworth.

Mowrer, O. H. (1947). On the dual nature of learning—a reinterpretation of conditioning and problem solving. *Harvard Educational Review, 17*, 102–148.

Mowrer, O. H. (1951). Two-factor learning theory: Summary and comment. *Psychological Review, 58*, 350–354.

Mowrer, O. H. (1956). Two-factor learning theory reconsidered, with special reference to secondary reinforcement and the concept of habit. *Psychological Review, 63*, 114–128.

Nesse, R. (2005). Evolutionary psychology. In D. Buss (Ed.), *The handbook of evolutionary psychology* (pp. 903–927). Hoboken, NJ: Wiley.

Nezu, A. M., & Nezu, C. M. (Eds.). (1989). *Clinical decision making in behavior therapy: A problem-solving perspective*. Champaign, IL: Research Press.

Nezu, A. M., Nezu, C. M., & D'Zurilla, T. J. (2013). *Problem-solving therapy: A treatment manual*. New York: Springer.

Nezu, A. M., Nezu, C. M., & Perri, M. G. (1989). *Problem-solving therapy for depression: Theory, research, and clinical guidelines*. New York: Wiley.

O'Donohue, W. T. (2009). A brief history of cognitive behavior therapy: Are there troubles ahead? In W. T. O'Donohue, J. Fisher, S. C. Hayes (Eds.), *General principles and empirically supported techniques of Cognitive Behavior Therapy* (2nd ed.) (pp. 1–14). New York: John Wiley & Sons, Inc.

O'Donohue, W. T. (2013). *Clinical psychology and the philosophy of science*. Switzerland: Springer International Publishing.

O'Donohue, W., & Benuto, L. (2011). Problems with the construct of cultural sensitivity. *Scientific Review of Mental Health Practice, 7*, 24–37.

O'Donohue, W. T., & Casselles, C. (1993). Homophobia: Conceptual, definitional, and value issues. *Journal of Psychopathology and Behavioral Assessment, 15*(3), 177–195.

O'Donohue, W. T., & Ferguson, K. E. (2001). *The psychology of B. F. Skinner.* Thousand Oaks, CA: Sage Publishing.

O'Donohue, W., Henderson, D. Hayes, S., Fisher, J., & Hayes, L. (Eds.) (2001). *The history of the behavioral therapies: Founders' personal histories.* Reno, NV: Context Press.

Pavlov, I. P. (1927). *Conditioned reflexes: An investigation of the physiological activity of the cerebral cortex.* (Trans. and Edited by G. V. Anrep). London: Oxford University Press.

Pavlov, I. P. (1928). *Lectures on conditioned reflexes* (Vol. 1). New York: International Universities Press.

Pierce, W. D., & Epling, W. F. (1999). *Behavior analysis and learning* (2nd ed.). Upper Saddle River, NJ: Prentice Hall.

Popper, K. R. (1959). *The logic of scientific discovery.* New York: Basic Books.

Popper, K. R. (1962). *Conjectures and refutations: The growth of scientific knowledge.* New York: Basic Books.

Popper, K. R. (1972). *Objective knowledge.* Oxford: Clarendon Press.

Quine, W. V., & Ullian, J. S. (1970). *The web of belief.* New York: Random House.

Rodrigues, S. M., Schafe, G. E., & LeDoux, J. E. (2004). Molecular mechanisms underlying review emotional learning and memory in the lateral amygdala. *Neuron, 44*, 75–91.

Skinner, B. F. (1945a). The operational analysis of psychological terms. *Psychological Review, 52*, 270–277, 291–294.

Skinner, B. F. (1945b, October). Baby in a box (The machine age comes to the nursery! Introducing the mechanical baby-tender). *Ladies Home Journal, 62*, 30–31, 135–136, 138.

Skinner, B. F. (1948). *Walden two.* London: Macmillan.

Skinner, B. F. (1953). *Science and human behavior.* New York: Macmillan.

Skinner, B.F. (1956). A case history in scientific method. *American Psychologist, 11*, 221–233.

Skinner, B. F. (1957). *Verbal behavior.* New York: Appleton-Century-Crofts.

Skinner, B. F. (1960). Teaching machines. *Review of Economics and Statistics, 42*(Suppl.), 189–191.

Skinner, B. F. (1966). The phylogeny and ontogeny of behavior. *Science, 153*, 1205–1213.

Skinner, B. F. (1969). *Contingencies of reinforcement: A theoretical analysis.* New York: Appleton Century.

Skinner, B. F. (1971). *Beyond freedom and dignity.* New York: Knopf.

Skinner, B. F. (1972). Some issues concerning the control of human behavior. In B. F. Skinner (Ed.), *Cumulative record* (3rd ed., pp. 25–38). New York: Appleton-Century-Crofts.

Skinner, B. F. (1974). *About behaviorism.* New York: Vintage.

Skinner, B. F. (1981). Selection by consequences. *Science, 213*, 501–504.

Skinner, B. F. (1984). Selection by consequences. *Behavioral and Brain Sciences, 7*, 477–510.

Skinner, B. F. (1988). Reply to J. Schull's, "Selectionism, mentalisms, and behaviorism." In A. C. Catania & S. Hamad's (Eds.), *The selection of behavior: The operant behaviorism of B. F. Skinner* (p. 65). Cambridge and New York: Cambridge University Press.

Skinner, B. F. (1990). Can psychology be a science of the mind? *American Psychologist, 45*, 1206–1210.

Smith, L. D. (1986). *Behaviorism and logical positivism: A reassessment of the alliance.* Stanford, CA: Stanford University Press.

Wittgenstein, L. (2009). *Philosophical investigations* (4th ed.). P.M.S. Hacker and Joachim Schulte (Eds. and trans.). Oxford: Wiley-Blackwell.

Wolpe, J. (1958). *Psychotherapy by reciprocal inhibition.* Stanford, CA: Stanford University Press.

Wolpe, J. (1976). *Theme and variations: A behavior therapy casebook.* New York: Pergamon Press.

Wolpe, J. (1990). *The practice of behavior therapy* (4th ed.). New York: Pergamon Press.

Competencies in Cognitive and Behavioral Interventions

Christine Maguth Nezu, Sarah Ricelli, *and* Arthur M. Nezu

Abstract

This chapter briefly describes the history of the competency movement in professional psychology and the development of competency benchmarks across various levels of professional development. With regard to applied psychology, we define the specialty of cognitive and behavioral psychology, and the application of the core competency areas. The areas of competency included in this chapter are relevant for psychologists who define themselves as specialists in the area of cognitive and behavioral psychology and who provide independent psychological services. Moreover, these competencies have been defined and elaborated through professional consensus to the specialty of cognitive and behavioral psychology as one of 15 psychology specialty areas recognized by the American Board of Professional Psychology (ABPP). Examples of both foundational and functional competencies required for best practices in the specialty of cognitive and behavioral psychology are provided and discussed.

Key Words: cognitive and behavioral psychology, professional competencies, assessment, intervention, foundational competencies, functional competencies

Over the past 20 years, professional psychology has devoted increasing attention to the identification and description of core competencies to inform and measure learning outcomes of psychology trainees (Fouad et al., 2009). For example, the APA-sponsored task force on Assessment of Competence in Professional Psychology has put forth published guidelines for the assessment of competence. These guidelines and benchmarks for the evaluation of competence are based, in part, on a review of the competency assessment models developed both within (e.g., Assessment of Competence Workgroup from Competencies Conference; Roberts, Borden, Christiansen, & Lopez, 2005) and outside (e.g., Accreditation Council for Graduate Medical Education, and American Board of Medical Specialties, 2015) the profession of psychology (Kaslow et al., 2007).

Moreover, additional psychological organizations have contributed to this national discussion,

including various entities primarily interested in credentialing professional psychologists, such as the American Board of Professional Psychology (ABPP), the Association of State and Provincial Psychology Boards (ASPPB), and the National Register of Health Service Providers in Psychology (Nezu & Nezu, 2004). This widespread interest and importance of the issue of competence can be especially appreciated, given the attention and collaboration afforded to this effort by professional groups from around the world.

From the earliest models of competence in professional education and training programs developed by the National Council of Schools and Programs in Professional Psychology (NCSPP) in 1986 (Peterson, Peterson, Abrams, Stricker, & Ducheny, 2010) to the current competencies delineated by the Assessment of Competency Benchmarks Workgroup authorized by the APA Board of Educational Affairs (BEA; Fouad et al.,

2009), much effort in professional psychology has been devoted to defining and assessing competence. Nelson has described the move toward defining and measuring the learning outcomes of trainees, referred to as competencies, as a "major pedagogical shift" (Nelson, 2007) as clinical educational programs and credentialing communities have embraced the need for this type of evaluation.

More recently, psychology specialties have adapted the core competencies defined by the field to postlicensure, specialty psychology practice. As an applied discipline, psychology has increasingly recognized the distinct and unique nature among various orientations, modalities, and approaches with regard to professional practice. These specialty areas represent distinct ways of practicing one's profession across various domains of activities that are based on specific bodies of scientific literature and particular populations or problems. For example, the American Psychological Association (APA) established the Commission on the Recognition of Specialties and Proficiencies in Professional Psychology (CRSPPP) in order to define the criteria by which a psychology specialty could be recognized. The Council of Credentialing Organizations in Professional Psychology (CCOPP), an interorganizational entity, was formed in reaction to the need to identify criteria and guidelines regarding the types of training programs related to education, training, and professional development of individuals seeking specialization. Finally, the Council of Specialties in Professional Psychology (CoS) was formed in 1997, independent to APA, to foster communication among established specialties, so that a unified position to the public regarding specialty education, training, credentialing, and practice standards could be communicated and applied to all specialties. Cognitive and behavioral psychology is one of 15 specialty boards currently recognized in the field. A brief history of the specialty is described in the next section.

Brief History of the Specialty of Cognitive and Behavioral Psychology

Cognitive and behavioral psychology was recognized as a specialty by the American Board of Professional Psychology (ABPP) in 1992 (originally titled the American Board of Behavioral Psychology when first incorporated in 1987 with support from the Association of Behavior and Cognitive Therapies, which was then known as the Association for Advancement of Behavior Therapy). Later, in 1994, the American Board of Cognitive and Behavioral

Psychology (ABCBP) adopted its current name to reflect the growing breadth of the field and to be consistent with similar name changes by organizations that promoted cognitive and behavioral therapies around the world, including the *Association for Behavioral and Cognitive Therapies* and *World Congress of Behavioral and Cognitive Therapies*. In 2000, the specialty was recognized by the CRSPPP, associated with the APA. Briefly described in the previous section, the mission of this commission involves reviewing petitions for specialty recognition within professional psychology and making recommendations to the APA regarding issues concerning psychology specialties and proficiencies. Additionally, a representative from the specialty of cognitive and behavioral psychology participates in the CoS, which is recognized by the APA and the ABPP to meet and consider policies affecting specialization in professional psychology.

Although there is no specific APA division that exclusively represents the specialty of cognitive and behavioral psychology, many specialists in this area are active in APA Divisions dedicated to behavioral analysis (APA Division 25), clinical psychology (Division 12, Section III, Society for a Science of Clinical Psychology), and developmental disabilities (Division 33). The postlicensure board certification process is administered by the American Board of Cognitive and Behavioral Psychology (ABCBP), and fellowship membership for board-certified cognitive and behavioral psychologists is offered through the American Academy of Cognitive and Behavioral Psychology. Related organizations that are multidisciplinary and include physicians, social workers, and other mental health professionals include the Association for Behavioral and Cognitive Therapies, the Behavior Analyst Certification Board, the Association for Behavior Analysis, and the Academy of Cognitive Therapy. Cognitive-behavioral psychologists are also very involved in the development of assessment and treatment strategies that cross over to other areas of professional psychology specialization, including (but not limited to) clinical, clinical child and adolescent, clinical health, geropsychology, school, organization and business consulting, couple and family, and rehabilitation areas.

Definition and Unique Characteristics of the Specialty

The specialty of cognitive and behavioral psychology emphasizes an experimental-clinical approach regarding the application of behavioral and cognitive sciences to understanding human behavior and developing interventions to enhance the human condition. Cognitive and behavioral psychologists engage in research, education, training, and clinical practice regarding a wide range of problems and populations. The specialty's distinct focus is two-fold: (a) its heavy reliance on empiricism and an evidence-based approach; and (b) its theoretical grounding in learning theories, broadly defined, including classical (respondent) learning models, such as associative and single stimulus conditioning, operant learning models, social learning, and information processing models (American Board of Cognitive and Behavioral Psychology, 2015).

With regard to education and training, cognitive and behavioral psychology has not been associated with a specific, specialty-affiliated, APA-accredited doctoral program. However, along with its emergence as a specialty, clinical, school, and counseling psychology training programs have historically included behavioral and cognitive courses, as well as training experiences, such as supervised clinical practicum. These have included theories of learning, neuroscience, cognitive psychology, and experimental analyses of behavior. Additionally, courses focused on learning theories were typically included in training programs for education, special education, clinical health, and behavioral economics.

Currently, there are four major subareas of the specialty that share their theoretical foundations in learning theory and a common approach to case conceptualization. These include applied behavior analysis, behavior therapy, cognitive-behavioral therapy, and cognitive therapy. While familiar with all subareas, cognitive and behavioral specialists most often focus their particular expertise on one of these focus areas. Additionally, there are many evidence-based therapeutic interventions and systems, as well as individual therapy techniques that fall under each subarea. For example, cognitive-behavioral therapy may include therapeutic interventions such as dialectical behavior therapy (DBT; Linehan, 1993) or cognitive processing therapy (CPT; Resick, Monson, & Chard, 2007), systems of psychotherapy such as problem-solving therapy (PST; D'Zurilla & Nezu, 2007; Nezu, Nezu, & D'Zurilla, 2013), acceptance and commitment therapy (ACT; Hayes, Strosahl, & Wilson, 1999), or behavioral activation treatment (BA; Dimidjian, Barrera, Martell, Munoz, & Lewinsohn, 2011; Jacobsen, Martell, & Dimidjian, 2001), as well as specific therapy techniques such as virtual systematic desensitization (Rothbaum et al., 1995), exposure and response prevention (ERP; Wilhelm & Steketee, 2006), cognitive hypnotherapy (Dowd, 2000), or progressive relaxation training (Bernstein, Borkovec, & Hazlett-Stevens, 2000). Moreover, learning is understood to occur on both a conscious and nonconscious level of awareness. Applied behavioral analysis may include assessment systems such as functional analysis or interventions such as token economies, time-out procedures, or differential reinforcement of incompatible behavior (Kazdin, 2000). The construct of "behavior" in the specialty of cognitive and behavioral psychology is very broadly defined to include overt actions, as well as private phenomena, such as cognitions, affect, emotional arousal, and physiological events (Dowd, Chen, & Arnold, 2010). In summary, the definition of cognitive-behavioral therapy is wide ranging and has its historic roots in behavior therapy, cognitive therapy, and experimental analysis of behavior, as well as contemporary learning approaches, physiologic psychology, neurocognitive models, and research concerning multiculturalism and theories of emotion. The specialty remains focused on clinical problems and clinical solutions associated with learning.

Application of the Core Competencies to Cognitive and Behavioral Psychology

As mentioned previously, the APA-sponsored Assessments of Competency Benchmarks Work Group has defined the essential components of core competencies for psychologists. This workgroup was the outcome of a proposal from the CCTC to the relevant APA board (BEA). The document developed by this workgroup identified and defined the core competency areas and created benchmarks for various levels of education and training (Fouad et al., 2009). Each area of competency is defined as under the rubric of two main competency areas: foundational and functional competencies. Foundational competencies represent important abilities and perspectives such as professional identity, self-reflection, and ethics that are incorporated into all of the day-to-day functional skills required of professional psychologists. Functional skills include important professional tasks such as assessment, treatment, consultation, or supervision. The ABPP has incorporated and adapted these areas of competence as a heuristic for all specialties under its organizational umbrella to define best practice across postlicensure specialty practice. The competencies, adapted from Fouad and colleagues (2009), are listed next.

- Foundation competencies
  - Professionalism
  - Reflective practice
  - Scientific knowledge and methods
  - Relationships
  - Interdisciplinary systems
  - Individual and cultural diversity
  - Ethical and legal standards and policy
- Functional competencies
  - Assessment
  - Intervention
  - Consultation
  - Research and evaluation
  - Supervision
  - Teaching
  - Management and administration
  - Advocacy

The following sections will describe the competencies for the specialty of cognitive-behavioral psychology with regard to each of these competency areas. Where relevant, competency areas may be combined to provide the most accurate description of the actualization of these competencies in this specialty.

Professional Identification

The professional values of the cognitive and behavioral specialty in psychology are derived from the vast amounts of scientific literature to construct a comprehensive bio-psycho-social-neural understanding of how these various components all result in our learned patterns of emotional reactivity, thoughts, and behavior. The hallmark value of empiricism that originally defined the specialty has been maintained throughout its development, and this preference for reliance on assessment and treatment interventions with a strong evidence base characterizes the professional identity of the cognitive and behavioral specialist.

With regard to a cognitive-behavioral identification with professional organizations, the specialty has no specific psychology division within the APA; however, it has maintained specialty recognition by the CRSPPP since 2000. Board certification through the ABCBP, under the umbrella of the ABPP, provides an assurance to both the public and the profession that the specialist in cognitive and behavioral psychology has met the education, training, and experience requirements, as well as demonstrating the advanced competencies required by the specialty through an individual, face-to face, peer-reviewed examination. The

ABPP continues to remain a "gold standard" for peer assessment of competency across all of its recognized specialties.

Meaningful involvement with the profession of psychology in general and the specialty field of cognitive and behavioral psychology, in particular, is an important part of the continued professional development of the cognitive and behavioral specialist. Several organizations provide especially meaningful opportunities for cognitive and behavioral specialists to learn of advances in the field, network with other professionals, and engage in continuing education opportunities. A few of these organizations are mentioned next.

ASSOCIATION FOR BEHAVIORAL AND COGNITIVE THERAPIES (HTTP://WWW.ABCT.ORG/HOME)

This multidisciplinary organization provides a major vehicle for collegial interaction and professional development for cognitive and behavioral specialists. The stated mission of this organization is a commitment "to the advancement of scientific approaches to the understanding and improvement of human functioning through the investigation and application of behavioral, cognitive, and other evidence-based principles to the assessment, prevention, treatment of human problems, and the enhancement of health and well-being."

THE AMERICAN PSYCHOLOGICAL SOCIETY (HTTP://WWW.PSYCHOLOGICALSCIENCE.ORG/)

APS was founded in 1988 to promote, protect, and advance scientific psychology at the national and international levels. Many cognitive-behavioral specialists who are committed to promoting practice with a strong evidence base are members of APS, and it has shown a strong growth since it was founded in 1988.

JOURNALS RELEVANT TO THE SPECIALTY

Numerous journals and published therapy manuals are relevant to the specialty, and many clinical psychology journals also provide information concerning the latest research with regard to cognitive and behavioral psychology. Additionally, there are various relevant journals from other fields or specialties that may spotlight the importance of learning-based theories and interventions to better understand psychological phenomena associated with the journal.

INTERNATIONAL ASSOCIATIONS

There are cognitive and behavioral specialists practicing all over the world, and organizations have been developed in North America (ABCT), Latin America (Asociación Latinoamericana de Análisis, Modificación del Comportamiento y terapia cognitivo conductual; ALAMOC), Asia (Asia Cognitive Behavioral Therapy Association, ACBTA), the United Kingdom (British Association for Behavioural and Cognitive Psychotherapies; BABCP), and Europe (European Association of Cognitive and Behavioural Therapies; EACBT). Every 3 years, six organizations that promote education and dissemination of cognitive and behavioral therapies internationally sponsor a World Congress for Behavioral and Cognitive Therapies (WCBCT), which provides an opportunity for researchers and clinicians from around the world to meet and discuss "state of the art" cognitive and behavioral psychotherapies across its many applications throughout the fields of mental health.

APPLIED BEHAVIORAL ANALYSIS

Specific to the methods and technology of applied behavior analysts, there are organizations, such as the Behavior Analyst Certification Board®, Inc. (BACB®), that were developed to credential professionals and require review and evaluation of their training and skills to protect the integrity of such interventions. With regard to a worldwide focus, there is also an Association for Behavior Analysis, International (ABAI), which is a nonprofit organization with a mission that supports the growth and vitality of the science of behavior analysis through research, education, and practice.

Self-Reflection, Relationships, and Continuing Professional Development

Competent practice requires personal self-awareness and reflection. Similar to other specialties, cognitive and behavioral psychologists learn to be aware of their own internal processes, such as emotional reactions, thoughts, and patterns of behavior, much in the way they instruct their patients. When psychotherapists are mindful of their own reactions, they may be better prepared to connect with the populations they are serving. This is important, in that whatever the approach or specific intervention employed, the therapeutic relationship remains one of the most powerful determinants of positive outcome in therapy (Norcross, Beutler, & Levant, 2007. Cognitive-behavioral psychologists have

recognized the central importance of the therapeutic relationship to their specialty (Gilbert & Leahy, 2007). This underscores the recognition of self-awareness and self-reflection and, as such, specialists' engagement in peer supervision and consultation. Such practice helps cognitive and behavioral psychologists learn how to identify their own challenges in relationships with others, especially those that may reflect habituated ways of responding to various social, environmental, and emotional interpersonal stimuli.

Another aspect of competency regarding relationships is that psychologists relate meaningfully and effectively with individuals, groups, and communities. Without self-reflection, empathic understanding, and the ability to understand alternative perspectives, this competency is compromised. Finally, as a part of the process of self-reflection, cognitive and behavioral psychotherapists will also remain attuned to changes in the specialty and engage in a lifelong learning process.

Although the theories upon which the specialty was originally grounded have a long history, cognitive and behavior specialists are committed to a lifelong learning process, recognizing that the paradigms of scientific study shift over time and that communication innovations contribute to a continual surge of new information. New technologies in brain imaging, virtual reality, and other phenomena add to a deepening understanding of how people learn, and cognitive-behavioral specialists must remain current in their knowledge of the science related to their professional work if they are to provide the most competent patient care possible.

As indicated in the preceding paragraphs, the actual knowledge base subsumed under the rubric of cognitive and behavioral psychology is derived from a wide range of experimental and applied research areas. Specifically, the knowledge core that is common to all four subareas includes the full spectrum of learning theories, theories of human development, biological bases of behavior, neurocognitive aspects of behavior, affective aspects of behavior, principles of measurement, ethics, case formulation, clinical decision making, theories of individual differences regarding ethnic and cultural diversity issues, and research methods, including both group and single-subject experimental designs. Cognitive and behavioral psychologists are also concerned with how the various behavioral, cognitive, affective, biological, and social factors interact and impact each other (Dowd, Chen, & Arnold, 2010); they assume a biopsychosocial view of human physical and mental health and illness (Nezu, Nezu, & Lombardo, 2001) and embrace a reflective multi-cultural perspective.

Scientific Research Foundations

Bieschke, Fouad, Collins, and Halonen (2004), members of the Competencies Conference Scientific Foundations and Research Competencies Workgroup, posited that the core competency of scientific practice is comprised of the following activities and responsibilities: access and apply current scientific knowledge habitually and appropriately, contribute to the scientific knowledge base, critically evaluate interventions and their outcomes, practice vigilance about how sociocultural variables influence scientific practice, and routinely subject one's work to the scrutiny of colleagues, stakeholders, and the public.

This foundational competency requires that psychologists understand research, research methodology, techniques of data collection and analysis, biological bases of behavior, cognitive-affective bases of behavior, and development across the life span. Functional competencies that are developed by competent cognitive and behavioral psychologists include the day-to-day use of these methodologies toward scientific investigations, program evaluation, or measurement of outcome in one's clinical practice. The research literature that provides for a sound scientific base of cognitive and behavioral psychology is evident in the hundreds of psychotherapy outcome studies and meta-analyses that directly test a given psychotherapeutic intervention. Additionally, there are over 20 English-language journals devoted to the ever-growing evidence base for cognitive and behavioral treatments (Nezu, Martell, & Nezu, 2014).

Cognitive and behavioral psychology has defined itself as being "insistent on the empirical verification of its various interventions" (Nezu, Nezu, & Cos, 2007, p. 350), and as such, scientific knowledge and methods are a foundational competency with high priority for the specialty.

Interpersonal Interactions with Interdisciplinary Systems

Competent cognitive and behavioral practice often involves work with related disciplines and larger organizational systems. Knowledge of key issues and concepts in related disciplines is an important part of developing competent skills in this area. Specifically, specialists focus their learning and knowledge toward increasing their abilities to interact collegially and collaboratively with other health care professionals or colleagues in different disciplines (Newman, 2010). It is important to adopt a competent interpersonal style that balances assertive communication of specialty expertise with openness to other opinions and models of treatment, a respect for the approaches of other disciplines, and a rational view that reduces a tendency to personalize a collegial disagreement.

Individual and Cultural Diversity

Essential components of competency with regard to individual and cultural diversity have been outlined by Fouad and colleagues (2009), and they include an awareness of the self and others as shaped by individual and cultural diversity, in addition to awareness of the interaction of self and others. Multicultural competence for the cognitive and behavioral specialist requires ongoing study, review of research data on cognitive and behavioral assessment and intervention strategies conducted with relevant population samples, ongoing training and supervision, ongoing self-reflection, and, perhaps, self-directed change (Nezu et al., 2014).

Foundational Competencies in Ethics and Legal Foundation

It can be argued that the practice of cognitive and behavioral treatment, based on empirical evidence of the efficacy of treatments consisting of, for the most part, carefully described therapeutic techniques, meets the ethical principles of doing no harm, respecting patient's autonomy, and doing good. However, psychologists must abide by the ethical standards set forth by the profession, and the practice of cognitive-behavioral interventions may lead to inevitable "gray" areas, in which a careful case formulation and review of all relevant factors is required as part of one's ethical decision making. For example, exposure-based treatment may involve accompanying a patient in his or her environment to confront feared stimuli. Additionally behavioral observations in natural, real-life settings may require a behaviorally oriented psychologist to conduct an observation in a patient's home or other environmental setting. The importance of documenting a best practice rationale for such therapist actions is important to ethical practice.

Functional Competencies in Assessment

One of the most important clinical tasks presented by assessment is to construct learning-based explanations that may help cognitive and behavioral clinicians to understand, predict, and ultimately change a challenging mental health problem by creating a new learning experience for the patient. To accomplish this task, the competent specialist utilizes behavioral assessment, which may include an array of evaluation procedures that cover a range of methods, and case formulation.

Behavioral Assessment

According to Steven Haynes (Haynes & O'Brien, 2000), behavioral assessment aims to increase the validity of clinical judgments, particularly judgments about the clinical case formulation. A "funnel" approach to assessment has been recommended (Haynes & O'Brien, 2000), which involves starting with broadly focused assessment instruments and then conducting a more focused assessment as a clinician begins to discern hypotheses concerning possible target areas. The various assessment strategies described next are designed to aid the clinician in answering these questions with maximal effectiveness, as well as to develop an explanatory model of a patient's current difficulty through a case formulation.

BEHAVIORAL ANALYSIS

Applied behavior analysis is designed to provide a learning-based explanation for the etiology, selectivity, and maintenance of the target behavior by focusing on objectively defined, observable behaviors and social significance. Information obtained through assessment, which often involves varying the conditions to demonstrate the function of the behavior, is then used to guide the intervention by direct alteration of the conditions that sustain behavior.

OTHER MEASURES OF OVERT BEHAVIOR

Separate from the specific applied behavior analysis procedures, there are other commonly used measures of observable behaviors that constitute an important part of a comprehensive assessment. These include observation of interview behavior, interpersonal interactions, and specific tests that have been designed to observe overt behavior under structured conditions.

BEHAVIORAL ASSESSMENT
OF COVERT PROCESSES

Over the past few decades, cognitive and behavioral psychologists have also included the identification of thoughts and emotions as part of a behavioral

assessment because they are learned and maintained (or extinguished) through the same processes as overt behaviors. While covert behaviors can be measured through the use of patient self-monitoring and patient self-reports, they are susceptible to subjective factors and therefore may be less reliable than direct observation.

STRUCTURED AND SEMISTRUCTURED INTERVIEWS

Structured and semistructured interviews provide the cognitive and behavioral specialist with additional standardized ways to clarify diagnostic impressions, identify the presence of a particular syndrome or several comorbid syndromes, and often help identify the specific aspects of a diagnostic syndrome on which to focus. For example, a cognitive behavioral specialist might use a structured or semistructured interview to determine if individuals meet diagnostic criteria for a disorder and then funnel down their further assessment by direct observation, self or other report, or standardized tests concentrating on the clinical target or area of interest.

PHYSIOLOGIC ASSESSMENT

Physiologic assessment methodologies that are traditionally associated with other specialties serve as important sources of information for the cognitive-behavioral specialist who seeks to develop a biopsychosocial case formulation to guide evidence-based treatment. They provide an important component of assessment, particularly when physiologic arousal, sexual arousal, brain injury or impairment, or metabolic processes such as hormone changes and immune functioning are relevant to patient symptoms or behavior.

Physiologic assessment of autonomic nervous system arousal may provide an important comparison with both subjective self-report of arousal and observation of behavior, including measurements of heart rate (HR), blood pressure (BP), electrodermal responses such as galvanic skin response (GSR), and stress hormone levels, such as cortisol, a common measure of stress reactivity. Physiologic measures are often a component of cognitive and behavioral assessment, particularly when mood or personality challenges occur in reaction or simultaneously with a stress-related medical condition, because the role of various behaviors, thoughts, and emotional phenomena to neuroendocrine changes and physical inflammation may have significant implications for treatment.

Assessment through brain imaging is increasingly important to cognitive and behavioral research, in that imaging studies have shown cognitive-behavioral therapy interventions seem to affect clinical recovery in syndromes such as depression and anxiety by modulating the functioning of specific sites in the brain. While brain imaging is rarely a tool used by cognitive and behavioral practitioners in day-to-day settings, this research provides important information for specialists to communicate to their patients as a means of instilling hope that learned habits of information processing are not hard-wired or impossible to change.

The overall assessment of sleep disorders by cognitive-behavioral specialists is likely to incorporate physiologic measures such as a "sleep study" or polysomnography, which consists of a test that records a variety of body functions during sleep, such as the electrical activity of the brain, eye movement, muscle activity, heart rate, respiratory effort, air flow, and blood oxygen levels. Polysomnography is used to diagnose the presence of comorbid conditions, such as sleep apnea, that can contribute to insomnia and require attention in the development of a treatment.

Physiologic assessment employed by cognitive and behavioral psychologists has included the use of measures of sexual functioning such as phallometric assessment or penile plethysmography, which may be used in the assessment of sexual dysfunction or, more typically, sexually deviant responses. This information provides specific areas of learning with regard to extinction of deviant associations such as preferential sexual arousal to children, as well as new learning, such as sexual arousal toward adults.

Standardized psychological tests with a strong evidence base, such as intelligence and achievement tests, specialized tests for individuals with sensory deficits, well-validated personality tests, and neuropsychological tests, are often integrated with cognitive-behavioral assessment as a way of determining the presence of individual strengths and vulnerabilities that can impact a learning situation. The information obtained from standardized testing may guide the clinician in identifying the types of interventions that will be more effective or less effective for each individual.

CULTURALLY RELEVANT BEHAVIORAL ASSESSMENT

Culture is an important consideration for clinicians conducting cognitive-behavioral assessment because cultural differences can impact self-report

(Okazaki & Tanaka-Matsumi, 2006), as well as the way a clinician might interpret a behavioral observation made during assessment (Cohen & Gunz, 2002, as cited in Okazaki & Tanaka-Matsumi, 2006). A strong multicultural focus should be maintained throughout all phases of the assessment process, and Hays (2001) provides a useful framework for doing so that integrates multicultural factors using the acronym "ADDRESSING," which represents the following areas: age and generational influences; developmental, which includes the areas of age and generational influences; developmental and acquired disabilities; religion; ethnic and racial identity; socioeconomic status; sexual orientation; indigenous heritage; national origin; and gender.

Case Formulation

Competent cognitive and behavioral practice often involves treating people with comorbidities from an individualized approach and in a multicultural context; therefore, it is important for therapists to have a model to guide their decision making during the assessment and treatment process. An "idiographic approach" focuses on each individual's unique clinical assessment and comorbid areas in need of change to guide a "best match" of techniques from various evidence-based interventions to achieve the ultimate outcomes for which therapy was undertaken (Nezu, Nezu, & Cos, 2007; Rosen & Proctor, 1981).

Several models provide a method for developing a cognitive-behavioral case formulation. The model by Nezu and Nezu (Nezu et al., 2007) focuses on the clinician's information processing and advocates a problem-solving approach to clinical decision making, including adoption of a multicausal and systemic worldview. Persons' model (Persons, 1989), which was initially aligned with a traditional cognitive therapy approach, has evolved to focus more on conditioning theories and emotion (Persons & Thompkins, 2006). Koerner (2006) has focused a case formulation model on the specific approach to assessment for clinicians theoretically grounded in dialectical behavior therapy (DBT; Linehan, 1993) for patients with borderline personality disorder (BPD). Haynes and Williams (2003) follow a functional analytic systems framework and quantify the potential strength of functional relationships between hypothesized etiological factors and psychological problems. Kuyken, Padesky, and Dudley (2009) integrate collaborative empiricism and identification of strengths with functional analysis, and Tarrier and Calam (2002) propose a probabilistic model in which idiographic characteristics of a patient's life and experience were identified through various vulnerability and risk factors.

Similarities among all of the cognitive and behavioral case formulation models include a multiple-causal hypotheses perspective, an emphasis on functional analysis, the development of positive treatment goals, and strategies to reduce biases in clinical judgment (Eells, 2006).

Functional Competencies in Intervention

The challenge to describing competent deployment of the vast number of cognitive-behavioral interventions found in competent clinical practice is to provide an overview of interventions without the appearance of the specialty consisting of a menu of techniques applied to specific problems. Development of effective treatments involves the selection of cognitive and behavioral strategies and techniques based on an individualized assessment, often involving a careful case formulation, and guided by the scientific evidence. Although the emphasis on behavioral or cognitive explanations for treatment depends on the theoretical leanings of the therapist or researcher, and his or her interpretation of the literature, the assumption is that behaviors, thoughts, and feelings all are important factors and collectively account for the amelioration of difficulties through learning. This section will provide a brief overview of the variety of interventions developed within cognitive and behavioral psychology, which reflect the core principles of change that currently define the specialty.

Interventions Originating from Learning and Conditioning Theories

Fear, worries, anxiety, and the unpleasant states associated with these emotional experiences seem to represent the "common cold" of behavioral syndromes. Such problems are learned and they are common. Without treatment they are often chronic in nature and have been the focus of many cognitive and behavioral interventions. Several of these intervention components or systems are highlighted next.

SYSTEMATIC DESENSITIZATION

Wolpe's systematic desensitization was an early behavioral treatment requiring patients to face feared stimuli in order to reduce the fear by imagining a fear-producing situation for 5 seconds after their anxiety began to rise and then practicing relaxation. This procedure would continue until the patient could imagine the situation with no reported increase in anxiety and then progressively move up to a situation that was higher on the hierarchy of fear-producing imagined situations (i.e., would produce a stronger fear response; Wolpe, 1990).

PROGRESSIVE RELAXATION TRAINING

Relaxation procedures include progressive relaxation training (Jacobson, 1928), wherein a patient alternates between tensing specific muscles and then letting go of the tension. Bernstein, Borkovec, and Hazlett-Stevens (2000) recommend starting with 16 muscle groups, beginning with the dominant hand and arm, and reducing the number of muscle groups used in training as the patient gains competence over time. Breathing retraining is another form of relaxation training, which consists of teaching a patient to breathe from the diaphragm rather than from the chest and to slow the pace of the breathing.

AUTOGENIC TRAINING

Another form of relaxation that does not consist of tensing or relaxing muscles is autogenic training, first introduced in the early 20th century by Schultz as an aspect of self-hypnosis according to Yardakul, Holttum, and Bowden (2009). In autogenic training the individual imagines a particular area of the body feeling heavy and warm, while repeating phrases such as "my right arm is heavy" or "my forehead is cool" (Yardakul et al., 2009, p. 404). As a form of self-hypnosis, or self-instructed relaxation, it is considered by many to be a forerunner of biofeedback.

BIOFEEDBACK

A process that helps individuals learn how to modify their physiologic activity for purposes of managing stress and improving their health and overall performance, biofeedback involves use of physiologic devices to measure internal activities such as brain waves, heart functions (e.g., blood pressure, heart rate variability), breathing, muscle activity, temperature, and skin conduction. This "feedback" is often integrated with learning ways to change or focus on new ways of thinking or managing feelings that support desired physiologic changes. Over time, the body learns how to achieve physiologic changes without the use of such instruments (Association for Applied Psychophysiology and Biofeedback; AAPB http://www.aapb.org/i4a/pages/index.cfm?pageid=1).

VISUALIZATION

Visualization is the conscious and intentional creation of impressions that use all of your senses (seeing, hearing, smelling, touching, emotional experience) for the purpose of creating a positive image of calmness and tranquility (Nezu & Nezu, 2004). Frequently referred to as traveling to one's "safe place" in many visualization instructions, an individual is guided through the use of instructions by the therapist, an audio product, or covert self-instruction to create a positive and peaceful image on which to focus when experiencing negative emotional reactions or a sense of hopelessness.

EXPOSURE TREATMENT

Perhaps the most frequent principle used to treat psychological disorders when avoidance is a prominent feature, exposure involves the patient willingly and intentionally encountering the feared image, memory, or actual situation. Exposure therapy allows new learning to take place through imagery "in vitro" or "in vivo," meaning that it occurs in the actual situation, helping patients to overcome their fears. Two exposure procedures, prolonged exposure (PE) for treatment of posttraumatic stress disorder or exposure with response prevention (ERP) for treatment of obsessive-compulsive disorder, have demonstrated efficacy in the treatment outcome literature.

Prolonged Exposure

Prolonged exposure (PE) allows for emotional processing of a traumatic memory to ameliorate PTSD symptoms (Foa, Hembree, & Rothbaum, 2007), with general procedures that include psychoeducation, breathing retraining, in vivo exposure, and prolonged exposure to imagined scenes of the trauma (Foa et al., 2007). The therapist collaborates with the patient to develop a hierarchy of in vivo situations that the patient avoids and assigns exposure to a safe lower level fear situation, during which the patient stays in the situation until fear is reduced somewhat. The patient then works up the hierarchy, with each successive exposure becoming less frightening to the individual.

Exposure with Response Prevention

Exposure with response prevention (ERP) is similar to PE and is often used in the treatment of obsessive-compulsive disorder (OCD) and other anxiety disorders. Exposure is graduated from less feared to most feared situations with the use of both imaginal and in vivo exposure, and as exposure occurs, ritual behaviors are blocked so that patients do not utilize compulsive rituals as safety behaviors.

Interventions Originating from Information-Processing Theory

The specialty of cognitive and behavioral psychology followed an evolution of theory, assessment, and intervention, and particularly during the 1960s and 1970s, an emerging interest in the development of techniques that targeted modification of cognitions and were rooted in information-processing theory. Early writings by Albert Ellis, the developer of rational emotive behavioral therapy (REBT), and by Aaron T. Beck, a pioneer of cognitive therapy (CT), described the focus of their respective treatments on changing distortions in thinking that resulted in negative states such as depression and worry (Beck, 1976; Ellis, 1962). The majority of cognitive therapy treatments also incorporate behavioral elements (Beck, Rush, Shaw, & Emery, 1979; Persons, 2008).

RATIONAL EMOTIVE BEHAVIOR THERAPY

As stated by Ellis and Bernard (1985), "The main sub-goals of RET consist of helping people to think more rationally (scientifically, clearly, flexibly); to feel more appropriately; and to act more functionally (efficiently, undefeatingly) in order to achieve their goals of living longer and more happily" (p. 5). REBT is based on an existential/humanistic philosophy that stresses the importance of individuals reaching their highest potential or "self-actualizing."

COGNITIVE THERAPY TECHNIQUES

Cognitive therapy, as it has developed based on Beck's work, endorses the premise that emotional reactions to various environmental stimuli are mediated by conscious and, more recently, nonconscious meaning attached to the stimulus (Beck, 1976). Cognitive therapists help patients identify the times when their thinking is biased or distorted, with the goal of working collaboratively with patients to find more accurate and broader ways of thinking to improve mood or shift behavior patterns. Throughout the treatment, therapists use various strategies, including guided discovery, Socratic dialogue in cognitive reappraisal, looking for the evidence, assessing the utility of a given thought, developing coping strategies, and using behavioral experiments for hypothesis testing.

COGNITIVE PROCESSING THERAPY

Based upon a cognitive therapy protocol, cognitive processing therapy (CPT) is an evidence-based treatment for posttraumatic stress disorder (Resick & Schnicke, 1992), in which individuals learn about their PTSD symptoms, become more aware of thoughts and feelings, and are taught how to think about or process the trauma that occurred in their life in a different way than they did previously. In addition to a cognitive restructuring component that provides an opportunity to learn new skills and understand changes in beliefs, the treatment may involve exposure to memories and recollections of the trauma.

More Recent Developments in Cognitive and Behavioral Therapies

Intellectual curiosity and research have contributed to several paradigm shifts in cognitive and behavioral interventions, with an initial emphasis on observable behavior, which led to the development of behavior therapies from respondent and operant conditioning theories. As the work of Bandura, Lazarus, Ellis, Beck, Meichenbaum, Mahoney, and others influenced the practice of behavior therapy, there was a shift in focus on the impact of beliefs on emotion and behavior, which is sometimes referred to as a "cognitive revolution" in behavior therapy. Contemporary cognitive and behavioral interventions incorporate and extend the behavioral theories but have a distinct focus on balancing change techniques with strategies for helping patients accept negative emotional states.

ACCEPTANCE AND COMMITMENT THERAPY

A contextual therapy that incorporates mindfulness and a behavioral theory of verbal behavior and cognition known as "relational frame theory" (Hayes, Barnes-Holmes, & Roche, 2001), acceptance and commitment therapy (ACT; Hayes, Strosahl, & Wilson, 1999) has an existential emphasis on helping people to have highly valued lives despite pain and suffering. Harris (2009) suggests that there are six "core processes" of ACT: contacting the present moment; defusion (or watching thoughts but not buying into them); acceptance or "making room for painful feelings, sensations, urges, and emotions" (p. 9); self-as context, or being aware of the observing self; values; and committed action (see also Hayes, Luoma, Bond, Masuda, & Lillis, 2005).

BEHAVIORAL ACTIVATION

A contemporary therapy that was developed for the treatment of major depressive disorder, behavioral activation (BA; Martell, Addis, & Jacobson, 2001; Martell, Dimidjian, & Herman-Dunn, 2010) is based on a behavioral theory associated with traditional behavioral therapy—specifically, that not enough environmental reinforcement or too much environmental punishment can contribute to depression—and the goal of the intervention is to increase reinforcement in an individual's life. Its incorporation of acceptance and view of rumination as behavior rather than changing beliefs has occasioned its inclusion among the contemporary behavior therapies.

CONTEMPORARY PROBLEM-SOLVING THERAPY

Problem-solving therapy (PST) is a cognitive-behavioral and integrated cognitive, emotional, and behaviorally focused intervention. The PST therapist teaches individuals a series of adaptive problem-solving strategies geared to foster their ability to cope effectively with stressful life circumstances in order to reduce psychopathology and negative physical symptoms (Nezu, Nezu, & D'Zurilla, 2013). The clinical components of PST include several foci that the authors often refer to as "toolkits," each of which is directed toward a possible barrier to effective problem solving under stress, including cognitive overload, emotional dysregulation, negative thinking, poor motivation, and ineffective problem-solving strategies. The intervention incorporates therapeutic strategies aimed at information processing, mindful awareness of negative arousal, decreased avoidance of negative emotions, cognitive and behavioral skills development, skills to increase emotional regulation, and specific planful or rational problem-solving skills to make needed life changes consistent with one's values and life goals.

DIALECTICAL BEHAVIOR THERAPY

Originally developed as a treatment for chronic parasuicidal behavior, but extended to treatment for borderline personality disorder by Linehan (1993), dialectical behavior therapy (DBT) is a contemporary cognitive-behavioral approach that integrates empirically based techniques such as problem solving, social skills training, and chain analysis. The intervention applies functional analytic principles to understand, predict, and ultimately change patients' therapy-interfering behaviors, and it provides the addition of mindfulness techniques, the notion of "radical acceptance," and the interpersonal nature of the therapeutic relationship, with an emphasis on validation and teaching skills for managing strong, negative emotions.

FUNCTIONAL ANALYTIC PSYCHOTHERAPY

Functional analytic psychotherapy (FAP; Kohlenberg & Tsai, 1993) emphasizes the therapeutic relationship in behavior therapy, encouraging the therapist to be aware of clinically relevant behaviors (CRBs) that occur in session and to assess the function of such behaviors. Depending on the context in which it occurs, similar behaviors can serve a different function for the same patient at different times.

MINDFULNESS-BASED COGNITIVE THERAPY

The practice of being fully present to momentary experience, or mindfulness, is used in many of the contemporary approaches to behavior therapy such as DBT (Linehan, 1993) and ACT (Hayes, Strosahl, & Wilson, 1999), as well as cognitive-behavioral addictions treatments (Marlatt & Marques, 1977) and stress reduction and pain management (Grossman, Niemann, Schmidt, & Walach, 2004). The incorporation of cognitive reappraisals has led to the development of mindfulness-based cognitive therapy for depression (Segal, Williams, & Teasdale, 2002) and has also been applied to the treatment of anxiety disorders (Orsillo & Roemer, 2011; Roemer & Orsillo, 2006).

METACOGNITIVE THERAPY

Metacognitive therapy is based on the view that people may experience distress such as anxiety and depression because their metacognitions cause a pattern of responding to inner experiences that maintain their distressful emotion and strengthen negative ideas (Wells, 2009). The goal of this intervention is to remove the pattern, also called the cognitive attentional syndrome, by helping patients develop new ways of controlling their attention, new ways of relating to negative thoughts and beliefs, and by modifying metacognitive beliefs that give rise to unhelpful thinking patterns.

Use of Treatment Manuals

Within the specialty, there are differing schools of thought with regard to the use of treatment manuals for cognitive and behavioral treatment. Some individuals recommend the use of a manual by a therapist who is competent in general counseling skills when the relevant clinical target is a focus of treatment, while other therapists believe that adaptation of effective interventions and manuals

is required since no two people are alike and one manual is not a "one size fits all." The suggestion of Nezu, Martell, and Nezu (2014) is to consider a manual-driven treatment in the limited number of cases when there is a specific problem to address without any idiosyncratic features or other treatment barriers.

Applied Behavioral Analytic Interventions

There are many interventions that have been shown to systematically change the contingencies of a target behavior, such that it is no longer reinforced, or an alternative behavior is learned through reinforcement. However, it is important for treatment to logically flow from the learning-based explanation of the behavior, with competent intervention requiring a sound behavioral assessment and functional analysis to precede the use of the intervention. An effective intervention plan should provide for new learning opportunities for a patient, which may include ways to increase the likelihood of a patient learning new associations or functional contingencies, inhibition of a patient's previous associations through extinction learning, reduction or extinction of a patient's behaviors that have been previously reinforced, or fostering a patient's learning of new skills or adaptive behavior.

Increasing adaptive behavior is the focus of treatment when a particular adaptive skill is not present in an individual's repertoire because it has not previously been learned. Many interventions have been developed and tested through both group and case designs that can be used to effectively teach new behavior, and a few examples are provided next. Those individuals who wish to extend their competencies to focus on interventions derived from behavioral analysis principles will require more extensive texts, such as those by Barker (2000), Kazdin (2000), Mittenberger (2012), or Ramnero and Torneke (2008).

SHAPING AND PROMPTING

Shaping refers to training and reinforcing successive approximations to an ultimate target behavior, a procedure that is used to establish a new topography or a new dimension of a more complex behavior (Mittenberger, 2012). It involves identifying a series of steps that can be reinforced, until the ultimate target behavior is reached. Another common procedure to teach new behavior involves the use of prompts, which can be provided verbally, physically, or environmentally to increase the likelihood that one will engage in the correct behavior at the correct time.

CONTINGENCY MANAGEMENT

When a relationship exists between a specific response and a consequence such that the consequence is presented if (and only if) the behavior occurs, it is referred to as a contingency, and in such cases, the consequence is said to be contingent on the response (Kazdin, 2000; Mittenberger, 2012). Although contingencies may be pleasant (positive) or unpleasant (punishing), the establishment of contingencies is a basic part of teaching new behavior or modifying existing behavior.

In addition to teaching new skills and increasing adaptive behavior, many clinical referrals to cognitive and behavioral specialists who focus their work on interventions associated with applied behavior analysis are often expected to develop effective interventions for decreasing challenging, problematic, or dangerous behavior. These strategies have been employed for decades with particular regard to decreasing the incidence of behavior that either impedes a patient's learning process or places the patient in a position of risk to herself or others.

PUNISHMENT

Mittenberger (2012) defines punishment as "the process by which a behavior is followed by a consequence that results in the future reduced probability of the behavior" (p. 102). Most behavioral clinicians, trainers, and writers provide important ethical and clinical guidelines with regard to the use of punishment-based procedures because of the distress that is associated with an individual experiencing a negative, unpleasant, or painful consequence. This includes specifying that the behavior or response—*not* the individual—is being punished and making it a practice not to use punishment strategies without a programmed use of reinforcement-based strategies in conjunction with the punishment procedure, in order to teach new behavior.

Other Functional Competencies
Consultation

Because of the historic focus that cognitive-behavioral psychologists have placed on measured changes in overt behavior as well as the empirical support that has accumulated with regard to cognitive-behavioral interventions, they are frequently consulted with regard to changing problematic behavior in many different contexts.

The incorporation of cognitive and behavioral interventions has become ubiquitous with regard to their integration into health care settings, and they are often viewed as adjunctive to traditional Western medical treatments because they can improve life quality and mood, and help people to cope with, or adapt to, physical problems. Additionally, consultation is frequently sought in school settings, correctional facilities, and other forensic rehabilitative settings; in private-sector areas, such as advertising and political campaigns (Gorn, 1982); by the leisure industry; and by the military, police, and public safety officials (Novaco, 1977).

Cognitive and behavioral psychologists who competently provide consultation to other psychology specialties, other disciplines, and the private sector follow several important heuristics to increase the success of their consultation experience. These are consistent with competencies in consultation services developed by a consensus task force (Fouad et al., 2009) and include recognizing situations in which consultation is appropriate, providing effective advice, feedback, and recommendations, and implementing interventions that meet the goals of the consultation request.

Supervision

Professional activities involving supervision and training in the specialty of cognitive and behavioral psychology are most effective when they are competency based and involve the use of strategies geared to shape the behavior of a trainee, such as behavioral observation, modeling, role play, guided practice, and use of audio and videotape. There is a common philosophy among cognitive and behavioral specialists that actually demonstrating how to interview, assess, intervene, and consult is an important part of clinical teaching and supervision, and additionally, reinforcement is seen as a key training strategy.

Newman (2010) has described supervision competencies in cognitive and behavioral therapies, including a "high level" of professional functioning in which a supervisor possesses significant skills in diagnosis, responsibility for patient care and records, and communication skills in order to provide clear, concise, and sensitive feedback to his or her supervisees. He also underscores the importance of cultural awareness and insight regarding how such factors influence both patient care and supervisory relationships. Additionally, Newman discusses the importance of recognizing the power differential inherent in the supervisory relationship and the impact of each supervision experience on a trainee's future career, stating that supervisors must rise to the occasion by "creating, communicating, and sustaining a safe, growth-enhancing climate in which their supervisees can learn optimally to conduct therapy more and more competently"(p. 17).

Teaching

Although many specialists do not require teaching competencies in the traditional sense of classroom teaching, competencies in teaching skills are necessary because their role is often as a teacher, providing new learning experiences in their day-to-day work with regard to patient care, consultation, and supervision. In addition to providing information, it is important to make use of the strategies that were developed within the specialty with regard to demonstration, guided instruction, prompting, shaping, and fading, and apply such concepts to teaching and training situations. Ultimately, the pedagogical process of increasing motivation and eagerness to learn, guiding and encouraging rather than doing and rescuing, and finally reinforcing successive approximations are all competencies required by the teaching process.

Management and Administration

For psychologists who manage the direct delivery of services and or the administration of organizations, programs, or agencies, the use of behavioral learning principles to competently complete the tasks would be consistent with the specialty. This would involve assuming a learning-based approach to establishing leadership, setting goals, and defining expectations of one who holds administrative or management authority. A learning-based approach would lend itself to clear definitions of objectives and job responsibilities for staff members, as well as having a motivational system of rewards in place.

Advocacy

Competencies in advocacy are required in situations where cognitive and behavioral psychologists are called upon to target the impact of social, political, economic, or cultural factors to promote positive change. For example, behavioral interventions focused on promoting positive behavior change with regard to protection of the environment, increasing public access to evidence-based interventions, reduction of violence, and promotion of cooperation and peace may have significant impact on the health and well-being of the population as a whole. This type of change requires strong competencies in advocacy to disseminate evidence-based methods for behavioral change and work toward adoption of policies based upon sound behavioral principles.

Summary

Over the past two decades the movement in professional psychology to develop, define, and assess professional competencies has aligned well with the development of the specialty of cognitive and behavioral psychology. The competencies developed through consensus of professional stakeholders such as the APA, training programs, licensing jurisdictions, and the ABPP regarding board certification has provided a useful heuristic by which cognitive and behavioral psychologists can delineate a best practices model of treatment.

References

American Board of Cognitive and Behavioral Psychology (ABCBP) (2015). Retrieved May 15, 2015, from http://www.abpp.org/i4a/pages/index.cfm?pageid=3315

ABCT (2012). Retrieved September 25, 2012, from The Association for Behavioral and Cognitive Therapies: www.abct.org/Home/

Accreditation Council for Graduate Medical Education (2015). Retrieved March 1, 2015, from https://www.acgme.org/acgmeweb

American Board of Medical Specialties (2015). Retrieved March 1, 2015, from http://www.abms.org

Barker, L. M. (2000). *Learning and behavior: Biological, psychological, and sociological perspectives* (3rd ed.). Englewood Cliffs, NJ: Prentice Hall.

Beck, A. T. (1976). *Cognitive therapy and the emotional disorders.* New York: Penguin Books.

Beck, A. T., Rush, A. J., Shaw, B. F., & Emery, G. (1979). *Cognitive therapy of depression.* New York: Guilford Press.

Bernstein, D. A., Borkovec, T. D., & Hazlett-Stevens, H. (2000). *New directions in progressive relaxation training: A guidebook for helping professionals.* Westport, CT: Praeger.

Bieschke, K. J., Fouad, N. A., Collins, F. L., & Halonen, J. S. (2004). The scientifically minded psychologist: Science as a core competency. *Journal of Clinical Psychology, 80,* 713–724.

Cohen, D., & Gunz, A. (2002). As seen by the other . . .: Perspectives on the self in the memories and emotional perceptions of easterners and westerners. *Psychological Science, 13,* 55–59.

Dimidjian, S., Barrera, M., Jr., Martell, C., Munoz, R. F., & Lewinsohn, P. M. (2011). The origins and current status of behavioral activation treatments for depression. *Annual Review of Clinical Psychology, 7,* 1–38.

Dowd, E. T. (2000). *Cognitive hypnotherapy.* New York: Jason Aronson.

Dowd, E. T., Chen, S. L., & Arnold, K. D. (2010). The specialty practice of cognitive and behavioral psychology. *Professional Psychology: Research and Practice, 41,* 89–95.

D'Zurilla, T. J., & Nezu, A. M. (2007). *Problem solving therapy: A positive approach to clinical intervention* (3rd ed.). New York: Springer.

Eells, T. D. (Ed.). (2006). *Handbook of psychotherapy case formulation*. New York: Guilford Press.

Ellis, A. (1962). *Reason and emotion in psychotherapy*. Oxford: Lyle Stuart.

Ellis, A., & Bernard, M. E. (Eds.). (1985). *Clinical applications of rational emotive therapy*. New York: Plenum.

Foa, E. B., Hembree, E. A., & Rothbaum, B. O. (2007). *Prolonged exposure therapy for PTSD. Emotional processing of traumatic experiences. Therapist guide*. New York: Oxford University Press.

Fouad, N. A., Grus, C. L., Hatcher, R. L., Kaslow, N. J., Hutchings, P. 5., Madson, M. B.,…Crossman, R. E. (2009). Competency benchmarks: A model for understanding and measuring competence in professional psychology across training levels. *Training and Education in Professional Psychology*, *3*, 5–26.

Gilbert, P., & Leahy, R. L. (2007). *The therapeutic relationship in the cognitive behavioral psychotherapies*. New York: Routledge/Taylor & Francis Group.

Gorn, G. J. (1982). The effects of music in advertising on choice behavior: A classical conditioning approach. *Journal of Marketing*, *46*, 94–101.

Grossman, P., Niemann, L., Schmidt, S., & Walach, H. (2004). Mindfulness-based stress reduction and health benefits: A meta-analysis. *Journal of Psychosomatic Research*, *57*, 35–43.

Harris, R. (2009). *ACT made simple*. Oakland, CA: New Harbinger.

Hayes, S. C., Barnes-Holmes, D., & Roche, B. (Eds.). (2001). *Relational frame theory. A post Skinnerian account of human language and cognition*. New York: Kluwer Academic/Plenum Publishers.

Hayes, S. C., Luoma, J. B., Bond, F. W., Masuda, A., & Lillis, J. (2005). Acceptance and commitment therapy: Model, processes, and outcomes. *Behaviour Research and Therapy*, *44*, 1–25.

Hayes, S. C., Strosahl, K. D., & Wilson, K. G. (1999). *Acceptance and commitment therapy: An experiential approach to behavior change*. New York: Guilford Press.

Haynes, S. N., & O'Brien (Eds.) (2000). *Principles and practice of behavioral assessment*. New York: Kluwer Academic/Plenum Publishers.

Haynes, S. N., & Williams, A. E. (2003). Case formulation and design of behavioral treatment programs: Matching treatment mechanisms to causal variables for behavior problems. *European Journal of Psychological Assessment*, *19*, 164.

Hays, P. A. (2001). *Addressing cultural complexities in practice: A framework for clinicians and counselors*. Washington, DC: American Psychological Association.

Jacobsen, E. (1928). *Progressive relaxation*. Chicago: University of Chicago Press.

Jacobsen, N. S., Martell, C. R., & Dimidjian, S. (2001). Behavioral activation treatment for depression: Returning to contextual roots. *Clinical Psychology: Science and Practice*, *8*, 256–270.

Kaslow, N. J., Rubin, N. J., Forrest, L., Elman, N. S., Van Horne, B. A., Jacobs, S. C.,…Thorn, B. E. (2007). Recognizing, assessing, and intervening with problems of professional competence. *Professional Psychology: Research and Practice*, *38*, 479.

Kazdin, A. E. (2000). *Behavior modification in applied settings* (6th ed.). Belmont, CA: Wadsworth.

Koerner, K. (2006). Case formulation in dialectical behavior therapy. In T. D. Eells (Ed.), *Handbook of psychotherapy case formulation* (pp. 317–348). New York: Guilford.

Kohlenberg, R. J., & Tsai, M. (1993). *Functional analytic psychotherapy: Creating intense and curative therapeutic relationships*. New York: Plenum.

Kuyken, W., Padesky, C., & Dudley, R. (2009). *Collaborative case conceptualization: Working effectively with clients in cognitive-behavioral therapy*. New York: Guilford Press.

Linehan, M. M. (1993). *Cognitive-behavioral treatment of borderline personality disorder*. New York: Guilford Press.

Marlatt, G. A., & Marques, J. K. (1977). Meditation, self-control, and alcohol use. In R. B. Stuart (Ed.), *Behavioral self-management: Strategies, techniques, and outcomes* (pp. 117–153). New York: Brunner-Mazel.

Martell, C. R., Addis, M. E., & Jacobson, N. S. (2001). *Depression in context: Strategies for guided action*. New York: Norton.

Martell, C. R., Dimidjian, S., & Herman-Dunn, R. (2010). *Behavioral activation for depression: A clinician's guide*. New York: Guilford Press.

Mittenberger, R. G. (2012). *Behavior modification: Principles and procedures* (5th ed.). Belmont, CA: Wadsworth.

Nelson, P. D. (2007). Striving for competence in the assessment of competence: Psychology's professional education and credentialing journey of public accountability. *Training and Education in Professional Psychology*, *1*(1), 3.

Newman, C. F. (2010). Competency in conducting cognitive-behavioral therapy: Foundational, functional, and supervisory aspects. *Professional Psychology: Research and Practice*, *47*, 12–19.

Nezu, C. M., Martell, C. R., & Nezu, A. M. (2014). *Specialty competencies in cognitive and behavioral psychology*. New York: Oxford University Press.

Nezu, A. M., Nezu, C. M., & Cos, T. A. (2007). Case formulation for the behavioral and cognitive therapies: A problem-solving perspective. In T. D. Eells (Ed.), *Handbook of psychotherapy case formulation* (2nd ed., pp. 349–378). New York: Guilford Press.

Nezu, A. M., Nezu, C. M., & D'Zurilla, T. J. (2013). *Problem-solving therapy: A treatment manual*. New York: Springer.

Nezu, A. M., Nezu, C. M., & Lombardo, E. R. (2001). Cognitive-behavior therapy for medically unexplained symptoms: A critical review of the treatment literature. *Behavior Therapy*, *32*, 537–583.

Nezu, C. M., & Nezu, A. M. (2004). *Awakening self-esteem: Spiritual and psychological techniques to improve your well-being*. Oakland, CA: New Harbinger.

Norcross, J. C., Beutler, L. E., & Levant, R. F. (2007). *Evidence-based practices in mental health*. Washington, DC: American Psychological Association.

Novaco, R. W. (1977). A stress inoculation approach to anger management in the training of law enforcement officers. *American Journal of Community Psychology*, *5*, 327–346.

Okazaki, S., & Tanaka-Matsumi, J. (2006). Cultural considerations in cognitive-behavioral assessment. In P. A. Hayes & G. Y. Iwamasa (Ed.), *Culturally responsive cognitive-behavioral therapy* (pp. 257–266). Washington, DC: American Psychological Association.

Orsillo, S. M., & Roemer, L. (2011). *The mindful way through anxiety: Break free from chronic worry and reclaim your life*. New York: Guilford Press.

Persons, J. B. (1989). *Cognitive therapy in practice: A case formulation approach.* New York: Norton.

Persons, J. B. (2008). *The case formulation approach to cognitive-behavior therapy.* New York: Guilford Press.

Persons, J. B., & Tomkins, M. A. (2006). Cognitive-behavioral case formulation. In T. D. Eells (Ed.), *Handbook of psychotherapy case formulation* (pp. 290–316). New York: Guilford Press.

Peterson, R. L., Peterson, D. R., Abrams, J. C., Stricker, G., & Ducheny, K. (2010). The National Council of Schools and Programs of Professional Psychology: Educational Model 2009. In M. B. Kenkel & R. L. Peterson (Eds), *Competency-based education for professional psychology* (pp. 13–42). Washington, DC: American Psychological Association.

Ramnero, J., & Torneke, N. (2008). *The ABCs of human behavior.* Oakland, CA: New Harbinger.

Resick, P. A., Monson, C. M., & Chard, K. M. (2007). *Cognitive processing therapy: Veteran/ military version.* Washington, DC: Department of Veterans Affairs.

Resick, P. A., & Schnicke, M. K. (1992). Cognitive processing therapy for sexual assault victims. *Journal of Consulting and Clinical Psychology, 60,* 748–756.

Roberts, M. C., Borden, K. A., Christiansen, M. D., & Lopez, S. J. (2005). Fostering a culture shift: Assessment of competence in the education and careers of professional psychologists. *Professional Psychology: Research and Practice, 36*(4), 355.

Roemer, L., & Orsillo, S. M. (2006). An open trial of an acceptance-based behavior therapy for generalized anxiety disorder. *Behavior Therapy, 38,* 72–85.

Rosen, A., & Proctor, E. K. (1981). Distinctions between treatment outcomes and their implications for treatment evaluation. *Journal of Consulting and Clinical Psychology, 49,* 418–425.

Rothbaum, B. O., Hodges, L. F., Kooper, R., Opdyke, D., Williford, J., & North, M. (1995). Virtual reality graded exposure in the treatment of acrophobia: A case report. *Behavior Therapy, 26,* 547–554.

Segal, Z. V., Williams, J. M., & Teasdale, J. M. (2002). *Mindfulness-based cognitive therapy for depression.* New York: Guilford Press.

Tarrier, N., & Calam, R. (2002). New developments in cognitive-behavioural case formulation. Epidemiological, systemic, and social context: An integrative approach. *Behavioural and Cognitive Psychotherapy, 30,* 311–328.

Wells, A. (2009). *Metacognitive therapy for anxiety and depression.* London: Guilford Press.

Wilhelm, S., & Steketee, G. S. (2006). *Cognitive therapy for obsessive compulsive disorder: A guide for professionals.* Oakland, CA: New Harbinger Publications.

Wolpe, J. (1990). *The practice of behavior therapy* (4th ed.). New York: Pergamon Press.

Yardakul, L., Holttum, S., & Bowden, A. (2009). Perceived changes associated with autogenic training for anxiety: A grounded theory study. *Psychology and Psychotherapy: Theory, Research and Practice, 82,* 403–419.

Behavioral Assessment and the Functional Analysis

William H. O'Brien, Stephen N. Haynes, *and* Joseph Keawe'aimoku Kaholokula

Abstract

Behavior therapists must often design treatments for individual patients who present with a wide array of behavior disorders. Behavioral assessment is a learning-based, empirically focused, and systematic evaluation approach. The functional analysis, which is an important outcome of a behavioral assessment, is a set of decisional strategies that are used to systematically gather, integrate, and summarize information about the form and function of a client's behavior problems. The functional analysis is a critically important outcome of assessment because it informs treatment design. The objectives of this chapter are to: (a) present a review of the conceptual foundations of behavioral assessment and the functional analysis; (b) outline steps required to generate a functional analysis; (c) explain simple decisional and statistical procedures that can be used to assist with the assessment and functional analysis; and (d) describe how functional analyses can be used to design interventions using graphic causal models.

Key Words: behavioral assessment, functional analysis, case formulation, clinical decision making, behavior therapy

Chapter Overview

Every day, thousands of persons find themselves or a loved one experiencing distressing cognitive, emotional, and behavioral states that create severe impairments in social, occupational, educational, and family functioning. A subset of these persons will seek help from a mental health professional. Upon arrival at the first appointment, the person (who we will hereafter refer to as the "client") will engage in a dialogue and information-sharing interaction with the professional (hereafter referred to as the "clinician") in an effort to explain the nature of his or her difficulties. The clinician, in turn, will engage in a series of actions (e.g., listen carefully and empathically, ask questions designed to expand on certain areas of information and/or clarify ambiguous information, make decisions about where to focus the assessment, determine the severity of the problems, assess risk for harm, etc.) that are designed to better understand the nature

of the client's difficulties. Importantly, as noted by O'Brien, Kaplar, and McGrath (2004), a vast amount of information about problem behaviors and possible causes for these problem behaviors will be described during initial few moments of the assessment interview. As the interview proceeds, even more information is made available through verbal and nonverbal behaviors. Further, as the assessment unfolds, the clinician may administer psychological tests, self-report inventories, rating scales, and/or behavioral observation strategies to augment interview information. An important assessment question thus becomes apparent: How can clinicians sort through this large and complex array of information in order to develop a valid model of the behavior problems and their causes?

In this chapter, we present an approach to assessment that is based on behavioral theory and is designed to aid in causal model construction for the purposes of intervention design. First, we will review the conceptual foundations of a behavioral approach to assessment. Following that, we will summarize the features of behavior problems and causal variables that are particularly relevant to behavioral assessment. Next, we will describe how the information obtained from a behavioral assessment can be used to develop a case conceptualization, which is referred to as a functional analysis in the behavioral assessment literature. Finally, we will show how functional analyses can be summarized using graphical modeling techniques.

Conceptual Foundations of Behavioral Assessment and the Functional Analysis

The core characteristics of behavioral assessment are clarified when they are compared to the psychodynamic and personality-oriented approaches to assessment. The prototypical psychodynamic approach hypothesizes that dysfunctional internal psychological processes (e.g., unconscious conflicts, impaired ego strength) are the principal causes of behavioral problems. Thus, psychodynamic assessments focus on the measurement in inferred internal states and processes, whereas measurement of external contextual factors is deemphasized.

The Rorschach is an example of how psychodynamic assessment emphasizes measurement of inferred internal dysfunctional psychological processes. In a Rorschach assessment, clients are presented with ambiguous inkblots and asked to describe what they perceive. The client's descriptions are then coded along a number of dimensions such as form (e.g., it looks like a bat), texture (e.g., it looks fuzzy), movement (e.g., it looks like people dancing), color (e.g., it looks like blood), and the like. These coded responses are then aggregated in various ways to derive indices of the client's internal processes (Exner, 1986, 1991). For example, based on the color-affect hypothesis, which is derived from psychodynamic theory about emotional regulation, if a client explicitly reports color in his or her description, it is thought that the client has poor ego control and is apt to be impulsive or suffer from impaired reality testing under emotionally activating circumstances (Frank, 1993). In sum, internal processes are inferred from verbal descriptions of the inkblots.

Personality assessment is similar to the Rorschach in that client responses to written questions are thought to yield information about internal psychological processes. The Minnesota Multiphasic Personality Inventory (MMPI) is a commonly used personality measure that illustrates this approach.

Items on the MMPI are carefully worded to avoid linking them to a specific situation or time. For example, a client can only respond "true" or "false" to broadly worded items such as "I like to read detective novels." Then, his or her response to this item is interpreted as an index of a personality characteristic such as masculinity, anxiety, paranoia, depression, and so forth.

Behavioral assessment differs from psychodynamic and personality approaches in two fundamental ways. First, instead of restricting itself to measurement of internal dispositional factors, behavioral assessments will examine a much wider array of responses including observable behavior, emotional reactions, physical reactions, and cognitive experiences. Second, rather than using global nonsituational measurement, behavioral assessments seek to measure *behavior in context*. That is, there is a key emphasis on identifying how the onset, maintenance, and termination of a particular behavior arise from interactions among behavior and environmental events. These characteristics, broad foci and behavior-context interactions, are two of the most critical foundations of the behavioral assessment and functional analysis. There are, however, a number of additional conceptual foundations and assumptions that underlie a behavioral approach to assessment and the functional analysis. These additional conceptual foundations and assumptions are reviewed next.

Learning Theories Provide a Sound Framework for Understanding Behavior Disorders and Formulating Interventions

The theories, assumptions, techniques, and goals of behavioral assessment have evolved across the past four decades. Hayes (2004) argues that this evolution can be broadly partitioned into three "waves." In the first wave, behavioral assessment and the functional analysis were largely based on principles of classical and operant conditioning. In the second wave, cognitive variables were incorporated into behavioral assessment and the functional analysis as important variables. In the third wave, functional contextualism was refined and added to behavioral assessments and functional analyses. We will briefly present the learning principles contained in each wave of behavior therapy and describe how they are relevant to behavioral assessment and the functional analysis.

Classical and operant conditioning in behavioral assessment and functional analysis. Many of the early behavior therapy researchers conducted studies demonstrating that classical conditioning principles could account for the onset, maintenance, and change in many problem behaviors. For example, Wolpe (1952a, 1952b) found that anxiety states could be induced with classical conditioning procedures. He then showed that anxiety states could be made less intense using systematic desensitization, which combined graded exposure with relaxation (Wolpe, 1958; 1963; Wolpe & Lazarus, 1966; Wolpe, Salter, & Reyna, 1964). Coinciding with Wolpe's research and shortly thereafter, other researchers began exploring how classical conditioning could explain the acquisition, maintenance, and remediation of other problem behaviors. Their findings supported the position that classical conditioning processes were highly relevant to the assessment and treatment of many disorders encountered in clinical settings.

The other major learning theory associated with the early years of behavior therapy was operant conditioning. Drawing upon the theoretical and empirical works of learning theorists such as Watson (1919), Skinner (1938, 1974), and Hull (1952), researchers began to evaluate how principles of stimulus control, reinforcement, and punishment could account for the acquisition, maintenance, and change of problem behaviors. Many of behavioral interventions were then developed using these same operant principles. Results indicated that many of these investigations were effective for a very wide array of behavioral problems.

The sound theoretical framework, scholarship, and success of the early years of behavioral therapy laid the groundwork for the entire behavior therapy movement and radically changed the mental health assessment and treatment landscape. Grounded in empiricism and careful experimentation, behavioral pioneers also strongly argued that behavioral assessment and the functional analysis should emphasize the measurement of observable target behaviors (target behaviors refers to any response that is the focus of assessment) and specific environmental events that preceded, co-occurred, and/or followed them.

Cognitive and emotional variables incorporated into behavioral assessment and functional analysis. Recognizing that important areas of unobservable human responding such as thoughts and emotions were inadequately represented in some of the early classical and operant conceptualizations of behavior disorders, researchers began incorporating cognitive variables into behavioral assessment and the functional analysis. The essential position

forwarded by these researchers was that cognitive variables acted as critically important mediators between observable problem behaviors and situational variables.

A classic example of cognitive mediation is Beck's cognitive model of depression (cf. Beck, Rush, Shaw, & Emery, 1979). According to Beck and colleagues, a person with depression may encounter an aversive event (e.g., a critical comment from a colleague). This event then prompts a number of dysfunctional thoughts about the self (e.g., "I am a loser"), the world (e.g., "people are coldhearted"), and the future (e.g., "I will never be accepted"). These dysfunctional thoughts can then promote a number of problematic behaviors such as avoidance, helplessness, and passivity. Thus, the problematic behaviors (e.g., avoidance) are thought to arise not from the aversive environmental event per se, but the person's interpretation of the event. As such, the interpretation (a cognitive event) is construed as a primary cause of problematic behavior.

Given that cognitive variables were conceptualized as critically important causes of problem behavior, behavioral-assessment techniques were developed to measure them. Additionally, therapy techniques were designed to help clients identify, stop, confront, and/or replace problematic cognitions. Thus, the term *behavior therapy* was gradually replaced with the term *cognitive-behavioral therapy* in many quarters.

In summary, during what is sometimes referred to as the second wave of behavior therapy, cognitive variables were added to behavioral assessment. This brought about a broad and important expansion of clinical research and the development of many new assessment methods and tools. Additionally, researchers and clinicians developed new intervention techniques aimed at modifying cognitive variables using principles of classical and operant conditioning. The tremendous success of cognitive-behavioral interventions developed during this expansion of behavior therapy is without dispute, and the vast majority of empirically supported treatments use cognitive-behavioral principles and techniques (e.g., Butler, Chapman, Forman, & Beck, 2006).

Functional contextualism. In recent years, a number of novel behavioral-assessment procedures and interventions have been developed. Examples of these "third-wave" interventions include: Acceptance and Commitment Therapy (ACT; Hayes, Strosahl, & Wilson, 1999), Dialectical Behavior Therapy (DBT; Linehan, 1993; Linehan et al., 2006), Functional Analytic Psychotherapy (FAP; Kohlenberg et al., 2004; Tsai et al. 2008) and Mindfulness-Based Cognitive Therapy (MBCT; Segal, Williams, & Teasdale, 2002). These new approaches diverge from earlier ones in terms of philosophical stance, theoretical formulations, and treatment aims.

As noted by Hayes (2004), this most recent expansion of behavior therapy represents a departure from the strong positivism and cognitivism found in the earlier cognitive-behavioral approaches and a recommitment to the more foundational tenets of classical and operant conditioning labeled *functional contextualism*. The philosophical divergence of third-wave approaches from earlier approaches are substantial (Fletcher & Hayes, 2005). The positivistic and mechanistic stance associated with the first- and second-wave points of view takes the position that cognitive events and other "private experiences" (e.g., emotional reactions) can be dismantled or broken down into their constituent "parts," and the relationships among these various "parts" can be studied and analyzed individually. It thus is logical to take the position that, for example, a thought such as "I am a loser" can *lead to* or *cause* a problematic behavioral response such as social avoidance. The thought itself is, therefore, labeled as "dysfunctional" because it causes maladaptive behavior. Further, it is important to stop, alter, or otherwise control the occurrence of dysfunctional thoughts in order to control problem behavior.

In contrast to the positivistic and mechanistic stance just described, functional contextualism takes the position that cognitive, emotional, and overt motor responses occur in *relation to, and derive meaning from,* historical and ongoing internal and external events (Hayes, 2004, Hayes, Luoma, Bond, Masuda, & Lillis, 2006). Consider again, the thought, "I am a loser." From a functional-contextual perspective, the thought itself is neither functional nor dysfunctional. It is simply a cognitive event. What is important to assess from a functional-contextual perspective is the *relationship* between the thought and other responses and/or environmental events. Further, the relationships that are particularly important are those derived from classical and operant conditioning. These varied relationships between a particular behavior (cognitive experience, emotional experience, or overt-motor response) and the antecedent, concurrent, and consequent stimuli are its context.

As discussed in O'Brien and Carhart (2011), a client who presented with major depression symptoms provides an illustration of the functional contextual approach to cognitive experiences. The client reported that he was experiencing very persistent and severely negative thoughts about himself, the future, and the world in general. For example, he noted that whenever he observed people interacting happily, he would experience positive and negative thoughts about the possibility for happiness in his own life. These thoughts then led to feelings of sadness. Shortly after experiencing sadness, he reported that he would oftentimes find himself dwelling on how the world was "bad and unjust" and that it was selfish and immoral to bring children into such a dysfunctional world. This second set of thoughts tended to create feelings of relief from sadness.

The structure of the relationship between environmental events (observing happy people), cognitive experiences, and emotional reactions can be analyzed from a functional-contextual perspective. The initial event, observing happy people, triggers hopeful/ hopeless predictions about his own future happiness. This internal cognitive dialogue brings about sadness. The sadness prompts a second set of thoughts ("the world is bad"). This second set of seemingly dysfunctional thoughts actually allows the client to momentarily escape from sadness. Additionally, these thoughts about the world also make it far less likely that the client will take action to improve his situation (if the world is bad, it is illogical to engage in actions for the purpose of achieving happiness), which would require effort and exposure to possible failure. Importantly, although the thoughts about the world would be labeled "maladaptive" from an earlier cognitive-behavioral perspective, a functional-contextual perspective would classify them according to their operant function. In this case, they would be viewed as negatively reinforced escape responses because they provide momentary relief from aversive emotional states.

The occurrence of worry can also be used to illustrate a functional-contextual approach. Persons experiencing worry often report that they cannot control the frequency and intensity of worry in various circumstances. They also typically report that the worry is associated with aversive emotional states. From a functional-contextual perspective, it *must be* that any behavior (thought, feeling, overt-motor response) that occurs at a high frequency and intensity is being reinforced. The question becomes, what is the reinforcer?

Borkovec and colleagues explored this question in a series of investigations (Borkovec, Alcaine & Behar, 2004; Sibrava & Borkovec, 2006). According to Borkovec, worry is a negatively reinforced response because it allows a person to escape from a more aversive cognitive and emotional state. Specifically, Borkovec argued that worry is a verbal-linguistic form of cognition. It essentially involves talking with oneself and engaging in problem-solving formulations. The more highly aversive cognitive and emotional states that precede worry according to Borkovec are negative visual-imaginal experiences.

Consider an example of a person waiting for his or her loved one to arrive home late in the evening. When it becomes evident that the loved one is late, according to Borkovec, the waiting person may generate a very negative image of his or her loved one in a severe car crash. This negative image brings about anxious activation. Worrisome thoughts are then generated by the person. These worrisome thoughts are verbal and problem-solving in nature. For example, the person might think "Maybe there was a traffic jam. I will check the news to see." This act of verbal problem solving according to Borcovek allows the person to momentarily escape from the disturbing visual image (because verbal processing interferes with visual processing) and associated anxiety. Hence, worrisome thoughts are negatively reinforced. Hayes et al. (1999) and Hayes et al. (2006) refer to these types of cognitive escape processes as "experiential avoidance."

From an earlier cognitive-behavioral perspective, the depressed client's thoughts and the worry described earlier would be classified as dysfunctional cognitions. Further, the client would be encouraged to identify, stop, and challenge/control these thoughts when they occur. From a functional-contextual perspective, however, these thoughts are simply cognitive responses that are negatively reinforced by a reduction in aversive states. Further, they will tend to continue as long as they are being negatively reinforced. Therefore, efforts to stop and/or control them using self-talking or thought management strategies will be unsuccessful because another set of negatively reinforced verbal responses or thoughts will simply be added to a behavioral chain. Instead, from a functional-contextual perspective, an effective intervention would involve exposure to the feared stimulus (the sadness, disturbing images, anxiety) and acquisition of competing behavioral responses (e.g., social activation in the presence of sadness, preventing excessive checking behavior in the presence of anxiety). As Hayes et al. (2004, 2006) have noted, this type of approach is congruent with Skinner's radical behaviorism (1974, 1987).

Functional contextualism is a key element of behavioral assessment because it reminds us that many internal events (thoughts, emotional states) and overt-motor behaviors are maintained by classical conditioning principles and operant conditioning principles. Thus, a principle goal of behavioral assessment is to focus on the function of the many cognitive, emotional, and overt-motor responses that are identified as the evaluation proceeds.

The implications of functional contextualism associated innovations for behavioral assessment and therapy are evolving. A great deal of research, however, is needed. First, there is a need to develop reliable and valid measures of the functional properties of thoughts and emotional experiences. Second, there is a need to develop and validate case conceptualizations and/or functional analyses based on a functional-contextual perspective. Finally, there is a need for a better understanding of how important principles derived from first and second wave approaches can be integrated with third-wave assessments and interventions.

Empiricism Is a Critically Important way to Learn about the Nature of Behavior Problems

A second key foundation of behavioral assessment is empiricism. Thus, there is an emphasis on obtaining unambiguous and specific measures of problem behaviors, contextual factors, and the relationships among them (Haynes & O'Brien, 2000). The emphasis on empiricism helps reduce the probability that dispositionally biased case conceptualizations are generated by a clinician because there is a tendency for human judges to impute personality constructs as causal variables when attempting to explain why problem behaviors occur. The essential difficulty with this is that the inferred personality constructs are typically unverified and frequently incorrect.

By adopting an empirical perspective, the clinician must obtain explicit measures of problem behaviors and any other variables that are believed to be important for a particular client. In essence, the behavioral assessment and the functional analysis will emphasize articulating relationships between the *observable* environmental events and *observable* behavioral responses (note that internal events such as thoughts and emotional experiences can be made observable using well-validated self-report inventories and psychophysiological recording). This focus on empirical strategies, in turn, permits the behavior therapist to generate testable hypotheses about behavior and then collect data that can plausibly confirm or disconfirm them.

The Hypothetico-Deductive Method Is an Important and Appropriate Decisional Strategy in Assessment

The hypothetico-deductive method is a third foundation of behavioral assessment and an important element of the scientist-practitioner model of clinical psychology. A model of the hypothetico-deductive method is provided in Figure 4.1. As shown in Figure 4.1, we begin with the construct level. All psychological phenomena and relationships among them are essentially ideas or constructs. For example, depression is not a "thing" with mass, velocity, and electrical charge. It is a concept or idea. Similarly, a causal relationship is not an observable "thing," but rather an idea based on observations of regularities in sequences of events (e.g., if event B consistently follows event A, we infer that B is caused by A). The first step of the hypothetico-deductive method is to carefully develop conceptual definitions of constructs.

Returning to depression, a clinician or researcher might decide that depression is a sad emotional state accompanied by thoughts of worthlessness, helplessness, and guilt. The clinician or researcher may also specify that depression is "caused" by exposure to "aversive and punishing interpersonal relationships."

The next step in the hypothetico-deductive method is to generate operational definitions of constructs. In a sense, operational definitions translate constructs into "real-world" measures and operations. This, of course, requires that the clinician or researcher consider all the threats to construct validity described in Cook and Campbell's seminal work on research design (Cook & Campbell, 1979). Again, in the aforementioned example, a clinician or researcher may decide that his or her operational definition of "depression" will be a score on the Beck Depression Inventory—II (Beck, Steer, & Brown, 1996), and that the operational definition of "interpersonal conflict" will be a report that interpersonal conflict was experienced within the past week on the Daily Stress Inventory (Brantley, Waggoner, Jones, & Rappaport, 1987). Finally, the operational definition of *cause* can be stated as a regression coefficient of .40 or higher in a path analysis. As is apparent in this example, the operational definitions used by clinicians and researchers are key elements of the hypothetico-deductive method.

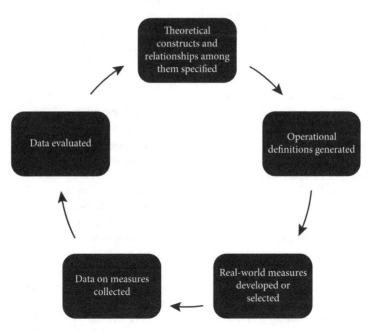

Figure 4.1 Hypothetico-deductive method.

After generating operational definitions, the clinician or researcher will then collect data using various measurement tools and strategies. These data can be collected using time-series approaches, experimentation, and/or self-report. As a rule, the measurements obtained on more than one occasion and/or under controlled settings will yield more internally valid and interpretable data.

Finally, data are evaluated and interpreted. The interpretation of data essentially involves determining whether the magnitude of relationships among measures supports an inference of a causal relationship among constructs. As Cook and Campbell noted (1979) this step of the decisional process requires that the researcher or clinician consider and rule out plausible threats to statistical conclusion validity.

It is important to restate that this process of construct development, operational definition generation, data collection, and data evaluation occur in both clinical and research contexts. In clinical contexts, the assessor typically explores the nature of behavior problems through interviewing, careful questioning, and observation. The assessor also pursues information about contextual factors that may be influencing the behavior problem. In essence, the clinician is developing and clarifying constructs at this point in the assessment. Later, in collaboration with the client, the clinician may opt to have the client collect daily ratings of the behavior problem and associated contextual variable occurrence. Here, the clinician has generated operational definitions and established a data collection strategy. When the client returns for subsequent sessions, the clinician will evaluate the daily ratings and determine whether there have been changes in the behavior problem and/or whether there are important relationships between behavior problems and contextual variables. Note that this decisional sequence is virtually identical to the one used by researchers to design studies and experiments.

Multivariate Models of Behavior Disorders and Contextual Variables Are Needed in Assessment

Persons who seek psychological interventions often have multiple behavior problems. Thus, a central tenet of behavioral assessment and the functional analysis is that behavior disorders must be approached from a multivariate perspective. This multivariate perspective assumes that a given client will often present with covarying sets of behavior problems that are influenced by many, and sometimes covarying, contextual variables. Further, these behavior problems and contextual variables have specific and qualitatively distinct aspects that are linked together in complex patterns and sequences.

Haynes, O'Brien, and Kaholokula (2011) noted that behavior problems covary when: (a) they are influenced by the same antecedent or consequent causal variable, such as when chronic pain interferes with sleep and mood; (b) one behavior problem acts as a causal variable for another behavior problem; such as when social avoidance leads to depressed mood; and (c) they are the result of two or more covarying causal variables, such as when the development of a medical condition leads to depressed mood, and the simultaneous use of a new medication leads to irritability. Additionally, a single causal variable can sometimes lead to multiple behavior problems. Examples of causal variables that bring about multiple behavior problems include: (a) avoidance of negative emotions that can lead to social withdrawal, alcohol use, and eating disorders; (b) life stressors that can lead to depressed mood, marital distress, and poor job performance; and (c) inappropriate response contingencies enacted by parents that can adversely affect child aggression, noncompliance, and antisocial behaviors.

Knowing that a person has multiple behavior problems that are affected by multiple contextual variables has a significant influence on the behavioral assessment process. A premature focus on a narrow set of behavior problems can preclude a more complete and accurate understanding of the nature of a client's difficulties. Thus, it is imperative to use assessment procedures that can capture a wide range of behaviors and potentially relevant contextual variables.

Behavior Problems Are Conditional and Vary across Time

An important concept in behavioral assessment and the functional analysis is that behavior problems vary systematically across contexts and are, therefore, conditional. For example, a client reporting alcohol abuse use may be more likely to drink heavily in response to interpersonal conflict relative to other types of life stressors. The behavior problems can also differ across persons. Returning to the prior example, one client experiencing alcohol abuse may be more likely to drink heavily in response to interpersonal conflict, whereas another may be more likely to drink heavily in response to peer encouragement.

The conditional assumption in behavioral assessment encourages the clinician to search for variation in the frequency, intensity, and/or duration of problem behaviors across contexts. Finding evidence of such variation can help the clinician identify causal variables that are important for intervention design. Consider, again, the client with alcohol difficulties. If the clinician finds that drinking occurs in response to interpersonal conflict but not other types of stressors, then he or she can systematically explore which specific elements of interpersonal stress lead to drinking urges and behaviors.

The characteristics of a client's behavior problem can also vary across time. That is, there can be variability across time in the dimensions, response modes, parameters, and causal relations of a behavior problem. For example, two people reporting a similar behavior problem such as insomnia may show different patterns of sleep difficulty across time. One may report persistent and chronic sleep disruption, whereas another may report that the sleep difficulties are more cyclical in nature.

As with the conditional nature of behavior problems, changes in the time-course of a behavior problem suggest that a causal variable might be operating. Haynes et al. (2011) outlined several means through which behavior problems can change over time as a function of variation in causal variables: (a) repeated or prolonged exposure to a causal variable can result in extinction, sensitization, or habituation; (b) new causal variables can emerge, whereas old causal variables cease to operate on a behavior problem; and (c) the actions of mediators and moderators can change over time.

The dynamic nature of behavior problems requires that a well constructed behavioral assessment and functional analysis will be based on information about behavior and contextual variables that has been collected across time. This time-series emphasis is a foundational method in behavioral assessment.

In summary, there are a number of conceptual assumptions associated with behavioral assessment and the functional analysis. First, there is an assumption that the theories, principles, and methods derived from the three waves of learning theory provide a solid foundation for understanding the onset, maintenance, and modification of problem behaviors. Second, empiricism is embraced as a means of learning about behavior problem-contextual variable interactions. Third, the hypothetico-deductive method is utilized as a decisional strategy that allows a clinician to translate psychological constructs and the relationships among them using deductive logic, operational definitions, careful measurement, and quantitative evaluation of collected data. Fourth, it is assumed that behavior problems and contextual factors are multidimensional and multidetermined. Fifth, behavior problems are conditional and are expected to vary across settings, persons, and time.

With these assumptions in mind, the clinician should approach each assessment armed with a well-developed knowledge of behavioral theories and principles, training in empirical methods, and experience with hypothetico-deductive reasoning. Further, the clinician will seek to collect wide-ranging information about multiple behavior and contextual variables with an awareness that the form and magnitude of relationships among these variables will vary across persons, settings, and time.

The Functional Analysis: A Primary Outcome of Behavioral Assessment

The functional analysis is defined as:

The identification of important, controllable, causal functional relations applicable to specified behaviors for an individual. (Haynes & O'Brien, 1990; 2000).

The functional analysis is a clinician's working model of a client's problem behaviors and the variables that affect them. There are several important aspects of the functional analysis. First, the functional analysis emphasizes *causal* functional relations among behavior problems and causal variables for an individual client. These causal functional relations are emphasized because they are the prime targets of interventions. For example, if marital distress is the key cause of depressed mood for a client, then the intervention would target marital distress in order to reduce depressed mood. Alternatively, if social-skills impairments are the primary cause of depressed mood, an appropriate intervention would target social-skills enhancements.

Second, the functional analysis emphasizes *important* behavior problems, causal variables, and functional relations. In the functional analysis, the clinician is most interested in identifying causal relations that have the strongest relations with, or effects on, a client's behavior problem. Modification of these important causal relationships should exert the largest impact on behavior problems.

Third, the functional analysis emphasizes causal variables that are *controllable*. Many important causal variables associated with that behavior problems (e.g., learning history, genetic characteristics) cannot be modified are, therefore, not particularly relevant to treatment design. Alternatively, important causal variables that can be changed are emphasized because of their utility in treatment planning.

Fourth, functional analyses are *idiographic*. There are likely to be important differences in the functional analyses of clients with the same behavior problem. This is in contrast to nomothetic models of behavior disorders that are based on patterns of data derived from many persons with the same behavioral problem. However, nomothetic models of a behavioral disorder can inform the clinician about causal variables that are more likely to be influencing a behavioral problem for an individual client.

Fifth, the conceptual foundations of the functional analysis and the assessment methods for it construction are not limited. Thus, functional relations can be estimated through a wide array of assessment techniques, tools, and measures. Additionally, many different types of behavior problems and causal variables can be incorporated into a functional analysis.

The construction of a functional analysis involves several interrelated steps. First, the clinician must identify and define important behavior problems. Second, the clinician must identify and define important, controllable, and relevant causal variables. These two steps are, respectively, referred to as the topographical analysis of behavior and the topographical analysis of contextual variables. After these initial steps are completed, the clinician will identify and evaluate the form and strength of functional relationships among behavior problems and contextual variables. Finally, the functional analysis can be summarized and integrated using functional analytic causal models.

Topographical Analysis of Behavior

A critical initial goal of the behavioral assessment and functional analysis is to generate clear and measurable operational definitions of behavioral problems. To accomplish this, the behavior therapist must initially conduct a broad inquiry of problem behaviors and possible contextual variables. A subset of more central problem behaviors and contextual variables will subsequently be identified and become the focus of the assessment and intervention.

Once a set of target behaviors has been identified, the behavior therapist must then identify their essential characteristics. Complex target behaviors can be divided into at least three modes of responding: cognitive-verbal behaviors, physiological-affective behaviors, and overt-motor behaviors. The cognitive-verbal mode includes cognitive experiences such as self-statements, images, irrational beliefs, and attitudes. The physiological-affective mode includes physiological responses and felt emotional states. Finally, the overt-motor mode includes observable actions.

The process of operationally defining a target behavior requires careful interviewing. For example, a client who is described as experiencing panic may present with many different cognitive-verbal, physiological-affective, and overt-motor behaviors such as catastrophic beliefs about dying, hypervigilance to physical sensations, sympathetic nervous system activation, muscle tension, and agoraphobic avoidance. However, another client with panic may present with a very different pattern of behaviors.

Once the mode of a given problem behavior has been operationalized, its parameters must be defined. The most commonly used parameters in behavioral assessment are frequency, duration, intensity, and latency. Frequency refers to how often the behavior occurs across a given interval (e.g., number per day, per hour, per minute). Duration refers to the time that elapses between the beginning point and endpoint of a problem behavior. Intensity refers to the "forcefulness" of a behavior. Intensity is often measured using rating scales, surveys, visual analog scales (e.g., fear thermometer), and psychophysiological recording devices (e.g., heart rate monitoring).

In summary, one of the initial goals of the behavioral assessment and functional analysis is to identify problem behaviors and then specify their modes and parameters. This initial step of operationalization allows the clinician and client to obtain a consensual and clear understanding of the key problem behaviors. Additionally, as this process unfolds, the clinician will have translated what are often informal descriptions of problem behaviors into terms that are consistent with contemporary psychological phrasing.

Topographical Analysis of Context

Subsequent to the topographical analysis of problem behaviors, the clinician will need to develop operational definitions of contextual variables. Contextual variables are internal and external events that precede, co-occur with, and/or follow the target behavior and exert important causal influences upon it based on classical conditioning and operant principles. Contextual factors can be broadly divided into environmental/situational variables and intrapersonal variables. Environmental/situational variables can be further divided into social variables (e.g., interactions with others) and physical variables (e.g., nonliving aspects of the environment such as temperature, noise, physical space, lighting levels, etc.). Intrapersonal variables include verbal-cognitive, affective-physiological, and overt-motor behaviors that may exert significant effects on onset, maintenance, and termination of problem behaviors. The contextual variable measurement parameters are similar to those used with problem behaviors. That is, frequency, duration, intensity, and latency are most often assessed.

In summary, the topographical analysis of problem behaviors and contextual variables are two of the initial goals of the behavioral assessment functional analysis. Problem behaviors can be divided into modes and measured along several dimensions. Similarly, contextual variables can be partitioned into classes and measured for several specific dimensions. This interaction between target behavior components and contextual variables is illustrated in Table 4.1.

Identifying Causal Functional Relationships among Variables in the Functional Analysis

After completing the topographical analysis of problem behaviors and contextual variables, the clinician must then estimate the magnitude of causal functional relationships among these variables. The decisional processes involved with causal relationship identification are complex, require careful deliberation, and are tied to centuries-old philosophical debates.

Many philosophers, including David Hume, an eighteenth-century Scottish philosopher, wrote extensively on the topic of causality. Hume emphasized three conditions that supported causal inferencing: (1) *contiguity* in time and space between the presumed cause and effect, (2) *temporal precedence* (i.e., causes precede effects), and (3) *constant conjunction* (whenever the effect is obtained, the cause must be present). It should be noted that Hume's requirement of temporal and spatial contiguity did not rule out the possibility of remote causes, if one could demonstrate that there was a causal chain between the remote cause and the more immediate effect (Beauchamp & Rosenberg, 1981).

Hume argued that because one must *infer* causal relationships from one's perceptions, there is no reason to believe that causality exists apart from our perceptions. Therefore "cause" is a mental construction. In order to illustrate his point, Hume used the billiard-ball example in his classic work, *A Treatise of Human Nature*: "Here is a billiard-ball lying on the table, and another ball moving towards it with rapidity. They strike; and the ball, which was formerly at rest, now acquires a motion ... There was no interval betwixt the shock and the motion" (Hume, as cited in Beauchamp & Rosenberg, 1981). Upon observing the billiard balls' interaction, most persons would conclude that the action of the first billiard ball *caused* the second billiard ball to move. Hume, however, pointed out that there was no directly observable evidence of this. The best that could be said, according to Hume was the there was a coincidence of time and space, temporal precedence (the first ball moves and then the second ball moves), and constant conjunction (the second ball does not move unless it is struck by the first ball).

A clinically relevant example can clarify this point. Suppose, for example, that a client's

Table 4.1 Target behavior modes and contextual variables

Contextual Variable Class	Target Behavior Modes		
	Cognitive-Verbal	Affective-Physiological	Overt-Motor
Social/Environmental			
Nonsocial/ Environmental			
Intrapersonal/ Cognitive-Verbal			
Intrapersonal/ Affective-Physiological			
Intrapersonal/ Overt-Motor			

depressive moods improve shortly after taking an antidepressant medication. It would seem quite reasonable to conclude that the medication caused the improvement. However, Hume would argue that this causal inference is based solely on the observation of coincidence in time and space. Further, this causal inference would be influenced by beliefs, expectations, prior experience, and many other psychological factors that are rooted in the mind of the observer.

As an empiricist, Hume did not find it logical to use unobserved and unmeasured phenomena in science (Skinner's radical behaviorism also embraced this position). Thus, he asserted that conclusions about causality can only be based on the observation of past coincidences or correlations among variables. However, this proves problematic because the mere fact that two variables were correlated in the past does not mean that they will continue to be correlated in the future. Thus, Hume voiced the difficult-to-accept opinion that all causal assertions are essentially tautological and ultimately illogical from an empirical perspective.

By examining the work of Hume, it is clear that causation cannot be directly observed, and it is, thus, impossible to empirically demonstrate causation. Instead, causal relationships must be based on inductive logic. That is, an individual concludes that one thing appears to cause another when: (a) the two are temporally and spatially close, (b) one precedes the other, and (c) one expects that this relationship will hold true in the future. Thus, in scientific and clinical contexts, it is important to acknowledge that the demonstration of a causal relationship is essentially a matter of persuasion using scientific methodology and data analysis.

In addition to Hume, John Stuart Mill, a nineteenth-century philosopher and radical empiricist, wrote extensively on the problem of demonstrating causal relationships. Mill (2012) argued that in order to infer causality three conditions must be met: (1) the cause must precede the effect (i.e., temporal precedence), (2) the cause and effect must be related, and (3) all other explanations of the cause-effect relationship must be eliminated. A key contribution of Mill's methodology is that it provided guidance about how to rule out threats to causal inference.

Mill proposed that three methods can be used to help rule out alternative cause-effect relationships. The Method of Agreement states that an effect must be present whenever the presumed cause is present. The Method of Difference states that the effect

will not be present when the cause is not present, and the Method of Concomitant Variation states that when both of the aforementioned methods are observed, alternative causal explanations can be logically ruled out.

These principles can be applied to Hume's billiard-ball example. Using the Method of Agreement, one observes whenever the second ball moves, the first ball has also moved. Using the Method of Difference, one observes that if the first ball does not move, the second ball does not move. Finally, using the Method of Concomitant Variation, one observes that the second ball will not move unless the first ball has struck it *and* whenever the first ball strikes the second ball, the second ball moves.

The previous depression and medication example can also be used to illustrate these important points. The Method of Agreement requires that the clinician would *always* observe a reduction in depressed mood whenever medication is taken. The Method of Difference would require that a reduction in depressed mood would *never* occur unless medication is first taken. Finally, the Method of Concomitant Variation would require that *all increases or decreases in depressed mood would be accounted for by variation in the presence or absence of the medication.* When we apply these standards to this example, it is clear that a casual assertion for the effectiveness of the medication is exceedingly weak.

Mill also strongly argued that correlation is not an adequate index of causality (even when there is temporal precedence) because a third variable may be responsible for the relationship. By studying Mill, one sees that the ability to rule out alternative explanations (such as the presence of a third variable), is crucial to inferring causal relationships. It is also clear that the empirical standards for causal assertion are rarely established in clinical contexts and psychological research in general.

Given the aforementioned philosophical perspectives, it is apparent that one can only infer causation on the basis of certain cues including covariation, temporal order, coincidence, and the ability to rule out plausible alternative explanations. Although the issue of whether causality exists apart from our perceptions of it was an important issue in eighteenth- and nineteenth-century philosophy; most behavioral scientists are willing to assume that causal relationships exist even though we cannot logically support such assertions (James, Mulaik, & Brett, 1982). This position is partially based on pragmatic concerns. If one can demonstrate that certain variables reliably produce important changes in the occurrence of a problem behavior, then identification and measurement of these "causal relationships" is a valid pursuit.

Contemporary standards that are currently used to guide the identification and estimation of causal relationships in clinical contexts incorporate much of Hume and Mill's thoughts about causality. Some of the more commonly accepted current standards for causal inference are:

1. *Covariation between variables:* Two variables must covary, meaning that they must have shared variance. The presence of covariation does not establish causality. However, the lack of correlation between variables is strong evidence against causality.

2. *Temporal precedence:* A hypothesized causal variable must reliably precede its effect. Without establishing that X precedes Y, it is difficult to rule out the possibility that X is the result of, rather than the cause of, Y or, alternatively, that both X and Y are caused by some common third variable.

3. *Logical basis for inferring causality:* For a variable to be considered causal, it must have a logical, scientifically-based, connection with the effect. This requires that one identify the causal mechanism, or the particular way that X causes Y.

4. *Exclusion of plausible alternative explanations:* It may be that two variables covary not because of a causal relationship between the two, but rather because of the presence of a third variable. Excluding plausible alternative explanations, such as the presence of a third variable, is perhaps the most difficult condition to meet, in part because so many hypothesized causal relationships in the behavioral sciences are open to alternative explanations.

Behavioral interviewing is the primary assessment method used by clinicians to explore the presence or absence of the aforementioned conditions for causal inference (O'Brien & Tabaczynski, 2009). Typically, the client is asked to describe sequences of events and provide reasons that the behavior problem is occurring. For example, the clinician might ask a client, "What do you think causes you to experience higher levels of depressed mood?" The client's response to this question is then treated as an index of the presence or absence of a *possible* causal relationship.

Although interviewing is the primary method used to identify causal relationships, interview-based causal assertions have very limited or unknown validity in most instances. Specifically, the interviewer cannot determine how well the client's reports of causation mirror causal relationships in real-world settings. Factors that influence the validity of client causal reports include ability to recognize and understand casual relationships, social desirability, capacity to verbalize the nature of causal relationships, and many commonly occurring human biases (e.g., illusory correlation, availability heuristic, confirmatory bias, anchoring effects, representativeness heuristic). In addition, the interviewer's own biases will influence how questions are posed and what information is encoded and recalled (Garb, 1996, 2005).

To enhance the validity of client reports of causal relationships, the interviewer should carefully and systematically enquire about covariation, temporal order, and plausible alternative explanations. To accomplish this, the interviewer can envision a 2 × 2 table (see Tables 4.2 and 4.3) and ask a series of questions that will provide information relevant to each cell. In Table 4.3, the interviewer is evaluating whether depressed mood is causally related to interpersonal conflict.

Functional analytic experimentation and observation can also be used to enhance client self-reports of causation. This strategy involves systematically modifying some aspect of the interview and observing consequent changes in behavior. This hypothesis-testing approach has been developed and validated by Kohlenberg (e.g., Kohlenberg et al., 2004). For example, as reported in O'Brien and Carhart (2011) a young man who was presenting with dysautonomia (heightened autonomic reactivity to stress) was interviewed alone, with his parents

Table 4.2 A 2 × 2 Table Illustrating Essential Conditions for Causal Inference

	Causal Variable Present	Causal Variable Absent
Target behavior present	Evidence Supporting Causation (Necessary Condition)	Evidence Against Causation
Target behavior absent	Evidence Against Causation	Evidence Supporting Causation (Sufficient Condition)

Table 4.3 Prototypical Questions That Pertain to Causal Inference

	Cause Variable Present	Causal Variable Absent
Behavior Problem Present	Conditional probability of occurrence questions: General format: "When the causal event occurs, what is the likelihood that the behavior problem will occur?" Example: "On a day with higher levels of interpersonal conflict, how likely is it that you experience depressed moods?"	Base rate of occurrence questions: General format: "When the causal event does not occur, what is the likelihood that the behavior problem will occur?" Example: "On a low-conflict day, how likely is it that you will experience depressed moods?"
Behavior Problem Absent	Conditional probability of nonoccurrence: General format: "When the causal event occurs, what is the likelihood that the behavior problem will not occur?" Example: "On a high-conflict day, how likely is it that you will not experience depressed moods?"	Base rate of nonoccurrence: General format: "When the causal event does not occur, what is the likelihood that the behavior problem will not occur?" Example: "On a low-conflict day, how likely is it that you will not experience depressed moods?"

present, alone again, and then with his parents present again. We observed that the frequency and intensity of symptom reporting and overt-motor expressions of distress covaried with each condition. Specifically, vivid and emphatic verbal reports of symptoms were more frequently verbalized when his parents were present relative to when the client was alone. Thus, it appeared that verbal reporting of symptoms (and potentially the client's experiencing of the symptoms) was being positively reinforced by parent behavior. Subsequent assessment indicated that the parental reinforcement was both social (comforting attention) and tangible (special meals and treats when the patient expressed discomfort).

A number of single-subject experimental designs have been developed that can help clinicians confirm or disconfirm hypotheses using this strategy. As illustrated in the disautonomia case example, we used an A-B-A-B design (where A = baseline, B = parental presence) to evaluate the relationship between symptom reporting and parental presence.

Evaluating Causal Functional Relationships in the Functional Analysis

Some researchers have argued that intuitive data evaluation such as visual inspection of a line graph is an appropriate method for evaluating behavioral assessment data. Arguments in favor of intuitive evaluation are based on convenience and clinical significance. In the latter case, it has been argued that visual inspection is conservatively biased, and one will only "see" a relationship between two variables when the relationship is of moderate to high magnitude.

We conducted an investigation on the adequacy of visual inspection using graduate students who had completed coursework in behavioral therapy. The students visually inspected a contrived set of self-monitoring data presented for three problem behaviors—headache frequency, intensity, and duration (O'Brien, 1995)—and three potential causal variables—hours of sleep, marital argument frequency, and stress levels. The data were constructed so that only a single causal factor was strongly correlated with a single problem behavior in the self-monitoring data.

Students were instructed to estimate the magnitude of correlation between each causal factor and target behavior and then select the most highly correlated causal factor for each problem behavior. Results indicated that the students consistently underestimated the magnitude of strong correlations and overestimated the magnitude of weak correlations. Additionally, their "hit rate" (i.e., correctly identifying the casual variable associated with each problem behavior) was very poor.

We further evaluated the potential limitations of intuitive data evaluation methods by surveying members of a large organization of behavior therapists (Association for Behavioral and Cognitive Therapies, ABCT). Similar to the O'Brien (1995) study, we created a data set that contained three target behaviors and three potential contextual factors in a 3 × 3 table. The correlation between a target behavior and three contextual factors was either low ($r = .1$), moderate ($r = .5$), or high ($r = .9$). Results again indicated that the participants were largely unable to accurately identify the causal variable most closely associated with each problem behavior or correctly estimate the magnitude of correlation among variables (O'Brien et al., 2004).

These two studies demonstrate that visual inspection and intuitive evaluation of behavioral assessment data is poorly suited for estimation of covariation, which, as noted earlier, is a critical requirement for establishing causal inference. As Garb (1996, 2005) noted, intuitive analysis of data similar to those described earlier often-times results in inaccurate interpretations of clinical data. One reason for this phenomenon is that confirmatory information or hits (i.e., instances in which the causal variable and hypothesized effect co-occur) are overemphasized, whereas disconfirming information such as false positive and misses are discounted.

Given the limitations of intuitive analyses, we recommend using statistical approaches for evaluating relationships among target behaviors and contextual variables. Given the complexity of most functional analysis models, it may be unwieldy to test all possible relationships among variables. However, it is workable to test the *key* causal relationships.

Conditional-probability analyses are easily applied statistical techniques. Conditional-probability analyses assume that functional relationships are evident in elevated conditional probabilities (Schlundt, 1985). To illustrate, let A = depressed mood (high\/low), B = daily stress level (high or low), and P = probability. A functional relationship between depression and stress level would be inferred if the probability of experiencing a depressed mood, *given* the presence of high stress (P[A|B]) is greater than the base-rate probability of experiencing a depressed mood (P[A]). Conditional-probability analyses have important strengths. First, a small number of data points can yield reliable estimates of association. Second, the statistical concepts underlying the methodology are easily understood. Third, many statistical programs can be used to conduct conditional-probability analyses or, if none are available, the computations can be easily done by hand using Bayes Theorem or Chi-Square analyses. Fourth, clients can be shown how to conduct such analyses using 2 × 2 tables and they are, therefore, more able to critically evaluate their assumptions about relationships between problem behaviors and causal variable occurrence.

As an example, we recently treated a young man with a psychosomatic disorder. He strongly believed that if he allowed his heart rate to exceed 150 beats per minute, he would experience severe fatigue symptoms 24 hours later. To test this possibility, we had the young man record levels of fatigue across a two-week interval. We also had the client record heart rate while exercising. He was then able to construct a 2 × 2 table (high/low heart rate × high/low fatigue 24 hours later). He was surprised to learn that heart rate was not reliably associated with fatigue even though he was convinced there was a relationship. This insight, promoted by a simple quantitative analysis, helped the client begin to increase activity levels with diminished fear of experiencing adverse effects.

Time series analyses can also be used to evaluate behavioral data. Typically, a time-series approach requires that the client collect data on the occurrence of the target behavior and contextual factor across time. The magnitude of causal functional relationships then can be estimated by calculating a measure of association between controlling variables and target behaviors after partitioning out the variance accounted for by autocorrelation. Structural equation modeling, ARIMA, and hierarchical linear modeling are all effective statistical approaches for analyzing times-series data for an individual client.

Putting it all Together: Integrating Assessment Information Using Functional Analytic Clinical Case Diagrams

Information about behavior problems, contextual variables, and the relationships among them will be complex. We have argued that causal modeling can be used to synthesize and organize assessment information. "Functional analytic clinical case diagrams" (FACCD) summarize the behavioral assessment and functional analysis using vector diagrams. Variables included in the FACCD include behavior problems, contextual variables, and the relationships among them (Haynes & O'Brien, 2000; Haynes et al., 2011).

The FACCD is a form of causal diagram that visually represents the functional analysis of a client's behavioral problems. All FACCDs have several central elements, usually represented by symbols for (a) "input" variables, (b) "output" variables, and (c) connections among variables (Haynes, et al., 2011). Input variables are generally causal variables for the client's behavioral problems. Output variables are usually the frequency, intensity, and duration intensity of a client's behavioral problems.

They can also include the effects of the behavioral problems on other behaviors. As noted earlier in this chapter, these input and output variables can vary in terms of modifiability (some may be more or less amenable to change) and importance.

The lines and arrows of a causal diagram describe the form and strength of relationships among inputs and outputs. These relationships can be unidirectional or bidirectional; causal or noncausal/correlational; mediated or direct; moderated or unmoderated; and weak, moderate, or strong. They can also be hypothesized or empirically confirmed.

A thorough description of the elements of FACCD and how they are constructed is beyond the scope of this chapter. However, Haynes et al. (2011) provide a comprehensive review of the foundations and methods of behavioral assessment along with a step-by-step guide on how the information derived from the behavioral assessment can be used to construct a FACCD.

Briefly, the development of a FACCD can be broken down into 22 steps. The first two steps are common to all assessments: (1) obtain informed consent and seek to establish a positive and collaborative relationship with the client and (2) evaluate the basic nature of the problem as well as level of risk to determine whether referral to another provider or agency is needed. In the third step, the clinician should engage in broadly focused assessment strategies (principally interviewing augmented by self-report inventories, rating scales, and observation) in order to identify behavior problems. Fourth, the clinician should specify the attributes and response modes of the behavior problems in order to render clearly defined operational definitions of each. Fifth, the dimensions (e.g., intensity, frequency, duration) of each behavior problem is determined. Sixth, the clinician should estimate the relative importance (low, medium, high) of each behavior problem. These importance ratings are based on a number of factors including: risk of harm; rate, severity, or duration of the behavior problem; impact on quality of life; and subjective reports from the client. Seventh, the clinician should identify the effects of the behavior problems on other aspects of client functioning (i.e., other behaviors, social relationships, work, quality of life indicators, etc.). Eighth, the form (correlational, causal, unidirectional, bidirectional) of relationships among behavior problems are articulated. Ninth, the strength of functional relationships (low, medium, high) among behavior problems are estimated. Tenth, causal variables associated with each behavior problem are identified.

Eleventh, the form of relationships among causal variables are articulated. Twelve, the strength of functional relationships among causal variables are estimated. Thirteenth, the modifiability (low, medium, high) of causal variables is estimated. This step of estimating causal variable modifiability is critically important because, as noted earlier, interventions typically seek to alter causal variables in order to change behavior problems. A causal variable that is not readily modified (e.g., traumatic brain injury) is helpful as an explanatory variable in a FACCD, but it is not targeted in an intervention. Fourteenth and fifteenth, the form and strength of functional relationships (low, medium, high) between causal variables and behavior problems are estimated. Sixteenth and seventeenth, moderator and mediator variables that are associated with the relationships among causal variables and behavior problems are identified. Eighteenth, the direction of effect (positive relationship, inverse relationship) for each functional relationship is estimated. Nineteenth, social systems variables (e.g., family member, other persons, social setting variables) are identified. Twentieth, functional response classes (i.e., behavior problems that are influenced by a common set of causal variables) are identified. In the twenty-first step, hypothetical causal variables and behavior problems are identified. These variables are added to the FACCD as indicators of areas that need further assessment. Finally, it is recommended that the FACCD be continually reevaluated and updated as new information is obtained.

Figure 4.2 is a simplified (a number of elements such as moderating and mediating variables are omitted for clarity. Haynes et al. (2011) provide several illustrations of complex multi-element FACCDs that include mediators, moderators, and hypothesized variables) FACCD for a patient with factitious disorder (sometimes referred to as Munchausen syndrome). The patient, a 22 year-old female (identifying information is changed to maintain confidentiality) was referred for evaluation in a regional medical hospital. The reason for referral was based on medical staff observations that the patient was engaging in behaviors that were designed to create symptom intensification (e.g., the patient was found to have foreign materials such as paper and cloth inserted into an abdominal wound, the patient was found to be in possession of a hypodermic needle with an unknown substance, the patient was suspected of self-inducing vomiting) and her overall reports of symptoms seemed to be highly exaggerated. The patient had a very extensive

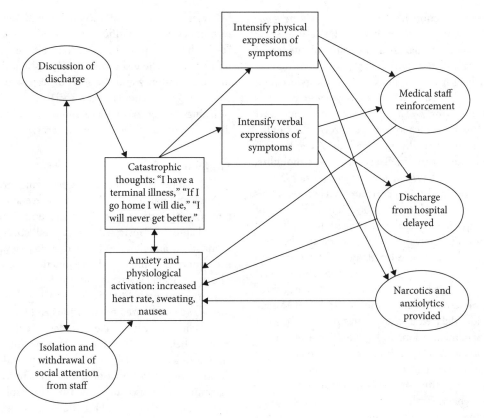

Figure 4.2 A functional analytic causal model of factitious disorder.

medical history, which included multiple hospitalizations for a variety of conditions that had vague symptom presentations and were not accompanied by a clear-cut medical diagnosis (e.g., chronic nausea and vomiting, chills, recurrent skin infections, recurrent diarrhea, reports of pain and fatigue).

The patient was interviewed. During the interview, the patient reported that she felt "anxious, depressed, and bored." She further volunteered that she was fearful of returning home from the hospital because no one at home could care for her. She further noted that she felt her home environment was unsafe (due to lack of supervision, living in a poor neighborhood, and severe family conflict from time to time). The patient also expressed a belief that she was very ill with an unknown terminal condition and that the medical doctors were not able to pinpoint her disease. This supported a fear that she was going to die if she returned home.

Behavioral observations were also conducted. It was noted by an observer who was stationed outside the patient's room (this was a requirement of the hospital's safety protocol given the patient's capacity for self-harm) that her social behavior varied as a function of the presence or absence of medical

staff. Specifically, the patient was observed to have animated conversations on the telephone when she was alone in her room. During these phone calls, the patient's mood tended to be appropriately varied and generally pleasant. However, when a medical staff member entered her room, the patient's expressed mood became somber and her affect was flat. Additionally, her voice rate and volume would diminish. Finally, the patient would close her eyes and become minimally responsive to verbal interactions with the staff. Finally, it was observed that the patient's symptoms would tend to intensify as she approached a discharge date.

An FACCD illustrates the essential model of behavior problem-contextual variable interaction for this client. Beginning at the left side of the diagram, it was hypothesized that two antecedent _contextual social and modifiable_ causal variables were exerting _important unidirectional causal_ influences on problem behaviors. One was discussion of discharge with her treatment team and the other was social isolation and staff withdrawal (over time, the staff would grow weary of her chronic complaints and avoid responding to the patient's requests and/or be more businesslike and less reinforcing in their interactions). These two events _were moderately correlated_ with each other (as indicated by thinner bidirectional arrows) because discussion of discharge and staff withdrawal tended to increase as her length of stay increased. These two causal variables elicited two sets of _important cognitive and physiological problem behaviors_ that were _highly correlated_ with each other: catastrophic thoughts (e.g., "I am terminally ill," "I will die if I go home") and anxious activation. The catastrophic thoughts, in turn, exerted a _strong unidirectional causal_ influence on two additional correlated sets of _important overt-motor problem behaviors_: intensification of verbal complaints and intensification of physical symptoms (using various means to create objective indicators of a physical malady such as infection, wound, or fever). Further, these two sets of overt-motor problem behaviors then brought about three types of responses from the medical staff: Social attention, delayed discharge, and provision of narcotic pain medications and anxiolytics. These social attention and delayed discharge, in turn, appeared to _strongly and positively_ reinforce (as indicated by thick bi-directional arrows) the symptom intensification behaviors while they did not exert as strong an influence on verbal complaints (staff were not highly responsive to verbal complaints but were highly responsive to physical symptom findings). The social attention also appeared to _strongly and negatively_ reinforce (as indicated by negative sign on arrow) anxious activation. Specifically, increased attention was associated with a reduction of anxious activation. Narcotic and anxiolytic medications were also hypothesized to be exerting important positive reinforcement effects on verbal complaints and symptom intensification behaviors and important negative reinforcement effects on anxious activation.

A behavioral intervention becomes apparent with examination of this FACCD. In order to dismantle the behavioral sequence of events, the reinforcement must be removed or competing behaviors must be acquired and reinforced. In this particular case, it was more workable to follow the latter course of action. Specifically, the staff members were encouraged to engage the client in nonmedical talk and provide social attention for improved physical health and non-self-injury. Additionally, the social work staff helped the client find an alternative place to live upon discharge. Third, the client was provided with outpatient vocational and educational counselors who were to assist her with pursuing education and job acquisition. Fourth,

behavior therapy using acceptance and defusion techniques, values clarification, graded exposure to "being healthy" (e.g., the client engaged in imaginal exposure where she envisioned "normal living" in the community and the sorts of fears and anxiety she would encounter), and social-skills training (learning to engage in social interactions without discussing medical and health concerns).

Summary

Behavioral assessment is an evolving area of research and practice that is based on several important assumptions and conceptual foundations. In this chapter we reviewed the central conceptual foundations and described how they are relevant to behavioral assessment and the functional analysis. The functional analysis was then introduced, and its primary elements were reviewed. Cutting across this review, we emphasized the decisions and judgments that a clinician must make in order to collect and evaluate behavioral data for the purposes of generating a functional analysis. Finally, we provided an illustration of how functional analytic clinical case diagrams can be used to summarize the results of a behavioral assessment and functional analysis.

References

Beauchamp, T. L., & Rosenberg, A. (1981). _Hume and the problem of causation._ New York: Oxford University Press.

Beck, A. T., Rush, A. J., Shaw, B. F., & Emery, G. (1979). _Cognitive therapy of depression._ New York: Guilford Press.

Beck, A. T., Steer, R. A., & Brown, G. K. (1996). _Manual for the Beck Depression Inventory:_ (2nd ed.). San Antonio: The Psychological Corporation.

Borkovec, T. D., Alcaine, O. M., & Behar, E. (2004). The avoidance theory of worry and generalized anxiety disorder. In R. G. Heimberg & C. Turk (Eds,), _Generalized anxiety disorder: Advances in research and practice_ (pp. 77–108). New York: Guilford Press.

Brantley, P. J., Waggoner, C. D., Jones, G. N., & Rappaport, N. B. (1987). A daily stress inventory: Development, reliability, and validity. _Journal of Behavioral Medicine, 10,_ 61–74.

Butler, A. C., Chapman, J. E., Forman, E. M., & Beck, A. T. (2006). The empirical status of cognitive-behavioral therapy: A review of meta-analyses. _Clinical Psychology Review, 26,_ 17–31.

Cook, T. D., & Campbell, D. T. (1979). _Quasi-Experimentation: Design & analysis issues for field settings._ Boston: Houghton Mifflin Company.

Exner, J. E. (1986). _The Rorschach: A comprehensive system._ (Vol. 1). New York: Wiley.

Exner, J. E. (1991). _The Rorschach: A comprehensive system._ (Vol. 2). New York: Wiley.

Fletcher, L., & Hayes, S. C. (2005). Relational frame theory, acceptance, and commitment therapy, and a functional analytic definition of mindfulness. _Journal of Rational-Emotive and Cognitive Therapy, 23,_ 315–336.

Frank, G. (1993). On the validity of hypotheses derived from the Rorschach: The relationship between color and affect. *Psychological Reports, 73*, 12–14.

Garb, H. N. (1996). *Studying the clinician: Judgment research and psychological assessment.* Washington, DC: American Psychological Association.

Garb, H. (2005). Clinical judgment and decision making. *Annual Review of Clinical Psychology, 1*, 67–89.

Hayes, S. C. (2004). Acceptance and commitment therapy, relational frame theory, and the third wave of behavioral and cognitive therapies. *Behavior Therapy, 35*, 639–665.

Hayes, S. C., Luoma, J. B., Bond, F. W., Masuda, A., & Lillis, J. (2006). Acceptance and commitment therapy: Model, processes and outcomes. *Behavior Research and Therapy, 44*, 1–25.

Hayes, S. C., Strosahl, K., & Wilson, K. G. (1999). *Acceptance and commitment therapy: An experiential approach to behavior change.* New York: Guilford Press.

Haynes, S. N., & O'Brien, W. H. (1990). The functional analysis in behavior therapy. *Clinical Psychology Review, 10*, 649–668.

Haynes, S. N., & O'Brien, W. H. (2000). *Principles and practice of behavioral assessment.* New York: Plenum Press.

Haynes, S. N., O'Brien, W. H., & Kaholokula, J. K (2011). *Behavioral assessment and case formulation.* New York: Wiley.

Hull, C. L. (1952). *A behavior system: An introduction to behavior theory concerning the individual organism.* New Haven, CT: Yale University Press.

James, L. R., Mulaik, S. A., & Brett, J. M. (1982). *Causal analysis: Assumptions, models, and data.* Beverly Hills: Sage.

Kohlenberg, R. J., Kanter, J. W., Bolling, M., Wexner, R., Parker, C., & Tsai, M. (2004). Functional analytic psychotherapy, cognitive therapy, and acceptance. In S. C. Hayes, V. M. Follette, & M. M. Linehan (Eds.), *Mindfulness and acceptance: Expanding the cognitive-behavioral tradition* (pp. 96–119). New York: Guilford Press.

Linehan, M. M. (1993). *Skills training manual for treating borderline personality disorder.* New York: Guilford Press.

Linehan, M. M., Comtois, K. A., Murray, A. M., Brown, M. Z., Gallop, R. J., Heard, H. L., … Lindenboim, N. (2006). Two-year randomized controlled trial and follow-up of dialectical behavior therapy versus therapy by experts for suicidal behaviors and borderline personality disorder. *Archives of General Psychiatry, 63*, 757–766.

Mill, J. S. (2012). A system of logic: *Ratiocinative and inductive, being a connected view of the principles of evidence, and the method of scientific investigation.* Calgary, CA: Thoephania Publishing.

O'Brien, W. H. (1995). Inaccuracies in the estimation of functional relationships using self-monitoring data. *Journal of Behavior Therapy and Experimental Psychiatry, 26*, 351–357.

O'Brien, W. H., & Carhart, V. (2011). Functional analysis in behavioral medicine settings. *European Journal of Psychological Assessment, 27*, 4–16.

O'Brien, W. H., Kaplar, M., & McGrath, J. J. (2004). Broadly-based causal models of behavior disorders. In M. Hersen, S. N. Haynes, & E. M. Heiby (Eds.), *Handbook of psychological assessment: Vol. 3: Behavioral assessment* (pp. 69–93). Hoboken, NJ: Wiley.

O'Brien, W. H., & Tabaczynski, T. (2009). *Unstructured interviewing.* In M. Hersen & J. Thomas (Eds.), *Handbook of Clinical Interviewing with Children* (pp. 16–29). New York: Sage.

Schlundt, D. G. (1985). An observational methodology for functional analysis. *Bulletin for the Society of Psychologists in Addictive Behaviors, 4*, 234–249.

Segal, Z. V., Williams, J. M., & Teasdale, J. D. (2002). *Mindfulness-based cognitive therapy for depression: A new approach to preventing relapse.* New York: Guilford Press.

Sibrava, N. J. & Borkovec, T. D. (2006) The cognitive avoidance theory of worry. In G. Davy & A. Wells (Eds.), *Worry and its psychological disorders: Theory, assessment and treatment* (pp. 239–256). Hoboken, NJ: Wiley.

Skinner, B. F. (1938). *The behavior of organisms: An experimental analysis.* Oxford, England: Appleton-Century.

Skinner, B. F. (1974). *About behaviorism.* Oxford, England: Knopf.

Skinner, B. F. (1987). Whatever happened to psychology as the science of behavior? *American Psychologist, 42*, 780–786.

Tsai, M., Kohlenberg, R., Kanter, J. W., Kohlenberg, B., Follette, W. C., & Callighan, G. M. (2008). *A guide to functional analytic psychotherapy: Awareness, courage, love, and behaviorism.* New York: Springer.

Watson, J. B. (1919). *Psychology from the standpoint of a behaviorist.* Philadelphia: Lippincott.

Wolpe, J. (1952a). Experimental neurosis as learned behavior. *British Journal of Psychology, 43*, 243–268.

Wolpe, J. (1952b). The formation of negative habits: A neurophysiological view. *Psychological Review, 59*, 290–299.

Wolpe, J. (1958). *Psychotherapy by reciprocal inhibition.* Oxford, England: Stanford University Press.

Wolpe, J. (1963). Psychotherapy: The nonscientific heritage and the new science. *Behavior Research and Therapy, 1*, 23–28.

Wolpe, J., & Lazarus, A. A. (1966). *Behavior therapy techniques: A guide to the treatment of neuroses.* Elmsford, NY: Pergamon Press.

Wolpe, J., Salter, A., & Reyna, L. J. (1964). *The conditioning therapies.* Oxford, England: Holt, Rinehart and Winston.

Case Formulation for the Cognitive and Behavioral Therapies: A Problem-Solving Perspective

Christine Maguth Nezu, Arthur M. Nezu, Sarah Ricelli, *and* Jessica B. Stern

Abstract

This chapter provides a discussion of the importance and usefulness of adopting a case formulation approach to the selection, integration, and idiographic application of multiple cognitive-behavioral interventions in clinical practice. The authors describe how one such case formulation model, based on problem-solving principles, may be adopted in clinical practice. This decision-making model focuses on three primary principles. They include functional analysis; use of the empirical literature as a means of identifying meaningful clinical targets and potential interventions intended to address such problems; and consideration of the cognitive-behavioral clinician as a "problem solver" in the context of a therapeutic relationship.

Key Words: case formulation, functional analysis, problem solving, clinical decision making, idiographic treatment

In this chapter we discuss the clinical importance of using a case formulation model for cognitive and behavioral psychotherapies. While the term "cognitive-behavioral therapy" is often used to refer to a specific therapeutic technique or orientation, the term serves as a wide umbrella for a large number of interventions, techniques, and clinical styles. The psychotherapies that are included under this cognitive and behavioral rubric share important characteristics. For example, these interventions are theoretically rooted in established learning principles and scientific investigation methods. More recently, however, cognitive and behavioral therapies have evolved to integrate contemporary research in neuroscience, implicit information processing, and theories of emotion and evolution (Nezu, Martell, & Nezu, 2014). Current therapies and systems referred to as cognitive and behavioral interventions include over 100 procedures (http://www.

commonlanguagepsychotherapy.org/), approaches, and techniques that target a very broad range of problems and populations. We advocate the use of a case conceptualization model as a "roadmap" for clinicians to use in taking on the task of integrating the large body of available scientific literature relevant to cognitive-behavioral interventions.

The Rationale for Cognitive-Behavioral Case Formulation

As the field of cognitive and behavioral therapies continues to grow, the number of specific treatments that address the same or similar clinical problems has also increased. Because clinical practice often involves treating people with comorbidities from an individualized and multicultural context, it is important for psychotherapists to have a set of heuristics that guide their decision making during the assessment and treatment process. In addition to what Barlow and colleagues (Barlow, Allen, & Choate, 2004) refer to as a "unified treatment approach," which involves distilling the common elements across effective treatments, a case formulation model provides a way for clinicians to remain committed to evidence-based procedures, yet flexible in applying these procedures with an individualized (versus manual-driven) treatment focus. This "idiographic approach" focuses on each individual's unique constellation of treatment targets, obstacles or therapy-interfering behaviors, and unique environmental and internal characteristics that are instrumental to the ultimate outcomes for which therapy was undertaken (Nezu, Nezu, & Cos, 2007; Rosen & Proctor, 1981).

Case formulation provides clinicians with a competent synthesis and integration of the many current assessment methods and measures available to them in their practice. Competent assessment in general has been described as a dynamic paradigm (Eells, 2007) that involves multiple methods, is culturally competent, reveals an awareness of the clinician's cognitive biases and common judgmental errors, employs a decision-making method to select tools, and employs a case formulation process to guide treatment (Fouad et al., 2009). Eells has defined case formulation as a "hypothesis" about the causes, precipitants, and maintaining influences of a person's psychological problems (cognitive and emotional), interpersonal problems, and behavioral problems. Moreover, a case formulation allows a clinician to organize the complex and contradictory information about an individual, identify therapy obstacles, accept what each patient may bring to treatment, and develop a blueprint for guiding treatment planning (Nezu, Martell, & Nezu, 2014).

Case Formulation Research

Until recently, very little was known about interrater reliability or predictive validity concerning therapy process and outcome with regard to the case formulation, and there are equivocal opinions about its impact in the literature (Tarrier & Calam, 2002). With regard to interrater reliability, one problem rests in the biases present in clinicians' information processing. There are many examples of the biases that exist with regard to human decision making, and behavioral clinicians are not exempt from engaging in these errors (Arkes, 1981; Arkes, Wortmann, Saville, & Harkness, 1981; Tversky & Kahnemann, 1981).

More recent research has shown that reliability and validity of case formulation is increased when a clinical judgment includes a focus on relationship interactions expressed in psychotherapy, when patient report is augmented with clinical judgment, when levels of inference remain close to observable statements or behaviors, when the formulation is broken down into components that can be measured, and when a diversity of viewpoints is taken into account (Eells, 2007). Flitcroft, James, and Freeston (2007) offer an explanation about why reliability among different clinicians' clinical formulations may be low. Specifically, they indicate that with any given clinical case, a therapist who is constructing a case formulation may attribute his or her observed phenomena to the existence of several different explanatory viewpoints. These include a focus on either situation specificity, functionality of problem behaviors or clinical targets, or trait features. The results of their research may partially explain why attempts to assess reliability in case formulation have been equivocal.

With regard to suggestions for competent case formulation in evidence-based practice settings, Tarrier and Calam (2002) underscore that assessment should be soundly based upon empirical evidence and hypothesis testing rather than on mere speculation. Lastly, they provide several suggestions for cognitive and behavioral clinicians. These authors underscore the importance of the conceptualization of a dysfunctional systems approach in the maintenance of clinical problems. They also advise that the historical background of a clinical problem should be described in terms of individualized vulnerabilities and an epidemiological evidence base. Finally, Tarrier and colleagues discuss the importance of the social behavioral context and recommend that it be emphasized in a case formulation (Tarrier & Calam, 2002).

Using a case formulation approach to treatment may reduce the likelihood that therapists, when confronted with obstacles in treatment, will be able to develop treatment revisions in a more systematic, rather than reactionary, manner. For example, Schulte and Eifert (2002) have observed that therapists who are implementing manualized treatments may tend to impulsively change treatments, concerned that the ongoing manualized treatment is not successful. They recommend that therapists should carefully consider the specific explanations regarding the lack of expected therapeutic change before changing an evidence-based strategy. Their suggestions are founded upon research suggesting that frequent therapy method changes are often associated with poorer treatment outcome. The authors speculate that treatment changes are not generally beneficial because therapists may incorrectly assess the state or progress of treatment. In other words, therapists may prematurely and impulsively abandon evidence-based, effective methods and adopt less appropriate or impactful strategies in an effort to prevent assumed failure. These authors note that the judgments of such therapists regarding session success and predictions of outcomes do not strongly correlate with actual treatment outcomes. On the other hand, adhering to manualized treatment programs is generally associated with more favorable treatment outcomes. Case formulation provides a systematic, less impulse-driven method for modifying one's treatment. A comprehensive case formulation may provide needed explanation for treatment challenges that a clinician may confront. Examples can include patient behavior such as diffuse treatment goals, lack of action orientation, lack of recognition of the relationship between symptoms and negative consequences, secondary gain from illness, low treatment expectations, or fear of change. In these instances, coauthors Shulte and Eiffert suggest that therapists consider such therapy-interfering behaviors as instrumental treatment targets in their own right. In these situations, a case formulation can provide a systematic path toward resolving these treatment obstacles. It is encouraging that the complex skills required in constructing a case formulation can be taught to clinical trainees with some success. For example Kendjelic and Eells (2007) demonstrated how training in case formulation can improve skills. Specifically, these coauthors reported a study in which clinicians who were trained in a case formulation model produced formulations rated as higher quality and better elaborated compared to clinicians who did receive training. Moreover, the reported effect sizes indicated that the average clinician in the training group produced a better formulation than 86% of those in the control group.

In summary, the more recent research regarding case formulation has suggested the following:

• Specific considerations in the case formulation process can improve accuracy and utility (Flitcroft, James, & Freeston, 2007; Tarrier & Calam, 2002).

• It has provided information concerning when it is most likely to improve patient care by considering a change from a manualized treatment to a more process-driven, case formulation model (Schulte & Eifert, 2002).

• It has demonstrated how training in case formulation can improve skills (Kendjelic & Eells, 2007).

Characteristics of a Case Formulation Model

With a current zeitgeist in the specialty of cognitive and behavioral therapies that recognizes the challenge of assessment and treatment of individuals with complex problems and histories, there are several models that have been proposed and offer methods to developing a case formulation. While there are differences between these various models, it may be most useful to focus on the similarities. Tracy Eells (2007) has accomplished this succinctly with the following points. First, all cognitive and behavioral case formulation models assume a multiple-causal hypotheses perspective. This is an important point, because regardless of the efficacy studies to support any one specific treatment for a particular problem, no one treatment is effective for every individual with the same diagnosis and no one etiological factor explains its presence in every individual. Additionally, individual factors such as temperament, social and cultural development, strengths, and comorbidities make every person unique.

Second, all of the cognitive and behavioral case formulation approaches place an emphasis on functional analysis as a way to understand what may be triggering or maintaining a problem. Functional analysis in behavioral psychology refers to the application of the laws of operant learning principles to establish relationships between internal and external stimuli and cognitive, behavioral, and affective responses.

Third, all cognitive and behavioral models of case formulation emphasize the need for positive treatment goals, such as the development of skills, as part of a constructional approach to intervention. In other words, in order for individuals to change the patterns of thoughts, feelings, and actions that are associated with their distress, and improve the quality of their lives, change will require the individual to practice new skills, intentionally "doing something different."

Finally, all cognitive and behavioral models underscore the ubiquity of cognitive errors and human decision-making bias, and therefore include strategies for therapists to employ as a means of reducing biases in clinical judgment. A competent cognitive and behavioral case formulation involves adopting a systematic approach to conducting assessment and integrating the results of assessment into a meaningful explanation of the likely etiologic, triggering, and maintaining factors regarding the symptoms for which people seek help. The result is that cognitive-behavioral intervention may be viewed as an individualized, methodologically driven treatment. Rather than a series of random techniques or manuals to be used whenever a therapist thinks they might be helpful, the approach assumes a strategic functional focus on the factors that appear to be maintaining clinical symptoms of distress. For the purpose of this chapter, we will focus on describing the problem-solving model of case formulation developed by Nezu and Nezu (Nezu & Nezu, 1989; Nezu et al., 2007). This model focuses on the clinician's information processing and advocates a problem-solving approach to clinical decision making, including adoption of a multicausal and systemic worldview. The Nezu and Nezu model of case formulation does not view any of cognitive, emotional, biologic, historic, or current functional factors as primary, but it underscores the importance of integrating and understanding all of these factors and their functional relations as contributory to understanding a person's individual "story." These authors view a case formulation approach as a "best practices" approach to translating the range of evidence-based cognitive-behavioral interventions to the problems of each individual patient.

Conceptual Framework of a Problem-Solving Model of Case Formulation

The problem-solving model of case formulation as we discuss in this chapter is centered on three primary principles as delineated by (1) employing functional analysis to understand and appreciate human functioning and psychopathology; (2) using empirical literature from a wide range of investigations as the primary source for the identification of meaningful clinical targets, along with interventions intended to address such problems; and (3) regarding the cognitive and behavioral clinician as the "problem solver" in the context of a therapeutic relationship (Nezu et al., 2007).

Functional Analysis

Functional analysis is a key tool to the successful development and implementation of a cognitive and behavioral case formulation. It is the process by which a clinician uses assessment methodologies to identify and integrate the important functional relationships among variables that an individual in

treatment may present (Eells, 2007). It is an analysis of the functional relations between a patient or client's problems and treatment goals with causal and mediating variables, and the functional relationships between these variables (Haynes & O'Brien, 2000).

In order to establish appropriate and well-defined treatment goals, we endorse the importance of distinguishing ultimate outcome goals from instrumental outcome goals as was initially conceptualized by Rosen and Proctor (1981). Ultimate outcome goals are general therapy goals that serve as a response to the concerns that initiate therapy and reflect the objectives for which treatment efforts are focused. Conversely, instrumental outcome goals represent the mechanisms (or *instruments*) by which more general treatment goals can be achieved. Depending on their functional relationships to other variables, instrumental outcomes may influence ultimate outcomes (e.g., increasing one's self-esteem can reduce depression) or other instrumental outcomes within a hypothesized causal chain (e.g., improving an individual's coping ability can increase his or her sense of self-efficacy, which in turn may decrease depression) (Eells, 2007).

Instrumental outcomes in a clinical context reflect the hypotheses a clinician forms based on the factors that are thought to be causally related to the ultimate outcomes. Ultimate outcomes can be viewed as dependent variables (DVs), while instrumental outcomes represent independent variables (IVs) (Eells, 2007). Instrumental outcome variables can serve as *mediators*, or factors that account for or explain the association between two other variables in a causal manner (i.e., the method by which an IV influences the DV) (Eells, 2007). Additionally, they can also serve as *moderators*, or factors that impact the strength and/or direction of the relationship between two or more variables (Eells, 2007; Haynes & O'Brien, 2000). Instrumental outcome goals can aid in targeting mechanisms of change, and thus, it is anticipated that generally, achieving instrumental outcome goals will lead to accomplishing the ultimate outcome goals.

Having an understanding and appreciation of instrumental outcome and ultimate outcome goals can direct the process of evaluation, treatment planning, and implementation (Nezu, Nezu, Friedman, & Haynes, 1997). Furthermore, it can aid a clinician in determining when treatment is stalled or unsuccessful and may need to be reconceptualized. Mash and Hunsley (1993) suggest that assessment should serve the purpose of early corrective feedback, rather than a mere evaluation at the conclusion of a path to a patient's ultimate outcome goal. If a problem-solving intervention, for example, is found to be ineffective in prompting changes in a depressed patient's coping ability, then assessment may provide for immediate feedback at that particular point. As such, assessment of success in achieving instrumental outcome goals (e.g., improvement in problem-solving ability) should be evaluated prior to the assessment of attainment of ultimate goals (e.g., decrease in depression) (Eells, 2007).

Evidence-Based Approach

While the interventions categorized under the cognitive and behavioral umbrella have unique characteristics, one of the unifying grounds on which these systems structure is the emphasis on an evidence-based approach to understanding and treating human problems. Well-controlled research studies advance the conceptualization of the etiology and development of psychological disorders, rather than merely collections of clinical cases and hypotheses. While nonexperimental study and observation serve an important piece in the theory and application of cognitive and behavioral principles, empirical sources of information serve as the basis for development of the field and its models.

While the cognitive and behavioral case formulation models strive to reflect evidence-based advancement, the current literature regarding the etiopathogenesis and treatment of psychological disorders is not yet expansive enough to provide idiographic recommendations and remedies for the vast multitude of problems that individuals may experience. Additionally, various causal hypotheses exist pertaining to the possible relationships between instrumental and ultimate outcome for a given psychological disorder. For example, several cognitive-behavioral theories exist regarding the etiopathogenesis of major depression (Eells, 2007). The differences in the emphasis they place on potential instrumental outcome variables, such as cognitive distortions (e.g., Beck, Rush, Shaw, & Emery, 1979), decreased levels of positive social and valued life experiences (e.g., Dimidjian, Barrera, Martell, Muñoz, & Lewinsohn, 2011), ineffective problem-solving ability and emotional dysregulation (Nezu, Nezu, & D'Zurilla, 2013), cognitive fusion and experiential avoidance (Hayes, 2004), or deficient social skills (e.g., Hersen, Bellack, & Himmelhoch, 1980), drive these various theoretical models. Although the relationships between instrumental and outcome variables proposed by these models are all empirically supported, studies have demonstrated that they are a result of unique, individual characteristics between individuals; therefore, no one theory can entirely explain the complex clinical symptoms and causal relationships in every individual case.

Additionally, the expectation for randomized controlled trials to be internally valid results in a limited understanding of how a given cognitive and behavioral approach can be implemented across populations, and whether or not efficacy can be achieved. For instance, even though cognitive therapy has been identified and confirmed as an efficacious treatment approach for individuals with depression, insufficient evidence exists to confirm that such efficacious results would be found across individuals with varying comorbid, cultural, demographic, or spiritual characteristics.

In summary, translating empirical findings involves more than reliance on a critical number of randomized trials to support a specific intervention. While important, empirical research concerning the theories underlying a specific approach, evidence-based investigations of mediators proposed as instrumental to outcome, comorbidities, and variables unique to a given individual must all be taken into account.

Therapy as Problem Solving

In conducting a case formulation based on problem-solving principles, the therapist adopts the role of a problem solver where the process of psychotherapy represents a series of problems to solve and the therapist's attempts to solve them. Problems are the patient's concerns and reasons for seeking treatment, and they may include the reduction of psychological symptoms or the achievement of positive goals. They are considered problems due to the presence of obstacles that prevent the individual from reaching such goals without the help of a therapist, contributing to a discrepancy between the patient's current state and the patient's desired state. Obstacles may include characteristics of the patient (e.g., affective, behavioral, cognitive, biologic, or socio-ethnic-cultural variables), characteristics of the therapist (e.g., training, specialization, relationship skills), and the environment (e.g., insufficient resources in the physical or social environment). Within this paradigm, effective problem solving is the process by which a clinician successfully aids patients in accomplishing their goals. Thus, the critical goal or problem to solve in therapy is the identification of the most effective treatment plan for an individual who is experiencing particular symptoms, given his or her unique history and current life situation at the present time, by a specific therapist.

The problem-solving approach to case formulation for cognitive-behavioral therapies is based on the prescriptive model of social problem solving that was developed by D'Zurilla, Nezu, and their colleagues (e.g., D'Zurilla & Nezu, 1996; Nezu, 2004; Nezu, Nezu, & D'Zurilla, 2013). This multidimensional model, which was adapted for the purpose of enhancing clinical decision making to foster the effectiveness and validity of cognitive and behavioral case formulation, is comprised of two interrelated problem-solving processes, problem orientation (PO) and problem-solving styles, which are discussed in the following section.

The Multidimensional Problem-Solving Model

According to contemporary problem-solving theory, problem-solving outcomes are influenced by two general, but partially independent, dimensions: (a) PO and (b) problem-solving style (D'Zurilla, Nezu, & Maydeu-Olivares, 2004). *PO* represents the set of cognitive-affective schemas regarding people's generalized beliefs, attitudes, and emotional reactions concerning real-life problems, as well as their ability to successfully cope with such difficulties. Originally thought of as being two ends of the same continuum (e.g., D'Zurilla & Nezu, 1982), research during the past several years has continued to characterize the two forms of POs as operating mostly independently of each other (Nezu, 2004). These two orientation components are positive PO and negative PO.

A *positive PO* involves the tendency for individuals to do the following:

- Perceive problems as challenges rather than major threats to one's well-being
- Be optimistic in believing that problems are solvable
- Have a strong sense of self-efficacy regarding their ability to handle difficult problems
- Believe that successful problem solving usually involves time and effort
- View negative emotions as important sources of information necessary for effective problem solving

A *negative PO* refers to the tendency of individuals to do the following:

- View problems as major threats to one's well-being

- Generally perceive problems to be unsolvable
- Maintain doubts about their ability to cope with problems successfully
- Become particularly frustrated and upset when faced with problems or when they experience negative emotions

As suggested by their content, both types of orientations can have a strong influence on people's motivation, either positive or negative, as well as on their ability to engage in focused attempts to solve problems and cope with stress. The importance of self-awareness of one's tendency toward a negative orientation, particularly when confronted with certain types of problems (e.g., an angry, blaming patient), as well as a commitment toward a positive orientation when facing clinical problems, is considered a key component of when assuming a problem-solving approach to case formulation.

As with other problem situations, in a clinical situation this refers to the set of orienting responses (e.g., beliefs, assumptions, appraisals, expectations, emotional reactivity) an individual clinician engages in when initially reacting to a problem. In other words, before one engages in any actual attempts to solve a challenging situation, there is an initial reaction. This may occur at a *nonconscious* level of classically *conditioned emotional arousal* or *implicit cognitive* reactions, as well as a more conscious *worldview* regarding problems. When applied to case formulation, the concept of PO represents the *clinician's own beliefs and worldview*, which guides efforts to understand, explain, predict, and change human behavior. It encompasses the clinician's own arousal, emotional responses, cognitive biases, and management of concerns and fears related to the problems presented by patients.

For this reason, the problem-solving model of case formulation promotes the adoption of a PO that underscores the importance of emotional processing and recognition of bias in the clinician (for a more complete description of the various types of heuristics involved in decision-making that can lead to errors of accuracy, see Nezu & Nezu, 1989 or Kahnemann, 2003). As an example, a therapist's own bias may lead him or her to attempt to quickly identify the answer to a patient's problem when one is not readily apparent or avoid clinical situations that involve material with which one is less familiar. The clinician's past experiences may also bias his or her assessment of the client and interpretations of different situations. Such a lack of awareness of clinicians' emotional reactions or biases may negatively impact how they respond to clients, hindering their ability to successfully address the client's concerns. For example, a patient who presents as extremely distressed and emotionally aroused may evoke a schema-driven response of a therapist's own fears of failure or criticism. As a result, the therapist may react with avoidance by changing the topic or turning his or her gaze away from the client, freeze up without validating the patient's concerns, or react impulsively with a hasty attempt to resolve the problem. Thus, the clinician will be required to make purposeful efforts to maintain a calm and flexible inner environment and to seek to understand his or her own biases, judgment, and emotional reactions in clinical situations in order to problem-solve effectively.

Mindfulness, described as the ability to be fully present in one's awareness of the current moment, is an important technique by which clinicians can foster increased awareness of their own reactions. A core component of dialectical behavior therapy (Robins, 2003), it has also been emphasized as an important strategy for therapists to become aware of their experience, facilitating the processing of their own emotions (Linehan, 1993; Manning & DuBose, 2010). Additionally, the importance of enhancing the mindfulness of the therapist has been highlighted in recent literature, which emphasizes the fundamental elements of presence and attunement in this process (Siegal, 2010). Being truly present with a patient, open to all possibilities, and attuned to the patient, fully receptive and letting go of expectations, is instrumental to fostering a *positive PO* and reducing a *negative PO*. Moreover, it enhances the therapist's flexibility, access to his or her knowledge base, and ability to make use of his or her problem-solving strengths.

Problem orientation regarding cognitive and behavioral case formulation also involves the recognition that behavior can have multiple causes and can occur within various systems. Most problems are complex and based on the person's history, deficits, and other causal variables interacting with one another, a perspective that is referred to as *planned critical multiplism* (Shadish, 1993). In accordance with this worldview, cognitive and behavioral clinicians identify empirically supported causal variables (e.g., cognitive distortions, medical-related difficulties, poor social skills, ineffective problem solving, low rates of positive reinforcement) for each symptom, and then seek both confirming and disconfirming evidence to determine the factors that are relevant for a particular client. Moreover, cognitive and behavioral clinicians employ a general systems perspective, which emphasizes the notion that instrumental outcome and ultimate outcome variables can relate to each other in interactive ways, rather than in a simple unidirectional and linear fashion (Nezu et al., 1997). For example, consistent with a biopsychosocial systems approach, various biological, psychological, and social factors can interact with each other in both initiating and maintaining biologically caused distressing physical symptoms, such as noncardiac chest pain, chronic fatigue syndrome, and fibromyalgia (Nezu, Nezu, & Lombardo, 2001). As such, the clinician evaluates the manner and degree with which different pathogenically involved variables interact with one another in order to develop a comprehensive understanding of the development and maintenance of a client's symptom. This approach allows the therapist to identify causal instrumental outcomes, which facilitates the prioritization of initial treatment targets. Additionally, this permits the possibility of addressing numerous clinical targets simultaneously in treatment, thereby maximizing the likelihood of achieving therapeutic progress regarding the client's symptoms.

PROBLEM-SOLVING STYLES

Problem-solving style, a second major dimension of problem-solving ability, refers to the core cognitive-behavioral activities in which people engage when attempting to solve stressful problems. Three differing styles have been identified (D'Zurilla, Nezu, & Maydeu-Olivares, 2004; D'Zurilla et al., 2004): *planful problem solving, avoidant problem solving*, and *impulsive-careless problem solving*. *Planful problem solving* is the constructive approach that involves the systematic and planful application of the following set of specific skills:

- *Problem Definition*—clarifying the nature of a problem, delineating a realistic set of problem-solving goals and objectives, and identifying those obstacles that prevent one from reaching such goals
- *Generation of Alternatives*—brainstorming a range of possible solution strategies geared to overcome the identified obstacles
- *Decision Making*—predicting the likely consequences of the various alternatives, conducting a cost-benefit analysis based on

these identified outcomes, and developing a solution plan that is geared to achieve the problem-solving goal

• *Solution Implementation and Verification*—carrying out the solution plan, monitoring and evaluating the consequences of such a plan, and determining whether one's problem-solving efforts have been successful or need to continue

In addition to planful problem solving, two social problem-solving styles have been further identified, both of which, in contrast, are generally found to be dysfunctional or maladaptive in nature (D'Zurilla et al., 2004). An *impulsive/careless style* is the problem-solving approach whereby an individual tends to engage in impulsive, hurried, and careless attempts at problem resolution. *Avoidant problem solving* is the maladaptive problem-solving style characterized by procrastination, passivity, and overdependence on others to provide solutions. In general, both styles are associated with ineffective or unsuccessful coping. Moreover, people who typically engage in these styles tend to worsen existing problems and even create new ones.

In the context of case formulation, the problem-solving styles reflect the actions of the therapist that are directed toward managing the problem presented by a patient, and they may be influenced by the therapist's PO. For example, a therapist who is unfamiliar with a particular area of difficulty that the patient is experiencing, and fearful of not having the answer, may react impulsively by rushing into a poorly chosen intervention or avoid addressing the concern by referring the client elsewhere (e.g., to a hospital or drug treatment). In contrast, we propose that a clinician who maintains a calm and positive orientation, and approaches the problem in a methodical and planful manner, is more likely to achieve improved patient outcomes.

We view this model to be suitable for varied sorts of patient or client problems and for all types of patient populations. However, we have found it to be especially helpful with complex cases where causal variables and intervention targets may not be easily identifiable, and solutions may not be readily apparent.

One particular area in which research and available references are scant is regarding minority populations, particularly those of minority cultural backgrounds and identification (Hall, 2001; Tanaka-Matsumi, Seiden, & Lam, 1996). Thus, it is important for a case formulation model to incorporate guidelines to account for such factors that may not be adequately addressed in the literature.

The model we have presented regards multicultural diversity as a crucial consideration in the process of conceptualizing a case formulation. This approach should be used when capturing information about sexual orientation, religious and spiritual affiliations, socioeconomic status, and medical history and disability. While this model for case formulation can be easily adapted to individuals of various identifications, the following factors should be assessed to determine whether they factor into the etiology or development of an individual's problem treatment target: (1) self-defined ethnic/racial/cultural identity; (2) self-identified cultural group; (3) immigration history; (4) acculturation status; (5) perceived minority status; (6) poverty level; (7) experience of discrimination; and (8) cultural-based values (Eells, 2007).

Steps in Case Formulation

The general objectives of case formulation are to obtain a detailed understanding of the patient's presenting problems; identify the factors that are functionally related to such problems; and delineate treatment targets, aims, and goals. The steps of this case formulation process, as well as the application of the various problem-solving activities that are integrated into this approach, are briefly outlined in this section (for a more comprehensive discussion of the conceptual foundations of this approach, see Nezu, Nezu, & Lombardo, 2004).

Step 1: Identify Ultimate Outcomes

The clinician uses a "funnel approach" to assessment (Mash & Hunsley, 1993), which initially involves the examination of a broad range of many areas, with the focus gradually narrowing down to the variables that are particularly salient to the client. To identify the ultimate outcomes, the therapist assesses various general life domains (e.g., interpersonal relationships, career, education, finances, physical health, spirituality, and leisure) and moves "down the funnel" as it is determined that a given area is not pertinent to a client's problems. This process facilitates the clinician's ability to pinpoint the client's specific difficulties and establish the objectives toward which treatment efforts are to be directed.

It is important to note that ultimate outcomes may be patient-defined goals that are expressed as the reasons for seeking treatment (e.g., a patient wants to feel less depressed or reduce binge-eating behavior), referral-defined goals that may be provided by a third party such as another health care provider (e.g., a physician refers a patient for the reduction of psychosomatic symptoms), or goals that are translated by the therapist as an increased understanding of the patient's problem develops (e.g., making a formal diagnosis of social anxiety disorder or identifying the outcome of increased self-esteem). Ultimate outcomes may be modified over the course of treatment as additional problems arise, goals change, or the patient exhibits improvement such that a problem is no longer a concern.

Step 2: Identify Potentially Relevant Instrumental Outcomes

The clinician then identifies instrumental outcomes that are potentially relevant to a given ultimate outcome, guided by the problem-solving orientation that advocates a critical multiplism worldview, in which complex problems have multiple causes. To address the wide-ranging scope of variables that are associated with a given ultimate outcome, it is recommended that the clinician consider the broad instrumental outcome dimensions related to the patient and to the environment. Patient-related variables include conscious and nonconscious affective factors (e.g., emotional experience, physiological sensations), behavioral factors (e.g., behavioral deficits, excesses, strengths), conscious and nonconscious cognitive factors (e.g., cognitive distortions, cognitive deficiencies, information processing styles, implicit beliefs, metacognitions), biological factors (e.g., age, gender, medical problems, biological vulnerability), and socio-ethnic-cultural factors (e.g., ethnicity, sexual orientation, sex roles, culture, socioeconomic status, religion/spirituality). Environment-related variables include physical environment factors (e.g., housing, crowding, climate, resources, health-related environmental variables) and social environment factors (e.g., partner, family, friends, coworkers, community, employment, culture/religion, early childhood, previous learning).

A brainstorming approach is recommended to increase the probability of identifying all possible variables that are linked with a given ultimate outcome, thus improving the likelihood of detecting those that are relevant to a specific patient. This involves initially conducting theory-driven and diagnosis-driven searches of the evidence-based literature for factors that are etiologically related to the ultimate outcome. For example, a comprehensive search of the research literature for depressed mood may identify the empirically supported instrumental outcome objectives of decreased dysfunctional thoughts, improved problem-solving ability, improved self-control skills, increased rate of positive reinforcement, and enhanced interpersonal skills (Nezu et al., 2004). The clinician should then apply brainstorming principles to the process of identifying additional variables that are potentially relevant to a specific patient but not found in the literature (e.g., cultural or other factors for which there is a dearth of research). The problem-solving principles for brainstorming include the following: quantity is important (i.e., the greater number of alternatives that are generated increases the probability of identifying those that are more effective), defer judgment (i.e., evaluation of the alternatives should be delayed until after a complete list of solutions has been generated because it increases one's ability to think creatively and produce higher quality solutions), and think of strategies versus tactics (i.e., identify general strategies and approaches, as well as specific tactics, to increase the production and variety of alternatives).

After the various possible instrumental outcomes have been identified, the clinician determines which instrumental outcomes are applicable to the specific client through continued assessment. Data are collected with clinical interviews and self-report measures to assess the relevance of each potential variable to the patient's presenting problem.

Step 3: Conduct a Functional Analysis

Next, a functional analysis of the ultimate outcomes and instrumental outcomes should be conducted, including both distal factors (i.e., past history) and proximal factors (i.e., immediate antecedents) that contribute to the client's problem. The purpose of this analysis is to establish the functional relationship between each of the variables, which refers to the covariation between two or more factors. The relationship may be causal, in that one variable causes another, or reciprocal, in that one variable changes in conjunction with another and vice versa. A variable that is reciprocally related to another variable may serve as a maintaining factor that perpetuates the occurrence of the other variable with which it is related.

The functional relationship between two variables can be viewed within a larger causal chain that links a stimulus, organismic variable, response, and consequence, represented by the acronym SORC. A clinician can use this framework to guide assessment of the variables that function as antecedents, consequences, and organismic mediators and moderators of the response that the patient is seeking to change (i.e., the patient's presenting problem). A variable can be labeled as a stimulus (S; intrapersonal or environmental antecedent), an organismic variable (O; biological, behavioral, affective, cognitive, socio-ethnic-cultural patient-related factor), a response (R; instrumental outcome or ultimate outcome variable), and/or a consequence (C; intrapersonal, interpersonal, or environmental effect produced by the response).

An example of SORC chaining is provided for the case of Laura, who presented with social anxiety. Her clinician conducted a functional analysis to determine the variables related to Laura's problem and identified the situation of meeting new people (i.e., stimulus) as a factor that caused an exacerbation of her anxiety (i.e., response). The clinician established that the stimulus triggered self-deprecating thoughts (i.e., organismic variable) associated with an increase in anxiety, which then resulted in increased self-statements regarding potential for social rejection (i.e., consequence). Moreover, these self-statements also served as a stimulus for further increased arousal (response) that was followed by avoidance (behavior). The avoidance behavior was negatively reinforced, because it was associated with a decrease in subjective arousal. However, another result of these functional sequences was a sense of failure and hopelessness that Laura experienced with regard to her ability to make meaningful changes in her life. This example demonstrates that it is important for clinicians to conduct a thorough analysis of the patient's presenting problem, as there are typically multiple causal chains occurring simultaneously and interacting with one another within a larger causal network. In this case, Laura's early environment and emotional learning experiences, which included isolation and harsh parental criticism, may have contributed to the development of a low threshold for arousal and early maladaptive schemas, resulting in a greater vulnerability to stressful situations.

Identification of the functional relationships among variables provides information to the clinician regarding potential target problems of the patient and aims one's decisions regarding interventions that may be used to address them. The clinician may then select intervention strategies that aim to address the specific factors in the causal chain (e.g., stimulus variables, organismic mediating variables, consequential variables) that cause or maintain the patient's ultimate outcomes. For example, in the case of Laura, the clinician identified Laura's low threshold for arousal as a clinical target because it resulted in increased negative self-evaluation, avoidant behavior, and a sense of hopelessness concerning her ability to change. The clinician was then able to select interventions that addressed the identified clinical targets that were viewed as instrumental to this patient's outcome. In this case, this included strategies to increase awareness of her physiologic arousal, practice strategies to manage her arousal, reframe thoughts to focus on the view that her symptoms were the result of her body's conditioning, and techniques to prevent her continued avoidance (exposure). This demonstrates the intricately linked relationship between functional analysis and case formulation, and it underscores the importance of these processes in a treatment design.

Step 4: Select Treatment Targets

The initial clinical targets, or instrumental outcome variables, that are selected are those that will have the greatest impact on the patient and maximize the success of treatment. The clinician's decision-making process involves evaluating the utility of each potential instrumental outcome target, which is determined by the likelihood that an alternative will achieve a particular goal and the value of that alternative.

LIKELIHOOD ESTIMATES

Estimates of likelihood are ascertained through assessing the probability that an alternative will achieve the desired goal, as well as the probability that the person implementing it will be able to do so optimally. This is determined by considering the following questions, in regard to a specific patient:

• Will addressing the instrumental outcome impact the desired ultimate outcome either directly or by means of addressing another related instrumental outcome?

• Based on the empirical literature, is the instrumental outcome amenable to treatment?

• Does the therapist have the expertise to implement the interventions that are aimed toward addressing the target?

• Is the treatment necessary to achieve the instrumental outcome goal actually available?

In determining the likelihood that the therapist will be able to effectively implement a treatment strategy to address a particular clinical target, the clinician must be aware of his or her own biases and schemas. The impact of these factors on the therapist's ability to provide optimal treatment is an important consideration that must not be overlooked.

VALUE ESTIMATES

The value of an alternative is estimated by considering the following four specific areas:

• Personal consequences (regarding both the therapist and patient)

  • Time, effort, or resources necessary to achieve the instrumental outcome
  • Emotional cost or gain involved in achieving the instrumental outcome
  • Consistency of the outcome with one's ethical values
  • Physical or life-threatening effects involved in changing the target problem
  • Effects of changing the problem area on other target problems

• Social consequences (i.e., effects on others, such as a significant other, family members, friends, or the community)
• Short-term effects (e.g., immediate consequences)
• Long-term effects (e.g., long-range consequences)

The clinician uses the likelihood and value estimates to conduct a cost-benefit analysis for each potential target. The instrumental outcome or set of instrumental outcomes that maximize positive effects and minimize negative effects has the highest degree of utility. This process guides the clinician in the selection of target problems and prioritization of problems to address initially.

Step 5: Develop a Clinical Pathogenesis Map

The next step of a cognitive and behavioral case formulation involves the construction of a clinical pathogenesis map (CPM; Nezu & Nezu, 1989; Nezu et al., 2004, 2007), which is a graphic depiction of the variables hypothesized to contribute to the initiation and maintenance of a patient's difficulties. It specifies the functional relationships among the all the variables using SORC nomenclature, and it can be viewed as an example of a path analysis or causal modeling diagram ideographically developed for a specific patient (Nezu et al.,

1997). The CPM offers a concrete statement of a therapist's initial causal hypotheses against which to test alternative hypotheses, and it can be modified as new information is obtained. It incorporates five elements, including distal variables, antecedent variables, organismic variables, response variables, and consequential variables (for examples of CPMs for multiple clinical cases, see Nezu & Nezu, 1989; Nezu et al., 2004, 2007).

DISTAL VARIABLES

Distal variables are historical and developmental variables that are hypothesized etiological factors regarding the initial emergence of specific vulnerabilities, symptoms, or psychological disorders. Examples include past trauma (e.g., rape, physical abuse), negative life events, the presence of chronic stressors, and other potential variables (e.g., tempermental or biologic vulnerability) that have contributed to the patient's current situation by increasing the patient's susceptibility to the difficulties he or she is experiencing. Identification of these factors is helpful for predicting the ways in which a patient will respond to certain stimuli.

ANTECEDENT VARIABLES

Antecedent variables refer to patient-related (e.g., behavioral, cognitive, affective, biological, socio-ethnic-cultural) and environment-related (e.g., social and physical environmental) factors, including recent major life events and daily problems, which can serve as proximal triggers or discriminative stimuli for other instrumental outcome factors or symptoms. An example of an environmental antecedent is being fired from a job, which may trigger thoughts of worthlessness that may then cause depressed mood.

MEDIATING VARIABLES

This category represents any of the various types of patient-related variables. These factors are response mediators (i.e., variables that explain a response that occurs in the presence of a certain antecedent) or response moderators (i.e., variables that influence the strength and/or direction of the relationship between the antecedent and response). Examples of mediating variables include cognitive distortions related to mistrust of other people (cognitive variable), heightened arousal and fear (emotional variable), coronary heart disease (biological variable), and ethnic background concerning one's understanding of the meaning of a particular set of symptoms (socio-ethnic-cultural variable). An example of a moderating variable is a characteristic, such as strong family supports or learned resilience, which has been found to reduce the likelihood of experiencing depression under high levels of stress (Nezu, 2004).

RESPONSE VARIABLES

This set of factors is comprised of either certain patient-related instrumental outcome variables that are closely associated with an ultimate outcome goal (e.g., social withdrawal is associated with loneliness) or the set of distressing symptoms that constitute the ultimate outcomes themselves (e.g., depression, chronic pain, substance abuse).

CONSEQUENTIAL VARIABLES

This category includes the full range of patient-related and environment-related variables that occur in reaction to a given response variable. Operant functional relationships are often involved, and as such, the relationship between a response and a consequence can serve to either increase or decrease the probability of the same response occurring in the future. Many challenging or distress-related behaviors are maintained over time due to consequential variables (e.g., the consequence of reduced anxiety is negatively reinforced when the patient avoids confronting a feared, phobic stimuli). Positive reinforcement may include attention or caring behavior from others, decreased responsibility, or perceptions of control.

Step 6: Evaluate the Validity of the CPM

The clinician determines the validity of the CPM through the processes of social validation and hypothesis testing. Social validation involves presenting the initial CPM to the patient and eliciting feedback regarding the relevance and importance of the selected target problems and treatment goals, which can be facilitated by having the CPM in pictorial form. Hypothesis testing can also be used to verify the CPM by seeking confirming and disconfirming support for the hypotheses generated by the CPM. For example, if a patient's CPM indicates that the presenting problem of anxiety is associated with interpersonal deficits and fears of social rejection, the therapist might predict that the patient would score high on measures on social avoidance and distress. Moreover, the clinician might predict that conducting a structured role play of a social situation would cause physical signs of anxiety, such as tension, as well as reported distress. Additional hypotheses regarding the effects of the treatment

strategies selected to address the clinical targets can be evaluated at a later time (for a detailed description of how case formulation drives treatment planning, see Nezu et al., 2004).

Application to Psychotherapy

Cognitive and behavioral case formulation is individualized to each patient, involving a series of functional analyses concerning precipitating internal and external events, behaviors, thoughts, and emotions that facilitates the identification of specific patient goals to target with treatment. It is predicated on the idiographic application of nomothetic principles, and therefore it assumes that no one treatment intervention or manual "fits all." As such, the case formulation model is integrally connected to the treatment plan, and the CPM can, thus, be used as a treatment map to actualize therapy goals.

Of equal importance is that the CPM is explained and shared with the patient to obtain initial feedback and ultimately establish a mutual agreement and consent regarding the treatments that will be used to work toward therapy goals. Additionally, the CPM can serve as a basis for dialogue and resolution of possible obstacles toward the attainment of those goals and the possible "side effects" that may be experienced. When sharing a case formulation, we have found that it serves as an important step in the therapeutic alliance. Through a discussion of the case formulation, a patient is provided with an empathic explanation offered by a clinician who has invested his or her knowledge into understanding the individual, learning his or her "story" and targeting help where it is likely to be most effective. Our collective clinical experience is that patients walk away form a case formulation feedback session with an understanding of their treatment and increased motivation. Particular considerations in sharing a case formulation with a patient might include reducing the elements of the CPM to those aspects that are most relevant to describing the recommended treatment, using words that represent everyday language, rather than scientific jargon, and asking for validation and feedback from the patient. For example, distal variables can be referred to as "how your background relates to your current problem areas," or mediators as "how you tend to react to stressful problems of this type," and even behavioral responses as "what you have learned to do when you experience these thoughts or feelings."

Although the scope of this chapter has been limited to the application of the problem-solving model to the process of cognitive and behavioral case formulation, the model can also be applied to treatment design (for a detailed description of this procedure, see Nezu et al., 2004).

What Are the Benefits of Case Formulation?

As we have explored throughout this chapter, case formulation can serve as a very useful tool for a clinician to assume a best practices approach in matching the extant evidence base from scientific studies and translate the use of these strategies to a given individual. Moreover, a case formulation can incorporate the unique characteristics each person brings to treatment, and it can encourage a clinician to engage in self-reflection, reduce errors of bias and clinical judgment, navigate treatment hurdles, and maintain a calm and present participation in the therapy relationship.

Just as case formulation serves as an important heuristic for experienced clinicians, it can function as a useful model for systematically teaching clinical trainees. It can aid trainees as an organizational tool for integrating their assessment and interview information, history taking, and understanding of interpersonal therapy behaviors. Lastly, a thorough CPM can lend itself to composing and reviewing progress notes, supervision review, and consultation management. A well-developed CPM provides a template for such notes that is clinically informed and prepared to consider therapeutic mechanisms of change.

References

Arkes, H. R. (1981). Impediments to accurate clinical judgment and possible ways to minimize their impact. *Journal of Consulting and Clinical Psychology, 49*(3), 323.

Arkes, H. R., Wortmann, R. L., Saville, P. D., & Harkness, A. R. (1981). Hindsight bias among physicians weighing the likelihood of diagnoses. *Journal of Applied Psychology, 66*(2), 252.

Barlow, D. H., Allen, L. B., & Choate, M. L. (2004). Toward a unified treatment for emotional disorders. *Behavior Therapy, 35*(2), 205–230.

Beck, A. T., Rush, A. J., Shaw, B. F., & Emery, G. (1979). *Cognitive therapy of depression.* New York: Guilford Press.

Dimidjian, S., Barrera, M. Jr., Martell, C., Muñoz, R. F., & Lewinsohn, P. M. (2011). The origins and current status of behavioral activation treatments for depression. *Annual Review of Clinical Psychology, 7*, 1–38.

D'Zurilla, T. J., & Nezu, A. M. (1982). Social problem solving in adults. *Advances in Cognitive-behavioral Research and Therapy, 1*(1), 201–274.

D'Zurilla, T. J., & Nezu, A. M. (1996). *Problem-solving therapy: A positive approach to clinical intervention* (3rd ed.). New York: Springer.

D'Zurilla, T. J., Nezu, A. M., & Maydeu-Olivares, A. (2004). Social problem solving: Theory and assessment. In E. C. Chang, T. J. D'Zurilla, & L. J. Sanna (Eds.), *Social problem solving: Theory, research, and training* (pp. 11–27). Washington, DC: American Psychological Association.

Eells, T. D. (Ed.). (2007). *Handbook of psychotherapy case formulation.* New York: Guilford Press.

Flitcroft, A., James, I. A., Freeston, M., & Wood-Mitchell, A. (2007). Determining what is important in a good formulation. *Behavioural and Cognitive Psychotherapy, 35*(03), 325–333.

Fouad, N. A., Grus, C. L., Hatcher, R. L., Kaslow, N. J., Hutchings, P. S., Madson, M. B., … Crossman, R. E. (2009). Competency benchmarks: A model for understanding and measuring competence in professional psychology across training levels. *Training and Education in Professional Psychology, 3*(4S), S5.

Hall, G. C. N. (2001). Psychotherapy research with ethnic minorities: Empirical, ethical, and conceptual issues. *Journal of Consulting and Clinical Psychology, 69*(3), 502.

Hayes, S. C. (2004). Acceptance and commitment therapy, relational frame theory, and the third wave of behavioral and cognitive therapies. *Behavior Therapy, 35*(4), 639–665.

Haynes, S. N., & O'Brien, W. H. (2000). *Principles and practice of behavioral assessment.* New York: Springer.

Hersen, M., Bellack, A. S., & Himmelhoch, J. M. (1980). Treatment of unipolar depression with social skills training. *Behavior Modification, 4*(4), 547–556.

Kendjelic, E. M., & Eells, T. D. (2007). Generic psychotherapy case formulation training improves formulation quality. *Psychotherapy: Theory, Research, Practice, Training, 44*(1), 66.

Kahneman, D. (2003). A perspective on judgment and choice: mapping bounded rationality. *American psychologist, 58*(9), 697.

Linehan, M. (1993). *Cognitive-behavioral treatment of borderline personality disorder.* New York: Guilford Press.

Manning, S. M., & DuBose, T. (2010). *DBT at a glance: An introduction to dialectical behavior therapy* [DVD]. Seattle, WA: Behavioral Tech, LLC.

Mash, E. J., & Hunsley, J. (1993). Assessment considerations in the identification of failing psychotherapy: Bringing the negatives out of the darkroom. *Psychological Assessment, 5*(3), 292.

Nezu, A. M. (2004). Problem solving and behavior therapy revisited. *Behavior Therapy, 35*, 1–33.

Nezu, A. M., & Nezu, C. M. (Eds.). (1989). *Clinical decision making in behavior therapy: A problem-solving perspective.* Champaign, IL: Research Press.

Nezu, A. M., Nezu, C. M., & Cos, T. A. (2007). Case formulation for the behavioral and cognitive therapies. In T. D. Eells (Ed.), *Handbook of Psychotherapy Case Formulation* (p. 349). New York: Guilford Press.

Nezu, A. M., Nezu, C. M., & D'Zurilla, T. (2013). *Problem-solving therapy: A treatment manual.* New York: Springer.

Nezu, A. M., Nezu, C. M., Friedman, S. H., & Haynes, S. N. (1997). Case formulation in behavior therapy: Problem-solving and functional analytic strategies. In T. D. Eells (Ed.), *Handbook of Psychotherapy Case Formulation* (pp. 368–401). New York: Guilford Press.

Nezu, A. M., Nezu, C. M., & Lombardo, E. R. (2001). Cognitive-behavior therapy for medically unexplained symptoms: A critical review of the treatment literature. *Behavior Therapy, 32*, 537–583.

Nezu, A. M., Nezu, C. M., & Lombardo, E. R. (2004). *Cognitive-behavioral case formulation and treatment design: A problem-solving approach.* New York: Springer.

Nezu, C. M., Martell, C., R., & Nezu, A. M. (2014). *Special competencies in cognitive and behavioral psychology.* New York: Oxford University Press.

Robins, C. J. (2003). Zen principles and mindfulness practice in dialectical behavior therapy. *Cognitive and Behavioral Practice, 9*(1), 50–57.

Rosen, A., & Proctor, E. K. (1981). Distinctions between treatment outcomes and their implications for treatment evaluation. *Journal of Consulting and Clinical Psychology, 49*(3), 418.

Schulte, D., & Eifert, G. H. (2002). What to do when manuals fail? The dual model of psychotherapy. *Clinical Psychology: Science and Practice, 9*(3), 312–328.

Shadish, W. R. (1993). Critical multiplism: A research strategy and its attendant tactics. In L. Sechrest (Ed.), *Program evaluation: A pluralistic enterprise* (pp. 13–57). San Francisco: Jossey-Bass.

Siegal, D. S. (2010). *The mindful therapist: A clinician's guide to mindsight and neural integration.* New York: W. W. Norton.

Tanaka-Matsumi, J., Seiden, D. Y., & Lam, K. N. (1996). The Culturally Informed Functional Assessment (CIFA) interview: A strategy for cross-cultural behavioral practice. *Cognitive and behavioral Practice, 3*(2), 215–233.

Tarrier, N., & Calam, R. (2002). New developments in cognitive-behavioural case formulation. Epidemiological, systemic and social context: An integrative approach. *Behavioural and Cognitive Psychotherapy, 30*, 311–328.

Tversky, A., & Kahneman, D. (1981). The framing of decisions and the psychology of choice. *Science, 211*(4481), 453–458.

Major Cognitive and Behavioral Therapy Approaches

Applied Behavior Analysis

Raymond G. Miltenberger, Bryon G. Miller, *and* Heather M. Zerger

Abstract

Applied behavior analysis (ABA) is the applied science and professional practice devoted to understanding and changing human behavior. The characteristics of applied behavior analysis include (a) a focus on socially important behavior; (b) demonstration of functional relationships between environmental events and behavior; (c) clear description of procedures; (d) connection to basic behavioral principles; and (e) production of meaningful, generalizable, and long-lasting changes in behavior. This chapter provides an overview of the field of ABA starting with issues in assessment and research design, followed by a review of basic behavioral principles that form the foundation of ABA procedures. Next, procedures to establish new behaviors are reviewed and the functional approach to assessing and changing problem behavior is described.

Key Words: applied behavior analysis, behavior, behavior analysis, functional assessment, functional interventions

Applied behavior analysis (ABA) is the applied science and professional practice devoted to understanding and changing human behavior (Miltenberger, 2016). In ABA, assessment procedures are used to record the target behavior and identify the factors that contribute to its occurrence, and intervention procedures are used to help people change their behavior. ABA procedures are based on basic principles of behavior discovered in experimental research with laboratory animals and humans over the past 80 years (e.g., Skinner, 1938; Ullmann & Krasner, 1965; Ulrich, Stachnik, & Mabry, 1966). The term *applied behavior analysis* was introduced by Baer, Wolf, and Risley in 1968 in the first issue of the *Journal of Applied Behavior Analysis*. Baer et al. (1968) identified a number of characteristics of ABA, including (a) a focus on socially important behavior; (b) demonstration of functional relationships between environmental events and behavior; (c) clear description of procedures; (d) connection to basic behavioral principles;

and (e) production of meaningful, generalizable, and long-lasting changes in behavior.

In ABA, there is an emphasis on observable behaviors, both behavioral excesses and behavioral deficits. Objective definition and measurement of behavior is a hallmark of ABA. Behavior change is accomplished by changing environmental events occurring at the time of the behavior; antecedents that evoke the behavior; and consequences that maintain the behavior. ABA is largely based on operant conditioning principles and to a lesser extent on respondent conditioning principles (Miltenberger, 2016). ABA has been successful in helping people of all ages and ability levels change a wide variety of socially significant behaviors in a wide variety of natural contexts (Cooper, Heron, & Heward, 2007; Fisher, Piazza, & Roane, 2011; Lerman, Iwata, & Hanley, 2013; Madden, 2013; Miltenberger, 2016).

This chapter provides an overview of the field of ABA, starting with issues in assessment and research design, and followed by a review of basic behavioral principles that form the foundation of ABA procedures. Next, procedures to establish new behaviors are reviewed and the functional approach to assessing and changing problem behavior is described.

Using Data in Applied Behavior Analysis

Observing, recording, and displaying data to evaluate treatment and make treatment decisions are important activities that help define ABA.

Observing and Recording Behavior

In ABA, emphasis is placed on objective measurement of behavior through direct observation procedures. A number of steps are involved in the process of recording behavior (Miltenberger, 2016; Miltenberger & Weil, 2013).

DEFINING THE BEHAVIOR

The first step in the process of recording behavior is to define the target behaviors in objective terms. Target behaviors are chosen based on their social importance (Baer et al., 1968; Wolf, 1978) and may include problematic behaviors to be decreased (behavioral excesses) and desirable behaviors to be increased (behavioral deficits). Target behaviors are defined using action verbs so that two independent observers could record their occurrence reliably.

LOGISTICS OF RECORDING

Once the target behaviors are defined, the next steps are to decide on the observer and the time and place of observation. The observer may be the person engaging in the behavior (self-monitoring) or a care provider (e.g., parent, teacher, staff member), therapist, or researcher. The observation period will be the time and place in which the behavior is most problematic or in which the behavior has the highest likelihood of occurrence.

RECORDING METHOD

The next step in the process of recording behavior is to decide on the use of continuous recording or a sampling procedure. With continuous recording, every instance of the behavior is recorded during the observation period. The four dimensions of behavior that can be measured include frequency (number of times the behavior occurred), duration (the time from onset to offset of the behavior), intensity (a measure of the force of the behavior), or latency (the time from some stimulus to the onset of the behavior). One or more dimensions are chosen for recording based on their relevance to the target behavior.

Sampling (discontinuous recording) procedures, including interval and momentary time sample recording, are not designed to record every instance of the behavior but rather to provide an estimate of the occurrence of the behavior (e.g., Devine, Rapp, Testa, Henrickson, & Schnerch, 2011; Meany-Daboul, Roscoe, Bouret, & Ahearn, 2007; Rapp, Colby-Dirksen, Michalski, Carroll, & Lindenberg, 2008). In interval recording, the observation period is divided into smaller consecutive intervals of time, and the behavior is recorded as occurring or not in each interval. Momentary time sample recording involves recording the occurrence of the behavior in brief intervals (e.g., 1–2 seconds) separated by longer intervals without observation. The outcome of interval or time sample recording is reported as the percentage of observation intervals in which the behavior occurred.

RECORDING INSTRUMENT

The final step is to choose a recording instrument. The most common recording instrument is a data sheet prepared for the particular client and target behaviors in question. The data sheet, designed to be convenient and easy to use, provides a space for recording each instance of the behavior as it is observed. Other recording instruments include the use of counters or timers, stop watches, smart phones or other handheld devices, laptop computers, and accelerometers or pedometers, to name a few. The recording instrument is designed to be practical, to minimize disruption of ongoing activities during behavior recording, and facilitate immediate recording of the behavior as it occurs.

Interobserver Agreement

Behavior recording procedures are designed to produce reliable information on the behavior. One index of reliability commonly used in ABA is interobserver agreement. Interobserver agreement is the degree to which two independent observers agree on the occurrence of the behavior during the same observation period. Interobserver agreement is a necessary component of research in ABA, although it is used less often in clinical applications of ABA. The reader is referred to Miltenberger (2016), Bailey and Burch (2002), Miltenberger and Weil (2013), or Cooper et al. (2007) for details on calculating interobserver agreement.

Indirect Measures

In ABA, emphasis is placed on direct observation of behavior. However, in some instances, indirect measures of behavior, including product measures and retrospective reports, are used. Product measures may be used when the target behavior produces permanent changes in the environment (products) that can be measured. Examples of product recording include number of assignments completed in an educational setting, number of units assembled in an employment setting, and number of hairs pulled by a person diagnosed with trichotillomania. Retrospective reports about the occurrence of behavior can be gathered through interviews or questionnaires. Retrospective reports of behavior are not used as the sole assessment method but are typically used during the initial phase of assessment to plan direct observation procedures (e.g., Hanley, 2011; Hanley, Jin, Vanselow, & Hanratty, 2014; Kelley, LaRue, Roane, & Gadaire, 2011).

Data Display and Research Design

In ABA the target behavior is recorded before, during, and after intervention is implemented. By recording before the intervention, a baseline level is established and the effects of the intervention can be assessed by looking at changes in the behavior. A graph is the tool used in ABA to identify changes in the behavior from baseline to intervention. In a graph, the level of the behavior is plotted on the vertical axis (y-axis) and time is plotted on the horizontal axis (x-axis) so that changes in behavior over time can be easily discerned.

In most clinical applications of ABA the target behavior is recorded and displayed on a graph in two phases, baseline and intervention. However, when research is conducted in ABA, more sophisticated research designs are used that demonstrate a functional relationship between environmental events (the intervention) and the target behavior. To demonstrate a functional relationship between intervention and the target behavior, the researcher must (a) reliably record the target behavior and show that it changes when (and only when) the intervention is implemented, and (b) provide a replication of the effect. In essence, the intervention is implemented two or more times and the behavior changes each time the intervention is implemented but only when the intervention is implemented.

A number of research designs are used in ABA to demonstrate a functional relationship. These include the reversal design; multiple baseline designs across behaviors, participants, or settings; alternating treatment design; and changing criterion design. See Iversen (2013), Miltenberger (2016), Bailey and Burch (2002), Kazdin (2011), or Cooper et al. (2007) for descriptions of these ABA research designs.

Basic Principles

ABA procedures are based on a core set of basic behavioral principles that describe functional relationships between specific types of environmental events and behavior. These basic behavioral principles include reinforcement, extinction, punishment, stimulus control, and respondent conditioning.

Reinforcement

Reinforcement is a fundamental principle that underlies many ABA procedures. First studied extensively by Skinner (1938) and Ferster and Skinner (1957), reinforcement is defined as the process in which the consequence of a behavior strengthens the future probability of the behavior. Understanding the principle of reinforcement is important for understanding the causes of behavior and for strengthening appropriate behavior. There are two forms of reinforcement: positive reinforcement, in which behavior is strengthened when it results in the delivery of a positive reinforcer; and negative reinforcement, in which behavior is strengthened when it results in escape from or avoidance of aversive stimuli. The consequences of the behavior involved in both positive and negative reinforcement may consist of changes in the physical environment or the behavior of others.

Reinforcement is influenced by a number of factors, including immediacy, contingency, motivating operations, individual differences, and magnitude (see Miltenberger, 2016 for discussion of these factors). One important factor that is increasingly utilized in ABA procedures is the motivating operation (e.g., Carbone, 2013; Miltenberger, 2016). A motivating operation (MO) is an antecedent event that alters the value of a reinforcer and influences the probability of a response that produces that reinforcer. Establishing operations (EO) and abolishing operations (AO) are two types of MOs. An EO makes a reinforcer more potent and evokes the behavior that produces that reinforcer, whereas an AO makes a reinforcer less potent and makes a behavior less likely to occur (Laraway, Snycerski, Michael, & Poling, 2003; Laraway, Snycerski, Olson, Becker, & Poling, 2014).

Extinction

Extinction occurs when the reinforcing consequence maintaining a behavior is no longer present following the behavior and, as a result, the behavior decreases and eventually stops occurring. For behavior maintained by positive reinforcement, extinction occurs when the positive reinforcer no longer follows the behavior. For behavior maintained by negative reinforcement, extinction occurs when escape or avoidance of the aversive stimulus no longer follows the behavior. In each case, when the behavior is no longer reinforced, it will stop occurring (Miltenberger, 2016; Thompson & Iwata, 2005).

One phenomenon frequently seen during extinction is an extinction burst (Lerman & Iwata, 1995). In an extinction burst, there is a temporary increase in one or more dimensions of the behavior or the occurrence of novel or emotional behaviors when the target behavior no longer produces the reinforcer. Although extinction temporarily increases response persistence and variability (e.g., Grow, Kelley, Roane, & Shillingsburg, 2008; MacDonald, Ahearn, Parry-Cruwys, Bancroft, & Dube, 2013), the target behavior will eventually stop occurring if the reinforcer continues to be withheld following the behavior. Understanding the extinction burst is important for the successful use of extinction in clinical practice.

Punishment

Punishment occurs when the consequence that follows a behavior decreases the future probability of the behavior. There are two variations of punishment: positive punishment and negative punishment. In positive punishment the behavior is followed by the addition of an aversive stimulus (also called a punisher), and in negative punishment, the behavior is followed by the removal of a positive reinforcer. In both cases, the behavior is weakened. As with reinforcement, punishment occurs naturally in our contact with the physical environment and in our interactions with others. Some ABA procedures are based on the principle of punishment (for example, time-out and response cost). The same factors that influence reinforcement influence punishment—immediacy, contingency, motivating operations, magnitude, and individual differences (Miltenberger, 2016). See Lerman and Vorndran (2002), Vollmer (2002), and Hanley, Piazza, Fisher, and Maglieri (2005) for discussion of punishment.

Stimulus Control

Although reinforcement, extinction, and punishment are the basic principles that determine whether a behavior will continue to occur, the effects of these operations are situation specific. Reinforcement strengthens behavior in situations that are similar to the ones in which the behavior was reinforced. Likewise, extinction and punishment weaken behavior in situations that are similar to the ones in which the behavior was subjected to extinction or punishment procedures. The increased probability that behavior will occur in specific situations (in the presence of specific stimuli) is referred to as stimulus control. A behavior is under the stimulus control of a specific stimulus when it is more likely to occur when that stimulus is present (Halle & Holt, 1991; Spradlin & Simon, 2011; Urcuioli, 2013).

Stimulus control is developed through stimulus discrimination training. In stimulus discrimination training (also called discrimination training), the behavior is reinforced in the presence of one stimulus (a discriminative stimulus or S^D) and is not reinforced in the presence of other stimuli. As a result, when the S^D is present in the future, the behavior is more likely to occur. The S^D has stimulus control over the behavior. The S^D will continue to have stimulus control over the behavior as long as the behavior continues to be reinforced in its presence.

Although discrimination training makes the behavior more likely to occur in the presence of the S^D, the behavior is also likely to occur in the presence of stimuli that are similar to the S^D. The more similar a stimulus is to the S^D, the more likely the behavior is to occur in its presence (Guttman & Kalish, 1956; Lalli, Mace, Livezey, & Kates, 1998; Miltenberger, 2016). The occurrence of behavior in the presence of stimuli that are similar to the S^D is called generalization.

Respondent Conditioning

Reinforcement, extinction, punishment, and stimulus control are all operant conditioning principles. In operant conditioning, behavior is controlled by its consequences (reinforcement strengthens behavior, and extinction or punishment weakens behavior). Although operant behavior comes under the stimulus control of antecedent stimuli (the S^D), stimulus control is developed through the differential consequences that are present when the S^D is present. Whereas operant behavior is controlled by its consequences, respondent behavior is controlled by antecedents. Respondent behavior is elicited by a prior stimulus: an unconditioned stimulus or a conditioned stimulus.

Respondent conditioning occurs when a neutral stimulus is paired with an unconditioned stimulus (US). The US elicits an unconditioned response

(UR) and, as a result of its pairing with the US, the neutral stimulus comes to elicit a response similar to the UR. The neutral stimulus is then called a conditioned stimulus and the response it elicits is called a conditioned response (Donahoe & Vegas, 2011; Lattal, 2013). Anxiety, anger, and inappropriate sexual arousal are examples of conditioned responses that may be targets of intervention in ABA procedures.

ABA procedures, the actual techniques used to help people change their behavior, are based on the basic principles described earlier. ABA procedures are used to establish new behaviors, to identify the variables contributing to the occurrence of problem behaviors, and to help people increase desirable behavior or decrease undesirable behaviors.

Procedures to Establish New Behaviors

When a desirable behavior is not currently in a person's repertoire, a number of procedures can be used to help the person acquire the behavior. These procedures include shaping, prompting and fading, chaining, and behavioral skills training procedures.

Shaping

Shaping is the differential reinforcement of successive approximations of a target behavior. Shaping is used to help an individual engage in a new behavior (e.g., a child saying a word for the first time), a new dimension of an existing behavior (e.g., a patient speaking with increasing voice volume), or a previously exhibited behavior that is no longer occurring (e.g., a stroke patient walking again) (e.g., Jackson & Wallace, 1974; Miltenberger, 2016; O'Neill & Gardner, 1983). To use shaping, the target behavior is defined and a starting behavior is chosen. The starting behavior (or first approximation, a behavior that already occurs at least occasionally) is reinforced a number of times until it occurs consistently. Then it is no longer reinforced (extinction) and the next approximation to the target behavior is reinforced instead. Once this behavior occurs a number of times, it is no longer reinforced and a closer approximation to the target behavior is reinforced. This process continues until the individual engages in the target behavior. Once the target behavior is exhibited, it is reinforced consistently to strengthen it and maintain its occurrence over time.

Shaping, a procedure that came from experimental research with laboratory animals (Skinner, 1938, 1951), has been used extensively in animal training (Pryor, 1985) and with humans to help individuals acquire a number of socially significant target behaviors in areas such as education, developmental disabilities, rehabilitation, and sports (Athens, Vollmer, & St. Peter Pipkin, 2007; Hagopian & Thompson, 1999; Hall, Maynes, & Reiss, 2009; Harrison & Pyles, 2013; Scott, Scott, & Goldwater, 1997). Shaping is used when more efficient behavioral acquisition strategies (e.g., prompting, instructions, modeling) are not possible or not effective.

Prompting and Fading

Prompting is used when a desired behavior is not currently occurring or not occurring in the correct circumstances (in the presence of the S^D). Prompting is a procedure in which an antecedent stimulus is delivered to evoke the behavior in the presence of the S^D so the behavior can be reinforced. Fading is the gradual elimination of the prompt once the behavior is occurring in the presence of the S^D. The prompt gets the correct behavior to occur at the right time, and fading eliminates the prompt to get the behavior under the stimulus control of the S^D.

Prompts can include the behavior of another person (response prompt) or a change in an antecedent stimulus (stimulus prompt). There are four types of response prompts: verbal, gestural, modeling, and physical. A verbal prompt involves the verbal behavior of another person. A gestural prompt involves a physical movement or gesture of another person. A modeling prompt involves a demonstration of the behavior. A physical prompt is when another person physically assists or guides a person to engage in the correct behavior. Physical prompting typically consists of hand-over-hand guidance.

When prompting is used to evoke the correct behavior, the trainer first presents the S^D and, if a response does not occur immediately, the trainer provides the prompt. When the prompted response occurs, the trainer provides a reinforcer. This sequence is referred to as a learning trial. Over a number of learning trials, the trainer gradually eliminates the prompt until the behavior occurs in the presence of the S^D without the prompt. This process is called fading. Once prompts are faded, the behavior is under the control of the S^D. See Noell, Call, and Adroin (2011); Cooper et al. (2007); Miltenberger (2016); and Mayer, Sulzer-Azaroff, and Wallace (2012) for more information on the use of prompting and fading.

Chaining

A chaining procedure is used to teach the learner to engage in a chain of behaviors. A behavioral chain (also called a stimulus-response chain) consists of a number of behaviors, each consisting of an S^D and a response, that occur together in a sequence. Each response in the chain creates the S^D for the next response in the chain (Miltenberger, 2016). For example, consider the behavior of getting a drink from a water fountain. There are at least three behaviors in the chain: pushing the handle for water, bending over the stream of water, and drinking the water. In this example, the water fountain is the S^D. The first response is turning on the water. This behavior creates the second S^D (the water stream). The second response is bending over the water stream. This behavior creates the third S^D (the water stream in proximity to or touching your mouth). The third response is drinking the water.

Before using a chaining procedure to teach a chain of behaviors, you must conduct a task analysis. A task analysis identifies every S^D and response in the chain of behaviors (e.g., Bellamy, Horner, & Inman, 1979; Williams & Cuvo, 1986). Careful observation of someone engaging in the chain of behaviors is used to develop the task analysis. Three procedures are used to teach a chain of behaviors: forward chaining, backward chaining, and total task presentation (Hur & Osborne, 1993; Jameson, Walker, Utley, & Maughan, 2012; Noell et al., 2011; Slocum & Tiger, 2011; Spooner, Weber, & Spooner, 1983).

FORWARD CHAINING

In forward chaining, you use prompting and fading to teach the first component in the chain. After the learner engages in the first response when the first S^D is presented without any prompts, prompting and fading are used to teach the first two components. At this time, the learner will engage in the first response when the first S^D is presented. When the first response creates the second S^D, the learner is prompted to engage in the second response. Once prompts are faded, the learner can now engage in the first two responses in the chain without prompts. Then prompting and fading are used to teach the first three components, and so on until all the component behaviors occur together.

BACKWARD CHAINING

In backward chaining, the last S^D is presented and prompting and fading are used to get the last response to occur. Once the last response is under the stimulus control of the last S^D, the next-to-last S^D is presented and the next-to-last response is

prompted. Once the next-to-last response occurs, it creates the last S^D and the learner will then engage in the last response. After the last two behaviors in the chain occur without prompts, the third-to-last S^D is presented, and prompting and fading are used until the last three responses occur without prompts. This process continues until the learner engages in the whole chain of behaviors without prompts.

TOTAL TASK PRESENTATION

In total task presentation, you present the first S^D and physically guide the learner through the entire chain of behaviors. Over trials, you fade the physical guidance to shadowing and then gradually eliminate shadowing until the physical prompt is eliminated. This fading method, in which physical prompting is faded to shadowing and eventually eliminated, is called graduated guidance. Total task presentation is typically used with more capable learners, while forward or backward chaining is used with learners with significant disabilities.

Behavioral Skills Training

Behavioral skills training (BST) is one final strategy for helping a learner acquire new skills. BST consists of instructions, modeling, rehearsal, and feedback (e.g., Himle & Miltenberger, 2004; Miltenberger, 2016). With instructions and modeling, the skills are described and demonstrated for the learner. Rehearsal is an opportunity for the learner to practice the skills in a simulation or role play. Finally, feedback consists of praise for correct performance of the skills and correction or further instruction when the skill is not performed correctly. BST is typically used for behaviors that can be demonstrated and practiced in a simulation or role-play format. Various skills have been taught with BST procedures, including social skills, parenting skills, job-related skills, child safety skills, and clinical interviewing skills, to name a few (e.g., Gunby & Rapp, 2014; Himle, Miltenberger, Flessner, & Gatheridge, 2004; Himle & Wright, 2014; Houvouras & Harvey, 2014; Johnson et al., 2005; Miltenberger, 2016; Miltenberger & Fuqua, 1985).

To conduct behavioral skills training, you first define the target behaviors and all of the situations in which the behaviors are to be performed. In teaching abduction prevention skills, for example, the target behavior consists of saying no, running away, and telling an adult when faced with an abduction lure. All of the different ways an adult might try to lure a child would then be identified and incorporated into training (e.g., offering the child candy or a toy to leave, asking for assistance, invoking authority). Once the target behaviors and S^Ds (situations) are identified, training begins with instructions and modeling. The trainer describes the behavior in detail and the situations in which the behavior is to be performed. The trainer then models the behavior in the context of a role play of one of the relevant situations.

After receiving instructions and modeling, the learner has the opportunity to rehearse the behavior. The trainer role-plays the same situation that was just modeled and the child practices the skill in response to the situation. For example, the trainer might tell a child to "pretend I am a stranger that walks up to you in your front yard and asks you to help me look for my puppy down the street. Show me what you would do if this happened." The trainer then role-plays the situation, delivers the lure, and observes the child's response. Immediately after the child rehearses the behavior, the trainer provides feedback. The trainer provides descriptive praise for any aspect of the behavior the child performed correctly and then tells the child how the behavior could be improved (if needed). The trainer then immediately conducts the same role play and provides the child the opportunity to rehearse the behavior again after receiving feedback. Once the child demonstrates the correct behavior in the role play, other situations are incorporated into role plays so that the full range of situations and responses is trained.

Functional Approach to Assessment and Intervention

A functional approach to assessment and intervention is used to help individuals decrease undesirable behaviors and increase desirable behaviors. The functional approach to assessment and intervention starts with a functional assessment to identify the antecedents and consequences influencing the behavior (e.g., Beavers, Iwata, & Lerman, 2013; Hanley, Iwata, & McCord, 2003; O'Neill et al., 1997). Functional interventions, designed to address the antecedents and consequences of the behavior, include extinction, differential reinforcement, and antecedent control procedures (Miltenberger, 2016). Changing the antecedents and consequences of the behavior and promoting functionally equivalent alternative behavior alter the conditions that influence the behavior, resulting in the greatest likelihood of lasting and generalized change in the behavior.

Functional Assessment

Functional assessment is a process of gathering information on the target behavior and the antecedents and consequences that are functionally related to the behavior (Lennox & Miltenberger, 1989). The outcome of a functional assessment is a hypothesis about the reinforcing consequences maintaining the behavior and the antecedents that evoke the behavior (O'Neill et al., 1997).

There are four categories of reinforcing consequences that could be maintaining a target behavior: social positive reinforcement (e.g., attention, tangible, or activity reinforcers provided by another person), automatic positive reinforcement (some form of stimulation or change in the environment arising directly from the behavior), social negative reinforcement (escape or avoidance of aversive activities or interactions mediated by another person), and automatic negative reinforcement (escape from aversive stimulation such as pain, discomfort, negative emotional responding, arising directly from the behavior) (Iwata, Vollmer, Zarcone, & Rodgers, 1993; Miltenberger, 2016). A functional assessment produces information that enables you to develop hypotheses about the type (or types) of reinforcement maintaining the problem behavior.

Antecedents that are identified in a functional assessment are the events, people, and circumstances reliably associated with the occurrence of the behavior. Antecedents can include S^Ds that occur immediately prior to the behavior and establishing operations (EO) whose onset may be proximal or more distal to the occurrence of the behavior. Identifying the S^D and EO associated with the behavior allows you to alter these antecedents to influence the problem behavior and promote alternative behaviors (Iwata, Smith, & Michael, 2000; McGill, 1999; Miltenberger, 2016; Smith & Iwata, 1997).

There are three methods for conducting a functional assessment: indirect assessment, direct assessment, and functional analysis.

INDIRECT ASSESSMENT

An indirect assessment involves interviews, questionnaires, or rating scales in which individuals who have frequent contact with the client (informants) provide information from their recall of antecedents and consequences associated with the behavior (Hanley, 2011; Hanley et al., 2014; Lennox & Miltenberger, 1989; O'Neill et al., 1997). O'Neill et al. (1997), for example, developed an interview format (the Functional Analysis Interview Format) that is structured to gather detailed functional assessment information. The advantages of an indirect functional assessment are that it is easy and convenient to administer and that it can provide information on a wide range of factors that might influence the target behavior. The limitation is that it does not involve direct observation of the behavior but instead relies on the informant's recall of events.

DIRECT OBSERVATION ASSESSMENT

A direct observation functional assessment (also called ABC recording) involves direct observation and recording of the behavior and its antecedents and consequences as they occur (Lennox & Miltenberger, 1989; O'Neill et al., 1997). Observations occur across a number of instances of the behavior until patterns in the antecedents and consequences are evident in the data. ABC recording can involve descriptive recording or the use of a checklist. In descriptive ABC recording, the observer writes down a description of antecedents, behavior, and consequences as they occur. To be of most value, the descriptions must be detailed and objective. In the checklist method, the observer has a checklist of possible target behaviors, antecedents, and consequences and places a checkmark in the appropriate column to designate the particular antecedents and consequences that were observed at the time of the behavior. The advantage of ABC recording is that the antecedents and consequences are observed as they occur, which results in objective (and likely more accurate) recording of the events. The limitation is that it takes more time to conduct multiple observations of the individual in the natural context (group home, school, etc.).

FUNCTIONAL ANALYSIS

A functional analysis involves direct observation of the target behavior as antecedents and consequences are systematically manipulated to identify their influence on the behavior (e.g., Beavers et al., 2013; Carr & Durand, 1985; Iwata, Dorsey, Slifer, Bauman, & Richman, 1982; Lydon, Healy, O'Reilly, & Lang, 2012; Mueller, Nkosi, & Hine, 2011; Wacker et al., 2013). For example, you could provide attention following each instance of the target behavior to see if the behavior increased, thus demonstrating that attention functioned as a reinforcer. Likewise, you could provide escape from demands contingent on the behavior or tangible reinforcers contingent on the behavior to see

whether these events functioned as reinforcers for the behavior.

A functional analysis might be used to test a hypothesis, in which case one reinforcer is manipulated, or a functional analysis might test a number of possible reinforcers. For example, to test the hypothesis that attention is reinforcing the target behavior, a functional analysis would alternate conditions in which attention is provided contingent on the behavior (test condition) and conditions in which attention is withheld contingent on the behavior (control condition). If attention is a reinforcer, the behavior will increase in the test condition relative to the control condition (e.g., Hanley, 2011; Hanley et al., 2014; Miltenberger, 2016). To test a number of reinforcers, you might alternate test conditions in which attention, escape, or tangible reinforcers are made contingent on the behavior and compare them to a control condition. An alone condition would also be used to see if the behavior persisted in the absence of social consequences (e.g., Iwata et al., 1982). The advantage of a functional analysis is that, because antecedents and consequences are manipulated and resulting changes in the target behavior are recorded, a functional relationship between the antecedents and consequences and the behavior is demonstrated. The limitation of a functional analysis is that it takes substantial time and expertise to conduct and requires temporarily reinforcing the undesirable behavior.

Once a functional assessment is conducted and firm hypotheses about the antecedents and consequences of the behavior have been developed, functional interventions (described later) are chosen based on the hypotheses. Functional interventions include extinction, differential reinforcement, and antecedent manipulations (Miltenberger, 2016).

Extinction

Extinction, as described earlier, is a basic principle of behavior. Extinction is also a behavioral procedure when it is used to help an individual stop engaging in an undesirable behavior (Iwata, Pace, Cowdery, & Miltenberger, 1994; Lerman & Iwata, 1996; Miltenberger, 2016). To use extinction, you must first conduct a functional assessment to identify the reinforcer maintaining the problem behavior. Once the reinforcer is identified, extinction involves eliminating the reinforcer after each instance of the behavior. If the behavior no longer gets reinforced, it will cease to occur. However, the successful use of extinction in clinical practice requires careful consideration of a number of questions (Miltenberger, 2016):

• Have you identified the reinforcer for the behavior? You cannot assume a particular reinforcer is maintaining a problem behavior; you must identify the reinforcer from a functional assessment. Sometimes multiple reinforcers are maintaining a problem behavior in different contexts.

• Can you eliminate the reinforcer? Eliminating the reinforcer can be a problem when the behavior is reinforced by other people and you do not have influence over those individuals or when the behavior is automatically reinforced.

• Is extinction safe to use? In some cases of aggressive or self-injurious behavior, if the parent or teacher no longer responds to the behavior, it might put individuals at risk for harm. Even though the adult's response to the behavior (i.e., attention) may be reinforcing the behavior, during extinction it may be necessary for the adult to respond to interrupt the behavior and assure the individual's safety. In such cases, the reinforcing consequence may be attenuated if it cannot be totally eliminated.

• Will individuals using extinction be able to deal effectively with an extinction burst? In most cases when extinction is used, the problem behavior temporarily worsens (increases in frequency, duration, or intensity) before it decreases. The parents, teachers, or others using extinction must be alerted to the probability of an extinction burst and be prepared to deal with it effectively. If they are not prepared, they might accidentally reinforce a more extreme problem behavior when it emerges during an extinction burst.

• Can consistency be maintained over time with all people? For extinction to be effective, it must be implemented each time the problem behavior occurs. If some instances of the behavior are reinforced at some times by some individuals, the behavior will likely persist and possibly worsen due to intermittent reinforcement.

When extinction is used clinically, it must be used with other functional interventions as well. Not only should the problem behavior result in extinction but differential reinforcement should be used to strengthen more desirable behavior. In addition, antecedent conditions should be altered to prevent the occurrence of the problem and evoke desired behaviors.

Differential Reinforcement

Differential reinforcement involves the use of reinforcement to increase desirable behavior and extinction to decrease the problem behavior (Hanley & Tiger, 2011). There are three variations of differential reinforcement: differential reinforcement of alternative behavior, differential reinforcement of other behavior, and differential reinforcement of low rates of behavior. In addition, differential reinforcement is utilized in token economies and behavioral contracts to promote desired behaviors (Miltenberger, 2016)

DIFFERENTIAL REINFORCEMENT OF ALTERNATIVE BEHAVIOR

In differential reinforcement of alternative behavior (DRA), reinforcement is provided for a desirable alternative behavior while extinction is used for the problem behavior. The goal of DRA is for the desirable behavior to increase in frequency and replace the problem behavior as it is decreased through extinction (e.g., Harper, Iwata, & Camp, 2013; Petscher, Rey, & Bailey, 2009; Travis & Sturmey, 2010). For DRA to be effective it is important to reinforce the desirable behavior each time it occurs while withholding reinforcement for every instance of the problem behavior. In addition, the reinforcer chosen for the desirable behavior should be a known reinforcer. When possible, it is best to reinforce the desirable behavior with the same reinforcer that was maintaining the problem behavior prior to the use of extinction. In this way, the desirable alternative behavior is functionally equivalent to the problem behavior because it produces the same outcome that previously reinforced the problem behavior (e.g., Carr, 1988).

DRA may involve positive reinforcement or negative reinforcement. In the case of positive reinforcement involving attention, attention no longer follows the problem behavior and instead is delivered following each occurrence of a desirable alternative behavior (Durand & Carr, 1991, 1992). In the case of negative reinforcement involving escape from aversive activities, escape is no longer contingent on the problem behavior and is delivered instead contingent on the occurrence of a desirable behavior (Allen & Stokes, 1987; Marcus & Vollmer, 1995). Steege et al. (1990) used DRA to decrease self-injurious behavior that was maintained by escape from grooming activities. In this case, a child with intellectual disabilities bit his wrist while an adult was brushing his teeth, and the biting was reinforced by the termination of tooth brushing. When DRA was used, wrist biting no longer resulted in termination of tooth brushing (extinction). Instead, the child was prompted to press a switch to activate a tape-recorded message asking for a break. When this alternative behavior occurred, it resulted in a break (termination of tooth brushing for a brief period of time). When pushing the button to activate the taped message was reinforced with escape but wrist biting was not, the child quit biting his wrist and engaged in the alternative behavior instead.

DIFFERENTIAL REINFORCEMENT OF OTHER BEHAVIOR

In differential reinforcement of other behavior (DRO), extinction is used for the problem behavior and reinforcement is delivered for the absence of the problem behavior (Miltenberger, 2016). If the problem behavior no longer produces a reinforcer and the reinforcer can only be acquired for the absence of the behavior, the behavior will decrease. Before using DRO you must first identify the reinforcer maintaining the problem behavior. Second, you identify the reinforcer to be delivered contingent on the absence of the problem behavior. In most cases, the reinforcer delivered for the absence of the problem behavior will be the reinforcer that was maintaining the problem. Third, you identify the interval for the delivery of the reinforcer. The interval will be based on the average time between occurrences of the problem behavior in baseline. For example, if a problem behavior occurs on average three times per minute, the average time between responses is 20 seconds and the DRO interval should be set at 20 seconds or less.

To use DRO, you provide the reinforcer after each interval in which the problem behavior does not occur. If the problem behavior occurs at any time, the reinforcer is withheld and the interval is reset. Again, the problem behavior must be absent for the entire interval for the reinforcer to be delivered. Once the problem behavior begins to decrease in frequency and the reinforcer is being delivered for its absence in the majority of intervals, the interval is gradually lengthened. As the interval is lengthened, the problem behavior must be absent for longer periods of time before the reinforcer is delivered. The goal when lengthening the DRO interval is to end up with an interval length that is practical for the parent or teacher. Although it will require the complete attention of the caregiver to deliver the reinforcer after every 20-second interval with the absence of the problem behavior, once the

interval is lengthened to a more manageable time (such as 30 minutes) the caregiver will be able to resume normal activities while implementing DRO (e.g., Cowdery, Iwata, & Pace, 1990; Iwata et al., 1994; Vollmer & Iwata, 1992; Watts, Wilder, Gregory, Leon, & Ditzian, 2013; Wilder, Chen, Atwell, Pritchard, & Weinstein, 2006).

DIFFERENTIAL REINFORCEMENT OF LOW RATES OF BEHAVIOR

In differential reinforcement of low rates of behavior (DRL), a reinforcer is delivered if a problem behavior happens fewer than a specified number of times in an observation period (e.g., Austin & Bevan, 2011; Jessel & Borrero, 2014). The goal is to provide a reinforcer for a lower rate of the behavior. Consider the case of a child with attention-deficit/hyperactivity disorder (ADHD) who gets up from the dinner table on average more than 10 times per meal. In a DRL procedure, the parent might arrange a contingency in which the child only gets dessert (a reinforcer) if she gets up from the table fewer than five times during the meal. Once the child is successful, the number of acceptable responses can be lowered to a more desired level. When using DRL, it is important to provide the child with a way to keep track of the number of responses that has occurred. In this case, the parent might bring to the table a chart with five boxes and place an X in a box each time the child gets up from the table. The child would have to have at least one blank box at the end of the meal to receive the reinforcer.

In another form of DRL, a reinforcer is delivered only if x amount of time has elapsed since the last response. In this form of DRL the timing of responses is important. As the interresponse time (IRT) increases, the response rate decreases (e.g., Anglesea, Hoch, & Taylor, 2008; Wright & Vollmer, 2002). An example of this form of DRL is from a study by Lennox, Miltenberger, and Donnelly (1987). The authors worked with adults with intellectual disabilities who engaged in rapid eating at meals. To decrease the rate of eating to make the individuals' eating more socially acceptable, the authors used a DRL procedure in which a bite of food was allowed in the mouth only if 15 seconds had elapsed since the last bite of food. If 15 seconds had not elapsed since the last bite, the authors blocked the participants from putting the bite in their mouth. In this way, the time between bites increased to more than 15 seconds (thus, eating rate decreased).

TOKEN ECONOMY

A token economy involves the systematic application of conditioned reinforcers called tokens to promote and maintain desirable behaviors (Ayllon & Azrin, 1968; Donaldson, Deleon, Fisher, & Kahng, 2014; Gilley & Ringdahl, 2014). In a token economy, tokens are delivered for desirable behaviors and later exchanged for backup reinforcers. Tokens maintain their effectiveness as conditioned reinforcers because they are paired with already established backup reinforcers. The following steps are involved in developing and implementing a token economy (Miltenberger, 2016).

- Identify and define the target behaviors you want to strengthen.
- Identify the objects that will be used as tokens. Tokens must be delivered to the client immediately following the desirable behavior. They can consist of anything that can be delivered and accumulated easily, such as poker chips, pennies, marbles, points, checkmarks, or hole punches in a card.
- Identify the backup reinforcers. It is important to choose items or activities that are known to be powerful reinforcers. Furthermore, it is best to have a variety of backup reinforcers available to help avoid satiation.
- Identify the number of tokens that will be delivered for each of the target behaviors. Typically more tokens are delivered for more difficult or more important behaviors.
- Identify the exchange rate for backup reinforcers. Determine how many tokens are exchanged for each backup reinforcer. Larger or more valued reinforcers will require more tokens.
- Identify a time and place for exchanging tokens for backup reinforcers. Clients will be receiving and accumulating tokens each day for engaging in desirable behavior. Unless a time and place is set for exchanging tokens, the clients may seek to purchase backup reinforcers numerous times daily, thus disrupting ongoing activities.

For a token economy to be effective, staff must be trained and supervised to carry out the program successfully. Furthermore, it is important to develop the token economy in such a way that (a) the tokens cannot be acquired in any way other than by engaging in the target behaviors and (b) the backup reinforcers cannot be acquired in any way other than with tokens. If tokens or backup reinforcers are freely available, individuals will not work to earn them.

BEHAVIORAL CONTRACT

A behavioral contract is a written agreement specifying a desired behavior and a reinforcing consequence for the behavior (e.g., Dallery, Meredith, & Glenn, 2008; Glenn & Dallery, 2007; O'Banion & Whaley, 1981). By writing a behavioral contract, a person is making a commitment to engage in the behavior in a specified time frame and arranging a consequence as a reinforcer for the behavior. Typically, a contract manager implements the contract with the person seeking behavior change. It is the contract manager's job to verify the occurrence of the behavior and carry out the consequence specified in the contract. For example, a student might agree to a behavioral contract with a school counselor in which the student commits to being on time for school each day for a week. When agreeing to the contract, the student gives the counselor five checks for $10 each. Each day the student gets to school on time (as verified by the teacher), she gets one of the checks back. If she is late, the check for that day is sent to charity. Knowing that she will avoid the loss of $10 by arriving on time helps motivate the student to engage in the behavior.

The essential components of a behavioral contract include (a) a clear description of the target behavior, (b) the time frame in which the target behavior should occur, (c) how the target behavior will be measured, (d) the consequence for engaging in the target behavior, and (e) signatures of the individual seeking behavior change and the contract manager (Miltenberger, 2016).

Antecedent Control

Antecedent control procedures involve the manipulation of S^Ds, EOs, or response effort to make the occurrence of a problem behavior less likely or evoke the occurrence of desirable behaviors (Miltenberger, 2016).

To use antecedent control to increase desirable behavior, you can present the S^D or an EO for the behavior or decrease response effort for the behavior. Presenting an S^D for a behavior makes the behavior more likely to occur because the behavior has been reinforced in the presence of the S^D. An example might be to send a student to a quiet room with textbooks on a desk to increase the likelihood of studying. Presenting an EO makes a behavior more probable because it increases the reinforcing value of the outcome of the behavior (Vollmer & Iwata, 1991). In the case of a training program with a child with autism in which small edible reinforcers are used (bits of favorite cereal), the trainer can run the training program just before meals when the child has not eaten in a few hours as a way to make the edible reinforcers more potent. The trainer can also make sure the child does not have access to the favorite cereal outside of the training session as a way to make the cereal more reinforcing. Decreasing response effort for a behavior makes the behavior more probable than a functionally equivalent alternative behavior that requires more effort (e.g., Horner & Day, 1991; Piazza, Roane, Keeney, Boney, & Abt, 2002). When a child with tantrum behavior maintained by attention is taught how to ask for attention, the child is more likely to ask for attention if asking takes less effort than engaging in the tantrum behavior and produces an equal amount of attention.

To use antecedent control to decrease a problem behavior, you can remove an S^D or EO for the behavior or increase response effort for the behavior. A behavior is less likely to occur in the absence of the S^D. If watching television and playing computer games interfere with doing homework, turning off the television and computer removes the S^Ds for these competing behaviors to make them less likely (and make doing homework more likely). If the EO for a particular reinforcer is removed, the reinforcer is no longer potent and the behavior producing that reinforcer will be less likely. In the case of the child whose tantrums are reinforced by parental attention, frequent noncontingent attention from the parent will make the tantrums less likely because the reinforcing value of parental attention for problem behavior is decreased through satiation (e.g., Vollmer, Iwata, Zarcone, Smith, & Mazaleski, 1993). Noncontingent reinforcement can make behavior maintained by various forms of reinforcement (attention, escape, tangibles) less likely by altering the EO through satiation (Wilder & Carr, 1998). Increasing response effort for a problem behavior makes the behavior less likely because the individual will be more likely to engage in a less effortful, functionally equivalent alternative behavior. For example, when a student with multiple disabilities in a special education classroom slapped students near him, the behavior was reinforced by teacher attention (the teacher came over to him, expressed concern, and explained why the behavior was inappropriate). In this case, the student was moved to a location in the classroom where other children were not within arm's reach. Because it now required more effort to slap another student, the student was more likely to engage in alternative behavior (e.g., raising his hand) for teacher attention.

To use antecedent control procedures successfully, you must identify relevant antecedents through a functional assessment and alter the antecedents that are functionally related to the target behaviors. Numerous studies have demonstrated the effectiveness of antecedent control procedures for problem behaviors maintained by positive reinforcement and negative reinforcement (e.g., Luiselli, 2006; Miltenberger, 2016).

Punishment

In ABA, problem behaviors are addressed first through a functional approach to assessment and intervention. After conducting a functional assessment, extinction, differential reinforcement, and antecedent control procedures are utilized, often with success. In cases where problem behaviors are not successfully treated with these functional interventions, punishment may be considered (Iwata, 1988; Miltenberger, 2016). The most commonly used punishment procedures are based on the principle of negative punishment and include time-out and response cost. Although positive punishment procedures involving the delivery of aversive stimulation have been used in the past, such procedures are rarely, if ever, used in contemporary ABA.

TIME-OUT

Time-out from positive reinforcement ("time-out" for short) is a procedure in which, contingent on a problem behavior, a child is removed from a reinforcing environment for a brief period of time. Time-out is a negative punishment procedure because the child is removed from all sources of positive reinforcement contingent on the problem behavior and the behavior decreases. The child is typically escorted to a nearby room or area devoid of access to any reinforcers. Time-out has been shown to be a successful intervention for a range of childhood problem behaviors (e.g., Donaldson & Vollmer, 2012; Donaldson, Vollmer, Yakich, & Van Camp, 2013; Mathews, Friman, Barone, Ross, & Christophersen, 1987; Porterfield, Herbert-Jackson, & Risley, 1976; Rortvedt & Miltenberger, 1994).

For time-out to be effective, a number of factors must be considered (Miltenberger, 2016):

• The environment from which the child is removed (the time-in environment) must be reinforcing (must contain positively reinforcing activities, interactions, and/or stimuli). If the time-in environment is not reinforcing, time-out will not function as negative punishment.

• Time-out must be initiated immediately contingent on the problem behavior.

• Time-out must be brief (a few minutes in duration) to provide minimal disruption of ongoing educational or other important activities.

• Attention or other reinforcers must not be available in the time-out area. If the time-out room or area is reinforcing, time-out will not be effective.

• The child should not get any attention while being taken to time-out. Contingent on the problem behavior, the parent should simply state that the child has to go to time-out for the behavior and proceed to escort the child to time-out without any further discussion.

• The child should not escape from time-out until released by the parent when time-out is over.

• The time-out room or area must be safe.

RESPONSE COST

Response cost is a procedure in which, contingent on the occurrence of the problem behavior, a specified amount of a reinforcer is removed to decrease the behavior. Losing the opportunity to have dessert contingent on problem behavior at supper, or loss of a portion of a child's allowance contingent on the occurrence of a problem behavior are examples of response cost that might be used by parents. In each case, the response-contingent loss of the reinforcer makes the problem behavior less likely in the future. Response cost procedures are used frequently by governments and other organizations (e.g., speeding tickets, fines for parking in handicapped parking spaces, fees for bounced checks, fees for late payments from credit card companies). Response cost is sometimes used in a token economy and involves the loss of tokens contingent on the occurrence of problem behavior. Likewise, response cost is sometimes used in a behavioral contract to decrease a problem behavior and involves the loss of a reinforcer (e.g., a $50 deposit) contingent on the behavior (Miltenberger, 2016). Response cost procedures are used effectively for a variety of child behavior problems as well. For example, response cost has been used to decrease noncompliance to parental requests (Little & Kelley, 1989), thumb sucking (Long, Miltenberger, & Rapp, 1999), hyperactive and disruptive behavior in children (McGoey & DuPaul, 2000; Rapport, Murphy, & Bailey, 1982), and stereotypy exhibited by children with autism (Watkins & Rapp, 2014), to name a few examples.

For response cost to be effective, the loss of the reinforcer (or a statement that the reinforcer will be lost) should occur immediately contingent on each instance of the problem behavior. The magnitude of the reinforcer loss should be sufficient to function as a punisher. Finally, ethical issues must be considered such that the loss of the reinforcer does not harm the child in any way or violate the child's rights (e.g., loss of meals, for example, is not an acceptable form of response cost).

Promoting Generalization

In ABA, generalization is defined as the occurrence of target behavior outside of the treatment or training setting in the natural environment. For example, if a child learns social skills in treatment sessions with the school psychologist, generalization occurs when the social skills are used with peers at school or in other natural settings. A number of strategies can be used to promote generalization (e.g., Miltenberger, 2016; Stokes & Baer, 1977; Stokes & Osnes, 1989).

• Provide reinforcement for the target behavior when it occurs in the natural environment. In the social skills example, the school psychologist could provide praise whenever she observes the child engaging in good social skills with peers.

• Teach skills that will contact natural contingencies of reinforcement. The child should be taught the kind of social skills likely to generate a reinforcing response from peers.

• Modify natural contingencies of reinforcement. The psychologist might have the student's teachers provide praise for the student's appropriate use of social skills.

• Incorporate a variety of relevant stimulus situations in training so that the child has practiced and received reinforcement for engaging in the correct behavior in a wide range of situations he might to encounter in the natural environment.

• Incorporate stimuli from the natural environment into the training situation (common stimuli). An example would be to have some same-age peers in the social skills training sessions so the student practices with the kinds of peers she is likely to encounter in school.

• Teach a variety of responses that may all achieve the same outcome for the client. Different responses that achieve the same outcome are called functionally equivalent responses.

• Provide cues or reminders in the natural environment that can make the target behavior more likely to occur in the correct circumstances. This might involve the teacher reminding or prompting the student to use the social skills when appropriate situations arise.

• Teach self-generated mediators of generalization. This strategy might include teaching the student some simple self-instructions that he could use in social situations to cue himself to use the social skills that he had learned.

Another form of generalization occurs when a problem behavior that decreased in treatment sessions also decreases in the natural environment. To promote a generalized reduction in problem behavior, it is important to reinforce a functionally equivalent alternative behavior so that the desirable behavior takes the place of the problem and produces the same type and amount of reinforcement that the problem behavior did before treatment (Carr, 1988). It is also important to maintain extinction or punishment contingencies across situations and over time in case the problem behavior occurs again for some reason (e.g., spontaneous recovery).

Summary

ABA emphasizes objective measurement of behavior before and after intervention to document the effects of the intervention. Intervention involves the application of behavioral principles to help people change socially significant behaviors. ABA procedures are aimed at changing aspects of the physical or social environment to bring about changes in behavior. ABA procedures are used to help people develop new behaviors (to overcome behavior deficits) and to help people stop engaging in undesirable behavior (to decrease behavioral excesses).

When using ABA procedures to help people address behavior problems, a functional approach to assessment and intervention is utilized. A functional assessment is conducted first to identify the variables contributing to the problem behavior. Interventions are then developed based on the results of the functional assessment information. Interventions seek to alter the antecedents and consequences that contribute to the problem behavior while promoting functionally equivalent alternative behavior to replace the problem behavior. ABA procedures are successful when they produce desired behavior changes that generalize to client's everyday environment and maintain over time.

References

Allen, K. D., & Stokes, T. F. (1987). Use of escape and reward in the management of young children during dental treatment. *Journal of Applied Behavior Analysis, 20,* 381–390.

Anglesea, M. M., Hoch, H., & Taylor, B. A. (2008). Reducing rapid eating in teenagers with autism: Use of a pager prompt. *Journal of Applied Behavior Analysis, 41,* 107–111.

Athens, E. S., Vollmer, T. R., & St. Peter Pipkin, C. C. (2007). Shaping academic task engagement with percentile schedules. *Journal of Applied Behavior Analysis, 40,* 475–488.

Austin, J. L., & Bevan, D. (2011). Using differential reinforcement of low rates to reduce children's requests for teacher attention. *Journal of Applied Behavior Analysis, 44,* 451–461.

Ayllon, T., & Azrin, N. (1968). *The token economy: A motivational system for therapy and rehabilitation.* New York : Appleton-Century-Crofts.

Baer, D. M., Wolf, M. M., & Risley, T. R. (1968). Some current dimensions of applied behavior analysis. *Journal of Applied Behavior Analysis, 1,* 91–97.

Bailey, J. S., & Burch, M. R. (2002). *Research methods in applied behavior analysis.* Thousand Oaks, CA: Sage.

Beavers, G. A., Iwata, B. A., & Lerman, D. C. (2013). Thirty years of research on the functional analysis of problem behavior. *Journal of Applied Behavior Analysis, 46,* 1–21.

Bellamy, G. T., Horner, R. H., & Inman, D. P. (1979). *Vocational habilitation of severely retarded adults.* Austin, TX: Pro-Ed.

Carbone, V. J. (2013). The establishing operation and teaching verbal behavior. *The Analysis of Verbal Behavior, 29,* 45–49.

Carr, E. G. (1988). Functional equivalence as a means of response generalization. In R. H. Horner, G. Dunlap, & R. L. Koegel (Eds.), *Generalization and maintenance: Lifestyle changes in applied settings* (pp. 221–241). Baltimore: Paul Brookes.

Carr, E. G., & Durand, V. M. (1985). Reducing behavior problems through functional communication training. *Journal of Applied Behavior Analysis, 18,* 111–126.

Cooper, J., Heron, T., & Heward, W. (2007). *Applied behavior analysis.* Upper Saddle River, NJ: Prentice Hall.

Cowdery, G. E., Iwata, B. A., & Pace, G. M. (1990). Effects and side-effects of DRO as treatment for self-injurious behavior. *Journal of Applied Behavior Analysis, 23,* 497–506.

Dallery, J., Meredith, S., & Glenn, I. M. (2008). A deposit contract method to deliver abstinence reinforcement for cigarette smoking. *Journal of Applied Behavior Analysis, 41,* 609–615.

Devine, S. L., Rapp, J. T., Testa, J. R., Henrickson, M. L., & Schnerch, G. (2011). Detecting changes in simulated events using partial-interval recording and momentary time sampling III: Evaluating sensitivity as a function of session length. *Behavioral Interventions, 26,* 103–124.

Donahoe, J. W., & Vegas, R. (2011). Respondent (Pavlovian) conditioning. In W. Fisher, C. Piazza, & H. Roane (Eds.), *Handbook of applied behavior analysis* (pp. 17–33). New York: Gilford Press.

Donaldson, J. M., DeLeon, I. G., Fisher, A. B., & Kahng, S. (2014). Effects of and preference for conditions of token earn versus token loss. *Journal of Applied Behavior Analysis, 47,* 537–548.

Donaldson, J. M., & Vollmer, T. R. (2012). A procedure for thinning the schedule of time-out. *Journal of Applied Behavior Analysis, 45,* 625–630.

Donaldson, J. M., Vollmer, T. R, Yakich, T. M., & Van Camp, C. (2013). Effects of reduced time-out interval on compliance with the time-out instruction. *Journal of Applied Behavior Analysis, 46,* 369–378.

Durand, V. M., & Carr, E. G. (1991). Functional communication training to reduce challenging behavior: Maintenance and application in new settings. *Journal of Applied Behavior Analysis, 24,* 251–264.

Durand, V. M., & Carr, E. G. (1992). An analysis of maintenance following functional communication training. *Journal of Applied Behavior Analysis, 25,* 777–794.

Ferster, C. B., & Skinner, B. F. (1957). *Schedules of reinforcement.* Upper Saddle River, NJ: Prentice Hall.

Fisher, W. W., Piazza, C. C., & Roane, H. S. (Eds.). (2011). *Handbook of applied behavior analysis.* New York: Gilford Press.

Gilley, C., & Ringdahl, J. E. (2014). The effects of item preference and token reinforcement on sharing behavior exhibited by children with autism spectrum disorder. *Research in Autism Spectrum Disorders, 8,* 1425–1433.

Glenn, I. M., & Dallery, J. (2007). Effects of Internet-based voucher reinforcement and a transdermal nicotine patch on cigarette smoking. *Journal of Applied Behavior Analysis, 40,* 1–13.

Grow, L. L., Kelley, M. E., Roane, H. S., & Shillingsburg, M. A. (2008). Utility of extinction-induced response variability for the selection of mands. *Journal of Applied Behavior Analysis, 41,* 15–24.

Gunby, K. V., & Rapp, J. T. (2014). The use of behavioral skills training and in situ feedback to protect children with autism from abduction lures. *Journal of Applied Behavior Analysis, 47,* 856–860.

Guttman, N., & Kalish, H. I. (1956). Discriminability and stimulus generalization. *Journal of Experimental Psychology, 51,* 79–88.

Hagopian, L. P., & Thompson, R. H. (1999). Reinforcement of compliance with respiratory treatment in a child with cystic fibrosis. *Journal of Applied Behavior Analysis, 32,* 233–236.

Hall, S. S., Maynes, N. P., & Reiss, A. L. (2009). Using percentile schedules to increase eye contact in children with fragile x syndrome. *Journal of Applied Behavior Analysis, 42,* 171–176.

Halle, J. W., & Holt, B. (1991). Assessing stimulus control in natural settings: An analysis of stimuli that acquire control during training. *Journal of Applied Behavior Analysis, 24,* 579–589.

Hanley, G. (2011). Functional analysis. In J. Luiselli (Ed.), *Teaching and behavior support for children and adults with autism spectrum disorder: A "how to" practitioner's guide* (pp. 22–29). New York: Oxford University Press.

Hanley, G. P., Iwata, B. P., & McCord, B. E. (2003). Functional analysis of problem behavior: A review. *Journal of Applied Behavior Analysis, 36,* 147–185.

Hanley, G., Jin, C., Vanselow, N., & Hanratty, L. (2014). Producing meaningful improvements in problem behavior of children with autism via synthesized analyses and treatments. *Journal of Applied Behavior Analysis, 47,* 16–36.

Hanley, G. P., Piazza, C. C., Fisher, W. W., & Maglieri, K. A. (2005). On the effectiveness of and preference for punishment and extinction components of function-based interventions. *Journal of Applied Behavior Analysis, 38,* 51–65.

Hanley, G. P., & Tiger, J. H. (2011). Differential reinforcement procedures. In W. Fisher, C. Piazza, & H. Roane (Eds.), *Handbook of applied behavior analysis* (pp. 229–249). New York: Guilford Press.

Harper, J. M., Iwata, B. A., & Camp, E. M. (2013). Assessment and treatment of social avoidance. *Journal of Applied Behavior Analysis, 46,* 147–160.

Harrison, A. M., & Pyles, D. A. (2013). The effects of verbal instruction and shaping to improve tackling by high school football players. *Journal of Applied Behavior Analysis, 46,* 518–522.

Himle, M. B., & Miltenberger, R. G. (2004). Preventing unintentional firearm injury in children: The need for behavioral skills training. *Education and Treatment of Children, 27,* 161–177.

Himle, M. B., Miltenberger, R. G., Flessner, C., & Gatheridge, B. (2004). Teaching safety skills to children to prevent gun play. *Journal of Applied Behavior Analysis, 37,* 1–9.

Himle, M. B., & Wright, K. A. (2014). Behavioral skills training to improve installation and use of child passenger safety restraints. *Journal of Applied Behavior Analysis, 47,* 549–559.

Horner, R. H., & Day, H. M. (1991). The effects of response efficiency on functionally equivalent competing behaviors. *Journal of Applied Behavior Analysis, 24,* 719–732.

Houvouras, A. J., IV, & Harvey, M. T. (2014). Establishing fire safety skills using behavioral skills training. *Journal of Applied Behavior Analysis, 47,* 420–424.

Hur, J., & Osborne, S. (1993). A comparison of forward and backward chaining methods used in teaching corsage making skills to mentally retarded adults. *British Journal of Developmental Disabilities, 77,* 108–117.

Iversen, I. H. (2013). Single-case research methods: An overview. In G. J. Madden (Ed.), *APA handbook of behavior analysis: Methods and principles* (pp. 3–32). Washington, DC: American Psychological Association.

Iwata, B. A. (1988). The development and adoption of controversial default technologies. *The Behavior Analyst, 11,* 149–157.

Iwata, B. A., Dorsey, M. F., Slifer, K. J., Bauman, K. E., & Richman, G. S. (1982). Toward a functional analysis of self-injury. *Analysis and Intervention in Developmental Disabilities, 2,* 3–20.

Iwata, B. A., Pace, G. M., Cowdery, G. E., & Miltenberger, R. G. (1994). What makes extinction work: Analysis of procedural form and function. *Journal of Applied Behavior Analysis, 27,* 131–144.

Iwata, B. A., Smith, R. G., & Michael, J. (2000). Current research on the influence of establishing operations on behavior in applied settings. *Journal of Applied Behavior Analysis, 33,* 411–418.

Iwata, B. A., Vollmer, T. R., Zarcone, J. R., & Rodgers, T. A. (1993). Treatment classification and selection based on behavioral function. In R. Van Houten & S. Axelrod (Eds.), *Behavior analysis and treatment* (pp. 101–125). New York: Plenum.

Jackson, D. A., & Wallace, R. F. (1974). The modification and generalization of voice loudness in a fifteen year old retarded girl. *Journal of Applied Behavior Analysis, 7,* 461–471.

Jameson, J. M., Walker, R., Utley, K., & Maughan, R. (2012). A comparison of embedded total task instruction in teaching behavioral chains to massed one-on-one instruction for students with intellectual disabilities: Accessing general education settings and core academic content. *Behavior Modification, 36,* 320–340.

Jessel, J., & Borrero, J. C. (2014). A laboratory comparison of two variations of differential-reinforcement-of-low-rate procedures. *Journal of Applied Behavior Analysis, 47,* 314–324.

Johnson, B. M., Miltenberger, R. G., Egemo-Helm, K., Jostad, C. M., Flessner, C., & Gatheridge, B. (2005). Evaluation of behavioral skills training for teaching abduction prevention skills to young children. *Journal of Applied Behavior Analysis*, 38, 67–78.

Kazdin, A. E. (2011). *Single-case research designs: Methods for clinical and applied settings*. New York: Oxford University Press.

Kelley, M. E., LaRue, R. H., Roane, H. S., & Gadaire, D. (2011). Indirect behavioral assessments: Interviews and rating scales. In W. Fisher, C. Piazza, & H. Roane (Eds.), *Handbook of applied behavior analysis* (pp. 182–190). New York: Guilford Press.

Lalli, J. S., Mace, F. C., Livezey, K., & Kates, K. (1998). Assessment of stimulus generalization gradients in the treatment of self-injurious behavior. *Journal of Applied Behavior Analysis*, 31, 479–483.

Laraway, S., Snycerski, S., Michael, J., & Poling, A. (2003). Motivating operations and terms to describe them: Some future refinements. *Journal of Applied Behavior Analysis*, 36, 407–414.

Laraway, S., Snycerski, S., Olson, R., Becker, B., & Poling, A. (2014). The motivating operations concept: Current status and critical response. *The Psychological Record*, 3, 601–623.

Lattal, K. M. (2013). Pavlovian conditioning. In G. J. Madden (Ed.), *APA handbook of behavior analysis: Methods and principles* (pp. 283–306). Washington, DC: American Psychological Association.

Lennox, D. B., & Miltenberger, R. G. (1989). Conducting a functional assessment of problem behavior in applied settings. *Journal of the Association for Persons with Severe Handicaps*, 14, 304–311.

Lennox, D. B., Miltenberger, R. G., & Donnelly, D. (1987). Response interruption and DRL for the reduction of rapid eating. *Journal of Applied Behavior Analysis*, 20, 279–284.

Lerman, D. C., & Iwata, B. A. (1995). Prevalence of the extinction burst and its attenuation during treatment. *Journal of Applied Behavior Analysis*, 28, 93–94.

Lerman, D. C., & Iwata, B. A. (1996). Developing a technology for the use of operant extinction in clinical settings: An examination of basic and applied research. *Journal of Applied Behavior Analysis*, 29, 345–382.

Lerman, D. C., Iwata, B. A., & Hanley, G. P. (2013). Applied behavior analysis. In G. J. Madden (Ed.), *APA handbook of behavior analysis: Methods and principles* (pp. 81–104). Washington, DC: American Psychological Association.

Lerman, D. C. & Vorndran, C. M. (2002). On the status of knowledge for using punishment: Implications for treating behavior disorders. *Journal of Applied Behavior Analysis*, 35, 431–464.

Little, L. M., & Kelley, M. L. (1989). The efficacy of response cost procedures for reducing children's noncompliance to parental instructions. *Behavior Therapy*, 20, 525–534.

Long, E., Miltenberger, R., & Rapp, J. (1999). Simplified habit reversal plus adjunct contingencies in the treatment of thumb sucking and hair pulling in a young girl. *Child and Family Behavior Therapy*, 21(4), 45–58.

Luiselli, J. (Ed.). (2006). *Antecedent assessment and intervention: Supporting children and adults with developmental disabilities in community settings*. Baltimore: Brookes.

Lydon, S., Healy, O., O'Reilly, M. F., & Lang, R. (2012). Variations in functional analysis methodology: A systematic review. *Journal of Developmental and Physical Disabilities*, 24, 301–326.

MacDonald, J. M., Ahearn, W. H., Parry-Cruwys, D., Bancroft, S., & Dube, W. V. (2013). Persistence during extinction: Examining the effects of continuous and intermittent reinforcement on problem behavior. *Journal of Applied Behavior Analysis*, 46, 333–338.

Madden, G. J. (Ed.). (2013). *APA handbook of behavior analysis: Methods and principles*. Washington, DC: American Psychological Association.

Marcus, B. A., & Vollmer, T. R. (1995). Effects of differential negative reinforcement on disruption and compliance. *Journal of Applied Behavior Analysis*, 28, 229–230.

Mathews, J. R., Friman, P. C., Barone, V. J., Ross, L. V., & Christophersen, E. R. (1987). Decreasing dangerous infant behavior through parent instruction. *Journal of Applied Behavior Analysis*, 20, 165–169.

Mayer, R. G., Sulzer-Azaroff, B., & Wallace, M. (2012). *Behavior analysis for lasting change*. Cornwall-on-Hudson, NY: Sloan Educational Publishing.

McGill, P. (1999). Establishing operations: implications for the assessment, treatment, and prevention of problem behavior. *Journal of Applied Behavior Analysis*, 32, 393–418.

McGoey, K. A., & DuPaul, G. J. (2000). Token reinforcement and response cost procedures: Reducing the disruptive behavior of preschool children with attention-deficit/hyperactivity disorder. *School Psychology Quarterly*, 15, 330–343.

Meany-Daboul, M. G., Roscoe, E. M., Bourret, J. C., & Ahearn, W. H. (2007). A comparison of momentary time sampling and partial-interval recording for evaluating functional relations. *Journal of Applied Behavior Analysis*, 40, 501–514.

Miltenberger, R. G. (2016). *Applied behavior analysis: Principles and procedures* (6th ed.). Boston: Cengage Learning.

Miltenberger, R. G., & Fuqua, R. W. (1985). Evaluation of a training manual for the acquisition of behavioral assessment interviewing skills. *Journal of Applied Behavior Analysis*, 18, 323–328.

Miltenberger, R. G., & Weil, T. M. (2013). Observation and measurement in behavior analysis. In G. J. Madden (Ed.), *APA handbook of behavior analysis: methods and principles* (pp. 81–104). Washington, DC: American Psychological Association.

Mueller, M. M., Nkosi, A., & Hine, J. F. (2011). Functional analysis in public schools: A summary of 90 functional analyses. *Journal of Applied Behavior Analysis*, 44, 807–818.

Noell, G. H., Call, N. A., & Adroin, S. P. (2011). Building complex repertoires from discrete behaviors by establishing stimulus control, behavioral chains, and strategic behavior. In W. Fisher, C. Piazza, & H. Roane (Eds.), *Handbook of applied behavior analysis* (pp. 250–269). New York: Guilford Press.

O'Banion, D. R., & Whaley, D. L. (1981). *Behavioral contracting: Arranging contingencies of reinforcement*. New York: Springer.

O'Neill, G. W., & Gardner, R. (1983). *Behavioral principles in medical rehabilitation: A practical guide*. Springfield, IL: Charles C. Thomas.

O'Neill, R. E., Horner, R. H., Albin, R. W., Sprague, J. R., Storey, K., & Newton, J. S. (1997). *Functional assessment and program development for problem behavior: A practical handbook*. Pacific Grove, CA: Brooks/Cole.

Petscher, E. S., Rey, C., & Bailey, J. S. (2009). A review of empirical support for differential reinforcement of alternative behavior. *Research in Developmental Disabilities*, 30, 409–425.

Piazza, C. C., Roane, H. S., Keeney, K. M., Boney, B. R., & Abt, K. A. (2002). Varying response effort in the treatment of pica maintained by automatic reinforcement. *Journal of Applied Behavior Analysis*, 35, 233–246.

Porterfield, J. K., Herbert-Jackson, E., & Risley, T. R. (1976). Contingent observation: An effective and acceptable procedure for reducing disruptive behavior of young children in a group setting. *Journal of Applied Behavior Analysis*, *9*, 55–64.

Pryor, K. (1985). *Don't shoot the dog: The new art of teaching and training*. New York: Bantam.

Rapp, J. T., Colby-Dirksen, A. M., Michalski, D. N., Carroll, R. A., & Lindenberg, A. M. (2008). Detecting changes in simulated events using partial-interval recording and momentary time sampling. *Behavioral Interventions*, *23*, 237–269.

Rapport, M. D., Murphy, H. A., & Bailey, J. S. (1982). Ritalin vs. response cost in the control of hyperactive children: A within subject comparison. *Journal of Applied Behavior Analysis*, *15*, 205–216.

Rortvedt, A. K., & Miltenberger, R. G. (1994). Analysis of a high probability instructional sequence and time-out in the treatment of child noncompliance. *Journal of Applied Behavior Analysis*, *27*, 327–330.

Scott, D., Scott, L. M., & Goldwater, B. (1997). A performance improvement program for an international-level track and field athlete. *Journal of Applied Behavior Analysis*, *30*, 573–575.

Skinner, B. F. (1938). *The behavior of organisms: An experimental analysis*. New York: Appleton-Century-Crofts.

Skinner, B. F. (1951). How to teach animals. *Scientific American*, *185*, 26–29.

Smith, R. G., & Iwata, B. A. (1997). Antecedent influences on behavior disorders. *Journal of Applied Behavior Analysis*, *30*, 343–375.

Slocum, S. K., & Tiger, J. H. (2011). An assessment of the efficiency of and child preference for forward and backward chaining. *Journal of Applied Behavior Analysis*, *44*, 793–805.

Spooner, F., Weber, L. H., & Spooner, D. (1983). The effects of backward chaining and total task presentation on the acquisition of complex tasks by severely retarded adolescents and adults. *Education and Treatment of Children*, *6*, 401–420.

Spradlin, J. E., & Simon, J. L. (2011). Stimulus control and generalization. In W. Fisher, C. Piazza, & H. Roane (Eds.), *Handbook of applied behavior analysis* (pp. 76–91). New York: Guilford Press.

Steege, M. W., Wacker, D. P., Cigrand, K. C., Berg, W. K., Novak, C. G., Reimers, T. M., . . . DeRaad, A. (1990). Use of negative reinforcement in the treatment of self-injurious behavior. *Journal of Applied Behavior Analysis*, *23*, 459–467.

Stokes, T. F., & Baer, D. M. (1977). An implicit technology of generalization. *Journal of Applied Behavior Analysis*, *10*, 349–367.

Stokes, T. F., & Osnes, P. G. (1989). An operant pursuit of generalization. *Behavior Therapy*, *20*, 337–355.

Thompson, R. H., & Iwata, B. A. (2005). A review of reinforcement control procedures. *Journal of Applied Behavior Analysis*, *38*, 257–278.

Travis, R., & Sturmey, P. (2010). Functional analysis and treatment of the delusional statements of a man with multiple disabilities: A four-year follow-up. *Journal of Applied Behavior Analysis*, *43*, 745–749.

Ullmann, L. P., & Krasner, L. (Eds.). (1965). *Case studies in applied behavior analysis*. New York: Holt, Rinehart, & Winston.

Urcuioli, P. J. (2013). Stimulus control and stimulus class formation. In G. J. Madden (Ed.), *APA handbook of behavior analysis: Methods and principles* (pp. 361–386). Washington, DC: American Psychological Association.

Ulrich, R., Stachnik, T., & Mabry, J. (Eds.). (1966). *Control of human behavior: Expanding the behavioral laboratory*. Glenview, IL: Scott Foresman.

Vollmer, T. R. (2002). Punishment happens: Some comments on Lerman and Vorndran's review. *Journal of Applied Behavior Analysis*, *35*, 469–473.

Vollmer, T. R., & Iwata, B. A. (1991). Establishing operations and reinforcement effects. *Journal of Applied Behavior Analysis*, *24*, 279–291.

Vollmer, T. R., & Iwata, B. A. (1992). Differential reinforcement as treatment for severe behavior disorders: Procedural and functional variations. *Research in Developmental Disabilities*, *13*, 393–417.

Vollmer, T. R., Iwata, B. A., Zarcone, J. R., Smith, R. G., & Mazaleski, J. L. (1993). The role of attention in the treatment of attention-maintained self-injurious behavior: Noncontingent reinforcement and differential reinforcement of other behavior. *Journal of Applied Behavior Analysis*, *26*, 9–22.

Wacker, D. P., Lee, J. F., Padilla Dalmau, Y. C., Kopelman, T. G., Lindgren, S. D., Kuhle, J. . . . Waldron, D. B. (2013). Conducting functional analyses of problem behavior via telehealth. *Journal of Applied Behavior Analysis*, *46*, 31–46.

Watkins, N., & Rapp, J. T. (2014). Environmental enrichment and response cost: Immediate and subsequent effects on stereotypy. *Journal of Applied Behavior Analysis*, *47*, 186–191.

Watts, A. C., Wilder, D. A., Gregory, M. K., Leon, Y., & Ditzian, K. (2013). The effect of rules on differential reinforcement of other behavior. *Journal of Applied Behavior Analysis*, *46*, 680–684.

Wilder, D. A., & Carr, J. E. (1998). Recent advances in the modification of establishing operations to reduce aberrant behavior. *Behavioral Interventions*, *13*, 43–59.

Wilder, D. A., Chen, L., Atwell, J., Pritchard, J., & Weinstein, P. (2006). Brief functional analysis and treatment of tantrums associated with transitions in preschool children. *Journal of Applied Behavior Analysis*, *39*, 103–107.

Williams, G. E., & Cuvo, A. J. (1986). Training apartment upkeep skills to rehabilitation clients: a comparison of task analytic strategies. *Journal of Applied Behavior Analysis*, *19*, 39–51.

Wolf, M. M. (1978). Social validity: The case for subjective measurement or how applied behavior analysis is finding its heart. *Journal of Applied Behavior Analysis*, *11*, 203–214.

Wright, C. S., & Vollmer, T. R. (2002). Evaluation of a treatment package to reduce rapid eating. *Journal of Applied Behavior Analysis*, *35*, 89–93.

Exposure-Based Interventions for Adult Anxiety Disorders, Obsessive-Compulsive Disorder, and Posttraumatic Stress Disorder

Seth J. Gillihan *and* Edna B. Foa

Abstract

In this chapter we provide an overview of exposure-based interventions for anxiety disorders, obsessive-compulsive disorder (OCD), and posttraumatic stress disorder (PTSD) among adults. We discuss the principles that underlie these interventions as described in emotional processing theory (Foa & Kozak, 1986), applications of exposure-based interventions for specific disorders, and the efficacy of existing exposure treatment programs. Although the majority of patients with anxiety disorders, OCD, and PTSD benefit significantly from these treatments, a significant percentage of patients continue to suffer from debilitating levels of symptoms; accordingly, we review efforts that have been made to increase the efficacy of exposure-based treatments, including combinations of exposure with psychopharmacological treatment and efforts to directly augment the efficacy of exposure. We conclude with a discussion of the gap between the development of effective treatments and their widespread use by clinicians, including a review of efforts to use technology to bridge this gap.

Key Words: exposure, cognitive-behavioral therapy, evidence-based treatment, anxiety, posttraumatic stress disorder, obsessive-compulsive disorder, specific phobia, social phobia, panic disorder, dissemination

In this chapter we will summarize and synthesize the knowledge base about effective exposure interventions for adult anxiety disorders, including panic disorder, social phobia, and specific phobia. We do not include generalized anxiety disorder here given that exposure-based interventions generally play a smaller role in efficacious treatments for this condition. The disorders we cover will also include OCD and PTSD because anxiety is a prominent aspect of these conditions and exposure-based interventions are very well validated for their treatment. For the sake of concision, when we refer hereafter to "anxiety disorders," we will be including OCD and PTSD with these conditions, even though they are no longer classified as anxiety disorders (American Psychiatric Association, 2013).

We begin with a description of exposure techniques, including in vivo, imaginal, and interoceptive exposure, and then summarize the relevant treatment literature for each disorder. We then review treatment outcome studies of combination therapies (exposure + medication) and conclude that, in general, supplementing exposure therapy with medication yields no marginal benefit. Finally, we discuss new directions in exposure-based treatments, including enhancement (pharmacological and behavioral) of exposure, the important issues of effectiveness research and dissemination, and new methods of treatment delivery (e.g., virtual reality, Internet). It is our hope that the current chapter will provoke further research in this area.

It is essential to understand not only how exposure is conducted but the mechanisms that are thought to underlie its efficacy. Therefore, we will ground our discussion of exposure interventions in the framework of emotional processing theory

(EPT; Foa & Kozak, 1986; Foa, Huppert, & Cahill, 2006). EPT integrates concepts from conditioning and extinction theory, cognitive therapy, and information processing, and provides a theoretical account of how exposure works in ameliorating pathological anxiety.

Emotional Processing Theory

PATHOLOGICAL FEAR STRUCTURES
IN ANXIETY DISORDERS

According to Foa and Kozak's (1986) emotional processing theory, fear is represented as a cognitive structure that contains information about fear stimuli, fear responses, and their meaning. For example, a combat veteran with PTSD may have a fear structure comprising representations of stimuli such as figures moving in the dark and representations of responses such as visually scanning the environment and one's heart beating fast. Of particular importance is the meaning of the figures as "dangerous" and the meaning of one's heart beating fast and eyes scanning the environment as "I am afraid." The representations of the stimuli, responses, and their meaning in the fear structure are related to each other such that a stimulus in the environment and/or a response that matches those represented in the fear structure will activate other elements in the structure. Thus, the perception of figures at night will activate the representation of the shadowy figures, the meaning associated with that representation ("danger"), and the physiological and behavioral fear responses (e.g., ducking to avoid being seen).

Foa and Kozak (1986) also distinguished between normal and pathological fear structures. In the earlier example, the combat veteran's fear structure is normal if it is restricted to settings that are actually dangerous such as a war zone; in these circumstances, activation of the fear structure will lead to adaptive responses such as moving stealthily or staying still. In contrast, the fear structure is pathological if it is activated by safe stimuli, for example, couples walking home from dinner in settings outside the war zone. Thus, a defining feature of pathological fear structures is the misinterpretation of safe stimuli and/or responses as dangerous. Pathological fear structures also include *excessive* response elements (e.g., hypervigilance in relatively safe settings).

Consider the example of a woman who is attacked by a rabid squirrel and subsequently develops a fear of all small mammals. The sight of a squirrel sitting in a tree reminds her of the squirrel that bit her, and she immediately associates this other squirrel with danger, which triggers an extreme fear response. She breaks out in a sweat, her heart pounds, and she trembles and breathes rapidly. She immediately crosses the street, going far out of her way to avoid the squirrel. This woman has a hard time believing that squirrels are safe and are unlikely to harm her, despite repeated reassurance. This scenario is repeated every time the woman encounters a squirrel, rabbit, chipmunk, and even domesticated animals like cats and dogs. She begins to avoid walking in the city out of fear that she will be attacked by one of these animals; her fear becomes so strong and pervasive that she ends up rarely leaving her home. The avoidance behavior causes so much interference in her life that she finally seeks treatment for her small animal phobia.

Conceptualization of Exposure as Modifying the Pathological Fear Structures

Clinicians can help the patient to decrease pathological fear through the use of exposure. Foa and Kozak (1986) proposed that two conditions must be met in order for treatment to reduce pathological fear: Treatment must (1) activate the fear structure and (2) provide corrective information that is incompatible with the existing pathological elements. Exposure therapy is an efficient and effective means of accomplishing both of these objectives. Exposure procedures activate the fear structure by encouraging the person to confront his or her feared situation or object. This confrontation provides an opportunity for new learning (i.e., corrective information) to be integrated into the memory of this situation, thus lessening the fear associated with it. For example, if the woman with the small animal phobia repeatedly approaches areas in the city where squirrels are found and does not flee when she sees a squirrel without being bitten or attacked by it, then she will learn that most squirrels are safe. This modification in the meaning of a squirrel from a "vicious, dangerous" to a "safe, harmless" animal comprises emotional processing, which underlies the reduction in pathological fear.

Effective exposure programs tailor interventions to the specific target disorder, and this tailoring requires understanding the core elements of the fear structure of each disorder. Panic disorder, for example, involves strong associations between fear responses and meaning of danger. For example, many patients with panic disorder experience physiological symptoms like a pounding heart (response) in specific situations like driving on an expressway (stimulus) and fear that they are dying of a heart attack (heart pounding means "heart attack"). Thus, the fear structure in panic disorder involves strong associations between response and meaning elements. For this reason, effective CBT for panic disorder will involve exposing the patient to the fear response by intentionally inducing that response (e.g., by climbing stairs; see "Interoceptive Exposure"). When the anticipated outcome (e.g., heart attack, fainting) does not occur, a new association is formed between "heart pounding" and "no danger," resulting in a new fear structure that more closely matches reality.

In contrast, patients with specific phobias generally are not afraid of their own fear response; rather, their fear is evoked by relatively safe external stimuli and situations such as being around nonpoisonous spiders. Therefore, CBT for specific phobia will focus on exposure to the feared, but safe, stimulus in order to modify the pathological association between nonpoisonous spiders and the meaning of danger.

The pathological fear structure in OCD tends to involve two sets of powerful erroneous associations. First, relatively harmless stimuli are associated with grave danger. For example, the patient might fear that touching a public toilet seat with a bare hand means that the person will contract a sexually transmitted disease; in this case there is an erroneous association between stimulus and meaning elements. Second, patients experience excessive distress in response to these meaning elements, resulting in avoidance of the stimulus and/or ritualizing that is intended to neutralize the feared consequences associated with the stimulus. This aspect of the fear structure represents an association between meaning elements and responses, such that compulsions become closely linked with reduction of distress. In light of this pattern of associations between stimulus, response, and meaning elements of the fear structure in OCD, effective treatment for this disorder requires exposure to feared stimuli in addition to prevention of the rituals (responses).

It is sometimes necessary to modify the exposure intervention in order to ensure disconfirmation of the erroneous elements in the patient's fear structure. Such modification often is required in the treatment of social phobia. In vivo exposure as it is typically practiced is often insufficient to adequately reduce social fear because the absence of social rejection or ridicule during in vivo exposure is not taken as disconfirmation of the patient's belief that he is socially awkward and inadequate. Individuals with social phobia commonly attribute the absence of overt rejection or criticism to the general social norm of not expressing direct criticism, rather than to the other person's positive regard for the patient. Additionally, high anxiety in social situations may prevent patients with social phobia from processing corrective feedback from others. For these reasons, CBT for social phobia often includes video feedback in which patients make specific predictions about how they will perform during a videotaped social interaction like a one-on-one conversation. In most cases patients will rate their behavior much more favorably after watching the video compared to their predictions before the interaction and compared to their subjective impressions of how the interaction went prior to seeing the video. Thus, supplementing the exposure with video feedback facilitates the patient's ability to incorporate corrective information that disconfirms his inaccurate association between the stimulus (the other person's behavior) and meaning ("criticism"), thereby modifying the pathological fear structure.

PTSD also requires tailoring the exposures to effect the necessary changes in the pathological fear structure. As discussed in the example of the combat veteran, PTSD patients generally have a wide array of dysfunctional associations between stimulus, response, and meaning elements of the fear structure. In addition to the excessive fear responses and the erroneous associations among stimulus, response, and meaning elements, the trauma memory tends to be fragmented in individuals with PTSD. Also, PTSD sufferers do not differentiate sufficiently between thinking about the trauma and "being retraumatized." Repeated revisiting of the trauma memory through imaginal exposure helps patients organize the traumatic memory and gain new perspectives on it, promotes differentiation between thinking about the trauma and being in the traumatic experience again, strengthens discrimination between the traumatic experience and similar situations (disconfirming the perception that the world is entirely dangerous), and disconfirms the patient's perception that he or she is unable to cope with stress (i.e., is incompetent).

Evidence for Efficacy of Exposure-Based Treatments

Patients and therapists alike appreciate the effectiveness of exposure treatments. An impressive number of scientifically rigorous studies have demonstrated that these treatments help the majority of patients with OCD (e.g., Foa et al., 2005),

PTSD (e.g., Foa et al., 2005), panic disorder (e.g., Barlow, Gorman, Shear, & Woods, 2000), specific phobia (e.g., Öst et al., 2001), and social phobia (e.g., Clark et al., 2006). In general, the effect sizes for these treatments are quite large. For example, a meta-analysis of the efficacy of prolonged exposure (PE) for PTSD versus control conditions reported an effect size of Hedges's $g = 1.07$, indicating that the average patient in the PE condition had better outcomes than 86% of individuals in the control conditions (Powers, Halpern, Ferenschak, Gillihan, & Foa, 2010). A large effect size (Cohen's $d = 1.13$) also was found for exposure and ritual prevention (EX/RP) in the treatment of OCD compared to control conditions (Rosa-Alcázar, Sánchez-Mecab, Gómez-Conesac, & Marín-Martínez, 2008); this effect size means that the typical EX/RP patient will have a better outcome than 87% of patients in the control condition.

A meta-analysis of randomized controlled trials (RCTs) for anxiety disorders including many exposure-based treatment programs (Hofmann & Smits, 2008) showed that cognitive-behavioral therapy (CBT) was highly effective for treating all anxiety diagnoses compared to pill placebo or non-specific treatments (e.g., supportive counseling). Effect size estimates were based on treatment programs that included varying amounts of exposure in combination with other elements such as cognitive restructuring and psychoeducation. Largest effect sizes were obtained for OCD ($g = 1.37$) and smallest for panic disorder ($g = 0.35$).

A crucial issue is whether exposure-based interventions translate well outside of the carefully controlled setting of RCTs in which their efficacy is established. A recent meta-analysis compared the effect sizes for exposure-based interventions delivered in nonresearch settings to effect sizes from RCTs (Stewart & Chambless, 2009). Analyses revealed a negligible reduction in efficacy for these therapies when they were used in community clinics and other non-RCT settings, which suggests that these treatment effects are robust across a range of clinic characteristics.

In the section that follows we describe the common techniques that are used in exposure-based interventions.

Description of Exposure Techniques
In Vivo Exposure

In vivo exposure is real-life confrontation with feared stimuli. Exposures are planned based on an in vivo exposure hierarchy—which the patient and therapist construct together—that comprises a list of situations or activities that the patient either endures with great distress or avoids altogether because of the patient's unrealistic concerns. Patients then assign each item a subjective units of distress (SUDS) rating from 0 (no distress or anxiety at all; e.g., "sitting on my boat last fall") to 100 (most distressed the person has ever been; e.g., "when our convoy was attacked"), which allows the items to be ordered from least to most distressing. It is important when constructing the hierarchy that the items span a range from ones that provoke moderate anxiety to ones that produce the most anxiety a patient can imagine. The items are then confronted systematically, beginning with items that were assigned moderate SUDS ratings and moving up the list to the more distressing items. As patients progress up their list, they gain confidence and a sense of self-efficacy through initial mastery experiences; furthermore, starting with moderately distressing exposure exercises is more tolerable to patients than is starting exposures with the highest-rated items on the hierarchy.

There are advantages to doing the first exposure during a treatment session, when possible, such that the therapist can demonstrate how to conduct the exposure, troubleshoot any difficulties that arise, and provide support for what is generally a challenging task. It sometimes will be necessary for the therapist to meet the patient outside of the office in order to conduct essential in vivo exposures. For example, if a patient with OCD is afraid that he will be contaminated in public places, a good first exposure would be touching keyboards and doorknobs in the therapist's clinic. Later in treatment it will be necessary to conduct exposure in places like train stations and supermarkets in order to promote disconfirmation of the patient's feared consequences. Additionally, it is critical that patients do exposures on their own between sessions, from the start of therapy. Some patients minimize success experiences that happen during in-session exposures. In the case of OCD, for example, patients might attribute the lack of negative consequences to the presence of the therapist, telling themselves that "it must not actually be dangerous if my therapist was complicit in the exposure." The patient with social phobia similarly might tell herself that exposure successes were a result of the benevolence of the therapist or other participants in the exposure, and thus unlikely to replicate in the "real world." In other anxiety disorders (e.g., panic disorder), clinicians may serve as safety cues, and it is crucial for patients to realize that they can confront their feared situations on their own and effectively manage their anxiety.

Exposure duration also is an important factor. Patients need to stay in contact with the feared stimuli long enough to realize that their feared outcomes do not materialize and that anxiety does not last forever but rather diminishes over time. Thus, therapy sessions generally need to be at least an hour long when exposure is conducted during the session. If an exposure is by nature very short (e.g., touching a dirty toilet), the patient should repeat the exposure exercise multiple times in a row. For example, a patient with PTSD who fears making eye contact with strangers (a behavior that takes just a couple of seconds) can be instructed to go to the mall and make eye contact with as many passersby as possible.

In the sections that follow we discuss the variants of in vivo exposure that are commonly used for panic disorder, social phobia, OCD, and PTSD.

IN VIVO EXPOSURE FOR PANIC DISORDER

Patients with panic disorder tend to fear situations in which they expect to experience a panic attack, and fortunately for the treating clinician, these kinds of situations often are readily available. Common to these situations is the patient's perception that he or she cannot leave the situations as soon as he or she wants or needs to in order to avoid a panic attack. Such exposures include riding the elevator, standing in long lines, riding the train or the subway, driving during rush hour, and going into crowded supermarkets. As discussed in the introduction to the in vivo section, it is important to have patients with panic disorder transition from doing exposures in the presence of the "safe" therapist to doing unaccompanied homework. A useful approach in this regard is to add intermediate steps to the hierarchy that involve phasing out the therapist's involvement. For example, a patient who was ready for more challenging driving exposures found that the next step in his hierarchy was unbearably anxiety inducing when done alone. To ease this transition, the therapist and patient drove the difficult route together, and then the patient immediately repeated the exposure by himself. Similar graded exposures can be done with friends or family members, who can be helpful early in treatment; as treatment progresses, these "safety nets" are phased out.

IN VIVO EXPOSURE FOR SOCIAL PHOBIA

As discussed earlier, in vivo exposure for social phobia may require adaptations in order to target the underlying fear that maintains the disorder. It may be necessary to design exposures that include other clinicians or staff members ("confederates"), which can range from one-on-one conversations to presentations in front of a group. Patients with social phobia often use "safety behaviors" during social interactions that they believe will prevent their feared outcome from happening (see McManus, Sacadura, & Clark, 2008). For example, an individual with social phobia might ask a lot of questions to avoid "awkward pauses" in the conversation, or he might keep his hands in his pockets so that nobody will see if his hands are shaking. Paradoxically, these behaviors often produce the exact outcome that the patients are trying to avoid. For example, the patient's attempt to keep still so as not to look "awkward" can appear odd and may draw others' attention to the person rather than producing the desired outcome of being inconspicuous. Moreover, these behaviors interfere with disconfirmation of the feared outcomes in social situations because patients can attribute positive outcomes to the safety behaviors.

For these reasons it is essential that therapists encourage patients with social phobia to participate in social interactions with and without safety behaviors, and to assess the extent to which the feared disaster comes true under each condition. To their surprise, most patients with social phobia report that they actually performed better when dropping safety behaviors. Given the difficulty that these patients often have with encoding information during high-stress social interactions, it may be necessary to use video feedback to disconfirm patients' expectations, thereby modifying their pathological fear structure. For example, patients can see objectively that their blushing may be rare and barely noticeable when their subjective impression was that they were constantly blushing bright crimson. Conversely, patients can see for themselves that safety behaviors intended to make them "look natural" in fact make them appear more awkward.

As in exposure treatment for panic disorder, it is essential that patients with social phobia plan with the therapist to continue exposure exercises between sessions. Exposures are tailored to domains in which the patient is having difficulty and progress gradually up the hierarchy. For example, a patient who is afraid to speak up in class may first make rehearsed statements and then make more spontaneous comments without rehearsing. Similarly, a patient who fears unstructured social interactions may first go out to dinner with a small group of friends, systematically working up the exposure hierarchy to the more challenging exercise of going to a party.

IN VIVO EXPOSURE FOR TREATMENT OF OCD

Most patients with OCD will require in vivo exposure in order to provide direct disconfirmation of their feared outcomes. In treating patients with OCD it is essential that exposure be combined with prevention of the rituals that patients perform to prevent their feared disasters from happening. Through exposure and ritual prevention, patients confront situations that raise obsessional concerns and learn that their feared consequences do not occur and that their distress and urge to ritualize decrease. For patients who perform mental rituals or whose rituals are very subtle, clinicians should remind the patient of the importance of complete ritual prevention before and during the exposure. When patients perform a ritual during or after an exposure, they should immediately re-expose themselves to the feared stimulus to minimize the negative reinforcement produced by the ritual.

The content of exposures for OCD varies widely in light of the diversity of obsessions and compulsions seen in this disorder. For a patient with contamination concerns, exposure can involve touching keyboards and the floor and then refraining from washing before eating food. For a patient with fears of burning down the house due to forgetting to turn off the stove, exposure might entail cooking with all four burners and then leaving the house without checking that the stove is off. Patients with blasphemy concerns might intentionally say and write things that are blasphemous (e.g., "I love Satan").

It is the nature of OCD to spread if "pockets" of it are left untreated, leading to relapse. For example, a patient with contamination concerns might progress up her exposure hierarchy and then refuse to carry out the highest items on it, such as eating without washing her hands. In this way the patient has denied herself an opportunity to disconfirm the erroneous belief that eating without washing her hands would result in contracting a terrible disease and becoming permanently ill. Thus, it is essential that in vivo exposure address all of the areas where the OCD "lives." An important intervention in this regard is to carry out home visits, particularly for patients whose homes are considered "safe" places. Home visits for patients with contamination concerns will focus on contaminating objects there. If patients have difficulty leaving the house because they worry about forgetting to lock the door, it is important that the therapist go to the patient's home and help her leave the house without checking the locks.

IN VIVO EXPOSURE FOR PTSD

As in the other disorders reviewed in this chapter, avoidance is a core symptom of PTSD. Trauma survivors often avoid places, people, and situations that remind them of their traumatic experience. Constructive modification of the pathological fear structure requires exposure to feared stimuli that do not realistically have a high risk of danger. Certainly, exposure to actually dangerous stimuli is not appropriate and would not have a positive therapeutic effect. Thus, it is not necessary for trauma survivors to confront their attacker or to go to the location of the trauma if that place is objectively unsafe (e.g., a dark street in a high-crime neighborhood at night).

Keeping this caveat in mind, other in vivo exposures are very beneficial in the treatment of PTSD. For example, a patient who was assaulted in a hotel now avoids being in any hotel out of fear that he will be attacked again; a reasonable goal is to incorporate staying in hotels into the exposure plan. If a patient survived a car crash and now avoids driving her car because she fears another accident, a good goal of treatment is to get the patient behind the wheel again. For other patients their avoidance may be driven not by fear of harm but rather by the desire to avoid distressing memories of the trauma that the stimuli trigger. For example, patients sometimes avoid wearing the clothes they had on at the time of their trauma, not because they think the clothes themselves are dangerous but because they evoke painful memories. For these patients, in vivo exposure would include wearing the avoided articles of clothing, thereby learning that they are strong enough to handle the distress that the clothes provoke and that the distress associated with the clothes does not last forever. They also form new associations between the clothes and outcomes other than the trauma, such that the clothes no longer provoke painful memories of the trauma.

Imaginal Exposure

In imaginal exposure the patient vividly imagines being in the presence of feared circumstances. The imagined scene generally includes a detailed description of the patient's thoughts, feelings, and physical sensations. Imaginal exposure is most commonly used in the treatment of OCD and PTSD, and also with social phobia. For each disorder the exposure is designed to address and modify the underlying pathological fear structure, as we will discuss in the subsections that follow.

IMAGINAL EXPOSURE FOR PTSD

In PTSD treatment, imaginal exposure (or "revisiting") is used to help the patient emotionally process and organize her traumatic memory. It is particularly important in PTSD treatment to provide a thorough rationale for the use of imaginal exposure in ameliorating PTSD symptoms, given the distress that revisiting the memory typically provokes. The therapist explains that the imaginal exposure promotes processing of the traumatic experience, which leads to greater coherence and organization of the memory, reduction in distress when thinking about the trauma, a realization that the memory per se is not dangerous and that anxiety does not last forever, and increased self-efficacy.

In standard imaginal exposure, the therapist instructs the patient to close his or her eyes and to describe aloud what happened during the trauma, while visualizing the events as vividly as possible. Patients use the present tense to describe the thoughts, feelings, and sensory experiences that occurred during the traumatic event. Imaginal exposure is continued for a prolonged period of time (30 minutes is typical) and includes multiple repetitions of the memory if necessary. The goal is to help the patient to emotionally engage with the trauma memory. Immediately after the imaginal exposure the patient and therapist discuss the experience and what it was like for the patient. Imaginal exposure is conducted in several treatment sessions until the anxiety and distress associated with the memory have subsided substantially. For homework, the patient listens daily to audio recordings of the imaginal exposure, which continues the work of emotionally processing the trauma (Foa et al., 2007). Patients often report that recounting the memory becomes "boring" as they near the end of their treatment, in contrast to the emotional arousal and distress that revisiting the memory initially elicited.

IMAGINAL EXPOSURE FOR OCD

In contrast to imaginal exposure for PTSD in which an actual horrifying event is recounted, imaginal exposure for OCD involves describing an event that has not happened and is unlikely to occur, namely the feared consequences of obsessions or of not performing rituals. As such, imaginal exposure for OCD has somewhat different aims. First,

imaginal exposure can address the thought-action fusion that often occurs in OCD; that is, the belief that thinking about something is equivalent to doing it (Shafran, Thordarson, & Rachman, 1996). By repeating the distressing ideas over and over, the person with OCD learns that dwelling on the thoughts does not make them occur. Second, patients experience a reduction in distress related to the imagined scenario as they encounter it over and over; as a result, patients may assign a lower cost to the feared outcome, which further reduces obsessions. Third, patients experience decreased distress after repeated imaginal exposure, which disconfirms their belief that confronting obsession-related material is always distressing and is so upsetting that patients "can't take it" or will "go crazy."

To conduct the imaginal exposure, the patient and therapist work together to develop the details of the imaginal scenario, which is written in the present tense and includes elaborate sensory and affective details to maximize the vividness of the story. The patient then engages in the imaginal exposure by imagining the event and its consequences while describing the scene that he or she is visualizing. The script is audio recorded and the patient listens to the scenario over and over while imagining that the events are actually happening. As with imaginal exposure for PTSD, the imaginal exposure is conducted over a prolonged interval and over successive days until the patient experiences a substantial reduction in distress and also realizes that thinking about disasters does not make them occur.

What follows is an imaginal exposure script for "Jane," an OCD patient with obsessions about causing a fire by leaving the stove on. The imaginal narrative aims to promote engagement with the OCD patient's feared consequences (causing a dangerous and destructive fire by carelessly leaving the stove on after cooking, and being blamed for her carelessness). Imaginal exposure is an effective way of allowing patients to confront feared situations and their unrealistic or excessive consequences.

> I make dinner for my family using all four burners because I'm making pasta, sauce, a vegetable, and am heating up other food for our baby. I'm nervous about having all the burners on at once as I see the blue flames and feel their heat. Seeing the flames triggers a moment of fear as I imagine the flames coming in contact with some paper in the kitchen and starting a dangerous or even deadly fire, and I think that maybe I should turn off the stove and order a pizza instead. I also want to make sure that

there are no papers in the kitchen that could blow into the flames and cause a fire, and want to close the window that I opened because it was getting hot in the kitchen from all the cooking. Instead of giving in to these urges to ritualize or avoid, I resolve to fight against my OCD in order to conquer these fears.

When the pasta is done, I turn off the stove, being careful not to check that it's off, and drain the water over the sink. As I'm draining the water, a gust of wind comes in through the open window and catches some papers that are next to the phone, blowing them toward the stove. I see some of the papers land on one of the burners that's still on and immediately burst into flames. I drop the pasta in the sink and rush to put out the fire, but I'm too late—the wind blows the burning papers against the cabinet which starts to burn. The dry wood burns fast and spreads to the other cabinets, and I'm being surrounded by flames. I feel helpless as I stand in the middle of the kitchen, too scared to move. The wood is making crackling sounds as it burns and the flames start to lick at the ceiling.

My husband, John, who was playing in the yard with our two kids, sees the smoke coming out the window and comes running inside, carrying our baby and our three-year-old. I can tell he's angry and scared as he looks at the flames and at me standing there helplessly. "What did you do?" he shouts at me. He hands the kids to me and grabs the fire extinguisher. Both of our kids are coughing from the smoke and crying in fear and bewilderment. I take the kids outside as my husband battles the flames with the fire extinguisher. John comes outside as the fire department arrives with their lights and sirens on. The firefighters talk with my husband, who gestures at me as he explains what happened and they go inside to make sure the fire is out. Neighbors are coming out of their houses and pointing, and I feel like they know that it's all my fault. The firefighters talk to me afterward and are very stern, saying I need to be more careful and not act so recklessly in the future.

When the fire trucks leave, I go back inside with my husband and kids. I can tell that John is furious. I feel completely worthless and terrified. Even my kids seem to look at me differently. Finally John says, "How could you have been so careless? Imagine if anything had happened to the kids!" I know he will always remember and judge me for causing the fire, and my kids will never feel safe around me. Neighbors who used to be friendly toward me now ignore me on the street because I could have set the whole neighborhood on fire through my actions. My

future holds only guilt and loneliness, and all because I selfishly tried to get over my OCD. The life I used to have is gone. I am miserable.

IMAGINAL EXPOSURE FOR SOCIAL PHOBIA

As with OCD treatment, imaginal exposure for social phobia involves a scenario that the patient greatly fears and yet is unlikely to actually happen. For many patients with social phobia, the threat of the feared event leads to high distress and avoidance behavior; imaginal exposure thus can be helpful in decreasing distress associated with the relevant social situations and decreasing avoidance. The patient and therapist collaboratively develop a script of the patient's concerns, again with plenty of vivid details. The content of imaginal exposure for social phobia generally involves receiving negative feedback in a social situation; the degree of negative feedback often is exaggerated to the point of being absurd. Through repeated listening to and imagining the exposure scenario, patients form more accurate appraisals of the likelihood of the event occurring. As a result, they begin to feel less anxious about approaching the relevant social situations and less likely to avoid them.

Interoceptive Exposure

Interoceptive exposure is used most often in the treatment of panic disorder, in which patients often fear their own bodily sensations because they attribute them to an impending disaster (e.g., racing heart = heart attack; see Goldstein & Chambless, 1978). In this form of exposure patients engage in activities that deliberately bring on the feared physical sensations, such as running in place, breathing through a straw, and hyperventilating. The goal of interoceptive exposure is to help patients learn new meanings of physical sensations—meanings that involve the absence of danger. Thus, patients can learn that these physical sensations need not be feared or viewed as a sign of imminent catastrophe.

Interoceptive exposure exercises should be chosen that address the patient's specific concerns, thereby activating the underlying fear structure. Patients who fear that dizziness or light-headedness signals a fainting episode, for example, could be instructed to spin around in a swivel chair, shake their head vigorously from side to side, or hyperventilate. Similarly, patients who fear that a strong and rapid heartbeat signals a heart attack can be asked to climb stairs to induce a pounding heart. Through repetition of these interoceptive exposures, patients form new associations between physical sensations and the absence of threat.

Studies of Exposure Plus Medication

As the studies reviewed earlier clearly demonstrate, exposure-based interventions are efficacious for the treatment of anxiety disorders. Nevertheless, a significant proportion of patients (which varies depending on the specific disorder) fails to respond to these treatments. Additionally, even many individuals who respond to the treatment may continue to experience significant symptoms. For these reasons there has been considerable interest in augmenting exposure-based treatments with other treatments that are known to work, particularly psychotropic medications. In the section that follows we review the major trials in this area. As this review will demonstrate, with few exceptions the addition of medications to exposure therapies does not result in any additional benefit; moreover, in some cases medication can be detrimental to exposure treatment outcomes.

OCD

Randomized trials that compared EX/RP alone to EX/RP plus medication have produced equivocal results. One study found a significant advantage for EX/RP plus the selective serotonin reuptake inhibitor (SSRI) fluvoxamine over EX/RP alone at the end of treatment (Hohagen et al., 1998). A trial by Cottraux et al. (1990) reported a trend toward better outcome in the combined condition versus EX/RP alone, which disappeared at follow-up. Similarly, Van Balkom et al. (1997) found no significant differences in outcome between EX/RP with and without fluvoxamine. In the largest trial to date in this area, Foa et al. (2005) found no additional benefit from adding clomipramine to EX/RP treatment. There is also evidence that patients already receiving open-label selective serotonin reuptake inhibitor (SSRIs) do no better in EX/RP than patients who are not on these medications (Franklin et al., 2002). Taken together, these results suggest that adding effective medication to an effective cognitive-behavioral treatment does not provide OCD patients with additional benefit.

Panic Disorder

A somewhat complex pattern of results has emerged from studies comparing CBT with and without medication. As with OCD, no consistent advantage has been found from the addition of medication to exposure-based treatments for panic disorder. Some studies have reported no difference between CBT with versus without medication; for example, Cottraux et al. (1995) found no significant differences between CBT plus buspirone and CBT plus placebo, either at the end of treatment or at follow-up. Other studies have reported better outcomes associated with adding medication to CBT. The combination of CBT and an SSRI (e.g., fluvoxamine, paroxetine) was found to be more effective at the end of a 9-month course of treatment compared to CBT alone (van Apeldoorn et al., 2008). In the largest study of its kind to date ($N = 312$), the combination of CBT plus imipramine (a tricyclic antidepressant) produced outcomes superior to CBT alone at the end of treatment and at the end of the maintenance phase (Barlow, Gorman, Shear, & Woods, 2000).

Although these findings from combination treatments were promising, multiple trials have reported that the addition of medication to CBT may actually have a detrimental effect on treatment outcome, particularly at follow-up. Marks et al. (1993) found no significant difference between exposure-based treatment with and without alprazolam at the end of treatment (71% responders in both conditions); at follow-up there were 62% responders in the exposure group and 36% in the combination treatment. In the follow-up period, Barlow et al. (2000) found that CBT alone was significantly better than the combination condition.

A meta-analysis of 20 trials of behavioral or cognitive-behavioral therapy alone versus with the addition of pharmacotherapy (primarily tricyclic antidepressants and SSRIs) revealed significantly better outcome for the combination treatment (Mitte, 2005). However, this advantage disappeared at follow-up, with no significant differences between psychotherapy with and without pharmacotherapy. In fact, Mitte (2005) reported that approximately two thirds of the effect sizes favored psychotherapy alone, which is in line with the findings by Barlow et al. (2000) and Marks et al. (1993). Very similar results were reported in a meta-analysis of 23 RCTs (Furukawa, Watanabe, & Churchill, 2006). Results from these studies suggest that although adding medication to effective CBT may be helpful in the short run for treatment of panic disorder, in the long run it is not helpful and may even hamper the effects of treatment.

Social Phobia

Mixed results also have emerged for the treatment of social phobia with CBT alone versus CBT plus medication. An early study in this area by Blomhoff and colleagues (2001) randomized 387 patients to treatment with the SSRI sertraline, placebo, exposure plus sertraline, or exposure plus placebo. At the end of treatment there were no significant differences between the active treatments. Similar results were reported by Davidson et al. (2004) from their study comparing the SSRI fluoxetine, group CBT either alone or with fluoxetine or placebo, and placebo; combined treatments were no more effective than the monotherapies. The addition of other classes of medications to CBT in the treatment of social phobia also has not consistently yielded results superior to CBT alone; Prasko et al. (2006) reported no significant outcome differences after 6 months of treatment between patients treated with CBT alone versus with the addition of moclobemide, a monoamine oxidase inhibitor (MAOI). Similarly, Clark and Agras (1991) reported no significant advantage of adding buspirone to CBT for performance anxiety in musicians. One study that appears to be an outlier in this literature found a significant advantage of group CBT plus the MAOI phenelzine over group CBT alone (Blanco et al., 2010). It is unclear why this study found different results than most other studies in this area; the results do not seem to be driven by a greater efficacy of phenelzine over medications used in other studies, as phenelzine alone was associated with a similar response rate at the end of treatment (approximately 55%) as other studies that found no advantage for the combination treatment (e.g., Davidson et al., 2004, 50.9% with fluoxetine alone).

As with some of the findings for combination treatment of panic disorder summarized earlier (e.g., Barlow et al., 2000), there is evidence that the addition of medication to exposure-based treatment may be harmful in the long run. Follow-up analyses of the patients from the study by Blomhoff et al. revealed that patients treated with exposure alone tended to continue to improve during the follow-up period, while patients who had received sertraline (with or without CBT) tended to worsen after treatment ended (Haug et al., 2003). Additional studies are needed to determine whether this finding is reliable and generalizes to other kinds of medication. Taken together, existing studies indicate that there is no reliable advantage in treatment outcome associated with adding medication to exposure-based treatments for social phobia.

Specific Phobia

Fewer studies have investigated the potential added benefit of medication to exposure-based treatment for specific phobia, in large part because exposure by itself is so efficacious in treating specific phobia. For example, Öst (1989) found that following a single session of exposure for specific phobias (average length = 2.1 hr), 90% of patients were "much improved" or recovered 4 years later. Nevertheless, it has been hypothesized that using benzodiazepines to lower patients' anxiety may allow them to progress more quickly up the exposure hierarchy, thereby resulting in more efficient treatment. To test this hypothesis, Coldwell and colleagues (2007) compared the outcomes for dental injection phobics who received systematic desensitization with alprazolam or pill placebo. In contrast to this hypothesis, taking alprazolam was not associated with a shorter duration of therapy; moreover, patients who had received alprazolam during treatment showed more anxiety during the behavioral test, which comprised an actual dental injection. Follow-up assessments at 3, 6, and 12 months revealed no significant differences between groups. Thus, with specific phobia as with other anxiety disorders, the addition of medication to exposure therapy appears to exert a neutral to negative effect on treatment outcome.

Summary

What might account for the relatively consistent finding that adding an efficacious medication to exposure-based treatments yields no reliable additional benefit? A possible explanation is that the medications that are commonly combined with exposure treatment (i.e., antidepressants and benzodiazepines) might interfere with the mechanisms whereby exposure works. For example, these medications suppress levels of glucocorticoids (e.g., cortisol), which are necessary for learning and memory consolidation involved in fear extinction (see Otto, McHugh, & Kantak, 2010). This explanation is consistent with the activation hypothesis of emotional processing theory (Foa & Kozak, 1986), which proposes that the pathological fear association must be activated in order to be modified; the cortisol suppression associated with concomitant medication use may dampen the effectiveness of exposure. Thus, any additional benefit provided by the pharmacotherapy may be washed out by this interference effect, resulting in no net benefit from combined treatment.

The replicated finding of a long-term disadvantage of combination treatment compared to exposure treatment alone also is consistent with the predictions of emotional processing theory and with what we have learned from animal studies of fear extinction. Patients who received CBT and also took medications may have experienced less effective learning from their treatment exposures; when the medication is withdrawn, the poorer fear extinction learning becomes apparent. These patients may attribute their treatment gains to the medication, leading them to believe that their symptoms will return when the medication is stopped. Additionally, state-dependent learning (Overton, 1985) may underlie the greater relapse associated with combination treatments in several trials. That is, learning in a medicated state may be less well recalled when the patient is no longer taking medication. Whatever the mechanism, it seems that combination treatment should not be recommended for most patients with anxiety disorders.

Frontier of Exposure Therapy

Thus far we have described exposure-based interventions, provided evidence for their efficacy, and shown that the addition of medication to these treatments results in no added benefit. In this section we present work that is being done at the frontier of exposure therapy. First, whereas additional treatments do not seem to augment the efficacy of exposure, there are several promising ways in which exposure itself may be enhanced. We then conclude with recent efforts to make exposure-based interventions more widely available.

Enhancement of Exposure

There have been many efforts to make exposure treatments more effective by enhancing the mechanisms by which exposure is believed to work (for a review see McGuire, Lewin, & Storch, 2014). These interventions differ from adding a stand-alone pharmacological treatment to exposure therapy in which there is no presumption that the medication will directly affect the action of the exposure. Efforts in this area have included both pharmacological and behavioral manipulations, which we will cover in turn.

PHARMACOLOGICAL
D-cycloserine

Laboratory studies of nonhuman animals have demonstrated that D-cycloserine (DCS), a partial agonist of N-methyl-D-aspartate receptors,

increases the speed and efficacy of extinction training. Although the precise mechanisms through which DCS exerts its effects are not currently known, it is believed to facilitate extinction learning and/or to disrupt reconsolidation of fear associations (Norberg, Krystal, & Tolin, 2008). There is evidence to support the utility of DCS in enhancing the extinction of conditioned fear. For example, Walker et al. (2002) reported that DCS administered both systemically and directly into the amygdala significantly enhanced fear extinction in rats as measured by reductions in fear-potentiated startle, with a large Cohen's *d* (1988) effect size of 1.17. Similarly, DCS administration after extinction training in rats led to reduced freezing in response to a conditioned stimulus (CS; in this case a light) during a post-extinction test phase compared to animals that received a saline injection (Parnas, Weber, & Richardson, 2005). A meta-analysis of DCS effects on enhancing extinction among nonhuman animals yielded a large and significant effect size of $d = 1.19$ (Norberg et al., 2008).

In light of its promising preclinical efficacy, several research groups have tested the ability of DCS to enhance exposure efficacy in humans. In the first such study, Ressler and colleagues (2004) administered DCS in the context of virtual reality exposure therapy for acrophobia (fear of heights). Individuals who were given DCS before therapy sessions experienced a greater reduction in phobia symptoms at the end of treatment and at 3-month follow-up. The promising results from this small pilot study ($N = 28$) with specific phobia have been replicated in social phobia (Guastella et al., 2008; Hofmann et al., 2006), panic disorder (Otto et al., 2010), and OCD (Kushner et al., 2007; Wilhelm et al., 2008). A meta-analysis of these findings (Norberg et al., 2008) revealed that in humans with anxiety disorders, DCS was associated with a significant advantage in symptom reduction, with medium-sized effects (Cohen, 1988) of $d = 0.60$ at post-treatment and $d = 0.47$ at follow-up. DCS was most beneficial when it was administered immediately before or after exposure; thus, Norberg et al. (2008) posit that DCS augments treatment outcomes by enhancing fear extinction memory consolidation.

The effect size associated with DCS administration tended to decrease across the course of treatment sessions (Norberg et al., 2008). Based on this finding, the authors concluded that the main advantage of DCS may be its ability to accelerate the speed of exposure by making it more efficient, as opposed to raising the ceiling on treatment effects.

More recent studies supported this idea; Siegmund et al. (2011) found that DCS did not improve treatment outcomes following in vivo exposure for panic disorder with agoraphobia, although there was a statistical trend for faster improvement among patients with more severe symptoms. Similarly, Chasson and colleagues (2010) reanalyzed the data from Wilhelm et al. (2008) and examined the symptom change slopes across treatment between DCS and the control group; they concluded that "DCS does not amplify the effects of [exposure therapy], but instead initiates treatment effects sooner in treatment" (p. 675; see also Kushner et al., 2007, who reported a similar pattern of results). These findings suggest that DCS may be used to decrease treatment costs and dropout rates since patients on average will experience faster improvement.

Yohimbine

As with DCS, animal studies of yohimbine showed that this selective competitive alpha2-adrenergic receptor antagonist facilitates fear extinction learning (e.g., Cain, Blouin, & Barad, 2004). Rats given yohimbine systemically showed reduced fear behavior (freezing) during extinction of a previously conditioned cue and during a test session (CS presented with no unconditioned stimulus [US]) 24 hours later (Morris & Bouton, 2007). These results led to efforts to translate the findings with nonhuman animals to the treatment of anxiety disorders.

The first study to examine the efficacy of yohimbine-augmented exposure in humans tested the effects of yohimbine versus placebo administered prior to exposure for claustrophobia (Powers, Smits, Otto, Sanders, & Emmelkamp, 2009). Although there was no significant effect of yohimbine on claustrophobia symptoms at the end of treatment, at 1-week follow-up there was a large and significant advantage for the yohimbine group, $d = 1.68$. These findings are consistent with the activation hypothesis of emotional processing theory, which posits that activation of the pathological fear structure is necessary for therapeutic changes to occur. Accordingly, the administration of an agent that increases noradrenergic function and leads to acute increases in physical and emotional anxiety symptoms (e.g., Charney, Heninger, & Breier, 1984) would be expected to lead to greater reductions in pathological fear responses.

However, results associated with the use of yohimbine have been mixed; a subsequent study that examined the efficacy of yohimbine among individuals with flying phobia found no significant effect of yohimbine on outcome (Meyerbroeker, Powers, van Stegeren, & Emmelkamp, 2012). An important caveat with this later study is that there was no follow-up assessment; thus, it cannot be known whether there were any group differences that emerged over time, as there were in the study by Powers et al. (2009). Powers and colleagues also investigated the effect of yohimbine in conjunction with CBT for social anxiety disorder (Smits et al., 2014). Results revealed a qualified advantage for those receiving yohimbine, which was apparent only on self-report measures and only among individuals who showed greater within-session habituation during exposures. Thus, additional research is needed to determine whether and under what circumstances yohimbine is an effective enhancer of fear extinction learning among individuals with anxiety disorders. Additional clinical trials are currently underway, including yohimbine added to prolonged exposure for veterans with PTSD.

Propranolol

The adrenergic system is also the target of the β-adrenergic blocker propranolol, which has been used in attempts both to prevent the occurrence of PTSD following a trauma and to augment exposure therapy for PTSD. Basic research in rodents established that the blockade of β-adrenergic receptors with propranolol interferes with the reconsolidation of fear memories (e.g., Debiec & LeDoux, 2004; Przybyslawski, Roullet, & Sara, 1999; but see Muravieva & Alberini, 2010). Therefore, it is reasonable to hypothesize that the administration of propranolol may reduce the occurrence of PTSD when administered acutely and may reduce PTSD symptoms when administered in conjunction with exposure to the trauma memory.

Results from prevention trials have been mixed, with initially promising results with small samples followed by larger trials that found less salutary effects of propranolol on PTSD prevention. A nonrandomized study of propranolol use in the acute post-trauma period (Vaiva et al., 2003) found a significantly lower rate of PTSD among a group of patients who had received propranolol (1 of 11) compared to individuals who had declined to receive propranolol (3 of 8). The very small sample and nonrandom assignment to propranolol render these results difficult to interpret. A larger double-blind randomized pilot study found promising results; although there was no significant difference in PTSD scores at either the 1- or 3-month post-trauma assessment, a significantly lower number of patients who received propranolol were above (two patients) versus below (nine patients) the control group's median (Pitman et al., 2002). A subsequent RCT failed to replicate these suggestive results; there were no significant differences in PTSD symptoms between the propranolol and placebo groups at the 1-month assessment ($d = 0.17$), and PTSD rates at the 4-month follow-up were equivalent at 25% (Stein, Kerridge, Dimsdale, & Hoyt, 2007). Taken together, there is limited evidence that administration of propranolol in the acute post-trauma phase prevents the development of PTSD.

More directly relevant to the topic of this chapter is the use of propranolol to enhance the effects of exposure therapy. Tollenaar et al. (2009) found in a preclinical analog study that propranolol had a significant effect on reactions to negative emotional memories in healthy adult men. In a small ($N = 19$) RCT, individuals with PTSD were randomized to receive either propranolol or placebo following a retelling of their traumatic events. Individuals who had received propranolol showed significantly less psychophysiologic responding during script-driven imagery 1 week later. Additional study is needed to determine whether propranolol reliably enhances the effects of exposure therapy on anxiety disorders.

Methylene Blue

One of the most recent developments in the enhancement of exposure therapy is the use of methylene blue (MB), a metabolic enhancer that has been found to improve memory retention (e.g., Martinez, Jensen, Vasquez, McGuinness, & McGaugh, 1978). MB appears to facilitate memory consolidation (Wrubel, Riha, Maldonado, McCollum, & Gonzalez-Lima, 2007), which led researchers to hypothesize that it would enhance fear extinction learning. Gonzalez-Lima and Bruchey (2004) tested this hypothesis in a fear learning and extinction paradigm with rats and found that MB administration resulted in less freezing following extinction compared to a saline control condition. Additional tests showed that the efficacy of MB was related to enhanced metabolism in brain regions that have been found to support the retention of extinction learning, including the prefrontal cortex. Similar findings were reported in a study of "congenitally helpless" rats who show greater fear learning and worse fear extinction than control animals (Wrubel, Barrett, Shumake, Johnson, & Gonzalez-Lima, 2007); this strain of rats has been proposed as an animal model of PTSD, given the extinction deficits present in that disorder (e.g., Milad et al., 2008). The administration of MB resulted in significant decreases in these animals' fear responses following extinction, supporting the hypothesis that MB can remediate deficient fear extinction.

These findings from animal studies have obvious potential applications to the treatment of pathological anxiety states, including PTSD. Clinical trials are underway to test whether these promising results in animals translate to enhanced exposure therapy outcomes in humans. Conclusions regarding the clinical utility of MB await the outcomes of these trials.

Cortisol

It may seem paradoxical that cortisol, a stress hormone, could be an effective exposure enhancer. Nevertheless, a growing number of studies have shown that glucocorticoids, including cortisol, may reduce pathological fear. One of the first such studies among individuals with PTSD (Aerni et al., 2004) was motivated by the recognition that excessive fear-memory retrieval drives many of the symptoms of PTSD, and by evidence that cortisol inhibits memory retrieval (e.g., de Quervain, Roozendaal, & McGaugh, 1998; de Quervain, Roozendaal, Nitsch, McGaugh, & Hock, 2000); additionally, some studies have found that PTSD is associated with low levels of cortisol (Yehuda, 2002). A small pilot study ($N = 3$) reported that patients with PTSD who received low doses of cortisol experienced significant reductions in their PTSD symptoms; exposure therapy was not a part of their treatment (Aerni et al., 2004). A more recent study found that veterans who received hydrocortisone—a glucocorticoid—had better outcomes following exposure therapy for PTSD (Yehuda et al., 2015). Interestingly the enhanced outcomes seemed to be driven by greater retention in the hydrocortisone group. More research is needed to determine if glucocorticoid administration reliably improves treatment retention and, if so, by what mechanism.

Subsequent work in this area built on findings from basic research showing that glucocorticoids like cortisol not only disrupt the retrieval of existing memories, including fear memories, but also can strengthen the consolidation of fear extinction learning (e.g., Barrett & Gonzalez-Lima, 2004). Thus, cortisol may not only weaken the retrieval of fear associations in anxiety disorders but might also enhance consolidation of fear extinction following exposure therapy (de Quervain & Margraf, 2008), suggesting that cortisol might be a powerful enhancer of exposure-based interventions. De Quervain and colleagues have carried out multiple tests of this hypothesis and have found support for the role of cortisol in enhancing the reduction of phobic fear. In a double-blind, placebo-controlled study of individuals with social or spider phobia (N = 60), participants who received cortisol administration 1 hour prior to exposure sessions showed less fear responding during the exposures sessions (Soravia et al., 2006). Individuals with social phobia who received placebo also experienced a significant heart-rate acceleration when informed about an impending stress test, whereas individuals who received cortisol demonstrated no such acceleration. Furthermore, spider phobics who received pre-exposure cortisol reported significantly less fear in response to spiders 2 days after the final treatment session, demonstrating that the cortisol-induced fear reduction persisted. Similar results were reported by de Quervain et al. (2011) in a study of virtual reality-based exposure treatment for acrophobia. Compared to individuals who received placebo, participants who received cortisol reported less fear of heights at post-treatment and at 1 month follow-up, as well as a smaller skin conductance response to a virtual reality-based height exposure at follow-up.

Although these results are promising for the enhancement of exposure treatments for anxiety disorders, they appear to present a challenge to the activation hypothesis of emotional processing theory (Foa & Kozak, 1986). How can cortisol-induced lower subjective fear during exposure and subsequently greater fear reduction be reconciled with the theoretical prediction that activation of the fear association, as indexed by subjective and autonomic fear responses, is necessary for the successful treatment of pathological fear? This apparent contradiction may be reconciled by distinguishing between *necessary conditions* for emotional processing and *indicators* of that processing. Emotional processing theory does not require that the CS-US association be recalled, but rather that the CS element of the memory be activated. In the absence of cortisol administration, the CS-US association may be strongly activated, whereas cortisol attenuates the recall of this learned association. Thus, an individual can bring online the CS and can more readily form and consolidate competing CS-NoUS associations through the dual effects of cortisol.

BEHAVIORAL

In addition to pharmacologic manipulations aimed to enhance exposure treatments, studies with humans and nonhuman animals have revealed behavioral manipulations that may lead to refinements in exposure treatments. Monfils et al. (2009) developed a behavioral paradigm in rats called reconsolidation update that substantially enhanced the reduction of conditioned fear via fear extinction learning. This paradigm introduced a single CS trial (e.g., a tone previously paired with shock) at a specified interval prior to extinction training. This isolated presentation of the CS led to a more prolonged attenuation of fear compared to animals that received extinction training without the isolated CS. These results were replicated in rodents by Clem and Huganir (2010).

The enhanced fear extinction produced by this behavioral manipulation is believed to depend on the memory reconsolidation that follows memory retrieval. During the initial encoding of events, memories are labile and subsequently consolidate into long-term storage. When retrieved, a memory becomes structurally labile again and requires *re*consolidation in order to endure (Misanin, Miller, & Lewis, 1968; Nader, Schafe, & LeDoux, 2000). Pharmacological or behavioral manipulations that enhance the molecular mechanisms involved in reconsolidation of fear memories strengthen existing fear associations, whereas manipulations that block the reconsolidation mechanisms weaken fear associations. Researchers continue to explore the behavioral, neural, and biochemical mechanisms that underlie the reconsolidation update effect.

These findings generated considerable enthusiasm among researchers interested in translating the reconsolidation update effect to the treatment of humans with anxiety disorders. The findings suggested that a simple behavioral manipulation could significantly increase the efficacy of exposure-based interventions, without the need for medications and their common side effects. A study by Schiller et al. (2010) represented an initial step toward translation to a clinical population. They adapted the experimental paradigm used by Monfils et al. (2009) to fear-conditioned healthy humans, and they also found evidence for enhanced extinction learning and suppression of the return of fear among the group that received the pre-extinction CS.

However, subsequent studies using similar paradigms have not replicated the findings of Schiller et al. (2010); Soeter and Kindt (2011) reported, for example, that fear responding returned from day 2 (end of extinction) to day 3 (start of re-extinction trials) even after subjects had been presented with the pre-extinction CS. Clinical applications of this paradigm similarly have produced mixed results. Telch, Monfils, and colleagues (unpublished data) applied the paradigm to exposure therapy in snake and spider phobics, with promising preliminary findings. Individuals in the Prime group received a single, brief (30 sec) exposure to a spider 30 minutes prior to the rest of the exposure sessions; each subsequent exposure lasted 3 minutes. Within-session peak fear was reduced in the Prime group compared to controls; there was a trend toward decreased peak fear in the Prime group at the 30-day follow-up. In contrast, Marks and Zoellner (2014) found that an adaptation of this procedure in the context of a distressing film paradigm actually resulted in *more frequent* intrusive thoughts about the film among the group that received the CS within the "reconsolidation window." This finding presents an important caveat for the potential adaptation of this approach in the treatment of PTSD, given that intrusive memories are a cardinal symptom of this disorder and may actually be worsened by this novel approach. Each of these studies differed in various ways (e.g., length and nature of CS) that make it difficult to determine why the findings are so discrepant. Clearly more work remains to be done in this area.

If the reported positive findings hold for the treatment of anxiety disorders, they would suggest a possible refinement of emotional processing theory; although the theory does state that activation of the CS-US association and incorporation of information that is inconsistent with the existing fear structure results in decreased fear responding, the theory does not account for how the introduction of an isolated CS and activation of the fear memory leads to greater fear attenuation following subsequent fear extinction/exposure. Future updates to the theory may incorporate a recognition that the timing of CS presentation can have important effects on the reduction of pathological fear.

VIRTUAL REALITY

The advent of technologically sophisticated computers made possible the development of computer-generated exposure, commonly known as virtual reality (VR) exposure therapy. Potential advantages of VR-based exposure include being able to conduct exposure exercises to a wide range of stimuli without having to leave the therapy office and the potential to construct exposure exercises

that would be difficult and/or expensive to implement in vivo. For example, individuals with a fear of flying can confront their feared stimuli (e.g., the inside of an airport, the airplane cabin) repeatedly without the considerable time and expense required to make several actual flights, and perhaps more vividly than is possible through imaginal exposure. Similarly, individuals with social phobia can give a talk to a large virtual audience in the setting of the therapist's office.

VR exposure therapy (VRET) has been designed to treat the majority of anxiety disorders, including specific phobia, social phobia, panic disorder, and PTSD. Stimuli for specific phobia VRET can include commonly feared animals like spiders and snakes, simulated height exposures for acrophobia, and exposure to a virtual flying experience for flying phobia. The latter can include entering the airport and checking in, going through security, hearing the announcements that frequently occur in airports, walking to the gate, and sitting in the airplane from takeoff to landing (perhaps including actual airplane chairs to sit in during the exposure; Meyerbröker & Emmelkamp, 2011). Social phobia stimuli in VRET have included presenting to a virtual audience (Anderson, Rothbaum, & Hodges, 2003) while stimuli for panic disorder VRET have included virtual environments that are often avoided (e.g., buses, a shopping mall) in combination with simulated panic-related interoceptive cues (e.g., heart palpitations, tunnel or blurred vision; Botella et al., 2007).

Based on emotional processing theory, one would predict that VRET would be at least as effective as in vivo exposure, given that VRET can be tailored to activate fear memories in a safe context, thereby leading to adaptive changes in pathological fear structures. The first RCT of VRET was for acrophobia; individuals who completed VR-based graded exposure to heights experienced significant improvement across the course of 8 weeks of treatment, whereas a waiting list control group experienced no significant change in phobic symptoms (Rothbaum et al., 1995). Subsequent studies have confirmed these positive results for the treatment of other specific phobias including flying (e.g., Rothbaum, Hodges, Smith, Lee, & Price, 2000) and spiders (Garcia-Palacios, Hoffman, Carlin, Furness, & Botella, 2002), and demonstrated the efficacy of VRET for the treatment of other anxiety disorders, including social phobia (e.g., Harris, Kemmerling, & North, 2002), PTSD (e.g., Difede et al., 2007), and panic disorder (Botella et al., 2007). Meta-analyses of findings from VRET RCTs have reported large effect sizes of approximately $d = 1.1$ when comparing VRET to waiting list controls (Opriş et al., 2012; Powers & Emmelkamp, 2008). Although the earlier of these two meta-analyses reported a small significant advantage of VRET over in vivo exposure ($d = 0.35$) based on 16 studies, the later meta-analysis by Opriş et al. (2012), which included an additional seven studies, found no significant difference between the two types of exposure ($d = 0.16$ in favor of VRET). Thus, it appears that VRET is as an efficacious treatment for anxiety disorders, but it is no more effective than traditional in vivo exposure.

Although VRET is unlikely to supplant traditional exposure therapy in the treatment of anxiety disorders, it may be useful in certain cases to reduce the time and cost required for exposure exercises. Additionally, it may be useful in RCTs for anxiety disorders, allowing for more precise control of exposure parameters and standardization of exposure across participants and settings.

Telehealth: Using Technology to Broaden Delivery of Exposure Treatment

Several aspects of traditional exposure therapy represent substantial challenges to disseminating it broadly. These challenges include the intensive investment of time required of a limited number of trained exposure therapists, the expense associated with therapist time, and the lack of access to exposure-trained therapists for patients in many (particularly rural) parts of the country. Furthermore, therapy sessions often require that patients repeatedly take time off from work in order to meet with a clinician during regular business hours.

Researchers and clinicians have begun to devise novel ways to use technology to address these challenges. The label "telehealth" comprises a broad range of interventions that are delivered remotely with the assistance of technology. In this section we will focus on interventions that facilitate remote access to exposure therapy, with varying degrees of therapist involvement. This area is rapidly expanding and an exhaustive review is beyond the scope of this chapter; here we review some of the recent efforts in this literature, which rely on the telephone, computers, and the Internet. We also highlight some of the important issues involved in these applications of exposure therapy.

VIDEOCONFERENCE TREATMENT

An approach that has exploited technology in the service of treatment delivery is videoconference (e.g., Skype). Videoconferencing provides many of the same advantages of in-person therapy—real-time interaction with a therapist, ability to detect and respond to facial and vocal cues—as well as some of the limitations such as demands on the therapist's time and scheduling constraints. A significant advantage of videoconferencing over traditional psychotherapy is the ability to deliver the treatment to anyone with a high-speed Internet connection. A distinct advantage of this modality for exposure-based interventions is the ability to work with the patient "where the anxiety lives." For many exposure-based treatment protocols, therapist visits to the patient's home are standard parts of the treatment (e.g., EX/RP for OCD; Foa et al., 2012). These visits require a lot of therapist time and may translate into more expensive treatment for the patient. Through the use of videoconference, the therapist can work in real time with the patient on home-based in vivo exposures, with no time lost for travel.

Researchers have begun to examine the efficacy of exposure therapy delivered through telehealth technology. Results from a pilot study of Prolonged Exposure for PTSD delivered via videoconferencing demonstrated the feasibility and acceptability of this approach (Tuerk, Yoder, Ruggiero, Gros, & Acierno, 2010). Rate of treatment completion was similar for telehealth PE (75%) and in-person PE (83%), and reductions in PTSD and depression symptoms were comparable between the two PE delivery modes. A larger subsequent study by the same research group found that PE delivered by telehealth was effective but less so than was in-person PE; the within-group effect size for PTSD symptom reduction was $d = 1.19$ for the telehealth group and 3.00 for the in-person group (Gros, Yoder, Tuerk, Lozano, & Acierno, 2010). Positive results were also reported for videoconference treatment of PTSD by Germain, Marchand, Bouchard, Drouin, and Guay (2009). Pilot work has been conducted for videoconference-delivered exposure treatment of OCD (Himle et al., 2006; Vogel et al., 2012), social anxiety disorder (Yuen et al., 2013), and panic disorder (Bouchard et al., 2000), also with promising results. Importantly, there is evidence that a positive therapeutic alliance is possible with therapy delivered via videoconference (Bouchard et al., 2000; Himle et al., 2006).

THERAPIST-GUIDED SELF-HELP

Several treatment trials have examined the efficacy of self-help materials in conjunction with guidance from an exposure therapist. Media for self-help materials have included primarily written materials and Web sites. An advantage of Web sites is that they are widely available and, once developed, are relatively inexpensive to make available to patients; additionally, they can decrease or eliminate the need for therapist involvement and the associated cost. They do require that patients have access to a computer with the Internet, which may exclude a certain percentage of patients from accessing these treatments. An additional advantage of Internet-delivered treatment is that it can be updated quickly in order to improve the treatment, which is not as easy with print material (Carlbring & Andersson, 2006).

Trials of self-help-based exposure with therapist contact primarily have used telephone- or e-mail-based communication between patient and therapist (for a review and meta-analysis, see Cuijpers et al., 2009). The telephone offers the advantage of "live" feedback from a therapist and for immediate clarification of issues that arise in the course of treatment. It also allows for the detection of prosody, affect, and other important cues that facilitate communication and the therapeutic relationship. On the other hand, e-mail allows both therapist and patient to communicate at their convenience, and it does not require their coordinating schedules (Carlbring & Andersson, 2006).

Therapist-guided self-help studies of exposure treatments have been conducted for a range of anxiety diagnoses. Internet-based CBT plus phone calls has been found to be efficacious compared to a waiting list control for the treatment of panic disorder, with 77% of patients who received the treatment no longer meeting criteria for the disorder (Carlbring et al., 2006). Positive results have also been obtained for the treatment of PTSD (e.g., Litz, Engel, Bryant, & Papa, 2007) and social phobia (e.g., Abramowitz, Moore, Braddock, & Harrington, 2009; Carlbring et al., 2007).

Despite the efficacy of these treatments, they still require regular contact with a therapist. Additional studies have tested the efficacy of technology-based self-help treatment without the guidance of a therapist.

SELF-HELP TREATMENT WITHOUT THERAPIST GUIDANCE

Several studies have found that self-guided exposure-based treatment can be effective for treating anxiety disorders. In a large trial (N = 218) of individuals with OCD, Greist et al. (2002) reported that computer-administered EX/RP was more effective than waitlist, with 38% versus 14%, respectively, meeting treatment responder criteria. Promising results also have been found for Internet-delivered treatment for panic disorder; Klein and Richards (2001) found that 1 week of the treatment produced greater reductions in panic frequency compared to a self-monitoring control condition. However, the effect sizes tended to be small. Unguided self-help treatment has also been found to be effective for treating OCD (Tolin et al., 2007). Other self-administered treatments have not been found to be efficacious, for example, a self-help booklet for the treatment of PTSD (Ehlers et al., 2003). It is important to note that the effect sizes for self-help treatments are reliably larger when delivered with therapist guidance; a meta-analysis of self-help treatments for anxiety with versus without therapist involvement revealed a significant advantage for the former (d = 0.34; Lewis, Pearce, & Bisson, 2012; see also Newman, Szkodny, Llera, & Przeworski, 2011).

STEPPED CARE

Taken together, the results from these telehealth studies suggest that stepped-care models may offer significant advantages in providing efficacious and cost-effective treatment, as some researchers have suggested (e.g., Tolin, Diefenbach, & Gilliam, 2011). The first step in care might involve the least expensive and most accessible treatment, such as self-directed care delivered via the Internet without therapist guidance. Individuals who do not respond to this treatment modality may then receive the next level of care, such as Internet-based treatment with regular phone calls or e-mail communication with a therapist, followed by in-person, one-on-one treatment for individuals who are not helped by the first two steps. Advantages of this approach include trying less expensive and generally more convenient treatment options first before moving to more expensive and labor-intensive treatments. As a result, clinician availability is maximized by reserving it for those individuals who may most need the intensive one-on-one efforts of a therapist. Importantly, preliminary studies of this approach have shown that stepped-care results in significant cost reductions without sacrificing efficacy or patient satisfaction (Tolin et al., 2011).

Conclusion

To summarize, exposure-based interventions include imaginal, in vivo, and interoceptive exposures. Treatments based around these interventions have been found to be highly efficacious in the treatment of anxiety disorders. Despite initial enthusiasm for the possibility of augmenting exposure-based interventions with psychopharmacological treatments, these combination treatments generally are no more effective than exposure therapy alone. Translational approaches that aim to enhance the effectiveness of exposure have shown initial promise. Challenges remain to disseminate these treatments broadly to the individuals who need them, and ongoing efforts to utilize technology in the service of treatment dissemination are addressing these challenges.

References

Abramowitz, J. S., Moore, E. L., Braddock, A. E., & Harrington, D. L. (2009). Self-help cognitive-behavioral therapy with minimal therapist contact for social phobia: A controlled trial. *Journal of Behavioral Therapy and Experimental Psychiatry, 40,* 98–105. doi:10.1016/j.jbtep.2008.04.004

Aerni, A., Traber, R., Hock, C., Roozendaal, B., Schelling, G., Papassotiropoulos, A., . . . de Quervain, D. J-F. (2004). Low-dose cortisol for symptoms of posttraumatic stress disorder. *American Journal of Psychiatry, 161,* 1488–1490.

American Psychiatric Association. (2013). *Diagnostic and statistical manual of mental disorders* (5th ed.). Washington, DC: Author.

Anderson, P., Rothbaum, B. O., & Hodges, L. F. (2003). Virtual reality exposure in the treatment of social anxiety. *Cognitive and Behavioral Practice, 10,* 240–247. doi:10.1016/S1077-7229(03)80036-6

Barlow, D. H., Gorman, J. M., Shear, M. K., & Woods, S. W. (2000). Cognitive-behavioral therapy, imipramine, or their combination for panic disorder: A randomized controlled trial. *Journal of the American Medical Association, 283,* 2529–2536.

Barrett, D. B., & Gonzalez-Lima, F. (2004). Behavioral effects of metyrapone on Pavlovian extinction. *Neuroscience Letters, 371,* 91–96.

Blanco, C., Heimberg, R. G., Schneier, F. R., Fresco, D. M., Chen, H., . . . Liebowitz, M. R. (2010). A placebo-controlled trial of phenelzine, cognitive behavioral group therapy, and their combination for social anxiety disorder. *Archives of General Psychiatry, 67,* 286–295.

Blomhoff, S., Haug, T. T., Hellström, K., Holme, I., Humble, M., Madsbu, H. P., & Wold, J. E. (2001). Randomised controlled general practice trial of sertraline, exposure therapy and combined treatment in generalized social phobia. *British Journal of Psychiatry, 179,* 23–30.

Botella, C., García-Palacios, A., Villa, H., Baños, R. M., Quero, S., Alcañiz, M., & Riva, G. (2007). Virtual reality exposure in the treatment of panic disorder and agoraphobia: A controlled study. *Clinical Psychology and Psychotherapy, 14,* 164–175. doi:10.1002/cpp.524

Bouchard, S., Payeur, R., Rivard, V., Allard, M., Paquin, B., Renaud, P., & Goyer, L. (2000). Cognitive behavior therapy for panic disorder with agoraphobia in videoconference: Preliminary results. *Cyberpsychology and Behavior, 3,* 999–1007.

Cain, C. K., Blouin, A. M., & Barad, M. (2004). Adrenergic transmission facilitates extinction of conditional fear in mice. *Learning and Memory, 11,* 179–187. doi:10.1101/lm.71504

Carlbring, P., & Andersson, G. (2006). Internet and psychological treatment: How well can they be combined? *Computers in Human Behavior, 22,* 545–553. doi:10.1016/j.chb.2004.10.009

Carlbring, P., Bohman, S., Brunt, S., Buhrman, M., Westling, B. E., Ekselius, L., & Andersson, G. (2006). Remote treatment of panic disorder: A randomized trial of internet-based cognitive behavior therapy supplemented with telephone calls. *American Journal of Psychiatry, 163,* 2119–2125.

Carlbring, P., Gunnarsdottir, M., Hedensjö, L., Andersson, G., Ekselius, L., & Furmark, T. (2007). Treatment of social phobia: Randomised trial of internet-delivered cognitive-behavioural therapy with telephone support. *British Journal of Psychiatry, 190,* 123–128. doi:10.1192/bjp.bp.105.020107

Charney, D. S., Heninger, G. R., & Breier, A. (1984). Noradrenergic function in panic anxiety. *Archives of General Psychiatry, 41,* 751–763.

Chasson, G. S., Buhlmann, U., Tolin, D. F., Rao, S. R., Reese, H. E., Rowley, T., . . . Wilhelm, S. (2010). Need for speed: Evaluating slopes of OCD recovery in behavior therapy enhanced with D-cycloserine. *Behaviour Research and Therapy, 48,* 675–679. doi:10.1016/j.brat.2010.03.007

Clark, D. B., & Agras, W. S. (1991). The assessment and treatment of performance anxiety in musicians. *American Journal of Psychiatry, 148,* 598–605.

Clark, D. M., Ehlers, A., Hackmann, A., McManus, F., Fennell, M., Grey, N., . . . Wild, J. (2006). Cognitive therapy versus exposure and applied relaxation in social phobia: A randomized controlled trial. *Journal of Consulting and Clinical Psychology, 74,* 568–578. doi:10.1037/0022-006X.74.3.568

Clem, R. L., & Huganir, R. L. (2010). Calcium-permeable AMPA receptor dynamics mediate fear memory erasure. *Science, 330,* 1108–1112.

Cohen, J. (1988). *Statistical power analysis for the behavioral sciences* (2nd ed.). Hillsdale: Lawrence Erlbaum Associates.

Coldwell, S. E., Wilhelm, F. H., Milgrom, P., Prall, C. W., Getz, T., Spadafora, A., . . . Ramsay, D. S. (2007). Combining alprazolam with systematic desensitization therapy for dental injection phobia. *Journal of Anxiety Disorders, 21,* 871–887. doi:10.1016/j.janxdis.2007.01.001

Cottraux, J., Mollard, E., Bouvard, M., Marks, I., Sluys, M., Nury, A. M., . . . Cialdella, P. (1990). A controlled study of fluvoxamine and exposure in obsessive-compulsive disorder. *International Clinical Psychopharmacology, 5,* 17–30. doi:10.1097/00004850-199001000-00002

Cottraux, J., Note, I. D., Cungi, C., Legeron, P., Heim, F., Chneiweiss, L., . . . Bouvard, M. (1995). A controlled study of cognitive behavior therapy with buspirone or placebo in panic disorder with agoraphobia. *British Journal of Psychiatry, 167,* 635–641. doi:10.1192/bjp.167.5.635

Cuijpers, P., Marks, I., van Straten, A-M., Cavanagh, K., Gega, L., & Andersson, G. (2009). Computer-aided psychotherapy for anxiety disorders: A meta-analytic review. *Cognitive Behaviour Therapy, 38,* 66–82.

Davidson, J. R. T., Foa, E. B., Huppert, J. D., Keefe, F. J., Franklin, M. E., Compton, J. S., . . . Gadde, K. M. (2004). Fluoxetine, comprehensive cognitive behavioral therapy, and placebo in generalized social phobia. *Archives of General Psychiatry, 61,* 1005–1013.

de Quervain, D. J-F., Bentz, D., Michael, T., Bolt, O. C., Wiederhold, B. K., Margraf, J., & Wilhelm, F. H. (2011). Glucocorticoids enhance extinction-based psychotherapy. *Proceedings of the National Academy of Sciences USA, 108*(16), 6621–6625.

de Quervain, D. J-F., & Margraf, J. (2008). Glucocorticoids for the treatment of post-traumatic stress disorder and phobias: A novel therapeutic approach. *European Journal of Pharmacology, 583*, 365–371.

de Quervain, D. J-F., Roozendaal, B., & McGaugh, J. L. (1998). Stress and glucocorticoids impair retrieval of long-term spatial memory. *Nature, 394*, 787–790. doi:10.1038/29542

de Quervain, D. J-F., Roozendaal, B., Nitsch, R. M., McGaugh, J. L., & Hock, C. (2000). Acute cortisone administration impairs retrieval of long-term declarative memory in humans. *Nature Neuroscience, 3*, 313–314.

Dębiec, J., & LeDoux, J. E. (2004). Disruption of reconsolidation but not consolidation of auditory fear conditioning by noradrenergic blockade in the amygdala. *Neuroscience, 129*, 267–272. doi:10.1016/j.neuroscience.2004.08.018

Difede, J., Cukor, J., Jayasinghe, N., Patt, I., Jedel, S., Spielman, L., . . . Hoffman, H. G. (2007). Virtual reality exposure therapy for the treatment of posttraumatic stress disorder following September 11, 2001. *Journal of Clinical Psychiatry, 68*, 1639–1647. doi:10.4088/JCP.v68n1102

Ehlers, A., Clark, D. M., Hackmann, A., McManus, F., Fennell, M., Herbert, C., & Mayou, R. (2003). A randomized controlled trial of cognitive therapy, a self-help booklet, and repeated assessments as early interventions for posttraumatic stress disorder. *Archives of General Psychiatry, 60*, 1024–1032. doi:10.1001/archpsyc.60.10.1024

Foa, E. B., Hembree, E. A., Cahill, S. P., Rauch, S. A. M., Riggs, D. S., Feeny, N. C., & Yadin, E. (2005). Randomized trial of prolonged exposure for posttraumatic stress disorder with and without cognitive restructuring: Outcome at academic and community clinics. *Journal of Consulting and Clinical Psychology, 73*, 953–964. doi:10.1037/0022-006X.73.5.953

Foa, E. B., Hembree, E. A., & Rothbaum, B. O. (2007). *Prolonged exposure therapy for PTSD: Emotional processing of traumatic experiences: Therapist guide.* New York: Oxford University Press.

Foa, E. B., Huppert, J. D., & Cahill, S. P. (2006). Emotional processing theory: An update. In B. O. Rothbaum (Ed.), *Pathological anxiety: Emotional processing in etiology and treatment* (pp. 3–24). New York: Guilford Press.

Foa, E. B., & Kozak, M. J. (1986). Emotional processing of fear: Exposure to corrective information. *Psychological Bulletin, 99*, 20–35.

Foa, E. B., Liebowitz, M. R., Kozak, M. J., Davies, S., Campeas, R., Franklin, M. E., . . . Tu, X. (2005). Randomized, placebo-controlled trial of exposure and ritual prevention, clomipramine, and their combination in the treatment of obsessive-compulsive disorder. *American Journal of Psychiatry, 162*, 151–161.

Foa, E. B., Yadin, E., & Lichner, T. K. (2012). *Exposure and response (ritual) prevention for obsessive-compulsive disorder: Therapist guide.* New York: Oxford University Press.

Franklin, M. E., Abramowitz, J. S., Bux, D. A., Jr., Zoellner, L. A., & Feeny, N. C. (2002). Cognitive-behavioral therapy with and without medication in the treatment of obsessive-compulsive disorder. *Professional Psychology: Research and Practice, 33*, 162–168.

Furukawa, T., Watanabe, N., & Churchill, R. (2006). Psychotherapy plus antidepressant for panic disorder with or without agoraphobia: Systematic review. *British Journal of Psychiatry, 188*, 305–312. doi:10.1192/bjp.188.4.305

Garcia-Palacios, A., Hoffman, H., Carlin, A., Furness, T. A., III, & Botella, C. (2002). Virtual reality in the treatment of spider phobia: A controlled study. *Behaviour Research and Therapy, 40*(9), 983–993.

Germain, V., Marchand, A., Bouchard, S., Drouin, M. S., & Guay, S. (2009). Effectiveness of cognitive behavioural therapy administered by videoconference for posttraumatic stress disorder. *Cognitive Behavioral Therapy, 38*, 42–53. doi: 10.1080/16506070802473494

Goldstein, A. J., & Chambless, D. L. (1978). A reanalysis of agoraphobia. *Behavior Therapy, 9*, 47–59. doi:10.1016/S0005-7894(78)80053-7

Gonzalez-Lima, F., & Bruchey, A. K. (2004). Extinction memory improvement by the metabolic enhancer methylene blue. *Learning and Memory, 11*(5), 633–640.

Greist, J., Marks, I. M., Baer, L., Kobak, K. A., Wenzel, K. W., Hirsch, M. J., . . . Clary, C. M. (2002). Behavior therapy for obsessive-compulsive disorder guided by a computer or by a clinician compared with relaxation as a control. *Journal of Clinical Psychiatry, 63*, 138–145.

Gros, D. F., Yoder, M., Tuerk, P. W., Lozano, B. E., & Acierno, R. (2010). Exposure therapy for PTSD delivered to veterans via telehealth: Predictors of treatment completion and outcome and comparison to treatment delivered in person. *Behavior Therapy, 42*, 276–283.

Guastella, A. J., Richardson, R., Lovibond, P. F., Rapee, R. M., Gaston, J. E., Mitchell, P., & Dadds, M. R. (2008). A randomized controlled trial of D-cycloserine enhancement of exposure therapy for social anxiety disorder. *Biological Psychiatry, 63*, 544–549. doi:10.1016/j.biopsych.2007.11.011

Harris, S. R., Kemmerling, R. L., & North, M. M. (2002). Brief virtual reality therapy for public speaking anxiety. *Cyberpsychology and Behavior, 5*, 543–550. doi:10.1089/109493102321018187

Haug, T. T., Blomhoff, S., Hellström, K., Holme, I., Humble, M., Madsbu, H. P., & Wold, J. E. (2003). Exposure therapy and sertraline in social phobia: 1-year follow-up of a randomized controlled trial. *British Journal of Psychiatry, 182*, 312–318. doi:10.1192/bjp.02.229

Himle, J. A., Fischer, D. J., Muroff, J. R., Van Etten, M. L., Lokers, L. M., Abelson, J. L., & Hanna, G. L. (2006). Videoconferencing-based cognitive-behavioral therapy for obsessive-compulsive disorder. *Behaviour Research and Therapy, 44*, 1821–1826. doi:10.1016/j.brat.2005.12.010

Hofmann, S. G., Meuret, A. E., Smits, J. A., Simon, N. M., Pollack, M. H., Eisenmenger, K., . . . Otto, M. W. (2006). Augmentation of exposure therapy with D-cycloserine for social anxiety disorder. *Archives of General Psychiatry, 63*, 298–304.

Hofmann, S. G., & Smits, J. A. J. (2008). Cognitive-behavioral therapy for adult anxiety disorders: A meta-analysis of randomized placebo-controlled trials. *Journal of Clinical Psychiatry, 69*, 621–632.

Hohagen, F., Winkelmann, G., Rasche-Räucle, H., Hand, I., König, A., Münchau, N., . . . Berger, M. (1998). Combination of behaviour therapy with fluvoxamine in comparison with behaviour therapy and placebo: Results of a multicentre study. *British Journal of Psychiatry, 173*(Suppl 35), 71–78.

Klein, B., & Richards, J. C. (2001). A brief Internet-based treatment for panic disorder. *Behavioural and Cognitive Psychotherapy, 29,* 113–117. doi:10.1017/S1352465801001138

Kushner, M., Kim, S. W., Donahue, C., Thuras, P., Adson, D., Kotlyar, M., ... Foa, E. B. (2007). D-cycloserine augmented exposure therapy for obsessive-compulsive disorder. *Biological Psychiatry, 62,* 835–838.

Lewis, C., Pearce, J., & Bisson, J. I. (2012). Efficacy, cost-effectiveness and acceptability of self-help interventions for anxiety disorders: Systematic review. *British Journal of Psychiatry, 200,* 15–21. doi:10.1192/bjp.bp.110.084756

Litz, B. T., Engel, C. C., Bryant, R. A., & Papa, A. (2007). A randomized, controlled proof-of-concept trial of an Internet-based, therapist-assisted self-management treatment for posttraumatic stress disorder. *American Journal of Psychiatry, 164,* 1676–1683. doi:10.1176/appi.ajp.2007.06122057

Marks, I. M., Swinson, R. P., Basoglu, M., Kuch, K., Noshirvani, H., O'Sullivan, G., ... Sengun, S. (1993). Alprazolam and exposure alone and combined in panic disorder with agoraphobia: A controlled study in London and Toronto. *British Journal of Psychiatry, 162,* 776–787. doi:10.1192/bjp.162.6.776

Marks, E. H., & Zoellner, L. A. (2014). Attenuating fearful memories: Effect of cued extinction on intrusions. *Emotion, 14,* 1143–1154. doi:10.1037/a0037862

Martinez, J. L., Jr., Jensen, R. A., Vasquez, B. J., McGuinness, T., & McGaugh, J. L. (1978). Methylene blue alters retention of inhibitory avoidance responses. *Physiological Psychology, 6,* 387–390.

McManus, F., Sacadura, C., & Clark, D. M. (2008). Why social anxiety persists: An experimental investigation of the role of safety behaviours as a maintaining factor. *Journal of Behavior Therapy and Experimental Psychiatry, 39,* 147–161. doi:10.1016/j.jbtep.2006.12.002

McGuire, J. F., Lewin, A. B., & Storch, E. A. (2014). Enhancing exposure therapy for anxiety disorders, obsessive-compulsive disorder and post-traumatic stress disorder. *Expert Review of Neurotherapeutics, 14,* 893–910. doi:10.1586/14737175.2014.934677

Meyerbröker, K., & Emmelkamp, P. M. G. (2011). Virtual reality exposure therapy for anxiety disorders: The state of the art. In S. Brahham & L. C. Jain (Eds.), *Advanced computational intelligence paradigms in healthcare 6: Virtual reality in psychotherapy, rehabilitation, and assessment* (pp. 47–62). Berlin: Springer-Verlag. doi:10.1007/978-3-642-17824-5_4

Meyerbroeker, K., Powers, M. B., van Stegeren, A., & Emmelkamp, P. M. G. (2012). Does yohimbine hydrochloride facilitate fear extinction in virtual reality treatment of fear of flying? A randomized placebo-controlled trial. *Psychotherapy and Psychosomatics, 81,* 29–37. doi:10.1159/000329454

Milad, M. R., Orr, S. P., Laskoa, N. B., Chang, Y., Rauch, S. L., & Pitman, R. K. (2008). Presence and acquired origin of reduced recall for fear extinction in PTSD: Results of a twin study. *Journal of Psychiatric Research, 42,* 515–520. doi:10.1016/j.jpsychires.2008.01.017

Misanin, J. R., Miller, R. R., & Lewis, D. J. (1968). Retrograde amnesia produced by electroconvulsive shock after reactivation of a consolidated memory trace. *Science, 160,* 554–555. doi:10.1126/science.160.3827.554

Mitte, K. (2005). Meta-analysis of cognitive-behavioral treatments for generalized anxiety disorder: A comparison with pharmacotherapy. *Psychological Bulletin, 131,* 785–795.

Monfils, M-H., Cowansage, K. K., Klann, E., & Ledoux, J. E. (2009). Extinction-reconsolidation boundaries: Key to persistent attenuation of fear memories. *Science, 324*(5929), 951–955.

Morris, R. W., & Bouton, M. E. (2007). The effect of yohimbine on the extinction of conditioned fear: A role for context. *Behavioral Neuroscience, 121,* 501–514.

Muravieva, E. V., & Alberini, C. M. (2010). Limited efficacy of propranolol on the reconsolidation of fear memories. *Learning and Memory, 17,* 306–313. doi:10.1101/lm.1794710

Nader, K., Schafe, G. E., & LeDoux, J. E. (2000). The labile nature of consolidation theory. *Nature Reviews Neuroscience, 1,* 216–220.

Newman, M. G., Szkodny, L. E., Llera, S. J., & Przeworski, A. (2011). A review of technology-assisted self-help and minimal contact therapies for anxiety and depression: Is human contact necessary for therapeutic efficacy? *Clinical Psychology Review, 31,* 89–103. doi: 10.1016/j.cpr.2010.09.008

Norberg, M. M., Krystal, J. H., & Tolin, D. F. (2008). A meta-analysis of D-cycloserine and the facilitation of fear extinction and exposure therapy. *Biological Psychiatry, 63*(12), 1118–1126.

Opriş, D., Pineta, S., García-Palacios, A., Botella, C., Szamosközi, S., & David, D. (2012). Virtual reality exposure therapy in anxiety disorders: A quantitative meta-analysis. *Depression and Anxiety, 25,* 89–93. doi:10.1002/da.20910

Öst, L-G. (1989). One-session treatment for specific phobias. *Behaviour Research and Therapy, 27,* 1–7. doi:10.1016/0005-7967(89)90113-7

Öst, L-G., Svensson, L., Hellström, K., & Lindwall, R. (2001). One-session treatment of specific phobias in youths: A randomized clinical trial. *Journal of Consulting and Clinical Psychology, 69,* 814–824.

Otto, M. W., McHugh, R. K., & Kantak, K. M. (2010). Combined pharmacotherapy and cognitive-behavioral therapy for anxiety disorders: Medication effects, glucocorticoids, and attenuated treatment outcomes. *Clinical Psychology: Science and Practice, 17,* 91–103. doi:10.1111/j.1468-2850.2010.01198.x

Otto, M. W., Tolin, D. F., Simon, N. M., Pearlson, G. D., Basden, S., Meunier, S. A., ... Pollack, M. H. (2010). Efficacy of D-cycloserine for enhancing response to cognitive-behavior therapy for panic disorder. *Biological Psychiatry, 67,* 365–370.

Overton, D. A. (1985). Contextual stimulus effects of drugs and internal states. In P. D. Balsam & A. Tomie (Eds.), *Context and learning* (pp. 357–384). Hillsdale, NJ: Erlbaum.

Parnas, A. S., Weber, M., & Richardson, R. (2005). Effects of multiple exposures to D-cycloserine on extinction of conditioned fear in rats. *Neurobiology of Learning and Memory, 83,* 224–231.

Pitman, R. K., Sanders, K. M., Zusman, R. M., Healy, A. R., Cheema, F., Lasko, N. B., & Orr, S. P. (2002) Pilot study of secondary prevention of posttraumatic stress disorder with propranolol. *Biological Psychiatry, 51,* 189–192.

Powers, M. B., & Emmelkamp, P. M. G. (2008). Virtual reality exposure therapy for anxiety disorders: A meta-analysis. *Journal of Anxiety Disorders, 22,* 561–569. doi:10.1016/j.janxdis.2007.04.006

Powers, M. B., Halpern, J. M., Ferenschak, M. P., Gillihan, S. J., & Foa, E. B. (2010). A meta-analytic review of prolonged exposure for posttraumatic stress disorder. *Clinical Psychology Review, 30*, 635–641. doi:10.1016/j.cpr.2010.04.007

Powers, M. B., Smits, J. A. J., Otto, M. W., Sanders, C., & Emmelkamp, P. M. G. (2009). Facilitation of fear extinction in phobic participants with a novel cognitive enhancer: A randomized placebo controlled trial of yohimbine augmentation. *Journal of Anxiety Disorders, 23*, 350–356.

Prasko, J., Dockery, C., Horácek, J., Houbová, P., Kosová, J., Klaschka, J., . . . Höschl, C. (2006). Moclobemide and cognitive behavioral therapy in the treatment of social phobia. A six-month controlled study and 24 months follow up. *Neuroendocrinology Letters, 27*, 473–481.

Przybyslawski, J., Roullet, P., & Sara, S. J. (1999). Attenuation of emotional and nonemotional memories after their reactivation: Role of β adrenergic receptors. *Journal of Neuroscience, 19*, 6623–6628.

Ressler, K. J., Rothbaum, B. O., Tannenbaum, L., Anderson, P., Graap, K., Zimand, E., . . . Davis, M. (2004). Cognitive enhancers as adjuncts to psychotherapy: Use of D-cycloserine in phobic individuals to facilitate extinction of fear. *Archives of General Psychiatry, 61*, 1136–1144.

Rosa-Alcázar, A. I., Sánchez-Mecab, J., Gómez-Conesac, A., & Marín-Martínez, F. (2008). Psychological treatment of obsessive-compulsive disorder: A meta-analysis. *Clinical Psychology Review, 28*, 1310–1325. doi:10.1016/j.cpr.2008.07.001

Rothbaum, B. O., Hodges, L. F., Kooper, R., Opdyke, D., Williford, J. S., & North, M. (1995). Effectiveness of computer-generated (virtual reality) graded exposure in the treatment of acrophobia. *American Journal of Psychiatry, 152*, 626–628.

Rothbaum, B. O., Hodges, L., Smith, S., Lee, J. H., & Price, L. (2000). A controlled study of virtual reality exposure therapy for the fear of flying. *Journal of Consulting and Clinical Psychology, 68*, 1020–1026. doi:10.1037/0022-006X.68.6.1020

Schiller, D., Monfils, M-H., Raio, C. M., Johnson, D. C., Ledoux, J. E., & Phelps, E. A. (2010). Preventing the return of fear in humans using reconsolidation update mechanisms. *Nature, 463*, 49–53.

Shafran, R., Thordarson, M. A., & Rachman, S. (1996). Thought-action fusion in obsessive compulsive disorder. *Journal of Anxiety Disorders, 10*, 379–391. doi:10.1016/0887-6185(96)00018-7

Siegmund, A., Golfels, F., Finck, C., Halisch, A., Räth, D., Plag, J., & Ströhle, A. (2011). D-cycloserine does not improve but might slightly speed up the outcome of in-vivo exposure therapy in patients with severe agoraphobia and panic disorder in a randomized double blind clinical trial. *Journal of Psychiatry Research, 45*, 1042–1047. doi:10.1016/j.jpsychires.2011.01.020

Smits, J. A. J., Rosenfield, D., Davis, M. L., Julian, K., Handelsman, P. R., Otto, M. W., . . . Powers, M. B. (2014). Yohimbine enhancement of exposure therapy for social anxiety disorder: A randomized controlled trial. *Biological Psychiatry, 75*, 840–846.

Soeter, M., & Kindt, M. (2011). Disrupting reconsolidation: Pharmacological and behavioral manipulations. *Learning and Memory, 18*, 357–366.

Soravia, L., Heinrichs, M., Aerni, A., Maroni, C., Schelling, G., Ehlert, U., . . . de Quervain, D. J-F. (2006). Glucocorticoids reduce phobic fear in humans. *Proceedings of the National Academy of Sciences USA, 103*, 5585–5590. doi:10.1073/pnas.0509184103

Stein, M. B., Kerridge, C., Dimsdale, J. E., & Hoyt, D. B. (2007). Pharmacotherapy to prevent PTSD: Results from a randomized controlled proof-of-concept trial in physically injured patients. *Journal of Traumatic Stress, 20*, 923–932. doi:10.1002/jts.20270

Stewart, R. E., & Chambless, D. L. (2009). Cognitive-behavioral therapy for adult anxiety disorders in clinical practice: A meta-analysis of effectiveness studies. *Journal of Consulting and Clinical Psychology, 77*, 595–606. doi:10.1037/a0016032

Tolin, D. F., Diefenbach, G. J., & Gilliam, C. M. (2011). Stepped care versus standard cognitive–behavioral therapy for obsessive-compulsive disorder: A preliminary study of efficacy and costs. *Depression and Anxiety, 28*, 314–323. doi: 10.1002/da.20804

Tolin, D. F., Hannan, S., Maltby, N., Diefenbach, G. J., Worhunsky, P., & Brady, R. E. (2007). A randomized controlled trial of self-directed versus therapist-directed cognitive-behavioral therapy for obsessive-compulsive disorder patients with prior medication trials. *Behavior Therapy, 38*, 179–191.

Tollenaar, M. S., Elzinga, B. M., Spinhoven, P., & Everaerd, W. (2009). Psychophysiological responding to emotional memories in healthy young men after cortisol and propranolol administration. *Psychopharmacology, 203*, 793–803.

Tuerk, P. W., Yoder, M., Ruggiero, K. J., Gros, D. F., & Acierno, R. (2010). A pilot study of prolonged exposure therapy for posttraumatic stress disorder delivered via telehealth technology. *Journal of Traumatic Stress, 23*, 116–123. doi: 10.1002/jts.20494

Vaiva, G., Ducrocq, F., Jezequel, K., Averland, B., Lestavel, P., Brunet, A., & Marmar, C. R. (2003). Immediate treatment with propranolol decreases posttraumatic stress disorder two months after trauma. *Biological Psychiatry, 54*, 947–949.

Van Apeldoorn, F. J., Van Hout, W. J. P. J., Mersch, P. P. A., Huisman, M., Slaap, B. R., Hale, W. W., III, . . . Den Boer, J. A. (2008). Is a combined therapy more effective than either CBT or SSRI alone? Results of a multicenter trial on panic disorder with or without agoraphobia. *Acta Psychiatrica Scandinavica, 117*, 260–270.

Van Balkom, A. J. L. M., Barker, A., Spinhoven, P., Blaauw, B. M. J. W., Smeenk, S., & Ruesink, B. (1997). A meta-analysis of the treatment of panic disorder with or without agoraphobia: A comparison of psychopharmacological, cognitive-behavioral, and combination treatments. *Journal of Nervous and Mental Disease, 185*, 510–516.

Vogel, P. A., Launes, G., Moen, E. M., Solem, S., Hansen, B., Haland, A. T., & Himle, J. A. (2012). Videoconference- and cell phone-based cognitive-behavioral therapy of obsessive-compulsive disorder: A case series. *Journal of Anxiety Disorders, 26*, 158–164.

Walker, D. L., Ressler, K. J., Lu, K-T., & Davis, M. (2002). Facilitation of conditioned fear extinction by systemic administration or intra-amygdala infusions of D-cycloserine assessed with fear-potentiated startle in rats. *Journal of Neuroscience, 22*, 2343–2351.

Wilhelm, S., Buhlmann, U., Tolin, D., Meunier, S. A., Pearlson, G. D., Reese, H. E., . . . Rauch, S. L. (2008). Augmentation of behavior therapy with D-cycloserine for obsessive-compulsive disorder. *American Journal of Psychiatry, 165*, 335–341.

Wrubel, K. M., Barrett, D., Shumake, J., Johnson, S. E., & Gonzalez-Lima, F. (2007). Methylene blue facilitates the extinction of fear in an animal model of susceptibility to learned helplessness. *Neurobiology of Learning and Memory, 87,* 209–217.

Wrubel, K. M., Riha, P. D., Maldonado, M. A., McCollum, D., & Gonzalez-Lima, F. (2007). The brain metabolic enhancer methylene blue improves discrimination learning in rats. *Pharmacology Biochemistry and Behavior, 86,* 712–717.

Yehuda, R. (2002). Post-traumatic stress disorder. *New England Journal of Medicine, 346,* 108–114.

Yehuda, R., Bierera, L. M., Pratchetta, L. C., Lehrner, A., Kocha, E. C., Van Manena, J. A., . . . Hildebrant, T. (2015). Cortisol augmentation of a psychological treatment for warfighters with posttraumatic stress disorder: Randomized trial showing improved treatment retention and outcome. *Psychoneuroendocrinology, 51,* 589–597.

Yuen, E. K., Herbert, J. D., Forman, E. M., Goetter, E. M., Juarascio, A. S., Rabind, S., . . . Bouchard, S. (2013). Acceptance based behavior therapy for social anxiety disorder through videoconferencing. *Journal of Anxiety Disorders, 27,* 389–397.

Cognitive Restructuring/Cognitive Therapy

Cory F. Newman

Abstract

The techniques that comprise cognitive restructuring are central to the practice of cognitive therapy, and they are a key component of the skills that clients learn in order to help themselves think in more hopeful, constructive ways. Clients learn to self-assess their cognitive biases and dysfunction in terms of *processes* (e.g., all-or-none thinking, disqualifying the positive, hopelessness) and *contents* (e.g., at the levels of automatic thoughts, intermediate beliefs, and schemas). Five chief methods of cognitive restructuring are reviewed: (1) rational responding, (2) the downward arrow, (3) role playing, (4) behavioral experiments, and (5) guided imagery. Additionally, the therapeutic relationship serves as fertile ground on which the clients may ascertain and modify their most common interpersonal misperceptions. The empirical status of cognitive therapy is reviewed across a wide range of clinical problems, and with regard to maintenance. Promising new applications of cognitive restructuring are also described, along with the importance of therapist self-reflection.

Key Words: rational responding, automatic thoughts, beliefs, schemas, homework, imagery, therapeutic relationship, prevention, dissemination, self-reflection

This chapter will focus largely on the area of cognitive-behavioral interventions known as "cognitive restructuring," also described by terms such as "rational responding" and "schema modification." This is the area of interest within the broader scope of cognitive-behavioral therapy approaches (CBT) that is most associated with the development of *cognitive therapy* as described and advanced by Aaron T. Beck and his associates (e.g., Beck, 1976; Beck, Freeman, Davis, & Associates, 2004; Beck, Rush, Shaw, & Emery, 1979; Beck, 2011; Clark, Beck, & Alford, 1999). Although the terms "cognitive therapy" and "CBT" are now often used interchangeably, and although it would be impractical and artificial to explicate the essentials of cognitive restructuring without drawing on CBT-related methods described elsewhere in this volume (e.g., behavioral activation, contemporary problem solving, relapse prevention), the present chapter will place special emphasis on interventions where the chief goals are to modify clients' problematic ways of thinking about themselves, their world, and their future (the "cognitive triad," see Beck, 1976).

The methods that comprise cognitive restructuring are first presented, demonstrated, and taught to clients by their therapists. Gradually, through a process of asking questions and assigning homework, cognitive therapists guide and nurture their clients in learning to make use of these techniques on their own, so that they attain greater self-efficacy in monitoring, modifying, and evaluating the functionality of their own thinking styles. Cognitive therapists teach clients a set of skills to think more flexibly (e.g., with fewer rigid, stereotyped ways of viewing situations), more objectively (e.g., less biased against themselves), more hopefully (e.g., less likely to experience despair), and with better problem-solving skills (i.e., not lapsing into helplessness in the face of stressors), taking into account the clients' learning histories that may have hindered the development of these psychological skills. An initial step in teaching the cognitive model to clients is simply to explain the important role that thinking plays in their emotional and behavioral functioning. For example, the therapist may say:

> In this treatment we're going to pay special attention to your thoughts, because a lot of research has demonstrated that how we think affects the way we feel, and it also influences what we do. By learning how to examine your thoughts, you will be in a better position to determine if there is a more hopeful and constructive way to think about yourself and whatever situation you are facing. This process can help you to improve your mood and general functioning.

Therapists go on to explain the phenomenon known as "automatic thoughts," which are spontaneous thoughts that arise without effort, and that tend to be taken at face value unless a person reflects upon them. These automatic thoughts can help people to size up situations quickly and efficiently; however, they can be problematic if they are erroneous, thus leading people to arrive at faulty conclusions, complete with emotions and actions that miss the mark and lead to more distress.

To ameliorate this problem, cognitive therapists teach their clients to engage in *metacognitive tasks* so that they can "think about their thinking" with a greater sense of objectivity. Stated another way, one of the chief goals of cognitive therapy is to teach clients to think like empiricists—to wit, to be social scientists about themselves, rather than to feel like helpless victims of their conditions. When clients learn to self-monitor their moods, behaviors, cognitions, and other processes in their lives, they achieve multiple gains, including a greater sense of personal empowerment, improved observational skills, reduced impulsivity, and an ability to see the "bigger picture" (looking at more data over longer periods of time).

Any discussion about the methods of cognitive restructuring begs the fundamental question, "What are the characteristics of the cognitions we are trying to restructure?" This question will be addressed in more detail later, but we may start by saying that therapists endeavor to assist clients in identifying and modifying both the *contents* and the *processes* of their thinking style that (1) seem to produce unnecessary levels of helplessness and hopelessness (as in the case of depression), (2) cause clients to avoid experiences that they would otherwise benefit from approaching and experiencing (as in the case of many anxiety disorders), (3) represent significantly flawed reality testing (as in mania, psychotic disorders, body dysmorphic disorder, obsessive-compulsive disorder, and related disorders), and that (4) interfere with healthy, constructive problem solving. The *content* of the clients' thinking is in regard to the question of *what* the clients are thinking, while the *process* of the clients' thinking pertains to the question of *how* the clients arrive at their hypotheses and conclusions. Cognitive therapists help their distressed clients make changes in both domains, such that the substance of their thinking is richer, more diverse, more hopeful, and less biased, and the manner in which they reason results in more functional behavior and a higher quality of emotional living.

Maladaptive Information Processing

A fundamental tenet in the realm of cognitive theory and therapy is that *errors* or *biases* in information processing play an important role in clients' emotional and behavioral problems (Beck, 1976). The following is a nonexhaustive list of categories of errors in thinking *process*:

All-or-None (Black Versus White) Thinking

Most things in life (outside the realm of quantum physics or matters of life and death) exist on a spectrum or continuum. Thinking in all-or-none, black-versus-white terms artificially limits people to only two choices, both of which may be extreme, statistically unlikely, and often less than optimally functional. Thinking in this manner as a general rule makes a person more vulnerable to extreme emotions and decisions, and inhibits creative problem solving. To counter this problem, cognitive therapists often teach their clients to use *subjective rating scales* to assess *levels or degrees* of their emotions, and/or their beliefs about themselves, life situation, and their future. For example, the client who habitually stirs herself into a frenzy with extreme self-statements such as "I'm completely overwhelmed and paralyzed about what to do!" would be encouraged to consider the possibility that even in this state of mind she may have a 5% or 10% capacity for making one small decision and taking one small step toward solving a problem.

Arbitrary Inference (Jumping to Conclusions)

This refers to the reaching of a conclusion without supporting evidence—indeed, even in the face of evidence to the contrary. An example is someone who becomes distraught when she learns that she has missed a call from her daughter's school, assumes that her child is ill or in trouble, and immediately worries that her delay in getting back to the school will be interpreted as her not caring and not being a competent mother. In reality, the school simply wanted to see if she was available at the last minute to fill in as a volunteer chaperone; they had other people on their call list, and *they* felt badly about having to scramble for help at the last minute. In cognitive therapy, this client would be helped to notice her tendency to make negative assumptions, and she would be encouraged to learn to reserve judgment until she obtained more information. If the client continued to think anxiously in terms of "What if [something bad has happened]?" she would be assisted in learning how to answer her own rhetorical question in a more practical manner—that is, with an eye toward problem solving.

Selective Abstraction (Seeing Things out of Context)

A person who often engages in the cognitive process of selective abstraction tends to miss "the big picture," instead focusing on a particularly negative (and/or unrepresentative) aspect of the situation. An example is a person who reads his job performance evaluation and focuses excessively on the one sentence that makes a suggestion for change, while paying scant attention to the majority of the letter that praises his work. In his cognitive therapy session, this client may report that his job position is "vulnerable," citing the minor nonpositive comment from his evaluation. The therapist might then ask to see a hard copy of the evaluation (to get the "raw data"), whereupon she may then help this client to carefully review the entire letter so as to "get the big picture," rather than simply zeroing in on one mildly negative aspect of the situation.

Mind Reading

While it is not unusual for people to surmise what others might be thinking, those who engage in the cognitive error of "mind reading" do so excessively, overestimating the accuracy of their assumptions, underestimating the validity of corrective feedback from others, and sometimes risking interpersonal discord by reading things into what others are saying or doing that are not necessarily true. Clients who are most apt to engage in this cognitive error are those who often talk about the motives of others with high certainty and may be prone to misread the therapist's thoughts as well (e.g., "You must think I sound stupid"). Cognitive therapists

will show such clients that by using good communication skills, they will be able to discuss (and hopefully clear up) important matters with others and relinquish their negative assumptions. These clients also learn how to give others "the benefit of the doubt" while considering that the other person may be thinking things that are innocent or irrelevant to the clients.

Emotional Reasoning

When clients arrive at what they believe to be factual conclusions based on their emotions, this is known as "emotional reasoning." For example, a man who says he "*feels* completely defeated" determines that there is no longer any point in trying to solve a pressing problem that has been troubling him, and so he abandons all productive activity and allows a potentially solvable problem to worsen. Similarly, a woman who says she "*feels* like a loser" owing to some recent disappointments translates this feeling into further assumptions that she is incapable of personal growth and future successes. Thus, she turns down opportunities to take on new personal projects (e.g., an exercise regimen, returning to classes part-time to finish her degree) based on the idea that a "loser" such as herself would simply be wasting her time by trying. Cognitive therapists offer such clients appropriate empathy in light of their negative emotional states. Feelings are important, and sensitive, competent cognitive therapists validate their clients' feelings *as feelings, but not as facts*. As one cognitive therapist put it to her client, "Emotions are a legitimate representation of your quality of life, and therefore they warrant care and attention. However, they should not necessarily dictate your most important decisions, or your most important ways of thinking about yourself, your life, and your future."

Catastrophizing (Magnification of the Negative)

When people catastrophize, they think about worst-case scenarios as if they are likely-case scenarios or only-case scenarios, and thus self-induce a great deal of emotional distress over anticipated hardships and losses that may in fact be unlikely and/or highly preventable. Clients who tend to magnify the negative are taught to consider how the situation could be manageable, or otherwise less harmful than they think. Again, good problem solving can be part of the plan, rather than succumbing to a sense of helplessness in the face of perceived disaster. For example, a student who becomes distraught when a midterm grade of "C" leads her to think that she will now lose her scholarship and have to leave school would be instructed to examine what steps she could actively take in order to maintain her high academic standing, rather than responding as if her worst fear has been realized and her life has been "ruined."

Disqualifying the Positive (Minimizing the Good, Hopeful Data)

People who are prone to this cognitive error typically give great weight to those facts that are unfavorable in some way but dismiss or ignore facts that would otherwise suggest something positive or hopeful. This type of thinking represents a double standard of sorts—negative data are seen as "real," but positive data are deemed irrelevant. Cognitive therapists begin by pointing out such positive data themselves, as if to say to the client, "I am taking some positive things into account when I think of you and your life, and I would like to point them out to you." The therapist goes on to demonstrate that in order to be objective and fair to themselves, clients need to consider *all* the information in their life—the favorable and the not so favorable alike—in order to have a balanced view that will promote more self-acceptance and hope.

With regard to all of the aforementioned points, cognitive therapists sometimes teach their clients the different categories of cognitive errors so that clients can identify and label them when they occur in their thinking. This is an academic exercise that some clients find interesting and engaging, but it is not essential that the clients become skilled in precisely defining each category of cognitive errors in order to benefit from understanding the overarching concept. In fact, many automatic thoughts are not so easily reducible to a single category. The main point is that it is important for clients to fathom that some of their routine ways of thinking are actually problematic, and that by noticing the flaws in their thinking the clients will have the opportunity to make some deliberate modifications in their viewpoints that may lead to an improved mood state, and more constructive actions.

Additional Areas of Cognitive Vulnerability

Related to the earlier short list of cognitive processing errors is a set of cognitive vulnerabilities that the empirical literature suggests are implicated as risk factors for (and/or accompanying manifestations of) emotional disorders, including suicidality. A brief set of descriptions is provided next:

Hopelessness and Helplessness

There is significant evidence that the depressive affect of clients is worsened if they believe they are unable to positively change their life situations (*helplessness*; see Alloy, Peterson, Abramson, & Seligman, 1984), and if their view of the future is dominated largely by the anticipation of unmitigated loss and misery (*hopelessness*; see Beck, Steer, Beck, & Newman, 1993). When clients evince this type of thinking, their risk for suicide increases, and therefore it becomes critically important for therapists to help them consider the possibility that their lot may improve, especially if they learn and enact useful coping skills. In order to keep tabs on this area of cognitive vulnerability, practitioners can ask clients to complete the Beck Hopelessness Scale (Beck, Weissman, Lester, & Trexler, 1974), along with the Beck Depression Inventory-II (Beck, Steer, & Brown, 1996). Even when clients are not actively depressed, it is still important to assess their levels of hopelessness, as "baseline hopelessness" (the client's view of the future even when he or she is euthymic) is still a predictor for future depressive and suicidal episodes (Young et al., 1996).

In response to this problem, cognitive therapists emphasize the importance of learning to envision more hopeful, positive outcomes—not simply to "wish upon a star," but to open the clients' minds to the possibility that things may not turn out as badly as they fear, that expecting the worst may not necessarily protect them from disappointment (as some clients fervently maintain), and that staying hopeful may translate to more constructive behaviors that may increase the clients' odds of actively improving their situation. Learning and applying problem-solving skills facilitates this therapeutic process.

Rigid Thinking Styles and Poor Problem Solving

Healthy, adaptive thinking, like a healthy, capable body, tends to be flexible. Rigid thinking styles often lead people to reject helpful suggestions, ignore new ideas, and to dismiss any attempt to use creative thinking to solve important problems (Ellis, 2006). Depressed, suicidal clients often perceive more problems but generate fewer solutions than their counterparts (Beck, Wenzel, Riskind, Brown, & Steer, 2006; Weishaar, 1996) and are similarly less apt to practice the principles of "damage control," essentially allowing bad situations to get worse (see Schotte & Clum, 1987). Again, an important therapeutic step is for clients to learn the process of constructive problem solving (Nezu, Nezu, & D'Zurilla, 2013).

One of the most ubiquitous exemplars of this cognitive problem is seen in clients who habitually, quickly say "I don't know" in response to important questions put forth by their therapists. It is as if the clients believe that if they do not know the answer to the question *for sure, in its entirety, right this instant*, then there is no benefit in pondering the matter. Thus, they lapse into a state of helpless passivity, which not only fails to address whatever problems they are facing but contributes to an ongoing sense of low self-efficacy to meet the psychological challenges of life. Cognitive therapists typically do not take "I don't know" for an answer. Instead, they encourage their clients to take educated guesses or otherwise come up with hypotheses, even if it requires some time. Cognitive therapists maintain that it is very important for clients to practice the self-respecting act of weighing in on their most important life questions, and not just to assume that they cannot generate ideas to help themselves.

Poor Autobiographical Recall

Clients with mood disorders have been found to have deficits in specific memories about their personal histories (Evans, Williams, O'Laughlin, & Howells, 1992; Gibbs & Rude, 2004; Scott, Stanton, Garland, & Ferrier, 2000). Consequently, they have more difficulty in learning useful lessons from past experiences when compared to nondepressed persons, and they similarly fail to acknowledge the importance of previous *positive* experiences that might otherwise weigh against their sense of general dissatisfaction. Cognitive therapists encourage and shape clients (via guided discovery questioning) to think with higher degrees of specificity and to perform exercises to improve their memories (e.g., writing successively more detailed accounts of important events in the past).

For example, a highly self-critical client who suffers from high anxiety, panic attacks, and agoraphobic avoidance may chastise himself for having difficulties in attending large meetings at work, saying, "What the heck is wrong with me? I used to do this all the time with no problem!" The therapist then takes this as a cue to ask, "What were the specific coping skills you used to use in order to attend and take part in these meetings?" When the client responds with a vague answer such as "I would just *deal* with it and not psych myself out," the therapist would then try to stimulate the client's more specific autobiographical accounts of previous coping

by saying, "Could you give me a detailed account of how you used to approach such meetings? What are the sorts of things you would say to yourself to prepare for the meetings? What would you say to yourself in order to stay in the meeting, even if you felt uncomfortable? How did you keep things in perspective, so that even if the meeting was stressful it didn't discourage you from attending further meetings? Let's learn from your own history of coping skills, because there is valuable information there, and we don't want to overlook or discount it." In taking this approach, the cognitive therapist helps the client to make use of his own history of psychological problem solving in order to provide specific ideas for coping with his symptoms in the here and now.

Perfectionism

Clients who are morbidly perfectionistic engage in excessive self-criticism if they do not meet the highest standards, thus effectively punishing themselves rather than encouraging their ambitions (Blatt, 1995; Hewitt, Flett, & Weber, 1994). Recently designed and tested self-report measures for assessing anxiogenic and depressogenic levels of perfectionism are the Evaluative Concerns Perfectionism Scale (ECPS) and the Self-Critical Perfectionism Scale (SCPS) (Wheeler, Blankstein, Antony, McCabe, & Bieling, 2011). Perfectionism interferes with self-acceptance and with achieving satisfaction through "good enough" solutions to problems. It can also get in the way of clients trying to pursue important goals from the start, as they "reason" to themselves that they cannot commence until they are certain of the best possible outcome. Cognitive therapists support clients in their desire to improve and advance themselves in life, but note when the clients' perfectionism is actually interfering with these goals, rather than promoting them. Therapists encourage clients to devise multiple solutions to problems (not just the best one), to see the merits in learning from mistakes (rather than trying desperately to avoid them), and in valuing themselves for both their strengths and their struggles.

Clients sometimes argue that perfectionism is a noble pursuit, and they may reject the idea that perfectionism is a problem that needs to be remedied. Such clients sometimes say, "I don't want to be average," or "I hold myself to a higher standard," or "I can't accept things that are not done right." When this happens, cognitive therapists realize that the client is misunderstanding the issue, and thus the therapists do not get embroiled in a power struggle over the false, black-and-white question of whether perfectionism is "good or bad." Instead, therapists validate the client's desire to succeed, and acknowledge that being ambitious in doing well is valued in our society. However, it is the *unforgiving, punitive* aspect of the client's thinking that makes the perfectionism a problem. Clients who are morbidly perfectionistic are not looking at the benefits of trial and error (i.e., successive approximations toward preferred outcomes), nor are they tolerating taking calculated risks in doing something less than optimally well as part of the natural learning curve (toward improved levels of performance). Instead, they are looking at the perfect outcome as *expected and necessary*, thus depriving themselves of the joy of ever exceeding their expectations, or the self-satisfaction that comes with struggling with and then overcoming a problem. They are focusing on the *punishment* aspect of learning, rather than the *rewards* of improving toward a goal. As one therapist explained, "The problem is not that you have high aspirations; it's that you are so willing to punish yourself severely for not attaining them completely, and so unwilling to reward yourself for working your way up the ladder."

"Levels" of Cognition

Now we turn to the *contents* of the clients' thinking. The literature on cognitive theory and therapy often describes the contents of clients' thinking in terms of "levels," including the following:

Automatic thoughts
Intermediate beliefs (including "conditional assumptions")
Core beliefs or maladaptive "schemas"

The division of these types of cognitions into discrete levels is not absolute (i.e., there are no veridical "quantum" levels of cognition), but this descriptive practice serves to indicate which types of thoughts tend to be more accessible to spontaneous self-awareness (higher levels) and which tend to be more difficult to change (lower levels).

Automatic Thoughts

At the "surface" level, the term "automatic thoughts" (Beck, 1976; Beck et al., 1979) pertains to the running commentary going through people's minds at any given point in time. These thoughts do not require deliberation or effort, but rather occur spontaneously, representing immediate reactions to what is happening in the client's sphere of experience at that moment, and/or the client's

recollections, ruminations, and the like. Automatic thoughts can come and go so rapidly that people sometimes are not very aware they are experiencing them, and yet such thoughts can have a significant impact on their emotions. Examples might be, "This is pointless," which may induce someone to quit trying to solve an otherwise manageable problem, and "How could I have been so selfish?" which may make someone feel ashamed, even when she didn't do anything wrong. Teaching clients to be aware of these automatic thoughts helps to reduce their potentially harmful impact, because the clients may then utilize strategic questions (e.g., "What are some other ways I can think about this situation?") to help modify their thoughts and therefore mitigate the emotional and behavioral consequences.

Intermediate Beliefs

At a deeper level of thought content we have intermediate beliefs, which are often in the form of general assumptions regarding oneself, others and the world, and the future (the "cognitive triad"), and "if-then" rules (also known as "conditional assumptions") that people implicitly follow. Although these intermediate beliefs typically are not part of the person's spontaneous running monologues in his or her mind (as are automatic thoughts), they have an impact on the types of automatic thoughts the person will be prone to have. One of the earliest attempts to identify and measure the maladaptive intermediate beliefs hypothesized to be implicated in clinical depression and anxiety disorders was the development of the Dysfunctional Attitudes Scale (DAS; Weissman & Beck, 1978). With this self-report questionnaire, clients were asked to endorse their degree of agreement (on a 7-point, Likert-type scale) with a wide range of beliefs hypothesized to be indicative of cognitive vulnerability to depression and anxiety. Items included the following:

People will think less of me if I make a mistake.
If I fail at work, then I am a failure as a person.
I am nothing if a person I love does not
love me.

There is evidence that with clients diagnosed with unipolar depression, moderations in and modifications of such negative assumptions are associated with positive outcome in treatment, as well as the reduction of symptomatic relapses in the future (Evans, Hollon, et al., 1992; Hollon, DeRubeis, & Seligman 1992; Parks & Hollon, 1988). Further, significant improvements in clients' mood during the course of cognitive-behavioral therapy have been found to follow sessions in which they made measurable changes in negative automatic thoughts and intermediate beliefs (Tang, Beberman, DeRubeis, & Pham, 2005; Tang & DeRubeis, 1999).

"Core Beliefs" or "Schemas"

At a deeper level still we have constructs known variously as "core beliefs" or "schemas," which denote the most basic, core dysfunctional beliefs that clients accept as fundamental truths in their lives, particularly clients with long-standing, cross-situational disturbance (Beck et al., 2004; Young, Klosko, & Weishaar, 2003). Rather than being conditional, schemas are hypothesized to be absolute. For example, the individual with an *unlovability* schema (see Layden, Newman, Freeman, & Byers, 1993) does not simply maintain that "I am lovable only if everyone loves me" but rather "I am unlovable (under all conditions, set in stone)." Similarly, a person with an *abandonment* schema does not hold that "I will be left alone by people unless I'm truly important to them" but rather "Everyone I care about is going to leave me (no matter what I do)."

The Young Schema Questionnaire (YSQ: see Schmidt, Joiner, Young, & Telch, 1995) uses a self-report, Likert-type scale to identify which of its 15 factor-analyzed schemas clients load on most heavily. These schemas include "mistrust," "defectiveness," "abandonment," "entitlement," and others, and they are hypothesized to be most prevalent in clients with the most severe personality disorders. A sample item is, "It is only a matter of time before someone betrays me" (mistrust schema). Another measure of deeper cognitive content, the Personality Beliefs Questionnaire (PBQ; Beck et al., 2001) is a self-report measure that also uses a Likert-type scale and comprises a clinically derived set of beliefs hypothesized to correspond to specific personality disorders. For example, the item "If I ignore a problem, it will go away" is hypothesized to reflect a part of the cognitive style of clients who meet the criteria for Avoidant Personality Disorder (*DSM-IV-TR*; American Psychiatric Association, 2000). Research on the PBQ indicates that clients with personality disorders preferentially endorse items theoretically linked to their specific diagnosis (Beck et al., 2001). Studies of serious mental health problems such as borderline personality disorder have looked at schema-level changes as indicative of the benefits of cognitive-behavioral approaches to treatment (e.g., Arntz, Klokman, & Sieswerda, 2005; Giesen-Bloo

et al., 2006; Spinhoven, Bockting, Kremers, Schene, & Williams, 2007), and recent texts have focused on explicating the theoretical, empirical, and clinical bases of schema work across a wide range of specific disorders (Riso, du Toit, Stein, & Young, 2007; Young et al., 2003).

Chief Methods of Cognitive Restructuring

It would be misleading to say that there are distinct, specialized cognitive restructuring techniques for each of the three levels of cognition, respectively. Most cognitive restructuring techniques (several of which are summarized next) can be applied appropriately to automatic thoughts, intermediate beliefs, and schemas. However, as will be described, methods that may be quickly and readily effective in modifying the higher level of automatic thoughts may require many repetitions, variations, and cross-situational applications in order to have comparable power in changing the client's intermediate beliefs. Similarly, techniques that employ tests of logical thinking that may be sufficient to make clients reconsider the validity and utility of their intermediate beliefs may come up short in loosening or modifying their schemas. In such instances, the cognitive restructuring methods may need to involve a strong emotional component—perhaps assisted by the use of guided imagery, role-play enactments, and other "experiential" devices—in order to help clients shift away from the negative absolutism of their schemas. Where appropriate, these nuances will be highlighted in the descriptions of the major cognitive restructuring methods that follow.

The following section provides an overview of some of the techniques most widely used by cognitive therapists to help their clients modify the contents and processes of their thinking so as to alleviate unnecessary suffering, broaden perspectives, and improve functional living. These techniques include (1) rational responding (often via the use of automatic thought records), (2) the downward arrow, (3) role playing, (4) behavioral experiments, and (5) imagery (for both reconstruction of past events and rehearsal of upcoming situations).

Rational Responding (and Automatic Thought Records)

A central, all-important skill that patients in cognitive therapy learn is *rational responding*. This concept may also be dubbed as *alternative responding* if the therapist does not wish to convey the message that the client is necessarily engaging in "irrational" thinking to begin with. Whichever name is used (and the author tends to use these names interchangeably), this skill entails a number of components that may be explained to clients as follows:

1. Being aware of your emotions when they seem excessive, problematic, disproportionate to or out of context with a given situation, and otherwise hindering of feeling or functioning well. An example is the person who notices that he is becoming very anxious and angry when someone does not return his text message right away.

2. Using this awareness as a *cue* to self-monitor the thoughts you may be having at the time that may be contributing to your emotional distress and/or behavioral problems. This means that you can then keep track of and document what is going through your mind, which will provide you with extremely useful information that you will need in order to help yourself.

3. Being a "healthy skeptic" of your own thinking, so that you do you not necessarily believe everything you think. This is *not* a matter of doubting your own perceptions in an invalidating way, but rather an exercise in thinking critically and constructively, rather than automatically succumbing to your automatic and/or stereotypic perceptions.

4. Using a set of questions to prompt alternative ways of thinking, so that your thoughts are more flexible, less hopeless, and more conducive to constructive problem solving. Such questions (see Beck, 2011; Newman, 2011) include the following:

a. What are some other plausible ways I can think about this situation? How can I look at this situation from other "angles" that may give me greater "depth perception"?

b. What concrete, factual evidence supports or contradicts my thinking? Is there is a *lack* of such evidence, and thus am I jumping to conclusions before I have the information I need? How can I obtain more data on this issue?

c. Even if my situation is objectively difficult to manage, what constructive action can I take to begin the process of problem solving?

d. Realistically, what is the worst thing that could happen in this situation? Could I cope with it? What is the *best* thing that could happen in this situation? Now that I have considered both extremes, neither of which has a high probability of occurring, what is the most *likely* thing that will happen? Is this more tolerable than what I was first assuming?

e. What are the pros and cons of believing my automatic thoughts without question? What are the pros and cons of trying to think in alternative ways?

f. What sincere advice would I give to a good friend if he or she were in my shoes? Would this advice be more compassionate and hopeful than what I typically tell myself? Could I try to talk to myself as if I am my own friend?

As one can see, such a process of asking oneself these sorts of questions can be quite an intellectual challenge. Indeed, this is a skill that requires clients to practice outside the therapy office and to receive feedback in the therapist's office. The upside, however, is considerable. First, anecdotally speaking, many clients in cognitive therapy comment that they have never been taught to reevaluate their thinking in this way, stating that they find the process interesting and productive. Second, when clients engage in the self-monitoring of their own automatic thoughts to which they then rationally respond, they are essentially behaving like social scientists, taking data on themselves. Thus, rather than just being passive sufferers, the clients are being active in learning about and helping themselves. This is potentially empowering to clients in itself, even before they produce rational responses per se. Third, clients who practice the skill of self-monitoring their automatic thoughts are less apt to act impulsively as they might on similarly unnoticed thoughts. Fourth, when clients routinely generate rational responses, they expand their worldview, breaking free from the limits of tunnel vision, engaging in less rumination, producing more creative solutions to problems, and generally having a better outlook. These are considerable advancements for clients who previously felt "stuck" in set ways of thinking and feeling that were simultaneously dissatisfying and all too familiar.

One of the ways that therapists help their clients to learn the methods of rational responding is to explain what it is *not*. First, rational responding does not mean that clients engage in rote affirmations out of the context of a careful, objective conceptualization of their respective situations. Clients are not asked to engage in idle positive thinking, as if this will be sufficient to solve real problems that they must confront in order to improve their lives. Yes, the tenor of rational responding is often positive in the sense that it is generally more hopeful, but it is not a simplistic approach that says, "Don't worry, be happy." Second, rational responding does not require clients to "forget about" or otherwise artificially stop thinking their automatic thoughts. Instead, rational responding (by definition) involves *responding* to automatic thoughts in ways that help clients gain a broader perspective, such that the automatic thoughts carry less weight and/or lose credibility, and new ideas—based on evidence, problem solving, and new hypotheses—give clients a fresh approach to understanding and coping with their concerns. Third, rational responding certainly does not require a denigration of the clients for entertaining their automatic thoughts in the first place, as if their upsetting thoughts are wrong, "ridiculous," or indicative of a lack of insight or intelligence. This last point is particularly important to emphasize to clients who are prone to feeling invalidated, and who may therefore be somewhat guarded in taking part in a treatment approach that questions the functionality and/or veracity of their thoughts. The following is a brief clinical illustration:

CLIENT: I'm so worried. I just keep thinking about all the things that could go wrong. I know I'm not supposed to do that. I'm supposed to stop thinking this way, and I'm really trying to stop, but the thoughts keep coming back. I'm sorry, but I just can't do the technique you want.

THERAPIST: I'm really sorry you've been so worried, and I believe you when you say you're trying hard to learn how not to buy into your worrisome thoughts, but you don't need to apologize, because you're allowed to have your own thoughts. The point of learning how to do *rational responding* is to notice your automatic thoughts and answer them, rather than just having them affect you without recourse. You don't have to *stop* having automatic thoughts, because we're going to work on ways to *respond* to your thoughts.

CLIENT: But I feel overwhelmed by my worries. I don't think I can just talk myself out of having them.

THERAPIST: You're right. You've had so much experience in thinking about worst-case scenarios that it's unrealistic for anyone to assume that you can just end that habit right away, as if your worries had no merit or basis whatsoever, and as if you can learn a new way of thinking on demand.

CLIENT: I'm not sure I follow. Are you saying that my worries really *are* real? I thought I was supposed to learn how to do rational responding.

THERAPIST: I'm making the point that we need to respect your original thoughts and try to understand how it is that you have come to have these thoughts. We're not going to just dismiss them. It's much better if we try to understand how you arrived at the interpretations and assumptions you're making, and then work together to see if we can look at them in a different way—a way that won't be so emotionally overwhelming, as you put it.

CLIENT: I guess I'm not sure how I'm going to make that change.

THERAPIST: It's a process. We'll go step by step, and you'll practice and get lots of repetitions. Like any new skill, you'll get better as you go along, and I'll help. Your current thought that you won't be able to learn a new thinking skill and that you will continue to be at the mercy of the thoughts that overwhelm you is itself a "worst-case scenario" thought that we can address like any other.

CLIENT: What if I don't believe the new thoughts that I try to have? What if the new thoughts don't affect how I feel?

THERAPIST: It's not an all-or-none situation. You won't have to believe your new rational responses totally, nor will you have to stop believing your old thoughts totally. You don't have to do an "extreme cognitive makeover" in order to benefit from this method. Also, if your use of rational responding helps just a little bit at first, this will be a big step forward. We're not going to get rid of all your old thoughts and replace them. We're just going to practice ways of thinking in more flexible and constructive ways.

A widely used method for helping clients document their self-assessment of their thoughts and their attempts at modifying them is the automatic thought record (ATR), a structured, multi-columned form that has been described in various ways, and with somewhat different names (e.g., "dysfunctional thought records," "daily thought records," "5-column technique") over the decades in which it has been employed (see Beck, 2011; Beck et al., 1979; Greenberger & Padesky, 1995, and many others). Therapists initially teach their clients to use ATRs in session, but then the clients learn that they can use ATRs as a staple of their cognitive therapy homework. By practicing this method between sessions, clients can use ATRs at key moments during the week when engaging in self-help is most needed. In doing so, clients solidify their sense of self-efficacy in employing this technique for the long run, thus improving maintenance of therapeutic gains. Figure 8.1 illustrates a sample ATR, in which a client tries to understand and modify his anger in response to a colleague's comment, then makes some deliberate changes in his outlook, consequently reducing his level of upset. Note that the client makes use of some of the prompting questions that are listed at the bottom of the ATR (similar to those described earlier).

The competent application of rational responding methods does *not* involve a heavy-handed attempt to argue clients out of their maintained ideas. For example, if a client says, "I have made so many mistakes in my life that I deserve to suffer," it does little good for the therapist simply to naysay with the comment, "You haven't made so many mistakes, and you do not deserve to suffer." Therapists need to consider the possibility that aspects of the client's thoughts and beliefs may be supported in fact and therefore may need to be validated in some reasonable way. It is considerably more empathic if the therapist is able to find points of agreement with their clients' comments, but to frame them in a compassionate way, and then help the clients craft reasonable alternatives.

Therapists who have a thorough understanding of their client's history and current life situation will be in an excellent position to choose the questions that are the best "fit" for the clients. In other words, a good case conceptualization naturally assists the processing of rational responding (Kuyken, Padesky, & Dudley, 2009). For example, if a client is prone to disqualify many positive events in his life, and instead concludes (on the basis of emotional reasoning) that he "feels like a loser," the therapist who is aware of the many ways this client has been successful in life will likely ask the client, "What is the evidence *against* the idea that you are a loser?" The therapist asks this question with the full knowledge that there will be many concrete examples on which to draw to make the point that the client has objective reason to feel more confident and self-efficacious. However, if a therapist knows that a client has indeed suffered many personal setbacks in her life and subsequently believes she is "cursed" and "doomed," the therapist is unlikely to ask a question about *evidence*, as the client's history is replete with examples of misfortune. Instead, the therapist may choose to ask the question "What positive actions can you take in spite of the past setbacks?" In other words, the therapist will help the client to look *forward* with a sense of hope and purpose, rather than look at the past as a necessary portent of things to come. Similarly, if a therapist knows that a given client typically is far more accepting of her friends' personal flaws than her own, she may ask her, "What sincere, caring, helpful advice would you give to a friend in the same situation?" This question likely will generate a benevolent response that the client can then be encouraged to apply to herself. The therapist would be less likely to use this question when working with a client who is less connected to and more cynical about others.

Downward Arrow—Toward Identification of Intermediate Beliefs and Schemas

Let us see how this technique could apply to Vance, the client from the earlier example. Vance recognized that his initial reaction of anger and shame was triggered by his colleague's ambiguous "cheer" upon hearing of the completed report. By doing the ATR, Vance realized that there were more benign ways he could have viewed the situation—ways that would not have led to such a magnified emotional reaction. However, the question remained, what accounted for Vance having such an extreme reaction in response to this trigger? In other words, why was his reaction disproportionate to the situation, and what does it suggest about his intermediate beliefs or schemas that underlie his automatic thoughts (as seen on the ATR)?

The downward arrow technique enables a client such as Vance to ascertain possible answers. Starting with an automatic thought that reflects what was going through his mind at the critical moments in question (when Tom reportedly said to Vance, "Yeah, the report is finally done!"), Vance then asks himself questions such as "What does that *mean*?" or "What would happen then?" These questions ostensibly call the client's attention to some of the assumed implications of his interpretation. As we see in Vance's downward arrow sheet (see Figure 8.2), the client hypothesizes a series of progressively worsening meanings about what just happened, going from the disappointment of not being appreciated, to the prospect of facing more criticism and consequences, to being seen as (and believing that he is) a failure, and being trapped in a job he hates with no place to go.

Directions: When you notice your mood getting worse, ask yourself, **"What's going through my mind right now?"** and as soon as possible jot down the thought or mental image in the Automatic Thoughts column.

DATE/TIME	SITUATION	AUTOMATIC THOUGHT(S)	EMOTION(S)	ALTERNATIVE RESPONSE	OUTCOME
	1. What event, daydream, or recollection led to the unpleasant emotion? 2. What (if any) distressing physical sensations did you have?	1. What thought(s) and/or image(s) went through your mind? 2. How much did you believe each one at the time?	1. What emotion(s) (sad, anxious, angry, etc.) did you feel at the time? 2. How intense (0–100%) was the emotion?	1. (optional) What cognitive distortion did you make? (e.g., all-or-nothing thinking, mind-reading, catastrophizing) 2. Use questions at bottom to compose a response to the automatic thought(s). 3. How much do you believe each response?	1. How much do you now believe each automatic thought? 2. What emotion(s) do you feel now? How intense (0–100%) is the emotion? 3. What will or did you do?
Tues. late afternoon at the office.	1. I told Tom that I finished the team report and he said, "Yeah, it's *finally done!*" 2. Felt tense, sweaty, "welling up."	1. "What a jerk! I don't need his sarcasm. I busted my butt to finish that report. Nobody else has any idea how hard it was to write this report. They just think I'm at fault for taking too long. I don't get any credit around this place, and I'm sick of it. I don't know why I do so much work anyway. It gets me nowhere. (I believe this at a level of 90%) 2. "I know I missed a couple of deadlines, and I feel terrible about this, and I was hoping that nobody was going to give me a hard time, but it looks like I'm still going to get criticized for being late. (I believe this at a level of 80%)	1. Angry (100%) 2. Ashamed (50%)	1. I am jumping to conclusions, catastrophizing, reading Tom's mind, and overgeneralizing to everybody else. I am also thinking in all or none terms. 2. Maybe Tom was just expressing relief or celebrating, but I'm taking it the wrong way. There is no evidence that Tom thinks badly of me or acts like a jerk. Even if I'm late, I still finished something very difficult and important.	1. Thoughts: 1st thought: 10% 2nd thought: 30% 2. Emotions: Angry (40%) Ashamed (20%) 3. Actions: I will not be sarcastic in return. I will be very professional and show pride in my work.

Questions to help compose an alternative response: (1) What is the evidence that the automatic thought is true? Not true? (2) Is there an alternative explanation? (3) What's the worst that could happen? Could I live through it? What's the best that could happen? What's the most realistic outcome? (4) What's the effect of my believing the automatic thought? What could be the effect of changing my thinking? (5) What should I do about it? (6) If _____ (friend's name) was in the situation and had this thought, what would I tell him/her?

Figure 8.1 Vance's "Automatic Thought Record."

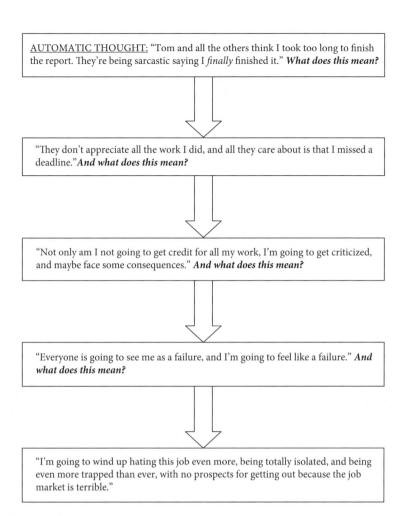

AUTOMATIC THOUGHT: "Tom and all the others think I took too long to finish the report. They're being sarcastic saying I *finally* finished it." **What does this mean?**

⬇

"They don't appreciate all the work I did, and all they care about is that I missed a deadline."**And what does this mean?**

⬇

"Not only am I not going to get credit for all my work, I'm going to get criticized, and maybe face some consequences." **And what does this mean?**

⬇

"Everyone is going to see me as a failure, and I'm going to feel like a failure." **And what does this mean?**

⬇

"I'm going to wind up hating this job even more, being totally isolated, and being even more trapped than ever, with no prospects for getting out because the job market is terrible."

Figure 8.2 Vance's Downward Arrow.

On the basis of these responses, Vance and his therapist may then hypothesize that the client may maintain an intermediate belief such as "Nobody is going to think well of me unless I do everything right," as well as deeper schemas of *incompetency, unrelenting standards*, and perhaps *vulnerability to harm*. At the very least, the downward arrow technique shows the client that his emotional reaction may have been out of proportion with the situation per se, but quite congruent with his own problematic schemas. This becomes a call to action to counteract the schemas, regardless of whether or not his work situation is changeable.

The Use of Role Playing as a Prime Mover in Modifying the Client's Thinking

When clients have some difficulties in using ATRs or otherwise report that they do not respond significantly well to tasks that largely involve writing, cognitive therapists can opt to use role playing in order provide an experiential vehicle by which clients can learn new, more constructive ways of thinking. For starters, the easier variation of this method (for the client) involves the client stating his or her automatic thought or counterproductive belief (e.g., "Nothing ever works out for me, so I might as well give up") to begin the role play, whereupon the therapist models a potential alternative response (e.g., "Yes, I have had some tough breaks, but there is some evidence that things can improve if I don't quit on myself"). Then, the client comes back with a typical way that he or she might negate the alternative response, followed by the therapist's modeling yet another alternative response. They continue in this fashion, as illustrated by the brief dialogue that follows:

CLIENT: (In the role of his or her own automatic thoughts) Whenever I try to have hope, life just slams me down. I can't deal with that anymore. I don't want to set myself up for more disappointment.

THERAPIST: (In the role of the client's potential alternative responses) It's very reasonable not to want to be disappointed again, and I shouldn't just blindly assume that everything is going to go well. That would be too black and white . . . going too far in the other direction. I'm just saying that there is reason to remain somewhat hopeful, and that being hopeful could actually help me, whereas giving up on myself too soon could needlessly keep me down. I don't want that either.

CLIENT: So that just means I'm trapped! If I expect the worst and just give up, that's bad for me, but if I let my guard down and try to be hopeful again, then I'm vulnerable to getting my expectations up again, only to then get crushed!

THERAPIST: That's the depressive way to look at it, and *that's* the real trap. To get out of being trapped, I need to be flexible about how I see things. For example, I could look at the upside of being more hopeful. If I refuse to quit, and I keep trying, I might actually do some things differently to improve my life, rather than just collapsing into helplessness. There is even some evidence from my own past that suggests that I can make some good things happen if I stay focused on my important goals. I could possibly do that again, but I'll never know if I stop myself.

CLIENT: It just sounds too scary, and too tiresome, and too impossible for me.

THERAPIST: I know that's the way it sounds, but that doesn't mean that's the way it has to be. I'm going to make a plan of action, and try it step by step, and try to stay hopeful, and see what happens. Then I can judge the results. But I'm not going to *pre-judge*.

At this point, the therapist may invite the client to come out of role and to process his or her reaction to the role play, asking questions such as:

What are your thoughts about that role play, and how do you feel right now?

Was there anything I said—in the role of your potential alternative responses—with which you can agree even a little bit?" Were there any things that you said—in the role of your automatic thoughts and depressive beliefs—that you would be even a little bit willing to modify in some way?

Which rational responses could you begin using for yourself? How would you modify them so that they could become useful to you in practice?

Which of my responses in the role play seemed to miss the mark for you? What makes them difficult to believe?

How would you alter these rational responses so they become more relevant or personalized for yourself?

Do you feel any more hopeful or encouraged than before?

On the other hand, was there anything about this role-play exercise or what I said in it that bothered you? Would you be willing to share your emotional reactions with me?

The next step may be for the therapist and client to try another role play, this time with the client role-playing the alternative responses (which is more challenging), while the therapist takes the role of devil's advocate. While doing this difficult but potentially skill-enhancing technique, therapists need to encourage those clients who might otherwise drop out of the role play to persevere beyond their first inclination to avoid and quit. Also, therapists need to take care not to sound as though they are portraying an unflattering caricature of the clients and their thought process. Competent therapists know how to enact role-play renditions of their client's typical thoughts with sensitivity and accurate empathy. Toward this goal, therapists often ask their clients for feedback following the completion of the devil's advocate role play, such as by saying, "I hope I was on target with my role play, that I said things to which you could relate, and that I sounded like I was respecting your views. What do you think?" When clients have success with this technique, it can be a very significant experience of empowerment. When clients flounder, the skilled, caring therapist simply states that this is a demanding technique, that more work is needed (perhaps in the form of more ATRs for homework), and that it is worth continuing to try.

Behavioral Experiments

Although the term "*cognitive* restructuring" would seem to imply a set of interventions that involves only abstract thinking and verbal discourse between therapist and client, the reality is more complex, as a person's behaviors, thoughts, emotionality, and physiological responses interact. Thus, when purely verbal techniques (such as the ATR) lack the necessary power to help clients make significant changes in how they construe themselves, their lives, and their future, it is advisable to add a behavioral component to the intervention. We saw this idea illustrated earlier in the description of role playing, where adding an interpersonal dialogue in which the clients must overtly express their thoughts and corresponding changes creates a more experiential form of discovery—one that may transcend passive thinking, and supplement a client's writing. Similarly, behavioral experiments involve *enactments*, in which clients are instructed to put their automatic thoughts, intermediate beliefs, and schemas to the test in an upcoming real-life situation, so as to gain more data in the context of in-vivo experiences (see Bennett-Levy, Fennell, Hackmann, Mueller, & Westbrook, 2004).

Behavioral experiments are often used in the context of the clients' negative expectations that reflect their intermediate beliefs and schemas. For example, a client with *dependency* and *abandonment* schemas may believe that she will not be able to tolerate her feelings of loneliness if she refrains from making demanding, desperate, and repeated phone calls to family members. However, with some support from the therapist, this client may agree to try the following behavioral experiment for homework—that the client will notice her urge to make a phone call, write down her automatic thoughts in her journal, respond rationally to those thoughts, and engage in an activity that has the potential to produce a sense of pleasure or accomplishment (examples of which can be generated in session), as a substitute for impulsively making phone calls that fray her relationships. Any degree of actual success in being able to implement this plan (e.g., reduced frequency of phone calls, reduced level of emotional distress) will have a direct positive bearing on the client's schema-driven assumption that she is unable to manage her emotions when she is alone. Any difficulties the client may have in following through on this behavioral experiment will provide useful in-vivo information about her schema activation that may help her and her therapist better conceptualize the problem and construct a revised behavioral experiment next time.

In sum, behavioral experiments are a valuable means by which to test clients' automatic thoughts, intermediate beliefs, and schemas in real-life situations. Through this method, clients come to recognize the importance of seeing *what really happens*, rather than *assuming* what is going to happen. This can happen within the therapy hour itself (as when the therapist encourages a client who believes he will not know how to do an ATR to work on one in session), or as part of the client's homework assignment, complete with instructions to document his thoughts, behaviors, and emotions, and to report in the next session how well things worked out compared to what he expected. It should be noted that many repetitions (and cross-situational applications) of behavioral experiments would often be required for the client to make changes at the level of schemas, as these are long-standing and engrained, and therefore are difficult to modify without investing much time, effort, and encouragement (Newman, 2011).

Imagery

When clients maintain problematic schemas—belief systems that are long-standing, core aspects of the fundamental ways in which they view themselves and their world—it is often helpful to augment rational responding methods with imagery techniques (Hackmann, Bennett-Levy, & Holmes, 2011). The use of imagery often involves either an attempt to re-experience and re-process important life events or a prospective attempt to "visually walk through" and otherwise cognitively rehearse ways for coping with anticipated stressful situations. The rationale for using imagery is two-fold. First, it makes use of another stimulus "channel" that supplements the verbal/auditory realm, thus helping clients to ascertain more experiential details about a past or expected life situation, and perhaps to retain the information more readily via supplemental systems processing. Second, imagery techniques can be quite affectively evocative, thus providing more of an "ocean of emotion" on which to carry the cognitions that are being addressed. Thus, rational responding methods that otherwise might seem intellectually dry in the face of deeply held, affectively charged schemas become enriched and energized by mental pictures that give more life to the words. This combination of imagery methods with rational responding is an important staple of schema-focused therapy (Young et al., 2003), and it is often associated with trauma work (see Layden et al., 1993; Resick & Schnicke, 1993). As can be ascertained from the following example, it is an advanced clinical method that requires a high level of competency and careful attention to the therapeutic relationship. Clients should be prepared for the technique in advance (rather than having it sprung on them), a strong rationale needs to be given, and the technique needs to be started early in a session so as to allow for sufficient processing and debriefing time. Repetitions over the course of several sessions, supplemented by related homework assignments (e.g., writing progressively more detailed narratives of the past experience being tapped by the imagery experiment) are often required in order to make inroads in modifying the clients' schema(s).

An example illustrates the aforementioned process. A young woman suffering from panic disorder with agoraphobia also presented with long-term, complicated grief and guilt owing to "not being there" for her father when he passed away in a hospital some years earlier. Although she made progress in reducing her panic attacks, becoming less avoidant, and expanding her travel mobility, she still maintained a schema that she was a "bad" person for not having visited her father in the hospital (she had not realized how seriously ill he was, and therefore procrastinated in making the potentially panic-inducing trip to see him). To deal with this rigid belief about her being a bad daughter, and to moderate her complicated bereavement, the therapist recommended an imagery induction, in which the patient (henceforth to be given the pseudonym "Hope") would undergo a standard relaxation exercise, and then imagine herself (with the therapist's guided instructions) visiting her father in the hospital, and having the conversation she wished she would have had while her father was still alive. The therapist felt on solid ground to recommend this intervention because he knew that Hope and her father had had a very close, loving relationship, and therefore there was great reason to believe that an imaginal conversation between Hope and her father would be very positive. One of the goals of this intervention was to induce a sense of forgiveness—both from the father (in Hope's imagination) and within Hope herself (as she would remember in an emotionally evocative manner how devoted she was to her father). Hope was fully apprised of this exercise and its components (including the preliminary relaxation induction) in advance of the actual session. Following 10 minutes of relaxed breathing and pleasant imagery (with the client's eyes closed), the therapist imaginally walked Hope through the steps of arriving at the hospital and approaching her father in his room, and moderated a hypothetical conversation between Hope and her father, a part of which follows:

THERAPIST: Hope, what do you want to say to your father?

HOPE: I love you, Dad. I'm so sorry I wasn't here for you earlier. I didn't realize how sick you were. I'm so sorry (tearful).

THERAPIST: What do you think your father would say to you if he saw that you were so upset and felt so guilty?

HOPE: He would tell me it's okay, that I don't have to be sorry, and that he knows I love him.

THERAPIST: What if he knew that you thought you were a bad person because you didn't make it to the hospital in time?

HOPE: He would tell me I'm a wonderful girl. He always said that (crying).

THERAPIST: Actually imagine him saying that right now. Look at him and hear his voice.

HOPE: (Crying)

THERAPIST: Tell your father how you feel about him and what he means to you.

HOPE: You're such a great father. I miss you so much (crying). I wish you were here right now. All the good things I've done in life I've done because you encouraged me and made me believe in myself. You would be so proud of me that I'm traveling so much more now, and I'm not as anxious anymore. I would love to take you and Mom on a long, faraway vacation. I can't do that now. I wish you were here (sighing).

THERAPIST: What if your father said that he felt like a "bad" person because he couldn't be here today to see how well you're doing?

HOPE: I would tell him that it's not his fault that he left. It's nobody's fault. He's a great person.

THERAPIST: Would he say the same to you— that it's nobody's fault that you're apart, and that you're a great person?

HOPE: Yes (crying).

THERAPIST: Actually try to hear him say that right now. Imagine it as accurately as you can.

After the imagery induction was over, the therapist allowed for a 20-minute "debriefing," which led to his and Hope's devising homework assignments that would continue the process of changing her belief that she was a "bad" daughter. These included ATRs in which Hope produced rational responses (against her excessively self-reproachful automatic thoughts) that her father would have endorsed, Hope writing little stories of times that she had "been there" for her father (such as being in charge of his surprise 60th birthday party), and looking at evidence of Hope's "goodness" as a person across many scenarios in her life, not just in her role as a loving daughter. These assignments carried more emotional weight in the aftermath of the guided imagery exercise; thus, the cognitive restructuring was more potent, and Hope indeed felt more forgiving and charitable toward herself.

Cognitive Restructuring in the Context of the Therapeutic Relationship

The therapeutic relationship is extremely valuable in providing clients—many of whom are emotionally vulnerable, sensitive to signs of interpersonal judgment and rejection, and perhaps prone to being guarded and mistrustful—with a safe interpersonal environment in which to feel validated and free to discuss highly personal matters they would be loath to mention elsewhere. There is an extensive empirical literature supporting the notion that a positive, healthy therapeutic relationship contributes significantly to the positive power of psychotherapy as practiced across theoretical models (see Norcross & Lambert, 2011). Further, there is evidence that the experience of directly addressing and solving a problem with a therapist can be a highly positive learning experience, giving hope to clients that interpersonal issues *can* be worked out. A study by Strauss et al. (2006), which studied the relationship between the therapeutic alliance and clinical outcomes for a population of clients receiving a year of cognitive therapy for avoidant and obsessive-compulsive personality disorders, lends support to this hypothesis. Here, the authors found that clients had the best outcomes when they experienced a strain in the therapeutic relationship that was well managed and resolved. On the other hand, the worst outcomes (including premature terminations) occurred when there were problems in the therapeutic relationship that were not resolved. Such findings suggest that moments of tension or conflict between client and therapist represent critical crossroads for the course of treatment.

Also, from the perspective of cognitive therapy case conceptualization, the therapeutic relationship is an excellent testing ground for clients to assess and modify some of their most problematic views relevant to their interpersonal lives (Gilbert & Leahy, 2007; Safran & Muran, 2000; Safran & Segal, 1990).

The Cognitive Therapy Scale (Blackburn et al., 2001; Young & Beck, 1980), the single most widely used general measure of therapist competence in applying cognitive therapy across populations (Trepka, Rees, Shapiro, Hardy, & Barkham, 2004), includes several items that measure aspects of the therapeutic relationship (e.g., "understanding," "interpersonal effectiveness," "collaboration"). These components of cognitive therapy are important in their own right, but they go even further in terms of helping clients to have "corrective experiences" that counter their negative expectations and interpretations about relationships—including their relationship with their cognitive therapist (Strauss et al., 2006). At times, clients make faulty interpretations of their therapist's comments or behaviors that unfortunately and unnecessarily lead them to feel belittled, rejected, abandoned, and other negative schema-fueled feelings. Here, the astute and sensitive cognitive therapist recognizes the client's signs of distress, empathically inquires, and tries to give feedback to clear up the misunderstanding. At such moments, it is critically important for the therapists to openly examine their own contribution to the problem—in the spirit of collaboration—so that the clients' concerns are given due consideration. Otherwise, the clients may feel that the process of cognitive therapy is being misused to trivialize their perceptions about the therapeutic relationship (Cummings, Hayes, Newman, & Beck, 2011). The following example illustrates how a cognitive therapist may handle this sort of situation. The vignette shows the therapist addressing the client's negative thoughts about what is transpiring in the therapeutic relationship—helping the client to make changes in her viewpoints so as to repair the alliance strain, while minimizing the risk of invalidating her concerns.

In the following dialogue, a therapist expresses his concern that the client's scores on the Beck Depression Inventory are climbing over the course of the previous three sessions, thus indicating an exacerbation of her condition. The therapist brings up this topic in the hope of doing some problem solving, with the client's best interest in mind. The client misinterprets this exchange, believing instead that the therapist is stating that therapy is failing and must end, thus stirring up her fears of being abandoned by the therapist.

THERAPIST: One of the things I would like to put on our agenda today is a discussion about your progress in therapy. I've been noticing that in spite of our best efforts, your scores on the Beck Depression Inventory and Beck

Hopelessness Scale are actually climbing, and this concerns me. I would like to deal with this head on, because it's very important for us to examine how this treatment is helping you, or not, and how to respond.

CLIENT: Well, you know I've been going through a terrible time, and I've been feeling awful.

THERAPIST: I know, and I want to make sure that you're getting the care that you need so that you can experience some improvement. I want to make sure that this is the right treatment plan for you, and maybe consider what else can be done.

CLIENT: (Becoming tearful)

THERAPIST: Oh my, I didn't mean to say something that would upset you. (Hands her the box of tissues) May I ask you what you're thinking about right now?

CLIENT: I'm sorry if I'm not doing what I'm supposed to be doing in this therapy. I know I haven't been doing the homework, and it's probably my fault that I'm not getting better, but I *really* need this therapy, and I don't want you send me someplace else. I don't know what I would do if you gave up on me.

THERAPIST: Oh dear! We're having an unfortunate miscommunication here. Please, please don't jump to the conclusion that I'm giving up on you and sending you elsewhere (tries to laugh in an engaging, friendly way). If you are finding this treatment to be helpful, then of course I am committed to helping you further.

CLIENT: But I thought you were saying that because my scores are getting worse you're going to conclude that therapy is failing and I have to leave.

THERAPIST: No, no, not at all. I am very motivated to help you. You know, I think this might be a little cognitive therapy teaching moment right now!

CLIENT: You mean I'm distorting things again?

THERAPIST: Oh, I definitely would *not* put it that way, because that sounds like we're blaming you for your perceptions. I think we can be much nicer to *both* of us for our little miscommunication and still learn something in the process. For starters, I want to acknowledge that I could have been much clearer from the start that my agenda for today is all about caring about how you're doing, and wanting to improve our work together in

whatever way we can so as to help you achieve your therapeutic goals. Your worsening scores on your Beck inventories were my cue that we needed to do some problem solving, and not at all a sign that we needed to end working together as a therapy team. We may just need to update our treatment plan together, that's all.

CLIENT: It just sounded like you were saying that I needed a different treatment altogether, and that you and I had to stop our sessions because I was failing to improve.

THERAPIST: And that's where I needed to be clearer from the start. I apologize for that.

CLIENT: Well, I apologize for jumping to conclusions. I should have trusted that you wouldn't just walk out on me, but that's what I expect from people in my life.

THERAPIST: Yes, we've talked about that. What are the schemas that get activated for you when you perceive that a current situation is going to result in the same sort of outcomes you have experienced in the past?

CLIENT: It's that abandonment schema, I think. Also, it's the unlovability schema. I just feel like nobody cares, and why should they? It's just for me, and who am I? I guess this is also an emotional deprivation schema as well, because I assume that my emotional needs will never be met.

THERAPIST: That's excellent. I think your assessment of your own cognitive processing is right on target.

CLIENT: And if I want to be totally honest with myself, and you, I have to admit that I probably had a little bit of an activation of my mistrust schema too, because I jumped to the conclusion that you were giving up on me, rather than trusting that you wanted to help me.

THERAPIST: Now that you recognize how your deepest, most core negative beliefs were triggered by our conversation, what could you say to yourself to rationally respond?

CLIENT: (Pauses to think) I could think of all the evidence about how you have been trying to help me, and always being kind and respectful to me. But then I just blame myself and say that even though you have been helpful and caring, I am a failure as a client.

THERAPIST: And what would be your rational responses to *that*?

CLIENT: (Pauses again) Ummm, that's harder (laughs). Ummm, I could remind myself that I have been coming every week, doing *some* homework, learning some useful things, and that my bad mood is more about my life situation—which you know has been one bad thing after another lately—and that maybe if I hadn't been working so hard to learn to do cognitive therapy techniques I would be even worse.

THERAPIST: That's an excellent point! You have indeed been working hard in treatment, and we have to remember that your life outside of this office has not exactly been kind to you these last few months, but you are doing your best to cope and to be hopeful.

CLIENT: Maybe the change we have to make in our work is to get me another life, rather than a different therapy (laughs along with the therapist). No, really, maybe I just need to come more than once a week, or maybe I should be on a medication, too. I don't know. What do you think?

THERAPIST: Well, those are options we can certainly discuss. I was also thinking that maybe we could do some more problem-solving interventions on the one hand, and perhaps also do some mindfulness and acceptance work on the other hand. That might sound a little bit contradictory, but let's talk about it.

CLIENT: Okay, that sounds fine. You know I want to do everything I can to get well.

THERAPIST: I know. I'm super motivated to help you, too. In this vignette the therapist recognizes that the client has misinterpreted his concerns about the treatment plan to mean that he is going to unilaterally end their work together. In response, the therapist decides to clarify the situation in order to help the client change her interpretation and therefore to be less distressed, defining this as a "cognitive therapy teaching moment." At the same time—and this point cannot be stated strongly enough—the therapist does not *blame* the client for making a faulty assumption pertinent to the therapeutic relationship (see Cummings et al., 2011). In the spirit of collaboration that is central to cognitive therapy, the therapist takes partial ownership of the problem, saying (without being dysfunctionally self-reproachful) that he could have been clearer, and that if they could discuss the matter further they would come to a more hopeful outcome.

Empirical Support for Cognitive Restructuring

There is a far greater body of empirical support for the full package of cognitive-behavioral treatments (as detailed in official, comprehensive manuals) than there is for the more discrete area of interventions subsumed under the category of "cognitive restructuring." On the one hand, one could state that cognitive restructuring is inextricably intertwined and identified with cognitive theory and therapy; hence, we may simply refer to the data on the efficacy of "full-package" cognitive therapy as a guide to understanding the level of empirical support for the more circumscribed area of cognitive restructuring. On the other hand, the cognitive-behavioral treatment known as *behavioral activation* is predicated on data from some studies suggesting that the behavioral components of the treatment are most relevant, with the cognitive aspects being more or less superfluous (e.g., Coffman, Martell, Dimidjian, Gallop, & Hollon, 2007; Jacobson et al., 1996). These findings necessarily make us more cautious in drawing firm conclusions about the centrality of cognitive restructuring. However, by contrast, findings from other studies seem to indicate that clients who make clinically significant cognitive changes—including those at the levels of intermediate assumptions and early maladaptive schemas—are apt to evince improvements in cognitive therapy, whether the problem is syndromal depression (Evans, Hollon, et al., 1992; Hollon et al., 1992; Tang et al., 2005) or more pervasive, longitudinal problems such as borderline personality disorder (Giesen-Bloo et al, 2006.). Further, there are several studies that seem to indicate that clients who learn to apply cognitive restructuring methods on themselves in a competent way tend to get more out of treatment as a whole (Jarrett, Vittengl, Clark, & Thase, 2011; Strunk, DeRubeis, Chiu, & Alvarez, 2007). Similarly, there is research showing that clients who do cognitive therapy homework—more regularly and with better quality—gain more from their participation in cognitive therapy, both in the short term and well after therapy has terminated (Burns & Splangler, 2000; Kazantzis, Whittington, & Dattilio, 2010; Rees, McEvoy, & Nathan, 2005). Because cognitive therapy homework assignments very commonly include cognitive restructuring exercises, these data give us more confidence about the importance of including cognitive restructuring in the treatment package, including using the ATR and other methods described earlier.

We must remember that it is very difficult and somewhat artificial to evaluate the efficacy of cognitive restructuring out of the context of a good case conceptualization and a positive therapeutic relationship. Without the "roadmap" that the case conceptualization supplies, the techniques of cognitive therapy can sometimes seem to get "lost" in the delivery process. Similarly, if the therapeutic relationship does not provide a sufficiently smooth "path" for the delivery of the techniques, the latter may "fall off the cart" and therefore never reach their destination. Once again, we see that in order to evaluate the efficacy of clinical methods such as cognitive restructuring, we need to study them in their natural context, or we lose something valuable in the process.

This idea takes us back to the argument that determining the efficacy of cognitive restructuring is best accomplished by examining the efficacy of the entirety of cognitive therapy as provided in real-life practice. Here, the data are broadly favorable (Butler, Chapman, Forman, & Beck, 2006). In a review of 16 methodologically rigorous meta-analyses on outcomes in cognitive (and cognitive-behavioral) therapy that included over 300 studies and nearly 10,000 clients, Butler et al. (2006) calculated a comparison-weighted grand mean effect size of 0.95 (standard deviation = 0.08) for the treatment of unipolar depression (child, adolescent, and adult); childhood anxiety disorders; adult anxiety disorders, including generalized anxiety disorder, social anxiety disorder, and panic disorder with and without agoraphobia; and PTSD. For cognitive therapy of bulimia, the authors report effect sizes significantly greater than those found for pharmacotherapy (mean effect size = 1.27; standard deviation = 0.11). When combined with medication, cognitive therapy has shown promising results in the treatment of schizophrenia, in which improving clients' reality testing skills via cognitive restructuring is one of the defining features of the treatment (Beck, Rector, Stolar, & Grant, 2009; Perivoliotis, Grant, & Beck, 2009). Here, Butler and his colleagues report an average within-groups (uncontrolled) effect size of 1.23 compared to an average within-groups (uncontrolled) effect size of 0.17 for schizophrenic clients who received treatment as usual. In direct comparison with alternative treatments, cognitive therapy was modestly superior to antidepressants (effect size = 0.38) and equally efficacious as behavior therapy in the treatment of adult, unipolar depression and obsessive-compulsive disorder. The meta-analyses also demonstrated the robust maintenance of gains promulgated by cognitive therapy, with relapse rates being approximately only half those found in the pharmacologic treatment of adult clients with depression and panic disorder.

In a multisite, randomized, controlled trial involving cognitive therapy for moderate to severe depression, cognitive therapy was equally efficacious as antidepressant medication with a trend toward superiority in terms of long-term maintenance (DeRubeis et al., 2005; Hollon et al., 2005). Cognitive therapy also provides added value when combined with medication for early-course bipolar spectrum illness, producing better adherence to pharmacotherapy, longer periods of inter-episode wellness (including higher global adaptive functioning scores), and decreased hospitalization (Lam, Hayward, Watkins, Wright, & Sham, 2005). Also, there are data supporting cognitive therapy for the reduction of suicide attempts in a very high-risk population. For example, a 10-week cognitive therapy intervention with recently hospitalized suicide attempters lowered the rate of suicide attempts over the following 18 months by 50% (Brown et al., 2005). In a major randomized, controlled trial involving another high-risk population (clients with borderline personality disorder), a 3-year course of schema-focused cognitive therapy produced outcomes superior to transference-focused therapy (Giesen-Bloo et al., 2006). In a previous open study, a 1-year course of cognitive therapy produced favorable outcomes in a cohort of clients with borderline personality disorder in terms of improved mood, decreased hopelessness and suicidality, and therapeutic modifications in dysfunctional beliefs typical of borderline personality disorder (Brown, Newman, Charlesworth, Crits-Christoph, & Beck, 2004). For more information that goes beyond the scope of this review, the reader is referred directly to the Butler et al. (2006) study, as well as the volume by Dobson and Dobson (2009).

Future Directions in Cognitive Restructuring

As described next, some of the future directions of cognitive therapy in general (and the methods of cognitive restructuring in particular) are more accurately presented as *further developments and expansions* of new means of delivery of these techniques that have already shown promise on a limited scale. Exciting new paths include the following:

1. The application of cognitive restructuring to populations that had previously been considered to be unresponsive to cognitive techniques, including those afflicted with psychotic disorders such as schizophrenia

2. The dissemination of cognitive therapy methods to practitioners in settings that treat the special-needs populations alluded to earlier, such as community mental health centers, where practitioners from all levels of training must deal with the challenges of implementing efficacious therapy in groups and to inpatients whose length of stay is highly uncertain and variable

3. Helping more patients gain access to cognitive therapy, even when practitioners are in short supply, waitlists are long, and therapists' offices are far away, via the use of computer-assisted models of cognitive therapy and

4. The teaching of cognitive self-monitoring and self-help to children and adolescents as a part of their educational curriculum to help *prevent* the potential onset of mood and/or anxiety disorders.

Application of Cognitive Therapy to the Treatment of Schizophrenia

Cognitive therapy for clients with chronic psychotic disorders has emerged as an empirically supported treatment (Grant, Huh, Perivoliotis, Stolar, & Beck, 2012; Perivoliotis et al., 2009, 2010). There is a growing body of evidence suggesting that even clients with low insight are capable of learning to shift their attention and modify their cognitions so that they find their delusions and hallucinations *less compelling and bothersome.* Therapists working with this population are instructed to use less Socratic dialogue and less directive focusing on evidence, and instead to help their clients to improve psychosocial functioning in spite of their entrenched beliefs. Clients are taught to view their delusions and hallucinations as having less importance when compared to new, adaptive skills they can learn, and they are helped to view their heretofore dominant symptoms as mere "background noise" in their lives. Rather than risking the extremes of confronting clients on their idiosyncratic beliefs and perceptions on the one hand, or passively validating them on the other hand, cognitive therapy for schizophrenia encourages open-mindedness to a range of hypotheses, both within and outside the clients' delusional beliefs. In the process, the clients often gradually begin to question their investment in their own delusions and hallucinations, and they become more receptive to more direct methods of cognitive restructuring, such as generating rational responses (often written down on "flashcards") that refute the contents of their psychotic thinking as being false and unimportant.

Dissemination of Cognitive-Behavioral Therapy to a Wider Range of Practitioners

Even though cognitive-behavioral interventions have gained a great deal of empirical support and consequently have become more prevalent in graduate and postgraduate programs across mental health care disciplines, not all practitioners have had sufficient exposure to the full range of cognitive-behavioral methods in their training. Dissemination research suggests that providing one-time workshops for such clinicians is insufficient to raise their levels of competence in and fidelity to cognitive-behavioral procedures to adequate levels (Sholomskas et al., 2005). What is needed is a more repeated, ongoing training experience, such as via consultation and supervision, and via a change in "climate" within institutional settings such that cognitive-behavioral applications become the accepted norm (including case conferences that illustrate how therapists are conducting such interventions as cognitive restructuring with real clients). This is especially important in settings where traditional approaches to treatment have involved primarily pharmacotherapy, group therapy, and inpatient "milieu therapy," but perhaps not as much cognitive-behavioral therapy.

An excellent model for the dissemination of cognitive-behavioral therapy to practitioners in this type of setting is the *Beck Initiative*, a partnership between the University of Pennsylvania and the city of Philadelphia's Department of Behavioral Health and Mental Retardation (Stirman, Buchhofer, McLaulin, Evans, & Beck, 2009). The therapists in the Beck Initiative serve as trainers and ongoing consultants to a range of mental health professionals at all levels of educational background, working collaboratively with established teams within community mental health agencies, helping them to apply best practices of cognitive-behavioral therapy with seriously ill clients, including those diagnosed with schizophrenia (Riggs, Wiltsey-Stirman, & Beck, 2012; Stirman et al., 2010). In this model, participants are provided with workshops, ongoing supervision, and collegial feedback and evaluation of their progress as cognitive-behavioral therapists over a 6-month period. In return, the therapists-in-training also provide the clinicians of the Beck Initiative with feedback as well. The more widespread use of this training model holds promise in bringing the evidence-based methods of cognitive-behavioral therapy to more treatment settings, and consequently to more clients in need.

Facilitating Access via the Use of Computer-Assisted Cognitive Therapy

Related to the dissemination issue discussed earlier is the issue of client *access* to cognitive therapy. As there is still a paucity of appropriately trained therapists to provide cognitive therapy to the large numbers of clients who are currently underserved, the use of computer-assisted cognitive therapy is an exciting development in the efficacious delivery of treatment to wider populations of clients, with reduced cost and waitlist time (Wright et al., 2005). Perhaps the most well-known, established application of this model is the *Good Days Ahead* multimedia, computer-assisted form of cognitive therapy with reduced therapist contact (Wright, Wright, & Beck, 2004). This program (in the form of a DVD) engages clients through a variety of interactive self-help exercises designed to help them build the self-help skills central to cognitive and behavioral therapies. "Video, audio, graphics, and checklists are used extensively throughout the program" (Wright et al., 2005, p. 1158).

Clients who utilize the *Good Days Ahead* program do in fact see a therapist in the early stages of treatment; however, most of the sessions are relatively short (approximately 25 minutes), and during this time they are already being educated in the proper use of the computer system so as to gain autonomy once they no longer see their therapists. The contents of the computer-assisted learning modules are derived from authoritative manuals on cognitive therapy such as *Cognitive Therapy: Basics and Beyond* (Beck, 1995). Wright et al. (2005) report findings that strongly support the viability of this treatment approach. They write that "Both negative core beliefs and automatic thoughts—specific targets of cognitive therapy—were significantly reduced for patients who received computer-assisted cognitive therapy" (p. 162), and that this represented an *improvement* over the results for those who received standard cognitive therapy without the computerized component. The authors add that their data indicated that "participants in the computer-assisted cognitive therapy condition . . . retained knowledge of the core concepts of cognitive therapy throughout the study" (p. 162). In sum, the future proliferation of computer-assisted cognitive therapy may help more clients in more locations to gain access to learning the concepts and skills of cognitive therapy by reducing waitlist time, treatment time, logistical obstacles, and cost, all while maintaining efficacy.

Teaching Cognitive Therapy to Children as Basic Education to Prevent Mental Illness

An important further development of clinical methods such as cognitive restructuring is its power to *prevent* psychological disorders by promoting psychological resiliency, particularly in childhood and adolescence. For example, the *Penn Resiliency Project* (PRP) has shown that by teaching children in early adolescence to apply cognitive monitoring and cognitive interventions on themselves, they can improve their levels of optimism and self-efficacy in ways that reduce their vulnerability to mood disorders (Gillham & Reivich, 2004). Early findings from this group showed that PRP halved the rates of moderate to severe depressive symptoms in their study sample of 11- to 14-year-olds over a 2-year follow-up, including reducing depressive symptoms in those children who presented with mood problems at the outset, and preventing depressive symptoms from developing in other children (Gillham, Reivich, Jaycox, & Seligman, 1995).

The cognitive therapy methods that the PRP teaches children are delivered with the help of cartoons that ask them to guess what the protagonists in the illustrated story might be saying to themselves, which is followed by applying this method to understanding their own self-talk. Children learn such skills as the "putting it into perspective" method (to decatastrophize) and the "one step at a time" method (to be more hopeful and confident about solving problems). The PRP serves as a model for what can be accomplished on a larger scale if school-based cognitive therapy were to become a more routine part of a child's educational curriculum, perhaps reducing the incidence and severity of psychological disorders in adolescence, with longitudinal benefits into adulthood as well.

Across the globe, the *Friends Project* in Queensland, Australia, similarly has focused on preventing the development of full-blown mood and anxiety disorders in at-risk children ages 7–14 (Barrett, Farrell, Ollendick, & Dadds, 2006). Here, cognitive-behavioral principles are imparted to students by their teachers (with assistance from postgraduate psychology students) over a 12-session course (with parents also receiving four sessions of psychoeducation). Results have been very promising, with implications for promoting universal early-prevention projects.

Epilogue: Cognitive Restructuring and Self-Reflective Practice

Cognitive restructuring is not just for clients—therapists themselves can benefit greatly by applying the skills of self-monitoring to their troublesome thoughts and flexibly thinking of more adaptive alternative responses. When therapists actively use cognitive therapy methods on themselves, they gain valuable practice to assist them in expertly delivering these techniques to their clients, they gain a better sense of empathy for their clients regarding the trial-and-error process of learning to make cognitive changes, and they benefit by improving their own morale and sense of self-efficacy as well. Further, therapists who employ cognitive therapy techniques for themselves may serve as better role models for their clients, especially if they choose to share their automatic thoughts and alternative responses in session, and they may also be more adept at remaining empathic when at first their thoughts may otherwise lead them to be angry with their clients (see Newman, 2012). Additionally, such therapists demonstrate humility (as if to communicate that "We are not above using our own techniques"), as well a desire to learn and grow (as if to say, "Like everybody else, our perceptions are evolving over time"). This sort of "self-reflective" practice is an essential part of developing expertise in conducting cognitive therapy (Bennett-Levy & Thwaites, 2007).

In order for cognitive therapists to maximize their levels of competency in applying the methods of cognitive restructuring—to their clients as well as themselves—it is important that the process begin with clinical supervisors fostering the development of their trainees' self-reflection skills. Supervisors can do this best by creating a safe, accepting environment in which their trainees can share their own automatic thoughts and deeper beliefs (e.g., about their own work, or how they feel about their clients) without fear of disapproval and censure (Newman, 2013). With practice, the cognitive therapy trainees then become that much more adept at encouraging their clients to do the same, thus leading to more productive therapy sessions and a better transfer of skills to the clients. As we have already seen, this readily results in therapeutic gains that endure.

References

Alloy, L. B., Peterson, C., Abramson, L. Y., & Seligman, M. E. P. (1984). Attributional style and the generality of learned helplessness. *Journal of Personality and Social Psychology, 46,* 681–687.

American Psychiatric Association. (2000). *Diagnostic and statistical manual of the mental disorders* (4th ed., text rev.). Washington, DC: American Psychiatric Association.

Arntz, A., Klokman, J., & Sieswerda, S. (2005). An experimental test of the schema mode model of borderline personality disorder. *Journal of Behavior Therapy and Experimental Psychiatry, 36,* 226–239.

Barrett, P. M., Farrell, L. J., Ollendick, T. H., & Dadds, M. (2006). Long-term outcomes of an Australian Universal Prevention Trial of Anxiety and Depression Symptoms in Children and Youth: An evaluation of the FRIENDS program. *Journal of Clinical Child and Adolescent Psychology, 35,* 403–411.

Beck, A. T. (1976). *Cognitive therapy and the emotional disorders.* New York: International Universities Press.

Beck, A. T., Butler, A. C., Brown, G. K., Dahlsgaard, K. K., Newman, C. F., & Beck, J. S. (2001). Dysfunctional beliefs discriminate personality disorders. *Behaviour Research and Therapy, 39,* 1213–1225.

Beck, A. T., Freeman, A., Davis, D., & Associates. (2004). *Cognitive therapy of personality disorders* (2nd ed.). New York: Guilford Press.

Beck, A. T., Rector, N. A., Stolar, N., & Grant, P. G. (2009). *Schizophrenia: Cognitive theory, research, and therapy.* New York: Guilford Press.

Beck, A. T., Rush, A. J., Shaw, B., & Emery, G. (1979). *Cognitive therapy of depression.* New York: Guilford Press.

Beck, A. T., Steer, R. A., Beck, J. S., & Newman, C. F. (1993). Hopelessness, depression, suicidal ideation, and clinical diagnosis of depression. *Suicide and Life-Threatening Behavior, 23,* 139–145.

Beck, A. T., Steer, R. A., & Brown G. K. (1996). *Manual for the Beck Depression Inventory II.* San Antonio, TX: Psychological Corporation.

Beck, A. T., Weissman, A., Lester, D., & Trexler, L. (1974). The measurement of pessimism: The Hopelessness Scale. *Journal of Consulting and Clinical Psychology, 42,* 499–505.

Beck, A. T., Wenzel, A., Riskind, J. H., Brown, G., & Steer, R. A. (2006). Specificity of hopelessness about resolving life problems: Another test of the cognitive model of depression. *Cognitive Therapy and Research, 30,* 773–781.

Beck, J. S. (1995). *Cognitive therapy: Basics and beyond.* New York: Guilford Press.

Beck, J. S. (2011). *Cognitive behavior therapy: Basics and beyond* (2nd ed.). New York: Guilford Press.

Bennett-Levy, J., Butler, G., Fennell, M., Hackmann, A., Mueller, M., & Westbrook, D. (2004). *The Oxford guide to behavioural experiments in cognitive therapy.* Oxford, UK: Oxford University Press.

Bennett-Levy, J., & Thwaites, R. (2007). Self and self-reflection in the therapeutic relationship: A conceptual map and practical strategies for the training, supervision, and self-supervision of interpersonal skills. In R. L. Leahy & P. Gilbert (Eds.), *The therapeutic relationship in the cognitive behavioral psychotherapies* (pp. 255–281). London: Routledge.

Blackburn, I. M., James, I. A., Milne, D. L., Baker, C., Standart, S., Garland, A., & Reichelt, F. K. (2001). The revised cognitive therapy scale (CTS-R): Psychometric properties. *Behavioural and Cognitive Psychotherapy, 29,* 431–446.

Blatt, S. J. (1995). The destructiveness of perfectionism: Implications for the treatment of depression. *American Psychologist, 50,* 1003–1020.

Brown, G. K., Newman, C. F., Charlesworth, S. E., Crits-Christoph, P., & Beck. A. T. (2004). An open trial of cognitive therapy for borderline personality disorder. *Journal of Personality Disorders, 18,* 257–271.

Brown, G. K., Ten Have, T., Henriques, G. R., Xie, S. X., Hollander, J. D., & Beck, A. T. (2005). Cognitive therapy for the prevention of suicide attempts: A randomized controlled trial. *Journal of the American Medical Association, 294,* 563–570.

Burns, D. D., & Spangler, D. L. (2000). Does psychotherapy homework lead to improvements in depression in cognitive-behavioral therapy or does improvement lead to increased homework compliance? *Journal of Consulting and Clinical Psychology, 68,* 46–56.

Butler, A. C., Chapman, J. E., Forman, E. M., & Beck, A. T. (2006). The empirical status of cognitive-behavioral therapy: A review of meta-analyses. *Clinical Psychology Review, 26,* 17–31.

Clark, D. A., Beck, A. T., & Alford, B. A. (1999). *Scientific foundations of cognitive theory and therapy of depression.* Hoboken, NJ: Wiley.

Coffman, S. J., Martell, C. R., Dimidjian, S., Gallop, R., & Hollon, S. D. (2007). Extreme non-response in cognitive therapy: Can behavioral activation succeed where cognitive therapy fails? *Journal of Consulting and Clincial Psychology, 75,* 531–541.

Cummings, J. A., Hayes, A. M., Newman, C. F., & Beck, A. T. (2011). Navigating therapeutic alliance ruptures in cognitive therapy for avoidant and obsessive-compulsive personality disorders and comorbid Axis-I disorders. *International Journal of Cognitive Therapy, 4,* 397–414.

DeRubeis, R. J., Hollon, S. D., Amsterdam, J. D., Shelton, R. C., Young, P. R., Salomon, R. M., . . . Gallop, R. (2005). Cognitive therapy vs. medications in the treatment of moderate to severe depression. *Archives of General Psychiatry, 62,* 409–416.

Dobson, D., & Dobson, K. S. (2009). *Evidence-based practice of cognitive-behavioral therapy.* New York: Guilford Press.

Ellis, T. E. (Ed.). (2006). *Cognition and suicide: Theory, research, and therapy.* Washington, DC: American Psychological Association.

Evans, J., Williams, J. M., O'Laughlin, S., & Howells, K. (1992). Autobiographical memory and problem-solving strategies of parasuicide clients. *Psychological Medicine, 22,* 399–405.

Evans, M. D., Hollon, S. D., DeRubeis, R. J., Piasecki, J. M., Grove, W. M., Garvey, M. J., & Tuason, V. B. (1992). Differential relapse following cognitive therapy and pharmacology for depression. *Archives of General Psychiatry, 49,* 802–808.

Gibbs, B. R., & Rude, S. S. (2004). Overgeneral autobiographical memory as depression vulnerability. *Cognitive Therapy and Research, 28,* 511–526.

Giesen-Bloo, J., van Dyck, R., Spinhoven, P., van Tilburg, W., Dirksen, C., van Asselt, T., . . . Arntz, A. (2006). Outpatient psychotherapy for borderline personality disorder: A randomized trial of schema-focused vs. transference-focused psychotherapy. *Archives of General Psychiatry, 63,* 649–658.

Gilbert, P., & Leahy, R. L. (Eds.). (2007). *The therapeutic relationship in the cognitive-behavioral psychotherapies* (pp. 106–142). New York: Routledge.

Gillham, J., & Reivich, K. (2004). Cultivating optimism in childhood and adolescence. *Annals of the American Academy of Political and Social Science, 591,* 146–163.

Gillham, J. E., Reivich, K. J., Jaycox, L. H., & Seligman, M. E. P. (1995). Preventing depressive symptoms in schoolchildren: Two year follow-up. *Psychological Science, 6,* 343–351.

Grant, P. M., Huh, G. A., Perivoliotis, D., Stolar, N. M., & Beck, A. T. (2012). Randomized trial to evaluate the efficacy of cognitive therapy for low-functioning patients with schizophrenia. *Archives of General Psychiatry, 69,* 121–127.

Greenberger, D., & Padesky, C. A. (1995). *Mind over mood.* New York: Guilford Press.

Hackmann, A., Bennett-Levy, J., & Holmes, E. A. (2011). *Oxford guide to imagery in cognitive therapy.* New York: Oxford University Press.

Hewitt, P. L., Flett, G. L., & Weber, C. (1994). Dimensions of perfectionism and suicidal ideation. *Cognitive Therapy and Research, 10,* 439–460.

Hollon, S. D., DeRubeis, R. J., & Seligman, M. E. P. (1992). Cognitive therapy and the prevention of depression. *Applied and Preventive Psychiatry, 95,* 52–59.

Hollon, S. D., DeRubeis, R. J., Shelton, R. C., Amsterdam, J. D., Salomon, R. M., O'Reardon, J. P., . . . Gallop, R. (2005). Prevention of relapse following cognitive therapy vs. medications for moderate to severe depression. *Archives of General Psychiatry, 66,* 417–422.

Jacobson, N. S., Dobson, K. S., Truax, P. A., Addis, M. E., Koerner, K., Gollan, J. K., . . . Prince, S. E. (1996). A component analysis of cognitive-behavioral treatment for depression. *Journal of Consulting and Clinical Psychology, 64,* 295–304.

Jarrett, R. B., Vittengl, J. R., Clark, L. A., & Thase, M. E. (2011). Skills of cognitive therapy (SoCT): A new measure of patients' comprehension and use. *Psychological Assessment, 23,* 578–586.

Kazantzis, N., Whittington, C., & Dattilio, F. (2010). Meta-analysis of homework effects in cognitive and behavior therapy: A replication and extension. *Clinical Psychology: Science and Practice, 17,* 144–156.

Kuyken, W., Padesky, C. A., & Dudley, R. (2009). *Collaborative case conceptualization: Working effectively with clients in cognitive-behavioral therapy.* New York: Guilford Press.

Lam, D. H., Hayward, P., Watkins, E., Wright, K., & Sham, P. (2005). Relapse prevention in patients with bipolar disorder: Cognitive therapy outcome after two years. *American Journal of Psychiatry, 162,* 324–329.

Layden, M. A., Newman, C. F., Freeman, A., & Byers, S. B. (1993). *Cognitive therapy of borderline personality disorder.* Boston: Allyn & Bacon.

Newman, C. F. (2011). Cognitive behavior therapy for depressed adults. In D. W. Springer, A. Rubin, & C. G. Beevers (Eds.), *Clinician's guide to evidence-based practice: Treatment of depression in adolescents and adults* (pp. 69–111). Hoboken, NJ: Wiley.

Newman, C. F. (2012). *Core competencies in cognitive-behavioral therapy: Becoming a highly effective and competent cognitive-behavioral therapist.* New York: Routledge.

Newman, C. F. (2013). Training CBT supervisors: Didactics, simulated practice, and "meta-supervision." *Journal of Cognitive Psychotherapy, 27,* 5–18.

Nezu, A. M., Nezu, C. M., & D'Zurilla, T. J. (2013). *Problem-solving therapy: A treatment manual.* New York: Springer.

Norcross, J. C., & Lambert, M. J. (2011). Psychotherapy relationships that work II. *Psychotherapy, 48,* 4–8.

Parks, C. W., Jr., & Hollon, S. D. (1988). Cognitive assessment. In A. S. Bellack & M. Hersen (Eds.), *Behavioral assessment: A practical handbook* (3rd ed., pp. 161–212). Elmsford, NY: Pergamon Press.

Perivoliotis, D., Grant, P. M., & Beck, A. T. (2009). Advances in cognitive therapy for schizophrenia: Empowerment and recovery in the absence of insight. *Clinical Case Studies, 8*, 424–437.

Perivoliotis, D., Grant, P. M., Peters, E. R., Ison, R., Kuipers, E., & Beck. A. T. (2010). Cognitive insight predicts favorable outcome in cognitive behavioral therapy and psychosis. *Psychosis, 2*, 23–33.

Rees, C. S., McEvoy, P., & Nathan, P. R. (2005). Relationship between homework completion and outcome in cognitive behaviour therapy. *Cognitive Behaviour Therapy, 34*, 242–247.

Resick, P. A., & Schnicke, M. K. (1993). *Cognitive processing therapy for rape victims: A treatment manual.* London: Sage.

Riggs, S. E., Wiltsey-Stirman, S., & Beck, A. T. (2012). Training community mental health agencies in cognitive therapy for schizophrenia. *The Behavior Therapist, 35*, 34–39.

Riso, L. P., du Toit, P. L., Stein, D. J., & Young, J. E. (2007). *Cognitive schemas and core beliefs in psychological problems: A scientist-practitioner guide.* Washington, DC: American Psychological Association.

Safran, J. D., & Muran, J. C. (2000). *Negotiating the therapeutic alliance: A relational treatment guide.* New York: Guilford Press.

Safran, J. D., & Segal, Z. V. (1990). *Interpersonal process in cognitive therapy.* Lanham, MD: Jason Aronson.

Schmidt, N. B., Joiner, T. E., Jr., Young, J. E., & Telch, M. J. (1995). The Schema Questionnaire: Investigation of psychometric properties and the hierarchical structure of a measure of maladaptive schemata. *Cognitive Therapy and Research, 19*, 295–321.

Schotte, D., & Clum, G. (1987). Problem-solving skills in suicidal psychiatric clients. *Journal of Consulting and Clinical Psychology, 55*, 49–54.

Scott, J., Stanton, B., Garland, A., & Ferrier, N. (2000). Cognitive vulnerability to bipolar disorder. *Psychological Medicine, 30*, 467–472.

Sholomskas, D. E., Syracuse-Siewart, G., Rounsaville, B. J., Ball, S. A., Nuro, K. F., & Carroll, K. M. (2005). We don't train in vain: A dissemination trial of three strategies of training clinicians in cognitive-behavioral therapy. *Journal of Consulting and Clinical Psychology, 73*, 106–115.

Spinhoven, P., Bockting, C. L. H., Kremers, I. P., Schene, A. H., & Williams, J. M. G. (2007). The endorsement of dysfunctional attitudes is associated with an impaired retrieval of specific autobiographical memories in response to matching cues. *Memory, 15*, 324–338.

Stirman, S. W., Bhar, S. S., Spokas, M., Brown, G. K., Creed, T. A., Perivoliotis, D., . . . Beck. A. (2010). Training and consultation in evidence-based psychosocial treatments in public mental health settings: The access model. *Professional Psychology: Research and Practice, 41*, 48–56.

Stirman, S. W., Buchhofer, R., McLaulin, J. B., Evans, A. C., & Beck, A. T. (2009). The Beck Initiative: A Partnership to implement cognitive therapy in a community behavioral health system. *Psychiatric Services, 60*, 1302–1304.

Strauss, J. L., Hayes, A. M., Johnson, S. L., Newman, C. F., Barber, J. P., Brown, G. K., . . . Beck, A. T. (2006). Early alliance, alliance ruptures, and symptom change in cognitive therapy for avoidant and obsessive-compulsive personality disorders. *Journal of Consulting and Clinical Psychology, 74*, 337–345.

Strunk, D. R., DeRubeis, R. J., Chiu, A. W., & Alvarez, J. (2007). Patients' competence in and performance of cognitive therapy skills: Relation to the reduction of relapse risk following treatment for depression. *Journal of Consulting and Clinical Psychology, 75*, 523–530.

Tang, T. Z., Beberman, R., DeRubeis, R. J., & Pham, T. (2005). Cognitive changes, critical sessions, and sudden gains in cognitive-behavioral therapy for depression. *Journal of Consulting and Clinical Psychology, 73*, 168–172.

Tang, T. Z., & DeRubeis, R. J. (1999). Sudden gains and critical sessions in cognitive-behavioral therapy for depression. *Journal of Consulting and Clinical Psychology, 67*, 894–904.

Trepka, C., Rees, A., Shapiro, D. A., Hardy, G. E., & Barkham, M. (2004). Therapist competence and outcome of cognitive therapy for depression. *Cognitive Therapy and Research, 28*, 143–157.

Weishaar, M. E. (1996). Cognitive risk factors in suicide. In P. M. Salkovskis (Ed.), *Frontiers of cognitive therapy* (pp. 226–249). New York: Guilford Press.

Weissman, A. N., & Beck, A. T. (1978, November). *Development and validation of the Dysfunctional Attitudes Scale: A preliminary investigation.* Paper presented at the Annual Meeting of the American Educational Research Association, Toronto, Canada.

Wheeler, H. A., Blankenstein, K. R., Antony, M. M., McCabe, R. E., & Bieling, P. J. (2011). Perfectionism in anxiety and depression: Comparisons across disorders, relations with symptom severity, and role of comorbidity. *International Journal of Cognitive Therapy, 4*, 66–91.

Wright, J. H., Wright, A. S., Albano, A. M., Basco, M. R., Goldsmith, L. J., Raffield, T., & Otto, M. W. (2005). Computer-assisted cognitive therapy for depression: Maintaining efficacy while reducing therapist time. *American Journal of Psychiatry, 162*, 1158–1164.

Wright, J. H., Wright, A. S., & Beck, A. T. (2004). *Good days ahead: The multimedia program for cognitive therapy.* Louisville, KY: Mindstreet.

Young, J. E., & Beck, A. T. (1980). *Cognitive Therapy Rating Scale Manual.* University of Pennsylvania, Philadelphia, PA.

Young, J. E., Klosko, J. S., & Weishaar, M. E. (2003). *Schema therapy: A practitioner's guide.* New York: Guilford Press.

Young, M. A., Fogg, L. F., Scheftner, W., Fawcett, J., Akiskal, H., & Maser, J. (1996). Stable trait components of hopelessness: Baseline and sensitivity to depression. *Journal of Abnormal Psychology, 105*, 155–165.

Rational Emotive Behavior Therapy

Monica E. O'Kelly *and* James J. Collard

Abstract

Rational emotive behavior therapy (REBT) was developed by Albert Ellis. He first presented his work in the 1950s and was a pioneer in the field of cognitive-behavioral therapy. The underlying tenet of REBT is that it is not the activating event that causes an emotional reaction but the associated thoughts and beliefs. His theory had a strong philosophical base, and he distinguished between functional and dysfunctional emotions. He also emphasized the importance of secondary emotional reactions in the development of disturbed thoughts, feelings, and behaviors. He highlighted the importance of disputing irrational demands and evaluations in therapy, rather than focusing on inferences. To date, there has been a weight of evidence supporting the relationship between irrational beliefs and psychological dysfunction. The research into clinical applications of REBT has been studied to a lesser degree, but the findings have supported its effectiveness in treating a range of psychological disturbances.

Key Words: rational emotive behavior therapy, Ellis, irrational beliefs, disputing, research base, REBT

Rational emotive behavior therapy (REBT), developed by Albert Ellis, is an active-directive therapy focusing on the here and now, with a philosophical and empirical basis. It aims to resolve an individual's emotional and behavioral problems and, by doing so, to enable the individual to lead a happier and healthier life, achieving one's objectives. The underlying tenet of REBT is that it is not the situation that causes an individual's problems but the view or cognition that he or she has of the situation.

Albert Ellis, in developing his theory on the relationship between an environmental event and a person's emotional reaction, made claim in 1955 to being the first to practice cognitive-behavioral therapy, also teaching and publishing on the topic (Ellis, 1962). He subsequently refined his theory and wrote extensively. His major work, *Reason and Emotion in Psychotherapy*, which he wrote in 1962 and then revised in 1994 (Ellis, 1962, 1994), has remained a significant text for REBT practitioners. Although

the name has changed from the original "rational psychotherapy" (Ellis, 1958), to "rational emotive therapy" or "RET," and then to "rational emotive behavior therapy" or "REBT" (Ellis, 1994), the underlying cognitive tenets of the therapy remain the same. Ellis was a leader in what has come to be called "the cognitive revolution" (Dember, 1974, p. 161). He believed that he got better and quicker results with his REBT than traditional psychoanalysis did, emphasizing that his approach was not only cognitive but also philosophical (Ellis, 2010).

It has been claimed that Ellis was one of the most controversial figures of modern psychology, being on a par with Freud and Skinner in his ability to attract friends and adherents on one hand and opponents and detractors on the other (DiMattia & Lega, 1990). Many saw him as cold, brash, flippant, opinionated, lacking compassion for his clients, and having little care for his friends. He was forceful and dogmatic in therapy with frequent use of profanities. Others, in contrast, believed that his idiosyncratic personality was characterized by immense care and concern for his clients, being warm, kind, and gentle. He was a tireless worker with 18-hour days being the norm. He spent his time working in therapy with individuals and groups, supervising trainee therapists, giving lectures, and presenting at workshops as well as writing (DiMattia & Lega, 1990). By the time he died at the age of 93 he had written over 80 books and more than 800 articles.

Ellis's Biography

Ellis (2010), in his biography published posthumously, described himself in the following way: "I am a continual promoter. I am an incessant theorist. I am a steady proponent of REBT. In fact, in a sense, I am REBT" (p. 15).

Albert Ellis was born in Pittsburgh, Pennsylvania, on September 13, 1913, and he died on July 24, 2007. He was born into a family from a German-Jewish background and was the eldest of three with a younger brother and sister. He regarded himself from the start as independent and curious with a thirst for learning but needlessly shy. He felt that his parents were neglectful. He saw his mother as a doer—one who was helpful but superficial. On the other hand, he considered his father to be a thinker—irritable, opinionated, and critical of others.

At the age of 5 years, Albert became ill, initially with tonsillitis and then nephritis (diagnosed later as acute nephrosis), leading to recurrent and severe headaches and also pneumonia. Between the ages of 5 to 7 years he had repeated hospitalizations, on one occasion for 10 months, but usually for 1 or 2 weeks. In later life Ellis (2010) made claim that the young Albert started to practice the use of fledgling REBT techniques, particularly those of distraction, to cope with his condition, the unpleasant medical procedures, and what he regarded as his parents' neglect in not visiting for prolonged periods of time. He was not concerned about the lack of attention from his parents because he enjoyed the freedom that it gave him. He was a good student and did not fall behind with his schoolwork in spite of his hospitalization. He was an avid reader from an early age and developed a passion for reading in the areas of psychology and philosophy.

In his autobiography Ellis (2010) repeatedly saw himself favorably and in many ways superior to others—more intelligent than other children in the class, sociable, and at least as athletic as other boys his age. This was despite also noting that he did not

socialize with boys his age but preferred to mix with those a couple of years younger.

In his late teens and early twenties, Ellis (2010) was an individualist and politically and economically a radical, being critical of capitalism and an ardent collectivist. He had a leadership role in the Young America movement. At about 24 years he became disillusioned with this movement and instead became a radical sexual revolutionary. He had a reputation for being outspoken and unconventional.

Ellis regarded himself as pathologically shy with a fear of public speaking and a fear of relating to women. His involvement in the Young America movement with a leadership role led to him being in a position where he had to speak in public often, thus leading to a reduction in his anxiety. His reading of psychology led to his much cited experiment to extinguish his fear of women. He visited the Bronx Botanical Gardens and in 1 month approached 130 women sitting on a park bench by themselves. He reportedly spoke to 100 of those women and realized that nothing really bad happened. Of the women that he spoke to he actually made three dates and went on to see one of those three for several dates.

Ellis considered himself an authority on sex, love, and emotions. He was forced to abandon his initial dissertation at Columbia University on the love emotions of college-age women. In his autobiography he reported that he had many liaisons with women. He married three times, although it appeared that his first two marriages had tensions due to his lack of interest in socializing, and had one other long-term relationship. He listed a number of people in his autobiography as friends but also noted that they did not consider him friendly enough. After his death it became known that he had three children as a result of an unconventional arrangement with his first wife. He made an arrangement to father the children some time after they separated when she was married to her subsequent husband. Ellis agreed to the arrangement, given that it was kept confidential.

He was self-admittedly impatient, disgusted at peoples' stupidities and inefficiencies, and kept order at his workshops firmly and at times harshly.

Influences on Development of Ellis's Ideas

From the age of 15 years, the young Albert developed an interest in philosophy, reading the stoic Greek and Roman philosophers such as Zeno of Citium from the fourth century BC, Epictitus in the first century, and Marcus Aurelius (121–180BCE). These philosophers were among the first to state that it is not the things that happen but our view of them that upsets us (Ellis, 2010, p. 56). Ellis was open about the influences to his thinking. He had read widely and considered that his ideas were not really new. In addition to the Greek and Roman philosophers, he read Asian philosophers such as Confucius, Gautama Buddaha, and Lao-Tsu. Modern philosophers who influenced Ellis included Kant, Dewey, and Russel. Ellis considered that REBT had a strong humanistic and existential base. He acknowledged the incorporation of ideas from Kierkegaard, Heidegger, Buber, Sartre, Tillich, and Horney. He was also influenced by the experiential and encounter movement, incorporating both the ideas and methods of Schultz, Perls, and others. Erhard's intensive groups procedures were also an influence.

Ellis trained initially in psychoanalytic therapy, reading Freud's works as well as his followers (Ellis, 1994). He underwent 2 years of analysis before embarking on the role of a psychoanalytical therapist in 1949. Over time he became disillusioned with the approach, noting that insight did not change his clients' behavior. He became more active-directive, using behavioral interventions based on Pavlovian classical conditioning, claiming that this brought better results. By 1954 he was bringing in the influences of philosophy, particularly the views of Epictetus, to his therapy and becoming more aware of his clients' cognitions and belief systems. He believed that some cognitions arose from biological predisposition, and many were learned from parents and other environmental influences. Ellis furthermore acknowledged that both psychoanalysts and radical behaviorists referred to verbal conditioning, with individuals learning to think dysfunctionally because they are told self-defeating ideas. He believed, however, that they, the analysts and behaviorists, were not aware of self-talk and the personal construction of meanings by which people disturb themselves.

Ellis viewed Pierre Janet, Paul Dubois, and Alfred Adler as partly espousing a cognitive approach, with Janet and Dubois using methods of disputing the irrational beliefs similar to those used by Ellis. In addition, George Kelly's theory outlined how humans construct their own thoughts, feelings, and behaviors and that these were not actually taught. Kelly, however, did not develop direct approaches to disputing the unhelpful cognitive construction but rather used the behavioral technique of roleplay. Ellis was a forerunner in using and advocating the active-directive, information-gathering and cognitive-restructuring methods (Ellis, 1994).

He acknowledged the concepts of Piaget and Kelly in suggesting that people actively construct ideas and rules rather than passively adopting them. He then saw causation of disturbance as philosophical rather than psychodynamic (Ellis, 1994). The therapeutic implication was that his focus then shifted from undoing the past to changing clients' current self-talk or thinking. Ellis (1994) reported that he became aware of the work of George Kelly two years after he had commenced using REBT. While he agreed with Kelly's ideas and incorporated his technique of fixed roleplay, Ellis also used methods of cognitive disputing similar to Janet and Dubois.

Ellis saw himself as the first cognitive-behavioral therapist, vociferously advocating an active-directive, information-gathering and cognitive-restructuring approach from 1955. He believed that other cognitive-behavioral therapists who developed and presented their theories after him basically agreed with his view that thoughts were influential in developing feeling and behavior, rather than the activating events themselves. He listed Glasser's espousal of reality therapy; Beck's publication of his work on cognitive therapy of depression; Bandura's presentation of social learning theory; and Lazarus, Michenbaum, Goldfried, and Maultsby, all publishing their approaches to cognitive-behavioral therapy in the late 1960s and early 1970s, as being influenced by his theory (Ellis, 1994).

REBT Theory

Ellis (1962, 1994) postulated that the most important "cause" of distress or neurosis was not the environmental trigger or activating events (A's) but our dysfunctional or irrational beliefs (iB's) about these events. Thus, undesirable environmental events could lead either to what was considered appropriate or healthy emotional consequences (C's), such as feelings of regret, annoyance, or sadness, or unhealthy negative consequences (C's), such as feelings of guilt, anger, or depression. It was when the feelings were mediated by dysfunctional irrational beliefs that disturbance occurred. Ellis (1994) asserted that people created their emotional reaction.

> I stated and implied that when people have the
> goals and values (G's) of remaining alive and
> making themselves happy, and when Activating

Events or Activating Experiences (A's) block and thwart these Goals, they have a choice of making themselves feel *healthily* or *self-helpingly* sorry, regretful, frustrated, or disappointed at point C, their emotional Consequence; or they can (consciously or unconsciously) *choose* to make themselves feel *unhealthily* or *neurotically* panicked, depressed, horrified, enraged, self-hating, or self-pitying at C. (p. 17)

He further pointed out that healthy feelings were created by functional or rational beliefs (rB's), such as "I don't like this situation, but I can cope with it and do my best to change it." On the other hand, unhealthy feelings were created by dysfunctional or irrational beliefs (iB's), such as "This situation shouldn't be like this. It's horrible and awful and I can't stand it." The theory is summarized in Figure 9.1.

While the aforementioned description of Ellis's theory seemed to assume that thoughts "cause" feelings, Ellis (1962, 1994) acknowledged an interaction between events, thoughts, and feelings. "Thinking brings about and assesses emotions and behaviors. Emotions motivate thoughts and feelings. Then thoughts and feelings *circularly* create and influence each other and hardly ever are completely disparate or independent" (1994, p. 21). Changing beliefs is a significant part of REBT, as with other cognitive therapies; however, Ellis (1962, 1994) pointed out that disturbed feelings and/or behavior can be changed by changing A's, B's, or C's.

A (Activating event)	B (Beliefs)	C (Consequence)
	iB's	Extreme feelings
		Difficulty in managing
	irrational beliefs	Inappropriate behavior
		Block achievement of goals
	rB's	Functional feelings
		Ease in managing
	rational beliefs	Appropriate behavior
		Enables achievement of goals

Figure 9.1 Summary of Ellis's ABC of rational emotive behavior therapy (REBT).

A major factor that set REBT apart from traditional therapies was its lack of attention to past events and feelings, claiming that because these were in the past they could not be changed. The focus of REBT was on current thoughts, feelings, and behaviors, but could, however, include current thoughts, feelings, and behaviors in response to past events (Ellis, 1962, 1994).

The stress on irrational beliefs was a major factor that set REBT apart from other forms of cognitive-behavioral therapy. Beck (1976), in his cognitive therapy, coined the terms "automatic thoughts" and "cognitive distortions" for the self-talk that leads to disturbance. Meichenbaum (1977) referred to "self statements." Ellis (1962, 1994) went further in his conceptualization, claiming that the real source of disturbance was not such surface-level, automatic thoughts or self statements but deeper level evaluations that may not be in the individual's conscious awareness. For example, a person may tell himself or herself, "I am going to fail at this task, and *I should not fail*. If I do, *it will be awful*, and *I'm an incompetent person*." The evaluations are shown in italics. Of most significance was a dogmatic insistence by Ellis that REBT, more than other cognitive-behavioral therapies, held that underlying all irrational beliefs leading to disturbance were grandiose and absolutely held demands in the form of "shoulds," "musts," and "oughts" (for example, "I should do well"). Ellis (1994) claimed that our nature "impels! (*sic*) us to preserve and enjoy ourselves. But, alas, it also strongly encourages us to foolishly raise our strong goals, desires, and preferences, into unrealistic, overgeneralised, self- (and social-) sabotaging absolutistic shoulds, oughts, musts, and commands" (p. 16). He further stated "REBT almost uniquely holds that when people become—or *make themselves*—emotionally disturbed, they almost always have conscious and unconscious, overt and tacit absolutistic *musts* that spark their other disturbance-creating irrationalities" (Ellis, 1994, p. 142). Others writing in the REBT field also asserted that demands were the basic cause of emotional distress (Bernard & DiGiuseppe, 1989; Wolfe & Naimark, 1991).

While Ellis (1962, 1994) initially spoke about 12 irrational beliefs, over time he simplified these to three major categories of demands:

1. I must do well and win the approval of others or else I am not good.

2. Others must do the right thing or else they are no good and deserve to be punished.

3. Life must be easy, without discomfort or inconvenience.

Ellis (1977) also referred to four irrational thought processes, "demandingness" being included as one of these. The others were the evaluative processes of "awfulizing," low frustration tolerance or "I can't stand it-itis," and generalized negative ratings of either self or others. In contrast to the latter, Ellis emphasized the importance of developing unconditional acceptance of self and others, in particular rating the goodness and badness of how you and others think, feel, and behave but not the goodness and badness of one's entire self or being. The four irrational processes were considered to be enduring, generalized cognitive structures that were philosophical in nature and broad in scope with application to many areas of life (Smith, 1982). The notion of a sequence of the processes was developed by Campbell and his colleagues (Campbell, Law, & Burgess, unpublished data; Campbell, 1985), who suggested that demands and the other evaluative processes occur together. In contrast to Ellis's (1994) view of the demands as the primary source of disturbance, Campbell (1985) stated that "a focus on the demand by itself may predispose one to, but does not contain, an emotional concomitance" (p. 160). Awfulizing has been proposed by others (Wessler & Wessler, 1980) as the major evaluative component of irrational beliefs leading to disturbance. Research has supported the notion that it is not so much the demand that leads to disturbance but the evaluation that is made if the demand is not met (O'Kelly, Joyce, & Greaves, 1998).

In further refinement of his theory, Ellis (1994) alluded to the depth of beliefs, pointing out that a "client's self-*meanings* and self-*philosophies*, . . . may not be held in the form of self-sentences or self-talk but in more complex or more tacit kinds of self communication" (p. 39). He refers to such irrational demands and evaluations as core beliefs. They can be likened to the schemas referred to by Beck and others (Beck, Freeman, & Associates, 1990; Young & Klosko, 1994). Such irrational or non-functional beliefs are in many ways like the air we breathe in that both are continually present but we are not always aware that they are there. It is frequently the role of the REBT to bring these core beliefs into conscious awareness.

Points of Difference

Ellis's REBT (Ellis, 1962, 1994) and Beck's cognitive therapy (CT)(Beck, 1963, 1976), the longest standing and most commonly used forms of cognitive-behavioral therapy, have much in common. They both share the underlying tenet connecting beliefs with feelings. Both of these therapies also use a range of cognitive, emotive, and behavioral techniques. Many of the techniques used are the same in each therapy. Understanding the points of difference between these two therapies enriches an understanding of REBT. Many of the difference are not absolute but are more differences in emphasis.

Many years ago the senior author had the privilege of attending a workshop in Copenhagen with Aaron Beck. At the end of the workshop, she asked him the question, "What do you see as the difference between your approach to therapy and that of Albert Ellis?" He responded with a smile, "I really think you should ask Albert Ellis that, and I dare say if you did he would say that you should ask Tim." ("Tim" was Dr. Beck's second name, as he was called by his friends.) Fortunately, a visit to New York and the Albert Ellis Institute was on the itinerary for the trip, so this topic was discussed with Albert Ellis. He was very clear and succinct, mentioning five aspects that he considered the most significant (Albert Ellis, personal communication):

1. REBT emphasizes the prominence of demands as central to disturbance.
2. REBT differentiates between constructive and unconstructive negative emotion.
3. REBT emphasizes the need for forceful disputation, rational emotive imagery, and shame attacks to challenge hot cognitions that may be understood intellectually as irrational but the client still holds onto them.
4. REBT uses a range of behavioral, invivo disputations to challenge beliefs.
5. REBT is very actively directive.

These difference and those evident from the literature and observation of therapy are explored more fully next.

Difference in Conceptualization of Cognitions

REBT and CT, although similar in referring to layers of cognitions, differ in their conceptualization of unhelpful beliefs.

If we have a look at Figure 9.2, the manner in which Beck categorizes cognitions is listed. He talks first about automatic thoughts; these are the thoughts that initially come into a person's mind. They are those that float by and form much of the chatter of our conscious awareness. Assumptions,

REBT	CT

• *Inferences*
   Person's interpretation of events
   For example, "other people will think
   I'm strange"
 	
 • *Demands*
   For example, "other people should approve of me"
 	
 • *Evaluations*
   Awfulizing
   I can't stand it-itis
   Globalizing or negative
   rating of self or others
   For example, "I'm no
   good," "He's no good"
	• *Automatic thoughts*
	   Initial thought that comes into a person's mind
	   For example, "Other people will think I'm strange"
	
	 • *Intermediate belief*
	   These are assumptions and rules
	   For example, "Other people should approve of me."
	   "If others don't approve of me, it is awful."
	
	 • *Core evaluations, beliefs, or schemas*
	   For example,
	   "If others don't approve of me, I'm no good."
	   "I'm hopeless and helpless."

Figure 9.2 Categories of beliefs: rational emotive behavior therapy (REBT) versus cognitive therapy (CT).

rules, and core beliefs, on the other hand, may not be in a person's conscious awareness to the same extent. They may be implied. As can be seen in Figure 9.2, Ellis talks about inferences, demands, and evaluations. In a fashion similar to that of Beck, Ellis is aware of the initial level of beliefs but labels them inferences. Again, this is the person's interpretation of the event or the conscious chatter that is going on in the mind. He then has an emphasis on demands, followed by the evaluations that emanate if demands are not met. Ellis's evaluations are "awfulizing" or "catastrophizing," low frustration tolerance in the form of "I can't stand it-itis," and globalizing. This can involve negative rating of self or others based on one feature. For example, " 'I failed my exam; therefore, I am hopeless."

In observing the different categorization of cognitions, it is evident that there are a lot of similarities between the conceptualization of Beck and Ellis. Both have three layers of cognition and both differentiate between the first conscious level of thought that comes to mind, automatic thoughts for Beck and inferences for Ellis, and deeper beliefs. The demands in REBT parallel the rules in CT, and the evaluations in REBT to some extent parallel the core beliefs in CT.

However, some of the REBT evaluations, particularly "awfulizing" and low frustration tolerance, would not be considered core beliefs in CT but are regarded as attitudes and assumptions under intermediate beliefs. "Awfulizing" in CT is often referred to as catastrophic misinterpretation. Core beliefs in CT tend to be self-referent evaluations of helplessness and unlovability (Beck, 1995). As such, they differ from the evaluations of REBT, which in

addition to "awfulizing" and "I can't stand it-itis" includes negative rating of self and of others.

Another difference in terminology relates to the general labels used. To Ellis the B's were all the levels of cognition. In CT the automatic thoughts are called thoughts and the label beliefs is reserved for the deeper intermediate and core beliefs.

Difference in Origin: Philosophical Versus Empirical

As outlined in earlier sections of this chapter, REBT was developed by Ellis from his reading of philosophy and his own therapy practice, which could be seen as a number of N=1 studies. In contrast, Beck developed CT based on his research with depressed patients. This has a number of implications for the underlying theory of each therapy.

Conceptualization of the deeper beliefs, core beliefs or evaluations, differs. As can be seen in Figure 9.2, Ellis talks about awfulizing, low frustration tolerance, and globalizing, which can be either negative self-rating or negative other rating. These beliefs were developed by taking into account the range of negative emotion, not only depression but also anxiety and anger. On the other hand, in CT, variations of the core belief are "I'm unlovable and helpless," which relate to depression. It is with regard to anger that this difference in core beliefs or evaluations is most relevant. Recent research indicates that demands on others and negative rating of others are significant cognitions that need to be addressed in anger (Tafrate, Kassinove, & Dundin, 2002). Furthermore, research indicates that anger is an emotion in its own right that needs to be addressed. It is erroneous to consider that it is the underlying anxiety that only needs to be addressed. This evaluation related to anger is included in REBT conceptualization but is not included in CT.

Difference in Importance of Demands

Ellis (1962, 1994) forcefully stated that the "shoulds" or demands are the primary source of disturbance. Ellis believed that Beck did not acknowledge the importance of demands. Ellis was clear in claiming that the demands or shoulds were the cognitive basis of disturbance, the other processes of awfulizing, low frustration tolerance, and globalizing being secondary to the shoulds.

Given this, challenging the demands is often a significant focus of many REBT therapists. The same focus on demands as the primary source of disturbance is not evident in CT. Although rules are elicited and explored in CT, the assumption is made that individuals differ in regard to which beliefs are actually the most relevant and disturbing for them.

Difference in Level of Belief Reevaluated or Disputed

REBT and CT differ in the emphasis they place on disputing different levels of belief. CT places considerable importance on disputing the automatic thoughts. It is assumed that in doing so changes can occur in the core beliefs. Ellis would consider such a focus to be inelegant and, in contrast, would focus attention on disputing the demands and evaluations. Ellis saw his theory as having a strong philosophical basis, with the therapy directed toward exploring and challenging a person's underlying philosophy of life. The REBT therapist is therefore encouraged to cut to the chase quickly and focus on the demands and evaluation that are considered to be the more philosophical beliefs.

This is not to say that REBT does not dispute inferences or automatic thoughts or that CT does not dispute core beliefs or evaluations. It is simply that the emphasis differs in each therapy. There are theoreticians in the REBT school, however, that regard automatic thoughts or inferences as activating events and do not bother to dispute them at all (Dryden, 2000).

One of the problems with working at the inference or automatic thought level is that these cognitions may, in fact, be true. A thought that "My mother doesn't love me" might in fact be true. In this case eliciting only inferences or automatic thoughts may leave the therapist with nowhere to go in working with the client.

Another point that needs to be made is that inferences or automatic thoughts tend to be situationally specific. Although changing those automatic thoughts as in CT may lead to indirect change at the core evaluations level, changing inferences or automatic thoughts, in fact, helps a client develop the ability to deal with a specific situation. Focusing on demands, evaluations, or core beliefs, as in REBT, on the other hand, leads to therapy that generalizes across a number of different settings by focusing on the person's deeper philosophy of life.

Difference in Nature of Disputing

In contrast to REBT, CT places a greater emphasis on empirical disputation. Considerable time is spent exploring support for or against a belief, a technique that is particularly useful in disputing automatic thoughts. In contrast, REBT, while also using empirical disputation, places a greater emphasis on pragmatic and logical disputation. Underlying this logical disputation are strong philosophical assumptions about characteristics that are necessary to be a happy and healthy individual (Bernard, 1986; Ellis, 1994).

Those that have seen Albert Ellis in action are often struck by his idiosyncratic style, which is characterized frequently by a didactic and forceful approach, often with colorful language, as in the Gloria tapes. The term *disputation* was used when he challenged beliefs. It needs to be remembered that this is Albert's style and not necessarily a characteristic of REBT. Other REBT therapists aspire to develop a more Socratic style (Dryden, 2002) common with CT therapists and may consider that, as with CT, they are reevaluating or exploring the beliefs.

Difference in Focus on Emotions

CT and REBT differ with regard to the emphasis placed on emotion. REBT draws a distinction between helpful and unhelpful negative emotions. It acknowledges that there are negative emotions that are understandable, adaptive reactions to obnoxious situations, such as sadness, annoyance, and concern. They are in contrast to unhelpful emotions that block the individual's achievement of goals, such as depression, anger, and anxiety. In REBT constructive and unconstructive negative emotions are placed on two different continua. Other therapies do not differentiate between these different types of emotions, putting them on a single continuum (Dryden, 2000). REBT considers that only the unhelpful emotions need to be the focus of therapy (Dryden & DiGiuseppe, 1990). In REBT, focus is therefore directed to assessing the emotions and their behavioral consequences and associated physical sensation to ascertain if the emotion is unhelpful. This differentiation is not evident in CT (Beck, 1995).

In the practice of REBT, time is also spent in explicitly drawing connections between the client's specific beliefs and emotions (Dryden & DiGiuseppe, 1990) rather than general psychoeducation—a process called "making the B-C connection." Again, this feature is not evident in CT (Beck, 1995).

A further difference may occur in eliciting the unhelpful beliefs. A common practice in REBT is to anchor the cognitions being elicited to the disturbed emotion, for example, "When your mother yells at you and you feel angry, what are you thinking?" This is in contrast to saying, "What are you thinking when your mother yells at you?" which is a more likely question in CT.

Difference in Focus on Secondary Emotion or Cognition

From the early days of REBT, Ellis stressed the importance of exploring clients' thoughts about their thoughts and their thoughts and feelings about their feelings (Ellis, 1994). This latter he called symptom disturbance. For example, while a person might be anxious about succeeding at a love relationship, he then might be demanding that he not be anxious in the situation and furthermore think that he is worthless if he does make himself depressed. Panic is seen by the REBT therapist as a secondary emotion. The REBT therapist as a matter of course not only looks for the primary emotion but also looks for emotions about the emotion. Ellis's views were the forerunner to more recently developed metacognitive therapy and acceptance and commitment therapy.

REBT in Practice

In going from theory to practice, Ellis (1994) extended his ABCs of REBT by adding D for dispute, referring to challenging or exploring the unhelpful beliefs, and E for developing effective thinking. This led to F for the resulting functional feeling.

Ellis was known for performing REBT in public, particularly at the Albert Ellis Institute in New York on Friday nights. His performance, with an entry fee of $5, was considered by many to be the cheapest therapy or entertainment in town. Due to his public presentations, Ellis (Ellis & Joffe, 2002) believed

that most REBT therapists followed his style to help clients in a fast and thorough way. From observing Ellis's style it is evident that he was frequently didactic and forceful and used profanities in therapy. This is a style that may not sit well with many therapists. It is evident that while REBT therapists share the underlying theory and philosophy, the execution of REBT varies from therapist to therapist with idiosyncratic styles apparent (Dryden, 2002).

A number of REBT therapists follow a sequential process, systematically taking the client step by step through cognitive restructuring (Dryden, DiGiuseppe, & Neenan, 2010). Furthermore, the REBT competency scale (Dryden, Beal, Jones, & Trower, 2010) has been developed to enable researchers and clinicians to assess adherence to this REBT treatment model.

An REBT sequence adapted from Dryden, DiGiuseppe, and Neenan (2010) is summarized in Figure 9.3.

Identifying the Activating Event or A

The A or activating event is anything that we react to, the trigger. It can be an event, behavior of self or others, a thought that we have, or even a feeling. While some therapists look for concrete occurrences as activating events, others focus on the person's inference as the actual A.

Identifying the Emotional Consequence or C

It is an important part of therapy to assist the client in identifying his or her emotional reaction to the activating event. Clients often present who "don't do feelings." They may need to be encouraged to allow themselves to explore their emotions and then may have trouble labeling them and therefore require help with this task. It is evident that an

---

1. Identify the activating events (A or situation).
2. Identify the consequences (C or feelings).
3. Evaluate the consequences (C).
4. Evaluate the presence of secondary emotions.
5. Elicit the thoughts and beliefs.
6. Make the B-C connection.
7. Clarify goals
8. Explore the unhelpful beliefs.
9. Develop helpful beliefs.
10. Set homework.
Throughout therapy there is a need to ensure that both therapist and client are working on collaboratively set goals.

Figure 9.3 The rational emotive behavior therapy (REBT) sequence.

individual may have a range of feelings in response to one situation. For example, after an accident a person may be feeling both anxious and angry. It is easier to address one situation and one emotional response at a time. Drawing the connection between beliefs and emotional consequences, a later step in the sequence, is made a much easier task if this is done.

Exploring the Emotional Consequences or Feeling

Focusing on the client's feeling and exploring the severity, behavioral consequence, and physical sensations can help the client to be more in touch with his or her emotion and give the therapist an indication of the severity of the client's problem. A client can be asked to rate the strength of his or her emotion on a 10-point SUDS scale (Wolpe, 1969). The client can be asked to describe the behavior he or she engages in when that emotion arises and to describe the accompanying physical sensations. There are a number of advantages for the therapy in doing this:

1. By assessing the congruence between the expressed emotion, behaviors, and physical sensations, the therapist can more fully understand the client's emotional and behavioral experience and indicate whether the client's emotional label was an accurate expression of his or her feeling.

2. This information enables the therapist to ascertain if the emotion is helpful or unhelpful. This is a characteristic that was previously mentioned as setting REBT and the work of Ellis apart from other cognitive-behavioral therapists. There are many situations where emotional responses are to be expected and are part of being human. Given this, not all emotions require therapy. It is those emotions that are excessively strong that block the ability of the individual to achieve his or her goals that are considered the focus of REBT. The therapist is well advised to explore whether an emotion the client presents with is a normal, healthy emotion or if it is an inappropriately strong emotion. If the emotion is healthy and appropriate, it needs to be acknowledged and affirmed, with the client given permission to have that emotion and to accept it as healthy. If the emotion is excessively strong, with the client blocked in his or her ability to achieve goals, then therapy is required. Self-defeating behaviors and unhealthy physical sensation are the data that give the therapist insight as to the helpfulness of the emotion.

3. Evaluating the consequence or feeling also helps in assessment of therapeutic intervention with before and after intervention comparisons being made.

Detailed attention to emotion can also be a constructive and effective way for the therapist to build an alliance with the client.

Evaluating the Presence of Secondary Emotions

A secondary emotion or meta-emotion involves being distressed about being distressed. Ellis (1994) referred to this as symptom stress, again another distinguishing feature of REBT. This can be relevant to any emotion; for example, clients can be depressed about being depressed, leading to more severe depression, or they can feel anxious about being angry. It is also conceptualized in REBT that panic is anxiety about being anxious.

If we talk in terms of helpful and unhelpful emotions, it is possible that the primary emotion is a helpful emotion and the secondary emotion is an unhelpful emotion. This is the case after the death of a loved one when the primary emotion may be sadness, which is considered healthy grief, but then with unhelpful cognitions about the sadness, such as "I should not be this way; I'm useless" the unhelpful secondary emotion, depression, can develop. It was Ellis's opinion that the secondary emotion, if unhelpful, is stronger than the primary emotion and needs to be addressed first.

If the client does have an unhelpful secondary emotion, the therapist would start the sequence again with the primary emotion as the activating event or A and the secondary emotion as the C. Once the secondary emotion has been addressed, then therapy would continue by addressing the primary emotion if required.

Secondary emotions may not always be present. It is helpful, however, to always be looking for them, because if they are present, they need to be addressed. A good indication of a secondary emotion being present is if there does not appear to be logical consistency or congruence between cognitions and the emotion expressed.

The simplest way to explore the presence of secondary emotions is to simply ask, "How do you feel about being angry/anxious/depressed?"

Eliciting Beliefs

By this stage the therapist and client should have a clear understanding of the activating event or

A that is the target and the emotional and behavioral consequence or C that is the focus of this sequence. The emotion has been explored and affirmed and understood.

Drawing out the unhelpful beliefs that are often not in conscious awareness can require considerable skill. One needs to be careful not to feed the cognitions to the client but to draw them out. Using a hypothetico-deductive approach and keeping in mind Ellis's layers of cognitions, that is, the inferences, demands, and evaluations, the therapist has a relatively good hunch regarding what cognitions are present with each emotion. Rather than tell the client, however, a Socratic question exploring the cognitions is likely to be more constructive. Figure 9.4 gives a number of questions that can be helpful.

Drawing the B-C Connection

Drawing the B-C connection is a vital part of REBT. In essence what is done at this step is helping the client understand and accept that beliefs lead to feelings. This is the core of the REBT model, and in fact the general CBT model, and enables the client to take emotional responsibility.

Therapists may teach clients theoretically about the ABCs in a didactic manner. Alternatively, a therapist might use the client's problem, teasing out the thoughts and feelings and helping the client see the connection. This can be done directly or through drawing comparisons with other responses.

Exploring or Disputing the Beliefs

Now that the client understands that his or her thoughts lead to his or her emotional reaction, the REBT therapist goes on to explore the client's beliefs, to reevaluate them, or, in Ellis's words, to dispute them. The skill in doing this is to explore the beliefs in a manner that challenges but does not threaten or rupture the therapeutic alliance.

To elicit inferences

You feel depressed because….

What is going through your head when you are depressed?

What are you thinking when you are depressed?

To elicit demands

What do you expect?

What do you think should happen?

To elicit evaluations

What does that mean to you/ about you/ about them?

Figure 9.4 Examples of questions to elicit beliefs; the same questions can be use with other emotions.

Four styles are used in REBT to challenge the thoughts (DiGiuseppe, 1991), the two most common styles being didactic and Socratic challenges. The other two styles are the use of metaphor and the use of humor. When a therapist works didactically, he or she tends to take on the role of teacher by telling the client what negative thoughts he or she has and the resulting negative emotional consequence. More constructive alternative thoughts along with the more constructive consequence are pointed out. Alternatively, a Socratic approach involves asking questions, most of which the therapist knows the answers to. This process can help the client explore cognitions and alternatives. The Socratic approach involves the client being more active in the cognitive restructuring process. When using metaphor, both common metaphors that have shared collective meaning and idiosyncratic metaphors that are fitting for the individual client can be used. It is common practice when using metaphors to discuss with the client the meaning and its relevance to him or her and the situation. Finally, the use of humor can give life to therapy. Not only can it lift the mood of therapy but it also enhances the possibility of restructuring and remembering the more constructive thought.

The REBT therapist disputes the thoughts in three major ways: empirically, logically or philosophically, and pragmatically.

Empirically

"Where is the evidence?' is a typical example of empirical disputation used in REBT? Using the empirical approach, the therapist helps the client explore evidence that is observable, experienced, or measured in an experiment to support or disconfirm a belief. The belief is tested to see if it is a fact or an assumption. Clients are encouraged to develop knowledge based on their experience rather than assumptions that have no basis in fact.

Logically or Philosophically

Logical or philosophical disputation involves exploring the logic of a belief. It is frequently the case that the logic of unhelpful beliefs does not stand up to rigorous evaluation. Because Ellis believes that shoulds are the primary source of disturbance, the absoluteness of the should is challenged in REBT with the aim to shift the demand to a preference. The leap of logic in globally rating self and others in response to a specific event is pointed out with the philosophical position of self and other acceptance being explored. The black-and-white thinking in catastrophizing is challenged to help the client see that there are shades of gray, and low frustration tolerance in the form of I can't stand it-itis is questioned to help the client see that not liking a situation does not equate with not being able to stand it.

Pragmatically

Pragmatic disputation explores whether a particular belief is helping the person. Simple question such as "Where does it get you thinking this way?" are used in pragmatic disputing. A further approach involves asking, "If your best friend was in this situation, would you tell him that he is no good, that he is hopeless, that he is useless?"Many clients are horrified to think they would talk to another person in the manner they are "talking" to themselves and readily see that their beliefs are not helpful.

Developing More Effective Beliefs

The REBT therapist finally works with the client to develop more constructive beliefs that lead to healthier emotional responses. Some clients can do this without assistance. With others the REBT therapist may need to be more active in formulating the summary with or for the client.

Setting Homework

Finally, the REBT therapist encourages the client to walk the talk to consolidate the new helpful belief. Setting homework is therefore an essential part of REBT. While behavioral assignments can be suggested for the client to do between sessions, the therapist can also incorporate behavioral tasks into the therapy session.

Homework can take many forms. The following are examples:

• Written homework—in which a client can be asked to challenge a particular belief
• Reading coping statements
• Behavioral tasks—systematic desensitization, flooding, behavioral rehearsal, behavioral experiments, and so on
• Reading—clients can be encouraged to read relevant books and articles
• Recording—the therapy session can be recorded for the client to listen to between sessions
• Using interactive digital material in the form of interactive CD ROM or DVDs where the clients are challenged to actively change their thinking
• Working on recording sheets or thought/feeling diaries

Research Evidence for REBT

It is at times put forth that REBT is largely a philosophical therapy, with little research support for its effectiveness in treating psychological conditions. This, however, is incorrect. There is, in fact, a considerable amount of research on REBT. This has taken the form of research investigating the theory underpinning REBT and research into the efficacy and effectiveness of REBT as a form of treatment for psychological dysfunction.

Research into the theory of REBT has investigated the relationship between irrational beliefs and feelings, physiological indicators, behaviors, and other cognitions. It has been conducted in both therapeutic and experimental contexts. Clinical studies of applied REBT as a treatment for psychological disturbance have also been conducted with clinical and subclinical populations. These encompass qualitative reviews through to meta-analyses of the utility of REBT.

Ellis also pulled on research investigating the effectiveness of other forms of cognitive-behavioral therapy to support the use of REBT. He argued that there were in fact two ways of conceptualizing REBT practice; he labeled these as "elegant REBT" and "inelegant REBT" (1979). Elegant REBT was concerned with the identification of clients' dysfunctional beliefs hypothesized by REBT philosophy to be at the core of emotional and behavioral disturbance (e.g., demanding and awfulizing). Inelegant or general REBT was instead considered to encompass a large variety of cognitive, behavioral, and emotive techniques included within the cognitive-behavioral framework. He did not consider such interventions to be elegant REBT as they did not directly focus on changing dysfunctional demands, evaluations, or life philosophy. Interventions fitting with this conceptualization of inelegant REBT included cognitive restructuring of distorted inferences, behavioral experiments, exposure tasks, and skills training activities (Ellis, 1979). This inclusive definition enabled Ellis to pull on evidence supporting other forms of cognitive-behavioral therapy to bolster claims for the effectiveness of REBT.

Dryden and David (2008) claim that this strategy by Ellis to incorporate a broader range of cognitive-behavioral research findings has contributed to confusion about what REBT does specifically entail. They also contend, however, that in general cognitive-behavioral interventions can all fall within the province of REBT, but that they may differentially target inferences, core beliefs, or behavior change. They contend that specifically targeting the client's dysfunctional demands and evaluations is merely the preferred method of therapy, but that it may be more pragmatic to utilize other interventions with some clients (Dryden & David, 2008).

The research specifically supporting REBT will be reviewed in the following sections.

Evidence in Support of REBT Theory

IRRATIONAL BELIEFS AND DYSFUNCTION

Considerable research has been conducted examining the ability for rational and irrational thinking to explain human functioning. Such studies have tended to investigate the relationship between emotional states, behavior, and somatic responses in relation to different thinking styles.

Irrational beliefs have been found to be associated with a range of negative emotions, including depression, anxiety, and anger. For instance, studies by Cash (1984) and Prud'homme and Barron (1992) both demonstrated associations between measures of irrational thinking and depression. Such studies were interpreted with caution, however, as early measures of irrational beliefs (e.g., the Rational Behaviour Inventory and the Irrational Beliefs Test) were found to have little discriminant validity, as they correlated highly with negative emotional states (David, Szentagotai, Eva, & Macavei, 2005; McDermut, Haaga, & Bilek, 1997). More recently, McDermut, Haaga, and Bilek (1997) found that depressed people scored higher than nondepressed people on irrational beliefs even once negative affect had been controlled for. A range of specific beliefs have also been shown to be associated with depression. While McDermut et al. (1997) found that a demand for achievement was associated with depression, Prud'homme and Barron (1992) found that a demand for approval was central to depression, and both found that low frustration tolerance also impacted upon participants' levels of depression. A sense of helplessness/external locus of control was also associated with depression in the studies by Cash (1984) and Prud'homme and Barron (1992).

With regard to anxiety, irrational beliefs have been found to be associated with a range of clinical and nonclinical forms of anxiety. For example, irrational beliefs have been associated with anxiety disorders (e.g., Goldfried & Sobocinski, 1975; Himle, Himle, & Thyer, 1989; Himle, Thyer, & Papsdorf, 1982), test anxiety (e.g., Boutin & Tosi, 1983; Wong, 2008), specific phobias (e.g., Thyer, Papsdorf, & Kramer, 1983), and health anxiety

(e.g., Fulton, Marcus, & Merkey, 2011). Irrational beliefs have also been found to be associated with a tendency to worry. Lorcher (2003) found that a demand for approval and other beliefs possibly representing a sense of helplessness over one's future and "should" were the most prominent beliefs in predicting worry.

Similarly, anger has been associated with irrational beliefs (Eckhardt & Jamison, 2002; Muran, Kassinove, Ross, & Muran, 1989). For example, Eckhardt and colleagues (e.g., Eckhardt & Jamison, 2002; Eckhardt, Barbour, & Davison, 1998) have demonstrated that the number of irrational beliefs reported during an anger episode was not only associated with the level of anger reported but also could help differentiate between those that would act more aggressively and even violently. They further discovered that arbitrary inferences and demandingness were the primary beliefs associated with domestic violence (Eckhardt & Jamison, 2002).

Irrational beliefs have also been associated with what could be described as more rigid thinking patterns. Tobacyk and Milford (1982) found that those who demonstrated a greater endorsement of irrational beliefs showed a higher level of dogmatism and were less critical of their inference making. Ziegler and Hawley (2001) further report that the possession of more irrational beliefs is related to greater levels of pessimism.

A range of dysfunctional behaviors have been related to irrational beliefs. Behaviors demonstrating a positive association with irrational beliefs include domestic violence (Eckhardt & Jamison, 2002), pathological gambling (Lund, 2011), disordered eating habits (Mizes, 1988; Möller & Bothma, 2001), procrastination (Beswick, Rothblum, & Mann, 1988; Bridges & Roig, 1997), less assertiveness (Cash, 1984), and disruptive behavior in children (Gonzalez et al., 2004).

Finally, irrational beliefs have been shown to be associated with physiological indicators of emotional states (Goldfried & Sobocinski, 1975; Harris, Davies, & Dryden, 2006). In a meta-analytic review, Lyons and Woods (1991) found that physiological markers of distress and somatic disorders were associated with irrational beliefs.

THE BINARY MODEL OF EMOTIONS

Ellis's proposal that there are qualitative differences between functional and dysfunctional emotions (e.g., sadness vs. depression, concern vs. anxiety, guilt vs. remorse, anger vs. annoyance) has received limited attention in psychological research.

This idea contends with the traditional view that the movement from functional into dysfunctional emotions is largely a quantitative difference, based more on the intensity of emotional arousal (e.g., Watson & Clark, 1984).

Initial examination of Ellis's binary model of emotions was conducted by Cramer and colleagues (Cramer, 1985; Cramer & Fong, 1991; Cramer & Kupshik, 1993). They found that irrational beliefs demonstrated a positive association with both functional and dysfunctional emotional experiences, in the contexts of imagined stressful situations and when irrational statements were repeatedly rehearsed. This was interpreted as being evidence in support of the unitary model of depression. Such a conclusion has been criticized on a number of accounts. First, REBT theory does not suggest that functional and dysfunctional emotions cannot co-occur, so it is possible that high levels of functional emotions, dysfunctional emotions, and irrational beliefs can demonstrate an association without disconfirming Ellis's theory (Ellis & DiGiuseppe, 1993). Ellis and DiGiuseppe (1993) also queried how functional and dysfunctional emotions were defined and identified in the research. Furthermore, the use of imaginary situations as stressors and the mere repetition of irrational thoughts have also been criticized as possibly having little validity for inducing true emotional states (David, Montgomery, Macavei, & Bovbjerg, 2005).

Preliminary evidence in support of the model has appeared in research conducted by David, Schnur, and Belloiu (2002). From a retrospective recall of actual stressful events, they found that high levels of irrational beliefs were related to the experience of dysfunctional emotions, while low levels of irrational beliefs related to the experience of functional emotions. It has also been found that measures of arousal do not differentiate between functional and dysfunctional emotional experiences (David et al., 2004). This contradicts the unitary model's sole focus on emotional intensity as the factor differentiating functional and dysfunctional emotions. Furthermore, David, Montgomery, et al. (2005) provided further support of the binary model of emotions when studying the experience of distress in women about to undergo surgery for breast cancer. They found that the women reporting a higher level of irrational beliefs reported experiencing a greater level of dysfunctional emotions. In contrast, there was no difference in reports of functional emotions between high and low endorsement of irrational beliefs (David, Montgomery, et al., 2005).

These results were consistent across a sample from the United States and a sample from Romania, suggesting the results may be universal across cultures.

Thus, while supporting the binary model of emotions, the results of the research to date may also indicate that the experience of rational beliefs and irrational beliefs may be independent of one another (Bernard, 1998). That is, a high level of irrational beliefs may co-occur with any level of rational belief, from high to low, and vice versa.

Evidence for Applied REBT

Empirical studies into the efficacy and effectiveness of REBT have occurred in three stages over time. Prior to 1970 there was little research conducted specifically on REBT. There was then a stage of qualitative studies, conducted in the 1970s and 1980s, which made way for more recent quantitative outcome studies (David, Szentagotai, et al., 2005). These outcome studies are either general, with REBT subsumed into a group with other cognitive-behavioral therapies, or specific, with the efficacy of REBT itself as a stand-alone therapy examined.

The general outcome studies in which REBT studies have been included (e.g., Norton & Price, 2007; Wampold et al., 1997) have largely demonstrated positive outcomes for cognitive-behavioral therapy. This, of course, does have positive implications for REBT, but such research tends not to indicate to what degree REBT contributed to overall findings. In an early comparative study of psychotherapies, however, REBT demonstrated the second highest effect size (ES = 0.77), with only systematic desensitization demonstrating a greater effect size (Smith & Glass, 1977).

With regard to research specifically investigating the efficacy of REBT, two meta-analytic studies were conducted in the early 1990s (i.e., Engels, Garnefski, & Diekstra, 1993; Lyons & Woods, 1991). A more recent meta-analysis has also been conducted on the use of REBT with children and adolescents (i.e., Gonzalez et al., 2004). Table 9.1 provides a summary of the meta-analyses for the effectiveness of REBT for various diagnostic groups and by outcomes studied.

From the earlier meta-analytic studies, REBT was shown to have a moderate to strong effect size for a range of psychological problems, both clinical and nonclinical. Lyons and Woods (1991) reported that REBT had strong comparative effect sizes in relation to baseline (Mean ES = 1.37, SD = 0.87), no treatment control groups (Mean

Table 9.1 Summary of Mean Effect Sizes by Diagnostic Groups and Treatment Measures

	Lyons & Woods (1991)	Engels et al. (1993)	Gonzalez et al. (2004)* (no standard deviations reported)
Treatment effect based on diagnostic groups:			
- Neurotic	ES = 0.99, SD = 1.0	ES = 1.75, SD = 1.83	NA
- Phobic	ES = 0.81, SD = 0.73	NA	NA
- Normal	ES = 0.52, SD = 0.29	NA	NA
- Emotional/somatic	ES = 1.92, SD = 1.26	ES = 2.54, SD = 1.79	NA
- Anxiety	NA	ES = 1.71, SD = 1.49	NA
- Unclassified	ES = 0.95, SD = 0.84	ES = 1.04, SD = 0.81	NA
Based on outcome measures:			
- Anxiety	ES = 0.77, SD = 0.74	ES = 1.52, SD = 1.44	ES = 0.48
- Standard test measures	ES = 0.81, SD = 0.61	NA	NA
- Physiological measures	ES = 2.90, SD = 1.20	NA	NA
- Rationality	NA	ES = 2.15, SD = 1.67	ES = 0.51
- Performance or behavior	NA	ES = 2.48, SD = 1.78	ES = 1.15 (disruptive behavior)
- Neuroticism	NA	ES = 1.95, SD = 2.65	ES = .049 (grade point average)
- Self concept	NA	NA	NA
- Unclassified	ES = 2.15, SD = 1.42	ES = 1.28, SD = 1.40	ES = 0.38 NA

* Indicates study utilized weighted mean.
NA, not available, as it was not included as a category in the particular paper.

ES = 0.98, SD = 0.91), and waitlist controls (Mean ES = 1.02, SD = 0.85). These results indicated that for the baseline and control groups the pretherapy clinical improvement rate was between 20% and 30%, whereas the improvement rate following REBT intervention was between 70% and 80%. Specifically for children and adolescents, Gonzalez et al. (2004) also found that REBT produced greater effects than no-treatment control groups (Mean ES = 0.49), indicating that 69% of children receiving REBT scored better on outcome measures than untreated controls.

In comparison to placebo groups, Lyons and Woods (1991) found that REBT was more effective (Mean ES = 0.80, SD = 0.74). Engels et al.

(1993) also compared REBT to placebo groups. They found that when compared to placebo groups there was only a trend toward REBT being a more effective treatment (p = .07). Post hoc analysis did indicate, however, that this was due to therapeutic effects on rationality.

Interestingly, the strongest effects were reported for physiological and performance-related (e.g., grade point average) variables, which tend not to be the focus of "elegant REBT." The impact on physiological markers may be due to REBT's focus on reducing dysfunctional secondary emotional reactions. For behavioral performances, it is possible that functional behavior is easier to implement and may improve at a faster rate than that required for the extinction of habitual irrational beliefs, and that REBT also gives strategies to help the individual improve his or her functioning despite the continued presence of such beliefs.

In comparison to other cognitive and behavioral therapies, Lyons and Woods (1991) reported that there was a trend toward REBT being more effective, but this was not statistically significant. Similarly, Engels et al. (1993) found that while REBT (Mean ES = 1.72, SD = 1.29) demonstrated a stronger effect size than systematic desensitization (Mean ES = 1.35, SD = 0.74), this again was not statistically significant. Lyons and Woods (1991) also compared REBT to "other therapies" (e.g., psychodynamic, Gestalt, undifferentiated counseling). This did show that REBT was comparatively more effective than the "other therapies" (Mean ES = 0.85, SD = 1.31). Similarly, Gonzalez et al. (2004) found that REBT outperformed alternative treatments (e.g., human relations education, self-concept enhancement training) for children and adolescents (Mean ES = 0.57). To collect such heterogeneous groups of therapies together, however, may unfairly discriminate against some forms of therapy included under the general titles of "other therapies" and "alternative therapies."

Postdating the meta-analytic studies for adults has been research investigating the effectiveness of REBT with medication and in comparison to it. For instance, Macaskill and Macaskill (1996) compared the use of Lofepramine, a tricyclic antidepressant, against REBT and Lofepramine in the treatment of unipolar depression. They found that only the combined treatment group improved on measures of depression (i.e., the Beck Depression Inventory and the Hamilton Depression Rating Scale) and on the Dysfunctional Attitudes Scale. While both groups also improved on the Social Adjustment Scale, the improvement for the combined group was significantly better than the medication-only group.

More recently, David and colleagues (David, Szentagotai, Lupu, & Cosman, 2008; Sava, Yates, Lupu, Szentagotai, & David, 2009) have compared the use of REBT to that of fluoxetine (Prozac), a selective serotonin reuptake inhibitor (SSRI), in the treatment of major depressive disorder (MDD). The study (David et al., 2008) compared the outcome of a 14-week treatment course whereby participants were either provided with REBT, CT, or fluoxetine. At the end of the treatment period all three forms of therapy were found to be equally

efficient; however, at 6-month follow-up the REBT treatment group scored significantly better on the Hamilton Rating Scale for Depression than the fluoxetine treatment group (David et al., 2008). The CT group's score was also better than the fluoxetine group, but it did not achieve significance (David et al., 2008). This suggests that such cognitive-behavioral therapies, and REBT in particular, have enduring effects that persist after treatment is ceased.

Other factors influencing the effectiveness of REBT in the research were the duration of treatment and the level of therapist training, with greater therapy duration (Gonzalez et al., 2004; Lyons & Woods, 1991) and higher levels of therapist training contributing to stronger effect sizes from REBT (Lyons & Woods, 1991). On the other hand, factors such as group versus individual therapy, gender, age, and clinical versus nonclinical symptamatology have not been shown to be related to the effectiveness of REBT (Dryden & David, 2008; Engels et al., 1993; Gonzalez et al., 2004; Lyons & Woods, 1991).

Recommendations for Future Research and Practice

There is now a weight of evidence behind REBT; however, this is predominantly of a correlational nature. Thus, while the relationships discovered to date are all promising for REBT, they do not establish any causal pathways. As noted by David, Montgomery, et al. (2005), there is not yet any research demonstrating a specific link between a reduction in dysfunctional emotions and improved mental and physical health. Similarly, the links between rational and irrational beliefs and physiological indicators of arousal are not well established. Ideally such research would make use of real stressful situations and distress, rather than experimental stressors and induced distress.

While it had been assumed that rationality had been a bipolar construct from highly rational thinking to highly irrational thinking, research now suggests that the relationship between rational and irrational thoughts and beliefs may be more complex than first presumed. Thus, future research into the relationship between rational and irrational thoughts is warranted. This would likely require the development of scales to assess independently the different types of thoughts and beliefs (Dryden & David, 2008). REBT research would also benefit from a more in-depth understanding of the interactions between specific cognitions and the different levels of thoughts and beliefs (i.e., inferences, demands, and evaluations) and on the impact of specific cognitive changes.

Such research could also help to further inform investigation of the binary model of emotions. Although recent studies have provided promising support for the qualitative distinction between functional and dysfunctional emotions, this area requires further investigation. It is still yet to be determined whether the differences are qualitative, quantitative, or even a combination of qualitative and quantitative factors.

Further study of the clinical applications of REBT would also be beneficial. To date, much of the research has been conducted with young, highly functional individuals, and it has included subclinical populations (Dryden & David, 2008), which limits the generalization of their findings to clinical practice. Consequently, future research would be enhanced by research into the efficacy and effectiveness of REBT in the treatment of a range of clinical disorders. Subsequent meta-analyses could then also be conducted to assess recent empirical studies of REBT and to determine if recent developments in REBT have resulted in any changes to the previous research findings. It would be beneficial to include in such research a measure of therapists' fidelity to REBT.

REBT has already moved into fields outside of mental health, into organizational and educational fields. Further research is required to ascertain the efficacy of its use in these areas.

References

Beck, A. T. (1963). Thinking and depression: Idiosyncratic content and cognitive distortion. *Archives of General Psychiatry, 9*, 324–444.

Beck, A. T. (1976). *Cognitive therapy and emotional disorders.* New York: International Universities Press.

Beck, A., Freeman, A., & Associates (1990). *Cognitive therapy of personality disorder.* New York: Guilford Press.

Beck, J. (1995). *Cognitive therapy: Basics and beyond.* New York: Guilford Press.

Bernard, M. E. (1986). *Staying rational in an irrational world: Albert Ellis and rational emotive therapy.* Carlton, Australia: McCullock Publishing.

Bernard, M. E. (1998). Validation of the General Attitude and Belief Scale. *Journal of Rational-Emotive and Cognitive-Behavior Therapy, 16*(3), 183–196.

Bernard, M., & DiGiuseppe, R. (Eds.). (1989). *Inside rational-emotive therapy: A critical appraisal of the theory and therapy of Albert Ellis.* San Diego, CA: Academic Press.

Beswick, G., Rothblum, E. D., & Mann, L. (1988). Psychological antecedents of student procrastination. *Australian Psychologist, 23*(2), 207–217.

Boutin, G. E., & Tosi, D. J. (1983). Modification of irrational ideas and test anxiety through rational stage directed hypnotherapy (RSDH). *Journal of Clinical Psychology, 39*(3), 382–391.

Bridges, R. K., & Roig, M. (1997). Academic procrastination and irrational thinking: A re-examination with context controlled. *Personality and Individual Differences, 22*(6), 941–944.

Cash, T. F. (1984). The Irrational Beliefs Test: Its relationship with cognitive-behavioral traits and depression. *Journal of Clinical Psychology, 40*(6), 1399–1405.

Campbell, I. M. (1985). The psychology of homosexuality. In A. Ellis & M. E. Bernard (Eds.), *Clinical applications of rational-emotive therapy* (pp. 153–180). New York: Plenum Press.

Cramer, D. (1985). Irrational beliefs and strength versus inappropriateness of feeling. *British Journal of Cognitive Psychotherapy, 3*, 81–92.

Cramer, D., & Fong, J. (1991). Effect of rational and irrational beliefs on intensity and "inappropriateness" of feelings: A test of rational-emotive theory. *Cognitive Therapy and Research, 15*(4), 319–329.

Cramer, D., & Kupshik, G. (1993). Effect of rational and irrational statements on intensity and "inappropriateness" of emotional distress and irrational beliefs in psychotherapy patients. *British Journal of Clinical Psychology, 32*(3), 319–325.

David, D., Montgomery, G. H., Macavei, B., & Bovbjerg, D. H. (2005). An empirical investigation of Albert Ellis's binary model of distress. *Journal of Clinical Psychology, 61*(4), 499–516.

David, D., Schnur, J., & Belloiu, A. (2002). Another search for the "hot" cognitions: Appraisal, irrational beliefs, attributions, and their relationship to emotion. *Journal of Rational-Emotive Cognitive-Behavior Therapy, 20*(2), 93–131.

David, D., Schnur, J., & Birk, J. (2004). Functional and dysfunctional feelings in Ellis' cognitive theory of emotion: An empirical analysis. *Cognition and Emotion, 18*(6), 869–880.

David, D., Szentagotai, A., Eva, K., & Macavei, B. (2005). A synopsis of rational-emotive behavior therapy (REBT): Fundamental and applied research. *Journal of Rational Emotive Cognitive Behavior Therapy, 23*(3), 175–221.

David, D., Szentagotai, A., Lupu, V., & Cosman, D. (2008). Rational emotive behavior therapy, cognitive therapy, and medication in the treatment of major depressive disorder: A randomized clinical trial, post treatment outcomes, and six-month follow-up. *Journal of Clinical Psychology, 64*(6), 728–746.

Dember, W. N. (1974). Motivation and the cognitive revolution. *American Psychologist, 29*, 161–168.

DiGiuseppe, R. (1991). Comprehensive cognitive disputing in RET. In M. Bernard (Ed.), *Using rational-emotive therapy effectively* (pp. 173–196). New York: Plenum Press.

DiMattia, D., & Lega, L. (1990). *Will the real Albert Ellis please stand up?* New York: Institute for Rational-Emotive Therapy.

Dryden, W. (2000). *Invitation to rational emotive behavioural psychology.* London: Whurr Publishers.

Dryden, W. (2002). *Idiosyncratic rational emotive behaviour therapy.* Ross-on-Wye, UK: PCCS Books.

Dryden, W., Beal, D., Jones, J., & Trower, P. (2010). The REBT competency scale for clinical and research applications. *Journal of Rational-Emotive and Cognitive-Behavior Therapy, 28*, 165–216.

Dryden, W., & David, D. (2008). Rational emotive behavior therapy: Current status. *Journal of Cognitive Psychotherapy, 22*(3), 195–209.

Dryden, W., DiGiuseppe, R., & Neenan, M. (2010). *A primer on rational-emotive behaviour therapy.* Champaign, IL: Research Press.

Eckhardt, C., & Jamison, T. R. (2002). Articulated thoughts of male dating violence perpetrators during anger arousal. *Cognitive Therapy and Research, 26*(3), 289–308.

Eckhardt, C. I., Barbour, K. A., & Davison, G. C. (1998). Articulated thoughts of maritally violent and nonviolent men during anger arousal. *Journal of Consulting and Clinical Psychology, 66*, 259–269.

Ellis, A. (1958). *Sex without guilt.* New York: Hillman.

Ellis, A. (1962). *Reason and emotion in psychotherapy.* Secaucus, NJ: The Citadel Press.

Ellis, A. (1977). The basic clinical theory of rational-emotive therapy. In A. Ellis & R. Greiger (Eds.), *Handbook of rational-emotive therapy* (pp. 3–34). New York: Springer.

Ellis, A. (1979). Rational-emotive therapy. In A. Ellis & J. M. Whiteley (Eds.), *Theoretical and empirical foundations of rational-emotive therapy* (pp. 101–173). Monterey, CA: Brooks/Cole.

Ellis, A. (1994). *Reason and emotion in psychotherapy.* New York: Birch Lane Press.

Ellis, A. (2010). *All out: An autobiography.* Amherst, NY: Prometheus Books.

Ellis, A., & DiGiuseppe, R. (1993). Are inappropriate or dysfunctional feelings in rational-emotive therapy qualitative or quantitative? *Cognitive Therapy and Research, 17*(5), 471–477.

Ellis, A., & Joffe, D. (2002). A study of volunteer clients who experience live sessions o REBT in front of a public audience. *Journal of Rational Emotive and Cognitive Behavior Therapy, 20*(2), 151–158.

Engels, G. I., Garnefski, N., & Diekstra, R. F. (1993). Efficacy of rational-emotive therapy: A quantitative analysis. *Journal of Consulting and Clinical Psychology, 61*(6), 1083–1090.

Fulton, J. J., Marcus, D. K., & Merkey, T. (2011). Irrational health beliefs and health anxiety. *Journal of Clinical Psychology, 67*(6), 527–538.

Goldfried, M. R., & Sobocinski, D. (1975). Effect of irrational beliefs on emotional arousal. *Journal of Consulting and Clinical Psychology, 43*(4), 504–510.

Gonzalez, J. E., Nelson, J. R., Gutkin, T. B., Saunders, A., Galloway, A., & Shwery, C. S. (2004). Rational emotive therapy with children and adolescents: A meta-analysis. *Journal of Emotional and Behavioral Disorders, 12*(4), 222–235.

Harris, S., Davies, M., & Dryden, W. (2006). An experimental test of a core REBT hypothesis: Evidence that irrational beliefs lead to physiological as well as psychological arousal. *Journal of Rational-Emotive and Cognitive-Behavior Therapy, 24*(2), 101–111.

Himle, D. P., Thyer, B. A., & Papsdorf, J. D. (1982). Relationships between rational beliefs and anxiety. *Cognitive Therapy and Research, 6*(2), 219–223.

Himle, J. A., Himle, D. P., & Thyer, B. A. (1989). Irrational beliefs and the anxiety disorders. *Journal of Rational Emotive Cognitive Behavior Therapy, 7*(3), 155–165.

Lorcher, P. S. (2003). Worry and irrational beliefs: A preliminary investigation. *Individual Differences Research, 1*(1), 73–76.

Lund, I. (2011). Irrational beliefs revisited: Exploring the role of gambling preferences in the development of misconceptions in gamblers. *Addiction Research and Theory, 19*(1), 40–46.

Lyons, L. C., & Woods, P. J. (1991). The efficacy of rational-emotive therapy: A quantitative review of the outcome research. *Clinical Psychology Review, 11*(4), 357–369.

Macaskill, N. D., & Macaskill, A. (1996). Rational-emotive therapy plus pharmacotherapy versus pharmacotherapy alone in the treatment of. *Cognitive Therapy and Research, 20*(6), 575–592.

McDermut, J. F., Haaga, D. A. F., & Bilek, L. A. (1997). Cognitive bias and irrational beliefs in major depression and dysphoria. *Cognitive Therapy and Research, 21*(4), 459–476.

Meichenbaum, D. (1977). *Cognitive-behavior modification: An integrative approach.* New York: Plenum.

Mizes, J. S. (1988). Personality characteristics of bulimic and non-eating-disordered female controls: A cognitive behavioral perspective. *International Journal of Eating Disorders, 7*(4), 541–550.

Möller, A. T., & Bothma, M. E. (2001). Body dissatisfaction and irrational beliefs. *Psychology Reports, 88*(2), 423–430.

Muran, J. C., Kassinove, H., Ross, S., & Muran, E. (1989). Irrational thinking and negative emotionality in college students and applicants for mental health services. *Journal of Clinical Psychology, 45*(2), 188–193.

Norton, P. J., & Price, E. C. (2007). A meta-analytic review of adult cognitive-behavioral treatment outcome across the anxiety disorders. *Journal of Nervous and Mental Disease, 195*(6), 521–531.

O'Kelly, M., Joyce, M., & Greaves, D. (1998). The primacy of the shoulds: Where is the evidence? *Journal of Rational—Emotive and Cognitive Behaviour Therapy, 16*, 223–234.

Prud'homme, L., & Barron, P. (1992). The pattern of irrational beliefs associated with major depressive disorder. *Social Behavior and Personality, 20*(3), 199–212.

Sava, F. A., Yates, B. T., Lupu, V., Szentagotai, A., & David, D. (2009). Cost-effectiveness and cost-utility of cognitive therapy, rational emotive behavioral therapy, and fluoxetine (prozac) in treating depression: a randomized clinical trial. *Journal of Clinical Psychology, 65*(1), 36–52.

Smith, M. L., & Glass, G. V. (1977). Meta-analysis of psychotherapy outcome studies. *American Psychologist, 32*, 752–760.

Smith, T. W. (1982). Irrational beliefs in the cause and treatment of emotional distress: A critical review of the rational emotive model. *Clinical Psychology Review, 2*, 505–522.

Tafrate, R., Kassinove, H., & Dundin, L. (2002). Anger episodes in trait anger community adults. *Journal of Clinical Psychology, 58*, 1573–1590.

Thyer, B. A., Papsdorf, J. D., & Kramer, M. K. (1983). Phobic anxiety and irrational belief systems. *Journal of Psychology, 114*(2), 145.

Tobacyk, J., & Milford, G. (1982). Criterion validity for Ellis' irrational beliefs: Dogmatism and uncritical inferences. *Journal of Clinical Psychology, 38*(3), 605–607.

Wampold, B. E., Mondin, G. W., Moody, M., Stich, F., Benson, K., & Ahn, H-N. (1997). A meta-analysis of outcome studies comparing bona fide psychotherapies: Empiricially, "all must have prizes." *Psychological Bulletin, 122*(3), 203–215.

Watson, D., & Clark, L. A. (1984). Negative affectivity: The disposition to experience aversive emotional states. *Psychological Bulletin, 96*(3), 465–490.

Wessler, R. A., & Wessler, R. L. (1980). *The principles and practice of rational-emotive therapy.* San Francisco: Jossey-Bass.

Wolfe, J., & Naimark, H. (1991). Psychological messages and social context: Strategies for increasing RET's effectiveness with women. In M. Bernard (Ed.), *Using rational-emotive therapy effectively* (pp. 265–301). New York: Plenum Press.

Wolpe, J. (1969). *The practice of behavior therapy.* New York: Pergamon Press.

Wong, S. (2008). The relations of cognitive triad, dysfunctional attitudes, automatic thoughts, and irrational beliefs with test anxiety. *Current Psychology, 27*(3), 177–191.

Young, J. E., & Klosko, J. S. (1994). *Reinventing your life.* New York: Plume Books.

Ziegler, D. J., & Hawley, J. L. (2001). Relation of irrational thinking and the pessimistic explanatory style. *Psychological Reports, 88*(2), 483–488.

Contemporary Problem-Solving Therapy: A Transdiagnostic Intervention

Arthur M. Nezu, Alexandra P. Greenfield, *and* Christine Maguth Nezu

Abstract

This chapter describes problem-solving therapy, a cognitive-behavioral intervention that teaches individuals a set of adaptive problem-solving activities geared to foster their ability to cope effectively with stressful life circumstances in order to reduce negative physical and psychological symptoms. This approach is based on the notion that what is often conceptualized as psychopathology and behavioral difficulties is a function of ineffective coping with life stress. Research addressing differences between effective and ineffective problem solving and the role of social problem solving as a moderator of the stress–distress relationship is presented. In addition, studies that support the efficacy of problem-solving therapy interventions are provided. A brief overview of the clinical components of problem-solving therapy is described that address problems of cognitive overload, emotional dysregulation, negative thinking, poor motivation, and ineffective problemsolving. Future directions for clinical practice, training, and research are included.

Key Words: social problem solving, problem-solving therapy, diathesis-stress models, stress–distress relationship, problem-solving strategies

Problem solving has traditionally been conceptualized as a major component of executive functioning that involves higher order mental or cognitive processes. In this context, research in experimental psychology has predominantly addressed the question of how humans solve problems of a cognitive or intellectual nature, such as a mathematical calculation or logic puzzle. However, these do not generally reflect the complexity of problems that people face in the real world, which are different than such cognitive problems in that they are (a) often stressful, (b) caused by or engender emotional difficulties, and (c) frequently involve other individuals. It was not until the second half of the twentieth century that research began to focus on those factors that impact one's ability to solve the types of problems that are typically encountered in everyday life (D'Zurilla & Nezu, 2007). This also led to the question of whether individuals can be trained to become better problem solvers as a means of

decreasing emotional difficulties and improve their overall quality of life. It was from this context that problem-solving therapy was developed.

Problem-solving therapy (PST) is a psychosocial intervention developed within a social learning framework and based on a biopsychosocial, diathesis-stress model of psychopathology. In general, this intervention involves training individuals in a set of skills aimed to enhance their ability to cope effectively with a variety of life stressors that have the potential to generate negative health and mental health outcomes, such as chronic medical conditions, depression, and anxiety. Life stressors can include both major negative life events (e.g., death of a loved one, diagnosis and treatment of a chronic illness, loss of a job, incarceration, military combat) and chronic daily problems (e.g., continuous tension with coworkers, reduced financial resources, discrimination, marital difficulties).

PST assumes that much of what is conceptualized as psychopathology and behavioral difficulties, including significant emotional problems, is a function of continuous ineffective coping with life stressors. As a result, it is hypothesized that teaching individuals to become better problem solvers can serve to reduce extant physical and mental health difficulties. The overarching goal of PST is to promote the successful adoption of adaptive problem-solving attitudes (i.e., optimism, enhanced self-efficacy) and the effective implementation of certain behaviors (i.e., adaptive emotional regulation, planful problem solving) as a means of coping with life stressors and thereby attenuating the negative effects of stress on physical and mental well-being.

The origins of PST from a social learning perspective can be traced back to the seminal article by D'Zurilla and Goldfried (1971), who developed a prescriptive model of training for individuals to enhance their ability to cope effectively with problems encountered in daily living. Early research applying this model to clinical populations focused on PST as a treatment for adults with major depressive disorder (e.g., Nezu, 1986). Subsequently, researchers and clinicians all over the world have successfully applied variations of this model to a wide range of psychological disorders, medical problems, and clinical populations (see D'Zurilla & Nezu, 2007). In addition, PST has been effective across different modes of implementation (e.g., individual, group, telephone, Internet) and has been applied as a means of enhancing one's adherence to other medical or psychosocial interventions (Nezu, Nezu, & Perri, 2006).

As new research improves our understanding of problem solving and stress, we have continuously revised and updated the basic PST model to incorporate findings from the outcome literature, as well as basic research from the fields of affective neuroscience, cognitive psychology, and clinical psychology. As such, we refer to the current model of treatment as "contemporary PST." This chapter will provide a broad overview of the conceptual and empirical underpinnings of this cognitive-behavioral intervention, as well as a brief description of clinical guidelines.

Problem, Solution, and Social Problem Solving

We begin by defining the constructs of problems, solutions, and social problem solving, the latter term used to describe the type of problem solving that occurs in real-life settings rather than problems of a more intellectual or academic nature.

Problem

We define a problem as a life situation, present or anticipated, that requires an adaptive response in order to prevent negative consequences from occurring but where an effective response or solution is not immediately obvious or available to the individual experiencing the situation due to the existence of various obstacles. The problem can arise from a person's social or physical environment (e.g., conflict with a family member, poor living conditions). It can also originate internally or intrapersonally (e.g., desire to make more money, confusion about life goals).

The barriers that make the situation a problem for a given individual or set of individuals can involve a variety of factors. These can include (a) novelty (e.g., beginning a new romantic relationship); (b) ambiguity (e.g., uncertainty about how one is perceived by his or her coworkers); (c) unpredictability (e.g., lack of control over one's job stability); (d) conflicting goals (e.g., difference between spouses/partners with regard to child-rearing philosophies); (e) performance skills deficits (e.g., difficulties with communication); (f) lack of resources (e.g., limited finances); and (g) significant emotional arousal (e.g., prolonged grief over the loss of a loved one).

An individual may recognize that a problem exists almost immediately based on one's overall reactions (e.g., physical symptoms, negative thoughts, urge to aggress) or only after repeated attempts to cope with the situation have failed. A problem can be a single, time-limited event (e.g., misplacing one's keys; forgetting to set one's alarm clock), a series of similar or related events (e.g., repeated disagreements between friends; not having a job that pays well), or a chronic, ongoing situation (e.g., a serious medical illness; persistent depressive symptoms).

According to this view, a problem is not a product of either the environment or the person alone. Rather, it is best understood as a person–environment relationship represented by a real or perceived discrepancy between the demands of the situation and one's coping ability and reactions. Problems are therefore idiographic and can be expected to change in difficulty or significance over time, depending on changes in the person, environment, or both. In other words, what a problem is for one person may not be a problem for someone else. In addition, what serves as a problem for a given person at one time may not be a problem for this same person at another point in time.

Solution

We define a solution as a situation-specific coping response that is the outcome of the problem-solving process when it is applied to a specific situation. An effective solution achieves the problem-solving goal while simultaneously maximizing positive consequences and minimizing negative consequences. The potential outcomes to consider may include possible impacts on the self and others, as well as short-term and long-term effects. Different individuals across different environments may vary in their evaluation of solutions based on the particular norms, values, and goals of the problem solver.

Social Problem Solving

Social problem solving (SPS) is the process by which individuals attempt to identify, discover, or create adaptive means of coping with a wide variety of stressful problems, both acute and chronic, encountered during the course of living (D'Zurilla & Nezu, 2007). It reflects the process whereby people direct their coping efforts at altering the problematic nature of a given situation, their reactions to such problems, or both. Rather than representing a singular type of coping behavior or activity, SPS represents the multidimensional metaprocess of ideographically identifying and selecting various coping responses to implement in order to match adequately the unique features of a given stressful situation at a given time (Nezu, 2004).

The construct of social problem solving should be differentiated from that of problem-focused coping. The term *coping* generally refers to the cognitive and behavioral activities that an individual uses to manage stressful situational demands, as well as the emotions they generate. Two major types of coping have been described in the literature: problem-focused coping and emotion-focused coping (Lazarus & Folkman, 1984). Problem-focused coping includes those activities that are directed at changing the stressful situation for the better (i.e., meeting, changing, or controlling situational demands). On the other hand, emotion-focused coping includes those activities aimed at managing the negative emotions generated by a stressful situation.

Within this context, SPS has, at times, been misrepresented as being equivalent to a form of problem-focused coping, suggesting that SPS goals include only mastery goals or attempts to control the environment (e.g., change another's behavior).

However, we define SPS as a broader, more versatile coping strategy that often includes both problem-focused and emotion-focused objectives. Regardless of whether the objective is articulated as problem focused or emotion focused, the ultimate goal is to minimize the negative effects of stressful life events on well-being. It is likely that particularly stressful problems require both problem-focused and emotion-focused objectives to be successfully resolved.

A Multidimensional Model of Social Problem Solving

According to contemporary SPS theory, problem-solving outcomes are largely determined by two general, but partially independent, dimensions: (a) problem orientation and (b) problem-solving style (D'Zurilla, Nezu, & Maydeu-Olivares, 2004). *Problem orientation* (PO) represents the set of cognitive-affective schemas regarding individuals' generalized beliefs, attitudes, and emotional reactions about real-life problems, as well as their ability to cope successfully with such difficulties. Whereas the original model suggested that the two types of problem orientations represented opposite ends of the same continuum (e.g., D'Zurilla & Nezu, 1999), subsequent research suggests that they operate somewhat independent of each other (Nezu, 2004). These two orthogonal orientation components are positive problem orientation and negative problem orientation.

A *positive problem orientation* involves the tendency for individuals to (a) perceive problems as challenges rather than major threats to one's well-being, (b) be optimistic in believing that problems are solvable, (c) have a strong sense of self-efficacy regarding their ability to handle difficult problems, (d) believe that successful problem solving usually involves time and effort, and (e) view negative emotions as important sources of information necessary for effective problem solving.

A *negative problem orientation* refers to the tendency of individuals to (a) view problems as major threats to one's well-being, (b) generally perceive problems to be unsolvable, (c) maintain doubts about their ability to cope with problems successfully, and (d) become particularly frustrated and upset when faced with problems or when they experience negative emotions.

An individual's problem orientation can have a strong influence on his or her motivation and ability to engage in focused attempts to solve problems. As such, the importance of assessing and addressing one's dominant orientation is considered a key component of the overall PST approach. For this reason, it is very important to include a specific and comprehensive focus on orientation variables when conducting PST. Unfortunately, some researchers have equated PST solely with "rational or logical" problem-solving skills and have de-emphasized or ignored problem-orientation variables. Because PST aims to help people cope effectively with real-life stressful problems, we firmly believe that attention must be paid to individuals' general beliefs, attitudes, and emotional reactions to real-world problems.

In support of this point, two recent meta-analytic reviews of the extant literature of PST, in addition to a randomized, controlled trial that directly posed this question (Nezu & Perri, 1989), support the notion that excluding a specific focus on problem-orientation variables consistently leads to significantly less efficacious outcome as compared to protocols that do include such training (Bell & D'Zurilla, 2009; Malouff, Thorsteinsson, & Schutte, 2007).

The second major dimension of SPS, *problem-solving style*, refers to the core cognitive-behavioral activities that people engage in when attempting to solve stressful problems. Three styles have been identified (D'Zurilla, Nezu, & Maydeu-Olivares, 2002; D'Zurilla et al., 2004): planful or rational problem solving, avoidant problem solving, and impulsive-careless problem solving.

Planful problem solving is the constructive approach that involves the systematic and planful application of the following set of specific skills: (a) *problem definition and formulation* (i.e., clarifying the nature of a problem, delineating a realistic set of problem-solving goals and objectives, and identifying those obstacles that prevent one from reaching such goals); (b) *generation of alternatives* (i.e., brainstorming a range of possible solution strategies geared to overcome the identified obstacles); (c) *decision making* (i.e., predicting the likely consequences of these various alternatives, conducting a cost-benefit analysis based on these identified outcomes, and developing a solution plan that is geared to achieve the problem-solving goal); and (d) *solution implementation and verification* (i.e., carrying out the solution plan, monitoring and evaluating the consequences of the plan, and determining whether one's problem-solving efforts have been successful or need to continue).

In addition to planful problem solving, two problem-solving styles have been further identified, both of which, in contrast, are frequently ineffective in nature (D'Zurilla et al., 2002, 2004). An *impulsive/careless style* is the problem-solving approach whereby an individual tends to engage in impulsive, hurried, and careless attempts at problem resolution. *Avoidant problem solving* is the problem-solving style characterized by procrastination, passivity, and overdependence on others to provide solutions. In general, both styles are associated with ineffective or unsuccessful coping. Moreover, people who typically engage in these styles tend to worsen existing problems and even create new ones.

It should be noted that this model does not suggest that individuals should be characterized exclusively by either type of orientation or problem-solving style across all situations. Rather, each represents a strong tendency to either view or react toward problems from a particular perspective based on one's learning experiences. For example, it is possible for individuals to be characterized as having a positive orientation when dealing with one type of problem (e.g., work-related difficulties), while simultaneously having a negative orientation when addressing other types of problems (e.g., relationship difficulties).

In addition, it should be noted that this five-component model of SPS (i.e., positive orientation, negative orientation, planful problem-solving style, impulsive/careless style, and avoidant style) has been cross-validated numerous times across various populations, ethnic minority cultures, and age groups (D'Zurilla & Nezu, 2007).

Social Problem Solving and Psychopathology

A large assumption underlying the relevance of PST as a psychosocial intervention is the notion that SPS represents a set of strategies that fosters effective coping with various forms of life stress. In support of this theory, research over the past several decades has consistently identified many pathology-related differences between individuals characterized as "effective" versus "ineffective" problem solvers across a range of age groups, populations, and cultures, and using differing measures of SPS (see D'Zurilla & Nezu, 2007; Nezu, Wilkins, & Nezu, 2004, for overviews of this literature). In general, when compared to their effective counterparts, ineffective problem solvers report a greater number of life problems, more health and physical symptoms, more anxiety, more depression, and more psychological maladjustment. Moreover, a negative problem orientation has been found to be associated with negative moods under routine and stressful conditions in general, as well as significantly related to pessimism, negative emotional experiences, and clinical depression (Nezu, 2004). Persons with a negative orientation also tend to worry and complain more about their health (Elliott, Grant, & Miller, 2004).

In addition, problem-solving deficits have been found to be significantly related to poor self-esteem, hopelessness, suicidal risk, self-injury, anger proneness, increased alcohol intake and substance risk taking, personality difficulties, criminal behavior, alcohol dependence, physical health problems, and diminished life satisfaction (D'Zurilla & Nezu, 2007).

A Problem-Solving/Stress Model of Psychopathology

Elsewhere, we have described in detail a diathesis-stress model of psychopathology that posits how SPS interacts with various biological, psychological, and social variables to influence how a given individual will respond to various life stressors and, consequently, what the outcome of this process might be (see Nezu, Nezu, & D'Zurilla, 2013 for a more detailed description of this model, particularly the distal, proximal, and immediate roles that various neurobiological, immune, and brain chemistry factors play in this process).

According to this model, certain distal factors, in the form of genetic predispositions and early life stress, have been found to produce both biological (e.g., increased stress sensitivity leading to lowered thresholds for triggering depressive reactions later in life; Nugent, Tyrka, Carpenter, & Price, 2011) and psychosocial (e.g., lack of opportunity to develop effective problem-solving skills due to stress-related overtaxed efforts to cope; Wilhelm et al., 2007) vulnerabilities that can further make one more susceptible to negative health and mental health outcomes during adolescence, adulthood, and older adulthood.

Focusing on more proximal variables, substantial research has documented the causal role of stress (in the form of major negative life events and chronic daily problems) in causing the initial onset and/or exacerbating preexisting psychopathology (e.g., depression) and certain medical disorders (e.g., heart disease, diabetes) (Pandey, Quick, Rossi, Nelson, & Martin, 2011). In addition to the presence of stress as a contributor to psychopathology, there may be important biological, developmental, sociodemographic, and psychological factors that

play a role in how individuals respond to stressors. Experiencing stress in the absence of effective coping can lead to increased levels of stress and distress (termed "stress generation") and a cyclical pattern of negative symptoms. Individuals who have experienced larger amounts of early life stress and/or possess a genetic vulnerability, in the face of this stress generation process, are then *especially* vulnerable to negative health outcomes (e.g., Monroe et al., 2006).

SPS is considered to be a key component of successful coping and is therefore hypothesized to serve as an important moderator of the overall stress–distress relationship. In other words, the manner in which people cope with extant stressful events via effective SPS may affect the degree to which they will experience both acute and/or long-term psychological distress. In general, studies directly exploring this question provide evidence that SPS, in fact, is a significant moderator of the stress–distress relationship. For example, under similar levels of high stress, individuals with ineffective or poor SPS have been found to experience significantly higher levels of psychological distress as compared to individuals characterized by effective SPS (Londahl, Tverskoy, & D'Zurilla, 2005; Nezu & Ronan, 1988; Ranjbar, Bayani, & Bayani, 2014).

The model further suggests that if one's problem-solving ability is unable to adequately cope with life stress, not only is it likely that he or she will experience negative health outcomes and psychological distress, but such outcomes can also subsequently produce further life stress, as well as continuously undermine one's problem-solving attempts. We suggest that this reciprocal "downward spiral" of stress-distress generation can lead to long-term clinical disorders.

Efficacy of Problem-Solving Therapy

PST has been applied, both as the sole intervention strategy and as part of a larger treatment package, to a wide variety of patient populations and clinical problems. In the past several years, three major meta-analyses of PST randomized, controlled trials have been published and provide support for the overall efficacy of this approach. For example, Malouff et al. (2007) conducted a meta-analysis of 32 studies, including close to 3,000 participants, that evaluated the efficacy of PST across a variety of mental and physical health problems. These authors found that PST was (a) equally as effective as other psychosocial treatments, and (b) significantly more effective than both no-treatment and attention-placebo control conditions. In addition, the inclusion of training in problem orientation and the assignment of homework led to larger effect sizes in treatment outcome.

A second meta-analysis published in the same year was conducted by Cuijpers, van Straten, and Warmerdam (2007). This investigation focused exclusively on trials of PST for the treatment of depression. Specifically, they focused on 13 randomized, controlled trials that collectively included over 1,100 participants. Based on their results, they concluded that although additional research is needed due to an identified variability in outcomes across studies, "there is no doubt that PST can be an effective treatment for depression" (p. 9). Note that one possible explanation for such variability involves the lack of a focus on problem-orientation variables in some of the studies characterized by lower effect sizes.

A third meta-analysis that also focused exclusively on PST for depression was conducted by Bell and D'Zurilla (2009) and included seven additional studies beyond those in the Cuijpers et al. (2007) meta-analysis. These authors came to similar conclusions when looking at both post-treatment and follow-up results across investigations. Specifically, PST was found to be equally effective for the treatment of depression as compared to both alternative psychosocial therapies and psychiatric medication, and more efficacious as compared to supportive therapy and attention-control conditions. In addition, Bell and D'Zurilla found that significant moderators of treatment effectiveness included whether the PST protocol included problem-orientation training and whether all four planful problem-solving skills were included.

Although not focusing exclusively on PST, three additional meta-analyses provide further support for PST as an evidenced-based treatment. One investigation involved both a meta-analysis and metaregression of randomized, controlled trials of brief psychological therapies for adult patients with anxiety, depression, or mixed common mental health problems treated in primary care (Cape, Whittington, Buszewicz, Wallace, & Underwood, 2010). Across 34 studies, involving close to 4,000 patients, it was concluded that PST for depression and mixed anxiety/depression was an effective treatment. Controlling for diagnosis, a metaregression analysis found no difference in efficacy between cognitive-behavioral therapy and PST. Another systematic review and meta-analysis evaluated the relative efficacy of various brief psychotherapy

approaches (eight or fewer sessions) for depression and again found PST to be an efficacious intervention (Nieuwsma et al., 2012). A more recent meta-analysis focused on different types of psychotherapy for adult depression and similarly found PST to be characterized by robust effects (Barth et al., 2013). These systematic reviews provide for substantial evidence in support of the efficacy of PST-based interventions for treating a wide range of mental disorders, particularly depression.

PST as a Transdiagnostic Intervention

Because PST has been found to be an effective treatment for a wide variety of populations and clinical problems, it can be viewed as a transdiagnostic approach. Conceptually, because stress plays a significant role, either as an etiological and/or maintaining variable, regarding many forms of psychopathology and patient problems, it stands to reason why this would be the case. A brief listing of problems and populations for which PST has been found to be effective include the following: adults with major depressive disorder (Nezu, 1986); medical patients also diagnosed with depression (Harpole et al., 2005); adults attempting suicide (Hatcher et al., 2011); adults with intellectual disabilities and comorbid psychiatric diagnoses (C. M. Nezu, Nezu, & Arean, 1991); young offenders with intellectual disabilities (Langdon et al., 2013); caregivers of patients with dementia (Garand et al., 2013), traumatic brain injury (Rivera et al., 2008), and stroke (Grant et al., 2002); adolescents with conduct disorder and substance abuse problems (Azrin et al., 2001); older adults with major depression and executive dysfunction (Alexopoulos et al., 2011); cancer patients and their significant others (Nezu, Nezu, Felgoise, McClure, & Houts, 2003); adults with hypertension (García-Vera, Labrador, & Sanz, 1997); patients with lower back pain (van den Hout, Vlaeyen, Heuts, Zijlema, & Wijen, 2003); low-income, Latino adults diagnosed with cancer (Ell et al., 2008); and adults with type 2 diabetes (Katon et al., 2004).

PST has also been used as an adjunct approach to foster the effectiveness of other behavioral intervention strategies (Nezu et al., 2006). It has been found to be effective if provided individually (Nezu et al., 2003), in a group format (Nezu & Perri, 1989), over the telephone (Allen et al., 2002), via the Internet (Choi et al., 2014), and as part of a collaborative care model of health care delivery (Unützer et al., 2002). More recently, PST has been applied to a US veteran population as a means of fostering their resilience in order to prevent future psychopathology (Tenhula et al., 2014).

Problem-Solving Therapy: Overview of Clinical Guidelines

In this next section, we provide a brief overview of the clinical components of contemporary PST. According to the model, we suggest that several major obstacles can potentially exist for a given individual when attempting to resolve real-life stressful problems successfully. These include the following:

1. The ubiquitous human presence of "brain overload," especially under stressful circumstances
2. Limited or deficient ability to engage in effective emotional regulation
3. Biased cognitive processing of various emotion-related information (e.g., negative automatic thoughts, poor self-efficacy beliefs, difficulties in disengaging from negative mood-congruent autobiographical memories)
4. Poor motivation due to feelings of hopelessness
5. Ineffective problem-solving strategies

PST focuses on training individuals in four major problem-solving "toolkits" that address each of the aforementioned general barriers. These toolkits include (a) problem-solving multitasking; (b) the "stop, slow down, think, and act" (SSTA) method of approaching problems while under stress; (c) healthy thinking and positive imagery; and (d) planful problem solving.

Note that a client's specific problem-solving strengths and weaknesses should determine whether *all* strategies in *all* toolkits are taught and emphasized. In addition, when choosing which training activities to engage in, the therapist should use clinical judgment regarding the relevance of other related factors, such as the anticipated length of treatment, the severity of negative symptoms, and the subsequent progress (or lack of) being made by the individual. In other words, not all materials across all four toolkits are mandatory to employ during treatment. Rather, the therapist should use assessment and outcome data to inform the inclusion and subsequent emphasis of particular PST activities.

Problem-Solving Multitasking: Overcoming Brain Overload

This set of tools is geared to help an individual overcome the ubiquitous human limitation when attempting to cope with stressful situations in real life: "brain or cognitive overload" (Rogers & Monsell, 1995). Due to basic human limitations in our ability to manipulate large amounts of information in our working memory simultaneously while attempting to solve complex problems or make effective decisions, especially when under stress, individuals are taught to use three "multitasking enhancement" skills: externalization, visualization, and simplification. These skills are considered foundational to effective problem solving, similar to those skills that may be taught as basic to effective aerobic exercise, such as stretching, breathing, and maintaining a healthy diet.

Externalization involves displaying information "externally" as often as possible. More specifically, clients are taught to write ideas down, draw diagrams or charts to determine relationships, draw maps, make lists, and audiotape ideas. In this manner, one's working memory is not overly taxed and can allow one to concentrate more on other activities, such as creatively thinking of various solutions. The *visualization* tool is presented as using one's "mind's eye" or visual imagery to help (a) better clarify the nature of a problem, (b) practice carrying out a solution (imaginal rehearsal), and (c) reduce high levels of negative arousal (i.e., a form of guided imagery whereby one is directed imaginally to go on a peaceful vacation). *Simplification* involves "breaking down" or simplifying problems in order to make them more manageable. Clients are taught to break down complex problems into more manageable smaller problems, and to translate complex, vague, and abstract concepts into more simple, specific, and concrete language.

"Stop, Slow Down, Think, and Act" (SSTA): Overcoming Emotional Dysregulation and Ineffective Problem Solving under Stress

This toolkit becomes especially important to emphasize in situations where the primary goal of PST for a particular individual involves the decrease of clinically significant emotional distress (e.g., depression, suicidal ideation, generalized anxiety). It is also useful for training individuals as a means of preventing extant emotional concerns from becoming particularly problematic. In essence, clients are taught a series of steps to enhance their ability to modulate (as opposed to "eradicate") negative emotional arousal in order to more effectively apply a systematic approach to solving problems (i.e., to be able to optimally use the various planful problem-solving skills). It is also presented to individuals as the overarching "map" to follow when attempting to cope with stressful problems that engender strong emotional reactions and is included as the major treatment strategy geared to foster adaptive emotional regulation skills. It is also included in PST as a means of minimizing impulsive/careless attempts at problem solving, as well as avoidance of the problem.

According to the SSTA method, clients are first taught to become "emotionally mindful" by being more aware of, and specifically focusing on, when and how they experience negative emotional arousal. Specifically, they are taught to notice changes in physical (e.g., headache, fatigue, pain), mood (e.g., sadness, anger, tension), cognitive (e.g., worry, thoughts of negative outcomes), and/or behavioral (e.g., urge to run away, yelling, crying) indicators. For certain individuals, additional training may be necessary to increase the accuracy by which they attempt to identify and label emotional phenomena. Next, they are taught to "Stop" and focus on what is happening in order to become more aware of what is engendering this arousal. More specifically, they are directed to engage in behaviors (e.g., shouting out loud, raising one's hands, holding up a stop sign) that help them to "put on the brakes" in order to better modulate their emotional arousal (i.e., prevent the initial arousal from evoking a more intense form of the emotion together with its "full-blown" concomitant negative thinking, state-dependent negative memories, negative affect, and maladaptive behaviors).

Next, in order to meaningfully be able to "Stop," clients are further taught to "Slow Down"; that is, to decrease the accelerated rate at which one's negative emotionality can occur. Various specific techniques are provided and practiced with clients in order to offer them a choice among a pool of potentially effective "slowing-down tools." These include counting down from 10 to 1, diaphragmatic breathing, guided imagery or visualization, "fake smiling" (in keeping with the potential positive impact related to the facial feedback hypothesis; Havas, Glenberg, Gutowski, Lucarelli, & Davidson, 2010), "fake yawning" (in keeping with recent neuroscience research demonstrating the efficacy of directed yawning as both a stress management strategy and a means to enhance cognitive awareness; Newberg & Waldman, 2009), meditation, exercise, talking to others, and prayer (if relevant to a particular individual). Individuals are also encouraged to use strategies that have been helpful to them in the past.

The "Thinking" and "Acting" steps in SSTA refer to applying the four specific planful problem-solving tasks (i.e., defining the problem and setting realistic goals, generating alternative solutions, decision making, solution implementation and verification) once one is "slowed down," in attempting to resolve or cope with the stressful problem situation that initially evoked the negative emotional stress reaction.

Healthy Thinking and Positive Imagery: Overcoming Negative Thinking and Reduced Motivation

This toolkit is included to specifically address additional problem orientation issues if relevant to a particular individual, that is, negative thinking and feelings of hopelessness. Similar to cognitive restructuring strategies, clients are taught that "how one thinks can affect how one feels." In essence, this toolkit entails a variety of cognitive change techniques geared to enhance optimism and enhanced self-efficacy. For example, clients are taught to use the "ABC Model of Thinking" (where "A" = the *a*ctivating or triggering event, "B" = a given *b*elief, attitude, or viewpoint, and "C" = the emotional *c*onsequence that is based on that belief, as compared to "reality") in order to determine whether one needs to change such negative beliefs. They are provided with a series of "healthy thinking" rules (e.g., "Nothing is 100% perfect…problems are a normal part of life…everyone makes mistakes…every minute I spend thinking negatively takes away from enjoying my life"), as well as a list of "realistically optimistic self-statements" (e.g., "I can solve this problem;" "I'm okay—feeling sad under these circumstances is normal;" "I can't direct the wind, but I can adjust the sails;" "Difficult and painful does not equal hopeless!"), as more optimistic examples of ways to think in order to readjust their orientation.

In addition, if a given individual has particular difficulty with changing his or her negative thinking, we also advocate having the PST therapist conduct a "reverse advocacy role play" exercise surrounding a given individual's unique negative thinking patterns. In this exercise, a given maladaptive attitude is temporarily "adopted" by the therapist using a role-play format. The individual, who now has to adopt the role of "counselor," has to provide reasons or arguments for why such an attitude is incorrect, maladaptive, or dysfunctional. In this manner, the client is influenced to begin verbalizing those aspects of a positive problem orientation. The process of identifying a more appropriate set of beliefs toward problems and providing justification for the validity of these attitudes helps the individual to begin to personally adopt such an orientation.

The second tool in this toolkit focuses on using visualization to enhance motivation and to decrease feelings of hopelessness. The use of visualization here, which is different than that described within the multitasking toolkit, is to help the client to sensorially experience what it "feels" like to successfully solve a difficult problem; in other words, to "see the light at the end of the tunnel or the crossing ribbon at the finishing line." With this strategy, the therapist's goal is to help patients create the experience of success in their "mind's eye" and vicariously experience the potential reinforcement to be gained. Clients are specifically taught to *not* focus on "how" the problem got solved; rather, to focus on the feelings associated with having *already* solved it. The central goal of this strategy is to have individuals create their own positive consequences (in the form of affect, thoughts, physical sensations, and behavior) associated with solving a difficult problem as a major motivational step toward overcoming low motivation and feelings of hopelessness, as well as minimizing the tendency to engage in avoidant problem solving.

Planful Problem Solving: Fostering Effective Problem Solving

This last toolkit provides training in the four planful problem-solving tasks, the first being *problem definition*. This activity involves having clients separate facts from assumptions when describing a problem, delineate a realistic and attainable set of problem-solving goals and objectives, and identify those obstacles that prevent one from reaching such goals. Note that this model advocates delineating both *problem-focused goals*, which include objectives that entail changing the nature of the situation so that it no longer represents a problem, as well as *emotion-focused goals*, which include those objectives that involve moderating one's cognitive-emotional reactions to those situations that cannot be changed. Strategies that might be effective in reaching such emotion-focused goals might include stress management, forgiveness of others, and acceptance that the situation cannot be changed.

The second task, *generating alternatives*, involves creatively brainstorming a range of possible solution strategies geared to overcome the identified obstacles to their goals using various brainstorming techniques. *Decision making*, the third planful problem-solving task, involves predicting the likely consequences of the various alternatives previously generated, conducting a cost-benefit analysis based on these identified outcomes, and developing a solution plan geared to achieve the articulated problem-solving goal. The last activity, *solution implementation and verification*, entails having the person optimally carry out the solution plan, monitor and evaluate the consequences of the plan, and determine whether his or her problem-solving efforts have been successful or need to continue.

Guided Practice

A major part of the PST intervention involves providing feedback and additional training to individuals in the four toolkits as they continue to apply the model to current problems they are experiencing. In addition, PST encourages individuals to "forecast" future stressful situations, whether positive (e.g., getting a promotion and moving to a new city) or negative (e.g., the break-up of a relationship) in order to anticipate how such tools can be used in the future to minimize potential negative consequences.

Future Directions

The need to address problems effectively is a fundamental part of the human experience across time and environments. Therefore, the importance of problem solving as a construct in psychology and psychotherapy is significant. In this last section, we outline several ideas about potential future directions across clinical practice, training, and research arenas.

Clinical Practice

Patients' self-management of chronic illnesses, such as diabetes, cancer, and heart disease, has received increasing attention as a means of enhancing one's sense of self-efficacy and the ability to deal with the difficult exigencies associated with ongoing medical illness (Bodenheimer, Lorig, Holman, & Grumbach, 2002). Within this context, teaching patients to become better problem solvers as a means of improving their self-management skills can be a potentially valuable approach.

Because ineffective problem solving has continuously been associated with mental health problems and poor adjustment to stressful events, focusing on the enhancement of problem solving *prior* to the experience of a stressful event can serve an important prevention role. Providing training in effective problem solving to individuals about to engage in a potentially stressful role, job, or activity may prevent them from experiencing consequent distress. For example, similar to the rationale for teaching critical thinking skills to college students as a basis for general learning, becoming a more effective problem solver may represent an important preventive approach provided to students at various educational levels as a means of enhancing overall adjustment. Additional examples can include training military personnel, firefighters, and police officers as a way to prevent burnout and ineffective adjustment to traumatic events. This concept can also apply to helping family members to become more effective caregivers when a loved one suffers from a chronic illness or dementia. All such situations represent ongoing difficult problems that can potentially be better handled through a more planful approach.

Further, it would be worthwhile for problem-solving-based approaches to be disseminated and integrated more effectively into standard health and behavioral health care delivery systems. For example, an initial evaluation of a national rollout of a PST-based intervention by the Department of Veterans Affairs, entitled Moving Forward (Nezu & Nezu, 2014), has shown promising results regarding its impact on decreasing depression, enhancing problem solving, and fostering resilience among veterans (Tenhula et al., 2014).

Training

Problem-solving and causal reasoning skills are core competencies in the scientific practice of professional psychology (Layne, Steinberg, & Steinberg, 2014; C. M. Nezu & Nezu, 1995). Effective problem solving, within a therapy context, is represented by a clinician's ability to define the problem validly (i.e., assessment, diagnosis, and case conceptualization), identify potentially effective means of reaching treatment goals (i.e., intervention strategies), make multiple decisions about conducting therapy (e.g., which intervention to carry out and when, when to terminate therapy), and evaluate the outcomes of the treatment subsequent to its implementation.

Problem solving, in this context, can be viewed as important skills to learn as part of an overall approach to competency-based training in applied psychology (Beck et al., 2014). Students at various levels of training and education in applied psychology fields can be taught problem-solving skills to apply in relation to a wide range of professional activities, including assessment, intervention, consultation, interpersonal relationships, ethical dilemmas, and research.

Research

Possible future research directions regarding PST involve testing the validity of the previously suggested applications of problem solving in clinical practice and training via rigorous research protocols. In addition, future studies could evaluate the value of adding PST to other forms of medical and psychotherapy interventions to enhance adherence to such treatments by overcoming various barriers (e.g., poor motivation, stress). Investigating possible moderators, such as personality characteristics, age, comorbid disorders, and intellectual functioning, of the effects of PST represents another major area of needed research in the future. Another research priority should be the continued determination of whether the established association between SPS and distress, as well as the efficacy of PST, is valid among other cultures. Last, similar to other psychotherapy research endeavors, it would be important to identify mediators of PST (i.e., mechanisms of action) in order to strengthen further the effectiveness of this intervention approach.

References

Alexopoulos, G. S., Raue, P. J., Kiosses, D. N., Mackin, R. S., Kanellopoulos, D., . . . Arean, P. A. (2011). Problem-solving therapy and supportive therapy in older adults with major depression and executive dysfunction: Effect on disability. *Archives of General Psychiatry, 68*, 33–41.

Allen, S. M., Shah, A. C., Nezu, A. M., Nezu, C. M., Ciambrone, D., Hogan, J. & Mor, V. (2002). A problem-solving approach to stress reduction among younger women with breast carcinoma: A randomized controlled trial. *Cancer, 94*, 3089–3100.

Azrin, N. H. D., Teichner, G. A., Crum, T., Howell, J., & DeCato, L. A. (2001). A controlled evaluation and description of individual-cognitive problem solving and family-behavior therapies in dually-diagnosed conduct-disordered and substance-dependent youth. *Journal of Child and Adolescent Substance Abuse, 11*, 1–43.

Barth, J., Munder, T., Gerger, H., Nüesch, E., Trelle, S., Znoj, H., . . . Cuijpers, P. (2013). Comparative efficacy of seven psychotherapeutic interventions for patients with depression: A network meta-analysis. *PLoS Medicine, 10*, e10001454.

Beck, J. G., Castonguay, L. G., Chronis-Tuscano, A., Klonsky, E. D., McGinn, L. K., & Youngstrom, E. A. (2014). Principles for training in evidenced-based psychology: Recommendations for the graduate curricula in clinical psychology. *Clinical Psychology: Research and Practice, 21*, 410–424.

Bell, A. C., & D'Zurilla, T. J. (2009). Problem-solving therapy for depression: A meta-analysis. *Clinical Psychology Review, 29*, 348–353.

Bodenheimer, T., Lorig, K., Holman, H., & Grumbach, K. (2002). Patient self-management of chronic disease in primary care. *Journal of the American Medical Association, 288*, 2469–2475.

Cape, J., Whittington, C., Buszewicz, M., Wallace, P., & Underwood, L. (2010). Brief psychological therapies for anxiety and depression in primary care: Meta-analysis and meta-regression. *BMC Medicine, 8*, 38.

Choi, N. G., Marti, C. N., Bruce, M. L., Hegel, M. T., Wilson, N. L., & Kunik, M. E. (2014). Six-month post-intervention depression and disability outcomes of in-home telehealth problem-solving therapy for depressed, low-income homebound older adults. *Depression and Anxiety, 31*, 653–661.

Cuijpers, P., van Straten, A., & Warmerdam, L. (2007). Problem solving therapies for depression: A meta-analysis. *European Psychiatry, 22*, 9–15.

D'Zurilla, T. J., & Goldfried, M. R. (1971). Problem solving and behavior modification. *Journal of Abnormal Psychology, 78*, 107–126.

D'Zurilla, T. J., & Nezu, A. M. (1999). *Problem-solving therapy: A social competence approach to clinical intervention* (2nd ed.). New York: Springer.

D'Zurilla, T. J., & Nezu, A. M. (2007). *Problem-solving therapy: A positive approach to clinical intervention* (3rd ed.). New York: Springer.

D'Zurilla, T. J., Nezu, A. M., & Maydeu-Olivares, A. (2002). *Manual for the Social Problem-Solving Inventory-Revised.* North Tonawanda, NY: Multi-Health Systems.

D'Zurilla, T. J., Nezu, A. M., & Maydeu-Olivares, A. (2004). Social problem solving: Theory and assessment. In E. C. Chang, T. J. D'Zurilla, & L. J. Sanna (Eds.), *Social problem solving: Theory, research, and training* (pp. 11–27). Washington, DC: American Psychological Association.

Ell, K., Xie, B., Quon, B., Quinn, D. I., Dwight-Johnson, M., & Lee, P. (2008). Randomized controlled trial of collaborative care management of depression among low-income patients with cancer. *Journal of Clinical Oncology, 26*, 4488–4496.

Elliott, T. R., Grant, J. S., & Miller, D. M. (2004). Social problem-solving abilities and behavioral health. In E. C. Chang, T. J. D'Zurilla, & L. J. Sanna (Eds.), *Social problem solving: Theory, research, and training* (pp. 117–134). Washington, DC: American Psychological Association.

Garand, L., Rinaldo, D. E., Alberth, M. M., Delany, J., Beasock, S. L., Lopez, O. L., . . . Dew, M. A. (2013). Effects of problem solving therapy on mental health outcomes in family caregivers of persons with a new diagnosis of mild cognitive impairment or early dementia: A randomized controlled trial. *American Journal of Geriatric Psychiatry, 22*, 771–778.

García-Vera, M. P., Labrador, F. J., & Sanz, J. (1997). Stress-management training for essential hypertension: A controlled study. *Applied Psychophysiology and Biofeedback, 22*, 261–283.

Grant, J. S., Elliott, T. R., Weaver, M., Bartolucci, A. A., & Giger, J. N. (2002). Telephone intervention with family caregivers of stroke survivors after rehabilitation. *Stroke, 33*, 2060–2065.

Harpole, L. H., Williams, J. W., Jr., Olsen, M. K., Stechuchak, K. M., Oddone, E., Callahan, C. M., . . . Unutzer, J. (2005). Improving depression outcomes in older adults with comorbid medical illness. *General Hospital Psychiatry, 27*, 4–12.

Hatcher, S., Sharon, C., Parag, V., & Collins, N. (2011). Problem-solving therapy for people who present to hospital with self-harm: Zelen randomised controlled trial. *British Journal of Psychiatry, 199*, 310–316.

Havas, D. A., Glenberg, A. M., Gutowski, K. A., Lucarelli, M. J., & Davidson, R. J. (2010). Cosmetic use of botulinum toxin-A affects processing of emotional language. *Psychological Science, 21*, 895–900.

Katon, W. J., Von Korff, M., Lin, E. H. B., Simon, G., Ludman, E., Russo, J., . . . Bush, T. (2004). The Pathways Study: A randomized trial of collaborative care in patients with diabetes and depression. *Archives of General Psychiatry, 61*, 1042–1049.

Langdon, P. E., Murphy, G. H., Clare, I. C., Palmer, E. J., & Rees, J. (2013). An evaluation of the EQUIP treatment programme with men who have intellectual or other developmental disabilities. *Journal of Applied Research on Intellectual Disabilities, 26*, 167–180.

Layne, C. M., Steinberg, J. R., & Steinberg, A. M. (2014). Causal reasoning skills training for mental-health practitioners: Promoting sound clinical judgment in evidenced-based practice. *Training and Education in Professional Psychology, 8*, 292–302.

Lazarus, R. S., & Folkman, S. (1984). *Stress, appraisal, and coping.* New York: Springer.

Londahl, E. A., Tverskoy, A., & D'Zurilla, T. J. (2005). The relations of internalizing symptoms to conflict and interpersonal problem solving in close relationships. *Cognitive Therapy and Research, 29*, 445–462.

Malouff, J. M., Thorsteinsson, E. B., & Schutte, N. S. (2007). The efficacy of problem solving therapy in reducing mental and physical health problems: A meta-analysis. *Clinical Psychology Review, 27*, 46–57.

Monroe, S. M., Torres, L. D., Guillaumont, J., Harkness, K. L., Roberts, J. E., Frank, E., & Kupfer, D. (2006). Life stress and the long-term treatment course of recurrent depression: III. Nonsevere life events predict recurrence for medicated patients over three years. *Journal of Consulting and Clinical Psychology, 74*, 112–120.

Newberg, A., & Waldman, M. R. (2009). *How God changes your brain.* New York: Ballantine Books.

Nezu, A. M. (1986). Efficacy of a social problem-solving therapy approach for unipolar depression. *Journal of Consulting and Clinical Psychology, 54*, 196–202.

Nezu, A. M. (2004). Problem solving and behavior therapy revisited. *Behavior Therapy, 35*, 1–33.

Nezu, A. M., & Nezu, C. M. (2014). *Moving forward: A problem-solving approach to achieving life's goals. Instructor's manual.* Unpublished treatment manual, Department of Veterans Affairs, Washington, DC.

Nezu, A. M., Nezu, C. M., & D'Zurilla, T. J. (2013). *Problem-solving therapy: A treatment manual.* New York: Springer.

Nezu, A. M., Nezu, C. M., Felgoise, S. H., McClure, K. S., & Houts, P. S. (2003). Project Genesis: Assessing the efficacy of problem-solving therapy for distressed adult cancer patients. *Journal of Consulting and Clinical Psychology, 71*, 1036–1048.

Nezu, A. M., Nezu, C. M., & Perri, M. G. (2006). Problem solving to promote treatment adherence. In W. T. O'Donohue & E. R. Levensky (Eds.), *Promoting treatment adherence: A practical handbook for health care providers* (pp. 135–148). New York: Sage Publications.

Nezu, A. M., & Perri, M. G. (1989). Social problem solving therapy for unipolar depression: An initial dismantling investigation. *Journal of Consulting and Clinical Psychology, 57*, 408–413.

Nezu, A. M., & Ronan, G. F. (1988). Stressful life events, problem solving, and depressive symptoms among university students: A prospective analysis. *Journal of Counseling Psychology, 35*, 134–138.

Nezu, A. M., Wilkins, V. M., & Nezu, C. M. (2004). Social problem solving, stress, and negative affective conditions. In E. C. Chang, T. J. D'Zurilla, & L. J. Sanna (Eds.), *Social problem solving: Theory, research, and training* (pp. 49–65). Washington, DC: American Psychological Association.

Nezu, C. M., Greenberg, J., & Nezu, A. M. (2006). Project STOP: Cognitive-behavioral assessment and treatment for sex offenders with intellectual disability. *Journal of Forensic Psychology Practice, 6*, 87–103.

Nezu, C. M., & Nezu, A. M. (1995). Clinical decision making in everyday practice: The science in the art. *Cognitive and Behavioral Practice, 2*, 5–25.

Nezu, C. M., Nezu, A. M., & Arean, P. A. (1991). Assertiveness and problem-solving training for mildly mentally retarded persons with dual diagnosis. *Research in Developmental Disabilities, 12*, 371–386.

Nieuwsma, J. A., Trivedi, R. B., McDuffie, J., Kronish, I., Benjamin, D., & Williams, J. W. (2012). Brief psychotherapy for depression: A systematic review and meta-analysis. *International Journal of Psychiatry and Medicine, 43*, 129–151.

Nugent, N. R., Tyrka, A. R., Carpenter, L. L., & Price, L. N. (2011). Gene-environment interactions: Early life stress and risk for depressive and anxiety disorders. *Psychopharmacology, 214*, 175–196.

Pandey, A., Quick, J. C., Rossi, A. M., Nelson, D. L., & Martin, W. (2011). Stress and the workplace: 10 years of science, 1997-2007. In R. J. Contrada & A. Baum (Eds.), *The handbook of stress science: Biology, psychology, and health* (pp. 137–149). New York: Springer.

Ranjbar, M., Bayani, A. A., & Bayani, A. (2014). Social problem solving ability predicts mental health among undergraduate students. *International Journal of Preventive Medicine, 4*, 1337–1341.

Rivera, P. A., Elliott, T. R., Berry, J. W., & Grant, J. S. (2008). Problem-solving training for family caregivers of persons with traumatic brain injuries: A randomized controlled trial. *Archives of Physical and Medical Rehabilitation, 89*, 931–941.

Rogers, R. D., & Monsell, S. (1995). The cost of predictable switch between simple cognitive tasks. *Journal of Experimental Psychology: General, 124*, 207–231.

Tenhula, W. N., Nezu, A. M., Nezu, C. M., Stewart, M. O., Miller, S. A., Steele, J., & Karlin, B. E. (2014). Moving forward: A problem-solving training program to foster veteran resilience. *Professional Psychology: Research and Practice, 45*, 416–424.

Unützer, J., Katon, W., Callahan, C., Williams, J. W., Hunkeler, E. M., Harpole, L., . . . Langston, C. A. (2002). Collaborative care management of late-life depression in the primary care setting: A randomized controlled trial. *Journal of the American Medical Association, 288*, 2836–2845.

van den Hout, J. H. C., Vlaeyen, J. W. S., Heuts, P. H. T., Zijlema, J. H. L., & Wijen, J. A. G. (2003). Secondary prevention of work-related disability in nonspecific low back pain: Does problem-solving therapy help? A randomized clinical trial. *Clinical Journal of Pain, 19*, 87–96.

Wilhelm, K., Siegel, J. E., Finch, A. W., Hadzi-Pavlovic, D., Mitchell, P. B., Parker, G., & Schofield, P. R. (2007). The long and the short of it: Associations between 5-HTT genotypes and coping with stress. *Psychosomatic Medicine, 69*, 614–620.

Mindfulness- and Acceptance-Based Cognitive and Behavioral Therapies

Susan M. Orsillo, Sara B. Danitz, *and* Lizabeth Roemer

Abstract

Across theoretical orientations, attempts to avoid and suppress difficult psychological content are presumed to interfere with psychological functioning and diminish well-being. Thus, a common theme in psychotherapy, which transcends theoretical orientation, is the promotion of acceptance. Recently, the use of mindfulness practices, and other experiential exercises aimed at increasing acceptance, to enhance existing cognitive and behavioral therapies has gained considerable attention. The goal of this chapter is to describe the theory underlying these efforts, provide a brief history of their development, describe the clinical strategies used with these approaches, and review the research that supports these efforts. We will also suggest future directions aimed at stimulating additional research literature and informing clinical practice.

Key Words: mindfulness, acceptance, behavior therapy, acceptance and commitment therapy, mindfulness-based cognitive therapy

Ask not that events should happen as you will, but let your will be that events should happen as they do, and you shall have peace.

—*Epictetus*

Through our daily experiences, joys, and struggles, humans come to know the personal benefits of accepting oneself and one's circumstances. This knowledge has deep historical roots, as is illustrated in a broad range of religious, philosophical, and literary works (Williams & Lynn, 2010). Yet, despite our cultural acknowledgment of this inherent truth, human suffering generally, and the psychological distress that drives many to therapy more specifically, is evidence of our continued struggle against what we cannot control. Thus, it is not surprising that a common theme in psychotherapy, which transcends theoretical orientation, is the promotion of acceptance.

Many of the most influential psychologists and psychiatrists of the twentieth century acknowledged the key role of acceptance (as opposed to denial or avoidance) in psychological functioning and overall well-being. William James is credited with saying, "Be willing to have it so: Acceptance of what has happened is the first step to overcoming the consequence of any misfortune." Freud (1910, 1965) proposed that neurotic patients hold on to emotional experiences from the past in a way that prevents them from freely focusing on, and engaging with, the realities of the present. Carl Jung, known for integrating spirituality with psychoanalysis, wrote, "We cannot change anything unless we accept it. Condemnation does not liberate, it oppresses" (1933, p. 240). Finally, Carl Rogers (1940) is credited with emphasizing the importance of promoting self-acceptance in psychotherapy. He proposed that when a therapist genuinely accepts a client, the client can move toward freely acknowledging and accepting the entirety of his or her own internal experience.

Mindfulness practice has long been acknowledged as a means of cultivating acceptance. Jon Kabat-Zinn has provided both a definition of mindfulness and a description of many of the key characteristics of this stance. According to Kabat-Zinn (1994), mindfulness involves "paying attention in a particular way: on purpose, in the present moment, and non-judgmentally" (p. 4). This attention is characterized by an "affectionate, compassionate quality. . . . a sense of openhearted, friendly presence and interest" (Kabat-Zinn, 2003, p. 145). Although the capacity to be mindful is an inherently human quality, and contemplative practices are at the core of many spiritual and philosophical traditions, the systematic cultivation of mindfulness has its origins in traditional Buddhist meditation, a practice that has been in existence for over 2,500 years (Kabat-Zinn, 2003).

This chapter will describe the recent integration of acceptance and mindfulness with cognitive-behavioral therapy, which we refer to as acceptance-based behavioral therapies (ABBT) and others have coined "third or new wave therapies" (Hayes, 2004), focusing primarily on acceptance and commitment therapy (Hayes, Strosahl, & Wilson, 1999, 2012), mindfulness-based cognitive therapy (Segal, Williams, & Teasdale, 2002), integrative behavioral couples therapy (Christensen, Jacobson, & Babcock, 1995; Jacobson & Christensen, 1996), and other acceptance-based behavioral approaches. Although dialectical behavior therapy (DBT; Linehan, 1993a, 1993b) also falls into this category, due to the extensive theoretical and empirical literature on DBT, it is described and reviewed more fully in the Chapter 12 devoted to this approach. The theoretical foundations of contemporary behavioral activation (Martell, Addis, & Jacobson, 2001) and contemporary problem-solving therapy (PST; Nezu, Nezu & D'Zurilla, 2013) also include significant components of mindfulness and emotional acceptance and are also covered under separate chapters. Finally, we will briefly discuss mindfulness-based stress reduction (MBSR; Kabat-Zinn, 2005), particularly focusing on the ways in which this program has influenced the integration of mindfulness with cognitive-behavioral therapy. However, since MBSR is not considered a form of cognitive-behavioral therapy, it will not be fully reviewed here (interested readers may refer to Kabat-Zinn, 2005, for a book-length description of the program).

In this chapter, we will describe the theoretical/conceptual underpinnings of these approaches, provide a brief history of their development within the cognitive-behavioral tradition, and describe the clinical strategies characteristic of each approach. We will also provide an overview of research literature in support of this approach across multiple problems and/or populations, and discuss future directions.

Theoretical/Conceptual Underpinnings of Therapies Integrating Acceptance and Mindfulness with Cognitive-Behavioral Psychotherapy
Acceptance and Commitment Therapy

Acceptance and commitment therapy (ACT; Hayes et al., 1999, 2012) is an approach to psychotherapy that integrates acceptance and mindfulness strategies with behavior change strategies with the goal of increasing psychological flexibility. From an ACT perspective, psychological problems stem from psychological inflexibility, a state presumed to be characterized by six core processes (cognitive fusion, inflexible attention, disruption of chosen values, inaction or impulsivity, attachment to a conceptualized self, and experiential avoidance; described in more detail later). The assumption underlying the model is that although pain is inevitable, human suffering is increased when psychological rigidity prevents a person from adapting and responding flexibly to context.

ACT is based on a pragmatic philosophy of science called functional contextualism (e.g., Biglan & Hayes, 1996; Hayes, Hayes, Reese, & Sarbin, 1993; Hayes et al., 2012) that extends Skinner's radical behaviorism by adopting a functional approach to understanding the whole organism in context. The goal of functional contextualism is "the prediction and influence of psychological events with precision, scope, and depth" (Hayes, 1993, p. 252). Thus, this approach takes a pragmatic approach, in that behavior can only be viewed as successful or effective relative to its intended consequences.

From an ACT perspective, language (or verbal processes) is assumed to play a core role in human suffering. ACT is informed by the principles of a contextual, behavioral theory of human language and learning known as relational frame theory (RFT). Although this theory is very briefly described next, interested readers are directed to a fuller account (Hayes, Barnes-Holmes, & Roche, 2001; Törneke, 2010).

According to RFT, human language and thinking are characterized by our unique, contextually controlled ability to derive arbitrary relations among stimuli in a way that transforms their function. In other words, we are systematically reinforced by our social environment for making complex, but arbitrary, associations between objects, events, and experiences. This process is referred to as relational framing. A simple example would be the positive reinforcement that Dad provides his daughter when she learns to associate the sound of the word "red" with a block that is a particular color. The sound of the word "red" is in no way innately related to the color of the block; the word and the object do not share physical properties. Thus, the relationship between the two is arbitrary. But our social culture has agreed to associate that particular sound and that specific color. Thus, the daughter will be routinely reinforced by Dad, Mom, Grandma, and the babysitter for making that association.

According to RFT, a core feature of language development is that ability to engage in mutual and combinatorial entailment. Mutual entailment is the process by which a reciprocal relationship is established between two stimuli, even when only one direction of association is directly reinforced. In other words, if a child is taught through reinforcement that the sound of the word "red" is associated with a particularly colored block, she will also learn that the particularly colored block is associated with the sound of the word "red." Combinatorial entailment suggests that reciprocal relationships develop among stimuli as a result of their relationship with another intermediary stimulus. For example, if the relationship between the sound of the word "red" and a particular color block is reinforced, and the relationship between the sound of the word "red" and an apple is reinforced, the child will develop an association between the red colored block and the apple.

One final characteristic of language that is central to RFT is the transformation of stimulus functions that occurs as a consequence of relational framing. When a stimulus is associated with another, it is presumed to acquire a similar psychological function. Take the example of a man who is physically attacked in a parking garage. Through its association with the physical attack, the parking garage itself can come to elicit a fear response. Further, this verbally derived relation may persist in the absence of direct experience that the city block is safe.

The normative language development processes are assumed to play a central role in promoting psychological inflexibility through the following six core processes.

COGNITIVE FUSION

Humans are often immersed in their "internal" world, planning, remembering, worrying, ruminating, describing, and evaluating events and experiences. Cognitive fusion is defined as "a process by which verbal events exert strong stimulus control over responding, to the exclusion of other contextual variables" (Hayes et al., 2012, p. 69). When people fuse with, or define themselves by, internal content (e.g., "If I have the thought 'I am a failure,' it must be so") or they rigidly adhere to unworkable verbal rules (e.g., "Avoiding people will keep me safe from pain"), several negative outcomes may occur.

For instance, cognitive fusion can interfere with attention to stimuli and contingencies in the present moment, which diminishes one's ability to respond flexibly. For example, if a man is fused with the belief that avoiding people is the way to reduce pain, he may not be fully aware of, and responsive to, the painful emotions that arise when he is alone. Or, despite a pleasant encounter with a neighbor, he may continue to avoid social contact.

Cognitive fusion can also increase the probability that internal experiences elicit considerable distress. For example, if a woman is fused to the belief "I am a failure," and she associates failure with "undesirable characteristics," she is likely to experience shame, sadness, and other painful emotions each time that thought arises. A failure experience is not required to trigger this response; simply having the thought is sufficient.

From an RFT perspective, verbal events that are associated with pain elicit pain. Simply remembering a past breakup or worrying about the possibility of failing at a future project can elicit the same shame and sadness as actually experiencing the event. When we are fused with internal events, the psychological pain they can inflict is increased. Under these conditions, it is not surprising that people engage in a number of strategies aimed at avoiding and escaping potentially painful experiences. Thus, fusion with painful internal content is proposed to motivate experiential avoidance, the second process underlying psychological inflexibility.

EXPERIENTIAL AVOIDANCE

Experiential avoidance is defined as attempts to change the form and frequency of private events, such as thoughts, emotions, physiological sensations, and memories (Hayes & Wilson, 1994). Although the urge to avoid or escape pain is innately human, there is compelling experimental evidence that attempts to avoid or suppress thoughts and emotions often fail, increasing the frequency of, and distress associated with, the unwanted internal experience (Dalgleish, Yiend, Schweizer, & Dunn, 2009; Najmi & Wegner, 2009). Efforts to dampen or avoid internal experiences may also reduce our ability to attend to and learn from the present moment. Moreover, behavioral efforts aimed at facilitating experiential avoidance, such as using drugs to dampen negative feelings, or avoiding social situations to prevent unwanted thoughts about failure and rejection, also carry considerable costs.

ATTACHMENT TO THE CONCEPTUALIZED SELF

The ACT model proposes that humans create a conceptualized self once they begin to acquire language. The conceptualized self is comprised of the verbal content we use to define ourselves and differentiate ourselves from others. For example, Mia might define herself as a 35-year-old, single, female who is an only child, quiet and shy, unlovable, and an overall failure in life. Conceptualized selves are often richly elaborated and they contain information about the causes and consequences of self-attributes (Hayes et al., 2012). For example, Mia may attribute her shyness to growing up as an only child in a rural area, and she may believe that her decision to attend the local community college ruined her chances of achieving a successful life.

Although it is adaptive and helpful to be able to describe one's demographic and physical attributes, and we are reinforced by our social community for having a consistent self-description, there are negative consequences to being fused with one's conceptualized self. First, the desire to maintain a consistent self-description can restrict our ability to notice and accept inconsistent information. For example, Mia may ignore or refuse social contact with people who show interest in her, because it is inconsistent with the idea that she is unlovable. Attachment to the conceptualized self can also limit behavioral options, increasing the possibility of a self-fulfilling prophecy. Mia is unlikely to take on the necessary risks and challenges to succeed in her career if she is bound by her view of herself as a failure. Thus, it is unlikely that she will have new, life-fulfilling experiences because of her narrowed behavioral repertoire.

INFLEXIBLE ATTENTION

In addition to the conceptualized self, sometimes referred to as "self as content," ACT describes two other forms of self-knowledge. The first is "self as process," which refers to ongoing awareness of internal experiences and immediate behavioral events (e.g., noticing "I feel an itch on my back," "I am experiencing feelings of sadness," and "I am sitting in a coffee shop").

A third form of self-knowledge is "self as context," also referred to as a "transcendent sense of self" or the "observer self." This is essentially the stable point of view from which one observes or experiences life. As one ages and matures, experiences physical changes in the body, feels a full range of emotions, and thinks a multitude of thoughts, there is still presumed to be a constant self for which all of these events occur and unfold.

From an ACT perspective, rigidly attending to limited content can decrease self-knowledge and maintain psychological inflexibility.

PERSISTENT INACTION, IMPULSIVITY, OR AVOIDANCE

The combined effects of cognitive fusion, experiential avoidance, attachment to a conceptualized self, and inflexible attention can take a toll on effective, approach behavior. These processes compel people to rigidly adhere to unworkable verbal rules and prevent them from attending to the present moment, which diminishes the ability to respond flexibly to environmental contingencies and erodes quality of life. When purely internal avoidance efforts, such as distraction or self-talk, fail to suppress painful internal content, behavior strategies aimed at avoiding eliciting situations and activities may increase, adding to psychological inflexibility. When individuals engage in avoidance, motivated by fusion, their behavior comes under aversive control. In other words, actions are primarily aimed at decreasing and avoiding pain rather than engaging in meaningful life activities.

LACK OF VALUES CLARITY

In ACT, valuing involves voluntarily constructing and engaging in dynamic patterns of activity that are intrinsically reinforcing (Wilson & Dufrene, 2008). For example, valuing could involve making the choice to be deeply intimate with others and involve staying in contact with friends, disclosing private thoughts and feelings, and engaging in shared activities. Such activities are ongoing and inherently reinforcing. In contrast, one might seek friends as a way of proving his or her own self-worth and popularity. From an ACT perspective, psychological inflexibility and suffering arise when one tries to adhere to socially prescribed rules for how to live a successful life, rather than constructing, and acting consistently with, personally held values.

Mindfulness-Based Cognitive Therapy

As described in more detail later, mindfulness-based cognitive therapy (MBCT) was originally developed as a method of decreasing the relapse and reoccurrence of major depressive disorder (MDD) among those who successfully completed treatment (Segal et al., 2002). Although several evidence-based treatments for MDD exist—including antidepressant medication, cognitive-behavioral therapy, behavioral activation, problem-solving therapy, and interpersonal therapy—approximately one quarter of those treated relapse within 1 year of treatment (Kanai et al., 2003; Keller, Lavori, Mueller, & Endicott, 1992). Moreover, the probability of reoccurrence increases with each relapse (Mueller et al., 1999).

Maintenance antidepressant therapy is considered to be the clinical standard for preventing depressive relapse or recurrence, but the preventative effects only persist as long as patients continue taking the medication. Unfortunately, less than one third of patients adhere to recommended guidelines for antidepressant medication maintenance (ten Doesschate, Bockting, & Schene, 2009). Given the effectiveness of cognitive therapy as a treatment for depression, and the fact that it reduces the probability of relapse by 22% compared with pharmacotherapy (Vittengl, Clark, Dunn, & Jarrett, 2007), a maintenance form of cognitive therapy could have promise. Yet, given the prevalence of MDD, and the scarcity and geographic inequity in the availability of CBT-trained therapists (Shapiro, Cavanagh, & Lomas, 2003), Segal and colleagues (2002) sought an approach that would be easier to disseminate. Thus, they turned to the literature to identify the factors that contribute to depressive relapse, as well as the mechanism of action CT, to inform their development efforts (Segal, Teasdale, & Williams, 2004).

FACTORS CONTRIBUTING
TO DEPRESSIVE RELAPSE

Beck's original theory of depression (1967; Kovacs & Beck, 1978) suggested that dysfunctional attitudes and negative schemas cause and maintain depression. However, research has not supported this hypothesis (Ilardi, Craighead, & Evans, 1997); instead, it appears that dysfunctional attitudes fluctuate with mood, suggesting they are a result, not a cause, of depression (Lewinsohn, Steinmetz, Larson, & Franklin, 1981; Peselow, Robins, Block, & Barouche, 1990).

An alternative theory, the "cognitive reactivity hypothesis," states that vulnerability to relapse and reoccurrence is caused by a pattern of negative, self-critical thinking that is easily reactivated by depressed mood (Persons & Miranda, 1992; Teasdale, 1983, 1988). A strong association between depressed mood and this style of thinking is proposed to form and strengthen during depressive episodes (Segal, Williams, Teasdale, & Gemar, 1996; Teasdale & Barnard, 1993), particularly among those with several previous episodes of depression.

Cognitive reactivity is proposed to reflect one of three particular "modes of mind" theorized to be available to individuals for processing information (Barnard & Teasdale, 1991). The *mindless emoting* mode is characterized by purely reactive, sensory-driven responses. The *conceptualizing-doing* mode is associated with processing that involves content and analysis. Finally, the *mindful-experiencing* mode involves recognizing experiences such as sensations, thoughts, and emotions in a manner that promotes present moment awareness. Cognitive reactivity is proposed to be one form of the *mindless emoting* mode.

Segal and colleagues (2002) further hypothesize that the "mode of mind" that is activated by sad mood involves both negative *content* (e.g., self-critical thoughts) and a problematic *process*, specifically ruminative thought patterns. In an attempt to reduce depression, individuals may engage in a ruminative process aimed at better understanding or gaining insights about the self or situation. Unfortunately, this ruminative process can backfire, increasing both the intensity and duration of the depressed mood.

Support for this theory comes from several related streams of research. A large body of research conducted by Susan Nolen-Hoeksema (1991) links rumination, a mode of thinking that involves repetitively and passively focusing on symptoms of distress and on the possible causes and consequences of these symptoms, with depression. Ironically, although ruminators often hold positive beliefs that ruminating will help them reduce their depression, it actually prolongs depression and reduces one's capacity to effectively problem-solve (Watkins & Moulds, 2005). Further, although rumination itself does decrease with the remission of depression, the tendency to ruminate pre-treatment is still correlated with the tendency to ruminate post-treatment, suggesting some stability in this response style (Bagby, Rector, Bacchiochi, & McBride, 2004).

MECHANISM UNDERLYING COGNITIVE THERAPY

Beck and his colleagues (Beck, Rush, Shaw, & Emery, 1979) proposed that cognitive therapy provided an opportunity for clients to gain some distance from their thoughts. However, from a traditional "Beckian" perspective, the notion of distancing or "decentering" is typically viewed as a means toward changing the *content* of thoughts (Segal et al., 2002). Other theorists have emphasized the importance of "decentering" as a metacognitive *process* that could be taught during cognitive therapy and applied by clients in challenging or distressing situations (Ingram & Hollon, 1986). Decentering involves experiencing thoughts as transient, passing events in the field of awareness, rather than as inherent aspects of self or valid reflections of reality (Teasdale, 1999).

There is some evidence that decentering may be an underlying mechanism in CBT for depression. Fresco, Segal, Buis, and Kennedy (2007) demonstrated that, among patients with depression treated to remission, CBT responders exhibited greater gains in decentering than did medication responders. Further, post-treatment levels of decentering and low cognitive reactivity in response to an emotion challenge were associated with the lowest rates of relapse in the 18-month follow-up period (Fresco et al., 2007). Decreased decentering in response to a mood induction also seems to predict depressive relapse (Teasdale et al., 2002). Thus, Segal and colleagues (2002) proposed that mindfulness practice could be a cost-effective, easier to disseminate method of increasing decentering, decreasing cognitive reactivity, and reducing the risk of depressive relapse among those successfully treated for depression.

Integrative Behavioral Couple Therapy

Integrative behavioral couple therapy (IBCT) aims to address couples' relational distress by fostering both acceptance and change of each partner's behaviors. The theory underlying IBCT assumes that incompatibilities between partners are not inherently problematic, but instead a characteristic common to all couples (Jacobson & Christensen, 1996; McGinn, Benson, & Christensen, 2011). However, when these incompatibilities are associated with existing vulnerabilities in either or both partners, the couple is at increased risk for significant distress. For example, Serena, an extremely responsible and organized woman, may have initially been attracted to Jim because his carefree and spontaneous manner complemented her style. Over time these differences in "control versus responsibility" will be more likely to ignite conflict if Serena fears that Jim will abandon her, the way her father did, and Jim finds Serena's style similar to his overbearing mother.

Certain "themes," such as demand-withdraw and closeness-independence, are theorized to polarize couples and create discord (Jacobson & Christensen, 1996). Repeated emergence of these interactional themes can increase polarization, causing couples to fall into a "mutual trap" wherein both partners feel that there is no solution and/or the only solution is for their partner to change.

As described in more detail later, whereas traditional behavior therapy focuses exclusively on helping members of a couple to negotiate change and problem-solve, IBCT takes a different tact. From this perspective, it is assumed that individuals bring specific learning histories and related vulnerabilities to their relationships that may not be easily amenable to change. Thus, IBCT aims to promote closeness and acceptance of those aspects of the relationship that may reflect unresolvable differences, while also supporting change efforts aimed at improving the relationship.

Acceptance-Based Behavioral Therapy

Although efficacious individual cognitive-behavioral therapies (CBT) have been developed for generalized anxiety disorder (GAD), a large proportion of individuals treated fail to meet criteria for high end-state functioning (Waters & Craske, 2005). Informed by recent research on the potential mechanisms proposed to cause and maintain GAD, as well as the promising effects of treatments like DBT, ACT, and MBCT, we developed an acceptance-based behavioral therapy (ABBT) for GAD (Roemer & Orsillo, 2002).

We use the term "ABBT" as a general label to describe a theoretical orientation toward case conceptualization and treatment that is informed by behavioral and mindfulness principles. In other words, ABBT is not a new treatment to be compared and contrasted with ACT, MBCT, or DBT. Instead, it reflects the way in which we integrated clinical methods and strategies from these different treatment approaches in an attempt to address specific characteristics thought to underlie GAD.

A similar, integrative approach may be beneficial for treating a wide range of presenting problems.

Our ABBT for GAD is informed by the theory that GAD is characterized by three problematic styles.

PROBLEMATIC RELATIONSHIP WITH INTERNAL EXPERIENCES

Individuals with GAD tend to have a *restricted or narrowed field of attention that is biased toward negative content* (Mogg & Bradley, 2005). A number of experimental studies that demonstrated that those with GAD preferentially attend to threat-relevant stimuli over neutral stimuli when the two compete for processing resources (Bar-Haim, Lamy, Pergamin, Bakermans-Kranenburg, & van IJzendoorn, 2007). They also describe *a critical, negative, and fearful stance toward their internal experiences*. For example, individuals with GAD report a heightened negative reactivity toward their emotions (Lee, Orsillo, Roemer, & Allen, 2010; Mennin, Heimberg, Turk, & Fresco, 2005; Turk, Heimberg, Luterek, Mennin, & Fresco, 2005), they view their worrisome thoughts as more dangerous and uncontrollable (Wells & Carter, 1999), and report intolerance of thoughts and feelings related to uncertainty (Dugas, Gagnon, Ladouceur, & Freeston, 1998).

EXPERIENTIAL AVOIDANCE

If individuals with GAD have a fearful and critical relationship with their thoughts and emotions, it stands to reason that they would be motivated to escape and avoid their internal experiences using strategies such as self-talk and distraction. Research has demonstrated that individuals diagnosed with GAD report more experiential avoidance than demographically matched, nonanxious controls (Lee et al., 2010) and that deficits in the ability to accept emotions is associated with GAD symptom (Salters-Pedneault, Roemer, Tull, Rucker, & Mennin, 2006). Moreover, there is evidence that worry itself can serve an avoidant function (Borkovec & Hu, 1990), and individuals with generalized anxiety symptoms are more likely to report that they worry to distract themselves from more emotional topics (Borkovec & Roemer, 1995).

Unfortunately, as noted earlier, distress can be paradoxically increased by experiential avoidance. Thus, a self-perpetuating cycle of anxiety can develop in which critical, avoidant reactions to internal experiences trigger attempts to suppress and avoid, which compound distress, cuing more negative reactions and stronger avoidance efforts.

BEHAVIORAL CONSTRICTION: FAILURE TO ENGAGE IN VALUED ACTION

Critical, avoidant reactions to internal experiences can also elicit behavioral avoidance of anxiety-provoking situations. Because behavioral avoidance is immediately negatively reinforced by a reduction in anxiety, it can become a habitual way of responding. This is particularly problematic when behavior becomes more strongly directed toward avoiding potentially uncomfortable internal experiences than pursuing personally meaningful experiences. Some support for this theory comes from the finding that individuals diagnosed with GAD report living less consistently with what matters to them than individuals not diagnosed with GAD (Michelson, Lee, Orsillo, & Roemer, 2011). Additionally, GAD symptoms are associated with a decreased ability to engage in goal-directed behaviors when distressed (Salters-Pedneault et al., 2006). As an added obstacle to living an engaged life, the intense cognitive effort associated with monitoring and managing one's internal experience can make it difficult to notice and appreciate the present moment.

We proposed that if symptoms of GAD are maintained through problematic and reactive relationships with internal experiences, experiential avoidance, and behavioral constriction, then a treatment that directly addresses these components should be efficacious (Roemer & Orsillo, 2002). We (Roemer & Orsillo, 2007, 2009) developed an ABBT aimed at helping clients to modify their relationship with their internal experiences, decrease rigid, habitual avoidance, and increase flexibility and action in valued domains.

A Historical Overview of the Integration of Acceptance and Mindfulness into Cognitive-Behavioral Psychotherapy

The centrality of acceptance in psychological well-being is apparent throughout the history of psychotherapy. Within the cognitive-behavioral tradition, Albert Ellis (1996; Ellis & Harper, 1961) conceptualized psychological distress and problems in functioning as arising from an unwillingness to accept difficult or painful life circumstances, a judgmental and critical stance toward one's thoughts and emotions, and the behavioral avoidance or passivity that accompanies this cognitive perspective. Although rational emotive behavior therapy

(REBT) was aimed at involved changing irrational beliefs, the ultimate goal of this approach was to promote, unconditional acceptance of self, other, and circumstance.

The importance of identifying and changing irrational beliefs was central to the development of Beck's theory of depression and the methods and strategies used in CBT. However, as noted earlier, Beck identified the process of cognitive distancing as "the first, critical step" in cognitive therapy (Hollon & Beck, 1979), which enables clients to respond to their negative thoughts as beliefs rather than facts. Presumably, this approach would allow clients to replace irrational, dysfunctional beliefs with more rational, balanced thoughts.

Marsha Linehan integrated acceptance and mindfulness with traditional behavioral approaches in order to develop a therapy that would be effective for chronically suicidal individuals (1987). She recognized that although it was critical to teach chronically suicidal clients change strategies, too much emphasis on change could leave clients feeling blamed and criticized for their problems (Robins & Rosenthal, 2011). Thus, the defining characteristic of DBT (Linehan, 1993a, 1993b) is that it balances both change strategies (drawn from traditional behavioral therapy) with acceptance strategies (informed by Eastern philosophy and mindfulness).

A Brief History of Acceptance and Commitment Therapy

Zettle (2005) provided a history of acceptance and commitment therapy (ACT) documenting three major stages in the development of this approach to treatment. According to Zettle, the foundations of the theoretical framework were laid in the late 1970s through 1985, in response to growing frustration with the cognitive-behavioral movement and its treatment of private events such as thoughts. Zettle and Hayes (1982) proposed a radical behavioral account of cognitive-behavioral therapy that reconceptualized cognitive control of behavior as a behavior-behavior relationship supported by arbitrary, social-verbal contingencies.

At that time, from a cognitive perspective, thoughts were assumed to be causal agents that could exert control over emotions and behaviors (Beck, 1967). In contrast, from a radical behavioral perspective, causal factors are limited to those factors that can be directly shown to predict and control behavior. Thus, thoughts are classified as "private" behaviors with no unique causal properties (Zettle & Hayes, 1982).

Zettle and Hayes (1982) argued that while thoughts could be part of a causal sequence, like any other behavior, there would have to be some environmental cause for the behavior–behavior relationship. Extending Skinner's (1957, 1969) basic conceptual work in verbal and rule-governed behavior, Zettle and Hayes proposed that thought–behavior relationships (best understood as behavior–behavior relationships) were established through social contingencies. For example, one might be reinforced by one's social community for describing an emotion or thought as a cause for behavior (e.g., I can't go to the party tonight because I am too anxious). From this perspective, it is not the anxiety that is preventing the person from attending the party, nor is it her thought. Instead, the avoidance behavior is controlled by a verbal rule that has been established through social contingencies that suggests that avoiding social events for emotional reasons is acceptable and expected. According to Zettle (2005), this theoretical framework influenced the development of an early form of ACT called "comprehensive distancing" that contained many of the defusion exercises considered core to ACT, but that did not emphasize values articulation or the cultivation of valuing as a process.

According to Zettle (2005), the mid to late 1980s are notable in that a detailed account of RFT was presented for the first time in a public, scientific forum (Hayes & Brownstein, 1985 as cited in Zettle, 2005), and a chapter describing the " contextual approach to therapeutic change" it informed was published (Hayes, 1987). The first book-length description of ACT was published by Hayes and colleagues in 1999, and this version included RFT-informed methods of values identification and clarification.

A Brief History of Mindfulness-Based Cognitive Therapy

As described earlier, MBCT was developed to decrease the relapse and reoccurrence of depression among those who had successfully achieved remission as a result of treatment (Segal et al., 2002). Based on the extant research, Segal and colleagues sought to develop clinical strategies that would increase defusion and decrease cognitive reactivity.

Segal and colleagues (2002) credit Marsha Linehan's work incorporating mindfulness with cognitive-behavioral therapy in the treatment of borderline personality disorder as one of their initial inspirations for considering a mindfulness-based relapse prevention program. This led them to consult with Jon Kabat-Zinn, then director of the Stress Reduction Clinic at the University of Massachusetts Medical Center, to learn more about the ways in which mindfulness-based stress reduction might inform their risk reduction efforts.

Attentional control training was the earliest version of MBCT. In this initial treatment, mindfulness was taught to clients through brief (20-minute) audiotapes of Jon Kabat-Zinn directing specific practices. Although some clients reported positive benefits from this approach, others continued to struggle, particularly when painful affect or more severe and persistent thoughts arose. Segal and colleagues (2002) report that at this stage in their treatment development, they were uncertain how mindfulness could be used under these conditions. Instead, they felt they would need to revert to cognitive therapy to deal with the most difficult content, something that was not feasible or cost-effective under the risk reduction model. Thus, they returned to the University of Massachusetts to gain more direct experience with, and understanding of, MBSR.

Segal and colleagues (2002) note that this second visit increased their awareness of the importance of cultivating a "welcoming, accepting" stance toward painful content. Rather than simply encouraging clients to engage in brief mindfulness practices as a strategy to help them to decenter from ruminative thoughts, mindfulness was aimed at completely changing the experience one has with the entirety of internal experiences. At this time in the development of MBCT, Segal and colleagues become convinced of the importance of therapist practice. Specifically, they came to believe that in order to have the skill and experience they needed to help clients struggle with the difficult experiences that can arise with mindfulness practice, they would need to commit to a sustained practice.

A Brief History of Integrative Behavioral Couples Therapy

Traditional behavioral couples therapy, based on social learning theory (Jacobson & Margolin, 1979), is aimed at improving couples' functioning and decreasing distress through the use of behavior exchange and the training of communication and problem-solving skills. Despite the demonstrated efficacy of this approach (Shadish & Baldwin, 2005), approximately one third of couples do not experience improvement in relationship quality (Jacobson & Follette, 1985). Moreover, among those who do improve, approximately 30% relapsed

within a 2-year period (Jacobson, Schmaling, & Holtzworth-Munroe, 1987), particularly more severely and chronically distressed couples (Baucom & Hoffman, 1986), who are more polarized on particular issues (Jacobson, Follette, & Pagel, 1986).

In an attempt to improve treatment for these difficult couples, Christensen and Jacobson developed IBCT, an approach aimed at helping clients to cultivate an accepting stance toward one's partner and those aspects of the relationship unlikely to change and to increase closeness and collaborative problem solving (Christensen et al., 1995; Jacobson, 1992; Jacobson & Christensen, 1996).

A Brief History of Integrative Acceptance-Based Behavior Therapy for GAD

Similarly, research from the 1990s demonstrated that although CBT was more efficacious than other approaches in treating GAD (Borkovec & Ruscio, 2001), only a proportion of those treated experienced sustained, clinically significant improvement. The most efficacious treatments for anxiety typically use exposure therapy to target the specific feared object (e.g., social situations, interoceptive cues, trauma reminders). However, the feared object in GAD is much more elusive as feared outcomes are often diffuse and transient. Some case studies found systematic, controlled exposure to worry to be helpful in conjunction with other CBT methods (Forsyth & McNeil, 2002), but the research supporting this approach is limited.

Drawing from Tom Borkovec's conceptualization of worry as a form of avoidance (1994) and the supporting research, we proposed that an acceptance-based behavioral treatment might be indicated for GAD. Heavily informed by acceptance-based treatments such as ACT (Hayes et al., 2012), MBCT (Segal et al., 2002), and DBT (Linehan, 1993b), our approach targets habitual responding and encourages mindfulness, acceptance of internal experience, and mindful action as a replacement for the habitual restrictions in action that accompany worry.

An Overview of Clinical Strategies
Acceptance and Commitment Therapy

As noted earlier, the goal of ACT is to increase psychological flexibility, which is characterized by an open, centered, and engaged response style (Hayes et al., 2012). Several clinical strategies and methods are described by Hayes and colleagues (2012) to cultivate this stance.

The first stage of treatment is aimed at creating a context in which meaningful change is possible. From an ACT perspective, most clients enter treatment with firmly established assumptions about the nature of their problems and the required solution. Specifically, clients often believe that their inability to suppress or change unwanted internal content (e.g., sad feelings, thoughts of inadequacy, memories of painful experiences) represents an inherent flaw that is preventing them from living a fulfilling life. In ACT, the goal is to encourage clients to look at their actual experience to determine the legitimacy of these assumptions and to see whether the client is willing to consider an alternative approach.

In ACT, the term *creative hopelessness* refers to the state in which a client "gives up" on *strategies* that are not working and opens up to the possibility that real, clinically significant change is possible. Relatively young clients who are new to therapy may be easily amenable to adopting a new perspective on change, whereas chronically stuck clients with a long-established, for the most part ineffective, treatment history may be more resistant. In either case, the goal is not to convince the client to adopt another view, but instead to persuade the client to objectively evaluate his or her own experiences with control efforts.

For example, clients are encouraged to consider the effectiveness and cost of different change strategies they have tried in the past. For example, a client with panic disorder might carefully evaluate whether her "self-reprimanding" strategy of dealing with fear and avoidance has been helpful in an enduring and life-changing way. It may be the case that she "believes" this approach could or should work, and that it has on occasion been enough to propel her out of her home and into a crowd, but the goal of treatment in this phase is to encourage the client to evaluate whether this approach has been uniformly helpful. Some clients may have control strategies that are quite effective in reducing pain and difficult internal content, such as substance use or behavioral avoidance. With these clients, it is critical to examine the personal and interpersonal costs of these strategies.

Rather than relying on didactic, psychoeducational methods, ACT underscores the importance of exercises and metaphors that allow clients to use experience rather than reason to evaluate strategies aimed at improving well-being. For example, the *Polygraph Metaphor* is used to illustrate that even when the stakes are at their highest, no human can override innate biological processes. Specifically,

the client is asked to imagine being attached to a machine with acute sensitivity to fear and that he or she will be severely harmed or killed if fear is detected. Most clients respond by recognizing that even under conditions of life threat, humans cannot modify or suppress our internal responses.

Several strategies are used to cultivate psychological flexibility in ACT. Mindfulness practice is used to promote a decentered response style and to enable a present-moment flexible awareness that is not dominated by thoughts of past or future (Hayes & Sandoz, 2012). Clients are asked to adopt a "sunset mode of mind" aimed at noticing and appreciating the present moment and to consider how it contrasts with "problem-solving mode of mind," which is aimed at automatically categorizing and evaluating objects and experiences.

Several strategies are used to increase a client's awareness of the conceptualized self and the ways in which this perspective can undermine psychological flexibility. For example, in the *Storyline* exercise clients are asked to write about how key historical events and experiences have shaped their lives. For example, a client might write about how her mother's alcoholism caused her to turn to substances as a method of coping with distress. After the initial writing, the client is asked to rewrite the story, maintaining the objective facts (e.g., "My mother got drunk and missed my high school graduation") and the psychological reactions (e.g., "I was extremely sad and disappointed"), but changing the ending (e.g., "Thus, I vowed to never abuse substances"). The client can be asked to rewrite the story again, this time retaining the facts, but changing the psychological reactions. The goal of this exercise is not to find the "correct" story. Instead, it demonstrates the ways our mind searches for explanations and reasons and how easily we can become attached to our life stories. Like all clinical strategies, it is critical that the therapist approach this exercise with clinical sensitivity and an understanding that we all engage in the development and defense of a conceptualized self.

Clinical methods aimed at promoting cognitive defusion are also core to ACT. The goal is to help clients observe the process of thinking and feeling rather than just responding to the content. Deliteralization strategies such as repeating a neutral (milk) or emotionally salient (failure) word over and over until the meaning of the word is reduced can be one method of demonstrating the arbitrary nature of language. The limits of verbal instruction in activities such as learning to walk or playing a sport are also demonstrated to increase clients' appreciation of experiential learning.

The cultivation of an accepting stance toward internal experiences is also critical in promoting psychological flexibility. Once clients have some experience with the paradoxical nature and costs of holding an escape/avoidance/controlling stance, acceptance of internal experiences can be considered as an alternative. Clients may misunderstand acceptance and believe it means resignation, failure, or toleration. They may equate the idea of being willing to experience painful thoughts and emotions as wanting them. Thus, it is important to convey the notion that acceptance is an active, purposeful stance that involves embracing whatever is present, in the service of living an engaged life. One complicating aspect of acceptance is that it is not readily rule governed. Instructions to accept can seem to inherently carry a problem-solving purpose (if you accept painful thoughts and emotions, they are more likely to diminish or subside).

The final characteristic of psychological flexibility is an active and engaged response style. ACT assumes that clients already possess everything they need to live a fulfilling life. Clients do not have to be anxiety-free or have "high self-esteem" in order to engage in the activities they care about. Instead, ACT assumes that cognitive fusion and avoidance are the main obstacles that prevent clients from living in accordance with the things they value. In ACT, valuing is viewed as a process (e.g., connecting with others in an intimate way), rather than being defined by a goal or outcome (e.g., committing to a partner), and an emphasis is placed on the fact that values reflect individual choices and that they are not derived from logical analysis. A number of writing or imaginal exercises can be used to help clients to articulate their values. A bull's-eye target can help clients to graphically represent how closely they are living in accordance with specific values. Encouraging and supporting clients as they commit to engage in valued activities is a core behavioral strategy in ACT.

Mindfulness-Based Cognitive Therapy

MBCT (as described by Segal et al., 2002) assumes that there are different modes of mind that can be entered either automatically or intentionally. When the mind is in a "doing" mode, we evaluate and see discrepancies between what the situation *is* and what we *want it to be*, which promotes problem-solving efforts. If the discrepancy is easily addressed (e.g., one is hungry and chooses to eat a snack), the situation is resolved. But, if the discrepancy is not easily resolvable (I feel sad and I want to feel happy), impulsively employing rational problem-solving efforts can trigger rumination and promote negative mood.

When the mind is in a "being" mode, there is no need to evaluate one's experience or take action. The mind is focused on the present moment and thoughts; emotions and other experiences are simply "observed" instead of "listened to." It is important to recognize that these modes of mind are not simply defined by motor action or passivity. One can be sitting still and trying to "meditate to achieve calmness," which reflects a "doing mode." Alternatively, one could be fully engaged in an activity (like walking) and still be in a mindful "being" mode.

The goal of mindfulness training in MBCT is to increase awareness of one's mode of mind and develop the skills necessary to disengage and intentionally process information in a different way. MBCT is most typically delivered in eight weekly group sessions with up to 12 participants, with four booster sessions offered in the year following treatment. Each session has a theme and planned curriculum, which is supplemented with handouts.

Sessions 1–4 are aimed at helping participants to become acquainted with the habits of their minds and to develop basic attention skills. For example, practices like the *Raisin Exercise*, which involves eating one raisin at a time using all of one's senses, help participants to learn how little we actually attend to our moment-to-moment experience. The *Body Scan*, a 40- to 45-minute exercise that involves intentionally directing attention to different parts of the body and noticing sensations, can be helpful in teaching participants how to return their attentional focus back to a target when the mind inevitably starts wandering. Active practices like *mindful walking* and *yoga* are also introduced in these early sessions. In each session, therapists model a curious stance by eliciting comments from, and providing validation to, participants as they share their experience with mindfulness practice.

Sessions also include traditional CBT techniques such as psychoeducation on the nature of depression, identification of automatic thoughts, and pleasant events monitoring.

Sessions 5–8 are aimed at teaching participants how to use the mindfulness when mood shifts arise. Specifically, participants are taught to acknowledge, accept, and allow painful thoughts and emotions. *Inviting a Difficulty In* is a practice that can be helpful in facilitating this stance. As they deliberately bring a difficult problem to mind, participants are asked to note the region of the body affected by the image (e.g., tightness in chest, nausea in the stomach) and are encouraged to bring a sense of "opening" and "softening" to these sensations as a way to allow what is already present.

These latter sessions also include the practice of sitting with thoughts as "thoughts." Participants are encouraged to "stand behind the waterfall" and watch thoughts as events unfolding in the mind. Consistent with traditional cognitive-behavioral therapy, clients are also introduced to some of the questions that can be used to consider negative thoughts such as "Am I confusing a thought with a fact?" or "Am I overestimating disaster?" Participants are encouraged to notice the link between activity and mood and to engage in activities that bring mastery and pleasure.

Integrative Behavioral Couples Therapy

A central tenant of IBCT that differentiates this approach from traditional behavioral couples therapy is the assumption that not all aspects of a couple's relationship are amenable to negotiated change. Thus, IBCT is directed toward helping couples to identify, and accept, potentially unresolvable differences (but not issues such as domestic violence), and to promote a closeness that can persist despite the presence of these differences.

As described by Jacobson and Christensen (1996), IBCT consists of three major phases. During the assessment/evaluation phase, the therapist meets with the couple to assess their presenting concerns, obtain a brief relationship history, and observe their patterns of communication. Next, the therapist meets with each partner separately to assess each of the partner's individual relationship concerns, commitment to the relationship, and historical factors that could be impacting current relationship difficulties.

In the second phase of treatment, the therapist shares a formulation of the couples presenting problems and presents a plan for treatment. The formulation typically includes a description of the major theme proposed to drive the couple's struggles, the understandable, historical reasons the couple has this struggle, and the ways in which previous efforts to resolve the struggles have paradoxically worsened the situation. From an IBCT perspective, it is the ways couples *respond to each other* when they disagree, not the disagreement itself, which is viewed as the core problem. Thus, this phase of treatment is aimed at helping the couple to develop a "collaborative set," or shared perspective from which they can see how they contribute to problematic patterns.

In the treatment phase of therapy, the couple is encouraged to describe positive and negative interactions from the previous week (which are typically reflective of the couple's major theme) using *soft emotions*. Hard emotional expressions include accusatory messages and communicate hostility, anger, contempt, and intolerance. Not surprisingly, hard expressions frequently evoke defensive or retaliative responses. In contrast, soft emotions, which include the expression of insecurity, vulnerability, and feelings such as sadness, fear, and love, are more likely to elicit understanding and help to cultivate *empathic joining*. Through these discussions, behavioral patterns initially viewed as character flaws, or purposeful, malevolent actions, are reformulated as differences in response style, largely influenced by different learning histories. In early sessions, the therapist plays a more active role by eliciting partners' unstated feelings and encouraging the expression of soft emotions. But over time, as members of the couple begin to treat each other more compassionately, soft emotional expression may increase naturally.

The therapist also tries to promote a state of *unified detachment* from which couples can view their difficulties with some emotional distance. Thus, couples are encouraged to step back and describe the sequence of how a particular conflict unfolded in objective, nonblaming ways. IBCT also aims to *build tolerance* of frustrating responses. For example, a client who is annoyed by her partner's tendency to spontaneously commit to last-minute social plans might be asked to describe the way this sociable tendency first attracted her to him.

After the couple has developed a more collaborative stance, traditional behavioral methods such as behavioral exchange, communication training, or problem solving can be used, if necessary, to address specific issues that may be responsive to intervention.

Acceptance-Based Behavioral Therapy for GAD

From an ABBT perspective, GAD is characterized by a problematic relationship with one's internal experiences (narrowed attention, critical stance, entanglement), experiential avoidance, and behavioral restriction. Thus, treatment is aimed at helping clients to cultivate an open, curious, compassionate, and unentangled stance toward internal experiences, encouraging them to allow painful thoughts, emotions, and images, and promoting engagement in personally meaningful activities (for a book-length description of the treatment, see Roemer & Orsillo, 2009).

We have typically delivered ABBT in the context of 14 weekly individual therapy sessions, followed by two biweekly sessions (Roemer & Orsillo, 2007; Roemer, Orsillo, & Salters-Pedneault, 2008). Although there is some evidence that the concepts can be adapted to group therapy (Orsillo, Roemer, & Barlow, 2003), which may be beneficial and cost-effective for psychoeducation and mindfulness practice, we found it difficult to fully explore each individual client's obstacles and barriers to valued action with this mode of therapy.

ABBT generally consists of two phases of treatment. In the first, sessions are fairly structured. Both the therapist and client engage in a planned formal mindfulness practice and discuss the experience. We follow a progression when choosing the practices, initially focusing on the mindfulness of the breath and other physical sensations and gradually moving toward more challenging targets such as emotions and thoughts. Next, we briefly review out-of-session practices (described in more detail later) as well as any questions or concerns from the previous session. Each week a new concept (described in more detail later) is introduced in multiple ways to facilitate didactic and experiential learning. For example, we frequently provide psychoeducation and handouts, use experiential exercises and metaphors, and engage the client in a discussion of the ways in which the concept does or does not relate to his or her own experience. Finally, each session ends with the client making a commitment to practice specific elements of the therapy over the course of the week.

In the second phase of treatment, clients are encouraged to choose the mindfulness practice that starts each session. The remainder of the session is focused on successes and struggles with applying the concepts learned in the first phase of therapy to the client's life. No new concepts are introduced, although concepts are often revisited as needed. The goal of this phase of treatment is to promote engagement in valued life activities and to address any obstacles that may prevent such behavior. Finally, two biweekly sessions are aimed at consolidating learning and planning for future challenges and lapses in mindfulness practice and values engagement.

Several specific clinical methods and strategies are used to address each of the three goals of treatment. The development of a strong, genuine therapeutic relationship is vital in helping clients to develop a compassionate and accepting stance toward internal experiences. Through appropriate disclosure, therapists demonstrate the universality of painful emotions and critical and avoidant processes. Validation is used to normalize and accept the client's full experience as it is.

Psychoeducation is also used to help change the relationship clients have with their anxiety and reduce experiential avoidance. Specifically, we share our models of anxiety and worry, underscoring how anxiety and fear are often normal responses to the challenges we engage in to enrich our lives. We teach clients about negative reinforcement and explore the ways in which worry may be playing an avoidant function, aimed at reducing fear about the uncontrollable nature of the future and distracting the client from other emotionally evocative issues. Psychoeducation is also aimed at teaching clients about the function of different emotions and differentiating between "clear" and "muddy" states. We define clear emotions as those that arise as a direct result of a particular experience, such as the sadness we feel when we lose a loved one. In contrast, muddy emotions, often characterized by intense, confusing periods of general distress, may arise if we engage in poor self-care, imagine future threats, or remember past conflicts, and are often intensified by a critical, judgmental, and avoidance stance. Finally, we provide psychoeducation about the limits and costs of internal control efforts.

Mindfulness practice plays a major role in helping clients to cultivate a compassionate and curious stance toward internal experiences and to enhance acceptance. In addition to the formal practices described earlier, we encourage clients to bring mindfulness to everyday activities and actions, focusing first on neutral contexts, such as mindfulness of walking, and gradually moving toward more challenging contexts, such as mindfulness during a difficult interpersonal interaction. Self-monitoring is, of course, a key component of traditional cognitive-behavioral therapy, but it can also be used to promote a curious, decentered stance toward internal experiences. We use a progression of monitoring sheets aimed at helping clients increase their awareness of thoughts, emotions, urges to avoid, and efforts to control.

Multiple strategies are also used to help clients engage in valued action. We provide psychoeducation differentiating values from goals and clarifying concepts such as willingness. We invite clients to complete a variety of writing exercises designed to promote deep, emotional processing of issues related to values. Clients are asked to write about the ways in which anxiety and worry hold them back from fully engaging in relationships, work/school, and self-nurturance/community involvement to articulate their personal values in each of the three domains. Prompt questions include "How open or private do you want to be in your intimate relationships?" and "How important is it for you to take on challenges in the workplace?" Finally, clients are invited to write about their stance on making a commitment to engage in valued actions, which allows them to explore barriers to change, including past experiences they have had with making, and breaking, commitments.

Self-monitoring is also used to enhance engagement in valued activities. First, clients monitor opportunities that arise where they could engage in a valued activity and describe whether they mindfully engaged in, or opted to avoid, the opportunity. In later sessions, clients monitor their engagement in valued activities and any barriers they faced.

Empirical Support

Over the last decade, there has been an explosion of research examining the efficacy of acceptance- and mindfulness-based cognitive and behavioral therapies. It is beyond the scope of this chapter to provide a comprehensive review of all acceptance and mindfulness-based approaches for every psychological and physical health outcome, but we attempt to give readers a sense for the scope and quality of the extant literature.

Mindfulness-Based Cognitive Therapy

MBCT was originally developed to prevent the relapse of depression among patients who had previously been successfully treated for depression. The first trial (Teasdale et al., 2000) revealed that number of previous episodes moderated the effect of treatment on relapse. Specifically, MBCT significantly reduced the rate of relapse compared to treatment as usual (66% vs. 37%), but only among patients with three or more previous MDEs. This finding was replicated by Ma and Teasdale (2004) in a study of similar design, and it was extended by Kuyken and colleagues (2008), who found a significantly lower relapse rate in those who received MBCT compared to maintenance antidepressant medication (47% vs. 60%).

More recently, MBCT has been applied as a treatment for a broad array of clinical problems. Studies have demonstrated the positive effects of MBCT for depressive symptoms (Kenny & Williams, 2007), anxiety symptoms (Craigie, Rees, Marsh, & Nathan, 2008; Kim et al., 2009), bipolar symptoms (Miklowitz et al., 2009; Weber et al., 2010), and hypochondriasis (Lovas & Barsky, 2010), but many of these preliminary studies failed to include a control group. Several authors have conducted reviews and meta-analyses of the impact of MBCT, or mindfulness more generally (MBCT and MBSR), on psychological and physical conditions (Chiesa & Serretti, 2011; Coelho, Canter, & Ernst, 2007; Fjorback, Arendt, Ørnbøl, Fink, & Walach, 2011; Hollon & Ponniah, 2010; Piet & Hougaard, 2011). However, there is considerable overlap in the studies examined in each review. Thus, here we focus on the Chiesa and Serretti meta-analysis.

Chiesa and Serretti (2011) specifically investigated the efficacy of MBCT compared to an active or inactive control among individuals with, or recovering from, a psychological disorder. MBCT was found to be significantly more efficacious than usual care in reducing relapse in patients with three or more depressive episodes. Further, MBCT with the gradual tapering of maintenance antidepressants produced similar relapse rates to maintenance antidepressant care. MBCT also reduced residual symptoms of depression in patients with major depression, and anxiety in patients with bipolar or anxiety disorders. However, as noted by the authors, there was considerable variability in the quality of studies included in the meta-analysis. Many studies are characterized by small sample size and the majority use treatment as usual as the primary comparison group.

Hofmann and colleagues (Hofmann, Sawyer, & Fang, 2010) conducted a meta-analysis that differed in several keys ways from Chisea and Serretti. First, the focus was specifically on anxiety and depression as outcome variables. Second, they expanded the scope to include studies of patients with physical disorders. Finally, they examined the impact of mindfulness more broadly, rather than focusing specifically on the integration of mindfulness and CBT. However, they did report effects by treatment type and found moderate to large pre-post effect sizes for MBCT on both depression and anxiety in this broader sample.

Several additional randomized controlled trials have been published since these reviews. Segal and colleagues compared the efficacy of MBCT in reducing the risk of relapse among patients with three of more previous episodes who were successfully treated with antidepressants to both maintenance antidepressant medication and placebo (Segal et al., 2010). Patients were treated with antidepressants, followed for a minimum of 7 months to ensure that their symptoms had remitted (acute phase), and then randomly assigned to one of the three maintenance therapies. Notably, the impact of MBCT was different between patients who were classified as stable (no periods of elevated symptoms) versus unstable (at least one period of elevated symptoms) remitters during the acute phase. Unstable remitters in the maintenance antidepressant and MBCT groups both showed a decreased risk of relapse relative to those in the placebo group. In contrast, neither maintenance medication nor MBCT influenced the rate of relapse relative to placebo in the stable remitters group.

Geschwind and colleagues (Geschwind, Peeters, Drukker, van Os, & Wichers, 2011) examined how MBCT might increase positive emotionality among patients with residual symptoms of depression after at least one episode of depression. Participants were randomly assigned to either MBCT or a wait list control. MBCT participation was associated with an increased experience of momentary positive emotions and a greater appreciation of, and responsiveness to, pleasant daily events above and beyond the effects of decreased depression.

Recent randomized controlled trials of MBCT have also expanded beyond mood and anxiety as potential targets of treatment. For example, Semple and colleagues (Semple, Lee, Rosa, & Miller, 2010) explored the impact of MBCT, relative to wait list, on the social-emotional resiliency of primarily ethnic minority children enrolled in a remedial reading program. Although participation decreased attentional problems, with gains that were retained at 3-month follow-up, there were no differences between the groups with regard to changes in self-report of anxiety or behavior problems.

Finally, Langer and colleagues (Langer, Cangas, Salcedo, & Fuentes, 2012) examined the feasibility and effectiveness of MBCT in patients with psychosis. Relative to a wait list control, those who completed MBCT reported a greater ability to respond mindfully to stressful internal events, although the groups did not significantly differ in their report of psychotic symptoms or experiential avoidance.

Integrative Behavioral Couples Therapy

A number of studies have compared the effectiveness of integrative behavioral couple therapy (IBCT; Jacobson & Christensen, 1996) with traditional behavioral couple therapy (TBCT; Jacobson & Margolin, 1979). Cordova, Jacobson, and Christensen (1998) provided some preliminary support for the differences in these two approaches. They found that couples in IBCT expressed more nonblaming descriptions of problems and used more soft emotions than those in TBCT during later sessions of therapy.

The first preliminary randomized controlled trial comparing the two treatments was conducted by Jacobson and colleagues (Jacobson, Christensen, Prince, Cordova, & Eldridge, 2000). Both husbands and wives in the IBCT condition reported greater increases in marital satisfaction than couples in the TBCT condition. Moreover, a greater percentage of couples in IBCT improved or recovered.

Christensen and colleagues (2004) extended these findings by conducting a large randomized controlled trial comparing the efficacy of TBCT and IBCT in seriously and stably distressed couples. Couples in both treatments experienced statistically and clinically significant improvements in relationship satisfaction, stability, and affective communication over the course of therapy. However, those in TBCT improved more quickly at the beginning of therapy and then plateaued, whereas couples in IBCT made steady improvement over the course of therapy. At 2-year follow-up, approximately two thirds of the couples reported clinically significant improvements (69% of IBCT couples and 60% of TBCT couples) with few differences between the two groups (Christensen, Atkins, Yi, Baucom, & George, 2006). At 5-year follow-up, 50.0% of IBCT couples and 45.9% of TBCT couples showed clinically significant improvement (Christensen, Atkins, Baucom, & Yi, 2010).

Acceptance and Commitment Therapy

The research on ACT has increased exponentially over the past decade. Three meta-analyses have found that ACT is associated with changes of moderate effect size (Hayes, Luoma, Bond, Masuda, & Lillis, 2006; Öst, 2008; Powers, Zum Vörde, & Emmelkamp, 2009). Not surprisingly, effect sizes were largest for comparisons against wait list, treatment as usual, and placebo (e.g., Hayes et al., 2006). Powers and colleagues (2009) found no significant differences between ACT and other active treatments; however, Levin and Hayes (2009) argued that these findings were inaccurate since a treatment they considered active in one study was classified as treatment as usual. A revised meta-analysis reclassifying this treatment condition found ACT to be superior to established treatments (Levin & Hayes, 2009), although Powers and Emmelkamp (2009) maintained that their original classification was more accurate.

Next we provide a very brief description of some of the key randomized controlled trials included, and published after, these meta-analytic reviews to provide the reader with an overview of this literature. For a narrative review of the ACT literature including studies with a wide range of designs, see Ruiz (2010).

DEPRESSION

Two early studies compared the efficacy of an early version of ACT to cognitive therapy for depression and found it to be equivalent to (Zettle & Rains, 1989) or more effective than (Zettle & Hayes, 1986) cognitive therapy. More recently, ACT has been shown effective in reducing depression among adults with mild to moderate symptoms, relative to a wait list condition (Bohlmeijer, Prenger, Taal, & Cuijpers, 2010). Additionally, patients in a chemical dependency unit, who also met criteria for depressive disorder, improved whether they received ACT or treatment as usual (Petersen & Zettle, 2009). Finally, in a recent randomized controlled trial, Louise Hayes and colleagues (Hayes, Bach, & Boyd, 2010) found ACT to be better than treatment as usual for reducing symptoms in depressed adolescents. Based on this evidence, ACT has been classified as having modest support for depression by Division 12 of the American Psychological Association (APA).

ANXIETY

Twohig and colleagues (Twohig, Whittal, Cox, & Gunter, 2010) compared the efficacy of ACT, without exposure, to progressive relaxation training for obsessive-compulsive disorder. More patients experienced clinically significant responses in OCD in the ACT condition (56%) than in the relaxation condition (15%). While this study established that ACT could impact OCD symptoms, research is needed to see whether it can either enhance, or serve as a credible alternative to, previously established evidence-based approaches. In a similar vein, ACT in conjunction with habit reversal produced positive results for clients diagnosed with trichotillomania relative to a wait list control (Woods, Wetterneck, & Flessner, 2006).

Block and Wulfert (2000) conducted a randomized controlled trial comparing ACT to CBT for subclinical social anxiety disorder. Although both groups produced positive changes, participants in the ACT condition did better on a behavioral measure of public speaking. Randomized controlled trials have also established that ACT is equivalent to systematic desensitization for math anxiety (Zettle, 2003) and that an acceptance-based behavioral therapy integrating ACT with mindfulness and elements of DBT is as effective as cognitive therapy in reducing test anxiety (Brown et al., 2011). Of note, students with test anxiety in the ABBT condition scored significantly better than the cognitive therapy group on their final exam.

An ABBT for generalized anxiety disorder produced significant reductions in clinician-rated and self-reported GAD symptoms relative to a wait list control that were maintained at 3- and 9-month follow-up assessments (Roemer et al., 2008). At post-treatment assessment 78% of participants no longer met criteria for GAD and 77% achieved high end-state functioning. Moreover, preliminary results from our current trial suggest that both ABBT and applied relaxation produce large effect size changes in GAD severity, anxiety symptoms, worry, depressive symptoms, and number of additional diagnoses, while significantly increasing quality of life. Further, in a completer sample, 80% of clients in ABBT and 64% in the applied relaxation (AR) group met criteria for high end-state functioning at 6-month follow-up.

GENERAL DISTRESS

Two randomized controlled trials examined the efficacy of ACT on depression, anxiety, or general distress in a student outpatient sample. In these studies, ACT produced greater improvement in general distress than cognitive therapy (Lappalainen et al., 2007) and similar improvement to CBT (Forman, Herbert, Moitra, Yeomans, & Geller, 2007).

PSYCHOSIS

A brief ACT intervention plus treatment as usual significantly reduced inpatients' believability in their hallucinations and delusions compared to treatment as usual (Bach & Hayes, 2002; Gaudiano & Herbert, 2006). Both studies also resulted in fewer rehospitalizations, but this difference only reached levels of statistical significance in the Bach and Hayes's trial. More recently, White and colleagues (2011) found that ACT produced significantly more change in negative, but not positive, psychotic symptoms and fewer crisis contacts than treatment as usual.

BORDERLINE PERSONALITY DISORDER

Gratz and Gunderson (2006) conducted a randomized controlled trial examining the efficacy of an ABBT therapy integrating ACT and DBT relative to treatment as usual with clients diagnosed with borderline personality disorder. Those in the ABBT condition reported significantly decreased self-harm, emotion dysregulation, experiential avoidance, anxiety, depression, and stress relative to those receiving treatment as usual.

ADDICTIVE BEHAVIORS

Hayes and colleagues (Hayes, Wilson et al., 2004) randomly assigned polysubstance-abusing clients on methadone maintenance to methadone maintenance alone, or with added ACT or intensive 12-step facilitation. No group differences were found post-treatment, but at 6-month follow-up ACT had a significantly greater decrease in opiate use than methadone maintenance alone. Smout and colleagues (2010) found that both ACT and CBT produced significant decreases in self-reported methamphetamine use, methamphetamine dependence, and negative consequences of use. However, only the CBT group had significant increases in methamphetamine hair samples. Recently, ACT was shown to reduce shame, decrease substance use, and increase attendance at follow-up treatment relative to treatment as usual in a sample of patients completing a 28-day residential treatment program (Luoma, Kohlenberg, Hayes, & Fletcher, 2012). Finally, ACT has been shown to produce significantly better long-term quit rates among smokers than nicotine replacement (Gifford et al., 2004).

PAIN

A considerable proportion of the randomized controlled trials on ACT have been conducted on physical health conditions. ACT is considered to have strong research support for chronic pain as noted on the APA Division 12 list of empirically based treatments. Compared to treatment as usual, ACT has been shown to reduce sick days and use of medical treatment resources (Dahl, Wilson, & Nilsson, 2004) and reduce pain disability/interference both in adults (Wicksell, Ahlqvist, Bring, Melin, & Olsson, 2008) and children (Wicksell, Melin, Lekander, & Olsson, 2009) 6 or more months post-treatment. Moreover, ACT appears to be equivalent to other CBT approaches in reducing pain (Vowles, Wetherell, & Sorrell, 2009; Wetherell et al., 2011).

Veehof and colleagues (Veehof, Oskam, Schreurs, & Bohlmeijer, 2011) recently conducted a meta-analysis of the impact of acceptance and mindfulness on chronic pain. They included controlled and uncontrolled studies of ACT and mindfulness-based approaches to treatment. Analysis of pre to post changes in pain and depression, anxiety, physical well-being, and quality of life yielded moderate effect sizes. Analysis of randomized controlled trials yielded small but significant effect sizes for pain, depression, and physical well-being. Specific effect sizes for ACT were not reported, but there were no significant differences between the two forms of treatment in the effects on pain or depression. One limitation, acknowledged by the authors, is that ACT is not necessarily aimed at reducing pain intensity, which was the primary outcome in the analysis.

WEIGHT AND PHYSICAL ACTIVITY

Compared to a wait list control, ACT has been shown to increase physical activity (Tapper et al., 2009), reduce self-stigma or body anxiety (Lillis, Hayes, Bunting, & Masuda, 2009; Pearson, Follette, & Hayes, 2012), and reduce body mass at 3-month follow-up (Lillis et al., 2009). Among patients who underwent bariatric surgery, ACT significantly decreased eating-disordered behavior and body dissatisfaction and increased quality of life relative to treatment as usual (Weineland, Arvidsson, Kakoulidis, & Dahl, 2012). ACT also increased physical activity compared to an educational workshop, but only among completers (Butryn, Forman, Hoffman, Shaw, & Juarascio, 2011). Finally, ACT produced significantly greater decreases in eating pathology than cognitive therapy (Juarascio, Forman, & Herbert, 2010).

OTHER HEALTH OUTCOMES

ACT has been shown to significantly reduce the number of seizures among those with epilepsy compared to supportive psychotherapy (Lundgren, Dahl, Melin, & Kies, 2006) and yoga (Lundgren, Dahl, Yardi, & Melin, 2008). Diabetes education plus ACT produced significant improvements in diabetic control, use of self-management, acceptance, mindfulness, and values relative to education alone (Gregg, Callaghan, Hayes, & Glenn-Lawson, 2007). Compared to a treatment as usual of relaxation, problem solving, and cognitive restructuring, ACT decreased psychological distress and increased quality of life among patients with Stage III or IV ovarian cancer (Rost, Wilson, Buchanan,

Hildebrandt, & Mutch, 2012). Finally, ACT reduced the negative impact of tinnitus relative to wait list control and tinnitus retraining therapy (Westin et al., 2011).

ACT IN THE WORKPLACE/STIGMA

ACT was more effective than an empirically supported program at improving worksite stress and anxiety (Bond & Bunce, 2000) and equivalent to stress inoculation training in reducing psychological distress among workers (Flaxman & Bond, 2010). Unemployed individuals on long-term sick leave due to depression significantly improved in depression and general psychological distress following an ACT intervention relative to a group that was unrestricted in the services they could seek out for help (Folke, Parling, & Melin, 2012).

ACT has also been used as an intervention to increase evidence-based practices and decrease stress and burnout among mental health providers. Eight weeks of an ACT and relapse prevention–informed supervision group and a 1-day workshop was more effective than the workshop alone in addressing barriers to using group drug counseling, an effective treatment for drug use (Luoma, Kohlenberg, Hayes, Bunting, & Rye, 2008). At 4-month follow-up, the ACT group maintained a significantly higher rate of implementation of the program and reported a higher sense of personal accomplishment. Similarly, Varra and colleagues (Varra, Hayes, Roget, & Fisher, 2008) found that a 1-day ACT workshop, compared to a 1-day educational workshop, in advance of a 2-day workshop on empirically supported treatments for substance abuse, increased willingness to refer, and actual referrals to pharmacotherapy at follow-up.

ACT has also been shown to decrease both burnout and stigmatizing attitudes toward clients held by alcohol and drug counselors 3 months after completion of the program, while an educational methamphetamine training had no significant results (Hayes, Bissett et al., 2004). The third condition examined in this randomized controlled trial, multicultural training, produced significant changes in stigmatizing attitudes post-workshop, but not at follow-up. Both ACT and an educational workshop reduced self-reported stigmatizing attitudes toward individuals with a psychological disorder among college students (Masuda et al., 2007). However, the educational workshop was only effective for those high in psychological flexibility at baseline. Finally, an ACT-based stress management workshop for social workers significantly reduced stress and burnout and increased general mental health compared to a wait list condition, but only among those who had high stress levels at baseline (Brinkborg, Michanek, Hesser, & Berglund, 2011).

Future Directions

Although there is growing evidence of the efficacy for mindfulness- and acceptance-based behavioral approaches to treatment, the field is still in its infancy. Future research, including studies of higher methodological quality, is needed to demonstrate the specific effects of these interventions relative to comparison approaches.

Öst (2008) raised several concerns regarding the methodological features of ACT studies. For example, he noted that often the ACT treatment and the comparison treatment were unequal in the number of contact hours. Öst was also concerned that clinical diagnoses to define participant samples and assess outcome were only used in about half of the studies he reviewed. Few studies conducted adherence and competency ratings or used independent assessors to evaluate outcome. Öst also criticized the use of a wait list control group and recommended that future studies move beyond the use of treatment as usual group as a comparison. Finally, Öst argued that ACT should be compared to active treatments with empirical support.

Some of these criticisms have been addressed by Gaudiano (2009). For example, he argued that the particular comparison group chosen for a study should be informed by the state of the particular literature. He also argued that ACT researchers are interested in improving a variety of outcomes; thus, studies need not be limited to diagnostic samples. Nonetheless, increased methodological rigor is necessary to adequately evaluate the impact of ACT and other ABBTs, and several more recently published studies do appear to have stronger designs.

Identification of the Mechanisms of Change Underlying ABBTs

According to Kazdin (2007), studies aimed at determining mechanisms of action can inform both science and practice. Understanding the factors that mediate change can lead to the development of more parsimonious, cost-effective, and easily disseminated forms of effective treatment. Research investigating the mechanisms of action underlying ACT have been a priority for the research community (Hayes, Levin, Plumb-Vilardaga, Villatte, & Pistorello, 2013), and thus a number of studies have been conducted demonstrating the statistical meditational effects of acceptance and psychological flexibility (e.g., Forman et al., 2007; Gifford et al., 2004, 2011; Gregg et al., 2007; Hesser, Westin, Hayes, & Andersson, 2009; Lundgren, Dahl, & Hayes, 2008; Varra et al., 2008; Vowles, McCracken, & O'Brien, 2011), cognitive defusion or believability of internal events (e.g., Hesser et al., 2009; Gaudiano, Herbert, & Hayes, 2010; Zettle, Rains, & Hayes, 2011), and values (e.g., Lundgren et al., 2008; Vowles et al., 2011) on treatment outcome. Similarly, reductions in rumination (Heeren & Philippot, 2011; Shahar, Britton, Sbarra, Figueredo, & Bootzin, 2010), increases in self-compassion (Kuyken et al., 2010), increases in curiosity (Bieling et al., 2012), and increases in mindfulness have been shown to mediate the effects of MBCT (Kuyken et al., 2010; Shahar et al., 2010).

However, several methodological features are required to truly demonstrate mediation, including temporality and specificity (Kazdin, 2007). Although these criteria are considered critical, they are rarely met in the extant treatment process and outcome literature (Kazdin, 2007). Within the ABBT literature, there is some preliminary evidence for the temporal precedence of mediators in studies of ACT/ABBT (e.g., Gifford et al., 2004; Lundgren et al., 2008; Wicksell, Olsson, & Hayes, 2011; Zettle et al., 2011) and MBCT (e.g., Bieling et al., 2012). However, more research in this area is clearly indicated.

Experimental or analogue studies can also provide some information about the specific action of different elements of treatment. The results of several lab-based studies underscore the benefits of acceptance (e.g., Campbell-Sills, Barlow, Brown, & Hofmann, 2006; Eifert & Heffner, 2003; Keogh, Bond, Hanmer, & Tilston, 2005; Levitt, Brown, Orsillo, & Barlow, 2004; Low, Stanton, & Bower, 2008; Najmi & Wegner, 2009). However, often experimental studies test the effects of instruction in acceptance, rather than the cultivation of an accepting stance, and thus their relevance to treatment may be limited (Ruiz, 2010). There are also a number of studies that have demonstrated the effects of brief mindfulness meditation on outcomes such as pain sensitivity (Zeidan, Gordon, Merchant, & Goolkasian, 2010), mood and cardiovascular response (Zeidan, Johnson, Gordon, & Goolkasian, 2010), positive emotions (Erisman & Roemer, 2010), and experiential avoidance (Hooper, Villatte, Neofotistou, & McHugh, 2010). Far fewer studies

have examined the specific effects of a values rationale in increasing participant willingness to engage in an unpleasant or painful task (Czech, Katz, & Orsillo, 2011; Gutiérrez, Luciano, Rodríguez, & Fink, 2004; Páez-Blarrina et al., 2008). Further, the clinical validity of the tasks used in many of these lab-based studies is limited.

Some have argued that in order to distinguish ABBTs from traditional CBT, research demonstrating mediators specific to each approach is needed (e.g., Arch & Craske, 2008; Hayes et al., 2011). There is a small body of research suggesting that the mechanisms underlying ACT differ from those underlying CBT (e.g., Forman et al., 2007) and multidisciplinary treatment and amitriptyline for pain (Wicksell et al., 2011) and that MBCT reduces the risk of relapse through a mechanism that is unique from the mechanism of action underlying medication (Bieling et al, 2012).

On the other hand, others suggest that research on mediators of ABBT may provide some insight into the mechanisms of action underlying traditional CBT. For example, Fresco and colleagues (2007) demonstrated that among those treated with CBT, high post-acute treatment levels of decentering and low cognitive reactivity were associated with the lowest rates of relapse in the 18-month follow-up period. Our preliminary data suggest applied relaxation may work through decentering (Hayes-Skelton, Roemer, & Orsillo, 2011). More research is needed to determine whether processes such as acceptance and decentering are common factors across different forms of CBT or specific to ABBTs.

Moderators

Very few studies have investigated whether particular baseline characteristics moderate the impact of ACT/ABBTs. There is some evidence that baseline experiential avoidance (e.g., Zettle, 2003) and baseline distress are predictors of outcome (Flaxman & Bond, 2010), whereas other studies have failed to identify baseline predictors of response (Vowles et al., 2011). Some studies have examined differential predictors of ACT versus other approaches to treatment. For example, Masuda et al. (2007) found that baseline psychological flexibility predicted the efficacy of psychoeducation, but not ACT, in reducing stigma toward mental illness.

Two studies demonstrated that number of previous episodes of major depression moderates the effect of MBCT on outcome. Specifically, MBCT was more effective than care as usual among people who had experienced three or more previous episodes of major depression (Ma & Teasdale, 2004; Teasdale et al., 2000).

Applicability of Treatment to Ethnically and Economically Diverse Populations

One concern about traditional CBT is that dominant cultural values are often implicit in many of these approaches (Benish, Quintana, & Wampold, 2011). For example, CBT often emphasizes individualism and rationality, values that may not be shared by some clients of nondominant cultural and/or marginalized backgrounds (Hays, 2009). In contrast, we (Fuchs, Lee, Roemer, & Orsillo, 2012) have argued that mindfulness- and acceptance-based behavioral approaches may be more relevant and acceptable to clients from marginalized and/or underserved populations.

For example, the stance inherent in these approaches that emotional distress is a universal, natural human response may be welcoming to clients who fear they will be blamed or stigmatized for their presenting difficulties. The use of metaphors, particularly those that are adapted to reflect a client's cultural context, may also help to normalize distress. Finally, many ABBTs balance acknowledging and validating painful situations that are out of a client's control with encouraging engagement in values-consistent actions. This perspective may be particularly relevant for clients who are struggling with distress due to systemic oppression and discrimination.

We (Fuchs et al., 2012) conducted a meta-analysis of 32 studies (2,198 participants) that examined the efficacy of acceptance- and mindfulness-based behavioral treatments among clients who were either (a) non-White, (b) non-European American, (c) older adults, (d) nonheterosexual, (e) low-income, (f) physically disabled, (g) incarcerated, and/or (h) individuals whose first language is not that of the dominant culture. The results yielded moderate effect sizes for studies that compared ABBTs to an active treatment.

Although ABBTs may hold promise for underserved cultural groups, some adaptations may be important. Hall and colleagues (Hall, Hong, Zane, & Meyer, 2011) recommended that ABBTs be modified to better align with the interdependent and allocentric orientations of Asian Americans. For example, they recommend considering mindfulness meditations such as loving-kindness, a practice that involves extending beyond the individual self and orienting acceptance and compassion toward others, as it may

be a more relevant practice. Similarly, they recommend values articulation exercises that help the client identify and prioritize social group values and consider the ways in which he or she can contribute to these groups.

Although some researchers have already started making cultural adaptations to ABBTs (Dutton, Bermundez, Matás, Majid, & Mylers, 2013; Hinton, Pich, Hofmann, & Otto, 2012), this research is in its infancy. We (Fuchs et al., 2012) recently collected qualitative data from clients of different ethnic backgrounds to obtain some preliminary information on the perceived appropriateness and cultural relevance of an ABBT for GAD that we hope will direct future research efforts. Until research establishes clear guidelines, therapists are urged to be culturally sensitive and responsive when using ABBTs with clients from nondominant cultural backgrounds.

Effectiveness, Dissemination, and Implementation

Our core challenge as mental health professionals is to reduce the prevalence and burden of psychological distress. However, need for services far outweighs our current resources. Thus, many (e.g., Kazdin & Blase, 2011; McHugh & Barlow, 2010) have called for a radical shift in intervention research and practice aimed at improving dissemination and implementation of evidence-based practices. The development of brief, cost-effective methods of flexibly delivering services through self-help books, telephone consultation, and the Internet are required to meet the growing need for mental health services (Kazdin & Blase, 2011).

Several studies have examined the potential effectiveness of self-directed ACT treatments with minimal therapist support. For example, an ACT-based self-help book for individuals with chronic pain has been shown to be effective in reducing anxiety, increasing quality of life (Johnston, Foster, Shennan, Starkey, & Johnson, 2010), and increasing acceptance (Thorsell et al., 2011). An Internet-delivered ACT program for tinnitus was as efficacious as an Internet-delivered CBT approach, both at post-treatment and at 1-year follow-up (Hesser et al., 2012).

Zindel Segal (2011) is currently developing and piloting an electronic version of MBCT as a cost-effective method of reducing relapse among those successfully treated for depression. Moreover, Thompson and colleagues (2010) found both an Internet and a telephone-delivered version of

MBCT to reduce depression among individuals with epilepsy.

Clearly, considerably more research is needed on how best to disseminate acceptance-based behavioral treatments in ways that are cost-effective, while maintaining effectiveness. This will be an important focus for future research moving forward.

Acceptance-based behavioral therapies (including ACT, MBCT, IBCT, ABBT for GAD, and DBT) show tremendous promise across a broad range of clinical problems. Additional research will help to clearly establish the presenting problems for which these approaches are efficacious, the mechanisms of action underlying these approaches, any contraindications or ways to enhance or adapt these approaches for particular populations or target problems, and how best to disseminate them and make them accessible to a broad range of people.

References

Arch, J. J., & Craske, M. G. (2008). Acceptance and commitment therapy and cognitive behavioral therapy for anxiety disorders: Different treatments, similar mechanisms? *Clinical Psychology: Science and Practice*, 15(4), 263–279.

Bach, P., & Hayes, S. C. (2002). The use of acceptance and commitment therapy to prevent the rehospitalization of psychotic patients: A randomized controlled trial. *Journal of Consulting and Clinical Psychology*, 70(5), 1129–1139. doi:10.1037/0022-006X.70.5.1129

Bagby, R. M., Rector, N. A., Bacchiochi, J. R., & McBride, C. (2004). The stability of the response styles questionnaire rumination scale in a sample of patients with major depression. *Cognitive Therapy and Research*, 28(4), 527–538. doi:10.1023/B:COTR.0000045562.17228.29

Bar-Haim, Y., Lamy, D., Pergamin, L., Bakermans-Kranenburg, M., & van IJzendoorn, M. H. (2007). Threat-related attentional bias in anxious and nonanxious individuals: A meta-analytic study. *Psychological Bulletin*, 133(1), 1–24. doi:10.1037/0033-2909.133.1.1

Barnard, P. J., & Teasdale, J. D. (1991). Interacting cognitive subsystems: A systemic approach to cognitive-affective interaction and change. *Cognition and Emotion*, 5(1), 1–39. doi:10.1080/02699939108411021

Baucom, B., & Hoffman, J. A. (1986). The effectiveness of marital therapy: Current status and application to the clinical setting. In N. S. Jacobson & A. S. Gurman (Eds.), *Clinical foundations of marital therapy* (pp. 597–620). New York: Guilford Press.

Beck, A. T. (1967). *Depression: Clinical, experimental, and theoretical aspects.* New York: Harper & Row.

Beck, A. T., Rush, A. J., Shaw, B. F., & Emery, G. (1979). *Cognitive therapy of depression.* New York: Guilford Press.

Benish, S. G., Quintana, S., & Wampold, B. E. (2011). Culturally adapted psychotherapy and the legitimacy of myth: A direct-comparison meta-analysis. *Journal of Counseling Psychology*, 58(3), 279–289. doi:10.1037/a0023626

Bieling, P. J., Hawley, L. L., Bloch, R. T., Corcoran, K. M., Levitan, R. D., Young, L. T.,.... Segal, Z. V. (2012). Treatment-specific changes in decentering following mindfulness-based cognitive therapy versus antidepressant medication or placebo for prevention of depressive relapse. *Journal of Consulting and Clinical Psychology*, 80(3), 365–372. doi:10.1037/a0027483

Biglan, A., & Hayes, S. C. (1996). Should the behavioral sciences become more pragmatic? The case for functional contextualism in research on human behavior. *Applied and Preventive Psychology*, 5(1), 47–57. doi:10.1016/S0962-1849(96)80026-6

Block, J., & Wulfert, E. (2000). Acceptance or change: Treating socially anxious college students with ACT or CBGT. *Behavior Analyst Today*, 1(3), 1–10.

Bohlmeijer, E., Prenger, R., Taal, E., & Cuijpers, P. (2010). The effects of mindfulness-based stress reduction therapy on mental health of adults with a chronic medical disease: A meta-analysis. *Journal of Psychosomatic Research*, 68(6), 539–544. doi:10.1016/j.jpsychores.2009.10.005

Bond, F. W., & Bunce, D. (2000). Mediators of change in emotion-focused and problem-focused worksite stress management interventions. *Journal of Occupational Health Psychology*, 5(1), 156–163. doi:10.1037/1076-8998.5.1.156

Borkovec, T. D. (1994). The nature, functions, and origins of worry. In G. C. L. Davey, F. Tallis, G. C. L. Davey, & F. Tallis (Eds.), *Worrying: Perspectives on theory, assessment and treatment* (pp. 5–33). Oxford, England: Wiley.

Borkovec, T. D., & Hu, S. (1990). The effect of worry on cardiovascular response to phobic imagery. *Behaviour Research and Therapy*, 28(1), 69–73. doi:10.1016/0005-7967(90)90056-O

Borkovec, T. D., & Roemer, L. (1995). Perceived functions of worry among generalized anxiety disorder subjects: Distraction from more emotionally distressing topics? *Journal of Behavior Therapy and Experimental Psychiatry*, 26(1), 25–30. doi:10.1016/0005-7916(94)00064-S

Borkovec, T. D., & Ruscio, A. M. (2001). Psychotherapy for generalized anxiety disorder. *Journal of Clinical Psychiatry*, 62, 37–42.

Brinkborg, H., Michanek, J., Hesser, H., & Berglund, G. (2011). Acceptance and commitment therapy for the treatment of stress among social workers: A randomized controlled trial. *Behaviour Research and Therapy*, 49(6–7), 389–398. doi:10.1016/j.brat.2011.03.009

Brown, L. A., Forman, E. M., Herbert, J. D., Hoffman, K. L., Yuen, E. K., & Goetter, E. M. (2011). A randomized controlled trial of acceptance-based behavior therapy and cognitive therapy for test anxiety: A pilot study. *Behavior Modification*, 35(1), 31–53. doi:10.1177/0145445510390930

Butryn, M. L., Forman, E., Hoffman, K., Shaw, J., & Juarascio, A. (2011). A pilot study of acceptance and commitment therapy for promotion of physical activity. *Journal of Physical Activity & Health*, 8(4), 516–522.

Campbell-Sills, L., Barlow, D. H., Brown, T. A., & Hofmann, S. G. (2006). Effects of suppression and acceptance on emotional responses of individuals with anxiety and mood disorders. *Behaviour Research and Therapy*, 44(9), 1251–1263. doi:10.1016/j.brat.2005.10.001

Chiesa, A., & Serretti, A. (2011). Mindfulness based cognitive therapy for psychiatric disorders: A systematic review and meta-analysis. *Psychiatry Research*, 187(3), 441–453. doi:10.1016/j.psychres.2010.08.011

Christensen, A., Atkins, D. C., Baucom, B., & Yi, J. (2010). Marital status and satisfaction five years following a randomized clinical trial comparing traditional versus integrative behavioral couple therapy. *Journal of Consulting and Clinical Psychology, 78*(2), 225–235. doi:10.1037/a0018132

Christensen, A., Atkins, D. C., Berns, S., Wheeler, J., Baucom, D. H., & Simpson, L. E. (2004). Traditional versus integrative behavioral couple therapy for significantly and chronically distressed married couples. *Journal of Consulting and Clinical Psychology, 72*(2), 176–191. doi:10.1037/0022-006X.72.2.176

Christensen, A., Atkins, D. C., Yi, J., Baucom, D. H., & George, W. H. (2006). Couple and individual adjustment for 2 years following a randomized clinical trial comparing traditional versus integrative behavioral couple therapy. *Journal of Consulting and Clinical Psychology, 74*(6), 1180–1191. doi: 10.1037/0022-006X.74.6.1180

Christensen, A., Jacobson, N. S., & Babcock, J. C. (1995). Integrative behavioral couple therapy. In N. S. Jacobson & A. S. Gurman (Eds.), *Clinical handbook of couple therapy* (pp. 31–64). New York: Guilford Press.

Coelho, H. F., Canter, P. H., & Ernst, E. (2007). Mindfulness-based cognitive therapy: Evaluating current evidence and informing future research. *Journal of Consulting and Clinical Psychology, 75*(6), 1000–1005. doi:10.1037/0022-006X.75.6.1000

Cordova, J. V., Jacobson, N. S., & Christensen, A. (1998). Acceptance versus change interventions in behavioral couple therapy: Impact on couples' in-session communication. *Journal of Marital and Family Therapy, 24*(4), 437–455. doi:10.1111/j.1752-0606.1998.tb01099.x

Craigie, M. A., Rees, C. S., Marsh, A., & Nathan, P. (2008). Mindfulness-based cognitive therapy for generalized anxiety disorder: A preliminary evaluation. *Behavioural and Cognitive Psychotherapy, 36*(5), 553–568. doi:10.1017/S135246580800458X

Czech, S. J., Katz, A. M., & Orsillo, S. M. (2011). The effect of values affirmation on psychological stress. *Cognitive Behaviour Therapy, 40*(4), 304–312. doi:10.1080/16506073.2011.585347

Dahl, J., Wilson, K. G., & Nilsson, A. (2004). Acceptance and commitment therapy and the treatment of persons at risk for long-term disability resulting from stress and pain symptoms: A preliminary randomized trial. *Behavior Therapy, 35*(4), 785–801. doi:10.1016/S0005-7894(04)80020-0

Dalgleish, T., Yiend, J., Schweizer, S., & Dunn, B. D. (2009). Ironic effects of emotion suppression when recounting distressing memories. *Emotion, 9*(5), 744–749. doi:10.1037/a0017290

Dugas, M. J., Gagnon, F., Ladouceur, R., & Freeston, M. H. (1998). Generalized anxiety disorder: A preliminary test of a conceptual model. *Behaviour Research and Therapy, 36*(2), 215–226. doi:10.1016/S0005-7967(97)00070-3

Dutton, M. A., Bermudez, D., Matás, A., Majid, H., & Mylers, N. L. (2013). Mindfulness-based stress reduction for low-income, predominantly african american women with PTSD and a history of intimate partner violence. *Cognitive and Behavioral Practice, 20*(1), 23–32.

Eifert, G. H., & Heffner, M. (2003). The effects of acceptance versus control contexts on avoidance of panic-related symptoms. *Journal of Behavior Therapy and Experimental Psychiatry, 34*(3–4), 293–312. doi:10.1016/j.jbtep.2003.11.001

Ellis, A. (1996). *Better, deeper, and more enduring brief therapy: The rational emotive behavior therapy approach.* Philadelphia, PA US: Brunner/Mazel.

Ellis, A., & Harper, R. A. (1961). *A guide to rational living.* Oxford, England: Prentice-Hall.

Erisman, S. M., & Roemer, L. (2010). A preliminary investigation of the effects of experimentally induced mindfulness on emotional responding to film clips. *Emotion, 10*(1), 72–82. doi:10.1037/a0017162

Fjorback, L. O., Arendt, M., Ørnbøl, E., Fink, P., & Walach, H. (2011). Mindfulness-based stress reduction and Mindfulness-based cognitive therapy—A systematic review of randomized controlled trials. *Acta Psychiatrica Scandinavica, 124*(2), 102–119. doi:10.1111/j.1600-0447.2011.01704.x

Flaxman, P. E., & Bond, F. W. (2010). Worksite stress management training: Moderated effects and clinical significance. *Journal of Occupational Health Psychology, 15*(4), 347–358. doi:10.1037/a0020522

Folke, F., Parling, T., & Melin, L. (2012). Acceptance and commitment therapy for depression: A preliminary randomized clinical trial for unemployed on long-term sick leave. *Cognitive and Behavioral Practice, 19*(4) 583–594.

Forman, E. M., Herbert, J. D., Moitra, E., Yeomans, P. D., & Geller, P. A. (2007). A randomized controlled effectiveness trial of acceptance and commitment therapy and cognitive therapy for anxiety and depression. *Behavior Modification, 31*(6), 772–799. doi:10.1177/0145445507302202

Forsyth, J. P., & McNeil, D. W. (2002). Mastery of your anxiety and worry: A multimodal case study of effectiveness of a manualized treatment for generalized anxiety disorder. *Cognitive and Behavioral Practice, 9*(3), 200–212. doi:10.1016/S1077-7229(02)80050-5

Fresco, D. M., Segal, Z. V., Buis, T., & Kennedy, S. (2007). Relationship of posttreatment decentering and cognitive reactivity to relapse in major depression. *Journal of Consulting and Clinical Psychology, 75*(3), 447–455. doi:10.1037/0022-006X.75.3.447

Freud, S. (1910). The origin and development of psychoanalysis. *American Journal of Psychology, 21,* 181–218.

Freud, S. (1965). *New introductory lectures on psychoanalysis.* Oxford, England: W.W. Norton.

Fuchs, C., Lee, J. K., Roemer, L., & Orsillo, S. M. (2012). Using mindfulness- and acceptance-based treatments with clients from nondominant cultural and/or marginalized backgrounds: Clinical considerations, meta-analysis findings, and introduction to the special series: Clinical considerations in using acceptance- and mindfulness-based treatments with diverse populations. *Cognitive and Behavioral Practice.* doi:10.1016/j.cbpra.2011.12.004

Gaudiano, B. A. (2009). Öst's (2008) methodological comparison of clinical trials of acceptance and commitment therapy versus cognitive behavior therapy: Matching apples with oranges? *Behaviour Research and Therapy, 47*(12), 1066–1070. doi:10.1016/j.brat.2009.07.020

Gaudiano, B. A., & Herbert, J. D. (2006). Acute treatment of inpatients with psychotic symptoms using acceptance and commitment therapy: Pilot results. *Behaviour Research and Therapy, 44*(3), 415–437. doi:10.1016/j.brat.2005.02.007

Gaudiano, B. A., Herbert, J. D., & Hayes, S. C. (2010). Is it the symptom or the relation to it? investigating potential mediators of change in acceptance and commitment therapy for psychosis. *Behavior Therapy, 41*(4), 543–554. doi:10.1016/j.beth.2010.03.001

Geschwind, N., Peeters, F., Drukker, M., van Os, J., & Wichers, M. (2011). Mindfulness training increases momentary positive emotions and reward experience in adults vulnerable to depression: A randomized controlled trial. *Journal of Consulting and Clinical Psychology, 79*(5), 618–628. doi:10.1037/a0024595

Gifford, E. V., Kohlenberg, B. S., Hayes, S. C., Antonuccio, D. O., Piasecki, M. M., Rasmussen-Hall, M., & Palm, K. M. (2004). Acceptance-based treatment for smoking cessation. *Behavior Therapy, 35*(4), 689–705. doi:10.1016/S0005-7894(04)80015-7

Gifford, E. V., Kohlenberg, B. S., Hayes, S. C., Pierson, H. M., Piasecki, M. P., Antonuccio, D. O., & Palm, K. M. (2011). Does acceptance and relationship focused behavior therapy contribute to bupropion outcomes? A randomized controlled trial of functional analytic psychotherapy and acceptance and commitment therapy for smoking cessation. *Behavior Therapy, 42*(4), 700–715. doi:10.1016/j.beth.2011.03.002

Gratz, K. L., & Gunderson, J. G. (2006). Preliminary data on acceptance-based emotion regulation group intervention for deliberate self-harm among women with borderline personality disorder. *Behavior Therapy, 37*(1), 25–35. doi:10.1016/j.beth.2005.03.002

Gregg, J. A., Callaghan, G. M., Hayes, S. C., & Glenn-Lawson, J. (2007). Improving diabetes self-management through acceptance, mindfulness, and values: A randomized controlled trial. *Journal of Consulting and Clinical Psychology, 75*(2), 336–343. doi:10.1037/0022-006X.75.2.336

Gutiérrez, O., Luciano, C., Rodríguez, M., & Fink, B. C. (2004). Comparison between an acceptance-based and a cognitive-control-based protocol for coping with pain. *Behavior Therapy, 35*(4), 767–783. doi:10.1016/S0005-7894(04)80019-4

Hall, G. C. N., Hong, J. J., Zane, N. W. S., & Meyer, O. L. (2011). Culturally competent treatments for asian americans: The relevance of mindfulness and acceptance—based psychotherapies. *Clinical Psychology: Science and Practice, 18*(3), 215–231. doi:10.1111/j.1468-2850.2011.01253.x

Hayes, L., Bach, P. A., & Boyd, C. P. (2010). Psychological treatment for adolescent depression: Perspectives on the past, present, and future. *Behaviour Change, 27*(1), 1–18. doi:10.1375/bech.27.1.1

Hayes, S. C. (1987). A contextual approach to therapeutic change. In N. S. Jacobson & N. S. Jacobson (Eds.), *Psychotherapists in clinical practice: Cognitive and behavioral perspectives.* (pp. 327-387). New York: Guilford Press.

Hayes, S. C. (1993). Analytic goals and the varieties of scientific contextualism. In S. C. Hayes, L. J. Hayes, H. W. Reese, & T. R. Sarbin (Eds.), *Varieties of scientific contextualism* (pp. 11–27). Reno, NV: Context Press.

Hayes, S. C. (2004). Acceptance and commitment therapy, relational frame theory, and the third wave of behavioral and cognitive therapies. *Behavior Therapy, 35*(4), 639–665. doi:10.1016/S0005-7894(04)80013-3

Hayes, S. C., Barnes-Holmes, D., & Roche, B. (2001). *Relational frame theory: A post-skinnerian account of human language and cognition* New York: Kluwer Academic/Plenum Publishers.

Hayes, S. C., Bissett, R., Roget, N., Padilla, M., Kohlenberg, B. S., Fisher, G.,. . . . Niccolls, R. (2004). The impact of acceptance and commitment training and multicultural training on the stigmatizing attitudes and professional burnout of substance abuse counselors. *Behavior Therapy, 35*(4), 821–835. doi:10.1016/S0005-7894(04)80022-4

Hayes, S. C., Hayes, L. J., Reese, H. W., & Sarbin, T. R. (Eds.). (1993). *Varieties of scientific contextualism.* Reno, NV: Context Press.

Hayes, S. C., Levin, M. E., Plumb-Vilardaga, J., Villatte, J. L., & Pistorello, J. (2013). Acceptance and commitment therapy and contextual behavioral science: Examining the progress of a distinctive model of behavioral and cognitive therapy. *Behavior Therapy, 44*(2), 180–198. doi:10.1016/j.beth.2009.08.002

Hayes, S. C., Luoma, J. B., Bond, F. W., Masuda, A., & Lillis, J. (2006). Acceptance and commitment therapy: Model, processes and outcomes. *Behaviour Research and Therapy, 44*(1), 1–25. doi:10.1016/j.brat.2005.06.006

Hayes, S. C. & Sandoz, E. K. (2012). Present moment awareness. In S. C. Hayes, K. D. Strosahl, & K. G. Wilson, Acceptance and commitment therapy: The process and practice of mindful change (2nd ed. pp. 201-219). New York, NY US: Guilford Press.

Hayes, S. C., Strosahl, K. D., & Wilson, K. G. (1999). *Acceptance and commitment therapy: An experiential approach to behavior change.* New York: Guilford Press.

Hayes, S. C., Strosahl, K. D., & Wilson, K. G. (2012). *Acceptance and commitment therapy: The process and practice of mindful change* (2nd ed.). New York: Guilford Press.

Hayes, S. C., & Wilson, K. G. (1994). Acceptance and commitment therapy: Altering the verbal support for experiential avoidance. *The Behavior Analyst, 17*(2), 289–303.

Hayes, S. C., Wilson, K. G., Gifford, E. V., Bissett, R., Piasecki, M., Batten, S. V.,. . . . Gregg, J. (2004). A preliminary trial of twelve-step facilitation and acceptance and commitment therapy with polysubstance-abusing methadone-maintained opiate addicts. *Behavior Therapy, 35*(4), 667–688. doi:10.1016/S0005-7894(04)80014-5

Hayes-Skelton, S., Roemer, L., & Orsillo, S. M. (2011). *Decentering as a common mechanism across two behavioral treatments for generalized anxiety disorder.* Alberta, Canada: Society for Psychotherapy Research.

Hays, P. A. (2009). Integrating evidence-based practice, cognitive–behavior therapy, and multicultural therapy: Ten steps for culturally competent practice. *Professional Psychology: Research and Practice, 40*(4), 354–360. doi:10.1037/a0016250

Heeren, A., & Philippot, P. (2011). Changes in ruminative thinking mediate the clinical benefits of mindfulness: Preliminary findings. *Mindfulness, 2*(1), 8–13. doi:10.1007/s12671-010-0037-y

Hesser, H., Gustafsson, T., Lundén, C., Henrikson, O., Fattahi, K., Johnsson, E.,. . . . Andersson, G. (2012). A randomized controlled trial of internet-delivered cognitive behavior therapy and acceptance and commitment therapy in the treatment of tinnitus. *Journal of Consulting and Clinical Psychology, 80*(4), 649–661. doi:10.1037/a0027021

Hesser, H., Westin, V., Hayes, S. C., & Andersson, G. (2009). Clients' in-session acceptance and cognitive defusion behaviors in acceptance-based treatment of tinnitus distress. *Behaviour Research and Therapy, 47*(6), 523–528. doi:10.1016/j.brat.2009.02.002

Hinton, D. E., Pich, V., Hofmann, S. G., & Otto, M. W. (2012). Acceptance and mindfulness techniques as applied to refugee and ethnic minority populations with PTSD: Examples from "culturally adapted CBT". *Cognitive and Behavioral Practice, 49*(2), 340–365.

Hofmann, S. G., Sawyer, A. T. & Fang, A. (2010). The empirical status of the "new wave" of cognitive behavioral therapy. *Psychiatric Clinics of North America, 33*(3), 701–710.

Hollon, S. D., & Beck, A. T. (1979). Cognitive therapy of depression. In P. C. Kendall & S. D. Hollon (Eds.), *Cognitive-behavioral interventions: Theory, research, and procedures* (pp. 153-203). New York: Academic Press.

Hollon, S. D., & Ponniah, K. (2010). A review of empirically supported psychological therapies for mood disorders in adults. *Depression and Anxiety, 27*(10), 891–932. doi:10.1002/da.20741

Hooper, N., Villatte, M., Neofotistou, E., & McHugh, L. (2010). The effects of mindfulness versus thought suppression on implicit and explicit measures of experiential avoidance. *International Journal of Behavioral Consultation and Therapy, 6*(3), 233–244.

Ilardi, S. S., Craighead, W. E., & Evans, D. D. (1997). Modeling relapse in unipolar depression: The effects of dysfunctional cognitions and personality disorders. *Journal of Consulting and Clinical Psychology, 65*(3), 381–391. doi:10.1037/0022-006X.65.3.381

Ingram, R. E., & Hollon, S. D. (1986). Cognitive therapy for depression from an information processing perspective. In R. E. Ingram & R. E. Ingram (Eds.), *Information processing approaches to clinical psychology* (pp. 259-281). San Diego, CA: Academic Press.

Jacobson, N. S. (1992). Behavioral couple therapy: A new beginning. *Behavior Therapy, 23*(4), 493–506. doi:10.1016/S0005-7894(05)80218-7

Jacobson, N. S., & Christensen, A. (1996). *Integrative couple therapy: Promoting acceptance and change.* New York: W. W. Norton.

Jacobson, N. S., Christensen, A., Prince, S. E., Cordova, J., & Eldridge, K. (2000). Integrative behavioral couple therapy: An acceptance-based, promising new treatment for couple discord. *Journal of Consulting and Clinical Psychology, 68*(2), 351–355. doi:10.1037/0022-006X.68.2.351

Jacobson, N. S., & Follette, W. C. (1985). Clinical significance of improvement resulting from two behavioral marital therapy components. *Behavior Therapy, 16*(3), 249–262. doi:10.1016/S0005-7894(85)80013-7

Jacobson, N. S., Follette, W. C., & Pagel, M. (1986). Predicting who will benefit from behavioral marital therapy. *Journal of Consulting and Clinical Psychology, 54*(4), 518–522. doi:10.1037/0022-006X.54.4.518

Jacobson, N. S., & Margolin, G. (1979). *Marital therapy: Strategies based on social learning and behavioral exchange principles.* New York: Brunner/Mazel.

Jacobson, N. S., Schmaling, K. B., & Holtzworth-Munroe, A. (1987). Component analysis of behavioral marital therapy: 2-year follow-up and prediction of relapse. *Journal of Marital and Family Therapy, 13*(2), 187–195. doi:10.1111/j.1752-0606.1987.tb00696.x

Johnston, M., Foster, M., Shennan, J., Starkey, N. J., & Johnson, A. (2010). The effectiveness of an acceptance and commitment therapy self-help intervention for chronic pain. *Clinical Journal of Pain, 26*(5), 393–402. doi:10.1097/AJP.0b013e3181cf59ce

Juarascio, A. S., Forman, E. M., & Herbert, J. D. (2010). Acceptance and commitment therapy versus cognitive therapy for the treatment of comorbid eating pathology. *Behavior Modification, 34*(2), 175–190. doi:10.1177/0145445510363472

Jung, C. G. (1933). *Modern man in search of a soul.* London: Kegan Paul Trench Trubner.

Kabat-Zinn, J. (1994). *Wherever you go, there you are: Mindfulness meditation in everyday life.* New York: Hyperion.

Kabat-Zinn, J. (2003). Mindfulness-based interventions in context: Past, present, and future. *Clinical Psychology: Science and Practice, 10*(2), 144–156. doi:10.1093/clipsy/bpg016

Kabat-Zinn, J. (2005). *Full catastrophe living: Using the wisdom of your body and mind to face stress, pain, and illness* (15th anniversary ed.). New York: Delta Trade Paperback/Bantam Dell.

Kanai, T., Takeuchi, H., Furukawa, T. A., Yoshimura, R., Imaizumi, T., Kitamura, T., & Takahashi, K. (2003). Time to recurrence after recovery from major depressive episodes and its predictors. *Psychological Medicine, 33*(5), 839–845. doi:10.1017/S0033291703007827

Kazdin, A. E. (2007). Mediators and mechanisms of change in psychotherapy research. *Annual Review of Clinical Psychology, 3*, 1–27. doi:10.1146/annurev.clinpsy.3.022806.091432

Kazdin, A. E., & Blase, S. L. (2011). Rebooting psychotherapy research and practice to reduce the burden of mental illness. *Perspectives on Psychological Science, 6*(1), 21–37. doi:10.1177/1745691610393527

Keller, M. B., Lavori, P. W., Mueller, T. I., & Endicott, J. (1992). Time to recovery, chronicity, and levels of psychopathology in major depression: A 5-year prospective follow-up of 431 subjects. *Archives of General Psychiatry, 49*(10), 809–816.

Kenny, M. A., & Williams, J. M. G. (2007). Treatment-resistant depressed patients show a good response to mindfulness-based cognitive therapy. *Behaviour Research and Therapy, 45*(3), 617–625. doi:10.1016/j.brat.2006.04.008

Keogh, E., Bond, F. W., Hanmer, R., & Tilston, J. (2005). Comparing acceptance- and control-based coping instructions on the cold-pressor pain experiences of healthy men and women. *European Journal of Pain, 9*(5), 591–598. doi:10.1016/j.ejpain.2004.12.005

Kim, Y. W., Lee, S., Choi, T. K., Suh, S. Y., Kim, B., Kim, C. M.,.... Yook, K. (2009). Effectiveness of mindfulness-based cognitive therapy as an adjuvant to pharmacotherapy in patients with panic disorder or generalized anxiety disorder. *Depression and Anxiety, 26*(7), 601–606. doi:10.1002/da.20552

Kovacs, M., & Beck, A. T. (1978). Maladaptive cognitive structures in depression. *American Journal of Psychiatry, 135*(5), 525–533.

Kuyken, W., Byford, S., Taylor, R. S., Watkins, E., Holden, E., White, K.,.... Teasdale, J. D. (2008). Mindfulness-based cognitive therapy to prevent relapse in recurrent depression. *Journal of Consulting and Clinical Psychology, 76*(6), 966–978. doi:10.1037/a0013786

Kuyken, W., Watkins, E., Holden, E., White, K., Taylor, R. S., Byford, S.,.... Dalgleish, T. (2010). How does mindfulness-based cognitive therapy work? *Behaviour Research and Therapy, 48*(11), 1105–1112. doi:10.1016/j.brat.2010.08.003

Langer, Á. I., Cangas, A. J., Salcedo, E., & Fuentes, B. (2012). Applying mindfulness therapy in a group of psychotic individuals: A controlled study. *Behavioural and Cognitive Psychotherapy, 40*(1), 105–109. doi:10.1017/S1352465811000464

Lappalainen, R., Lehtonen, T., Skarp, E., Taubert, E., Ojanen, M., & Hayes, S. C. (2007). The impact of CBT and ACT models using psychology trainee therapists: A preliminary controlled effectiveness trial. *Behavior Modification, 31*(4), 488–511. doi:10.1177/0145445506298436

Lee, J. K., Orsillo, S. M., Roemer, L., & Allen, L. B. (2010). Distress and avoidance in generalized anxiety disorder: Exploring the relationships with intolerance of uncertainty and worry. *Cognitive Behaviour Therapy, 39*(2), 126–136. doi:10.1080/16506070902966918

Levin, M., & Hayes, S. C. (2009). Is acceptance and commitment therapy superior to established treatment comparisons? *Psychotherapy and Psychosomatics, 78*(6), 380. doi:10.1159/000235978

Levitt, J. T., Brown, T. A., Orsillo, S. M., & Barlow, D. H. (2004). The effects of acceptance versus suppression of emotion on subjective and psychophysiological response to carbon dioxide challenge in patients with panic disorder. *Behavior Therapy, 35*(4), 747–766. doi:10.1016/S0005-7894(04)80018-2

Lewinsohn, P. M., Steinmetz, J. L., Larson, D. W., & Franklin, J. (1981). Depression-related cognitions: Antecedent or consequence? *Journal of Abnormal Psychology, 90*(3), 213–219. doi:10.1037/0021-843X.90.3.213

Lillis, J., Hayes, S. C., Bunting, K., & Masuda, A. (2009). Teaching acceptance and mindfulness to improve the lives of the obese: A preliminary test of a theoretical model. *Annals of Behavioral Medicine, 37*(1), 58–69. doi:10.1007/s12160-009-9083-x

Linehan, M. M. (1987). Dialectical behavior therapy for borderline personality disorder: Theory and method. *Bulletin of the Menninger Clinic, 51*(3), 261–276.

Linehan, M. M. (1993a). *Cognitive-behavioral treatment of borderline personality disorder.* New York: Guilford Press.

Linehan, M. M. (1993b). *Skills training manual for treating borderline personality disorder.* New York: Guilford Press.

Lovas, D. A., & Barsky, A. J. (2010). Mindfulness-based cognitive therapy for hypochondriasis, or severe health anxiety: A pilot study. *Journal of Anxiety Disorders, 24*(8), 931–935. doi:10.1016/j.janxdis.2010.06.019

Low, C. A., Stanton, A. L., & Bower, J. E. (2008). Effects of acceptance-oriented versus evaluative emotional processing on heart rate recovery and habituation. *Emotion, 8*(3), 419–424. doi:10.1037/1528-3542.8.3.419

Lundgren, T., Dahl, J., & Hayes, S. C. (2008). Evaluation of mediators of change in the treatment of epilepsy with acceptance and commitment therapy. *Journal of Behavioral Medicine, 31*(3), 225–235. doi:10.1007/s10865-008-9151-x

Lundgren, T., Dahl, J., Melin, L., & Kies, B. (2006). Evaluation of acceptance and commitment therapy for drug refractory epilepsy: A randomized controlled trial in South Africa—A pilot study. *Epilepsia, 47*(12), 2173–2179. doi:10.1111/j.1528-1167.2006.00892.x

Lundgren, T., Dahl, J., Yardi, N., & Melin, L. (2008). Acceptance and commitment therapy and yoga for drug-refractory epilepsy: A randomized controlled trial. *Epilepsy and Behavior, 13*(1), 102–108. doi:10.1016/j.yebeh.2008.02.009

Luoma, J. B., Kohlenberg, B. S., Hayes, S. C., Bunting, K., & Rye, A. K. (2008). Reducing self-stigma in substance abuse through acceptance and commitment therapy: Model, manual development, and pilot outcomes. *Addiction Research and Theory, 16*(2), 149–165. doi:10.1080/16066350701850295

Luoma, J. B., Kohlenberg, B. S., Hayes, S. C., & Fletcher, L. (2012). Slow and steady wins the race: A randomized clinical trial of acceptance and commitment therapy targeting shame in substance use disorders. *Journal of Consulting and Clinical Psychology, 80*(1), 43–53. doi:10.1037/a0026070

Ma, S. H., & Teasdale, J. D. (2004). Mindfulness-based cognitive therapy for depression: Replication and exploration of differential relapse prevention effects. *Journal of Consulting and Clinical Psychology, 72*(1), 31–40. doi:10.1037/0022-006X.72.1.31

Martell, C. R., Addis, M. E., & Jacobson, N. S. (2001). *Depression in context: Strategies for guided action.* New York: W. W. Norton.

Masuda, A., Hayes, S. C., Fletcher, L. B., Seignourel, P. J., Bunting, K., Herbst, S. A.,. . . . Lillis, J. (2007). Impact of acceptance and commitment therapy versus education on stigma toward people with psychological disorders. *Behaviour Research and Therapy, 45*(11), 2764–2772. doi:10.1016/j.brat.2007.05.008

McGinn, M. M., Benson, L. A., & Christensen, A. (2011). Integrative behavioral couple therapy: An acceptance-based approach to improving relationship functioning. In J. D. Herbert, E. M. Forman, J. D. Herbert, & E. M. Forman (Eds.), *Acceptance and mindfulness in cognitive behavior therapy: Understanding and applying the new therapies.* (pp. 210–232). Hoboken, NJ: Wiley.

McHugh, R. K., & Barlow, D. H. (2010). The dissemination and implementation of evidence-based psychological treatments: A review of current efforts. *American Psychologist, 65*(2), 73–84. doi:10.1037/a0018121

Mennin, D. S., Heimberg, R. G., Turk, C. L., & Fresco, D. M. (2005). Preliminary evidence for an emotion dysregulation model of generalized anxiety disorder. *Behaviour Research and Therapy, 43*(10), 1281–1310. doi:10.1016/j.brat.2004.08.008

Michelson, S. E., Lee, J. K., Orsillo, S. M., & Roemer, L. (2011). The role of values-consistent behavior in generalized anxiety disorder. *Depression and Anxiety, 28*(5), 358–366. doi:10.1002/da.20793

Miklowitz, D. J., Alatiq, Y., Goodwin, G. M., Geddes, J. R., Fennell, M. J. V., Dimidjian, S.,. . . . Williams, J. M. (2009). A pilot study of mindfulness-based cognitive therapy for bipolar disorder. *International Journal of Cognitive Therapy, 2*(4), 373–382. doi:10.1521/ijct.2009.2.4.373

Mogg, K., & Bradley, B. P. (2005). Attentional bias in generalized anxiety disorder versus depressive disorder. *Cognitive Therapy and Research, 29*(1), 29–45. doi:10.1007/s10608-005-1646-y

Mueller, T. I., Leon, A. C., Keller, M. B., Solomon, D. A., Endicott, J., Coryell, W.,. . . . Maser, J. D. (1999). Recurrence after recovery from major depressive disorder during 15 years of observational follow-up. *American Journal of Psychiatry, 156*(7), 1000–1006.

Najmi, S., & Wegner, D. M. (2009). Hidden complications of thought suppression. *International Journal of Cognitive Therapy, 2*(3), 210–223. doi:10.1521/ijct.2009.2.3.210

Nezu, A. M., Nezu, C. M., & D'Zurilla, T. J. (2013). *Problem-solving therapy: A treatment manual.* New York: Springer.

Nolen-Hoeksema, S. (1991). Responses to depression and their effects on the duration of depressive episodes. *Journal of Abnormal Psychology, 100*(4), 569–582. doi:10.1037/0021-843X.100.4.569

Orsillo, S. M., Roemer, L., & Barlow, D. H. (2003). Integrating acceptance and mindfulness into existing cognitive-behavioral treatment for GAD: A case study. *Cognitive and Behavioral Practice, 10*(3), 222–230. doi:10.1016/S1077-7229(03)80034-2

Öst, L. (2008). Efficacy of the third wave of behavioral therapies: A systematic review and meta-analysis. *Behaviour Research and Therapy, 46*(3), 296–321. doi:10.1016/j.brat.2007.12.005

Páez-Blarrina, M., Luciano, C., Gutiérrez-Martínez, O., Valdivia, S., Ortega, J., & Rodríguez-Valverde, M. (2008). The role of values with personal examples in altering the functions of pain: Comparison between acceptance-based and cognitive-control-based. *Behaviour Research and Therapy, 46*(1), 84–97. doi:10.1016/j.brat.2007.10.008

Pearson, A. N., Follette, V. M., & Hayes, S. C. (2012). A pilot study of acceptance and commitment therapy as a workshop intervention for body dissatisfaction and disordered eating attitudes. *Cognitive and Behavioral Practice, 19*(1), 181–197. doi:10.1016/j.cbpra.2011.03.001

Persons, J. B., & Miranda, J. (1992). Cognitive theories of vulnerability to depression: Reconciling negative evidence. *Cognitive Therapy and Research, 16*(4), 485–502. doi:10.1007/BF01183170

Peselow, E. D., Robins, C., Block, P., & Barouche, F. (1990). Dysfunctional attitudes in depressed patients before and after clinical treatment and in normal control subjects. *American Journal of Psychiatry, 147*(4), 439–444.

Petersen, C. L., & Zettle, R. D. (2009). Treating inpatients with comorbid depression and alcohol use disorders: A comparison of acceptance and commitment therapy versus treatment as usual. *The Psychological Record, 59*(4), 521–536.

Piet, J., & Hougaard, E. (2011). The effect of mindfulness-based cognitive therapy for prevention of relapse in recurrent major depressive disorder: A systematic review and meta-analysis. *Clinical Psychology Review, 31*(6), 1032–1040. doi:10.1016/j.cpr.2011.05.002

Powers, M. B., & Emmelkamp, P. M. G. (2009). Response to "is acceptance and commitment therapy superior to established treatment comparisons?" *Psychotherapy and Psychosomatics, 78*(6), 380–381. doi:10.1159/000235979

Powers, M. B., Zum Vörde, S. V., & Emmelkamp, P. M. G. (2009). Acceptance and commitment therapy: A meta-analytic review. *Psychotherapy and Psychosomatics, 78*(2), 73–80. doi:10.1159/000190790

Robins, C. J., & Rosenthal, M. Z. (2011). Dialectical behavior therapy. In J. D. Herbert, E. M. Forman, J. D. Herbert, & E. M. Forman (Eds.), *Acceptance and mindfulness in cognitive behavior therapy: Understanding and applying the new therapies.* (pp. 164–192). Hoboken, NJ: Wiley.

Roemer, L., & Orsillo, S. M. (2002). Expanding our conceptualization of and treatment for generalized anxiety disorder: Integrating mindfulness/acceptance-based approaches with existing cognitive-behavioral models. *Clinical Psychology: Science and Practice, 9*(1), 54–68. doi:10.1093/clipsy/9.1.54

Roemer, L., & Orsillo, S. M. (2007). An open trial of an acceptance-based behavior therapy for generalized anxiety disorder. *Behavior Therapy, 38*(1), 72–85. doi:10.1016/j.beth.2006.04.004

Roemer, L., & Orsillo, S. M. (2009). *Mindfulness- and acceptance-based behavioral therapies in practice.* New York: Guilford Press.

Roemer, L., Orsillo, S. M., & Salters-Pedneault, K. (2008). Efficacy of an acceptance-based behavior therapy for generalized anxiety disorder: Evaluation in a randomized controlled

trial. *Journal of Consulting and Clinical Psychology, 76*(6), 1083–1089. doi:10.1037/a0012720

Rogers, C. R. (1940). The processes of therapy. *Journal of Consulting Psychology, 4*(5), 161–164. doi:10.1037/h0062536

Rost, A. D., Wilson, K., Buchanan, E., Hildebrandt, M. J., & Mutch, D. (2012). Improving psychological adjustment among late-stage ovarian cancer patients: Examining the role of avoidance in treatment. *Cognitive and Behavioral Practice, 19*(4), 508–517. doi:10.1016/j.cbpra.2012.01.003

Ruiz, F. J. (2010). A review of acceptance and commitment therapy (ACT) empirical evidence: Correlational, experimental psychopathology, component and outcome studies. *International Journal of Psychology and Psychological Therapy, 10*(1), 125–162.

Salters-Pedneault, K., Roemer, L., Tull, M. T., Rucker, L., & Mennin, D. S. (2006). Evidence of broad deficits in emotion regulation associated with chronic worry and generalized anxiety disorder. *Cognitive Therapy and Research, 30*(4), 469–480. doi:10.1007/s10608-006-9055-4

Segal, Z. V. (2011). *What's next for mindfulness-based cognitive therapy? Moving beyond efficacy to mechanisms and Dissemination.* Toronto: Association for Behavioral and Cognitive Therapies.

Segal, Z. V., Bieling, P., Young, T., MacQueen, G., Cooke, R., Martin, L.,. . . . Levitan, R. D. (2010). Antidepressant monotherapy vs sequential pharmacotherapy and mindfulness-based cognitive therapy, or placebo, for relapse prophylaxis in recurrent depression. *Archives of General Psychiatry, 67*(12), 1256–1264. doi:10.1001/archgenpsychiatry.2010.168

Segal, Z. V., Teasdale, J. D., & Williams, J. M. (2004). Mindfulness-based cognitive therapy: Theoretical rationale and empirical status. In S. C. Hayes, V. M. Follette, & M. M. Linehan (Eds.), *Mindfulness and acceptance: Expanding the cognitive-behavioral tradition* (pp. 45–65). New York: Guilford Press.

Segal, Z. V., Williams, J. M., & Teasdale, J. D. (2002). *Mindfulness-based cognitive therapy for depression: A new approach to preventing relapse.* New York: Guilford Press.

Segal, Z. V., Williams, J. M., Teasdale, J. D., & Gemar, M. (1996). A cognitive science perspective on kindling and episode sensitization in recurrent affective disorder. *Psychological Medicine, 26*(2), 371–380. doi:10.1017/S0033291700034760

Semple, R. J., Lee, J., Rosa, D., & Miller, L. F. (2010). A randomized trial of mindfulness-based cognitive therapy for children: Promoting mindful attention to enhance social-emotional resiliency in children. *Journal of Child and Family Studies, 19*(2), 218–229. doi:10.1007/s10826-009-9301-y

Shadish, W. R., & Baldwin, S. A. (2005). Effects of behavioral marital therapy: A meta-analysis of randomized controlled trials. *Journal of Consulting and Clinical Psychology, 73*(1), 6–14. doi:10.1037/0022-006X.73.1.6

Shahar, B., Britton, W. B., Sbarra, D. A., Figueredo, A. J., & Bootzin, R. R. (2010). Mechanisms of change in mindfulness-based cognitive therapy for depression: Preliminary evidence from a randomized controlled trial. *International Journal of Cognitive Therapy, 3*(4), 402–418. doi:10.1521/ijct.2010.3.4.402

Shapiro, D. A., Cavanagh, K., & Lomas, H. (2003). Geographic inequity in the availability of cognitive behavioural therapy in

England and Wales. *Behavioural and Cognitive Psychotherapy*, *31*(2), 185–192. doi:10.1017/S1352465803002066

Skinner, B. F. (1957). *Verbal behavior*. New York: Appleton.

Skinner, B. F. (1969). *Contingencies of reinforcement: A theoretical analysis*. New York: Appleton.

Smout, M. F., Longo, M., Harrison, S., Minniti, R., Wickes, W., & White, J. M. (2010). Psychosocial treatment for methamphetamine use disorders: A preliminary randomized controlled trial of cognitive behavior therapy and acceptance and commitment therapy. *Substance Abuse, 31*, 98–107.

Tapper, K., Shaw, C., Ilsley, J., Hill, A. J., Bond, F. W., & Moore, L. (2009). Exploratory randomised controlled trial of a mindfulness-based weight loss intervention for women. *Appetite, 52*(2), 396–404. doi:10.1016/j.appet.2008.11.012

Teasdale, J. (1988). Cognitive models and treatments for panic: A critical evaluation. In S. Rachman & J. D. Maser (Eds.), *Panic: Psychological perspectives* (pp. 189-203). Hillsdale, NJ: Erlbaum.

Teasdale, J. D. (1983). Negative thinking in depression: Cause, effect, or reciprocal relationship. *Advances in Behaviour Research and Therapy, 5*(1), 3–25. doi:10.1016/0146-6402(83)90013-9

Teasdale, J. D. (1999). Metacognition, mindfulness and the modification of mood disorders. *Clinical Psychology and Psychotherapy, 6*, 145–155.

Teasdale, J. D., & Barnard, P. J. (1993). *Affect, cognition, and change: Re-modelling depressive thought*. Hillsdale, NJ: Erlbaum.

Teasdale, J. D., Moore, R. G., Hayhurst, H., Pope, M., Williams, S., & Segal, Z. V. (2002). Metacognitive awareness and prevention of relapse in depression: Empirical evidence. *Journal of Consulting and Clinical Psychology, 70*(2), 275–287. doi:10.1037/0022-006X.70.2.275

Teasdale, J. D., Segal, Z. V., Williams, J. M., Ridgeway, V. A., Soulsby, J. M., & Lau, M. A. (2000). Prevention of relapse/recurrence in major depression by mindfulness-based cognitive therapy. *Journal of Consulting and Clinical Psychology, 68*(4), 615–623. doi:10.1037/0022-006X.68.4.615

ten Doesschate, M. C., Bockting, C. L. H., & Schene, A. H. (2009). Adherence to continuation and maintenance antidepressant use in recurrent depression. *Journal of Affective Disorders, 115*(1–2), 167–170. doi:10.1016/j.jad.2008.07.011

Thompson, N. J., Walker, E. R., Obolensky, N., Winning, A., Barmon, C., DiIorio, C., & Compton, M. T. (2010). Distance delivery of mindfulness-based cognitive therapy for depression: Project UPLIFT. *Epilepsy and Behavior, 19*(3), 247–254. doi:10.1016/j.yebeh.2010.07.031

Thorsell, J., Finnes, A., Dahl, J., Lundgren, T., Gybrant, M., Gordh, T., & Buhrman, M. (2011). A comparative study of 2 manual-based self-help interventions, acceptance and commitment therapy and applied relaxation, for persons with chronic pain. *Clinical Journal of Pain, 27*(8), 716–723. doi:10.1097/AJP.0b013e318219a933

Törneke, N. (2010). *Learning RFT: An introduction to relational frame theory and its clinical application*. Oakland, CA: Context Press/New Harbinger.

Turk, C. L., Heimberg, R. G., Luterek, J. A., Mennin, D. S., & Fresco, D. M. (2005). Emotion dysregulation in generalized anxiety disorder: A comparison with social anxiety disorder. *Cognitive Therapy and Research, 29*(1), 89–106. doi:10.1007/s10608-005-1651-1

Twohig, M. P., Whittal, M. L., Cox, J. M., & Gunter, R. (2010). An initial investigation into the processes of change in ACT, CT, and ERP for OCD. *International Journal of Behavioral Consultation and Therapy, 6*(1), 67–83.

Varra, A. A., Hayes, S. C., Roget, N., & Fisher, G. (2008). A randomized control trial examining the effect of acceptance and commitment training on clinician willingness to use evidence-based pharmacotherapy. *Journal of Consulting and Clinical Psychology, 76*(3), 449–458. doi:10.1037/0022-006X.76.3.449

Veehof, M. M., Oskam, M., Schreurs, K. M. G., & Bohlmeijer, E. T. (2011). Acceptance-based interventions for the treatment of chronic pain: A systematic review and meta-analysis. *Pain, 152*(3), 533–542. doi:10.1016/j.pain.2010.11.002

Vittengl, J. R., Clark, L. A., Dunn, T. W., & Jarrett, R. B. (2007). Reducing relapse and recurrence in unipolar depression: A comparative meta-analysis of cognitive-behavioral therapy's effects. *Journal of Consulting and Clinical Psychology, 75*(3), 475–488. doi:10.1037/0022-006X.75.3.475

Vowles, K. E., McCracken, L. M., & O'Brien, J. Z. (2011). Acceptance and values-based action in chronic pain: A three-year follow-up analysis of treatment effectiveness and process. *Behaviour Research and Therapy, 49*(11), 748–755. doi:10.1016/j.brat.2011.08.002

Vowles, K. E., Wetherell, J. L., & Sorrell, J. T. (2009). Targeting acceptance, mindfulness, and values-based action in chronic pain: Findings of two preliminary trials of an outpatient group-based intervention. *Cognitive and Behavioral Practice, 16*(1), 49–58. doi:10.1016/j.cbpra.2008.08.001

Waters, A. M., & Craske, M. G. (2005). Generalized anxiety disorder. In M. M. Antony, D. R. Ledley, & R. G. Heimberg (Eds.), *Improving outcomes and preventing relapse in cognitive-behavorial therapy* (pp. 77-127). New York: Guilford Press.

Watkins, E., & Moulds, M. (2005). Positive beliefs about rumination in depression—A replication and extension. *Personality and Individual Differences, 39*(1), 73–82. doi:10.1016/j.paid.2004.12.006

Weber, B., Jermann, F., Gex-Fabry, M., Nallet, A., Bondolfi, G., & Aubry, J-M. (2010). Mindfulness-based cognitive therapy for bipolar disorder: A feasibility trial. *European Psychiatry, 25*(6), 334–337. doi:10.1016/j.eurpsy.2010.03.007

Weineland, S., Arvidsson, D., Kakoulidis, T. P., & Dahl, J. (2012). Acceptance and commitment therapy for bariatric surgery patients, a pilot RCT. *Obesity Research and Clinical Practice, 6*(1), 21–30.

Wells, A., & Carter, K. (1999). Preliminary tests of a cognitive model of generalized anxiety disorder. *Behaviour Research and Therapy, 37*(6), 585–594. doi:10.1016/S0005-7967(98)00156-9

Westin, V. Z., Schulin, M., Hesser, H., Karlsson, M., Noe, R. Z., Olofsson, U.,.... Andersson, G. (2011). Acceptance and commitment therapy versus tinnitus retraining therapy in the treatment of tinnitus: A randomised controlled trial. *Behaviour Research and Therapy, 49*(11), 737–747. doi:10.1016/j.brat.2011.08.001

Wetherell, J. L., Afari, N., Rutledge, T., Sorrell, J. T., Stoddard, J. A., Petkus, A. J.,.... Atkinson, J. H. (2011). A randomized, controlled trial of acceptance and commitment therapy and cognitive-behavioral therapy for chronic pain. *Pain, 152*(9), 2098–2107. doi:10.1016/j.pain.2011.05.016

White, R., Gumley, A., McTaggart, J., Rattrie, L., McConville, D., Cleare, S., & Mitchell, G. (2011). A feasibility study of acceptance and commitment therapy for emotional dysfunction following psychosis. *Behaviour Research and Therapy*, *49*(12), 901–907. doi:10.1016/j.brat.2011.09.003

Wicksell, R. K., Ahlqvist, J., Bring, A., Melin, L., & Olsson, G. L. (2008). Can exposure and acceptance strategies improve functioning and life satisfaction in people with chronic pain and whiplash-associated disorders (WAD)? A randomized controlled trial. *Cognitive Behaviour Therapy*, *37*(3), 1–14. doi:10.1080/16506070802078970

Wicksell, R. K., Melin, L., Lekander, M., & Olsson, G. L. (2009). Evaluating the effectiveness of exposure and acceptance strategies to improve functioning and quality of life in longstanding pediatric pain—a randomized controlled trial. *Pain*, *141*(3), 248–257.

Wicksell, R. K., Olsson, G. L., & Hayes, S. C. (2011). Mediators of change in acceptance and commitment therapy for pediatric chronic pain. *Pain*, *152*(12), 2792–2801. doi:10.1016/j.pain.2011.09.003

Williams, J. C., & Lynn, S. J. (2010). Acceptance: An historical and conceptual review. *Imagination, Cognition and Personality*, *30*(1), 5–56. doi:10.2190/IC.30.1.c

Wilson, K. G., & Dufrene, T. (2008). *Mindfulness for two: An acceptance and commitment therapy approach to mindfulness in psychotherapy*. Oakland, CA: New Harbinger.

Woods, D. W., Wetterneck, C. T., & Flessner, C. A. (2006). A controlled evaluation of acceptance and commitment therapy plus habit reversal for trichotillomania. *Behaviour Research and Therapy*, *44*(5), 639–656. doi:10.1016/j.brat.2005.05.006

Zeidan, F., Gordon, N. S., Merchant, J., & Goolkasian, P. (2010). The effects of brief mindfulness meditation training on experimentally induced pain. *Journal of Pain*, *11*(3), 199–209. doi:10.1016/j.jpain.2009.07.015

Zeidan, F., Johnson, S. K., Gordon, N. S., & Goolkasian, P. (2010). Effects of brief and sham mindfulness meditation on mood and cardiovascular variables. *Journal of Alternative and Complementary Medicine*, *16*(8), 867–873. doi:10.1089/acm.2009.0321

Zettle, R. D. (2003). Acceptance and commitment therapy (ACT) vs. systematic desensitization in treatment of mathematics anxiety. *The Psychological Record*, *53*(2), 197–215.

Zettle, R. D. (2005). The evolution of a contextual approach to therapy: From comprehensive distancing to ACT. *International Journal of Behavioral and Consultation Therapy*, *1*(2), 77–89.

Zettle, R. D., & Hayes, S. C. (1982). Rule governed behavior: A potential theoretical framework for cognitive behavior therapy. In P. C. Kendall (Ed.), *Advances in cognitive behavioral research and therapy* (pp. 73-118). New York: Academic.

Zettle, R. D., & Hayes, S. C. (1986). Dysfunctional control by client verbal behavior: The context of reason giving. *Analysis of Verbal Behavior*, *4*, 30–38.

Zettle, R. D., & Rains, J. C. (1989). Group cognitive and contextual therapies in treatment of depression. *Journal of Clinical Psychology*, *45*(3), 436–445. doi:10.1002/1097-4679(198905)45:3<436::AID-JCLP2270450314>3.0.CO;2-L

Zettle, R. D., Rains, J. C., & Hayes, S. C. (2011). Processes of change in acceptance and commitment therapy and cognitive therapy for depression: A mediation reanalysis of zettle and rains. *Behavior Modification*, *35*(3), 265–283. doi:10.1177/0145445511398344

Dialectical Behavior Therapy: A Comprehensive Multi- and Transdiagnostic Intervention

Anita Lungu *and* Marsha M. Linehan

Abstract

Dialectical behavior therapy (DBT) is a comprehensive multidiagnostic, modularized behavioral intervention designed to treat individuals with severe mental disorders and out-of-control cognitive, emotional, and behavioral patterns. It has been commonly viewed as a treatment for individuals meeting criteria for borderline personality disorder (BPD) with chronic and high-risk suicidality, substance dependence, or other disorders. However, over the years, data have emerged demonstrating that DBT is also effective for a wide range of other disorders and problems, most of which are associated with difficulties in regulating emotions and associated cognitive and behavioral patterns. This chapter both describes DBT and its associated empirical support as well as the origins and theoretical framework underpinning the treatment.

Key Words: dialectical behavior therapy, behavioral intervention, DBT, emotion regulation, cognitive and behavioral therapy

Formal development of dialectical behavior therapy (DBT) started in the early 1980s and has continued uninterrupted for more than three decades. Development of DBT emerged from efforts to apply outpatient cognitive-behavioral therapy to treat suicidal individuals with current high risk for suicide. By asking area hospitals to refer their most severe and difficult suicidal patients, the initial treatment efforts focused on individuals who were not only highly suicidal but also had severe and complex problems and met criteria for multiple mental disorders. The fundamental focus of treatment from the beginning (as well as now) was to help individuals build "lives worth living." The original treatment (as well as the first complete draft of the treatment manual) focused primarily on ameliorating suicidal behaviors. Subsequent grant funding, however, required adding a mental disorder diagnosis. This led to a series of clinical trials focused on chronically suicidal individuals meeting

criteria for BPD, a population with a known high rate of suicide (Leichsenring, Leibing, Kruse, New, & Leweke, 2011).

Development of DBT was primarily a trial-and-error clinical effort based originally on attempts to apply basic principles of behaviorism (Skinner, 1974), social learning theory (Staats, 1975; Staats & Staats, 1963) particularly as applied to suicidal behaviors (Linehan, 1981; Linehan & Egan, 1979), experimental findings from social psychology, and the traditional practices of cognitive-behavioral therapy (Goldfried & Davison, 1976; Wilson & O'Leary, 1980) that had led to the development of efficacious treatments for many other disorders. It rapidly became clear, however, that the available behavioral interventions were inadequate for the goal. Solving the various problems encountered in developing an effective intervention for such a high-risk, complex, and multidiagnostic population then shaped the treatment's subsequent theoretical and philosophical underpinning, its structure, and its specific treatment strategies.

The focus of treatment from the very beginning was on teaching clients how to more effectively problem-solve and build lives experienced as worth living. In practice, however, building such a life required clients to embrace and work toward making substantial changes in their lives. Such a focus on change, however, was routinely experienced by the client not only as invalidating some specific behaviors of theirs but as invalidating themselves as a whole. This often led to clients' subsequent attacks on the therapist, emotional shutdowns, storming out of therapy sessions, or abandoning therapy altogether. Research by Swann (Swann, Stein-Seroussi, & Giesler, 1992) may explain how such perceived invalidation leads to problematic behavior in therapy. Their research revealed that when an individual's basic self-constructs are not verified, the individual's arousal increases. The increased arousal then leads to dysregulation (cognitive, affective, and/or behavioral) and the failure to process new information.

Jumping to the other extreme in treatment, an approach focused primarily on acceptance and emotional support only led to clients again abandoning therapy, feeling misunderstood and invalidated, asking how can acceptance be the solution given the extent of their suffering and their need for a different life? To continue treating these clients effectively, it became clear that therapists had to both push for change to help clients transform their lives while at the same time accepting clients' often slow rate of progress with a risk of suicide while also communicating to clients acceptance of them as they were in that moment.

From a different perspective, clients had their own problems with both acceptance and change. Suicidal behaviors and other problem behaviors functioned to reduce pain experienced as intolerable. The complexity of their disorders, problems, and crises required an ability they did not have to accept and tolerate one set of problems in order to work on another problem. For many, the tragedy of their pasts and/or present lives elicited emotions that, untolerated, led them to a series of extreme and dysfunctional responses. At the time DBT was created the focus of the behavioral movement was on alleviating suffering rather than teaching individuals how to tolerate suffering. Something new was needed. It was clear that at its core, effective treatment had to provide a framework simultaneously pressing for the apparently opposite strategies of acceptance and change for both therapists and clients.

To balance the therapist's focus on helping clients change, a corresponding focus was required on what were valid client responses that did not need to change, finding the "kernel of gold in the cup of sand" so to speak. This led to a requirement that within each clinical interaction therapists find ways to balance problem-focused change strategies with validation strategies, changing focus as needed to keep progress on track.

To increase acceptance of both clients and therapists, Linehan began searching for a way to teach acceptance to both. Treatments that stressed acceptance, such as client-centered therapy (Rogers, 1946), inherently used acceptance to further change and, thus, did not address the problem at hand. Searching for individuals who could teach pure acceptance (without a linkage to a change-related goal) ultimately led to the study and practice of Zen and other contemplative practices in the mystical traditions (Aitken, 1982; Jager, 2005), both of which teach and encourage radical acceptance of the present moment without attempts to change it. Most important for the development of DBT, Zen as it moved west evolved into primarily a transconfessional practice applicable to individual of all faiths and of no faith (http: & willigisjaeger-foundation.com/zen.html) focusing on acceptance, validation, and tolerance, exactly what was needed to balance behavior therapy's emphasis on change.

Once it became clear that many of the individuals being treated simply could not meditate in silence (i.e., focus attention on their breath or inner sensations, etc.) a new approach to integrating contemplative and acceptance practices was needed. First, basic Zen practices along with aspects of other contemplative practices were translated into a set of behavioral skills that could be taught to both clients and therapists. Second, it was needed to create a focus on acceptance per se and not on religious/nonreligious names for the skills. The term *mindfulness* was used to describe the skills translated from Zen. The term was adopted from the work of both Ellen Langer (1989) and Thich Nhat Hanh (1976). The skills translating contemplative practices were labeled "reality acceptance skills" and drew heavily from the work of Gerald May (1987).

The tensions arising from this attempt to integrate the principles of behaviorism with those of Zen and contemplative practices required a framework that could house opposing views. The dialectical philosophy, which highlights the process of synthesizing oppositions, provides such a framework. Once dialecticts as a foundational philosophy was adopted, the entire treatment was scrutinized to be sure the manual was consistent with dialectics and the first final version of the treatment was published (Linehan, 1993a, 1993b). Through the continual resolution of tensions between theory and research versus clinical experience and between Western psychology versus Eastern practice, DBT continues to evolve in a manner similar to the theoretical integration model described by psychotherapy integration researchers (Arkowitz, 1989, 1992; Norcross & Goldfried, 2005; Prochaska & Diclemente, 2005; Ryle, 2005).

Theory Underpinning DBT

DBT is founded on three theoretical underpinnings: social behavioral theory, Zen practice, and dialectics. Behavior therapy, rooted in social behavioral theory, represents the technology of change so necessary to transform the lives of individuals experiencing extreme suffering such as those who are suicidal or meet criteria for severe mental disorders. However, as discussed earlier, to be effective with this population, a technology of change needs to be balanced by a technology of acceptance. In DBT the technology of acceptance comes from translating the fundamentals of Zen practice into behavioral terms. Dialectical philosophy is the framework that keeps the treatment together by containing the tension inherent in synthesizing a technology of change with one of acceptance.

Social Behavioral Theory and DBT

The behavioral model that underpinned the development of DBT was Staats's social behavioral model of personality (Staats & Staats, 1963; Staats, 1975). An important aspect of this model is the notion that it can be profitable to conceptualize human functioning as occurring in one response system or a combination of separate but interrelated response systems: the overt behavior response system, the cognitive response system, and the physiological/affective response system. The lines between the systems are not always clear, and many molar responses are best viewed as cross-system response patterns. Thus, emotions include simultaneous physiological arousal together with specified cognitive and overt behavioral contents. Because there is always a physiological aspect of any emotion, affect is defined as part of the physiological system.

An important aspect of this approach to behavioral analysis—a core component of any behavioral intervention, including DBT—is its emphasis on the interdependence of the three systems. Changes in one system effect changes within the other systems, thereby bringing about changes in the total organism. In a similar manner, from this theoretical vantage, people are viewed as dynamically related to their environments. Thus, not only do situational stimuli affect people, people also influence their own situational surroundings; people create their own environments, both cognitively by acting on the stimuli impinging on the senses and objectively by influencing events. The observed responses that people make are products of interactions both within the person (via the three response systems) and between the person and the environments in which he or she exists.

The importance of this theoretical approach to both suicidal behavior and to severe emotion dysregulation is fourfold. First, it links suicide and other dysfunctional behaviors, including behavioral dyscontrol and dysfunctional thoughts, beliefs, and appraisals to both emotion dysregulation and environmental factors. DBT as a treatment for emotion dysregulation is based on the view that emotions are complex, brief, involuntary, patterned, full-system responses to internal and external stimuli. DBT emphasizes the importance of the evolutionary adaptive value of emotions in understanding them today (Tooby & Cosmides, 1990). From this perspective, emotions can be viewed as arising from six transacting subsystems: (1) distal and proximal events that increase vulnerability; (2) internal and/or external events that serve as emotional cues; (3) appraisal/interpretations of cues; (4) emotional response tendencies, including physiological responses, cognitive processing, experiential responses, and action urges; (5) nonverbal/verbal expressive responses and actions; and (6) after-effects of the initial emotion, including secondary emotions (see Linehan, 1993a). Second, the model highlights those areas of functioning important for an adequate understanding of the phenomena in question. Third, it points to the potential impact of the environment on the person and the potential impact of the person on environmental contingencies. Finally, it suggests that interventions for the reduction of suicide and emotion dysregulation will be most effective if focused on the individual person as an integrated and dynamic system of behavioral-environment-linked patterns.

As mentioned earlier, the treatment was initially developed for chronically suicidal individuals, then for BPD, and is now expanding to target emotion dysregulation transdiagnostically. From DBT's perspective, suicide, BPD, and many other disorders can best be viewed as disorders of pervasive emotion dysregulation. Emotion dysregulation can be defined as the inability to change or regulate emotional cues, experiences, and actions even when desired and when best efforts are applied (Gross, 2009). Pervasive emotion dysregulation refers to cases when the dysregulation occurs across a wide array of emotions, adaptation problems, and situational contexts.

A specific biosocial model of emotion dysregulation (Crowell, Beauchaine, & Linehan, 2009) was developed by Linehan to better understand and articulate the developmental factors that likely led to and maintained the pervasive dysregulation of the clients being treated. Under the biosocial theory, pervasive emotion dysregulation is developed due to a transactional pattern being established, over time between an individual with a *biological vulnerability* for heightened emotional responses and an *invalidating social environment*. More precisely, the biological vulnerability refers to an array of biological causal factors (heredity, epigenetics; Henikoff & Matzke, 1997; Zhang & Meaney, 2010; intrauterine, childhood, or adult neural insults) that contribute to an individual being more sensitive to emotional cues as well as having a heightened and longer lasting response once the emotion unfolds. For example, developmental research has identified two dimensions of infant temperament: effortful control and negative affectivity that contribute to a propensity for developing emotion and behavioral dysregulation. Effortful control can be defined as "the ability to inhibit a dominant response to perform a subdominant response, to detect errors, and to engage in planning…and self regulation" and negative affectivity "is characterized by discomfort, frustration, shyness, sadness, and nonsoothability" (Rothbart & Rueda, 2005. p. 169, as cited in Crowell et al., 2009). Because the human emotion regulation system is complex, dysfunction in different parts of the system can result in vulnerability to develop emotion dysregulation.

The second developmental contributor to pervasive emotion dysregulation is an invalidating social environment. Such an environment is a poor fit to the child's biological makeup and is characterized by a tendency to invalidate emotions, to inappropriately model emotional expression, and to reinforce extreme emotional displays. Overall, the invalidating environment is ineffective in teaching the child how to label and modulate emotions, to tolerate distress, and to inherently trust his or her own understanding of events and responses. Within an invalidating environment normative displays of emotional distress are not acknowledged or reinforced until they escalate to extreme levels. The development of pervasive emotion dysregulation emerges thus within a system as a learning transaction over time between the biological vulnerability to emotion dysregulation and an invalidating environment. Ineffective behaviors such as extreme, impulsive, often destructive behaviors of suicidal or BPD individuals or avoidance behaviors in anxiety disorders are conceptualized in the context of high suffering as ways of regulating emotions that might work in the short term to bring negative emotion down but are ineffective strategies in the long term. Within a context of a client's significant emotion dysregulation the task of the therapy becomes, in large part, to teach the client to regulate emotion in an effective way, to better tolerate distress, and to build ability to self-validate his or her emotions, behaviors, and thoughts.

Dialectical Philosophy and DBT

As the name implies, dialectical philosophy is a critical underpinning of DBT. The principles of dialectics go back thousands of years; however, both Marx and Hegel have been associated with developing and applying dialectics to a more modern context. In the context of behavior therapy, dialectics can be understood and defined as both a method of persuasion and as a worldview (Basseches, 1984; Kaminstein, 1987).

Simplified, dialectics as persuasion represents a method of logic or argumentation by disclosing the contradictions (antithesis) in an opponent's argument (thesis) and overcoming them (synthesis). Further, the dialectical process of change unfolds when an idea or event (thesis) generates and is transformed into its opposite (antithesis) and then is persevered and fulfilled by it, leading to a reconciliation of opposites (synthesis). Thus, dialectics becomes particularly relevant to therapy if we understand it as the process of enacting change through persuasion. Within DBT, dialectics guides assumptions about the nature of reality, provides the conceptual foundation for understanding the pathogenesis of a biosocial etiology of disorder, and balances treatment goals and strategies.

Dialectics as worldview is comprised of three fundamental principles. The world is viewed as holistic, connected, and in continuous change. A "whole" is comprised of heterogeneous "parts" that cannot be understood in isolation but become meaningful only in relation to each other and as they together define the "whole." In this way, dialectical thinking is systemic; parts can only be understood as they function within a system, and the same part can change completely when it becomes attached to a different whole or system. For example, in DBT a client cannot be understood in isolation from his or her environment and the inherent transactions. The parts of a system are seen as complex, oppositional, and in polarity. An "inside" can only exist in relation to an "outside." The connected nature of reality together with the opposition and polarity of parts leads to a world of continual and transactional change. A stasis is not desirable because the only constant is change. Identity in such a system is also relational and in continuous change. As mentioned earlier, this worldview of understanding reality as systemic and interconnected matches well with the philosophy of behavioral science and Zen.

The dialectical worldview translates into case conceptualization and treatment in several ways. First, dialectics provides a foundation for biosocial etiology of disorder by emphasizing the transactional development and maintenance of disorder as well as its systemic nature, viewing disorder in an environmental context. Further, disorder is assumed to have multiple as opposed to singular causal factors. Second, disorder is also not seen as separated from normal functioning, but both are viewed along a continuum—a perspective that questions the utility of the current diagnostic system organized in a categorical fashion. Third, dialectics as a framework balances the treatment strategies of acceptance and change that are central to DBT. Indeed, the tension between acceptance and change that permeates treatment is the fundamental dialectic of DBT. When polarities occur between client and therapists, or among therapists during the treatment consultation team, the approach is for each party to search for "what is left out" such that a synthesis between the two poles can be reached. A specific characteristic of DBT treatment is that of maintaining "movement, speed, and flow" throughout therapy, coming back to the continuous change of reality, from a dialectical worldview. Related to this, DBT also allows and trusts in natural change to occur.

This dialectical worldview becomes apparent also in the perspectives and behaviors of DBT therapists as they work with their clients and other therapists. In their work with clients DBT therapists have to dialectically synthesize the capability model with the motivation model as explanatory for what is blocking the client's way toward a life worth living. The capability model views the client's lack of skills as the main factor interfering with progress, while the motivation model views lack of motivation toward change as the culprit. DBT therapists integrate the two models by viewing increasing client motivation as a treatment target in itself and also by relentlessly working on building needed skills through both group skills training and strengthening and generalizing skills in individual session and outside of session.

The most fundamental dialectic in DBT is that between acceptance and change. DBT therapists thus must fully accept their clients as they are moment by moment while at the same time being adamant about working with them toward change. Maintaining that balance between acceptance and change with clients is crucial for both keeping a client in treatment and ensuring he or she is making progress toward goals. Leaning too heavily toward acceptance leads to the clients feeling invalidated in that the therapists do not understand their emotional pain because if they did how could the therapists not help them change? Similarly, pushing for change too much leads to the clients again feeling invalidated and rejected because it communicates they are not acceptable as they are. This focus on change is probably responsible for the high dropout from therapy for which BPD clients are notorious.

Finally, as is the case for many of the DBT strategies used by therapists with clients in their individual sessions, clients are also specifically taught how to be dialectical themselves through a specific skill.

DBT Components and Organization
DBT as a Modular Treatment

Because DBT was built for high-risk, multidiagnostic, complex clients, the clinical problems that were addressed in therapy were complicated. Well-known strategies for approaching and resolving complex problems are modularity and hierarchy. Modularity can be used to separate the functions of a treatment/intervention into independent modules such that each module contains everything necessary to carry out one specific aspect of the desired treatment. At a conceptual level modularity infers separation of concerns by emphasizing logical boundaries between components. For modularity to work in solving a complex problem, each module needs to have clearly defined its goals, how to reach them, and throughout this process, how to communicate outcomes or difficulties and problems to be solved with the other modules. When decision making is also involved, modularity needs to be augmented with hierarchy to specify where the responsibility lies in making a decision.

DBT is conceptually modular at several levels. First, DBT clearly articulates, at a high level, the functions of treatment that it addresses, namely: (1) to enhance an individual's capability by increasing skillful behavior, (2) to improve and maintain a client's motivation to change and be engaged with treatment, (3) to ensure generalization of change occurring through treatment, (4) to enhance motivation of therapists to deliver effective treatment, and (5) to assist the individual in restructuring or changing his or her environment such that it supports and maintains progress and advancement toward goals (see Figure 12.1).

Second, to effectively provide these functions, treatment is delivered in a variety of modes (individual therapy or case management, family intervention, group and individual skills training, between session coaching, and regular team consultation for therapists), each having different targets and also different strategies available for reaching those targets (see Figure 12.2). There is also clarity in how the different modes of treatment communicate and collaborate.

Third, the skills training itself is modular in the focus of acceptance skills versus change skills such that both clients and therapists can remember that for any problem encountered, effective approaches can include acceptance as well as change (see Figure 12.3). Skills are further modular by the topics they address (mindfulness, emotion regulation, interpersonal effectiveness, and distress tolerance) such that clients can work on a single set of skills at a time, which limits being overwhelmed by all the things they need to learn and change (see Figure 12.3). At the same time, once clients have mastered or made progress in a set of skills, they can easily incorporate those

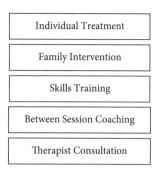

Figure 12.2 Modularity of treatment modes.

skills while working on a new module. Some of the more complex skills, such as the interpersonal assertiveness skills, are also modular in that they are comprised of smaller parts, taught separately to increase comprehension and accessibility (see Figure 12.3). The "DEAR MAN" skill, for example, is an interpersonal assertiveness skill that targets how to effectively ask for things and say no to demands, keeping in mind priorities for the interaction (achieving the objective, maintaining or improving relationships with others, as well as self-respect). The skill is comprised of several steps (Describe, Express, Assert, Reinforce, Mindful, Appear confident, Negotiate; see the original DBT manual [Linehan, 1993b] for more details). The skills training is modular also in following the same well-defined structure in how the skills training sessions unfold as a succession of steps.

Fourth, DBT strategies are divided into three sets: (1) acceptance strategies, (2) change strategies, and (3) dialectical strategies that incorporate both acceptance and change (see Figure 12.4). Strategies are then further divided into core strategies (*problem solving*, the main change strategy focused on addressing the specific problems that come up in the patient's day-to-day life versus *validation*, the main acceptance strategy focused on communicating to the patient that her behavior makes sense and is understandable in the current context), communication strategies (*irreverent*, meant to push the patient "off balance" so that rebalancing can occur vs. *reciprocal/warm* that incorporate responsiveness, self-disclosure, warm engagement, and genuineness), and environmental management strategies (teaching clients to manage their own environments vs. environmental intervention on behalf of the client). Furthermore, applications of both core strategies (problem solving and validation) are further broken down into smaller modules. Within the change strategies five sets of basic behavioral procedures are outlined and applied as needed: (1) behavioral

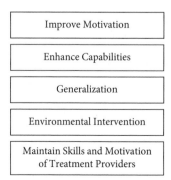

Figure 12.1 Functions of comprehensive treatment.

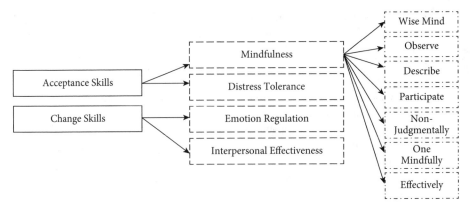

Figure 12.3 Modularity of dialectical behavior therapy skills training.

assessment (formulating the problem in terms of the patient's feelings, thoughts, or actions; Linehan, 1993a, 1993b, p. 254), (2) contingency management (Linehan, 1993a, 1993b, p. 353), (3) skills training (Linehan, 1993a), (4) exposure-based procedures (extended in DBT to treat emotions such as guilt, shame, and anger besides the fear-related problems traditionally treated with exposure (Linehan, 1993a, 1993b, p. 343), and (5) cognitive modification (aimed to change an individual's appraisals, rules, and cognitive style (Linehan, 1993a, 1993b, p. 358). Within the acceptance strategies, validation is further divided into six steps, each providing a stronger sense of validation than the previous step (see Figure 12.4).

The dialectical thesis that reality is change encourages DBT therapists to stay up to date in terms of the research with both acceptance and behavioral change procedures, changing the application of the procedures as the science changes. DBT also has a specified protocol for incorporating new or updated interventions and protocols once assessment has identified a specific largely self-contained problem that interferes with a client's reaching his or her goals, not ideally addressed with current DBT strategies and procedures. When this is the case, DBT remains a framework for treatment delivery, incorporating the ancillary intervention to address the target identified. The treatment team follows a specific protocol for transitioning ancillary procedures in and out of DBT. For example, part of this transitioning protocol specifies in what stage of disorder a particular intervention can be applied (see later for description of stages). Incorporating treatment for posttraumatic stress disorder (PTSD) for a population with high

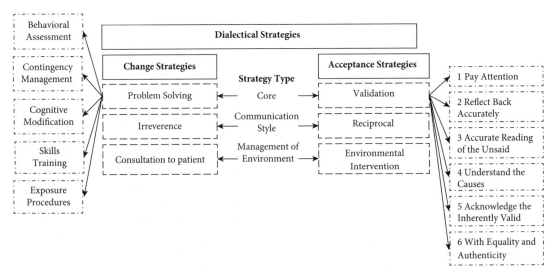

Figure 12.4 Modularity of dialectical behavior therapy strategies and procedures.

risk for suicide is an example where such a protocol needs to be in place. Recently such protocols have been devised, and research is emerging to support the efficacy of applying adapted versions of standard PTSD interventions (Foa, Keane, Friedman, & Cohen, 2009) for this group (Bohus et al., 2013; Harned & Linehan, 2008; Harned, Korslund, Foa, & Linehan, 2012).

DBT as a Hierarchical Treatment

The concept of hierarchy is apparent in DBT in several ways. First, DBT uses the notion of stages of disorder in conceptualizing the clinical presentation of a particular client. Introducing different stages of disorder captures the different levels of clinical complexity and difficulty that a client can be facing at a particular time. This is hierarchichal form and modularity. It organizes the treatment in terms of the main targets that need to be addressed in therapy and specific strategies for addressing them. The stages of treatment are based on the levels of disorder addressed and at each level treatment targets have a hierarchical organization dictated by clinical importance (see Figure 12.5), with serious behavioral dyscontrol at the top (Stage 1 disorder), followed by quiet desperation (severe emotional suffering with action under control) (Stage 2 disorder), basic problems in living and low-grade Axis 1 disorders (Stage 3 disorder), and addressing a sense of incompleteness or emptiness (Stage 4 treatment). Each level of disorder is then linked to a hierarchical set of specified targeted categories of behavior (see Figure 12.5). This hierarchical organization is used in structuring treatment both at the level of a more stable case conceptualization and in structuring each therapy session where the clinical content to be addressed can change from week to week.

Second, in comprehensive DBT where all four components of treatment are provided, hierarchy is present in structuring the treatment staff. At the top of the hierarchy is the client in the sense that all treatment staff is working for the client. From a clinical perspective the main decision maker in terms of treatment plan and interventions is the individual therapist, with the other treatment providers in a sense reporting to the individual therapist (see Figure 12.6).

Stages of Disorder and Treatment Targets

The concept of stages of disorder globally refers to the severity of the clinical presentation of a particular individual and incorporates the pervasiveness of dysfunction, the complexity of the problems that block the client's progress, and the extent of comorbidity of disorder. Taking stage of disorder into account is particularly important when we try to determine what treatment and treatment dose work for whom as well as to evaluate treatment outcomes (Chambless et al., 1998; Garfield, 1994). DBT conceptualizes four different stages of disorder, progressing from the most severe clinical presentation of behavioral dyscontrol (Stage 1), to less severe problems, quiet desperation (Stage 2), problems in living (Stage 3), and incompleteness (Stage 4). Stages of disorder largely organize case conceptualization for a client and determine the treatments targets. A client can progress through all stages or skip some of them; clients can also sometimes regress to a more severe stage. Also, the stage the client is in identifies the critical treatment targets to be working on, but additional less severe treatment targets can be added given sufficient therapy time.

The treatment is structured to accommodate treatment plans for Stage 1 individuals. However, as described earlier, DBT has a modular and flexible

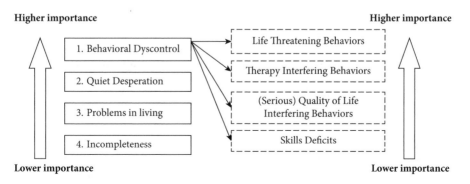

Figure 12.5 Modularity and hierarchy of dialectical behavior therapy stages of treatment and associated targeted behaviors.

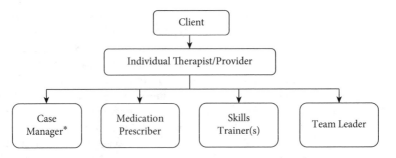

*The case manager can function as the individual provider if no individual therapist is available.

Figure 12.6 Dialectical behavior therapy treatment provider hierarchy.

structure and can be scaled down to also treat clients who start therapy with simpler clinical presentations or who progress in therapy to simpler problems. Also, as mentioned earlier, DBT takes an integrative approach to treating comorbidity by treating all problems within the context of the same treatment and by the same therapist (although potentially at different times). Different disorders are treated depending on a treatment hierarchy with protocols within DBT or protocols brought in from other treatments for specific contained problems (for example, formal exposure for specific phobias).

STAGE 1 DISORDER: BEHAVIORAL DYSCONTROL

Stage 1 is the most severe stage of disorder and refers to clients entering therapy with complex clinical presentations, meeting criteria for multiple DSM Axis I and/or Axis II diagnoses, being potentially actively suicidal or self-harming. The characteristic of this stage is a lack of behavioral control particularly when under emotion dysregulation. The main goal of this stage is to help the client gain control over his or her behaviors. However, multiple treatment targets must be followed to reach this goal. Treatment with Stage 1 individuals can be chaotic if the therapist does not maintain a hierarchy of treatment targets guiding therapy accordingly.

The highest treatment goal is to decrease life-threatening behaviors (such as suicidal and/or homicidal behaviors, accidental drug overdoses, aggressive behaviors, very high-risk behaviors, etc.) If such a behavior is present in a client's life, the therapist needs to target it, but this does not mean spending all therapy time on the behavior.

The next important target is therapy-interfering behavior, which refers to any behavior, on the side of the client or therapist that might interfere with

the client being in treatment. On the side of the client, these behaviors include noncollaborative behaviors, noncompliance, nonattending behaviors, behaviors that interfere with other clients receiving therapy, or behaviors that burn out the therapist (e.g., the client transgressing the therapist's limits in extent or content of out-of-session contact). Therapy-interfering behaviors of the therapist include behaviors that unbalance the therapy, such as extreme acceptance or change orientation, extreme flexibility or rigidity, extreme vulnerability or irreverence, or disrespectful behaviors. Additional barriers to therapy can include motivation, transportation, financial factors, the therapist's travel schedule, and so on. The reason for the high priority placed on this factor is obvious; if the client is not receiving therapy, no progress can be made in treatment.

Once there is no immediate danger to life or danger of discontinuing therapy treatment can target helping the client achieve control over behaviors that seriously interfere with quality of life. Assessment techniques like chain analyses are used to identify controlling variables of behavior, and treatment focuses on teaching and motivating (for example, using contingency management) alternative behaviors to replace ineffective, out-of-control ones. Once a reasonable level of control is achieved over behavior, the therapy progresses to teach the client at least a minimal level of skill needed for basic problem solving and goal achievement necessary to decrease quality-of-life-interfering behaviors. Such skills are primarily taught in DBT skills group training but are revisited (sometimes retaught), generalized, and reinforced in individual therapy. Quality-of-life-interfering behaviors can be incapacitating Axis I or II disorders (e.g., incapacitating PTSD), engaging in high-risk or unprotected sexual behaviors, extreme financial difficulties, criminal behaviors that might lead to jail, unemployment, and so on.

In summary, the goals of Stage 1 treatment are to *decrease* life-threatening behaviors, therapy-interfering behaviors, and quality-of-life-interfering behaviors and to *increase* core mindfulness, distress tolerance, interpersonal effectiveness, emotion regulation, and self-management skills. Once these treatment goals have been reasonably achieved, the client can progress to Stage 2 or skip to another stage. It is also possible for the client to return to Stage 1, although usually this happens only temporarily and while major life stressors emerge.

STAGE 2 DISORDER: QUIET DESPERATION

Overcoming Stage 1 assumes reasonable control has been achieved over overt behavior; however, the fact that external behavior is under control says nothing about control over internal experiencing of emotional pain. The name of this stage was chosen to reflect extreme emotional pain in the presence of controlled action. Globally the goal of this stage is to assist the individual in experiencing emotion in a nontraumatic way. Examples of this stage would be individuals with chronic PTSD, with sequelae from traumatic invalidation as children, severe depression, inhibited or complicated grieving, and a sense of being a perpetual outsider. When the emotional pain is experienced in response to trauma cues, an important treatment strategy is to coach the clients to expose themselves to new experiences that would provide corrective information and allow learning of new responses to trauma cues. Treatment at this stage thus largely consists of exposure to emotion and experiential emotional processing work. The goals for this stage are to get the client to experience emotion in a nontraumatic, nonanguished way (Garfield, 1994; Gross, John, & Richards, 2000; Gross & Levenson, 1993, 1997), to gain a sense of connection to the environment, and to gain a sense of essential goodness and personal validity as an individual.

It can be the case that individuals start treatment at Stage 2 or progress to Stage 2 from Stage 1. Unfortunately, it is often the case that individuals starting in Stage 1 take a long time in therapy to achieve behavioral control and then lack resources to continue therapy at Stage 2. However, even though the emotional suffering can be severe, the lack of external behaviors might not communicate to the environment its full extent and such an individual can deteriorate and then fall to Stage 1.

STAGE 3 DISORDER: PROBLEMS IN LIVING

A client can either reach this stage after having worked through severe behavioral dyscontrol (Stage 1) and traumatic emotional experiencing (Stage 2) or can start here when there was never any severe disorder. At this stage, therapy deals with problems in living that do not severely interfere with a reasonably functional life and do not lead to unacceptable unhappiness. Examples of clinical situations here could be uncomplicated or mild depression, mild to moderate severity Axis I disorders (anxiety, eating disorders) without significant comorbidity, significant interpersonal problems such as severe marital conflict, lack of significant relationships, and so on. The goal at this stage is to achieve an acceptable quality of life and an acceptable level of happiness, increased self-respect, mastery, and self-efficacy. This is a stage where it is highly probable for DBT to bring in outside protocols for treating specific contained Axis I disorders (interpersonal or cognitive therapy for depression or relationship problems, cognitive-behavioral therapy for eating disorders, exposure for specific phobias, etc.).

STAGE 4 DISORDER: INCOMPLETENESS

This stage is for individuals who, despite achieving a reasonable level of functioning, remain unhappy and unable to experience much joy in their lives. This can be the case, for example, for clients who have progressed from Stage 1 who are in search of some meaning for the past tragedy of their lives. Not finding this meaning can lead to a sense of incompleteness and dissatisfaction. This sense of meaningless and incompleteness though can also occur outside of a traumatic past in individuals who do not experience other clinical problems. A maladaptive way of satisfying this craving for meaning or peak experiencing can be consuming illicit drugs, which can simulate the "high" experience that sometimes follows intense spiritual practice. Many individuals, if not most do not need a Stage 4 of treatment. For those that do, however, the treatment goals can be expanded awareness of self and of others, spiritual fulfillment, and developing the capacity to have peak experiences. Such goals could be achieved through long-term insight-oriented psychotherapy, spiritual direction, mindfulness practice, and so on.

PRETREATMENT STAGE OF THERAPY

Regardless of stage of disorder, all treatment must begin with a pretreatment stage, where a negotiation takes place between the therapist and the client with respect to goals and responsibilities in therapy, treatment approach, fees and requirements, duration of therapy, and so on. This treatment stage is tremendously important as it can determine whether the client stays in treatment or drops out prematurely, as well as the specific treatment goals. The therapist and client need to reach agreement and commitment to goals and approach for treatment to have a high chance of success. The specific agreements that clients entering DBT have to agree to are to stay in therapy for the specified time period, attend scheduled therapy sessions, work toward changing targeted behaviors (as appropriate to level of disorder), work on problems that arise that interfere with progress in therapy, participate in skills training for the specified time period, abide by any research conditions of therapy, and pay agreed-upon fees. The therapist in standard DBT must also commit to a series of agreements: to make every reasonable effort to conduct competent and effective therapy; to obey standard ethical and professional guidelines; to be available to clients for weekly therapy sessions, phone consultations, and back-up; to respect confidentiality and integrity of clients; and to obtain consultation when needed.

Overview of Research across Multiple Problems and Populations
Comprehensive DBT Randomized Controlled Trials

Several randomized controlled trials (RCTs) have evaluated the efficacy of DBT for individuals meeting criteria for BPD recruited for high suicidality (Linehan, Armstrong, Suarez, Allmon, & Heard, 1991; Linehan et al., 2006; Mcmain et al., 2009; Pistorello, Fruzzetti, MacLane, Gallop, & Iverson, 2012). DBT was superior in decreasing *suicide attempts* compared to treatment as usual (Linehan et al., 1991), community treatment by experts (CTBE; Linehan et al., 2006), and psychodynamic treatment supervised by experts (Pistorello et al., 2012) but not general psychiatric management plus emotion-focused psychotherapy (Mcmain et al., 2009). Specifically, when comparing DBT to treatment by expert therapists in the community, participants in the DBT condition were half as likely to attempt suicide or to visit an emergency department for suicidality and were 73% less likely to be hospitalized for suicidality. Together these results provide evidence that DBT is an efficacious treatment for suicidal individuals. Although all studies have shown DBT results in significant reductions in *suicide ideation*, some RCTs find significant reductions

in DBT compared with usual treatment (Koons et al., 2001) while others have found no differences (Linehan et al., 1991, 2006).

Another high target in DBT is the decrease of nonsuicidal self-injury behaviors (NSSIs). Most studies found DBT to be superior in improving NSSI compared to the control condition (Bohus et al., 2004; Koons et al., 2001; Linehan et al., 1991; Pistorello et al., 2012; Turner, 2000; van den Bosch, Verheul, Schippers, & Van den Brink, 2002), with some studies finding no between-condition differences (Carter, Willcox, Lewin, Conrad, & Bendit, 2010; Feigenbaum et al., 2012; Linehan et al., 2006). As noted earlier, DBT has also been found effective in reducing the *use of crisis services* such as visits to the emergency rooms, hospital admissions, and length of stay (Koons et al., 2001; Linehan et al., 1991, 2006), although some studies found no differences compared to the control condition (Carter et al., 2010; Feigenbaum et al., 2012; Mcmain et al., 2009).

DBT has also been evaluated and found effective with individuals meeting criteria for BPD and comorbid *substance dependence* (Linehan et al., 1999, 2002). DBT has also been found effective in targeting and improving high prevalence, comorbid disorders such as *depression* and *anxiety* in some studies significantly more so than the control condition (Bohus et al., 2004; Koons et al., 2001; Koons, Betts, Chapman, O'Rourke, & Robins, 2004; Pistorello et al., 2012; Soler et al., 2005) while other studies found both treatments effective with no significant differences (Linehan et al., 1991, 2006; Mcmain et al., 2009). During 1 year of treatment there was similar remission from depression and anxiety for both DBT and the control condition, although remission from substance dependence was higher in DBT (Harned et al., 2008). Similarly, both DBT and the control condition were effective in decreasing anger, impulsivity, and irritability over 1 year of treatment (Bohus et al., 2004; Clarkin, Levy, Lenzenweger, & Kernberg, 2007; Feigenbaum et al., 2012; Linehan et al., 1999), with some studies finding DBT superior (Koons et al., 2001).

A common critique to behavioral therapies is that they only change symptoms of a particular disorder, without impacting any of the fundamental underpinnings of the disorder. Contradicting this hypothesis, DBT was found superior, compared to treatment by (nonbehavioral) community experts in the development of a positive introject, including greater self-affirmation, self-love, and self-protection, and less self-attack during a 1-year treatment (Bedics, Atkins, Harned, & Linehan, 2015).

Skills-Only RCTs

In an analysis of data from three independent RCTs, participants in the DBT condition have been found to increase their use of skillful behavior significantly more than participants in the control condition. Furthermore, increase in skillful behavior has been found to fully mediate main DBT outcomes such as decrease in number of suicide attempts and improvement in depression and anger control (Neacsiu, Rizvi, & Linehan, 2010). DBT skills training thus appears to be a mechanism of change in DBT. Interest in DBT skills-only interventions has increased significantly in recent years with RCTs evaluating and finding support for efficacy of such interventions with BPD (Soler et al., 2009), binge eating disorder (Hill, Craighead, & Safer, 2011; Safer, Robinson, & Jo, 2010; Safer, Telch, & Agras, 2001), treatment-resistant depression (Harley, Sprich, Safren, Jacobo, & Fava, 2008; Safer et al., 2001, 2010), incarcerated women with childhood abuse (Bradley & Follingstad, 2003), attention-deficit/hyperactivity disorder (Hirvikoski et al., 2011), bipolar disorder (Safer et al., 2001, 2010; Van Dijk, Jeffrey, & Katz, 2012), and transdiagnostic across mood and anxiety disorders (Neacsiu, 2012).

Future Directions for Research

The conceptual and theoretical tenets that have guided the initial development of DBT continue to be fundamental in envisioning the future of DBT research. At a high level, DBT's foundation in behavioral science implies keeping DBT flexible and open to change. However, changes need to be motivated by new advances in behavior research and rigorous evaluation of efficacy as opposed to by convenience or by desire to simply create a new treatment.

For decades, clinical psychology research has followed a single-disorder diagnosis system based on clinical symptoms (American Psychiatric Association, 1987, 1994). However, the categories thus identified have not been later validated in terms of common clinical course, separation of disorders, or further laboratory tests (Regier, Narrow, Kuhl, & Kupter, 2009). Treatment seekers often fall into the "Not Otherwise Specified" category, have "subsyndromal" levels of multiple problems, or meet criteria for multiple diagnoses (Biederman, Newcorn, & Sprich, 1991; Conway, Compton, Stinson, &

Grant, 2006; Howland et al., 2009). Following an increase in understanding psychopathology driven by behavioral studies and cognitive neuroscience, the field has witnessed the emergence of *transdiagnostic* treatments (Barlow, Allen, & Choate, 2004; McHugh, Murray, & Barlow, 2009) targeting general dysfunctional processes and mechanisms of change common across disorders.

From early on DBT has proposed pervasive emotion dysregulation as the fundamental mechanism underlying BPD. Further research has proposed emotion dysregulation as a transdiagnostic mechanism of disorder going beyond BPD to other disorders maintained by difficulty regulating emotion. DBT is well equipped with tools to treat emotion dysregulation transdiagnostically. Rigorous research needs to be conducted to understand how comprehensive DBT can most effectively change emotion dysregulation in terms of impacting different components of a model of emotion (such as factors behind vulnerability to emotion, emotion reactivity, return to baseline, etc.).

As reviewed earlier, the clinical research community has increased interest in adapting and evaluating skills-only interventions focused on different clinical presentations. However, this area is still in its infancy and often lacks rigor in systematically building skills curricula, making decisions on duration of intervention, deciding which DBT components to include (e.g., is there a consultation team or skills coaching included?), and monitoring and reporting adherence to the DBT model.

Another relatively new direction of clinical research is the emphasis on cost-effective treatment dissemination. Many individuals with mental health problems do not receive evidence-based treatments fitting their clinical profile, although effective treatments have been generated by research for many disorders (Kessler, Merikangas, & Wang, 2007; Shafran et al., 2009; Stobie, Taylor, Quigley, Ewing, & Salkovskis, 2007). Large-scale treatment dissemination remains a grand challenge for the field (Addis, 2002; Barlow, Levitt, & Bufka, 1999). Common barriers include the high cost of face-to-face treatment, mental health stigma (Lyons, Hopley, & Horrocks, 2009; Wright et al., 2009), and inaccessibility due to geographical locations. Fortunately, technology is undergoing fast advances in availability and interaction modalities and can become an effective vehicle for large-scale dissemination (Cartreine, Ahren, & Locke, 2010; Marks, Cavanagh, & Gega, 2007; Newman, 2004). Computerized psychotherapy treatments have been found efficacious in depression (Proudfoot et al., 2003; Richards & Richardson, 2012) and anxiety (Marks, Kenwright, McDonough, Whittaker, & Mataix-Cols, 2004) disorders, and some can be as efficacious as face-to-face interventions (Selmi, Klein, Greist, Sorrell, & Erdman, 1990). DBT, with its established efficacy in face-to-face interventions for a variety of clinical problems and populations and its structured skills training format is an ideal candidate for dissemination as a computerized intervention.

References

Addis, M. E. (2002). Methods for disseminating research products and increasing evidence-based practice: Promises, obstacles and future directions. *Psychology Science and Practice, 9*, 367–378.

Aitken, R. (1982). *Taking the path of zen.* San Francisco, CA: North Point Press.

American Psychiatric Association. (1987). *Diagnostic and statistical manual of mental disorders* (3rd ed., rev.). Washington, DC: American Psychiatric Association.

American Psychiatric Association. (1994). *Diagnostic and statistical manual of mental disorders* (4th ed.). Washington, DC: American Psychiatric Association.

Arkowitz, H. (1989). The role of theory in psychotherapy integration. *Journal of Integrative and Eclectic Psychotherapy, 8*, 8–16.

Arkowitz, H. (1992). Integrative theories of therapy. In D. Freedheim (Ed.), *The history of psychotherapy: A century of change* (pp. 261–303). Washington, DC: American Psychologic.

Barlow, D. H., Allen, L. B., & Choate, M. L. (2004). Toward a unified treatment for emotional disorders. *Behavior Therapy, 35*, 205–230.

Barlow, D. H., Levitt, J. T., & Bufka, L. F. (1999). The dissemination of empirically supported treatments: A view of the future. *Behaviour Research and Therapy, 37*, S147–S162.

Basseches, M. (1984). *Dialectical thinking and adult development.* Norwood, NJ: Ablex Publishing.

Bedics, J. D., Atkins, D. C., Harned, M. S., & Linehan, M. M. (2015). The Therapeutic Alliance as a Predictor of Outcome in Dialectical Behavior Therapy Versus Nonbehavioral Therapy by Experts for Borderline Personality Disorder. *Psychotherapy, 52*, 67–77.

Biederman, J., Newcorn, J., & Sprich, S. (1991). Comorbidity of attention deficit hyperactivity disorder with conduct, depressive, anxiety, and other disorders. *American Journal of Psychiatry, 148*, 564–577.

Bohus, M., Dyer, A. S., Priebe, K., Kruger, A., Kleindienst, N., Schmahl, C., … Steil, R. (2013). Dialectical behaviour therapy for post-traumatic stress disorder after childhood sexual abuse in patients with and without borderline personality disorder: A randomised controlled trial. *Psychotherapy and Psychosomatics, 82*, 221–233.

Bohus, M., Haaf, B., Simms, T., Limberger, M. F., Schmahl, C., Unckel, C., … Linehan, M. M. (2004). Effectiveness of inpatient dialectical behavioral therapy for borderline personality disorder: A controlled trial. *Behavioral Research and Therapy, 42*, 487–499.

Bradley, R. G., & Follingstad, D. R. (2003). Group therapy for incarcerated women who experienced interpersonal violence: A pilot study. *Journal of Traumatic Stress, 16*, 337–340.

Carter, G. L., Willcox, C. H., Lewin, T. J., Conrad, A. M., & Bendit, N. (2010). Hunter DBT project: Randomized controlled trial of dialectical behaviour therapy in women with borderline personality disorder. *Australia New Zealand Journal of Psychiatry, 44*, 162–173.

Cartreine, J. A., Ahren, D. K., & Locke, S. E. (2010). A roadmap to computer-based psychotherapy in the United States. *Harvard Review of Psychiatry, 18*, 80–95.

Chambless, D. L., Baker, M. J., Baucom, D. H., Beutler, L. E., Calhoun, K. S., Crits-Christoph, P., … McCurry, S. (1998). Update on empirically validated therapies, II. *Clinical Psychologist, 51*, 3–16.

Clarkin, J. F., Levy, K. N., Lenzenweger, M. F., & Kernberg, O. F. (2007). Evaluating three treatments for borderline personality disorder: A multiwave study. *American Journal of Psychiatry, 164*, 922–928.

Conway, K. P., Compton, W., Stinson, F. S., & Grant, B. F. (2006). Lifetime comorbidity of DSM-IV mood and anxiety disorders and specific drug use disorders: Results from the National Epidemiologic Survey on Alcohol and Related Conditions. *Journal of Clinical Psychiatry, 67*, 247–257.

Crowell, S. E., Beauchaine, T. P., & Linehan, M. M. (2009). A biosocial developmental model of borderline personality: Elaborating and extending Linehan's theory. *Psychological Bulletin, 135*, 495–510.

Feigenbaum, J. D., Fonagy, P., Pilling, S., Jones, A., Wildgoose, A., & Bebbington, P. E. (2012). A real-world study of the effectiveness of DBT in the UK National Health Service. *British Journal of Clinical Psychology, 51*, 121–141.

Foa, E. B., Keane, T. M., Friedman, M. J., & Cohen, J. A. (2009). *Effective treatments for PTSD: Practice guidelines from the International Society for Traumatic Stress Studies.* (2nd ed.) New York: Guilford Press.

Garfield, S. L. (1994). Research on client variables in psychotherapy. In A. E. Bergin & S. L. Garfield (Eds.), *Handbook of psychotherapy and behavior change.* (4th ed., pp. 190–228). New York: Wiley.

Goldfried, M. R., & Davison, G. C. (1976). *Clinical behavior therapy.* New York: Holt, Rinehart & Win.

Gross, J. J. (2009). *Handbook of emotion egulation.* New York: Guilford Press.

Gross, J. J., John, O. P., & Richards, J. M. (2000). The dissociation of emotion expression from emotion experience: A personality perspective. *Personality and Social Psychology Bulletin, 26*, 712–726.

Gross, J. J., & Levenson, R. W. (1993). Emotional suppression: Physiology, self-report, and expressive behavior. *Journal of Personality and Social Psychology, 64*, 970–986.

Gross, J. J., & Levenson, R. W. (1997). Hiding feelings: The acute effects of inhibiting negative and positive emotion. *Journal of Abnormal Psychology, 106*, 95–103.

Hahn, T. N. (1976). *The miracle of mindfulness: A manual of meditation.* Boston: Beacon Press.

Harley, R., Sprich, S., Safren, S., Jacobo, M., & Fava, M. (2008). Adaptation of dialectical behavior therapy skills training group for treatment-resistant depression. *Journal of Nervous and Mental Disease, 196*, 136–143.

Harned, M. S., Chapman, A. L., Dexter-Mazza, E. T., Murray, A., Comtois, K. A., & Linehan, M. M. (2008). Treating co-occurring Axis I disorders in recurrently suicidal women with borderline personality disorder: A 2-year randomized trial of dialectical behavior therapy versus community treatment by experts. *Journal of Consulting and Clinical Psychology, 76*, 1068–1075.

Harned, M. S., Korslund, K. E., Foa, E. B., & Linehan, M. M. (2012). Treating PTSD in suicidal and self-injuring women with borderline personality disorder: Development and preliminary evaluation of a Dialectical Behavior Therapy Prolonged Exposure Protocol. *Behaviour Research and Therapy, 50*, 381–386.

Harned, M. S., & Linehan, M. M. (2008). Integrating dialectical behavior therapy and prolonged exposure to treat co-occurring borderline personality disorder and PTSD: Two case studies. *Cognitive and Behavioral Practice, 15*, 263–276.

Henikoff, S., & Matzke, M. A. (1997). Exploring and explaining epigenetic effects. *Trends in Genetics, 13*, 293–295.

Hill, D. M., Craighead, L. W., & Safer, D. L. (2011). Appetite-focused dialectical behavior therapy for the treatment of binge eating with purging: A preliminary trial. *International Journal of Eating Disorders, 44*, 249–261.

Hirvikoski, T., Waaler, E., Alfredsson, J., Philgren, C., Holmstrom, A., Johnson, A., ... Nordström, A. L. (2011). Reduced ADHD symptoms in adults with ADHD after structured skills training group: Results from a randomized controlled trial. *Behavior Research and Therapy, 49*, 175–185.

Howland, P. H., Rush, A. J., Wisniewski, S., Trivedi, M., Warden, D., Fava, M., ... Berman, S. R. (2009). Concurrent anxiety and substance use disorders among outpatients with major depression: Clinical features and effect of treatment outcome. *Drug and Alcohol Dependence, 99*, 248–260.

Jager, W. (2005). *Mysticism for modern times: Conversations with Willigis Jager.* Liguori, MO: Liguori Publications.

Kaminstein, D. S. (1987). Toward a dialectical metatheory for psychotherapy. *Journal of Contemporary Psychotherapy, 17*, 87–101.

Kessler, R. C., Merikangas, K. R., & Wang, P. S. (2007). Prevalence, comorbidity, and service utilization of mood disorders in the United States at the beginning of the twenty-first century. *Annual Review of Psychology, 3*, 158.

Koons, C. R., Betts, B., Chapman, A. L., O'Rourke, B., & Robins, C. J. (2004). Dialectical behavior therapy for vocational rehabilitation. *Journal of Personality Disorders, 18*, 79.

Koons, C. R., Robins, C. J., Tweed, J. L., Lynch, T. R., Gonzalez, A. M., Morse, J. Q., & Bishop, G. K. (2001). Efficacy of dialectical behavior therapy in women veterans with borderline personality disorder. *Behavior Therapy, 32*, 371–390.

Langer, E. J. (1989). *Mindfulness.* Boston, MA: Merloyd Lawrence Books.

Leichsenring, F., Leibing, E., Kruse, J., New, A. S., & Leweke, F. (2011). Borderline personality disorder. *Lancet, 377*, 74–84.

Linehan, M. M. (1981). A social-behavioral analysis of suicide and parasuicide: Implications for clinical assessment and treatment. In H. Glazer & J. F. Clarkin (Eds.), *Depression: Behavioral and directive intervention strategies* (pp. 229–294). New York: Garland Press.

Linehan, M. M. (1993a). *Skills training manual for treating borderline personality disorder.* New York: Guilford Press.

Linehan, M. M. (1993b). *Cognitive-behavioral treatment of borderline personality disorder.* New York: Guilford Press.

Linehan, M. M., Armstrong, H. E., Suarez, A., Allmon, D., & Heard, H. L. (1991). Cognitive-behavioral treatment of chronically parasuicidal borderline patients. *Archives of General Psychiatry, 48*, 1060–1064.

Linehan, M. M., Comtois, K. A., Murray, A. M., Brown, M. Z., Gallop, R. J., Heard, H. L., ... Lindenboim, N. (2006). Two-year randomized controlled trial and follow-up of dialectical behavior therapy vs therapy by experts for suicidal behaviors and borderline personality disorder. *Archives of General Psychiatry, 63*, 757–766.

Linehan, M. M., Dimeff, L. A., Reynolds, S. K., Comtois, K. A., Welch, S. S., Heagerty, P., & Kivlahan, D. R. (2002). Dialectical behavior therapy versus comprehensive validation therapy plus 12-step for the treatment of opioid dependent women meeting criteria for borderline personality disorder. *Drug and Alcohol Dependency, 67*, 13–26.

Linehan, M. M., & Egan, K. J. (1979). Assertion training for women. In A. S. Bellack & M. Hersen (Eds.), *Research and practice in social skills training* (pp. 237–271). New York: Plenum Press.

Linehan, M. M., Schmidt, H., III, Dimeff, L. A., Craft, J. C., Kanter, J., & Comtois, K. A. (1999). Dialectical behavior therapy for patients with borderline personality disorder and drug-dependence. *American Journal of Addiction, 8*, 279–292.

Lyons, C., Hopley, P., & Horrocks, J. (2009). A decade of stigma and discrimination in mental health: Plus ca change, plus c'est la meme chose (the more things change, the more they stay the same). *Journal of Psychiatric and Mental Health Nursing, 16*, 501–507.

Marks, I. M., Cavanagh, K., & Gega, L. (2007). *Hands-on help: Computer-aided psychotherapy.* London, UK: Psychology Press.

Marks, I. M., Kenwright, M., McDonough, M., Whittaker, M., & Mataix-Cols, D. (2004). Saving clinicians' time by delegating routine aspects of therapy to a computer. A randomized controlled trial in phobia/panic disorder. *Psychological Medicine, 34*, 9–18.

May, G. G. (1987). *Will and spirit: A contemplative psychology.* San Francisco: Harper & Row.

McHugh, K. R., Murray, K., & Barlow, D. H. (2009). Balancing fidelity and adaptation in the dissemination of empirically supported treatments: The promise of thransdiagnostic interventions. *Behaviour Research and Therapy, 47*, 946–953.

Mcmain, S. F., Links, P. S., Gnam, W. H., Guimond, T., Cardish, R. J., Korman, L., & Streiner D. L. (2009). A randomized trial of dialectical behavior therapy versus general psychiatric management for borderline personality disorder. *American Journal of Psychiatry, 166*, 1365–1374.

Neacsiu, A. D. (2012). *A treatment mechanism for emotion dysregulation across mood and anxiety disorders.* Seattle: University of Washington.

Neacsiu, A. D., Rizvi, S. L., & Linehan, M. M. (2010). Dialectical behavior therapy skills use as a mediator and outcome of treatment for borderline personality disorder. *Behaviour Research and Therapy, 48*(9), 832–839.

Newman, M. G. (2004). Technology in psychotherapy: An introduction. *Journal of Clinical Psychology, 60*, 141–145.

Norcross, J. C., & Goldfried, M. R. (2005). *Handbook of psychotherapy integration.* (2nd ed.). New York: Oxford University Press.

Pistorello, J., Fruzzetti, A. E., MacLane, C., Gallop, R., & Iverson, K. M. (2012). Dialectical behavior therapy (DBT) applied to college students: A randomized clinical trial. *Journal of Consulting and Clinical Psychology, 80*, 982–994.

Prochaska, J. O., & Diclemente, C. C. (2005). The transtheo-retical approach. In J. C. Norcross & M. R. Goldfried (Eds.), *Handbook of psychotherapy integration* (pp. 147–171). New York: Oxford University Press.

Proudfoot, J., Goldberg, D., Mann, A., Everitt, B., Marks, I. M., & Gray, J. A. (2003). Computerized, interactive, multimedia cognitive-behavioural program for anxiety and depression in general practice. *Psychological Medicine, 33*, 217–227.

Regier, D. A., Narrow, W. E., Kuhl, E. A., & Kupter, D. J. (2009). The conceptual development of DSM-V. *American Journal of Psychiatry, 166*, 1–7.

Richards, D., & Richardson, T. (2012). Computer-based psychological treatments for depression: A systematic review and meta-analysis. *Clinical Psychology Review, 32*, 329–342.

Rogers, C. R. (1946). Significant aspects of client centered therapy. *American Psychologist, 1*, 415–422.

Rothbart, M. K., & Rueda, M. R. (2005). The development of effortful control. In U. Mayr, E. Awh, & S. Keele (Eds.), *Developing individuality in the human brain: A tribute to Michael I. Posner* (pp. 167–188). Washington, DC: American Psychological Association.

Ryle, A. (2005). Cognitive analytic therapy. In J. C. Norcross & M. R. Goldfried (Eds.), *Handbook of psychotherapy integration* (pp. 196–217). New York: Oxford University Press.

Safer, D. L., Robinson, A. H., & Jo, B. (2010). Outcome from a randomized controlled trial of group therapy for binge eating disorder: Comparing dialectical behavior therapy adapted for binge eating to an active comparison group therapy. *Behavioral Therapy, 41*, 106–120.

Safer, D. L., Telch, C. F., & Agras, W. S. (2001). Dialectical behavior therapy for bulimia nervosa. *American Journal of Psychiatry, 158*, 632–634.

Selmi, P. M., Klein, M. H., Greist, J. H., Sorrell, S. P., & Erdman, H. P. (1990). Computer-administered cognitive-behavioral therapy for depression. *American Journal of Psychiatry, 147*, 51–56.

Shafran, R., Clark, D. M., Fairburn, C. G., Arntz, A., Barlow, D. H., Ehlers, A., … Wilson, G. T. (2009). Mind the gap: Improving the dissemination of CBT. *Behavior Research and Therapy, 47*, 902–909.

Skinner, B. F. (1974). *About behaviorism*. Westminister, MD: Alfred Knoft.

Soler, J., Pascual, J. C., Campins, J., Barrachina, J., Puigdemont, D., Alvarez, E., & Perez, V. (2005). Double-blind, placebo-controlled study of dialectical behavior therapy plus olanzapine for borderline personality disorder. *American Journal of Psychiatry, 162*, 1221–1224.

Soler, J., Pascual, J. C., Tiana, T., Cebria, A., Barrachina, J., Campins, M. J., … Perez, V. (2009). Dialectical behaviour therapy skills training compared to standard group therapy in borderline personality disorder: A 3-month randomised controlled clinical trial. *Behaviour Research and Therapy, 47*, 353–358.

Staats, A. W. (1975). *Social behaviorism*. Homewood, IL: Dorsey Press.

Staats, A. W., & Staats, C. K. (1963). *Complex human behavior*. New York: Holt, Rinehart & Win.

Stobie, B., Taylor, T., Quigley, A., Ewing, S., & Salkovskis, P. M. (2007). "Contents may vary": A pilot study of treatment histories of OCD patients. *Behavioral and Cognitive Psycotherapy, 35*, 273–282.

Swann, W. B., Jr., Stein-Seroussi, A., & Giesler, R. B. (1992). Why people self-verify. *Journal of Personality and Social Psychology, 62*, 392–401.

Tooby, J., & Cosmides, L. (1990). The past explains the present: Emotional adaptations and the structure of ancestral environment. *Ethology and Sociobiology, 11*, 375–424.

Turner, R. M. (2000). Naturalistic evaluation of dialectical behavioral therapy-oriented treatment for borderline personality disorder. *Cognitive and Behavioral Practice, 7*, 413–419.

van den Bosch, L. M. C., Verheul, R., Schippers, G. M., & Van den Brink, W. (2002). Dialectical behavior therapy of borderline patients with and without substance use problems. Implementation and long-term effects. *Addictive Behaviors, 27*, 911–923.

Van Dijk, S., Jeffrey, J., & Katz, M. R. (2012). A randomized, controlled, pilot study of dialectical behavior therapy skills in a psychoeducational group for individuals with bipolar disorder. *Journal of Affective Disorders, 145*(3), 386–393.

Wilson, G. T., & O'Leary, K. D. (1980). *Principles of behavior therapy*. Engelwood Cliffs, NJ: Prentice Hall.

Wright, K. M., Cabrera, O. A., Bliese, P. D., Adler, A. B., Hoge, C. W., & Castro, C. A. (2009). Stigma and barriers to care in soldiers postcombat. *Psychological Services, 6*, 116.

Zhang, T. Y., & Meaney, M. J. (2010). Epigenetics and the environmental regulation of the genome and its function. *Annual Review of Psychology, 61*, 439–466.

Relapse Prevention

Katie Witkiewitz *and* Megan Kirouac

Abstract

The phrase "relapse prevention" has multiple meanings: It is a theory about behavior change attempts, a specific treatment approach, and a set of intervention strategies. The theory of relapse prevention acknowledges that behavior change is difficult and that cognitive-behavioral strategies can be useful for maintaining successful behavior changes. Relapse prevention treatment can be defined as either a treatment program or a set of intervention strategies with two specific aims: (1) to prevent an initial lapse and maintain treatment gains; and (2) to provide lapse management if a lapse occurs in order to prevent further relapse. The ultimate goal is to provide the skills to foster positive behavior change. In this chapter we review the conceptual background and history of relapse prevention, provide an example of a relapse prevention treatment protocol, review the latest research on relapse prevention approaches, and introduce numerous directions for future research and clinical practice.

Key Words: relapse prevention, addiction, cognitive-behavioral model of relapse, dynamic model of relapse, skills training, negative emotions, self-efficacy, abstinence violation effect

Lapses, defined as engaging in a previously problematic behavior following a successful behavior change attempt, are the modal outcome following treatment for addictive behaviors. More generally, the majority of individuals who attempt to change a specific behavior in a certain direction (e.g., lose weight, spend more time with family, stop smoking, etc.) will experience multiple lapses that can often lead to a full-blown "relapse" (defined as returning to the problematic behavior). For example, among cigarette smokers the ability to maintain abstinence following a smoking cessation attempt is rare, with approximately 70% of individuals who receive smoking cessation treatment returning to smoking within the first year (Fiore, 2000). Among smokers who quit without formal treatment, approximately 95%–98% will return to smoking within 6–12 months following a quit attempt (Hughes, Keely, & Naud, 2004).

Relapse prevention is an intervention and a treatment strategy that focuses on the problem of relapse through an integration of behavioral skills training, cognitive interventions, and lifestyle change procedures (Marlatt & Gordon, 1985). Based on a cognitive-behavioral framework, relapse prevention seeks to identify situations in which an individual is most at risk for a relapse and use both cognitive and behavioral strategies to prevent future relapses in similar situations. Relapse prevention can be described as an intervention strategy with two specific aims: (1) preventing an initial lapse and maintaining treatment gains; (2) providing lapse management if a lapse occurs, to prevent further relapse. The ultimate goal is to provide the skills to prevent a complete relapse, regardless of the situation or impending risk factors. Although initially developed for alcohol use disorders, the principles and concepts of relapse prevention have been adapted to many other addictive and nonaddictive disorders, including depression (Teasdale et al., 2000), eating disorders (Mitchell & Carr, 2001), erectile dysfunction (McCarthy, 2001), bipolar disorders (Lam et al., 2000), schizophrenia (Herz et al., 2000), and sexual offenses (Laws, 1995).

Relapse prevention begins with the assessment of the potential interpersonal, intrapersonal, environmental, and physiological risks for relapse and the factors or situations that may precipitate a relapse. Once potential relapse triggers and high-risk situations are identified, cognitive and behavioral approaches are implemented that incorporate both specific interventions and global self-management strategies. The primary component in the cognitive-behavioral model of relapse is the identification of high-risk situations, and the primary relapse prevention intervention strategies incorporate teaching the client to recognize high-risk situations and warning signs for them, then evaluating the client's ability to cope with the situation and, if necessary, encouraging more effective coping responses.

In addition to teaching effective coping responses, a major component of relapse prevention is the enhancement of self-efficacy. Self-efficacy is the extent to which an individual feels capable of performing a certain behavior (Bandura, 1977), and higher levels of self-efficacy are predictive of improved treatment outcomes. The collaboration between the client and therapist plays a critical role in the encouragement of efficacy, as clients who are active in the therapeutic process will have an increased sense of mastery over successful outcomes. Positive feedback from the therapist concerning substance use and non-substance-use-related tasks may help to increase a client's sense of general self-efficacy, which may further motivate the client's effort to change.

As in most cognitive-behavioral treatments, relapse prevention incorporates a significant psychoeducational component, as well as restructuring of misperceptions and maladaptive thoughts. Eliminating myths related to positive outcome expectancies and discussing the psychological components of substance use (e.g., placebo effects) may provide the client with opportunities to make more informed choices in high-risk situations. Positive outcome expectancies play an influential role in the relapse process. After a client has been abstinent for some period of time, a shift in attitudes and beliefs about the effects of the foregone substance or activity often occurs. Positive outcome expectancies for the immediate effects become an especially potent motivating force to resume drinking, drug use, or criminal conduct when the client is faced with a high-risk situation and is beginning to feel unable to cope effectively (low self-efficacy) or is reacting to an unbalanced lifestyle. In either case, the temptation to "give in" and relinquish control by indulging in the formerly taboo activity is a powerful influence.

Clients are taught to recognize and cope with high-risk situations that may precipitate a lapse and to modify cognitions to prevent a single lapse from developing into a full-blown relapse. Lapse management is presented as an emergency procedure to be implemented in the event a lapse occurs. Clients are taught to restructure their negative thoughts about lapses, to not view them as a "failure" or an indication of a lack of willpower. Education about the relapse *process* and the likelihood of a lapse occurring equips clients to navigate the rough terrain of behavior change.

Conceptual Underpinnings of Relapse Prevention

Relapse prevention is grounded in the cognitive-behavioral model of relapse, which defines the relapse process as a progression centered on "triggering" events, both internal and external. In this process, after experiencing a trigger, an individual will make a series of choices and have thoughts that will lead to being placed in a high-risk situation or not. There are two major types of high-risk situations, those with intrapersonal determinants, in which the person's response is physical or psychological in nature, and interpersonal determinants, those that are influenced by other individuals or social networks.

Based on a cognitive-behavioral model of relapse, it is proposed that when an individual encounters a high-risk situation, he or she can utilize either an effective or ineffective coping response. Effective coping skills can lead to increased self-efficacy and a decreased probability of a lapse. However, if one lacks skills, then the model predicts a decrease in self-efficacy and an increase in positive outcome expectancies for the effects of using the substance. This is a likely predecessor of giving into temptation in the initial use of a substance.

Despite the empirical support for many components of the cognitive-behavioral model, there have also been many criticisms of the model for being too static and hierarchical (Kadden, 1996; Lowman, Allen, & Stout, 1996). In response to these criticisms, Witkiewitz and Marlatt (2004) proposed a revision of the cognitive-behavioral model of relapse that incorporated both static and dynamic factors that are believed to be influential in the relapse process. The "dynamic model of relapse" builds upon several previous studies of relapse risk factors by incorporating the characterization of distal and proximal risk factors. Distal risks, which are thought to increase the probability of relapse, include background variables (e.g., severity of alcohol dependence) and relatively stable pretreatment characteristics (e.g., expectancies). Proximal risks actualize, or complete, the distal predispositions and include transient lapse precipitants (e.g., stressful situations) and dynamic individual characteristics (e.g., negative affect, self-efficacy). Combinations of precipitating and predisposing risk factors are innumerable for any particular individual and may create a complex system in which the probability of relapse is greatly increased, even after only slight changes in risk factors. For example, a client who has been successfully abstaining for several weeks and who experienced a stressful day at work might be more likely to give into the temptation to drink at dinner that evening after only a small disagreement with his or her spouse.

The revised dynamic model of relapse also takes into account the timing and interrelatedness of risk factors. For example, based on the dynamic model, it is hypothesized that changes in one risk factor (e.g., negative affect) influence changes in drinking behavior and that changes in drinking also influence changes in the risk factors (Witkiewitz & Villarroel, 2009). The dynamic model of relapse has generated enthusiasm among researchers and clinicians who have observed these processes in their data and their clients (Brandon, Vidrine, & Litvin, 2007; Hunter-Reel, McCrady, & Hildebrandt, 2009; Stanton, 2005).

Only a few empirical tests of the dynamic model of relapse have been conducted to date and the results are promising, albeit preliminary. Witkiewitz (2011) examined both distal and proximal risk factors as predictors of heavy drinking during the course of treatment and up to 1 year following treatment using data from the COMBINE study (Anton et al., 2006). Results indicated that higher levels of distal and proximal risk, as well as increased proximal risk over time, were significantly associated with significant increases in heavy drinking. Likewise, higher levels of distal risk and heavy drinking were associated with increased levels of proximal risk over time, suggesting a feedback loop whereby proximal risk increased drinking and heavy drinking predicted greater proximal risks. Consistent with the hypotheses of the dynamic model of relapse, Witkiewitz (2011) also found that proximal risk factors significantly mediated the association between certain distal risk factors (including psychiatric symptoms and treatment history) and changes in heavy drinking over time.

In a second study that tested the dynamic model using the COMBINE study data (Anton et al., 2006) with a different statistical modeling approach, Chow and colleagues (Chow, Witkiewitz, Grasman, & Maisto, in press) found that individuals with high distal risk showed a significantly greater increase in the probability for a lapse when proximal risk was high (i.e., from .15 to .54). In contrast, for those with low distal risk, the probability for a lapse actually decreased slightly on the days with high proximal risk. Overall, the detrimental effects of high proximal risk on triggering a lapse among those with high distal risk were clear throughout the treatment phase, providing support for the postulates of the dynamic model of relapse.

To date, the empirical tests of the dynamic model have focused on statistical associations between relapse risk factors and drinking outcomes following alcohol treatment. The critical next step is to put the dynamic model of relapse into clinical practice by using the postulates of the model to better predict client outcomes. Recent clinical textbooks on the subject of addiction counseling have attempted to guide clinicians in the application of the dynamic model (Miller, 2010; Mitcheson et al., 2010). For example, Mitcheson and colleagues (2010) concluded that "the implications of the model for clinical practice follow intuition and could, like its predecessor, become one of the central planks in the addictions field" (p. 34). In their description of the model, the authors specifically focused on the importance of the dynamic model for assessment and tailoring treatment to the interaction of various risk factors and an individual's environmental context. As such, they consider the dynamic model an improvement over the "washing machine concept" (p. 36) of treatment, whereby all individuals are put through the same treatment with the idea that a single washing machine will "clean" everyone equally. One of the problems with the original relapse prevention model was that it also subscribed to this washing machine formula. Revisions to the relapse prevention approach should, in drawing on the dynamic model of relapse, provide more tailored treatment to each individual's strengths and vulnerabilities. In other words, each individual case might require a unique case formulation.

History of Relapse Prevention
The history of relapse prevention is a relatively short one, considering relapse prevention did not

emerge into treatment practices until the 1980s. And, although relapse prevention has since been applied to several behavior changes (e.g., sexual offending, depression, and eating disorders), it originally applied to substance abuse. In that regard, in order to better understand the history of relapse prevention, it makes sense to briefly discuss the historical conceptual underpinnings of relapse as it applies to substance abuse first.

Traditionally, relapse had been viewed under the moral model of addiction where relapse was considered the result of one's own moral flaws and failure to remain abstinent. Because it was considered the result of one's own morality, it is not surprising that relapse was something many felt was beyond treatment. Consequently, relapse prevention was virtually nonexistent until researchers in the 1970s began to study relapse and relapse prevention techniques emerged (see review by Donovan, 2003).

Relapse then began to be viewed as part of a natural path to recovery, rather than a final endpoint to abstinence. Medical models of addiction cited endogenous factors such as withdrawal as the primary cause of relapse, while cognitive-behavioral approaches attributed relapse to contextual factors such as environment and coping skills (Donovan, 2003; Hendershot, Witkiewitz, George, & Marlatt, 2011). Marlatt was one of the first researchers on the cognitive-behavioral front, and one of the first techniques he applied to prevent relapse was to train clients to respond to alcohol-related cues with behaviors incompatible with alcohol use. Consequently, the identification of one's personal triggers for relapse emerged as one of the first relapse prevention techniques (Donovan, 2003). This technique was studied, honed, and added to until the model became what we know today as one of the first cognitive-behavioral relapse prevention models (Marlatt & Gordon, 1984).

The relapse prevention model developed by Marlatt and Gordon (1985) served as one of the first cognitive-behavioral approaches to relapse prevention treatment of addictive behaviors and viewed relapse as a multifaceted process in the course of behavior change. Accordingly, relapse prevention was used as a specific maintenance strategy to prevent relapse to a problematic behavior, or it was used in a broader behavior maintenance scope in which the therapist's primary goal is to teach the client how to achieve and maintain a balanced lifestyle by avoiding unhealthy habits. This model achieved abstinence through relapse prevention by focusing on two levels of an individual's situation preceding a relapse: the immediate, high-risk situation, and one's response to such a situation. Techniques such as identifying high-risk situations, knowing personal "warning signs" for relapse, practicing behavioral and cognitive coping strategies, and avoiding the abstinence violation effect evolved in Marlatt and Gordon's original model.

While the techniques developed in the 1970s and 1980s still remain the foundations of the relapse prevention techniques used today, clear changes have since been made to Marlatt and Gordon's original cognitive-behavioral model for relapse prevention. For example, the dynamic model of relapse prevention marks one of the largest changes to Marlatt and Gordon's original model (see previous section for more information; Witkiewitz & Marlatt, 2004). However, this addition to the original model is the result of many years and individuals' efforts and reflects a process whereby relapse prevention techniques are created, studied, implemented, and revised.

Accordingly, one key element in the history of relapse prevention has been the interaction between research and practice. It is through this interaction that relapse prevention techniques have been and continue to be adjusted and adapted to fit a variety of individual client needs. Consequently, relapse prevention has been adapted from a substance abuse treatment adjunct to an umbrella term for achieving the maintenance of a variety of behavior changes ranging from maintaining weight loss to reducing alcohol use to quitting smoking to maintaining abstinence from sexual offenses, and it is currently being adjusted, adapted, and improved for a variety of problem behaviors (Witkiewitz & Marlatt, 2007).

Description of a Relapse Prevention Protocol

The seminal text on relapse prevention by Marlatt and Gordon (1985) provided an overview of the cognitive-behavioral model of relapse and a theoretical description of relapse prevention as a treatment strategy, but it was not organized as a step-by-step treatment protocol or manual. In some ways the relapse prevention approach, as advocated by Marlatt and colleagues (Marlatt & Gordon, 1985; Witkiewitz & Marlatt, 2004), is not well suited as a manualized protocol because of the important focus on the high-risk situations of individual clients. For example a client who can only identify one specific high-risk situation would likely benefit from skills training around avoiding or coping with that specific situation. Another client who is experiencing craving and lapses across many situations would require numerous strategies for coping that may generalize across situations.

Nevertheless, Marlatt's research team found it necessary to develop a manualized protocol for relapse prevention in order to evaluate the treatment in a randomized controlled trial. The unpublished protocol, which we describe later, was an amalgamation of several existing empirically supported, manual-based, cognitive-behavioral treatments for substance use disorders. Much of the content was pulled directly from the Daley and Marlatt (2006) "Overcoming Your Alcohol or Drug Problem" manual and adapted for a group setting. An additional portion of the content was adapted from the Monti, Kadden, Rohsenow, Cooney, and Abrams (2002) "Coping Skills Training Guide." The protocol also incorporated content from the relapse prevention guidelines published online at www.bhrm.org/guidelines/RPT%20guideline.pdf (Marlatt, Parks, & Witkiewitz, 2002).

The randomized controlled trial of the relapse prevention protocol indicated that two different versions of relapse prevention, relapse prevention and mindfulness-based relapse prevention (described in more detail later; Bowen, Chawla, & Marlatt, 2010), resulted in better substance use outcomes 6 months following treatment than a standard aftercare program in a community substance abuse treatment agency (Bowen et al., 2014). The mindfulness-based relapse prevention program resulted in continued significant reductions in drug use days and probability of heavy drinking, compared to both relapse prevention and standard aftercare, at a 12-month follow-up (Bowen et al., 2014).

The relapse prevention protocol developed for the trial is a group-based closed cohort aftercare treatment for substance use disorders that consists of weekly 2-hour sessions over the course of 8 weeks. Each session builds on the prior session and all sessions are explicitly tied to the cognitive-behavioral model of relapse. All sessions include an assigned "home practice" exercise that clients are instructed to complete in between sessions. The home practice exercises are critical for individuals to have the opportunity to practice skills in their home environments. Importantly, many of the exercises were adapted to be as individualized as possible, with a specific focus on individual high-risk situations for relapse.

Session 1, "Introduction to Relapse Prevention," includes an introduction to relapse prevention theory and the cognitive-behavioral model of relapse. Clients are also assisted with an exercise of setting personal goals for treatment and the future. Session 2, "Managing Thoughts about Using Substances," focuses on people, situations, or events that can trigger urges and thoughts that may accompany these triggers. Session 3, "Coping Skills and Managing Emotions," extends the discussion of thought patterns with a specific focus on negative thinking, emotions, and the role of negative thinking and emotions in the relapse process. Session 4, "Dealing with High-Risk Situations," explicitly focuses on identifying common high-risk situations and relapse warning signs. The session also covers the "abstinence violation effect" and how to prevent a lapse from becoming a relapse. Session 5, "Self-Efficacy and Problem Solving," discusses the fact that many individuals have doubts about their ability to maintain treatment goals. Self-efficacy enhancement exercises and strategies for problem-solving skills training are reviewed and practiced in session. Session 6, "Thinking through the Drink/Drug," covers the "nuts and bolts" of recovery, including discussions of the reasons for recovery, ideas about how to succeed in recovery, and what to do in the event of a lapse (e.g., reaching out to important significant others who are supportive of recovery). Sessions 1 through 6 are the precursors to the core instructions and exercises of Session 7, "Lapse Management and Relapse Prevention Planning." In Session 7 the clients explore the possibility of lapses and relapses as "opportunities" for learning, and each client creates his or her own "relapse road map" to help identify possible twists, turns, or detours on the road to recovery. The final session, Session 8, "Building Support Networks and Lifestyle Balance," attempts to complete the circle by reexamining and updating personal goals that were identified at the beginning of the 8-week treatment. Session 8 also focuses on how clients can build a lifestyle that is supportive of preventing relapse by building supportive social networks and identifying pleasurable substance-free activities. This manualized eight-session relapse prevention protocol is just one example of a relapse prevention protocol that was developed explicitly for the treatment of substance use disorders. Numerous other protocols for other disorders have also been developed.

Overview of Research on Relapse Prevention across Problems and Populations

Since its emergence onto the scientific and clinical scenes in the 1970s and 1980s, relapse prevention has been adapted for the treatment of a variety of populations and for the maintenance of many different behaviors. Although detailed discussion of the past several decades' research of relapse prevention is beyond the scope of this chapter, the following will serve as a brief overview of the research to date across problems and populations.

In accordance with the history of relapse prevention stemming from substance abuse treatment, it makes sense to first discuss the research to date for the treatment of substance abuse. More specifically, relapse prevention originated for the treatment of alcohol abuse. Accordingly, it is for alcohol use disorders that relapse prevention has the strongest evidence to date (Carroll, 1996; Irvin, Bowers, Dunn, & Wang, 1999; Witkiewitz & Marlatt, 2007).

In addition to alcohol use disorders, relapse prevention has been supported for the treatment of other substance use disorders. For example, Carroll (1996) reviewed randomized controlled trials on the effectiveness of relapse prevention for the treatment of smoking, alcohol abuse, cocaine abuse, opiate abuse, and other substance abuse and found relapse prevention was more effective than no treatment across drug types and at least equally effective across other active treatments such as interpersonal psychotherapy. Furthermore, Irvin and colleagues (1999) found relapse prevention to be especially effective for the treatment of alcohol and polysubstance abuse.

Despite the support for the efficacy of relapse prevention for a variety of substance use disorders, there have been some limitations to the research conducted to date. First, there is little to no research on efficacy of relapse prevention for treatment for the abuse of noncocaine stimulants, club drugs, inhalants, hallucinogens, and steroids (Douaihy, Stowell, Park, & Daley, 2007; Kilmer et al., 2005). Second, there have been only modest effect sizes in long-term efficacy findings of relapse prevention for marijuana users, suggesting that interventions need to be better tailored for this population.

Despite some limitations across drug class, the literature generally supports relapse prevention as an effective strategy to enhance the recovery from a wide variety of substance use disorders. Furthermore, the literature generally supports relapse prevention for substance use disorders across treatment modalities (i.e., individual and group treatment) and treatment settings (i.e., inpatient and outpatient; Irvin et al., 1999). For example, the Focus on Families program incorporates relapse prevention techniques in a family-oriented, outpatient setting with both individual and group therapy sessions to address the needs of both methadone-treated parents and their children. Results from this program have found that parents in the Focus on Families group had stronger relapse prevention, coping, and general problem-solving skills in addition to lower overall drug use compared to the controlled condition (Catalano, Gainey, Fleming, Haggerty, & Johnson, 1999; Catalano, Haggerty, & Gainey, 2003; Catalano, Haggerty, Gainey, & Hoppe, 1997). These results are consistent with findings that support the efficacy of relapse prevention for adults with substance use disorders (Catalano, Haggerty, Fleming, & Skinner, 2007).

One point that should be made regarding the research of substance abuse relapse prevention across populations is the fact that the majority of this research has been conducted with adult populations. However, there is some emerging evidence that supports the use of relapse prevention for the treatment of substance abuse among other populations, including adolescents and older adults. Existing outcome studies on substance use disorders among adolescents provide some promise and suggest that researchers evaluate which relapse prevention interventions could be modified to make treatment more effective for adolescents and take into account some of the factors that have been shown to impact relapse for youth (e.g., neurocognitive development; Dennis et al., 2004; Ramo, Myers, & Brown, 2007).

Similar to research of relapse prevention among adolescent substance-abusing populations, there is only emerging evidence for relapse prevention for older adults' substance abuse disorders. Relapse prevention has been used for the treatment of alcohol use disorders among older adults, and emerging evidence suggests that older adults respond to such treatment similarly to younger adults with some differences that may be associated with age (Blow, Brockmann, & Barry, 2007). Some of these age-related factors potentially involved in relapse for this population in particular include comorbid medical conditions, more serious social and emotional problems than other populations face, and lower rates of engagement (Barrick & Connors, 2002; Oslin, Slaymaker, Blow, Owen, & Colleran, 2005). Each of these variables puts this population at higher risk of relapse and suggests the need for age-appropriate treatment protocols.

One successful adaptation of relapse prevention to the needs of those outside of adult, substance-abusing populations has been the adaptation of relapse prevention strategies to criminal offender populations to prevent recidivism (Dowden & Andrews, 2007). The Core Correctional Practice used the original relapse prevention model to augment the existing correctional treatment of criminal offenders. Certain elements of the relapse prevention model have been shown to have stronger, positive treatment effects than others. For example, identifying high-risk situations has been shown to have great importance in preventing recidivism, while teaching offenders how to deal with failure situations has been less effective for this population (Andrews & Carvell, 1998; Dowden & Andrews, 2004).

In addition to testing various relapse prevention elements against one another to create the most effective correctional treatment possible, research has also tested the addition of treatment components that were not in the original relapse prevention model. For instance, the addition of anger management, sexual education, and victim empathy components, delivered in a relapse prevention framework has been shown to improve treatment outcomes for criminal populations (Laws, 1999, 2003). In this sense, the correctional practices have adapted relapse prevention to the specific needs of their clients in two ways: by using the traditional relapse prevention model to augment their preexisting correctional treatment services, and by making relapse prevention the underlying framework upon which various treatment services are provided (Dowden & Andrews, 2007).

Although correctional services have had success in adapting traditional relapse prevention to criminal offender populations outside of traditional adult substance-abusing populations, there are still many other diverse populations with problems beyond substance abuse or criminal offense that need effective treatment options. However, these problems may not be as intuitively manageable as maintaining abstinence from substance use or criminal offenses—for example, the treatment of anxiety disorders. Although it may be difficult to conceptualize how one might remain "abstinent" from anxiety, there has been research conducted on the adaptation of relapse prevention techniques to anxiety disorder treatment. Specifically, studies have found that the cognitive-behavioral framework in which relapse prevention is delivered is more effective for symptom reduction maintenance than other forms of therapy (e.g., relaxation therapy) in individuals with generalized anxiety disorder (Dugas,

Rodomsky, & Brillon, 2004; Gould & Otto, 1996). For individuals with generalized anxiety disorder, the goal of relapse prevention is to prevent a return to pathological worry using many of the same cognitive-behavioral techniques from the original relapse prevention model, such as viewing lapses or relapses as an opportunity for learning to prevent the return to unwanted thoughts and behaviors (Whiteside et al., 2007).

Due to its focus on maintaining desired thoughts and behavior such as preventing a return to pathological worry, it is easier to understand how relapse prevention has been used for the treatment of other anxiety disorders, such as posttraumatic stress disorder (PTSD). One example of how relapse prevention has been implemented for treatment of PTSD is the Seeking Safety program developed by Najavits (2002), which was designed for treatment of individuals with dual diagnosis of PTSD and substance use disorders. Consequently, there is evidence supporting Seeking Safety as a treatment for dually diagnosed individuals with PTSD and substance use disorders (Najavits, 2007). Furthermore, although Seeking Safety differs from traditional relapse prevention in that it focuses intensely on trauma and PTSD (and related themes), it retains many of the same elements such as developing and rehearsing coping skills and its flexibility between treatment modalities and settings.

Similar to the process by which traditional relapse prevention has been modified for the treatment of anxiety disorders is the process by which it has been modified for the treatment of depression. This modification process integrated relapse prevention techniques to existing treatments much the same way that Seeking Safety augmented PTSD treatments with relapse prevention elements, as is seen in mindfulness-based cognitive therapy (MBCT) for treatment of depression. While traditional models of relapse prevention focused on the present in order to avoid giving in to substance cravings, mindfulness has been successfully used in treating individuals with depression to avoid depressive relapse (Ma & Teasdale, 2004; Teasdale et al., 2000). Additionally, there is emerging work being done to study the efficacy of MBCT in the treatment of recurrent suicidal ideation (Lau & Segal, 2007).

Along with suicide ideation, researchers are currently studying the efficacy of using relapse prevention techniques to prevent deliberate self-harm to augment existing dialectical behavior therapy (DBT). Although DBT has been widely supported for the treatment of individuals with chronic suicidal behaviors and self-injury, relapse prevention has been implemented in order to help maintain abstinence from deliberate self-harm. The relapse prevention strategies used have included preventing or modifying high-risk situations and reducing dysfunctional or crisis-generating behaviors, which may even apply to problems outside of deliberate self-harm (Brown & Chapman, 2007).

One example of a problem outside of deliberate self-harm for which the aforementioned relapse prevention strategies have been supported is the relapse prevention of disordered eating. Although there are only emerging data supporting relapse prevention for disordered eating, relapse prevention training has been incorporated into a number of cognitive-behavioral therapies for treating bulimia nervosa and anorexia nervosa through focusing on improving patient psychosocial functioning, practicing healthy behaviors learned in therapy sessions, and exercises to reinforce the maintenance of healthy behavior (Fairburn, 1995; Schlam & Wilson, 2007).

An area in which maintaining healthy behaviors can be particularly beneficial is for individuals with schizophrenia. As a disorder that often disrupts many elements of one's life ranging from social to financial problems, making small behavior changes can have large impacts for an individual with schizophrenia. Because relapse prevention emphasizes a focus on the present, enhancing coping and communication skills, and problem-solving skills training, it may not be surprising that relapse prevention techniques have been implemented in the context of cognitive-behavioral therapy for individuals with schizophrenia (Ziedonis, Yanos, & Silverstein, 2007). For example, focusing on identifying events and situations that may trigger unwanted thoughts or behaviors has been incorporated into existing interventions with success at preventing relapse for individuals with schizophrenia (Mueser et al., 2002). Additionally, relapse prevention techniques have been successfully used in this population to improve medication adherence (Cramer & Rosenheck, 1999).

In addition to improving medication adherence, relapse prevention techniques have been used for augmenting existing cognitive-behavioral treatments for individuals with schizophrenia in other ways. Social skills training is one example in which individuals who are in partial or full remission of florid psychotic symptoms are taught effective problem-solving techniques and communications skills with an emphasis on learning how to deal with high-risk situations in which stress and vulnerability may challenge the skills they have learned (Liberman & Kopelowicz, 2005). Also, relapse prevention has been used for improving treatment of individuals with comorbid schizophrenia and substance use disorders in a dual recovery therapy approach that combines psychosocial skills training of problem-solving and communication skills (Ziedonis et al., 2007).

While relapse prevention has had success in the treatment of disorders such as schizophrenia, other problems still remain largely unaided by relapse prevention. One obstacle that relapse prevention has faced in its use across problems and populations is that it was originally designed for adults with substance use disorders. Accordingly, relapse prevention was developed for individuals who wanted to be abstinent from substance use and wanted to maintain abstinence. These elements pose particular problems in the relapse prevention for sexual offenders. As Yates and Ward point out (2007), not all sexual offenders are homogenous in their motivation to change their behavior and to abstain from sexually deviant behavior (Laws, 2000). Additionally, the term "abstinence" applies poorly to this population as it becomes unclear if sexual offenders must remain sexually abstinent or abstinent only from sexually deviant behavior or fantasies. The role of negative affect also complicates the use of traditional relapse prevention for sexual offenders because the traditional model assumes that negative affect often plays a role in relapse, but sexual offenses can occur for individuals experiencing positive affect (Yates, 2005). Similarly, the traditional relapse prevention model fails to adapt to the varying degree of planning that is involved for some sexual offenders (i.e., some offenders go to great lengths to plan their offenses, and relapse prevention traditionally focuses on high-risk, unplanned events; Yates & Ward, 2007).

Despite the fact that relapse prevention was originally designed primarily for the treatment of adults with alcohol use disorders, and consequently faces challenges adapting to other problems and populations, relapse prevention has largely been successfully used for treating a variety of disorders and populations. Various cognitive-behavioral interventions have been augmented with elements of relapse prevention in order to positively impact the lives of many individuals. Similarly, research to date has shown largely supportive outcomes for the use of relapse prevention across populations and problems; however, there is still work that needs to be done in order to continue to improve the use of relapse prevention for a wider variety of problems and populations.

Future Directions

As discussed in the previous section, relapse prevention has been adapted from adult, treatment-seeking populations with substance use disorders to a variety of other problems and populations. However, the degree of success in such adaptations has been varied and yet other problems and populations remain largely unincorporated in relapse prevention treatment options. Although the list of all such needs for relapse prevention treatment adaptations is beyond the scope of this section, the following will serve as a guide for future directions in terms of the most promising areas for relapse prevention work to be done, or those areas in which relapse prevention is in greatest need for improvement.

One area in which relapse prevention research has generated early support for improving already existent treatment is mindfulness-based relapse prevention (MBRP; Bowen, Chawla, & Marlatt, 2010) for a variety of behavioral problems (including substance use disorders and problem gambling). The idea behind MBRP was to bring together Marlatt's early work on transcendental meditation as a treatment for alcohol use (Marlatt & Marques, 1977) with the skills training components of relapse prevention (Witkiewitz, Marlatt, & Walker, 2005) into a combined treatment for substance use disorders (Bowen et al., 2010). Bowen and her colleagues (2009, 2014) have completed two randomized controlled trials (RCTs) of MBRP for substance use disorders. Results from the first trial (Bowen et al., 2009), which randomized 168 individuals with substance use disorders to receive 8 weeks of group MBRP or 8 weeks of aftercare treatment as usual, indicated that MBRP was associated with significantly fewer days of alcohol or other drug use at 2 months following the interventions. The differences between MRBP and the treatment as usual group were not significant at 4 months. The results from the second trial (Bowen et al., 2014), described earlier, indicated that MBRP was associated with significantly fewer drug use days and lower probability of heavy drinking, as compared to both standard aftercare treatment as usual and relapse prevention, at 12 months following treatment. Likewise, Witkiewitz and colleagues (2014) found that MBRP resulted in significantly fewer

drug use days and significantly fewer legal and medical problems, as compared to a relapse prevention treatment, in a sample of women ($n = 105$) receiving treatment in a residential addictions treatment program for women referred by the criminal justice system.

Zgierska and colleagues (2009) conducted a narrative review of four studies that have examined the effectiveness of MBRP (or a modified MBRP approach) in the treatment of substance use disorders (Bowen et al., 2009; Brewer et al., 2009; Vieten, Astin, Buscemi, & Galloway, 2010; Zgierska et al., 2008) and concluded that MBRP appears to be associated with better substance use outcomes. The review also warned that the data on MBRP for a variety of disorders are still emerging and more randomized controlled trials are needed to fully understand the breadth of its application across problems and populations.

Another area in which relapse prevention shows promise but requires further work is the adaptation of relapse prevention for a variety of ethnic and racial minorities. As discussed in the "Overview of Research across Problems and Populations" section, relapse prevention has been adapted for adolescents, adults, and older populations. However, attempts to adapt relapse prevention within those age groups across culturally diverse populations have been limited. Castro, Nichols, and Kater (2007) describe a number of culturally relevant issues for substance use disorders but explain that these issues are often overlooked by treatment providers and are completely omitted from the National Institute of Drug Abuse's (NIDA) principles of drug addiction treatment (Castro et al., 2007). In that regard, cultural issues are often underrepresented in the substance abuse literature as a whole (not just relapse prevention), and there is much work to be done adapting treatment interventions for a wider variety of ethnic populations. Importantly, there is some evidence that certain aspects of relapse prevention may be more effective for certain ethnic minority groups. For example, Witkiewitz, Villarroel, Hartzler, and Donovan (2011) found that drink refusal skills training (which is often included in relapse prevention interventions) was associated with better alcohol treatment outcomes among African American clients, as compared to non-Hispanic White clients. Specifically, 80% of African American clients who received the specialized training could be classified as having a good clinical outcome (defined by non-heavy drinking and few alcohol-related problems) one year following treatment, whereas only

52% of non-Hispanic White clients received the same good clinical outcome classification.

There is also necessary work to be done for improving relapse prevention among sexual offenders. As discussed earlier, the adaptation of relapse prevention for sexual offenders has been met with limited success. One reason for this is because relapse prevention was originally designed for substance-using populations who wanted to remain abstinent from substance use while not all sexual offenders want to remain abstinent from sexually deviant behavior. Furthermore, despite its limited success, relapse prevention for sexual offenders remained essentially unchanged for the past 15 years (Yates & Ward, 2007). However, recent research has been done to improve relapse prevention for this population by developing a self-regulation model of the offense and relapse process that has promising support (Yates & Ward, 2007). Work is still needed to further refine this new model of relapse prevention for sexual offenders.

In addition to the specific problems and populations in which relapse prevention research is still needed, there are a number of more general areas in which future research should be conducted. One such area is the examination of genetic factors involved in relapse. Due to advances in technology, genetic variations can be studied as they relate to relapse as well as how they relate to pharmacotherapy interventions used in combination with relapse prevention (Hendershot et al., 2011). For example, studies have shown that the OPRM1 A118G polymorphism serves as a moderator of clinical response to naltrexone, a medication for alcohol dependence (e.g., Oslin et al., 2003). By understanding the underlying genetic components that effect relapse and relapse prevention processes (e.g., pharmacotherapy efficacy), we can continue to improve existing relapse prevention treatments for a variety of problems and populations.

Another example of a way in which we can improve our understanding of relapse to improve relapse prevention is through the use of nonlinear methods and other advanced statistical techniques for modeling relapse. As noted earlier, Chow and colleagues (in press) recently applied a mixture structural equation model with regime switching to the study of drinking states during and following treatment. The model was particularly useful for explicitly testing the lagged effects of previous drinking on current drinking, as well as the role of person- and time-specific covariates to predict the probability of transitioning between lapses, prolapses, and relapses within and between subjects over time. Similarly, Witkiewitz (2011) tested a dynamic latent difference score model of proximal and distal risks in the prediction of heavy drinking during and following treatment, which allowed for changes in drinking to feed back into the system and impact changes in proximal risks.

These modeling approaches are particularly important when we consider designing treatment strategies that are customized to each individual's mechanisms of behavior change, which is a key concept behind adaptive care—an alternative treatment protocol that has generated considerable interest among researchers and applied practitioners in recent years. Closely related to the advent of adaptive care is the increased prevalence of studies aimed at delivering *momentary interventions* to individuals in their own environments (i.e., in real world) during times when treatments are most needed (i.e., in real time) by means of electronic devices. Timely delivery of interventions can be greatly enhanced by having an automated real-time prediction model that can provide clinicians and applied practitioners with direct insights into the timing for implementing interventions and identify individual-specific antecedents/precipitants that may trigger an impending lapse. Advances in analytic techniques for modeling relapse will improve these real-time prediction models.

Integrating technology into the treatment of addictive behaviors is another recent advance that could improve relapse prevention interventions. There are at least two primary means for improving relapse prevention interventions via technology: computerized treatment and mobile interventions. With advances in computing technology, a number of researchers have developed interventions that can be administered on computers or mobile devices (see review by Heron & Smyth, 2010; also see Carroll et al., 2008; Newman, Consoli, & Taylor, 1997; Norton, Wonderlich, Myers, Mitchell, & Crosby, 2003). There are many advantages of computerized interventions, including 24-hour availability, anonymity, portability, and accurate data recording (when assessment is combined with intervention).

One of the most noteworthy advantages of mobile interventions is the considerable benefit of sending and receiving information in real time. Specifically, daily monitoring of proximal influences on real-time behavior via a smartphone or tablet computer could provide the opportunity for targeted relapse prevention interventions.

The dynamic model of relapse proposes that individual risk factors are constantly changing and that small changes in the environment (e.g., seeing your friend drinking at your favorite bar) could predict large changes in behavior (e.g., heavy drinking after 5 months of abstinence). The application of a real-time intervention could be incredibly useful for helping individuals prevent an initial lapse or reduce the severity of a lapse after the initial transgression.

There are numerous future directions for relapse prevention, in addition to those mentioned earlier, with an important emphasis on expanding the scope and dissemination of evidence-based relapse prevention interventions. It is particularly important for future research to address the following issues in the adaptation and delivery of relapse prevention.

1. Are there added benefits of combining relapse prevention and other evidence-based treatments for continuing care? Recent research has found that combining relapse prevention with abstinence incentives as part of a contingency management aftercare program for cocaine use disorders yielded better outcomes (defined as higher abstinence rates) at 6- and 9-month follow-ups than treatment as usual or relapse prevention only (McKay et al., 2010). More research is needed to determine which combinations of treatments are most effective at reducing long-term relapse rates.

2. How can we improve the dissemination of evidence-based relapse prevention? The dissemination of evidence-based treatments into routine clinical practice settings has been a recognized struggle of the addiction field (McGovern, Fox, Xie, & Drake, 2004). Interestingly, "relapse prevention" is commonly used to describe components of treatment programs across numerous clinical settings (i.e., residential, outpatient), which is surprising given the initial negative reaction to the idea of relapse prevention when it was first introduced by Marlatt and his colleagues in the early 1980s (see Donovan & Witkiewitz, 2012, for a review). Yet what constitutes "relapse prevention" in community treatment settings can often be a mixed bag and is generally more consistent with psychoeducation and 12-step groups. More important, it has been observed that many clinicians report that they routinely use evidence-based practices, but whether evidence-based practices are implemented effectively is an important empirical question for future research (Carroll, 2012). In general, we need more research on the dissemination of effective implementation strategies for evidence-based relapse prevention interventions.

3. How can we tailor relapse prevention treatment using the dynamic model of relapse? As noted earlier, the revised version of Marlatt's original cognitive-behavioral model of relapse (on which relapse prevention is largely based), called the dynamic model of relapse (Witkiewitz & Marlatt, 2004), has clear heuristic value for its acknowledgment of relapse as a complex process. The dynamic model of relapse has been lauded by clinicians (e.g., Mitcheson et al., 2010) and supported by empirical analyses (Chow et al., in press; Witkiewitz, 2011); yet the translation of the dynamic model into a relapse prevention intervention has not been fully realized. Future research should be conducted that attempts to utilize the tenets of the dynamic model of relapse to improve the probabilities of preventing relapse as part of an individualized relapse prevention program. Such research is currently under way by our research group, and we hope other researchers will consider pursuing applications of the dynamic model of relapse to improve clinical practice.

Summary and Conclusions

The 30th anniversary of the publication of the original text on relapse prevention (Marlatt & Gordon, 1985) is fast approaching. In the past 30 years we have learned a lot about the relapse process and the field has come far in the implementation of relapse prevention interventions (see Donovan & Witkiewitz, 2012 for a historical review). Yet there is considerably more research that needs to be conducted on the adaptation of relapse prevention interventions for other behaviors and different populations. The dissemination of relapse prevention into new settings (e.g., primary care, mobile interventions) and the effective implementation of relapse prevention in standard treatment settings are critical next steps.

References

Andrews, D. A., & Carvell, C. (1998). *Core correctional training—core correctional supervisión and counseling: Theory, research, assessment, and practice.* Unpublished training manual Carleton University, Ottawa, Canada.

Anton, R. F., O'Malley, S. S., Ciraulo, D. A., Cisler, R. A., Couper, D., Donovan, D. M.,…COMBINE Study Research Group. (2006). Combined pharmacotherapies and behavioral interventions for alcohol dependence: The COMBINE Study: A randomized controlled trial. *Journal of the American Medical Association, 295,* 2003–2017. doi: 10.1001/jama.295.17.2003

Bandura, A. (1977). Self-efficacy: Toward a unifying theory of behavioral change. *Psychological Review, 84*(2), 191–215.

Barrick, C., & Connors, G. J. (2002). Relapse prevention and maintaining abstinence in older adults with alcohol-use disorders. *Drugs and Aging, 19*, 583–594. doi: 10.2165/00002512-200219080-00004

Blow, F. C, Brockmann, L. M., & Barry, K. L. (2007). Relapse prevention with older adults. In K. A. Witkiewitz & G. A. Marlatt (Eds.), *Therapist's guide to evidence-base relapse prevention* (pp. 313–352). San Diego, CA: Elsevier Academic.

Bowen, S., Chawla, N., Collins, S. E., Witkiewitz, K., Hsu, S., Grow, J.,…Marlatt, A. (2009). Mindfulness-based relapse prevention for substance use disorders: A pilot efficacy trial. *Substance Abuse, 30*(4), 295–305. doi: 10.1080/08897070903250084

Bowen, S., Chawla, N., & Marlatt, G. A. (2010). *Mindfulness-based relapse prevention for addictive behaviors: A clinician's guide.* New York: Guilford Press.

Bowen, S., Witkiewitz, K., Clifasefi, S., Grow, J., Chawla, N., Hsu, S.,…Larimer, M. E. (2014). Relative long-term efficacy of mindfulness-based relapse prevention, standard relapse prevention and treatment as usual for substance use disorders. *JAMA Psychiatry, 71*, 547–565.

Brandon, T. H., Vidrine, J. I., & Litvin, E. B. (2007). Relapse and relapse prevention. *Annual Review of Clinical Psychology, 3*, 257–284. doi: 10.1146/annurev.clinpsy.3.022806.091455

Brewer, J. A., Sinha, R., Chen, J. A., Michalsen, R. N., Babuscio, T. A., Nich, C.,…Rounsaville, B. J. (2009). Mindfulness training and stress reactivity in substance abuse: Results from a randomized, controlled stage I pilot study. *Substance Abuse, 30*, 306–317. doi: 10.1080/08897070903250241

Brown, M. Z., & Chapman, A. L. (2007). Stopping self-harm once and for all: Relapse prevetnion in dialectical behavior therapy. In K. A. Witkiewitz & G. A. Marlatt (Eds.), *Therapist's guide to evidence-base relapse prevention* (pp. 191–214). San Diego, CA: Elsevier Academic.

Carroll, K. M. (1996). Relapse prevention as a psychosocial treatment: A review of controlled clinical trials. *Experimental and Clinical Psychopharmacology, 4*(1), 46–54. doi: 10.1037/1064-1297.4.1.46

Carroll, K. M. (2012). Dissemination of evidence-based practices: How far we've come and how much further we've got to go. *Addiction, 107*, 1031–1033. doi: doi:10.1111/j.1360 0443.2011.03755.x

Carroll, K. M., Ball, S. A., Martino, S., Nich, C., Gordon, M. A., Portnoy, G. A., & Rounsaville, B. J. (2008). Computer-assisted delivery of cognitive behavioral therapy for addiction: A randomized trial of CBT4CBT. *American Journal of Psychiatry, 165*, 881–889. doi: 10.1176/appi.ajp.2008.07111835

Castro, F. G., Nichols, E., & Kater, K. (2007). Relapse prevention with Hispanic and other racial/ethnic populations: Can cultural resilience promote relapse prevention? In K. A. Witkiewitz & G. A. Marlatt (Eds.), *Therapist's guide to evidence-base relapse prevention* (pp. 259–292). San Diego, CA: Elsevier Academic.

Catalano, R. F., Gainey, R. R., Fleming, C. B., Haggerty, K. P., & Johnson, N. O. (1999). An experimental intervention with families of substance abusers: One-year follow-up of the Focus on Families project. *Addiction, 94*, 241–254. doi: 10.1046/j.1360-0443.1999.9422418.x

Catalano, R. F., Haggerty, K. P., Fleming, C. B., & Skinner, M. L. (2007). Focus on families: Integration of relapse prevention and child drug abuse with parents in methadone treatment. In K. A. Witkiewitz & G. A. Marlatt (Eds.), *Therapist's*

guide to evidence-base relapse prevention (pp. 237–257). San Diego, CA: Elsevier Academic.

Catalano, R. F., Haggerty, K. P., & Gainey, R. R. (2003). Prevention approaches in methadone treatment settings: Children of drug abuse treatment clients. In W. J. Bukoski & Z. Sloboda (Eds.), *Handbook of drug abuse prevention. Theory, science, and practice* (pp. 173–196). New York: Kluwer Academic/Plenum.

Catalano, R. F., Haggerty, K. P., Gainey, R. R., & Hoppe, M. J. (1997). Reducing parental risk factors for children's substance misuse: Preliminary outcomes with opiate-addicted parents. *Substance Use and Misuse, 32*, 699–721. doi: 10.3109/10826089709039371

Chow, S-M., Witkiewitz, K., Grasman, R., & Maisto, S. A. (in press). The cusp catastrophe model as cross-sectional and longitudinal mixture structure equation models. *Psychological Methods.*

Cramer, J. A., & Rosenheck, R. (1999). Enhancing medication compliance for people with serious mental illness. *Journal of Nervous and Mental Disease, 187*(1), 53–55. doi: 10.1097/00005053-199901000-00009

Daley, D. C., & Marlatt, G. A. (2006) *Overcoming your alcohol or drug problem: Effective recovery strategies* (2nd ed.). New York: Oxford University Press.

Dennis, M., Godley, S. H., Diamond, G., Tims, F. M., Babor, T., Donaldson, J.,…Funk, R. (2004). The cannabis youth treatment (CYT) study: Main findings from two randomized trials. *Journal of Substance Abuse Treatment, 27*, 197–213. doi: 10.1016/j.jsat.2003.09.005

Donovan, D. M. (2003) Relapse prevention in substance abuse treatment. In J. L. Sorensen, R. A. Rawson, J. Guydish, & J. E. Zweben (Eds.), *Drug abuse treatment through collaboration: Practice and research partnerships that work* (pp. 121–137). Washington, DC: American Psychological Association. doi: 10.1037/10491-008

Donovan, D. M., & Witkiewitz, K. (2012). Relapse prevention: From radical idea to common practice. *Addiction Research and Theory, 20*, 204–217. doi: 10.3109/16066359.2011.647133

Douaihy, A., Stowell, K. R., Park, T. W., & Daley, D. C. (2007). Relapse prevention: Clinical strategies for substance use disorders. In K. A. Witkiewitz & G. A. Marlatt (Eds.), *Therapist's guide to evidence-base relapse prevention* (pp. 37–72). San Diego, CA: Elsevier Academic.

Dowden, C., & Andrews, D. A. (2004). The importance of staff practice in delivering effective correctional treatment: A meta-analytic analysis. *International Journal of Offender Therapy and Comparative Criminology, 48*, 203–214. doi: 10.1177/0306624X03257765

Dowden, C., & Andrews, D. A. (2007). Utilizing relapse prevention with offender populations: What works. In K. A. Witkiewitz & G. A. Marlatt (Eds.), *Therapist's guide to evidence-base relapse prevention* (pp. 339–352). San Diego, CA: Elsevier Academic.

Dugas, M. J., Rodomsky, A. S., & Brillon P. (2004). Tertiary intervention for anxiety and prevention of relapse. In D. J. A. Dozois & K. S. Dobson (Eds.), *The prevention of anxiety and depression: Theory, research, and practice* (pp. 161–184). Washington, DC: American Psychological Association.

Fairburn, C. G. (1995). *Overcoming binge eating.* New York: Guilford Press.

Fiore, M. C. (2000). A clinical practice guideline for treating tobacco use and dependence: A US Public Health Service

Report. *Journal of the American Medical Association, 283,* 3244–3254. doi: 10.1001/jama.283.24.3244

Gould, R. A., & Otto, M. W. (1996). Cognitive-behavioral treatment of social phobia and generalized anxiety disorder. In M. H. Pollac, M. W. Otto, & J. F. Rosenbaum (Eds.), *Challenges in clinical practice: Pharamacologic and psychosocial strategies* (pp. 171–200). New York: Guilford Press.

Hendershot, C. S., Witkiewitz, K., George, W. H., & Marlatt, G. A. (2011). Relapse prevention for addictive behaviors. *Substance Abuse Treatment, Prevention, and Policy, 6*(17), 1–17. doi: 10.1186/1747-597X-6-17

Heron, K., & Smyth, J. M. (2010). Ecological momentary interventions: Incorporating mobile technology into psychosocial and health behavior treatments. *British Journal of Health Psychology, 15,* 1–39. doi: 10.1348/135910709X466063

Herz, M. I., Lamberti, J. S., Mintz, J., Scott, R., O'Dell, S. P., McCartan, L., & Nix, G. (2000). A program for relapse prevention in schizophrenia: A controlled study. *Archives of General Psychiatry, 57,* 277–283. doi: 10.1001/archpsyc.57.3.277

Hughes, J. R., Keely, J. P., & Naud, S. (2004). Shape of the relapse curve and long-term abstinence among untreated smokers. *Addiction, 99,* 29–38. doi: 10.1111/j.1360-0443.2004.00540.x

Hunter-Reel, D., McCrady, B., & Hildebrandt, T. (2009). Emphasizing interpersonal factors: an extension of the Witkiewitz and Marlatt relapse model. *Addiction, 104,* 1281–1290. doi: 10.1111/j.1360-0443.2009.02611.x

Irvin, J. E., Bowers, C. A., Dunn, M. E., & Wang, M. C. (1999). Efficacy of relapse prevention: A meta-analytic review. *Journal of Counsulting and Clinical Psychology, 67,* 563–570. doi: 10.1037//0022-006X.67.4.563

Kadden, R. M. (1996). Is Marlatt's relapse taxonomy reliable or valid? *Addiction, 91* (Suppl), S139–S145. doi: 10.1111/j.1360-0443.1996.tb02334.x

Kilmer, J. R., Cronce, J. M., & Palmer, R. S. (2005). Relapse prevention for abuse of club drugs, hallucinogens, inhalants, and steroids. In G. A. Marlatt & D. M. Donovan (Eds.), *Relapse prevention* (2nd ed., pp. 208–247). New York: Guilford Press.

Lam, D. H., Bright, J., Jones, S., Hayward, P., Schuck, N., Chisholm, D., & Sham, P. (2000). Cognitive therapy for bipolar illness-a pilot study of relapse prevention. *Cognitive Therapy and Research, 24,* 503–520. doi: 10.1023/A:1005557911051

Lau, M. A., & Segal, Z. V. (2007). Mindfulness-based cognitive therapy as a relapse prevention approach to depression. In K. A. Witkiewitz & G. A. Marlatt (Eds.), *Therapist's guide to evidence-base relapse prevention* (pp. 73–90). San Diego, CA: Elsevier Academic.

Laws, D. R. (1995). Central elements in relapse prevention procedures with sex offenders. *Psychology, Crime and Law, 2,* 41–53. doi: 10.1080/10683169508409763

Laws, D. R. (1999). Relapse prevention: The state of the art. *Journal of Interpersonal Violence, 14,* 285–302. doi: 10.1177/088626099014003005

Laws, D. R. (2000). Relapse prevention: Reconceptualization and revision. In C. R. Hollin (Ed.), *Handbook of offender assessment and treatment* (pp. 297–307). Chichester, UK: Wiley.

Laws, D. R. (2003). The rise and fall of relapse prevention. *Australian Psychologist, 38,* 22–30. doi: 10.1080/00050060310001706987

Liberman, R. P., & Kopelowicz, A. (2005). Recovery from schizophrenia: A concept in search of research. *Psychiatric Services, 56*(6), 735–742.

Lowman, C., Allen, J., & Stout, R. L. (1996). Replication and extension of Marlatt's taxonomy of relapse precipitants: Overview of procedures and results. *Addiction, 91*(12), S51–S71. doi: 10.1111/j.1360-0443.1996.tb02327.x

Ma, S. H., & Teasdale, J. D. (2004). Mindfulness-based cognitive therapy for depression: Replication and exploration of differential relapse prevention effects. *Journal of Consulting and Clinical Psychology, 72,* 31–40. doi: 10.1037/0022-006X.72.1.31

Marlatt, G. A., & Gordon, J. R. (1984). Relapse prevention: Introduction and overview of the model. *British Journal of Addictions, 79,* 261–273. doi: 10.1111/j.1360-0443.1984.tb00274.x

Marlatt, G. A., & Gordon, J. R. (1985). *Relapse prevention: Maintenance strategies in the treatment of addictive behaviors.* New York: Guilford Press.

Marlatt, G. A., & Marques, J. K. (1977). Meditation, self-control, and alcohol use. In R. B. Stuart (Ed.), *Behavioral self-management* (pp. 117–153). New York: Brunner/Mazel.

Marlatt, G. A., Parks, G. A., & Witkiewitz, K. (2002). *Clinical guidelines for implementing relapse prevention therapy.* Peoria, IL: Behavioral Health Recovery Management Project.

McCarthy, B. W. (2001). Relapse prevention strategies and techniques with erectile dysfunction. *Journal of Sex and Marital Therapy, 27,* 1–8. doi: 10.1080/00926230152035804

McGovern, M. P., Fox, T. S., Xie, H., & Drake, R. E. (2004). A survey of clinical practices and readiness to adopt evidence-based practices: Dissemination research in an addiction treatment system. *Journal of Substance Abuse Treatment, 26,* 305–312. doi: 10.1016/j.jsat.2004.03.003

McKay, J. R., Lynch, K. G., Coviello, D., Morrison, R., Cary, M. S., Skalina, L., & Plebani, J. (2010). Randomized trial of continuing care enhancements for cocaine-dependent patients following initial engagement. *Journal of Consulting and Clinical Psychology, 78,* 111–120. doi: 10.1037/a0018139

Miller, G. (2010). *Learning the language of addiction counseling.* Hoboken, NJ: Wiley.

Mitchell, K., & Carr, A. (2001). Anorexia and bulimia. In A. Carr (Ed.), *What works for children and adolescents? A critical review of psychological interventions with children* (pp. 233–257). London: Routledge.

Mitcheson, L., Maslin, J., Meynen, T., Morrison, T., Hill, R., & Wanigaratne, S. (2010). *Applied cognitive and behavioral approaches to the treatment of addiction.* Hoboken, NJ: Wiley.

Monti, P. M., Kadden, R. M., Rohsenow, D. J., Cooney, N. L., & Abrams, D. B. (2002) *Treating alcohol dependence. A coping skills training guide* (2nd ed.). New York: Guilford Press.

Mueser, K. T., Corrigan, P. W., Hilton, D. W., Tanzman, B., Schaub, A., Gingerich, S., … Herz, M. I. (2002). Illness management and recovery: A review of the research. *Psychiatric Services, 20,* 253–262. doi: 10.1176/appi.ps.53.10.1272

Najavits, L. M. (2002). *Seeking safety: A treatment manual for PTSD and substance abuse.* New York: Guilford Press.

Najavits, L. M. (2007). Seeking safety: An evidence-based model for substance abuse and trauma/PTSD. In K. A. Witkiewitz & G. A. Marlatt (Eds.), *Therapist's guide to evidence-base relapse prevention* (pp. 141–167). San Diego, CA: Elsevier Academic.

Newman, M. G., Consoli, A., & Taylor, C. B. (1997). Computers in the assessment and cognitive-behavioral treatment of clinical disorders: Anxiety as a case in point. *Behavior Therapy, 28*, 211–235. doi: 10.1016/S0005-7894(97)80044-5

Norton, M., Wonderlich, S. A., Myers, T., Mitchell, J. E., & Crosby, R. D. (2003). The use of palmtop computers in the treatment of bulimia nervosa. *European Eating Disorders Review, 11*, 231–242. doi: 10.1002/erv.518

Oslin, D. W., Berrettini, W., Kranzler, H. R., Pettinati, H., Gelernter, J., Volpicelli, J. R., & O'Brien, C. P. (2003). A functional polymorphism of the mu-opioid receptor gene is associated with naltrexone response in alcohol-dependent patients. *Neuropsychopharmacology, 28*, 1546–1552. doi: 10.1038/sj.npp.1300219

Oslin, D. W., Slaymaker, V. J., Blow, F. C., Owen, P. L., & Colleran, C. (2005). Treatment outcomes for alcoho dependence among middle-aged and older adults. *Addictive Behaviors, 30*, 1431–1436. doi: 10.1016/j.addbeh.2005.01.007

Ramo, D. E., Myers, M. G., & Brown, S. A. (2007). Relapse prevention for adolescent substance abuse: Overview and case examples. In K. A. Witkiewitz & G. A. Marlatt (Eds.), *Therapist's guide to evidence-base relapse prevention* (pp. 293–312). San Diego, CA: Elsevier Academic.

Schlam, T. R., & Wilson, G. T. (2007). Relapse prevention for eating disorders. In K. A. Witkiewitz & G. A. Marlatt (Eds.), *Therapist's guide to evidence-base relapse prevention* (pp. 169–190). San Diego, CA: Elsevier Academic.

Stanton, M. (2005). Relapse prevention needs more emphasis on interpersonal factors. *American Psychologist, 60*, 340–341. doi: 10.1037/0003-066X.60.4.340

Teasdale, J. D., Segal, Z. V., Williams, J. M. G., Ridgeway, V. A., Soulsby, J. M., & Lau, M. A. (2000). Prevention of relapse/recurrence in major depression by mindfulness-based cognitive therapy. *Journal of Consulting and Clinical Psychology, 68*, 615–623. doi: 10.1037/0022-006X.68.4.615

Vieten, C., Astin, J. A., Buscemi, R., & Galloway, G. P. (2010). Development of an acceptance-based coping intervention for alcohol dependence relapse prevention. *Substance Abuse, 31*, 108–116. doi: 10.1080/08897071003641594

Whiteside, U., Nguyen, T., Logan, D. E., Fagan, C., Marlatt, G. A., & Witkiewitz, K. (2007). Relapse prevention for return of pathological worry in CBT-treated GAD. In K. A. Witkiewitz & G. A. Marlatt (Eds.), *Therapist's guide to evidence-base relapse prevention* (pp. 91–116). San Diego, CA: Elsevier Academic.

Witkiewitz, K. (2011). Predictors of heavy drinking during and following treatment. *Psychology of Addictive Behaviors, 25*, 426–438. doi: 10.1037/a0022889

Witkiewitz, K., & Marlatt, G. A. (2004). Relapse prevention for alcohol and drug problems: That was zen, this is tao. *American Psychologist, 59*(4), 224–235. doi: 10.1037/0003-066X.59.4.224

Witkiewitz, K., & Marlatt, G. A. (2007). Overview of relapse prevetnion. In K. A. Witkiewitz & G. A. Marlatt (Eds.), *Therapist's guide to evidence-base relapse prevention* (pp. 3–17). San Diego, CA: Elsevier Academic.

Witkiewitz, K., Marlatt, G. A., & Walker, D. (2005). Mindfulness-based relapse prevention for alcohol and substance use disorders. *Journal of Cognitive Psychotherap, 19*(3), 211–228. doi: 10.1891/jcop.2005.19.3.211

Witkiewitz, K., & Villarroel, N. (2009). Dynamic association between negative affect and alcohol lapses following alcohol treatment. *Journal of Consulting and Clinical Psychology, 77*, 633–644. doi: 10.1037/a0015647

Witkiewitz, K., Villarroel, N. A., Hartzler, B., & Donovan, D. M. (2011). Drinking outcomes following drink refusal skills training: Differential effects for African American and non-Hispanic white clients. *Psychology of Addictive Behaviors, 25*, 162–167. doi: 10.1037/a0022254

Witkiewitz, K., Warner, K., Sully, B., Barricks, A., Stauffer, C., Steckler, G., … Luoma, J. (2014). Randomized trial comparing mindfulness based relapse prevention with relapse prevention for women offenders at a residential addiction treatment center. *Substance Use and Misuse, 49*, 536–546. doi: 10.3109/10826084.2013.856922

Yates, P. M. (2005). Pathways to the treatment of sexual offenders: Rethinking intervention. *Forum, Summer*, 1–9.

Yates, P. M., & Ward, T. (2007). Treatment of sexual offenders: Relapse prevention and beyond. In K. A. Witkiewitz & G. A. Marlatt (Eds.), *Therapist's guide to evidence-base relapse prevention* (pp. 215–234). San Diego, CA: Elsevier Academic.

Ziedonis, D., Yanos, P. T., & Silverstein, S. M. (2007). Relapse prevention for schizophrenia. In K. A. Witkiewitz & G. A. Marlatt (Eds.), *Therapist's guide to evidence-base relapse prevention* (pp. 117–140). San Diego, CA: Elsevier Academic.

Zgierska, A., Rabago, D., Chawla, N., Kushner, K., Koehler, R., & Marlatt, A. (2009). Mindfulness meditation for substance use disorders: A systematic review. *Substance Abuse, 30*(4), 266–294. doi: 10.1080/08897070903250019

Zgierska, A., Rabago, D., Zuelsdorff, M., Miller, M., Coe, C., & Fleming, M. F. (2008). Mindfulness meditation for relapse prevention in alcohol dependence: A feasibility pilot study. *Journal of Addiction Medicine, 2*, 165–173. doi: 10.1097/ADM.0b013e31816f8546

Behavioral Activation

Derek R. Hopko, Marlena M. Ryba, Crystal McIndoo, *and* Audrey File

Abstract

Considered a third-wave behavior therapy, behavioral activation is a therapeutic process emphasizing structured attempts to increase overt behaviors likely to bring patients into contact with reinforcing environmental contingencies and corresponding improvements in thoughts, mood, and quality of life. In the past two decades, behavioral activation has emerged as an empirically supported treatment for depression that has effectively been provided to patients with diverse clinical presentations and in multiple therapeutic contexts. This chapter focuses on providing a brief historical context of behavioral activation, a description of the principles and procedures underlying contemporary behavioral activation therapies, a review of assessment strategies particularly relevant to this approach, a comprehensive analysis of treatment outcome studies, and a presentation of limitations and future directions that need to be addressed to further solidify the status of behavioral activation as an effective and feasible approach to treating clinical depression and other mental health problems.

Key Words: behavioral activation, behavior principles, assessment, treatment outcome review, clinical depression

The National Comorbidity Survey (NCS-R) suggested that major depression has a lifetime prevalence of 16% and 12-month prevalence of 7%, is associated with substantial life impairment, and adequate treatment occurs for less than 50% of individuals with depression (Kessler et al., 2003; Wang et al., 2005). Although there are many factors associated with this problem and the dissemination of efficacious and parsimonious treatments for depression in general (Collins, Westra, Dozois, & Burns, 2004; Voelker, 2003), one of the primary barriers is a lack of relatively uncomplicated and highly transportable interventions that have the potential to be administered by a variety of mental health and medical practitioners. Recent depression treatment outcome research shows that briefer and less complicated behavioral activation interventions might be as effective in reducing depression as more elaborate cognitive-behavioral approaches, making them a viable option toward resolving this

issue (Dimidjian et al., 2006; Hopko et al., 2011; Jacobson et al., 1996). Although the term *behavioral activation* is rooted in the biological basis of behavior (Gray, 1982), behavioral activation as a therapeutic process refers to structured attempts to increase overt behaviors likely to bring patients into contact with reinforcing environmental contingencies and produce corresponding improvements in thoughts, mood, and overall quality of life (Hopko, Lejuez, Ruggiero, & Eifert, 2003). Beginning with the pioneering work of Peter Lewinsohn and colleagues (Lewinsohn, 1974; Lewinsohn & Graf, 1973; Lewinsohn, Sullivan, & Grosscup, 1980), revitalized by the cognitive-behavioral therapy component analysis study (Jacobson et al., 1996), and culminating in its current status as an empirically validated treatment for depression (Cuijpers, van Straten, & Warmerdam, 2007; Ekers, Richards, & Gilbody, 2008; Mazzucchelli, Kane, & Rees, 2009; Sturmey, 2009), behavioral activation interventions have gained prominent status as an effective treatment modality across a range of clinical samples and settings. This chapter focuses on providing a brief historical context of behavioral activation, a description of the principles and procedures underlying contemporary behavioral activation therapies, a review of assessment strategies particularly relevant to this approach, a comprehensive analysis of treatment outcome studies, and a presentation of limitations and future directions that will need to be addressed to further solidify the status of behavioral activation as an effective and feasible approach to treating clinical depression and other mental health problems in a variety of clinical contexts.

Historical Context of Behavioral Activation

As highlighted in previous works (Dimidjian, Barrera, Martell, Munoz, & Lewinsohn, 2011; Hopko, Lejuez et al., 2003; Jacobson, Martell, & Dimidjian, 2001), the basic conceptual foundation for behavioral activation can be traced back to original behavioral models of depression that implicated decreases in response-contingent reinforcement for nondepressive behavior as the causal factor in eliciting depressive affect (Ferster, 1973; Lewinsohn, 1974; Lewinsohn & Graf, 1973). Detailed historical accounts of the evolution of behavioral activation have been nicely articulated (Jacobson et al., 2001; Kanter, Manos, et al., 2010; Martell, Addis, & Jacobson, 2001), including an interesting narrative depicting its initial development in the laboratory of Peter Lewinsohn at the University of Oregon (Dimidjian et al., 2011). Although Peter Lewinsohn should be considered the father of behavioral activation, his work was clearly influenced by B. F. Skinner, who initially proposed that depression was associated with an interruption of established sequences of healthy behavior that had been positively reinforced by the social environment (Skinner, 1953). In subsequent expansions of this model, the reduction of positively reinforced healthy behavior was attributed to a decrease in the number and range of reinforcing stimuli available to an individual for such behavior, a lack of skill in obtaining reinforcement, and/or an increased frequency of punishment (Lewinsohn, 1974; Lewinsohn, Antonuccio, Breckenridge, & Teri, 1984; Lewinsohn & Shaffer, 1971).

A functional analytic view of this paradigm suggests that continued engagement of depressed behavior must result from some combination of reinforcement for depressed behavior and/or a lack of reinforcement or even punishment of more healthy alternative behavior (Ferster, 1973; Hopko, Lejuez et al., 2003; Kanfer & Grimm, 1977; Kazdin, 1977). As degree of social reinforcement was an integral component of Lewinsohn's model (1974), it was also indicated that although depressed affect and behavior could initially be maintained through positive social reinforcement, depressed behavior also could ultimately result in aversive social consequences in the form of negative responses from significant others (Coyne, 1976). Accordingly, this behavioral model of depression highlighted the quantitative (number, level of gratification) and qualitative (type, function) aspects of reinforcing events, their availability, and an individual's instrumental behaviors as critical toward decreased levels of response-contingent positive reinforcement, particularly as it pertained to one's social environment (and related social avoidance). Using a number of research designs, these fundamental assertions generally have been strongly supported. For example, using home observations (Lewinsohn & Shaffer, 1971; Lewinsohn & Shaw, 1969) and self-monitoring paradigms (Grosscup & Lewinsohn, 1980; Lewinsohn & Graf, 1973; Lewinsohn & Libet, 1972), it was demonstrated that depressed mood was related to decreased positive reinforcement for healthy behaviors and less engagement in pleasurable activities. In a recent daily diary study, self-reported depression was inversely related to general activity level as well as the amount of reward or pleasure obtained through overt behaviors (Hopko, Armento, Cantu, Chambers, & Lejuez, 2003). Another study showed that mildly depressed college students also engaged less frequently in social, physical, and educational behaviors (Hopko & Mullane, 2008).

In terms of other model assertions, several studies demonstrated that depressed mood also was associated with an increased frequency of aversive events and experiences (Grosscup & Lewinsohn, 1980; Lewinsohn & Talkington, 1979; MacPhillamy & Lewinsohn, 1974; Rehm, 1977). Also supporting Lewinsohn's emphasis on decreased social reinforcement as a catalyst for depression, several studies highlighted the premise that social behaviors of depressed individuals were less likely to be reinforced relative to nondepressed individuals (Libet & Lewinsohn, 1973; Lewinsohn & Shaffer, 1971; Rehm, 1988; Youngren & Lewinsohn, 1980). Important to acknowledge, although it has accurately been pointed out that conclusions regarding the causal relationship between decreased response-contingent positive reinforcement and depression is limited due to the unavailability of statistical mediation analyses decades ago (Dimidjian et al., 2011), at least two recent studies support this causal association (Carvalho & Hopko, 2011; Carvalho, Trent, & Hopko, 2011). Similarly, although decreased social skills and diminished social reinforcement have been associated with depression (Dimidjian et al., 2011; Segrin, 2000), support for the causal link is equivocal (Segrin, 1999, 2000).

Behavioral Theory into Practice

Based on behavioral theories of depression, conventional behavioral therapy for depression was aimed at increasing access to pleasant events and positive reinforcers as well as decreasing the intensity and frequency of aversive events and consequences (Lewinsohn & Graf, 1973; Lewinsohn, Sullivan, & Grosscup, 1980; Sanchez, Lewinsohn, & Larson, 1980). In these pioneering efforts to examine the efficacy of behavioral activation strategies, Lewinsohn and colleagues demonstrated that through daily monitoring of pleasant/unpleasant events and corresponding mood states as well as behavioral interventions that included activity scheduling, social skills development, and time management training, depressive symptoms often were alleviated. Importantly, these early studies documented the potential efficacy of activation-based approaches in multiple contexts, including individual, group, family, and marital therapy settings (Brown & Lewinsohn, 1984; Lewinsohn & Atwood, 1969; Lewinsohn & Shaffer, 1971; Lewinsohn & Shaw, 1969; Zeiss, Lewinsohn, & Munoz, 1979). The study by Brown and Lewinsohn (1984) found that the efficacy of individual, group, and minimal contact (telephone) conditions was superior to a delayed contact control condition. Fundamental behavioral activation strategies (i.e., pleasant event scheduling) also were as effective as cognitive and interpersonal skills training approaches in treating depressed outpatients (Zeiss et al., 1979). Based on several of these early studies, what could be considered the first behavioral activation treatment manual was developed (Lewinsohn, Biglan, & Zeiss, 1976).

As support for behavioral therapies for depression accumulated, increased attention was being given to biological, interpersonal, and cognitive factors as etiologically associated with depression. For example, with increased interest in cognitive theory in the latter quarter of the twentieth century, interventions based exclusively on operant and respondent principles, once thought adequate, were viewed as insufficient, and the absence of direct cognitive

manipulations was widely regarded as a limitation of behavioral treatment. These changing perspectives, along with three highly influential studies, contributed to the de-emphasis of purely behavioral interventions as stand-alone treatments. In the first of these studies, Hammen and Glass (1975) demonstrated that mild to moderately depressed college students who increased their participation in events they had rated as pleasurable did not become less depressed. Second, Shaw (1977) published a multimethod assessment study with depressed college students and suggested the potential superiority of cognitive techniques over behavioral strategies in attenuating depression symptoms. In a third study published 2 years later, a component analysis revealed no differential effectiveness between activity scheduling, skills training, and cognitive techniques (Zeiss et al., 1979). In response to these studies and the changing zeitgeist that reflected a more integrative multidimensional model of depression, purely behavioral interventions generally were abandoned in favor of more comprehensive cognitive-behavioral approaches (Lewinsohn, Hoberman, Teri, & Hautzinger, 1985). The increasing popularity of cognitive therapy culminated in its inclusion (and exclusion of behavioral therapy) in the Treatment of Depression Collaborative Research Program (TDCRP; Elkin et al., 1989) funded by the National Institute of Health. This transition stated, however, the distinction among interventions for depression considered purely "cognitive" or "behavioral" has become blurred because of their significant conceptual and technical overlap (Barlow, Allen, & Choate, 2004; Hollon, 2001). Indeed, cognitive strategies have been integrated into more traditional behavioral approaches (Fuchs & Rehm, 1977; Rehm, 1977; Lewinsohn et al., 1980, 1984; Lewinsohn & Clarke, 1999; Lewinsohn, Munoz, Youngren, & Zeiss, 1986) and vice versa (Beck, Rush, Shaw, & Emery, 1979).

Despite the documented efficacy of cognitive and cognitive-behavioral therapies for depression (DeRubeis & Crits-Christoph, 1998; Hollon & Ponniah, 2010; Hollon, Thase, & Markowitz, 2002; Westen & Morrison, 2001), several recent findings along with evolving socioeconomic and professional developments raise the question as to whether "purely" behavioral approaches to treating clinical depression were abandoned too hastily. For example, managed care organizations and academic counseling centers have established the need to develop and utilize psychosocial interventions that are both time limited and empirically validated

(Peak & Barusch, 1999; Voelker, 2003), which are features typifying the behavioral model. Second, empirical data from carefully conducted clinical studies demonstrate that cognitive change may be just as likely to occur using environment-based manipulations or cognitive interventions (Jacobson et al., 1996; Jacobson & Gortner, 2000; Simons, Garfield, & Murphy, 1984; Zeiss et al., 1979). Third, it has been demonstrated that behavioral activation interventions have been effective with even difficult-to-treat medical and psychiatric samples (Dimidjian et al., 2006; Ekers, Richards, McMillan, Bland, & Gilbody, 2011; Hopko et al., 2011; MacPherson et al., 2010; Pagoto et al., 2008). Fourth, therapeutic benefits of cognitive-behavioral treatment packages for depression most often occur in the initial sessions of the treatment course (Hopko, Robertson, & Carvalho, 2009), a period in which behavioral components often are more prominent (Hollon, Shelton, & Davis, 1993; Otto, Pava, & Sprich-Buckminster, 1996). In response to these issues, research programs have continued to evolve that evaluate the feasibility, effectiveness, and efficacy of purely behavioral interventions for depression.

Contemporary Behavioral Activation Strategies

The revitalization of behavioral approaches to treating depression has been most evident in the development of two new interventions: behavioral activation (BA; Martell et al., 2001) and the brief behavioral activation treatment for depression (BATD; Lejuez, Hopko, & Hopko, 2001; BATD-R; Lejuez, Hopko, Acierno, Daughters, & Pagoto, 2011). Although these treatment protocols utilize somewhat different strategies, both are based on traditional behavioral models of the etiology and treatment of depression (Ferster, 1973; Lewinsohn, 1974) and to a greater or lesser degree include conventional behavioral therapy strategies designed to increase response-contingent positive reinforcement. These strategies include increasing pleasant or rewarding events, teaching relaxation skills, social and problem-solving skill training, contingency management, decreasing behavioral avoidance, and the incorporation of cognitive-behavioral methods such as self-instructional training and rumination-cued activation (Antonuccio, Ward, & Tearnan, 1991; Hersen, Bellack, Himmelhock, & Thase, 1984; Lewinsohn et al., 1986; Nezu, Nezu, & Perri, 1989). These treatment components, sometimes enhanced using exposure-based therapy techniques for coexistent anxiety conditions (Hopko et al., 2011; Hopko, Robertson, & Lejuez, 2006; Jakupcak et al., 2006), collectively fall under the rubric of behavioral activation.

Although contemporary behavioral activation approaches are consistent with the original etiological formulation and treatment approaches, these newer protocols entail important advancements over early behavioral approaches. First, current activation approaches are more idiographic, giving more attention to unique environmental contingencies maintaining depressed behavior, and in the case of BATD also incorporate an individualized life areas and value assessment (LAVA) that provides the foundation for activity identification and structured activation. Second, there has been a concerted movement from targeting pleasant events alone (Lewinsohn & Graf, 1973) toward understanding the *functional* aspects of behavior change (Martell et al., 2001). So rather than increasing exposure to events and behaviors presumed to be pleasant or rewarding, this functional analytic approach involves a detailed assessment of contingencies maintaining depressive behavior, idiographic assessment of patient values and goals, and the subsequent targeting of behavior that functionally is likely to attenuate depressive affect and improve quality of life. Accordingly, the appropriateness of any particular behavioral change is determined by ongoing assessment of whether the frequency and/or duration of that behavior increases over time and leads to a corresponding reduction in depressive symptoms. Although this process may involve several strategies as outlined earlier, the critical mechanism of change is to decrease avoidance behavior and increase reward via principles of extinction, fading, shaping, and differential reinforcement of healthy behaviors (Hopko, Lejuez, et al., 2003). Third, as elucidated in other works (Manos, Kanter, & Busch, 2010), unlike traditional behavioral treatments, BA focuses significantly more on the role of negative reinforcement in maintaining depressive symptoms. Consistent with the perspective that individuals with depression often experience aversive or punitive environmental events and stimuli, negative affect resulting from such experiences may result in extreme escape and avoidance behavior that cyclically may exacerbate depression and further increase the likelihood of avoidance behavior. Important to highlight, however, at this stage of research, behavioral activation methods more strongly focus on increasing response-contingent positive reinforcement and in a much less structured manner address aversive environmental events and the "deactivation" of patient behaviors that may elicit such events.

Fourth, behavioral activation approaches are unique from traditional behavior therapy in that along with dialectical behavior therapy (DBT; Linehan, 1993), acceptance and commitment therapy (ACT; Hayes, Strosahl, & Wilson, 1999), functional analytic psychotherapy (FAP; Kohlenberg & Tsai, 1991), mindfulness-based therapy (MBT; Kabat-Zinn, 1990; Segal, Williams, & Teasdale, 2002), and the cognitive-behavioral analysis system of psychotherapy (CBASP; McCullough, 2000), behavioral activation adheres to principles consistent with *third-wave behavioral therapies*. Where first- and second-wave therapies focused primarily on behavior modification of immediate problems, third-wave methods emphasize the broad constructs of values, spirituality, relationships, and mindfulness. Indeed, when the acceptance and mindfulness-based philosophies of behavioral activation are recognized in the context of emphasizing value-based behavior, and through overt behavioral change, reducing the discrepancy between the perceived and ideal self, it is not unreasonable to suggest behavioral activation shares many fundamental assertions of traditional humanistic therapy (Rogers, 1951). On many levels, activating is congruent with strides toward self-actualization. Third-wave behavioral therapy is particularly sensitive to the context and functions of psychological phenomena, not just their form, and thus tend to emphasize contextual and experiential change strategies in addition to more direct and didactic ones (Hayes, 2004). So where a second-wave cognitive-behavior therapist might identify and restructure cognitive errors, a third-wave therapist might focus more on encouraging patients to understand and accept the cognitions, learn their function, and how they associate with the patient's value system. Accordingly, differing from early behavioral therapies for depression, behavior activation is much more focused on a balanced acceptance-change model (Hayes, Strosahl, & Wilson, 1999). Based on this paradigm, behavioral activation partially involves teaching patients to formulate and accomplish behavioral goals irrespective of certain aversive thoughts and mood states they may experience. This focus on action makes it unnecessary to attempt to control and change such thoughts and mood states directly, as was more common with traditional behavioral interventions (Lewinsohn, Munoz et al., 1986; Rehm, 1977). Instead, changes in patterns of overt behavior are likely to coincide with changes in thoughts and mood, in most instances following rather than preceding behavior change.

Behavior activation models acknowledge that there continues to be significant controversy surrounding cause-effect relations among biological, cognitive, and behavioral components in the etiology and maintenance of depression (Eifert, Beach, & Wilson, 1998; Hopko, Lejuez et al., 2003; Martell et al., 2001; Plaud, 2001). As with other pathogenic models of depression, the importance of cognition in the genesis and maintenance of depression is acknowledged in activation-based approaches, but cognitions are not regarded as proximal causes of overt behavior to be targeted directly for change. Thus, behavioral activation procedures address cognitions and emotions indirectly by bringing the individual into contact with more positive consequences for overt behavior. In doing so, behavioral activation addresses the environmental constituent of depressive affect, a component deemed more external, observable, measurable, and capable of being modified. Finally, relative to traditional behavioral therapies, contemporary behavioral activation approaches are designed to more systematically address coexistent anxiety conditions (Hopko, Robertson, & Lejuez, 2006). In large part due to high rates of comorbidity and shared symptom patterns (Barlow, Allen, & Choate, 2004; Kessler et al., 2003), the contention has been made that heterogeneity of anxiety and depressive symptom patterns is but an inconsequential variant of what is more importantly a broader general neurotic or negative affect syndrome (Barlow, 2002; Barlow et al., 2004). Based on this functional analytic framework in which depressive and anxiety-based symptom patterns are viewed as conceptually parallel, behavioral avoidance is targeted within behavioral activation both as a means to increase response-contingent positive reinforcement and systematically extinguish anxiety-related fears and phobias. For a comprehensive review of treatment components of traditional and contemporary behavioral activation interventions, as well as a thoughtful discussion of the construct of behavioral activation and whether effective psychotherapies such as self-control therapy (Rehm, 1977) should fall under this category, the reader is referred to the work of Jonathan Kanter and colleagues (2010).

BA or Washington BA

BA directly evolved from a component analysis study comparing cognitive-behavioral therapy for depression, behavioral activation supplemented with automatic thought restructuring, and behavioral activation alone. Data indicated that the behavioral activation condition was just as effective as the comprehensive intervention in terms of both overall treatment outcome and the modification of negative thinking and dysfunctional attributional styles (Jacobson et al., 1996). Longer term maintenance of gains also was noted in that at 24-month follow-up, BA and the comprehensive cognitive-behavioral treatment were equally effective in preventing relapse (Gortner, Gollan, Dobson, & Jacobson, 1998). Predictor analyses indicated that positive outcome of BA was associated with pretreatment expectancies and inversely related to "reason giving," or the tendency to offer multiple explanations with respect to the etiology and maintenance of depression (Addis & Jacobson, 1996). Several years later, a BA treatment manual was published that clearly highlighted the underlying philosophy and treatment components of BA (Addis & Martell, 2004; Martell et al., 2001). The focus of BA is on the evolving transactions between the person and environment over time and the identification of environmental triggers and ineffective coping responses involved in the etiology and maintenance of depression (Martell et al., 2001). Much like traditional behavioral therapy, this approach conceptualizes depressed behavior (e.g., inactivity, withdrawal) as a coping strategy to avoid environmental circumstances that provide low levels of positive reinforcement or high levels of aversive control (Jacobson et al., 2001). Behavioral avoidance is central to the BA treatment model. Within the context of a collaborative patient–therapist relationship, the initial treatment objective is to increase patient awareness of how internal and external events (triggers) result in a negative emotional (response) that may effectively establish a recurrent avoidance pattern (i.e., TRAP; trigger, response, avoidance pattern). Once this pattern is recognized, the principal therapeutic objective is to assist the patient in reengaging in healthy behaviors through the development of alternative coping strategies (i.e., TRAC; trigger, response, alternative coping).

Along with increased patient awareness and progression from a TRAP- to TRAC-based coping philosophy, BA involves teaching patients to take ACTION. To reduce escape and avoidance behavior, patients are taught to assess the function of their behavior, and then to make an informed choice as to whether to continue escaping and avoiding or instead engage in behavior that may improve their mood, integrate such behavior into their lifestyle, and never give up. Additional treatment strategies are used to facilitate action and development of active coping, including rating mastery and pleasure of activities, assigning activities to increase mastery and pleasure, mental rehearsal of assigned activities, role-playing behavioral assignments, therapist modeling, periodic distraction from problems or unpleasant events, mindfulness training or relaxation, self-reinforcement, and skills training (e.g., sleep hygiene, assertiveness, communication, problem solving) (Martell et al., 2001). Rumination-cued activation also is an important intervention component in which patients are taught to recognize negative cognitions and to use this identification as a cue to reengage with the environment and behaviorally activate. The treatment duration of BA typically is between 20 and 24 sessions.

Behavioral Activation Treatment for Depression or Morgantown BA

At approximately the same time the BA treatment manual was released, our research team at West Virginia University published the brief behavioral activation treatment for depression (BATD: Lejuez, Hopko, & Hopko, 2001) based on behavioral matching theory. Applied to depression, matching theory suggests that the frequency and duration of depressed relative to nondepressed (or healthy) behavior is directly proportional to the relative value of reinforcement obtained for depressed versus nondepressed behavior (Herrnstein, 1970; McDowell, 1982). When the value (e.g., accessibility, duration, immediacy) of reinforcement for depressed behavior is increased through environmental change (e.g., increased accessibility to social attention, increased opportunity to escape aversive tasks), the relative value of reinforcement for healthy behavior decreases, increasing the likelihood of depressive behavior. Similarly, when the value of reinforcement for healthy behavior is decreased through environmental change (e.g., decreased availability of peers), the relative value of reinforcement for depressed behavior is simultaneously increased. The BATD model predicts that increased contact with reinforcement for healthy behavior (or reduced contact with reinforcement for depressed behavior) would have the effect of decreasing depressed behavior and increasing healthy behavior.

Based on this paradigm, BATD generally is conducted over an eight- to ten-session protocol, although two-session BATD has recently been shown to be effective in reducing symptoms of depression among moderately depressed under-graduate students (Armento, McNulty, & Hopko, 2012; Gawrysiak, Nicholas, & Hopko, 2009). Initial sessions consist of assessing the function of depressed behavior, efforts to weaken access to positive reinforcement (e.g., sympathy) and negative reinforcement (e.g., escape from responsibilities) for depressed behavior, establishing patient rapport, identifying the pros and cons of behavioral change, and introducing the treatment rationale. Patients begin with a weekly self-monitoring exercise that serves as a baseline assessment of daily activities, orients patients to the quality and quantity of their activities, and generates ideas about activities to target during treatment. The emphasis then shifts to the life areas and value assessment (LAVA), in which ideographic life values are identified and behavioral goals are established within major life areas: family, peer, and intimate relationships; daily responsibilities; education; employment; hobbies and recreational activities; physical/health issues; spirituality; and anxiety-eliciting situations (Hayes et al., 1999). Such goal setting has long been considered an important component in the behavioral treatment of depression (Rehm, 1977). Subsequent to goal selection, an activity hierarchy is constructed in which 15 activities are rated ranging from "easiest" to "most difficult" to accomplish. Using activity logs to monitor progress, the patient progressively moves through the hierarchy. For each activity, the therapist and patient collaboratively determine what the *weekly* and *final* goals will be in terms of the frequency and duration of activity. At the start of each session, the monitoring form is examined and discussed, with the following week's goals established as a function of patient success or difficulty with goals for the prior week. The BATD treatment manual recently was revised to simplify and clarify treatment components, procedures, and forms, with an additional emphasis on therapeutic alliance issues and applications of BATD for the cognitively impaired (Lejuez, Hopko, et al., 2011).

BA and BATD: Similarities and Differences

The most important similarity in BA and BATD is their direct focus on behavioral avoidance as the primary target of therapy. Both interventions strongly emphasize that behavioral avoidance is the pathognomonic feature of depression that inhibits exposure to response-contingent reinforcement and extinction of anxiety-related symptoms and behaviors. Based on this conceptual similarity, a primary and common treatment focus is facilitating approach behavior. In the context of BA, activities in graded task assignments are designed based on current activity level, likelihood of success, and importance of activities in meeting life goals. This process is quite open and the therapist has significant flexibility in assigning activities, how to assess life goals, and determining whether (and when) the remaining treatment components are to be implemented. With BATD, following the LAVA assessment and based on a model forwarded by Hayes and colleagues (1999), an activity hierarchy is systematically constructed that directly reflects life values and is followed by systematic movement through the hierarchy to achieve value-consistent life goals. The course of therapy is held relatively constant across all patients. Second, both BA and BATD researchers and clinicians would suggest that affective change and cognitive modification are directly attributable and secondary to relative increases in reinforcement for healthy relative to depressive behavior patterns. Third, both interventions focus on functional assessment of depressive behaviors to varying degrees. In the BA model, the TRAP/TRAC strategies are used to identify avoidance patterns and teach a functional analytic style of understanding and modifying behavior. In contrast, and consistent with traditional behavior therapies for depression, the BATD model does not focus significantly on assisting patients with functional analytic interpretations of behavior because precise functional analyses are difficult for even highly trained clinicians (Hayes, Wilson, Gifford, Follette, & Strosahl, 1996). Consequently, functional analytic strategies in BATD are deemed secondary to the primary overt activation component. Beyond the theoretical distinctions explicated earlier, the primary difference in the two approaches is that BA includes many strategies generally not incorporated within BATD, such as mental rehearsal, periodic distraction, mindfulness training, and skill-training procedures. BATD is based on the premise that systematic activation toward positive activities and situations will allow patients to develop skills in the natural environment, enhance generalizability of treatment gains beyond the clinic, and maximize maintenance of gains over time. That stated, the question of whether a multimodal strategy is superior to a pure activation-based approach must be answered empirically, and to date, the incremental benefits of treatment approaches included in BA beyond those of BATD are unstudied. In terms of practical applications, a clinician who desires a greater range of intervention strategies might prefer the BA method, whereas therapists and patients desiring greater structure and decreased interest in strategies beyond direct activation might prefer BATD. This is not to suggest, however, that BA cannot be organized more systematically or that BATD cannot be used flexibly. We merely assert that such efforts are less easily accomplished within the framework of the particular approaches and therefore likely would require greater practical and conceptual skill on the part of the therapist.

The Focus of Behavioral Activation: Behaviors Amenable to Activation

When discussing behavioral activation interventions, it is important to clearly operationalize the scope of behaviors amenable to activation. Toward this objective, it is useful to distinguish between nondepressive or healthy overt behaviors we are striving to activate and the depressive behaviors we are attempting to eliminate or deactivate. Nondepressive behavior is defined as overt behaviors that are generally value based, directed toward improving quality of life and life functioning, minimize aversive response-consequence contingencies, and are directed toward the attainment of some objective or rewarding consequence. Nondepressive behavior is directly incompatible and the antithesis of depressive behavior. Depressed behavior may occur as a function of some reward via positive (e.g., sympathy from friend or family member) or negative reinforcement (escape from responsibility), or in response to decreased availability of reinforcers for healthy behavior. Depressed behavior also is often a direct consequence of aversive or unpleasant life events or experiences, some of which are beyond human control and unpredictable (e.g., sexual or physical trauma, natural disasters, chronic medical illness, death of a loved one) and others where human accountability is more apparent (e.g., alcoholism and substance abuse, gambling, aggression, and other social indiscretions). In contrast with healthy behavior, depressive behavior generally is not consistent with one's value system and generally does not function to improve functioning or quality of life. Depressive behavior generally refers to responses associated with major depressive disorder (*DSM-IV-TR*; American Psychiatric Association, 2000).

Practitioners of behavioral activation conceptualize depressive behavior from a contextual perspective, which (a) considers behavior as a function of the environmental contingencies that shape and maintain its occurrence and (b) encourages the identification of environment–behavior relations that may be measured objectively and reliably. For example, lethargic and passive behavior associated with anhedonia as well as suicidal behavior largely is understood with reference to operant principles. Although these forms of behavior primarily occur as a function of environmental context, they also are considered "choice" behaviors insofar as the person has some degree of control over whether situations are approached or avoided. Social withdrawal, substance abuse, and other maladaptive actions (antagonistic social behavior, lack of work productivity) associated with depressive behavior may well be considered in the same category. Neurovegetative symptoms such as decreased eating and sleeping, on the other hand, though still a function of environmental contingencies, are perhaps more biologically based responses and less directly controllable (Benca, Obermeyer, Thisted, & Gillin, 1992). Yet even in this example "choice" (in a stochastic rather than mentalistic sense) plays a certain role in whether one eats or decides to sleep or awaken. Finally, symptoms such as negative cognitions and psychomotor agitation/retardation primarily are viewed as private (nonobservable) responses to environmental stimuli that are less controllable, difficult to manipulate therapeutically, and in the latter case biologically based. In conducting behavioral activation, patients and therapists target behavior that is within the realm of patient control and where the environmental context can be modified. In the case of BATD, multiple life domains are focused on simultaneously as a guideline to structured activation. Private behaviors (thoughts, feelings) do not fall into this category, are more difficult to observe and measure, and consequently are less often the focus of behavioral activation methods. Such behavior is not ignored, however, but rather is expected to alleviate following overt behavior modification that increases environmental reward. For example, although cognitions often are not targeted directly in behavioral activation strategies, covert change has been directly implicated as a transfer effect of activation (Jacobson et al., 1996; Simons et al., 1984). That stated, it is noteworthy that rumination-cued activation is a BA treatment component that focuses on recognition of maladaptive cognitions, their impact on life functioning, and the incorporation of activation as a viable coping mechanism by which ruminative behavior is replaced via engagement in rewarding overt behaviors (Addis & Martell, 2004).

Behavioral Activation as a Mechanism for Anxiety Exposure

As indicated earlier, behavioral activation provides a framework in which exposure strategies can easily be implemented. The theoretical basis for this integration has been highlighted in earlier works (Hopko, Robertson, & Lejuez, 2006) and is largely based on a unified model of internalizing disorders (Barlow, 2002; Barlow et al., 2004). Indeed, in addition to several case studies, a few randomized trials have demonstrated preliminary support for the efficacy of both BA and BATD in attenuating symptoms of anxiety (Hopko et al., 2011; Jakupcak et al., 2006). Nonetheless, the process of behavioral activation should be differentiated from that of in vivo exposure. In the latter procedure, exposing individuals to aversive conditioned stimuli while preventing an avoidance response is an application of extinction within a classical conditioning framework. Without experiencing the anticipated aversive or traumatic event, over time anxious responding in the presence of the conditioned stimuli is likely to extinguish. Although exposure strategies are not fundamental to the behavioral activation process, avoidance behaviors characteristic of depressed individuals may partially be a function of aversive contextual stimuli (e.g., situations or individuals). To the extent that avoidance behavior functions to minimize anxiety elicited by these contexts, the therapeutic effects of guided activity (or activation) and graduated systematic exposure might be functionally similar. Exploration of the relevance of behavioral activation in treating anxiety disorders is worthy of further investigation because of the interrelatedness of anxiety and depressive conditions (Barlow et al., 2004; Kessler et al., 2003; Mineka, Watson, & Clark, 1998), the potential transfer effects of treating one condition on the other (Hopko et al., 2011; Stanley et al., 2003), and increased focus on refining treatments for patients with mixed anxiety-depressive disorders (Barlow & Campbell, 2000). More systematic research clearly is needed to examine how activation strategies supplemented with graduated fear hierarchies, progressive muscle relaxation, and other behavioral strategies may enhance treatment of patients with coexistent anxiety and depressive symptoms.

Behavioral Activation Assessment Methods

Based on conceptual models of depression and proposed mechanisms of change linked to behavioral activation (Ferster, 1973; Hopko, Lejuez, et al., 2003; Lewinsohn, 1974; Manos et al., 2010; Martell et al., 2001), measurement of a number of constructs is relevant toward evaluating the process and outcomes associated with behavioral activation. Among these constructs are depression, environmental reinforcement and reward, behavioral avoidance, behavioral activation and inhibition, and aversive or unpleasant events. Organized on the basis of assessment methods, measurement of these constructs is presented next, with an important caveat to be acknowledged. Specifically, the fundamental principle of behavioral models of depression and the ultimate objective of behavioral activation is to increase response-contingent positive reinforcement. As highlighted in several works (Armento & Hopko, 2007; Carvalho et al., 2011; Manos et al., 2010), it is highly difficult to measure the process of reinforcement, in that by definition it refers to change in behavior frequency over time that is contingent upon the presentation of controlled stimuli. If a given behavior increases as a function of a consequence or stimulus presented, a positive reinforcer has been identified. Problematically, the direct measurement of reinforcement is pragmatically difficult in that it would necessitate extensive and microanalytical control over the patient's environment, lengthy observation periods, and careful assessment of a plethora of ongoing response-consequence contingencies across a breadth of life domains. Accordingly, many measures either do not purport to measure the process of reinforcement or, alternatively, attempt to measure reinforcement by means of proxy variables (e.g., environmental reward, pleasant events). The remainder of the section highlights assessment strategies relevant to assessing behavioral activation and depression. Although many resources are available, their appropriateness and clinical utility vary greatly across patient and assessment context. The level of skill and training required of the assessor to incorporate these strategies also is quite variable, ranging from minimal skill to administer a self-report measure, moderate skill to conduct a valid structured interview, and extensive skill to perform a comprehensive functional assessment of depressive behaviors.

Unstructured and Structured Interviews

Clinical interviews have significant utility, both in terms of evaluating symptoms of depression and actively engaging in behavioral activation therapy. Of course, clinical interviewing procedures can range from primarily unstructured and highly flexible approaches to structured methods that are more restrictive and goal directed. In terms of assessing depression, the most commonly used interviews include the Structured Clinical Interview for DSM-IV Patient Version (SCID-I/P; First et al., 1996), the Anxiety Disorders Interview Schedule (ADIS-IV; Brown, Di Nardo, & Barlow, 1994), the Schedule for Affective Disorders and Schizophrenia (SADS; Endicott & Spitzer, 1978), and the Diagnostic Interview Schedule (DIS; Robins, Helzer, Croughan, & Ratcliff, 1981). The 17-item Hamilton Rating Scale for Depression (HRSD; Hamilton, 1960) was designed as a postdiagnostic measure to assess the severity of depressive symptoms and to measure changes in patient functioning over time. The recommendation is that the HRSD be completed (in about10 minutes) following a clinical interview in which the necessary information is obtained to accurately assess the patient on dimensions such as mood, anhedonia, insomnia, and weight change. Following Hamilton's development of the HRSD, several alternative Hamilton rating scales have evolved with some instruments including as many as 29 items (Williams, Link, Rosenthal, & Terman, 1988). Interrater reliability coefficients of the HRSD generally are excellent (>0.84) and data suggest moderate convergent validity with several self-report measures of depression (Nezu, Ronan, Meadows, & McClure, 2000). Although recently criticized as conceptually and psychometrically flawed (Bagby, Ryder, Schuller, & Marshall, 2004), the HRSD generally is the most widely used and accepted outcome measure for the evaluation of depression and is the standard outcome measure in clinical trials (Kobak & Reynolds, 1999), including treatment outcome research in behavioral activation (Dimidjian et al., 2006; Hopko et al., 2011).

In addition to increasing diagnostic precision, interviewing strategies with the patient and significant others also can provide valuable assessment data at several stages of behavioral activation. For example, in assessing level of environmental reward, in addition to using daily self-monitoring strategies endorsed in both BA and BATD, the therapist is always encouraged to further explore activities and behaviors in the context of specific reward ratings and to strive to identify behavioral patterns, as well as stimulus and response classes and their associated reward or pleasure ratings. Interviewing and questioning are often critical toward facilitating this process, elaborating on self-monitoring data, and helping to ensure that the patient and therapist are conceptualizing behaviors and reward systems reliably. When possible, incorporating the observations of a spouse or significant friend also is recommended. Arguably at no other treatment phase is meticulous interviewing as crucial as it is during the life areas and values (LAVA) assessment; in the domains of family, social, and intimate relationships, education, employment and career, hobbies and recreation, volunteer work and charity, physical and health issues, spirituality, and avoidance behavior related to anxiety-eliciting situations. A *value* is defined as an ideal, quality, or strong belief that should translate into certain patterns of behavior. To assess values, patients are interviewed about which life domains are more or less important, what they would like to accomplish in each area, who would be involved in each area, what observable and measurable overt behaviors could be engaged in that would be consistent with life values and accomplish goals in life domains, and which possible obstacles might prevent engagement in behaviors. Patients are asked to identify values that are highly personal and not necessarily values of other people in their life or society in general. Based on this model, the therapist must not only be skillful at interviewing but also cognizant of possibilities for treatment failure. First, it is conceivable that patients are unable to articulate their life values due to misunderstandings about the purpose of the exercise (e.g., lack of therapist proficiency, patient cognitive impairment). Second, because discussion of life areas can be a highly sensitive exercise, patients may be unwilling to disclose due to emotional avoidance or personal discomfort. Third, and different from patient unwillingness, engaging in the value assessment may be difficult for some patients due to minimal insight or lack of psychological awareness. Finally, patients must be encouraged to focus on their unique values and life circumstances, embrace their individuality, and refrain from impulses to adopt other people's values and beliefs that might be common, yet markedly different from their own perspectives and value systems. Given these objectives, and the fact that the LAVA assessment serves as the foundation for guided activation, significant therapeutic interviewing skills are required to accurately assess patients' unique value systems with awareness of how this process could potentially become derailed. If conducted ineptly, the efficacy of behavioral activation could be greatly compromised.

In addition to the importance of proficient interviewing during behavioral activation treatment components, it is important to note that therapeutic alliance and associated therapist–patient communication patterns are strongly emphasized in behavioral activation and other third-wave behavioral therapies (Lejuez, Hopko, Levine, Gholkar, & Collins, 2005). In addition to assisting with the development of patient rapport, basic behavioral principles such as reinforcement, punishment, shaping, and fading are utilized within sessions to address patient adherence to behavioral activation and develop skills necessary to activate in the natural environment. In an interesting integration of FAP and behavioral activation, it was demonstrated that whereas the latter intervention largely focuses on activation out of session, FAP can utilize therapist interviewing skills and dyadic discussions to identify clinically relevant problem behaviors that can be behaviorally modified within session to promote increased access to naturalistic environmental reinforcement (Kanter, Manos, Busch, & Rusch, 2008; Manos et al., 2009). Strategies such as this may prove useful toward supplementing more traditional activation approaches.

Self-Report Measures

Self-report measures of depression, behavioral activation, inhibition, avoidance, environmental reward, and pleasant and unpleasant events have proven useful as screening instruments, auxiliaries in the diagnostic process, as tools for monitoring progress across treatment sessions, and as outcome measures assessing the efficacy and effectiveness of behavioral activation interventions. At present, there are over 100 measures designed to assess depression and related constructs, with the majority having adequate to excellent psychometric properties (Hopko, Lejuez, Armento, & Bare, 2004; Nezu et al., 2000). Because the strengths and limitations of self-report measures relevant to behavioral activation have nicely been presented (Manos et al., 2010), only a few of the most commonly utilized measures are presented here.

Depression

The Beck Depression Inventories (BDI; Beck & Steer, 1987; BDI-II; Beck, Steer, & Brown, 1996) assess the severity of depressive symptoms and each consists of 21 items. The instruments have excellent reliability and validity with depressed younger and older adults (Beck & Steer, 1987; Beck et al., 1996; Beck, Steer, & Garbin, 1988; Snyder, Stanley,

Novy, & Beck, 2000). Among younger clinical and nonclinical adults, the instruments have good internal consistency (α; = 0.73–0.95) and adequate test-retest reliability for nondepressed individuals (r = .60–.83) and psychiatric patients (r = .48–.93) (Beck et al., 1988, 1996). Concurrent and construct validity among the Beck inventories and other indices of depression ranges from moderate (r = .33 with DSM-III diagnosis of clinical depression; Hesselbrock et al., 1983) to strong (r = .86 with the Zung SDS; Turner & Romano, 1984; see Beck et al., 1988, 1996 for comprehensive reviews).

The Center for Epidemiological Studies' Depression Scale (CES-D; Radloff, 1977) is a 20-item self-report questionnaire of depressive symptoms that was designed as a survey instrument for assessing depressive affect in the general population. Although it was not intended for use as a diagnostic measure, CES-D totals have been shown to be moderately related to a diagnosis of clinical depression (Myers & Weissman, 1980) and some have argued for its utility as an initial depression screening measure (Roberts & Vernon, 1983). When used for screening, scores greater than 16 indicate that a patient may have clinical depression (Radloff, 1977). The CES-D has adequate psychometric properties in psychiatric and medical samples (Nezu et al., 2000).

Behavioral Avoidance and Activation

The Cognitive-Behavioral Avoidance Scale (CBAS; Ottenbreit & Dobson, 2004) is a self-report measure that assesses depression-related avoidance. The scale includes 31 items and includes four subscales: Behavioral Social, Cognitive Social, Behavioral Nonsocial, and Cognitive Nonsocial avoidance. Subscales demonstrate adequate to strong coefficient alphas (α; = .86, .78, .75, .80, respectively) and test-retest reliability (r = .86, .58, .88, .94, respectively). A total avoidance score also is calculated, which has excellent internal consistency (α; = .91) and test-retest reliability (r = .92). The CBAS also correlates moderately with other measures of avoidance as well as depression and anxiety scales (Kanter et al., 2007, 2009; Ottenbreit & Dobson, 2004). Sample items include "I try not to think about problems in my personal relationships" (Cognitive Social) and "I quit activities that challenge me too much" (Behavioral Nonsocial).

The Behavioral Activation for Depression Scale (BADS; Kanter et al., 2007) is a 25-item scale assessing behaviors targeted during behavioral activation treatment interventions. The measure includes four subscales: Activation, Avoidance/Rumination, Work/School Impairment, and Social Impairment. Sample items include "I engaged in a wide and diverse array of activities" (Activation subscale), "I did things to avoid feeling sadness or other painful emotions" (Avoidance/Rumination subscale), and "I stayed in bed for too long even though I had things to do (Work/School Impairment subscale). Internal consistency of the total score and subscales is adequate (α; = .76 to .87), and good 1-week test-retest reliability was established ($r = .74$). The BADS also correlated strongly with the BDI ($r = -.67$ to $-.70$), and had good discriminant validity as evidenced by a significant albeit weak relationship with the Beck Anxiety Inventory ($r = -.19$; Beck, Epstein, Brown, & Steer, 1988). Finally, there was some support for the predictive validity of the BADS in that individuals with higher scores on the Avoidance/ Rumination subscale were less likely to return for follow-up assessment (Kanter et al., 2007).

The *Behavioral Inhibition and Behavioral Activation Scale* (BIS/BAS; Kasch, Rottenberg, Arnow, & Gotlib, 2002) is a 20-item self-report questionnaire that assesses how people typically react to certain situations. The scale is subdivided into four subscales: Behavioral Inhibition, Behavioral Activation-Reward Responsiveness, Behavioral Activation-Drive, and Behavioral Activation-Fun-Seeking. Internal consistencies of all subscales are high (BIS = .78; BAS-RR = .80; BAS-Drive = .83; BAS-Fun = .69). The BIS/BAS scales also have good convergent and discriminant validity, with scores on the BAS scales typically relating to positive affect and extraversion and scores on the BIS scale generally being related to anxiety symptoms, negative affect, and neuroticism (Carver & White, 1994; Jorm et al., 1999).

Environmental Reward

The Reward Probability Index (RPI; Carvalho et al., 2011) is a 20-item self-report measure designed to measure the magnitude of environmental reward as an approximation of response-contingent positive reinforcement. The scale assesses RCPR's four dimensions via two factors: Reward Probability (potentially reinforcing events and instrumental behaviors in obtaining reinforcement) and Environmental Suppressors (availability of reinforcement in the environment and presence of punishing/aversive experiences). Sample items include "I consider myself to be a person with many skills" (Reward Probability) and "There are a lot of activities I might enjoy, but they just don't seem to

happen" (Environmental Suppressors). Participants rate each item on a 4-point Likert scale (1 = *strongly disagree* to 4 = *strongly agree*) for the time period of the "past several months," with higher scores indicating higher levels of reward. Psychometric properties of the RPI were established through three studies. The measure had strong internal consistency (α = .88 to .92) and very good 2-week test-retest reliability ($r = .69$). Convergent validity was established via strong correlations with measures of activity, avoidance, reward, and depression ($r = .65$ to .81). Discriminant validity was supported via smaller correlations with measures of social support and somatic anxiety ($r = -.29$ to $-.40$). Further, the RPI accounted for unique variance in daily diary-reported environmental reward above that accounted for by a preexisting reward measure (EROS) and self-reported depression (BDI-II).

The Environmental Reward Observation Scale (EROS; Armento & Hopko, 2007) is a 10-item measure that assesses environmental reward. The scale is intended to identify the magnitude of reinforcing events, the availability of reinforcement in the environment, and the ability of an individual to elicit reinforcement. Sample items include "A lot of activities in my life are pleasurable," "It is easy for me to find enjoyment in my life," and "The activities I engage in have positive consequences." The EROS has strong internal consistency (α = .85–.90) and excellent 1-week test-retest reliability ($r = .85$). The EROS also correlated strongly with other commonly administered and psychometrically sound self-report measures of depression and anxiety, as well as the Pleasant Events Schedule ($r = -.43$ to $-.71$; Armento & Hopko, 2007).

Pleasant and Unpleasant Events

The *Pleasant Events Schedule* (PES; MacPhillamy & Lewinsohn, 1982) is a 320-item measure assessing the frequency and subjective pleasure of potentially reinforcing events or activities. Each item has a frequency and enjoyability score, each of which is rated on a 0 ("not happened in last 30 days"; "not pleasant") to 2 ("happened often"; "very pleasant") Likert-type scale. Average frequency and pleasure ratings are multiplied to form a cross-product score, with higher cross-product scores indicating that activities have a higher level of reinforcement potential, considered a useful index of experienced positive reinforcement (Correia et al., 2002). The PES has strong psychometric properties (MacPhillamy & Lewinsohn, 1982; Nezu et al., 2000).

The Unpleasant Events Schedule (UES; Lewinsohn & Talkington, 1979) is a list of 320 unpleasant events that is used as an indicator of contact with punishers and negative reinforcers. Each item has a frequency and aversiveness score. Examples of items include "being alone," "attending funerals," and "performing in public." Like the PES, the UES uses the time frame of the past month and yields a frequency score on a 3-point scale, a subjective aversiveness score on a 3-point scale, and the crossproduct that is thought to approximate response-contingent punishment and negative reinforcement.

Factor analytic investigation by Lewinsohn et al. (1985) resulted in the following scales: Legal, Sexual–Marital-Friendship, Death Related, Controllable versus Uncontrollable, Life Changes, Self versus Other, and Most Discriminating Items.

The Life Experiences Survey (LES; Sarason, Johnson, & Siegel, 1978) is a 57-item measure that assesses stressful life changes over the past year and includes blank spaces for write-in events. Each experienced event is rated on a 7-point Likert scale ranging from "extremely negative impact" (–3) to "extremely positive impact" (+3). Sample items include "Death of a close family member," "Change of residence," and "Beginning a new school experience at a higher academic level." The LES has good reliability and is significantly related to several stress-related measures (Sarason et al., 1978).

Observational Methods

Observational methods of assessing depression, its overt manifestation, and related behavioral activation and avoidance patterns represent an additional valuable assessment tool. For example, the frequency and duration of observable (overt-motor) depressive behaviors may be monitored that include excesses such as crying, irritable/agitated behaviors, and even suicidal behaviors, or deficits such as minimal eye contact, psychomotor retardation, decreased recreational and occupational activities, and disruption in sleep, eating, and sexual behaviors (Bonierbale, Lancon, & Tignol, 2003; Rehm, 1988; Riemann, Berger, & Voderholzer, 2001; Thase, 2006). In the realm of verbal behavior (see Rehm, 1988, for a comprehensive discussion), several studies have demonstrated that depressed individuals generally exhibit slower and more monotonous speech (Gotlib & Robinson, 1982; Libet & Lewinsohn, 1973; Robinson & Lewinsohn, 1973). Individuals with depression also have longer response latencies to the verbal behavior of others

(Libet & Lewinsohn, 1973) and more commonly engage in self-focused negative remarks (Blumberg & Hokanson, 1983; Gotlib & Robinson, 1982) and use fewer "achievement" and "power" words in their speech (Andreasen & Pfohl, 1976). Nonverbal (motoric) differences between depressed and nondepressed individuals also are evident. In a pioneering investigation, Williams, Barlow, and Agras (1972) developed the Ward Behavior Checklist to assess smiling, motoric activities (e.g., reading, grooming), and "time out of the room" among a small group of depressed inpatients. These behaviors correlated moderately with depression, and other studies have suggested depressed individuals smile less frequently (Gotlib & Robinson, 1982), make less eye contact during conversation (Gotlib, 1982), and hold their head in a downward position more frequently (Ranelli & Miller, 1981). Depressed individuals also react differently to emotional facial experiences (Seidel, Hable, et al., 2010) and are sometimes rated as less competent in social situations (Dykman, Horowitz, Abramson, & Usher, 1991), although other studies have not supported this latter finding (Gable & Shean, 2000; Segrin, 1999). There also is couples research suggesting when one or both partners is clinically depressed, there is increased conflict and decreased marital satisfaction (Fincham, Beach, Harold, & Osborne, 1997; Hinchliffe, Hooper, & Roberts, 1978; Whisman, Uebelacker, & Weinstock, 2004).

Although such behavioral observations characteristic of depressed individuals are highly relevant insofar as assessment and treatment monitoring are concerned, observational assessment also has specific applications within behavioral activation. For example, in traditional behavioral treatments, daily diaries, activity monitoring logs, and home observations were utilized in the context of assessing patients' sources and degree of environmental reinforcement (Lewinsohn & Atwood, 1969; Lewinsohn & Libet, 1972; Lewinsohn & Shaffer, 1971). In the context of contemporary behavioral activation treatments, daily diaries and activity schedules are useful indicators of overt behavior and assist with case conceptualization in that they allow patients to topographically record behaviors over a given time interval and also permit recording of mood, mastery, and/or pleasure ratings. As detailed elsewhere, such strategies are typically used as indicators of environmental reinforcement in lieu of more detailed, functional analyses of reinforcement following specific activities (Manos et al., 2010). Nonetheless, in addition to serving useful purposes insofar as pretreatment assessment and treatment monitoring are concerned, daily diaries and activity logs have proven valuable in terms of quantitatively evaluating treatment adherence. For example, in our work with depressed cancer patients and college students, treatment compliance has been assessed using an adherence score that is formulated for each patient by dividing the number of behavioral assignments completed by those assigned (Gawrysiak et al., 2009; Hopko, Bell, Armento, Hunt, & Lejuez, 2005, 2008). These daily diaries can also be useful toward using mood and reward ratings to evaluate behavioral models of depression. For example, it has been demonstrated that the immediate and future reward value of current overt behaviors correlated highly with self-report measures of depression, with mildly depressed and nondepressed students distinguishable via response style (Hopko, Armento, Cantu, Chambers, & Lejuez, 2003). Compared to nondepressed college students, mildly depressed individuals also less frequently engaged in social, physical, and educational behaviors and more often in activities related to employment (Hopko & Mullane, 2008). In an interesting single-subject design that provided some support for the proposed mechanism of change in behavioral activation, it was shown that change in activity level predicted change in depression over time (Gaynor & Harris, 2008). Finally, an intriguing and emerging area of interest to explore mechanism of change issues in behavioral activation involves the use of therapist coding to more clearly decipher the relation between patient activation and attenuated depression (Dimidjian, Hubley, Martell, Herman-Dunn, &, Dobson, unpublished manuscript; Hubley, Dimidjian, & Gallop, unpublished manuscript). Although self-report measures and observational methods have much to offer toward establishing the merit of behavioral models of depression and behavioral activation therapy, the cross-sectional methodologies only allow for partial inferences to be drawn at present. More longitudinal work that incorporates enhanced technology and sophisticated statistical analysis will be essential toward assessing the causal relationships between response-contingent positive reinforcement, aversive (or punitive) environmental events, and their collective impact on depression.

Functional Assessment

Functional assessment generally refers to the process of identifying important, controllable, and causal environmental factors that may be related to the etiology and maintenance of depressive behavior(s), such as passivity, social withdrawal, crying, alcohol abuse, and suicidality. Strategies for conducting a functional assessment include interviews with the patient and significant others, naturalistic observation, the manipulation of specific situations that result in an increase or decrease of target behaviors, or some combination. Functional assessment is not to be equated with functional analysis, with the latter process being but one option to accomplish the former. Indeed, functional analysis refers to the manipulation of environmental events under highly controlled experimental conditions with systematic observation of behaviors (Horner, 1994; O'Neill, Horner, Albin, Storey, & Sprague, 1990). Functional assessment generally is less rigid, an ongoing process without the experimental constraints of functional analysis, and under certain conditions highly appropriate for clinical practice (Horner, 1994). With the exception of significant clinical research in childhood externalizing disorders that has relied heavily on functional analysis (Hanley, Iwata, & McCord, 2003), this specific assessment and intervention process is only infrequently used in clinical practice, including cognitive-behavioral treatment outcome research for depression. In addition to highly limited implementation in general, recurrent reference to behavioral activation as adopting this strategy is grossly inaccurate. Indeed, both BA and BATD researchers have erroneously endorsed functional analysis as a critical component of behavioral activation (Dimidjian et al., 2006; Hopko, Lejuez, et al., 2003; Jacobson et al., 2001), where functional assessment is the more operative term.

This important semantic issue acknowledged, functional assessment is integral to both BA and BATD. In particular, the shared perspective is that depressive behavior such as passivity and withdrawal functions as avoidance behavior as individuals minimize exposure to environments that lack positive reinforcement and/or have aversive or punitive consequences. So depressive behavior occurs because reinforcement for healthy behavior is minimal, positive and negative reinforcement for depressive behavior is excessive, healthy behavior is punished, or some combination of these factors. As avoidance behavior patterns are negatively reinforced via the short-term relief often experienced, in the longer term negative affect frequently heightens and a cyclical pattern is initiated (i.e., avoidance–depression–more avoidance). In the initial stages of behavioral activation and often incorporating some form of daily monitoring, patients may be asked to record depressive (target) behaviors, the context (time, place, surroundings) in which they occur, and the consequences that follow. With all functional assessment strategies, the therapist is concerned with identifying the function (or maintaining reinforcers) that depressed behavior produces for an individual, or put more simply, why the depressed behavior occurs. Communication with significant others also might facilitate this functional conceptualization. In the Washington BA model, the principal strategies of change involve teaching patients to identify avoidance patterns (i.e., TRAP and TRAC models described earlier), teaching a functional assessment style of understanding behavior, and focusing on guided activity to foster enduring changes in overt behavior. In contrast, the Morgantown BATD model does not focus to a similar degree on assisting patients with functional assessment interpretations of behavior. As mentioned earlier, functional assessment strategies in BATD are secondary to the primary value assessment and overt activation components. In addition to using functional assessment to conceptualize overt behavior, or lack thereof, this strategy can be used to identify specific thought patterns elicited by certain environmental events and how these cognitions may correspond with depressive mood states. Indeed, a unique feature of Washington BA is the use of rumination-cued activation (Addis & Martell, 2004), an assessment and intervention strategy that focuses on identifying the context and function of ruminative thought patterns and how to cope through guided activation. Intuitively, it is evident that functional assessment strategies should be useful in case conceptualization, generating specific treatment goals, and as a method of intervention. At this stage of outcome research, however, the incremental benefits of functional assessment, the structured value assessment of BATD, and the additional treatment strategies at the disposal of BA practitioners above and beyond the benefits of overt activation toward increasing RCPR are largely unknown.

Behavioral Activation Treatment Outcome Research

Behavioral activation interventions largely have been used to treat depressive disorders and symptoms, with three meta-analyses supporting their efficacy such that behavioral activation is now considered an empirically validated treatment for depression (Cuijpers et al., 2007; Ekers et al., 2008; Mazzucchelli et al., 2009; Sturmey, 2009). In one of the more compelling studies, behavioral

activation was comparable to antidepressant medication and superior to cognitive therapy in treating severe depression (Dimidjian et al. 2006), results that were maintained at 2-year follow-up (Dobson et al., 2008). In a recent study examining the relative efficacy of BATD and problem-solving therapy in treating depressed breast cancer patients, intent-to-treat analyses suggested both treatments were efficacious, with both evidencing significant pre-post treatment gains across a breadth of outcome measures assessing depression, environmental reward, anxiety, quality of life, social support, and medical outcomes (Hopko et al., 2011). Across both treatments, gains were associated with strong effect sizes, and based on response and remission criteria, a reliable change index, and numbers needed to treat analyses, approximately two thirds of patients exhibited clinically significant improvement. Importantly, treatment gains were maintained at 12-month follow-up. In addition to these studies, behavioral activation has been effectively used with depressed patients in a variety of settings and among samples with divergent medical and psychiatric problems (Daughters et al., 2008; Ekers et al., 2011; Gawrysiak et al., 2009; Hopko et al., 2005; Hopko, Lejuez, LePage, Hopko, & McNeil, 2003; Jacobson et al., 1996; Jakupcak et al., 2006; MacPherson et al., 2010; Pagoto et al., 2008).

As presented in Table 14.1, the efficacy of both traditional and contemporary behavioral activation interventions has been strongly supported. Although the overwhelming majority of these studies reflect applications of behavioral activation for depressed individuals, it is important to highlight its successful implementation among individuals with comorbid medical problems that include cancer, HIV, brain trauma, and obesity. In addition, albeit much more preliminarily than in the treatment of depression, behavioral activation outcome research supports its potential effectiveness in patients with coexistent anxiety problems (particularly posttraumatic stress disorder and generalized anxiety disorder), Alzheimer's disease, smoking and alcohol dependence, and possibly even schizophrenia and borderline personality disorder. Although most studies have examined the efficacy of behavioral activation with younger to middle-aged adults, more systematic research is beginning to assess its utility with younger adolescents and older adults.

In the first of three recent meta-analyses in this area (Cuijpers et al., 2007), the focus was on assessing the efficacy of activity scheduling as a behavioral treatment for depression. In an examination

Table 14.1 The Efficacy of Behavioral Interventions

Study	Sample	Interventions and Research Design	Duration	Primary Results
Conventional Behavioral Treatments				
Barrera (1979)	20 participants with MDD • Immediate treatment (IT) • Delayed treatment (DT) • Age: M = 33.9 years	Group (Design: RT): 1. IT: Self-instructional materials: monitoring pleasant activities and mood, daily activity goals, and graphing progress 2. DT: Self-instructional materials: monitoring pleasant activities and mood, and graph progress; daily activity goals after 4 weeks	• IT (4 weeks): individual session and group meeting in first week; 2-hour sessions for 3 weeks • DT (4 weeks): following training in self-monitoring, researcher called weekly to assess compliance with monitoring	• IT was not more effective than DT • After DT, participants successfully increased activities and decreased depression relative to IT • Increased self-monitoring may be necessary to facilitate progress in pleasant event scheduling
Biglan & Craker (1982)	4 participants • Females with MDD • Age: M = 33.5 years	Individual (Design: group time series): • Baseline • Activity goal setting • Self-reward • Reversal	• 4 days activity scheduling	• Increase in pleasant activities produced no improvement in self-monitored mood
Comas-Díaz (1981)	26 participants • Low-SES Puerto Rican women • Spanish-speaking • Age: M = 38 years	Group (Design: RCT): 1. Cognitive therapy 2. Activity scheduling 3. Wait list control	• 5 sessions	• Decreased depression in the cognitive therapy and activity scheduling groups relative to the wait list control
Fuchs & Rehm (1977)	36 participants • Females with MDD • Age: 18–38 years	Group (Design: RCT): 1. Self-control therapy (with activity scheduling) 2. Supportive therapy 3. Wait list control	• 6 sessions	• Self-control therapy group exhibited increased activity levels and decreased depression at posttreatment compared to other groups
Gardner & Oei (1981)	16 participants • Treatment groups matched on gender, age, and depression severity • Age = 19–65 years	Individual (Design: RT): 1. Activity scheduling 2. Cognitive: rational emotive therapy	• 8 sessions	• Both cognitive and behavior therapy effectively reduced depression (no difference between treatment groups • Rate of improvement faster in the cognitive therapy group

Study	Participants	Design/Conditions	Duration	Results
Hammen and Glass (1975)	40 participants • College students • Mild to moderate depression	Group (Design: RCT): 1. Activity scheduling 2. Self-monitoring 3. Control: dietary monitoring 4. No treatment	• 2 weeks	• Activity scheduling group engaged in more pleasurable activities • Increases in pleasant activities did not correspond to depression reduction • No differences between groups
Harmon, Nelson, and Hayes (1980)	6 participants • MDD • Age = 18–23 years • All previous outpatients	Individual (Design: group time series): 1. Self-monitoring activity 2. Self-monitoring of mood 3. Control group	• 5 weeks • Experimental groups intervention at weeks 2 and 4	• Self-monitoring of activity and self-monitoring of mood increased pleasant events and decreased depression
Lewinsohn and Libet (1972)	30 participants • Undergraduates students • Depressed (10) • Psychiatric control (10) • Normal control (10)	Individual (Design: OT): 1. Rate moods and indicate frequency of pleasant activities	• 30 days	• Significant association between pleasant activities and mood • Association between rate of pleasant activities and depression varied between groups, but not significant
McLean and Hakstain (1979)	196 patients • MDD • Age: M = 39.3 years	Group (Design: RT): 1. Activity scheduling 2. Brief psychodynamic 3. Relaxation training 4. Amitriptyline	• 8–12 sessions	• Behavior therapy superior to all other interventions at posttreatment • Results maintained at 3-month follow-up • Attrition lowest (5%) in activity scheduling group
McNamara and Horan (1986)	40 participants • BDI > 16 • HRSD > 20 • Age: M = 23.0 years	Group (Design: RT); 1. Activity scheduling 2. Cognitive therapy 3. Combined	• 8 sessions (groups 1,2) • 10 sessions (combined)	• All groups improved significantly and equally in terms of reduced depression (BDI)
Padfield (1976)	24 adult female participants • Living in rural area: Low SES • Moderately depressed as determined by the Grinker Interview Checklist (GIC) • Age = 21–56 years	Individual (Design: RT): 1. Activity scheduling 2. Supportive counseling	• 12 sessions	• Women of lowest SES status had the most significant depression reduction • Results concerning comparative effectiveness of interventions inconclusive, but GIC scores suggest behavior therapy was most effective
Rehm, Kaslow, and Rabin (1987)	104 participants • Age: M = 38.6 years	Group (Design: RT): 1. Self-control: behavioral target 2. Self-control: cognitive target 3. Combined target	• 10 sessions	• All groups improved significantly and equally

(continued)

Table 14.1 Continued

Study	Sample	Interventions and Research Design	Duration	Primary Results
Conventional Behavioral Treatments				
Scogin, Jamison, and Gochneaur (1989)	67 older adult participants • Mild and moderately depressed • Age: M = 68.3 years	Individual (Design = RT): 1. Cognitive bibliotherapy 2. Behavioral bibliotherapy	• 4 weeks	• Both groups improved significantly and equally
Shaw (1977)	32 participants • MDD • Age: 18–26 years	Group (Design: RCT): 1. Cognitive therapy 2. Activity scheduling 3. Supportive therapy 4. Wait list control	• 4 sessions	• Cognitive therapy most effective in reducing depression • Activity scheduling more effective than control condition
Taylor and Marshall (1977)	28 participants • BDI ≥ 14 • Age: M = 22.4 years	Individual (Design: RCT): 1. Cognitive therapy 2. Activity scheduling 3. Combined 4. Wait list control	• 6 sessions	• All treatment groups superior to control group in reducing depression • Combined treatment more effective than other active interventions • No significant differences between cognitive and activity scheduling groups
Teri, Logsdon, Uomoto, and McCurry (1997)	72 participants • MDD and Alzheimer's Disease	Group (Design: RCT) 1. Activity scheduling 2. Caregiver problem solving 3. TAU 4. Wait list control	• 9 sessions	• Patients in activity scheduling and problem solving had significantly reduced depression relative to other two groups • Same results for depressive symptoms of caregivers
Thompson, Gallagher, and Breckenridg (1987)	91 older adults • MDD • BDI ≥ 17 • HRSD ≥ 14 • Age 60 years or older	Individual (Design: RT): 1. Activity scheduling 2. Cognitive therapy 3. Brief psychodynamic	• 16–20 sessions	• Significant and equivalent depression reduction in all three groups • Response rates similar to younger samples
Wilson (1982)	64 participants • BDI ≥ 20 • Age = 20–55 years	Individual (Design: RCT): 1. Activity scheduling 2. Relaxation training 3. Minimal contact (each group was also randomized to either amitriptyline or placebo)	• 7 sessions • Minimal contact = 2 sessions for medication	• Reduced depression across all groups • No group differences • More rapid improvement in patients receiving amitriptyline • Participants in activity scheduling and relaxation training groups sought less additional treatment at follow-up

Study	Participants	Design	Sessions	Findings
Wilson, Goldin, and Charbonneau-Powis (1983)	25 participants • BDI ≥ 17 • Age: M = 39.5 years	Individual (Design: RCT): 1. Activity scheduling 2. Cognitive therapy 3. No treatment control	• 8 sessions	• Activity scheduling and cognitive therapy both effective in reducing depression and superior to control • Treatment effects maintained at 5-month follow-up
Zeiss et al. (1979)	66 participants • Outpatients with MDD • Age: M = 33.9 years	Individual (Design: RT): 1. Interpersonal skills therapy 2. Activity scheduling 3. Cognitive therapy	• 12 sessions	• All interventions reduced depression at posttreatment and no significant differences between treatments • There were no treatment-specific effects on a single class of behavior

Contemporary Behavioral Treatments

Based or modified from the Brief Behavioral Activation Treatment (BATD; Lejuez, Hopko, & Hopko, 2001)

Study	Participants	Design	Sessions	Findings
Alfonsson, Parling, and Ghaderi (2014)	96 participants • Severe obesity and binge eating disorder Age: M = 44.3 years BMI > 30	Group (Design: RCT): 1. BA 2. WL	• 10 sessions	• BA improved some aspects of disordered eating and reduced depressive symptoms • No significant difference between the groups in binge-eating behavior
Armento and Hopko (2009)	1 participant • MDD and GAD • White female with breast cancer • Age: 58 years	Individual (Design: CS): 1. BA for cancer patients	• 8 sessions	• Decreased depression and anxiety • Improvement in quality of life and psychosocial functioning
Armento, McNulty, and Hopko (2012)	50 participants • Undergraduate students • Age: M = 20.0 years • BDI-II > 14 • 78% with depressive disorder	Individual (Design: RT): 1. BA for religious behaviors 2. Supportive therapy	• 1 session (2 weeks)	• BA increased religious behaviors and attitudes • Significantly reduced depression and anxiety in BA group • Increased quality of life in BA group • Gains maintained at 1-month follow-up
Bailey and Arco (2010)	2 participants • 28 years old (BDI-II = 16) • 39 years old (BDI-II = 28)	Group (Design: CS): 1. BATD	• 8 sessions • Multiple baseline	• Decreased depression at posttreatment: 28 year olds (BDI-II = 6); 39 year olds (BDI-II = 1)

(continued)

Table 14.1 Continued

Study	Sample	Interventions and Research Design	Duration	Primary Results
Contemporary Behavioral Treatments				
Collado, Castillo, Maero, Lejuez, and MacPherson (2014)	• 10 participants • Limited English proficiency • Latino • BDI-II ≥ 10	Individual (Design: OT) 1. BATD	• 10-session, direct (i.e., literal) Spanish-language translation of BATD	• Decreased depression at posttreatment and increased activation and environmental reward • Increased activation corresponded with decreased depression and environmental reward preceded decreases in depression • Sustained clinical gains at follow-up.
Daughters et al. (2008)	• 44 participants • Diagnosis of substance dependence • BDI-II ≥ 10 • Inpatient setting	Group (Design: RCT): 1. Modified BATD 2. Treatment as usual	• 2 weeks (6 sessions)	• Significantly reduced depression, anxiety, and increased environmental reward at posttreatment in BATD • Lower attrition in BATD (4.5%) compared to TAU (22.7%)
Daughters, Magidson, et al. (2010)	• 3 participants • HIV-positive and MDD • Low-income African American • Residential substance abuse facility	Individual (Design: CS) 1. ACT HEALTHY (BATD + cognitive therapy for medication adherence)	• 8 sessions (4 weeks) as an inpatient, followed by 8 sessions (4 weeks) as an outpatient	• Decreased depression and improved medication adherence in all patients • Increased environmental reward in two of three patients
Dichter et al. (2009; Dichter, Felder, & Smoski 2010)	• 27 participants • 12 adults with MDD • Age: M = 39.0 years • 15 adults without MDD • Age: M = 30.8 years	Individual (Design: OT): 1. Participants received two fMRI scans 2. MDD patients received BATD between scans	• Average of 11 sessions	• 75% treatment responders HRSD ≤ 6 • BATD resulted in improved functioning of structures that mediate response to rewards • Magnitude of pretreatment activation in paracingulate gyrus responsive to BATD predicted depression symptom change
Egede et al. (2009)	• 224 participants • MDD • 40% African American • Age 60 or older	Individual (Design: RT): 1. BATD via in-home video conferencing 2. BATD via outpatient	• 8 sessions	• Both interventions equally effective in reducing depression
Ekers et al. (2011)	• 47 participants • MDD • Moderate–severe depression • Age: M = 47.7 years	Individual (Design: RCT): 1. BATD (via mental health nurses) 2. TAU	• 12 sessions	• Decreased depression in BATD group relative to TAU • Improved work and social adjustment in BATD group

Study	Participants	Treatment	Sessions	Outcomes
Freij and Mastri (2008)	8 participants • MDD • 87% female • Age: M = 40 years	Individual (Design: OT) 1. BATD	• 13 sessions (Mean)	• Reduced depression and life impairment • Improved quality of life
Gawrysiak et al. (2009)	30 participants • Undergraduate students • 80% women • BDI-II ≥ 14 • Age: M = 18.4 years	Individual (Design: RCT): 1. Modified BATD 2. No treatment control	• One 90-minute session • Two weeks activation	• Significantly reduced depression and increased environmental reward in BATD
Gros et al. (2012)	117 participants • Combat veterans diagnosed with PTSD • 28% diagnosed with MDD	Individual (Design: OT) 1. BA-TE	• Eight 90-minute sessions	• Improvements in symptoms of PTSD, and overlapping symptoms of PTSD and depression, but not in nonoverlapping symptoms of depression
Hopko et al. (2011)	80 participants • Diagnosed with breast cancer • Principal diagnosis of major depression of moderate severity • Age: M = 55.4 years	Individual (Design: RT): 1. BATD 2. PST	• 8 sessions	• Both interventions reduce depression and anxiety and improve medical outcomes and quality of life • Minimal differences between groups • Gains maintained at 12 months • Combined rates of response and remission based on the HRSD were 78% in BATD and 81% in PST
Hopko et al. (2005)	6 participants • Diagnosed with cancer • MDD • Age: M = 46.4 years	Individual (Design: OT): 1. BATD	• 9 sessions	• Significant reduction in depression, improved quality of life and medical outcomes • Gains maintained at 3-month follow-up • Moderate/large effect sizes $d = 0.5–2.3$
Hopko, Bell, Armento et al. (2008)	18 participants • Diagnosed with cancer • MDD • Age: M = 52.2 years	Individual (Design: OT): 1. BATD supplemented with brief cognitive therapy, relaxation training, PST, and sleep hygiene	• 9 sessions	• Significant reduction in depression and anxiety, improved quality of life and medical outcomes • Gains maintained at 3-month follow-up • Moderate/large effect sizes $d = 0.5–2.0$
Hopko, Lejuez, and Hopko (2004)	1 participant • 28-year old Caucasian female • Coexistent anxiety and depression	Individual (Design: CS): 1. BATD	• 10 sessions	• Decrease is anxiety and depression and increased quality of life at posttreatment

(continued)

Table 14.1 Continued

Study	Sample	Interventions and Research Design	Duration	Primary Results
Contemporary Behavioral Treatments				
Hopko, Lejuez, et al. (2003)	25 participants • Psychiatric inpatients • MDD • Age: M = 30.5 years	Individual (Design: RT): 1. BATD + antidepressant 2. Supportive therapy + antidepressant	• 6 sessions (2 weeks)	• Decreased depression in both groups • Significantly greater improvements in the BATD group
Hopko et al. (2013)	80 participants • Diagnosed with breast cancer • Principal diagnosis of MDD of moderate severity • Age: M = 55.4 years	Individual (Design: RT): 3. BATD 4. PST	• 8 sessions	• Decreased depression and suicidal ideation and increased hopefulness at posttreatment • Results maintained at 12-month follow-up
Hopko, Sanchez, Hopko, Dvir, and Lejuez (2003)	1 participant • 25 year-old Hispanic female • MDD, borderline PD	Individual (Design: Case Study): 1. BATD supplemented with DBT strategies	• 12 sessions	• Decreased depression and suicidal ideation
Lazzari, Egan, and Rees (2011)	3 older adult participants • Moderate depression • Age: 65–73 years	Group: (Design: CS) 1. BATD (Video conferencing)	• 5 sessions	• Reduced depression and improved positive affect at posttreatment • Gains maintained at 1-month follow-up
Lejuez, Hopko, et al. (2001)	3 participants • MDD • Caucasian females • Age: 29–43 years	Individual: (Design: CS) 1. BATD	• 9–12 sessions	• Reduced depression at posttreatment
MacPherson et al. (2010)	68 participants • 73% African American • 49% women • Smokers • Depression BDI-II ≥ 10	Group (Design: RT) 1. BATD + Standard treatment (ST) 2. ST	• 8 sessions	• Participants in BATD + ST reported greater smoking abstinence • Participants in BATD + ST significantly greater reduction in depression
Magidson et al. (2011)	58 participants • Adult substance users in residential treatment • BDI-II ≥ 12 • Age M = 43.8 years	Individual (Design: RT): 1. LETS ACT–BATD 2. Supportive counseling	• 5 sessions (2.5 weeks)	• Decreased depression in both groups at posttreatment • Decreased attrition in LETS ACT • Significant increase in behavior activation in LETS ACT group

Mairs, Lovell, Campbell, and Keeley (2011)	8 participants • All schizophrenia • Age: M = 33 years • Moderate negative symptoms	Individual (Design: OT) 1. BATD	• 15 sessions (Mean)	• Decreased depression, improved negative symptoms, and improved social adjustment at posttreatment • Moderate maintenance of gains at 6-month follow-up
McIndoo, File, Preddy, Clark, and Hopko (in press)	50 participants • College students • 67% diagnosed with MDD	Individual (Design: RCT) 1. BATD 2. MBT 3. WL	• 4 sessions • 1 month follow-up	• BATD and MBT of comparable efficacy and superior to the WL • Significant improvement in depression, rumination, stress, and mindfulness • Gains maintained at 1-month follow-up
Meeks, Looney, Van Haitsma, and Teri (2008)	25 participants • Nursing home residents • 1st phase: Pilot study included 5 depressed residents • 2nd phase: Randomized trial included 20 nursing homes residents • Age: M = 75 years	Individual (Design: OT) • 1st phase: 1. BE-ACTIV Individual (Design: RCT) • 2nd phase: 1. BE-ACTIV 2. TAU	• 6 sessions • 4 weeks maintenance • 12 week follow-up (Both 1st and 2nd phase)	• 1st phase: BE-ACTIV reduced institutional barriers to participation in activities, increased activities, and reduced depression • 2nd phase: Depressive reduced in BE-ACTIV group compared to TAU group and 75% recovery rate at follow-up in BE-ACTIV and 50% in TAU
Reynolds, MacPherson, Tull, Baruch, and Lejuez (2011)	71 participants • College freshmen • Moderate depression • Alcohol abuse	Group (Design: RT) 1. Standard orientation (SO) 2. BATD + SO	• 15 weeks (2 hours)	• Problem drinking significantly reduced in BATD + SO • No reduction in depression (possible floor effect)
Ruggiero, Morris, Hopko, and Lejuez (2007)	1 participant • 17 year-old European American in foster care	Individual (Design: CS) 1. BATD	• 9 sessions	• Reduced depression at posttreatment
Snarski et al. (2011)	50 participants • Older adults (>65 years) • Mild to moderate cognitive impairment • Residents of a geriatric psychiatric facility	Individual (Design: RCT) 1. BATD + TAU 2. TAU	• 8 sessions (4 weeks)	• Significantly reduced depression in the BATD + TAU group relative to the TAU group • Efficacy of BATD + TAU not impacted by cognitive impairment
Staley and Lawyer (2010)	1 participant • 46-year-old Japanese-American male • Coexistent depression and social anxiety • Diabetes	Individual (Design: CS) 1. BATD integrated within cognitive-behavior therapy	• 9 biweekly sessions	• Decreased depression and anxiety at posttreatment • Results maintained at 3-weeks follow-up

(continued)

Table 14.1 Continued

Study	Sample	Interventions and Research Design	Duration	Primary Results
Contemporary Behavioral Treatments				
Strachan, Gros, Ruggiero, Lejuez, and Acierno (2012)	31 participants • Military veterans • 93% male • 63% PTSD: 37% subthreshold PTSD • 23% MDD	Individual (Design: RT) 1. BATD + Exposure (outpatient) 2. BATD + Exposure (home-based telehealth)	• 8 sessions (90-minute)	• Reduced depression, somatic anxiety, and PTSD symptoms at posttreatment • No between-group differences
Based or modified from BA (Martell, Addis, & Jacobson, 2001; Jacobson et al., 2001)				
Chu, Colognori, Weissman, and Bannon (2009)	4 participants • 7th and 8th grade (Age: 12–14 years) • MDD and coexistent anxiety disorder • School setting	Group (Design: OT) 1. BA supplemented with exposure to address anxiety	• 13 sessions	• 75% of sample did not meet criteria for principal and secondary diagnosis at posttreatment
Cullen, Spates, Pagoto, and Doran (2006)	25 participants • MDD • Age: M = 38 years	Individual (Design: RCT) 1. BA 2. WL	• 10 sessions	• Reduced depression BA group relative to WL at posttreatment • Maintained at 3-month follow-up
Dimidjian et al. (2006); Coffman, Martell, et al. (2007); Dobson et al. (2008)	241 participants • MDD • BDI-II ≥ 20 • HRSD ≥ 14 • Age: 18–60 years	Individual (Design: RCT) 1. BA 2. CT 3. ADM 4. Placebo	• BA and CT 16 weeks (24 sessions) • ADM (Paroxetine) 16 weeks (36 sessions) • Placebo 8 weeks (12 sessions)	• Reduced depression in all four groups • Low depression severity group: No differences between groups • High depression severity group: BA and ADM more effective than CT • At 2-year follow-up, BA and CT patients less likely to relapse • Significantly more extreme nonresponders to treatment in BA relative to CT • Patients with severe depression and functional impairment may be more appropriate for BA relative to CT

Study	Participants	Design	Sessions	Outcomes
Jacob, Keeley, Ritschel, and Craighead (2013)	3 adolescent participants • Low-income African American • MDD • Age: 13–17 years	Individual (Design: OT) 1. Adapted BA for adolescents with inclusion of parents in intervention	• 14–17 sessions (6 months)	• 2 of 3 participants no longer met criteria for MDD at posttreatment • Depression and functional impairment decreased for all participants
Jacobson et al. (1996); Gortner et al. (1998)	150 participants • Outpatients with MDD • BDI-II ≥ 20 • HRSD ≥ 14	Individual (Design: RT) 1. BA 2. BA plus automatic thought modification 3. CT	• 20 sessions	• BA comparable to full CT at posttreatment in reducing depression • Results maintained at 2-year follow-up
Jakupcak et al. (2006)	9 participants • Veterans with PTSD • Veterans Administration outpatient PTSD clinic	Individual (Design: OT) 1. BA	• 16 sessions	• Reduction of PTSD severity at posttreatment based on the CAPS • Reduced depression and improved quality of life (not significant)
Jakupcak et al. (2010)	8 participants • Caucasian military Veterans • PTSD and 50% current MDD • Age: M = 25 years	Individual (Design: OT) 1. BA	• 8 sessions	• Reduction of PTSD severity at posttreatment • Reduced depression and improved quality of life (not significant)
Kanter et al. (2010)	10 Latina participants • Age: M = 40 years • At bilingual (English-Spanish) mental health clinic • HRSD ≥ 16; BDI-II ≥ 20 • MDD according to PRIME-MD	Individual (Design: RCT) 1. BA-Latino 2. TAU	• 12 sessions	• Reduced depression at posttreatment in the BA group • High attrition in the TAU group prohibited group comparisons
Mulick and Naugle (2004)	1 participant • Police officer/military veteran • PTSD and MDD • Age: 37 years	Individual (Design: CS) 1. BA	• 11 sessions	• Patient no longer met diagnostic criteria for PTSD and MDD at posttreatment

(continued)

Table 14.1 Continued

Study	Sample	Interventions and Research Design	Duration	Primary Results
Contemporary Behavioral Treatments				
Nixon and Nearmy (2011)	20 participants • PTSD and MDD • 35% coexistent anxiety • 85% female • Age: M = 45 years	Individual (Design: OT) 1. BA + exposure therapy	• 12–16 sessions • First 6 BA, then integration of exposure for up to 10 sessions	• Decreased PTSD and depression severity at posttreatment • Treatment gains maintained at 3 months follow-up with 60% and 70% no longer meeting diagnostic criteria for PTSD and MDD, respectively
Pagoto et al. (2008)	14 participants • Obese, BMI ≥ 30 • MDD • BDI-II ≥ 10; HDRS ≥ 10 • Age: M = 45 years	Group (Design: OT) 1. BA with nutrition counseling for weight loss, and groups led by dietician	• 12 sessions (6 biweekly, 90-minute)	• Reductions in body weight and daily caloric intake • Reduced depression at posttreatment • 10/14 patients had full depression remission at posttreatment
Porter, Spates, and Smitham (2004)	26 participants • MDD • Age: M = 44 years	Group (Design: RCT) 1. BA 2. Wait list control	• 10 sessions (95-minute)	• Significantly reduced depression in the BA group at posttreatment • Results maintained at 3-month follow-up
Ritschel, Ramirez, Jones, and Craighead (2011)	6 adolescent participants • MDD • BDI: M = 27.00 • Age: 14–17 years	Individual (Design: OT) 1. BA modified for adolescents with inclusion of parents	• 11–16 sessions	• Decreased depression at posttreatment
Santiago-Rivera et al. (2008)	1 male Latino participant • Monolingual Spanish-speaking • Age: 46 years	Individual (Design: CS) 1. BA: conducted in Spanish	• 45 sessions	• Significant reduction in depressive symptoms at posttreatment

Study	Participants	Design/Conditions	Sessions	Outcomes
Wagner, Zatzick, Ghesquiere, and Jurkovich (2007)	8 participants • MDD and PTSD • Physically injured survivors of traumatic injury • Glasgow Coma Scale <15 or Mental State Examination <7 • Age: 18–65 years	Individual (Design: RCT) 1. BA modified for physical injured trauma survivors 2. TAU	• BA: 4 sessions (60–90 minutes) • TAU: community referrals	• BA group showed decreased PTSD symptom severity, but not depression severity at posttreatment • BA group had improved physical functioning at posttreatment
Weinstock, Munroe, and Miller (2011)	10 participants • MDD with atypical features • IDS-C ≥ 30 • Age: M = 36 years	Individual (Design: OT) 1. BA	• 16 sessions	• Decreased depression and functional impairment and increased activity level at posttreatment

Assessment Measures: BDI, Beck Depression Inventory (Beck & Steer, 1987); BDI-II, Beck Depression Inventory-II (Beck, Steer, & Brown, 1996); BMI, body mass index; CAPS, Clinician-Administered PTSD Scale (Blake et al., 1995); HRSD, Hamilton Rating Scale for Depression (Hamilton, 1960); IDS-C, Inventory of Depressive Symptomatology-Clinician version (Rush, Guillon, Basco, Jarrett, & Trivedi, 1996); PRIME-MD, Primary Care Evaluation for Mental Disorders (Spitzer, Williams, Kroenke, & Linzer, 1994). *Treatment Condition Abbreviations:* ADM, antidepressant medication (Paroxetine); BATD, brief behavioral activation treatment for depression; BA-TE, behavior activation with therapeutic exposure; CT, cognitive therapy; DBT, dialectical behavior therapy; MBT, mindfulness-based therapy; PST, problem solving therapy; TAU, treatment as usual; WL, wait list. *Research Design Abbreviations:* CS, case study; OT, open trial; RCT, randomized controlled trial; RT, randomized trial. *Diagnostic Abbreviations:* GAD, generalized anxiety disorder; MDD, major depressive disorder; PTSD, posttraumatic stress disorder.

of 16 studies, the pooled effect size indicating the difference between activity scheduling and control conditions at posttreatment was large ($d = 0.87$ [95% CI: 0.60–1.15]). Comparisons with other psychological treatments at posttreatment resulted in a nonsignificant pooled effect size of 0.13, in favor of activity scheduling. In 10 studies where activity scheduling was compared to cognitive therapy, a nonsignificant pooled effect size of 0.02 was indicated. Importantly, the changes from posttreatment to follow-up for activity scheduling were nonsignificant, indicating that the benefits of treatment were retained at follow-up. In a second meta-analysis of 17 randomized controlled trials involving behavioral interventions (Ekers et al., 2008), posttreatment symptom assessment showed behavioral therapies were superior to control conditions (standardized mean difference [SMD] −0.70, 95% CI −1.00 to −0.39, $k = 12$, $n = 459$), brief psychotherapy (SMD −0.56, 95% CI −1.0 to −0.12, $k = 3$, $n = 166$), supportive therapy (SMD −0.75, 95% CI −1.37 to −0.14, $k = 2$, $n = 45$), and equal to cognitive behavioral therapy (SMD −0.08, 95% CI −0.14 to 0.30, $k = 12$, $n = 476$). Finally, in a third meta-analysis that assessed the impact of behavioral activation on subjective well-being and life satisfaction, a pooled effect size across 20 studies indicated a significant difference in well-being between behavioral activation and control conditions at posttreatment that was associated with a moderate effect size (Hedges's g = 0.52). This significant effect was found for both nonclinical individuals and those with elevated depression symptoms. Taken together, the studies highlighted in Table 14.1 and these three meta-analyses strongly support the efficacy of behavioral activation as a treatment for depression and suggest that the relatively uncomplicated and time-efficient approach may be adequate as a stand-alone intervention for a wide range of patients, including those with severe depression (Dimidjian et al., 2006).

Directions for Future Research

Based on accumulating data, behavioral activation interventions show promise as parsimonious and potentially cost-effective means to treat clinical depression. Given the current status of behavioral activation as an empirically validated treatment for depression, the foundation has been established to further explore important theoretical and empirical questions related to behavioral models of depression and the extrapolation of these models toward refining behavioral activation interventions. First,

more systematic longitudinal research is required to assess causality in terms of the degree that decreased response-contingent positive reinforcement is critical toward the etiology of depressive symptoms and disorders. Second, congruent with Lewinsohn's behavioral model (1974), increased specification of the relevance of reward probability (i.e., potentially reinforcing events and instrumental behaviors in obtaining reinforcement) and environmental suppression (i.e., availability of reinforcement in the environment and presence of punishing/aversive experiences) toward conceptualizing the onset and maintenance of depression will be useful toward treatment development and refinement. Third, at this stage of research, very little is known about how reinforcement value (i.e., magnitude, immediacy, duration, and certainty) is associated with the development of a depressive disorder or how these factors should be addressed within behavioral activation treatment protocols. Similarly, the qualitative (type, function) aspects of reinforcing events and an individual's reinforcement sensitivity are factors that may affect the efficacy of behavioral activation protocols but are generally unstudied. Fourth, more rigorous empirical testing is required to further assess the efficacy and effectiveness of behavioral activation relative to other well-established, empirically validated psychosocial and pharmacological interventions for depression, particularly newer generation antidepressants.

Fifth, a more sophisticated understanding of behavioral activation dose–response relationships is required. Because most sudden reductions in depressive symptoms are observed in the first four sessions of treatment (Hopko et al., 2009), and as few as 2 weeks have been shown as adequate toward reducing depression (Armento et al., 2012; Gawrysiak et al., 2009), future clinical trials might focus on determining the level of activation required to promote depression reduction and maintenance of gains over time. Considering that focusing on the single activation domain of spirituality significantly reduced depression symptoms in college students (Armento et al., 2012), understanding the relative importance of other behavioral domains in attenuating depression (across different samples) yields some exciting research opportunities. Sixth, dismantling studies that better isolate the intervention component(s) most essential to engendering nondepressive (healthy) behavior also are needed, as is an answer to the question of whether the more comprehensive 20–24 session BA protocol yields incremental treatment gains beyond those of the more streamlined 8–10 session BATD proto-col. Relatedly, how much do mindfulness training, mental rehearsal, and therapist modeling contribute to treatment outcome relative to guided activity? Is teaching patients the TRAC, TRAP, and ACTION models critical to treatment success? Similar concerns may be raised in regard to BATD. For example, what impact does behavioral contracting have on treatment outcome? How necessary is it to base the activity hierarchy on a life value (LAVA) assessment? Is it necessary to address all life domains or would transfer effects be evident by targeting fewer (or the most important) areas? There also are components common to the BA and BATD approaches that may moderate outcome and prove difficult to measure and control, such as the nature and quality of the therapeutic relationship. These questions all require further empirical attention.

Seventh, the relatively uncomplicated and time-efficient administration of behavioral activation strategies may allow for "real-world" effectiveness studies that may be conducted in primary care environments. Accordingly, focusing on quality improvement in primary care settings by incorporating behavioral activation interventions with an emphasis on treatment efficacy and cost-effectiveness is a pressing need (Coyne, 2000; Schoenbaum, Unutzer, Sherbourne, & Duan, 2001). Indeed, as recently demonstrated (Ekers et al., 2011), the structured and manualized behavioral activation approach may allow for implementation by health care providers such as physicians, nurses, and social workers. Eighth, although important strides have been made toward evaluating the potential transfer effects of behavioral activation treatment to other Axis I and II treatment conditions, much more systematic work is required in this area. Along these lines, we also need to identify potential patient-related variables associated with positive treatment outcome to make evaluations and recommendations as to which patients will be more or less likely to respond to behavioral activation interventions. Finally, although pioneering work has examined the potential utility of behavioral activation across the life span and across ethnic and racial minorities, this research is very much in its infancy.

In closing, as we indicated a decade ago (Hopko, Lejuez, et al., 2003), this continues to be an exciting time for researchers and practitioners involved with behavioral activation. The highly favorable treatment outcome data have renewed interest in behavioral treatment approaches once thought insufficient for treating clinical depression and have paved the way for a multitude of exciting research opportunities related to behavioral theory and treatment outcome. It has become evident that purely behavioral approaches to treating depression were in fact abandoned prematurely some 30 years ago. Instead of repeating history, the data collectively suggest that behavioral activation merits strong regard as a parsimonious and effective intervention with many applications supported, and hopefully many more to follow in the years ahead.

References

Addis, M. E., & Jacobson, N. S. (1996). Reasons for depression and the process and outcome of cognitive-behavioral psychotherapies. *Journal of Consulting and Clinical Psychology, 64,* 1417–1424.

Addis, M. E., & Martell, C. R. (2004). *Overcoming depression one step at a time: The new behavioral activation approach to getting your life back.* New York, NY: New Harbinger Press.

Alfonsson, S., Parling, T., & Ghaderi, A. (2014). Group behavioral activation for patients with severe obesity and binge eating disorder: A randomized controlled trial. *Behavior Modification.* Epub ahead of print.

Armento, M. E. A., & Hopko, D. R. (2007). The Environmental Reward Observation Scale (EROS): Development, validity, and reliability. *Behavior Therapy, 38,* 107–119.

Armento, M. E. A., & Hopko, D. R. (2009). Behavioral activation of a breast cancer patient with coexistent major depression and generalized anxiety disorder. *Clinical Case Studies, 8,* 25.

Armento, M. E. A., McNulty, J. K., & Hopko, D. R. (2012). Behavioral activation of religious behaviors: Treating depressed college students with a randomized controlled trial. *Psychology of Religion and Spirituality, 4,* 206–222.

American Psychiatric Association. (2000). *Diagnostic and statistical manual of mental disorders* (4th ed., text rev.). Washington, DC: Author.

Andreasen, N. J. C., & Pfohl, B. (1976). Linguistic analysis of speech in affective disorders. *Archives of General Psychiatry, 33,* 1361–1367.

Antonuccio, D. O., Ward, C. H., & Tearnan, B. H. (1991). The behavioral treatment of unipolar depression in adult outpatients. In M. Hersen, R. M. Eisler, & P. M. Miller (Eds.), *Progress in behavior modification* (Vol. 24, pp. 152–191). Newbury Park, CA: Sage.

Bagby, M. R., Ryder, A. G., Schuller, D. R., & Marshall, M. B. (2004). The Hamilton Depression Rating Scale: Has the gold standard become a lead weight? *American Journal of Psychiatry, 161,* 2163–2177.

Bailey, D. L., & Arco, L. (2010). Effects of a brief behavioural activation treatment on activities of various difficulty and depression. *Behaviour Change, 27,* 184–197.

Barlow, D. H. (2002). *Anxiety and its disorders: The nature and treatment of anxiety and panic* (2nd ed.). New York, NY: Guilford Press.

Barlow, D. H., Allen, L. B., & Choate, M. L. (2004). Toward a unified treatment for emotional disorders. *Behavior Therapy, 35,* 205–230.

Barlow, D. H., & Campbell, L. A. (2000). Mixed anxiety-depression and its implications for models of anxiety and mood disorders. *Comprehensive Psychology, 41,* 55–60.

Barrera, M. (1979). An evaluation of a brief group therapy for depression. *Journal of Consulting and Clinical Psychology*, *47*, 413.

Beck, A. T., Epstein, N., Brown, G., & Steer, R. A. (1988). An inventory for measuring clinical anxiety: Psychometric properties. *Journal of Consulting and Clinical Psychology*, *56*, 893–897.

Beck, A. T., Rush, A. J., Shaw, B. J., & Emery, G. (1979). *Cognitive therapy of depression*. New York, NY: Guilford Press.

Beck, A. T., & Steer, R. A. (1987). *Beck Depression Inventory: Manual*. San Antonio, TX: The Psychiatric Corporation.

Beck, A. T., Steer, R. A., & Brown, G. K. (1996). *Manual for Beck Depression Inventory-II*. San Antonio, TX: Psychological Corporation.

Beck, A. T., Steer, R. A., & Garbin, M. G. (1988). Psychometric properties of the Beck Depression Inventory: 25 years of evaluation. *Clinical Psychology Review*, 8, 77–100.

Benca, R. M., Obermeyer, W. H., Thisted, R. A., & Gillin, J. C. (1992). Sleep and psychiatric disorders: A meta-analysis. *Archives of General Psychiatry*, *49*, 651–668.

Biglan, A., & Craker, D. (1982). Effects of pleasant-activities manipulation on depression. *Journal of Consulting and Clinical Psychology*, *50*, 436–438.

Blake, D. D., Weathers, F. W., Nagy, L. M., Kaloupek, D. G., Gusman, F. D., Charney, D. S., & Keane, T. M. (1995) The development of a clinician-administered PTSD scale. *Journal of Traumatic Stress*, 8, 75–90.

Blumberg, S. R., & Hokanson, J. E. (1983). The effect's of another person's response style on interpersonal behavior in depression. *Journal of Abnormal Psychology*, *92*, 196–209.

Bonierbale, M., Lancon, C., & Tignol, J. (2003). The ELIXIR study: Evaluation of sexual dysfunction in 4,557 depressed patients in France. *Current Medical Research Opinions*, *19*, 1114–1124.

Brown, R. A., & Lewinsohn, P. M. (1984). A psychoeducational approach to the treatment of depression: Comparison of group, individual, and minimal contact procedures. *Journal of Consulting and Clinical Psychology*, *52*, 774–783.

Brown, T. A., Di Nardo, P., & Barlow, D. H. (1994). *Anxiety disorders interview schedule for DSM-IV*. San Antonio, TX: The Psychological Corporation.

Carvalho, J. P., & Hopko, D. R. (2011). Behavioral theory of depression: Reinforcement as a mediating variable between avoidance and depression. *Behavior Therapy and Experimental Psychiatry*, *42*, 154–162.

Carvalho, J. P., Trent, L. R., & Hopko, D. R. (2011). The impact of decreased environmental reward in predicting depression severity: Support for behavioral theories of depression. *Psychopathology*, *44*, 242–252.

Carver, C. S., & White, T. L. (1994). Behavioral inhibition, behavioral activation, and affective responses to impending reward and punishment: The BIS/BAS scales. *Journal of Personality and Social Psychology*, *67*, 319–333.

Chu, B. C., Colognori, D., Weissman, A. S., & Bannon, K. (2009). An initial description and pilot of group behavioral activation therapy for anxious and depressed youth. *Cognitive and Behavioral Practice*, *16*, 408–419.

Coffman, S. J., Martell, C. R., Dimidjian, S., Gallop, R., & Hollon, S. D. (2007). Extreme nonresponse in cognitive therapy: Can behavioral activation succeed where cognitive therapy fails? *Journal of Consulting and Clinical Psychology*, *75*, 531–541.

Collins, K. A., Westra, H. A., Dozois, D. J. A., & Burns, D. D. (2004). Gaps in accessing treatment for anxiety and depression: Challenges for the delivery of care. *Clinical Psychology Review*, *24*, 583–616.

Collado, A., Castillo, S. D., Maero, F., Lejuez, C. W., & MacPherson, L. (2014). Pilot of the brief behavioral activation treatment for depression in Latinos with limited English proficiency: Preliminary evaluation of efficacy and acceptability. *Behavior Therapy*, *45*, 102–115.

Comas-Díaz, L. (1981). Effects of cognitive and behavioral group treatment on the depressive symptomatology of Puerto Rican women. *Journal of Consulting and Clinical Psychology*, *49*, 627.

Correia, C. J., Carey, K. B., & Borsari, B. (2002). Measuring substance-free and substance-related reinforcement in the natural environment. *Psychology of Addictive Behaviors*, *16*, 28–34.

Coyne, J. C. (1976). Toward an interactional description of depression. *Psychiatry*, *39*, 28–40.

Coyne, J. C. (2000). Depression in primary care: Depressing news, exciting research opportunities. *American Psychological Society Observer*, *14*, 1–4.

Cuijpers, P., van Straten, A., & Warmerdam, L. (2007). Behavioral activation treatments of depression: A meta-analysis. *Clinical Psychology Review*, *27*, 318–326.

Cullen, J. M., Spates, C. R., Pagoto, S. L., & Doran, N. (2006). Behavioral activation treatment for major depressive disorder: A pilot investigation. *Behavior Analyst Today*, *7*, 151–166.

Daughters, S. B., Braun, A. R., Sargeant, M. N., Reynolds, E. K., Hopko, D. R., Blanco, C., & Lejuez, C. (2008). Effectiveness of a brief behavioral treatment for inner-city illicit drug users with elevated depressive symptoms: The Life Enhancement Treatment for Substance Use (LETS Act!). *Journal of Clinical Psychiatry*, *69*, 122–129.

DeRubeis, R. J., & Crits-Christoph, P. (1998). Empirically supported individual and group psychological treatments for adult mental disorders. *Journal of Consulting and Clinical Psychology*, *66*, 37–52.

Dichter, G. S., Felder, J. N., Petty, C., Bizzell, J., Ernst, M., & Smoski, M. J. (2009). The effects of psychotherapy on neural responses to rewards in major depression. *Biological Psychiatry*, *66*, 886–897.

Dichter, G. S., Felder, J. N., & Smoski, M. J. (2010). The effects of brief behavioral activation therapy for depression on cognitive control in affective contexts: An fMRI investigation. *Journal of Affective Disorders*, *126*, 236–244.

Dimidjian, S., Barrera, M., Martell, C., Munoz, R. F., & Lewinsohn, P. M. (2011). The origins and current status of behavioral activation treatments for depression. *Annual Review of Clinical Psychology*, *7*, 1–38.

Dimidjian, S., Hollon, S. D., Dobson, K. S., Schmaling, K. B., Kohlenberg, R. J., Addis, M. E., … Jacobson, N. S. (2006). Randomized trial of behavioral activation, cognitive therapy, and antidepressant medication in the acute treatment of adults with major depression. *Journal of Consulting and Clinical Psychology*, *74*, 658.

Dimidjian, S., Hubley, A., Martell, C. R., Herman-Dunn, A. &, Dobson, K. S. (2012). *The Quality of Behavioral Activation Scale (Q-BAS)*. Unpublished manuscript, University of Colorado, Boulder.

Dobson, K. S., Hollon, S. D., Dimidjian, S., Schmaling, K. B., Kohlenberg, R. J., Gallop, R. J., … Jacobson, N. S. (2008).

Randomized trial of behavioral activation, cognitive therapy, and antidepressant medication in the prevention of relapse and recurrence in major depression. *Journal of Consulting and Clinical Psychology, 76*, 468.

Dykman, B. M., Horowitz, I. M., Abramson, L. Y., & Usher, M. (1991). Schematic and situational determinants of depressed and nondepressed students' interpretation of feedback. *Journal of Abnormal Psychology, 100*, 45–55.

Egede, L. E., Frueh, C. B., Richardson, L. K., Acierno, R., Mauldin, P. D., Knapp, R. G., & Lejuez, C. (2009). Rationale and design: Telepsychology service delivery for depressed elderly veterans. *Trials, 10*, 22.

Eifert, G. H., Beach, B., & Wilson, P. H. (1998). Depression: Behavioral principles and implications for treatment and relapse prevention. In J. J. Plaud & G. H. Eifert (Eds.), *From behavior theory to behavior therapy* (pp. 68–97). Boston: Allyn & Bacon.

Ekers, D., Richards, D., & Gilbody, S. (2008). A meta-analysis of randomized trials of behavioural treatment of depression. *Psychological Medicine, 38*, 611–623.

Ekers, D., Richards, D., McMillan, D., Bland, J. M., & Gilbody, S. (2011). Behavioral activation delivered by the non-specialist: Phase II randomized controlled trial. *British Journal of Psychiatry, 198*, 66–72.

Elkin, I., Shea, M. T., Watkins, J. T., Imber, S. D., Sotsky, S. M., Collins, J. F., … Parloff, M. B. (1989). National Institute of Mental Health Treatment of Depression Collaborative Research Program: General effectiveness of treatments. *Archives of General Psychiatry, 46*, 971–982.

Endicott, J., & Spitzer, R. L. (1978). A diagnostic interview: The Schedule for Affective Disorders and Schizophrenia. *Archives of General Psychiatry, 35*, 837–844.

Ferster, C. B. (1973). A functional analysis of depression. *American Psychologist, 28*, 857–870.

Fincham, F. D., Beach, S. R. H., Harold, G. T., & Osborne, L. N. (1997). Marital satisfaction and depression: Different causal relationships for men and women. *Psychological Science, 8*, 351–357.

First, M. B., Spitzer, R. L., Gibbon, M., & Williams, J. (1996). *Structured clinical interview for DSM-IVaxis I disorders-patient edition (SCID-I/P, Version 2.0)*. New York, NY: New York Psychiatric Institute.

Freij, K., & Masri, N. (2008). The brief behavioral activation treatment for depression: A psychiatric pilot study. *Nordic Psychology, 60*, 129.

Fuchs, C. Z., & Rehm, L. P. (1977). A self-control behavior therapy program for depression. *Journal of Consulting and Clinical Psychology, 45*, 206–215.

Gable, S. L., & Shean, G. D. (2000). Perceived social competence and depression. *Journal of Social and Personal Relationships, 17*, 139–150.

Gardner, P., & Oei, T. (1981). Depression and self-esteem: An investigation that used behavioural and cognitive approaches to the treatment of clinically depressed clients. *Journal of Clinical Psychology, 37*, 129–135.

Gawrysiak, M., Nicholas, C., & Hopko, D. R. (2009). Behavioral activation for moderately depressed university students: Randomized controlled trial. *Journal of Counseling Psychology, 56*, 468.

Gaynor, S. T., & Harris, A. (2008). Single-participant assessment of treatment mediators: Strategy description and examples from a behavioral activation intervention for depressed adolescents. *Behavior Modification, 32*, 372–402.

Gortner, E. T., Gollan, J. K., Dobson, K. S., & Jacobson, N. S. (1998). Cognitive-behavioral treatment for depression: Relapse prevention. *Journal of Consulting and Clinical Psychology, 66*, 377–384.

Gotlib, I. H. (1982). Self-reinforcement and depression in interpersonal interaction: The role of performance level. *Journal of Abnormal Psychology, 91*, 3–13.

Gotlib, I. H., & Robinson, L. A. (1982). Responses to depressed individuals: Discrepancies between self-report and observer-rated behavior. *Journal of Abnormal Psychology, 91*, 231–240.

Gray, J. A. (1982). *The neuropsychology of anxiety: An enquiry into the functions of the septohippocampal system.* New York, NY: Oxford University Press.

Gros, D. F., Price, M., Strachan, M., Yuen, E. K., Milanak, M. E., & Acierno, R. (2012). Behavioral activation and therapeutic exposure: An investigation of relative symptom changes in PTSD and depression during the course of integrated behavioral activation, situational exposure, and imaginal exposure techniques. *Behavior Modification, 36*, 580–599.

Grosscup, S. J., & Lewinsohn, P. M. (1980). Unpleasant and pleasant events and mood. *Journal of Clinical Psychology, 36*, 252–259.

Hamilton, M. (1960). A rating scale for depression. *Neurology, Neurosurgery and Psychiatry, 23*, 56–61.

Hammen, C. L., & Glass, D. R. (1975). Depression, activity, and evaluation of reinforcement. *Journal of Abnormal Psychology, 84*, 718–721.

Hanley, G. P., Iwata, B. A., & McCord, B. E. (2003). Functional analysis of problem behavior: A review. *Journal of Applied Behavior Analysis, 36*, 147–185.

Harmon, T. M., Nelson, R. O., & Hayes S. C. (1980). Self-monitoring of mood versus activity by depressed clients. *Journal of Consulting and Clinical Psychology, 48*, 30–38.

Hayes, S. C. (2004). Acceptance and commitment therapy, relational frame theory, and the third wave of behavioral and cognitive therapies. *Behavior therapy, 35*, 639–665.

Hayes, S. C., Strosahl, K. D., & Wilson, K. G. (1999). *Acceptance and commitment therapy: An experiential approach to behavior change.* New York, NY: Guilford Press.

Hayes, S. C., Wilson, K. G., Gifford, E. V., Follette, V. M., & Strosahl, K. (1996). Experiential avoidance and behavioral disorders: A functional dimensional approach to diagnosis and treatment. *Journal of Consulting and Clinical Psychology, 64*, 1152–1168.

Herrnstein, R. J. (1970). On the law of effect. *Journal of the Experimental Analysis of Behavior, 13*, 243–266.

Hersen, M., Bellack, A. S., Himmelhock, J. M., & Thase, M. E. (1984). Effects of social skills training, amitriptyline, and psychotherapy in unipolar depressed women. *Behavior Therapy, 15*, 21–40.

Hesselbrock, M. M., Hesselbrock, V. M., Tenmen, H., Meyer, R. E., & Workman, K. L. (1983). Methodological considerations in the assessment of depression in alcoholics. *Journal of Consulting and Clinical Psychology, 51*, 399–405.

Hinchliffe, M., Hooper, D., & Roberts, F. J. (1978). *The melancholy marriage.* New York: Wiley.

Hollon, S. D. (2001). Behavioral activation treatment for depression: A commentary. *Clinical Psychology: Science and Practice, 8*, 271–274.

Hollon, S. D., & Ponniah, K. (2010). A review of empirically supported psychological therapies for mood disorders in adults. *Depression and Anxiety, 27*, 891–932.

Hollon, S. D., Shelton, R. C., & Davis, D. D. (1993). Cognitive therapy for depression: Conceptual issues and clinical efficacy. *Journal of Consulting and Clinical Psychology, 61*, 270–275.

Hollon, S. D., Thase, M. E., & Markowitz, J. C. (2002). Treatment and prevention of depression. *Psychological Science in the Public Interest, 3*, 39–77.

Hopko, D. R., Armento, M. E. A., Cantu, M. S., Chambers, L. L., & Lejuez, C. W. (2003). The use of daily diaries to assess the relations among mood state, overt behavior, and reward value of activities. *Behaviour Research and Therapy, 41*, 1137–1148.

Hopko, D. R., Armento, M. E. A., Robertson, S., Ryba, M. M., Carvalho, J. P., Colman, L. K., ... Lejuez, C. W. (2011). Brief behavioral activation and problem-solving therapy for depressed breast cancer patients: Randomized trial. *Journal of Consulting and Clinical Psychology, 79*, 834–849.

Hopko, D., Bell, J., Armento, M., Hunt, M., & Lejuez, C. (2005). Behavior therapy for depressed cancer patients in primary care. *Psychotherapy: Theory, Research, Practice, Training, 42*, 236–243.

Hopko, D. R., Bell, J. L., Armento, M. E. A., Robertson, S. M. C., Mullane, C., Wolf, N., & Lejuez, C. W. (2008). Cognitive-behavior therapy for depressed cancer patients in a medical care setting. *Behavior Therapy, 39*, 126–136.

Hopko, D. R., Funderburk, J. S., Shorey, R. C., McIndoo, C. C., Ryba, M. M., ... Vitulano, M. (2013). Behavioral activation and problem-solving therapy for depressed breast cancer patients: Preliminary support for efficacy in reducing suicidal ideation. *Behavior Modification, 37*, 747–767.

Hopko, D. R., Lejuez, C. W., Armento, M. E. A., & Bare, R. L. (2004). Depressive disorders. In M. Hersen (Ed.), *Psychological assessment in clinical practice: A pragmatic guide* (pp. 85–116). New York, NY: Taylor & Francis.

Hopko, D. R., Lejuez, C., & Hopko, S. D. (2004). Behavioral activation as an intervention for coexistent depressive and anxiety symptoms. *Clinical Case Studies, 3*, 37.

Hopko, D. R., Lejuez, C., Lepage, J. P., Hopko, S. D., & McNeil, D. W. (2003). A brief behavioral activation treatment for depression. *Behavior Modification, 27*, 458.

Hopko, D. R., Lejuez, C. W., Ruggiero, K. J., & Eifert, G. H. (2003). Contemporary behavioral activation treatments for depression: Procedures, principles, and progress. *Clinical Psychology Review, 23*, 699–717.

Hopko, D. R., & Mullane, C. M. (2008). Exploring the relation of depression and overt behavior with daily diaries. *Behaviour Research and Therapy, 45*, 1085–1089.

Hopko, D. R., Robertson, S., & Lejuez, C. W. (2006). Behavioral activation for anxiety disorders. *Behavior Analyst Today, 7*, 212–232.

Hopko, D. H., Robertson, S. M. C., & Carvalho, J. (2009). Sudden gains in depressed cancer patients treated with behavioral activation therapy. *Behavior Therapy, 40*, 346–356.

Hopko, D. R., Sanchez, L., Hopko, S. D., Dvir, S., & Lejuez, C. (2003). Behavioral activation and the prevention of suicidal behaviors in patients with borderline personality disorder. *Journal of Personality Disorders, 17*, 460–478.

Horner, R. H. (1994). Functional assessment: Contributions and future directions. *Journal of Applied Behavior Analysis, 27*, 401–404.

Hubley, S., Dimidjian, S., & Gallop, R. (2012). *Increasing activity and decreasing depression: Observational coding of patient reports of activation and the relationship to improvement in depression.* Unpublished manuscript.

Jacob, M., Keeley, M. L., Ritschel, L., & Craighead, W. E. (2013). Behavioural activation for the treatment of low-income, African American adolescents with major depressive disorder: A case series. *Clinical Psychology and Psychotherapy, 20*, 87–96.

Jacobson, N. S., Dobson, K. S., Truax, P. A., Addis, M. E., Koerner, K., Gollan, J. K., ... Prince, S. E. (1996). A component analysis of cognitive-behavioral treatment for depression. *Journal of Consulting and Clinical Psychology, 64*, 295–304.

Jacobson, N. S., & Gortner, E. T. (2000). Can depression be de-medicalized in the 21st century: Scientific revolutions, counter-revolutions and the magnetic field of normal science. *Behaviour Research and Therapy, 38*, 103–117.

Jacobson, N. S., Martell, C. R., & Dimidjian, S. (2001). Behavioral activation treatment for depression: Returning to contextual roots. *Clinical Psychology: Science and Practice, 8*, 255–270.

Jakupcak, M., Roberts, L., Martell, C., Mulick, P., Michael, S., & Reed, R. (2006). A pilot study of behavior activation for veterans with posttraumatic stress disorder. *Journal of Traumatic Stress, 19*, 387–391.

Jorm, A. F., Christensen, H., Henderson, A. S., Jacomb, P. A., Korten, A. E., & Rodgers, B. (1999). Using the BIS/BAS scales to measure behavioural inhibition and behavioural activation: Factor structure, validity and norms in a large community sample. *Personality and Individual Differences, 26*, 49–58

Kabat-Zinn, J. (1990). *Full catastrophe living: Using the wisdom of your body and mind to face stress, pain, and illness.* New York, NY: Delacorte.

Kanfer, F. H., & Grimm, L. G. (1977). Behavioral analysis: Selecting target behaviors in the interview. *Behavior Modification, 1*, 7–28.

Kanter, J. W., Manos, R. C., Bowe, W. M., Baruch, D. E., Busch, A. M., & Rusch, L. C. (2010). What is behavioral activation? A review of the empirical literature. *Clinical Psychology Review, 30*, 608–620.

Kanter, J. W., Manos, R. C., Busch, A. M., & Rusch, L. C. (2008). Making behavioral activation more behavioral. *Behavior Modification, 32*, 780–803.

Kanter, J. W., Mulick, P. S., Busch, A. M., Berlin, K. S., & Martell, C. R. (2007). The Behavioral Activation for Depression Scale (BADS): Psychometric properties and factor structure. *Journal of Psychopathology and Behavioral Assessment, 29*, 191–202.

Kanter, J. W., Rusch, L. C., Landes, S. J., Holman, G. I., Whiteside, U., & Sedivy, S. K. (2009). The use and nature of present-focused interventions in cognitive and behavioral therapies for depression. *Psychotherapy, 46*, 220–232.

Kanter, J. W., Santiago-Rivera, A. L., Rusch, L. C., Busch, A. M., & West, P. (2010). Initial outcomes of a culturally adapted behavioral activation for Latinas diagnosed with depression at a community clinic. *Behavior Modification, 34*, 120–144.

Kasch, K. L., Rottenberg, J., Arnow, B. A., & Gotlib, I. H. (2002). Behavioral activation and inhibition systems and the severity and course of depression. *Journal of Abnormal Psychology, 111*, 589–597.

Kazdin, A. E. (1977). Assessing the clinical or applied importance of behavior change through social validation. *Behavior Modification, 1*, 427–452.

Kessler, R. C., Berglund, P., Demler, O., Jin, R., Koretz, D., Merikangas, K. R., ... Wang, P. S. (2003). The epidemiology of major depressive disorder: Results from the National Comorbidity Survey Replication (NCS-R). *Journal of the American Medical Association, 289*, 3095–3105.

Kobak, K. A., & Reynolds, W. M. (1999). Hamilton Depression Inventory. In M. E. Maruish (Ed.), *The use of psychological testing for treatment planning and outcomes assessment* (2nd ed., pp. 935–969). Mahwah, NJ: Erlbaum.

Kohlenberg, R. J., & Tsai, M. (1991). *Functional analytic psychotherapy: Creating intense and curative therapeutic relationships.* New York, NY: Plenum.

Lazzari, C., Egan, S.J., & Rees, C.S. (2011). Behavioural activation treatment for depression in older adults delivered via videoconferencing: A pilot study. *Cognitive and Behavioural Practice, 18*, 555–565.

Lejuez, C., Hopko, D. R., Acierno, R., Daughters, S. B., & Pagoto, S. L. (2011). Ten year revision of the brief behavioral activation treatment for depression: Revised treatment manual. *Behavior Modification, 35*, 111–161.

Lejuez, C. W., Hopko, D. R., & Hopko, S. D. (2001). A brief behavioral activation treatment for depression: Treatment manual. *Behavior Modification, 25*, 255–286.

Lejuez, C. W., Hopko, D. R., Levine, S., Gholkar, R., & Collins, L. M. (2005). Therapeutic alliance in behavior therapy. *Psychotherapy: Theory, Research, Practice, Training, 42*, 456–468.

Lewinsohn, P. M. (1974). A behavioral approach to depression. In R. M. Friedman & M. M. Katz (Eds.), *The psychology of depression: Contemporary theory and research* (pp. 157–185). New York, NY: Wiley.

Lewinsohn, P. M., Antonuccio, D. O., Breckenridge, J. S., & Teri, L. (1984). *The "Coping with depression" course.* Eugene, OR: Castalia.

Lewinsohn, P. M., & Atwood, G. E. (1969). Depression: A clinical-research approach. *Psychotherapy: Theory, Research, and Practice, 6*, 166–171.

Lewinsohn, P. M., Biglan, A., & Zeiss, A. M. (1976). Behavioral treatment for depression. In P. O. Davidson (Ed.), *Behavioral management of anxiety, depression and pain* (pp. 91–146). New York, NY: Brunner/Mazel.

Lewinsohn, P. M., & Clarke, G. N. (1999). Psychosocial treatments for adolescent depression. *Clinical Psychology Review, 19*, 329–342.

Lewinsohn, P. M., & Graf, M. (1973). Pleasant activities and depression. *Journal of Consulting and Clinical Psychology, 41*, 261–268.

Lewinsohn, P., Hoberman, H., Teri, L., & Hautzinger, M. (1985). An integrative theory of depression. In S. Neiss & R. Bootzin (Eds.), *Theoretical issues in behavior therapy* (pp. 331-359). New York, NY: Academic Press.

Lewinsohn, P. M., & Libet, J. (1972). Pleasant events, activity schedules, and depressions. *Journal of Abnormal Psychology, 79*, 291.

Lewinsohn, P. M., & Shaffer, M. (1971). Use of home observations as an integral part of the treatment of depression: Preliminary report and case studies. *Journal of Consulting and Clinical Psychology, 37*, 87–94.

Lewinsohn, P. M., & Shaw, D. A. (1969). Feedback about interpersonal behavior change: A case study in the treatment of depression. *Psychotherapy and Psychosomatics, 17*, 82–88.

Lewinsohn, P. M., Sullivan, J. M., & Grosscup, S. J. (1980). Changing reinforcing events: An approach to the treatment of depression. *Psychotherapy: Theory, Research, and Practice, 47*, 322–334.

Lewinsohn, P. M., & Talkington, J. (1979). Studies on the measurement of unpleasant events and relations with depression. *Applied Psychological Measurement, 3*, 83–101.

Libet, J., & Lewinsohn, P. M. (1973). The concept of social skill with special reference to the behavior of depressed persons. *Journal of Consulting and Clinical Psychology, 40*, 304–312.

Linehan, M. M. (1993). *Cognitive-behavioral treatment of borderline personality disorder.* New York, NY: Guiford Press.

MacPherson, L., Tull, M. T., Matusiewicz, A. K., Rodman, S., Strong, D. R., Kahler, C. W.,...Lejuez, C. W. (2010). Randomized controlled trial of behavioral activation smoking cessation treatment for smokers with elevated depressive symptoms. *Journal of Consulting and Clinical Psychology, 78*, 55.

MacPhillamy, D. J., & Lewinsohn, P. M. (1974). Depression as a function of levels of desired and obtained pleasure. *Journal of Abnormal Psychology, 83*, 651–657.

MacPhillamy D. J., & Lewinsohn, P. M. (1982). The Pleasant Events Schedule: Studies on reliability, validity, and scale intercorrelation. *Journal of Consulting and Clinical Psychology, 50*, 363–380.

Mairs, H., Lovell, K., Campbell, M., & Keeley, P. (2011). Development and pilot investigation of behavioral activation for negative symptoms. *Behavior Modification, 35*, 486–506.

Magidson, J. F., Gorka, S. M., MacPherson, L., Hopko, D. R., Blanco, C., Lejuez, C. W., & Daughters, S. B. (2011). Examining the effect of the Life Enhancement Treatment for Substance Use (LETS ACT) on residential substance abuse treatment retention. *Addictive Behaviors, 36*, 615–623.

Manos, R. C., Kanter, J. W., & Busch, A. M. (2010). A critical review of assessment strategies to measure the behavioral activation model of depression. *Clinical Psychology Review, 30*, 547–561.

Manos, R. C., Kanter, J. W., Rusch, L. C., Turner, L. B., Roberts, N. A., & Busch, A. M. (2009). Integrating functional analytic psychotherapy and behavioral activation for the treatment of relationship distress. *Clinical Case Studies, 8*, 122–138.

Martell, C. R., Addis, M. E., & Jacobson, N. S. (2001). *Depression in context: Strategies for guided action.* New York, NY: W. W. Norton.

Mazzucchelli, T., Kane, R., & Rees, C. (2009). Behavioral activation treatments for depression in adults: A meta-analysis and review. *Clinical Psychology: Science and Practice, 16*, 383–411.

McCullough, J. P. (2000). *Treatment for chronic depression: Cognitive behavioral analysis system of psychotherapy.* New York, NY: Guilford Press.

McDowell, J. J. (1982). The importance of Hernstein's mathematical statement of the law of effect for behavior therapy. *American Psychologist, 37*, 771–779.

McLean, P. D., & Hakstain, A. R. (1979). Clinical depression: Comparative efficacy of outpatient treatments. *Journal of Consulting and Clinical Psychology, 47*, 818–836.

McIndoo, C. C., File, A. A. Preddy, T., Clark, G., & Hopko, D. R. (in press). Mindfulness-based therapy and behavioral activation: A randomized controlled trial with depressed college students. *Behavior Therapy.*

McNamara, K., & Horan, J. J. (1986). Experimental construct validity in the evaluation of cognitive and behavioral treatments for depression. *Journal of Counseling Psychology, 33*, 23–30.

Meeks, S., Looney, S. W., Van Haitsma, K., & Teri, L. (2008). BE-ACTIV: A staff-assisted behavioral intervention for depression in nursing homes. *Gerontologist, 48,* 105–114.

Mineka, S., Watson, D., & Clark, L. A. (1998). Comorbidity of anxiety and unipolar mood disorders. *Annual Review of Psychology, 49,* 377–412.

Mulick, P. S., & Naugle, A. E. (2004). Behavioral activation for comorbid PTSD and major depression: A case study. *Cognitive and Behavioral Practice, 11,* 378–387.

Myers, J. K., & Weissman, M. M. (1980). Use of a self-report symptom scale to detect major depression in a community sample. *American Journal of Psychiatry, 137,* 1081–1084.

Nezu, A. M., Nezu, C. M., & Perri, M. G. (1989). *Problem-solving therapy for depression: Theory, research, and clinical guidelines.* New York: Wiley.

Nezu, A. M., Ronan, G. F., Meadows, E. A., & McClure, K. S. (2000). *Practitioner's guide to empirically based measures of depression.* New York: Kluwer Academic/Plenum.

Nixon, R. D., & Nearmy, R. M. (2011). Treatment of comorbid posttraumatic stress disorder and major depressive disorder: A pilot study. *Journal of Traumatic Stress, 24,* 451–455.

O'Neill, R. E., Horner, R. H., Albin, R. W., Storey, K., & Sprague, J. R. (1990). *Functional analysis of problem behavior: A practical assessment guide.* Sycamore, IL: Sycamore.

Ottenbreit, N., & Dobson, K. (2004). Avoidance and depression: The construction of the cognitive–behavioral avoidance scale. *Behaviour Research and Therapy, 42,* 293–313.

Otto, M. W, Pava, J. A., & Sprich-Buckminster, S. (1996). Treatment of major depression: Application and efficacy of cognitive-behavioral therapy. In M. H. Pollack & M. W. Otto (Eds.), *Challenges in clinical practice: Pharmacologic and psychosocial strategies* (pp. 31–52). New York, NY: Guilford Press.

Padfield, M. (1976). The comparative effects of two counseling approaches on the intensity of depression among rural women of low socioeconomic status. *Journal of Counseling Psychology, 23,* 209–214.

Pagoto, S., Bodenlos, J. S., Schneider, K. L., Olendzki, B., Spates, C. R., & Ma, Y. (2008). Initial investigation of behavioral activation therapy for co-morbid major depressive disorder and obesity. *Psychotherapy: Theory, Research, Practice, Training, 45,* 410–415.

Peak, T., & Barusch, A. (1999). Managed care: A critical review. *Journal of Health and Social Policy, 11,* 21–36.

Plaud, J. J. (2001). Clinical science and human behavior. *Journal of Clinical Psychology, 57,* 1089–1102.

Porter, J. F., Spates, C. R., & Smitham, S. (2004). Behavioral activation group therapy in public mental health settings: A pilot investigation. *Professional Psychology: Research and Practice, 35,* 297–301.

Radloff, L. (1977). The CES-D scale: A self-report depression scale for research in the general population. *Applied Psychological Measurement, 1,* 385–401.

Ranelli, C. J., & Miller, R. E. (1981). Behavioral predictors of amitryptaline response in depression. *American Journal of Psychiatry, 138,* 30–34.

Rehm, L. P. (1977). A self control model for depression. *Behavior Therapy, 8,* 787–804.

Rehm, L. P. (1988). Assessment of depression. In A. S. Bellack and M. Hersen (Eds.), *Behavioral assessment: A practical handbook* (3rd ed., pp. 313–364). New York, NY: Pergamon.

Rehm, L. P., Kaslow, N. J., & Rabin, A. S. (1987). Cognitive and behavioral targets in a self-control therapy program for depression. *Journal of Consulting and Clinical Psychology, 55,* 60.

Reynolds, E. K., MacPherson, L., Tull, M. T., Baruch, D. E., & Lejuez, C. (2011). Integration of the Brief Behavioral Activation Treatment for Depression (BATD) into a college orientation program: Depression and alcohol outcomes. *Journal of Counseling Psychology, 58,* 555–564.

Riemann, D., Berger, M., & Voderholzer, U. (2001). Sleep and depression—Results from psychobiological studies: An overview. *Biological Psychology, 57,* 67–103.

Ritschel, L. A., Ramirez, C. L., Jones, M., & Craighead, W. E. (2011). Behavioral activation for depressed teens: A pilot study. *Cognitive and Behavioral Practice, 18,* 281–299.

Roberts, R. E., & Vernon, S. W. (1983). The Center for Epidemiologic Studies Depression Scale: Its use in a community sample. *American Journal of Psychiatry, 140,* 41–46.

Robins, L. N., Helzer, J. E., Croughan, J. L., & Ratcliff, K. S. (1981). National Institute of Mental Health Diagnostic Interview Schedule: Its history, characteristics, and validity. *Archives of General Psychiatry, 38,* 381–389.

Robinson, J. C., & Lewinsohn, P. M. (1973). Behavior modification of speech characteristics in a chronically depressed man. *Behavior Therapy, 4,* 150–152.

Rogers, C. R. (1951). *Client-centered therapy: Its current practice, implications, and theory.* London, England: Constable.

Ruggiero, K. J., Morris, T. L., Hopko, D. R., & Lejuez, C. (2007). Application of behavioral activation treatment for depression to an adolescent with a history of child maltreatment. *Clinical Case Studies, 6,* 64–78.

Rush, A. J., Guillon, C. M., Basco, M. R., Jarrett, R. B., & Trivedi, M. H. (1996). The Inventory of Depressive Symptomatology (IDS): Psychometric properties. *Psychological Medicine, 26,* 477–486.

Sanchez, V. C., Lewinsohn, P. M., & Larson, D. W. (1980). Assertion training: Effectiveness in the treatment of depression. *Journal of Clinical Psychology, 36,* 526–529.

Santiago-Rivera, A., Kanter, J., Benson, G., Derose, T., Illes, R., & Reyes, W. (2008). Behavioral activation as an alternative treatment approach for Latinos with depression. *Psychotherapy: Theory, Research, Practice, Training, 45,* 173–185.

Sarason, I. G., Johnson, J. H., & Siegel, J. M. (1978). Assessing the impact of life changes: Development of the Life Experiences Survey. *Journal of Consulting and Clinical Psychology, 46,* 932–946.

Schoenbaum, M., Unutzer, J., Sherbourne, C., & Duan, N. (2001). Cost effectiveness of practice-initiated quality improvement for depression: Results of a randomized controlled trial. *Journal of the American Medical Association, 286,* 1325–1330.

Scogin, F., Jamison, C., & Gochneaur, K. (1989). Comparative efficacy of cognitive and behavioral bibliotherapy for mildly and moderately depressed older adults. *Journal of Consulting and Clinical Psychology, 57,* 403–407.

Segal, Z. V., Williams, J. M. G., & Teasdale, J. D. (2002). *Mindfulness-based cognitive therapy for depression: A new approach to preventing relapse.* New York: Guilford Press.

Segrin, C. (1999). Social skills, stressful life events, and the development of psychosocial problems. *Journal of Social and Clinical Psychology, 18,* 14–34.

Segrin, C. (2000). Social skills deficits associated with depression. *Clinical Psychology Review, 20,* 379–403.

Seidel, E. M., Habel, U., Finkelmeyer, A., Schneider, F., Gur, R. C., & Derntl, B. (2010). Implicit and explicit behavioral tendencies in male and female depression. *Psychiatry Research*, *177*, 124–130.

Shaw, B. F. (1977). Comparison of cognitive therapy and behavior therapy in the treatment of depression. *Journal of Consulting and Clinical Psychology*, *45*, 543.

Simons, A. D., Garfield, S. L., & Murphy, G. E. (1984). The process of change in cognitive therapy and pharmacotherapy: Changes in mood and cognitions. *Archives of General Psychiatry*, *41*, 45–51.

Skinner, B. F. (1953). *Science and human behavior*. New York: The Free Press.

Snarski, M., Scogin, F., DiNapoli, E., Presnell, A., McAlpine, J., & Marcinak, J. (2011). The effects of behavioral activation therapy with inpatient geriatric psychiatry patients. *Behavior Therapy*, *42*, 100–108.

Snyder, A. G., Stanley, M. A., Novy, D. M., & Beck, J. G. (2000). Measures of depression in older adults with generalized anxiety disorder: A psychometric evaluation. *Depression and Anxiety*, *11*, 114–120.

Spitzer, R., Williams, J., Kroenke, K., & Linzer, M. (1994). Utility of a new procedure for diagnosing mental disorders in primary care: The PRIME-MD 1,000 study. *Journal of the American Medical Association*, *272*, 1749–1756.

Staley, C. S., & Lawyer, S. R. (2010). Behavioral activation and CBT as an intervention for coexistent major depression and social phobia for a biracial client with diabetes. *Clinical Case Studies*, *9*, 63.

Stanley, M. A., Beck, J. G., Novy, D. M., Averill, P. M., Swann, A. C., Diefenbach, G., & Hopko, D. R. (2003). Cognitive-behavioral treatment of late-life generalized anxiety disorder. *Journal of Consulting and Clinical Psychology*, *71*, 301–319.

Strachan, M. K., Gros, D. F., Ruggiero, K. J., Lejuez, C. W., & Acierno, R. (2012). An integrated approach to delivering exposure-based treatment for symptoms of PTSD and depression in OIF/OEF Veterans: Preliminary findings. *Behavior Therapy*, *43*, 560–569.

Sturmey, P. (2009). Behavioral activation is an evidence-based treatment for depression. *Behavior Modification*, *33*, 818–829.

Taylor, F. G., & Marshall, W. L. (1977). Experimental analysis of a cognitive–behavioral therapy for depression. *Cognitive Therapy and Research*, *1*, 59–72.

Teri, L., Logsdon, R. G., Uomoto, J., & McCurry, S. M. (1997). Behavioral treatment of depression in dementia patients: A controlled clinical trial. *Journal of Gerontology: Psychological Sciences*, *52B*, 159–166.

Thase, M. E. (2006). Depression and sleep: Pathophysiology and treatment. *Dialogues in Clinical Neuroscience*, *8*, 217–226.

Turner, J. A., & Romano, J. M. (1984). Self-report screening measures for depression in chronic pain patients. *Journal of Clinical Psychology*, *40*, 909–913.

Voelker, R. (2003). Mounting student depression taxing campus mental health services. *Journal of the American Medical Association*, *289*, 2055–2056.

Wagner, A. W., Zatzick, D. F., Ghesquiere, A., & Jurkovich, G. J. (2007). Behavioral activation as an early intervention for posttraumatic stress disorder and depression among physically injured trauma survivors. *Cognitive and Behavioral Practice*, *14*, 341–349.

Wang, P. S., Berglund, P., Olfson, M., Pincus, H. A., Wells, K. B., & Kessler, R. C. (2005). Failure and delay in initial treatment contact after first onset of mental disorders in the National Comorbidity Survey Replication. *Archives of General Psychiatry*, *62*(6), 603-613.

Weinstock, L. M., Munroe, M. K., & Miller, I. W. (2011). Behavioral activation for the treatment of atypical depression: A pilot open trial. *Behavior Modification*, *35*, 403–424.

Westen, D., & Morrison, K. (2001). A multi-dimensional meta-analysis of treatments for depression, panic, and generalized anxiety disorder: An empirical examination of the status of empirically supported treatments. *Journal of Clinical and Consulting Psychology*, *69*, 875–899.

Whisman, M. A., Uebelacker, L. A., & Weinstock, L. M. (2004). Psychopathology and marital satisfaction: The importance of evaluating both partners. *Journal of Consulting and Clinical Psychology*, *72*, 830–838.

Wilson, P. H. (1982). Combined pharmacological and behavioural treatment of depression. *Behavior Research and Therapy*, 20, 173–184.

Wilson, P. H., Goldin, J. C., & Charbonneau-Powis, M. (1983). Comparative efficacy of behavioral and cognitive treatments of depression. *Cognitive Therapy and Research*, *7*, 111–124.

Williams, J. B. W., Link, M. J., Rosenthal, N. E., & Terman, M. (1988). *Structured Interview Guide for the Hamilton Depression Rating Scale, Seasonal Affective Disorders Version (SIGHSAD)*. New York, NY: New York Psychiatric Institute.

Williams, J. G., Barlow, D. H., & Agras, W. S. (1972). Behavioral measurement of severe depression. *Archives of General Psychiatry*, *27*, 330–333.

Youngren, M. A., & Lewinsohn, P. M. (1980). The functional relation between depression and problematic interpersonal behavior. *Journal of Abnormal Psychology*, *89*, 333–341.

Zeiss, A. M., Lewinsohn, P. M., & Munoz, R. F. (1979). Nonspecific improvement effects in depressionusing interpersonal cognitive, and pleasant events focused treatments. *Journal of Consulting and Clinical Psychology*, *47*, 427–439.

Cognitive-Behavioral Approaches
to Stress Management

Sarah L. Mann *and* Richard J. Contrada

Abstract

This chapter provides an overview of cognitive-behavioral stress management techniques, which include some of the most effective means of stress reduction. We begin by briefly outlining major themes and approaches in the scientific study of stress and summarizing key constructs in psychologically oriented stress science. We then provide an overview of three major cognitive-behavioral stress management techniques: progressive muscle relaxation, breathing therapies, and guided imagery. The chapter concludes with a discussion of some of the contemporary scientific and clinical issues in cognitive-behavioral stress management, focusing on the advancement of research into physiological and cognitive mechanisms and the application of these stress management methods in institutional settings.

Key Words: stress management, cognitive-behavioral therapies, progressive muscle relaxation, breathing, guided imagery

For the lay public, stress is a highly familiar and reasonably well-understood phenomenon. The word "stress" and its variants are used frequently in conversation and various media. And although it is understood that stress can mean different things for different people, and despite significant differences between ethnic groups and across cultures, there is a good deal of commonality that runs through these meanings. Most people know (or think they know) what "stress" is, and its causes, manifestations, and consequences make up at least the outlines of a shared folk understanding of stress. Moreover, while a certain amount of stress is seen as an unavoidable aspect of life, there are many well-recognized ways of minimizing stress and its negative consequences, ranging from mental and behavioral activity of the individual to the functions performed by major social institutions such as medicine, religion, and the family, and to myriad commercial products marketed for their supposed stress-reducing properties.

In the field of stress science, things are less clear. To be sure, there is substantial agreement about what stress is, why it occurs, and how it affects the person. Indeed, the field of stress has shown considerable development and increased sophistication in the time since its inception. But there is ambiguity and controversy about definitional matters, regarding the relative importance of different aspects of stress, and concerning our understanding of the origins, immediate effects, and long-term consequences of stress. In part, this state of affairs reflects the fact that stress has been studied within different scientific disciplines and from various perspectives within those disciplines. As a consequence, what we demonstrably know about ways to avoid and to reduce stress, and about the benefits of doing so, is limited, qualified, and subject to debate. As such, understanding and managing stress are currently active and productive areas of inquiry, and they can be rewarding areas of involvement for basic research and clinical intervention.

This chapter provides an overview of the state of the art of cognitive-behavioral stress management. Cognitive-behavioral approaches have seen steady improvement and include some of the most effective means of stress reduction that are currently available. These techniques and the theoretical and empirical work on which they are based are highly compatible with the dominant perspectives in basic theory and research in the field of psychological stress, although these two bodies of work are not as well integrated as one might imagine.

We begin with a brief outline of major themes and approaches to the scientific study of stress and a summary of the current status of the main stress-related constructs employed by psychologically oriented stress scientists. Next, we provide a heuristic overview of a few major stress management techniques that fall within this perspective: progressive muscle relaxation, breathing therapies, and guided imagery. The chapter concludes with a discussion of some of the major conceptual and clinical issues in contemporary work on the cognitive-behavioral management of stress.

Theoretical Bases of Cognitive-Behavioral Stress Management

Effective stress management techniques reflect advances in at least two bodies of research. They are grounded in basic stress science, and they are developed, evaluated, and refined in research applying specific techniques in specific populations to address specific stress-related problems. Although it is useful to distinguish these two research areas, they are not entirely separable; for example, theoretical propositions regarding basic stress processes may be evaluated through experimental manipulations that incorporate elements of stress management techniques, and stress management research in specific populations and problem areas can and often should be designed in a way that informs basic stress science. With that caveat in mind, this section discusses some of the developments and challenges of basic stress research that have particular relevance to advancing the development and clinical implementation of methods for cognitive-behavioral stress management.

Environmental Stressors

Much stress involves stressors, that is, threatening or demanding environmental events and conditions that are ongoing, recalled, or anticipated. A major stream of stress research that emerged early on has focused on the experience of individual environmental events, or clusters of events, the demands or adjustments they require, and their relationship with negative mental or physical outcomes. An event-focused perspective remains a discernible paradigm for contemporary stress science (Cohen, Kessler, & Gordon, 1997). Accumulating research findings have increased understanding of the kinds of environmental events that activate stress responses. These include major events such as war, terrorism, natural and technological disasters, and other potentially traumatizing occurrences (Norris, Friedman, & Watson, 2002); more common social and environmental events such as divorce, bereavement, and physical illness (Anderson, Wethington, & Kamarck, 2011); routine, daily stresses encountered, for example, in the workplace and the home (Almeida, Stawski, & Cichy, 2011); and even more temporally circumscribed events that describe moment-to-moment experience (Schiffman, Stone, & Hufford, 2008).

An environmental focus also characterizes research on stressful conditions examining the impact of longer term exposures to ongoing circumstances of social life such as work (Pandey, Quick, Rossi, Nelson, & Martin, 2011) and the marital relationship (Kiecolt-Glaser & Newton, 2001); persistent features of the physical environment, including population density (Baum, 1987) and noise (Glass & Singer, 1972), stressors that are found together in certain geographic locations such as inner cities (Anderson & Armstead, 1995); demands and constraints created by organizations (Weinberg & Cooper, 2011; Zapf, Dormann, & Frese, 1996); life as experienced within different socioeconomic strata (Marmot & Brunner, 2005); and the experience of chronic medical conditions and the demands of illness management (Baum, Herberman, & Cohen, 1995; Nezu, Nezu, & Xanthopoulos, 2011).

Cognitive Appraisal and Coping Processes

For the most part, exposure to the events and conditions outlined earlier bears only a probabilistic relationship with negative outcomes. There are large, systematic individual differences in how different people respond, with some showing negative effects, some not, and others even showing benefits such as personal growth as a consequence of the encounter. Stress and its consequences appear to arise out of the relationship between environmental demands and constraints, on the one hand, and the adaptive resources of the individual, on the other. It is an imbalance in this equation that creates stress-related problems in living that require clinical intervention.

This premise, referred to as a transactional model of stress, seems necessary as a means of accounting for individual differences in both the short-term response and the long-term adaptive outcome of even the more extreme stressful events and conditions. It forms a basic assumption of a theory of psychological stress formulated by Richard S. Lazarus and his collaborators (Lazarus, 1966; Lazarus & Folkman, 1984; Smith & Lazarus, 1993).

The work of Lazarus and others concerning psychological processes that mediate the impact of exposure to stressful events and conditions represents a second major stream of stress research apart from that associated with the environmental approach described earlier. The psychological and environmental approaches are often integrated, but the two are separable and often pursued somewhat independently. The psychological perspective has placed a heavy emphasis on the processes of cognitive appraisal and coping (Lazarus & Folkman, 1984). Appraisal is a cognitive-evaluative process in which the individual judges the actual or potential impact of perceived events and conditions on his or her physical or mental well-being. Stress-promoting appraisals include the perception that harm or loss has already occurred, the threat of future harm or loss, and challenge, a mixed state that contains elements of threat in combination with the opportunity for positive outcomes. It is possible to distinguish a primary appraisal process, in which harm and loss are evaluated, from a secondary appraisal process, in which resources and options for coping are evaluated. Coping refers to mental and behavioral activity aimed at dealing directly with the person-situation imbalance that gave rise to a stressful appraisal, sometimes referred to as problem-focused coping, or at managing its impact on the person, sometimes referred to as emotion-focused coping. Several alternative conceptualizations have also been proposed that make different kinds of distinctions among various coping responses (Skinner, Edge, Altman, & Sherwood, 2003).

The Stress Response

Following exposure to demanding events and conditions and appraisal of harm/loss, threat, or challenge, there follow biological, psychological, and behavioral changes that, taken together, may be referred to as the stress response. A focus on biological aspects of the stress response constitutes a third major stream of stress research. It has its origins in the work of Walter B. Cannon (1929) on the fight-or-flight response, which emphasized the impact of physical emergencies, such as the presence of a predator, in activating sympathetic adrenomedullary activity as manifested by elevations in circulating levels of the catecholamines, epinephrine and norepinephrine, which are now recognized as major stress hormones. These substances (especially epinephrine) are secreted by the adrenal medullae, a pair of endocrine glands, and their heightened production is accompanied by increased activity of the sympathetic branch of the autonomic nervous system for which norepinephrine is a major neurotransmitter. Physiological consequences of this increased endocrine and nervous system activity include cardiovascular, respiratory, and other adjustments whose effects in mobilizing energy that support vigorous muscle activity confer survival advantage in situations of immediate physical danger.

A biological perspective on stress became crystallized and was given impetus as a result of the work of Hans Selye (1956). Selye described stress as a specific biological response that is nonspecifically elicited by a variety of noxious stimuli. This response, referred to as the general adaptation syndrome, features activity of the cortices of the adrenal glands, and it is described in terms of a triphasic pattern of alarm, resistance, and exhaustion marked by a rise and fall in the production of corticosteroids, most notably cortisol, a major stress hormone in humans. Selye popularized the use of the term "stress" and brought the stress concept to the attention of psychologists.

Biological activity produced by stress processes is not confined to mobilization of adrenal medullary and cortical activity, heighted sympathetic nervous system tone, and associated cardiovascular and metabolic changes. It may not be much of an exaggeration and certainly has heuristic value to think of the biological stress response as organism wide. Depending upon the severity and duration of exposure to the stressor, and on the nature of ensuing psychological responses, changes may be seen throughout the body.

Much has been learned about the brain mechanisms that mediate psychological processing of stressful events and conditions and that regulate behavioral and peripheral physiologic responses (Dedovic, D'Aguiar, & Pruessner, 2009; Gianaros & O'Connor, 2011), and about the effects of stress on the brain (Sapolsky, 1996). In short, acute stress induces neurochemical changes, including increased release of glucocorticoid hormones and the neurotransmitters dopamine and norepinephrine, which help shift the brain "from slow, thoughtful PFC [prefrontal cortical] regulation to the reflexive and rapid emotional responses of the amygdala and related subcortical structures" (Arnsten, 2009, p. 411). This regulatory shift often proves adaptive for facing mortal threats, but it can become problematic when circumstances instead require careful, controlled decision making. When chronic stress prolongs these neurochemical processes, they cause structural changes to the PFC and to subcortical structures such as the amygdala and hippocampus (Cerqueira, Mailliet, Almeida, Jay, & Sousa, 2007; Leuner & Gould, 2010; Roozendaal, McEwen, & Chattarji, 2009). Over time, these changes can effectively weaken the PFC's regulatory capacities while strengthening the subcortical stress response, leaving the organism vulnerable to heightened and prolonged responses to future stressors (Arnsten, 2009).

In addition to these stress-related neurological changes, psychophysiologists have documented stress-related changes in major physiologic systems, including electrodermal, respiratory, and skeletomotor systems, among other responses (Cacioppo, Tassinary, & Berntson, 2007). With regard to autonomic nervous system (ANS) processes that mediate many end-organ responses to stress, parasympathetic activity, and interactions between the sympathetic and parasympathetic branches of the ANS, also figure prominently in the bodily response to stressful encounters (Berntson et al., 1994; Berntson, Norman, Hawkley, & Cacioppo, 2008; Porges, 2009). And immunological/inflammatory responses to stress have received much attention, especially in light of their potential role in the development of acute infectious and chronic physical disease (Segerstrom & Miller, 2004) and in the production of emotional states through immune-to-brain pathways (Dantzer, O'Connor, Freund, Johnson, & Kelley, 2008).

Stress Moderators

Exposure to stressors and the psychological and biological responses that ensue do not occur in a vacuum. These processes are potentially shaped by a large number of factors that increase or decrease exposure to stressors and the magnitude of the stress response. Often referred to as stress moderators, they include aspects of the context in which stress occurs, including social, physical, organizational, and sociocultural factors, and characteristics of the person, including age, gender, and other sociodemographic variables, as well as personality, intellectual

capabilities, and mental and physical health. Stress moderators that reduce exposure to stressors or that modulate the effects of such exposures may be conceptualized as coping resources in that they inform, guide, and otherwise support the efforts of an individual to minimize stressful exposures and to manage their impact.

Stress Outcomes

At the individual level, consequences of stress may include unpleasant emotional reactions, including anxiety, anger, and sadness; development and exacerbation of mental and physical health problems; impairments in cognitive functioning; poor performance in a variety of domains, including occupational and academic activities; inability to manage physical illness and to benefit from associated rehabilitation regimens; and the acquisition of or relapse in behavioral problems, including unhealthy eating and use of nicotine, alcohol, and other substances. These outcomes may have negative consequences for social units ranging from married couples and families to companies, corporations, and the military. The wide scope and potential importance of the many possible negative outcomes of stress provide a strong rational and considerable impetus for developing improved methods of stress management.

Specific Techniques
Progressive Muscle Relaxation

BRIEF HISTORY

The technique of progressive muscle relaxation (PMR) was developed by the physiologist Edmund Jacobson and was based on two key psychophysiological innovations of his early career. First, in collaboration with A. J. Carlson, he found that the degree of psychological tension a patient was experiencing could be measured physiologically in terms of amplitude of the individual's knee-jerk reflex, and that when the patient relaxed, the reflex amplitude decreased (Jacobson, 1974). Second, working with Bell Telephone Laboratory scientists, Jacobson helped to improve the technology for measuring tension in electrical muscle action potentials, making these recordings easier, more direct, and unprecedentedly precise. This new technology, quantitative electromyography (EMG), provided him with a new method of exploring mind-body relations, which he used to document covert connections between mental life and the activity of the skeletal muscles.

Jacobson's subsequent investigations using EMG revealed that in a relaxed person, thoughts elicited measurable, low-amplitude responses in muscle groups corresponding to the person's mental activity. Thoughts of limb movements produced small EMG bursts in relevant muscles of the corresponding limb, whereas mental imagery or verbalizations registered EMG activity in the eye and the speech muscles, respectively. Jacobson summarized the resulting model of the mind-body connection in his description of thinking as "a series of acts, quite similar to the organism's overt relations to the environment but differing in that images more or less replace the direct sensory experiences, while the muscular tensions consist of relatively feeble contractions, with little or no effect on the environment" (Jacobson, 1974, p. 195). Based on this view, Jacobson developed progressive muscle relaxation as a course of training for relaxing the mind and body simultaneously by becoming highly sensitive to subtle skeletal muscle contractions and able to relax specific sites of tension at will.

THEORETICAL AND EMPIRICAL BASES

In clinical practice, PMR can be used either to help to control or to alleviate stress-related conditions—including both cognitive and somatoform symptoms—or to reduce susceptibility to this kind of problem. The technique utilizes the body's neuromuscular connections as a means of voluntarily decreasing physical and psychological stress. A key premise is that information is relayed from the skeletal muscles to the brain through neuromuscular circuits that project to the reticular formation. This central brain stem structure is involved not only in aspects of motor control but also in regulating autonomic activity (via connections with the hypothalamus) and cardiovascular control (Bernhaut, Gelhorn, & Rasmussen, 1953; Gelhorn, 1958; Gelhorn & Keily, 1972). Thus, sustained muscle tension effectively increases excitatory inputs to brain regions that can trigger a variety of physiological stress reactions via the sympathetic nervous system.

When a tense person relaxes his or her muscles, feedback loops connecting the muscles, the brain, and the sympathetic nervous system convey fewer excitatory impulses, with the result of calming the mind and body. Trainees in PMR learn to become sensitive to trace levels of muscle tension, called *control signals*, which reflect and reinforce their psychological stress. By becoming attuned to these control signals, people can develop refined abilities

to allow specific tensed, or contracted, groups of muscle fibers to lengthen, thereby "relaxing away" both the muscle tension and the associated stress.

Furthermore, within the psychophysiological model on which PMR is based, slight muscle tensions are thought to play an important role in generating thoughts and emotions. Covert contractions of the speech musculature have been recorded during many kinds of verbal cognition, including silent reading, verbal meditation, and silently processing the answer to a question (McGuigan, 1978; McGuigan, Culver, & Kendler, 1971). Similarly, mental visualization is associated with subtle movements of the eye muscles. The PMR model posits an intimate link between these mental and muscular activities, such that thoughts are generated by the rapid interactions between the brain and the particular skeletal muscles relevant to the thought content. In this view, decreasing muscle tension not only decreases widespread physiological arousal but also quiets the mind by reducing the neuromuscular reverberations that give rise to cognitive activity. Over the long term, individuals highly skilled at PMR develop automaticity, so that the release of unwanted physical tension and psychological stress becomes unconscious and effortless.

CURRENT PRACTICE

As its name suggests, PMR training systematically progresses through several muscle groups in a set order, typically beginning with the hands/arms, then moving to the feet/legs, trunk, neck, eyes, and speech musculature, though additional areas of focus can be added, depending on the learner's needs (McGuigan & Lehrer, 2007). The process begins with large muscle groups, where contractions are easiest to recognize and to control, and proceeds to smaller muscles in which sensation is fainter and voluntary control more challenging. During hour-long training sessions, the learner is guided in recognizing the control signal in each muscle group, one at a time. The process involves focusing on the subtle differences in proprioceptive sensation that occur as the muscles tense and relax during a simple repeated movement (McGuigan & Lehrer, 2007). The goal is to learn to sense the precise timing, location, and sensation of the control signal involved in initiating movements in each muscle group, and then to learn to relax the muscles involved completely. Although it is not always possible in practice, progress in treatment can be measured by comparing the learner's EMG profiles to her earlier, baseline recordings and/or to a standard set of goal measures representing normal, or normotensive, levels of muscle tension (McGuigan & Lehrer, 2007).

Preparation

To minimize distractions, training should take place in a quiet, dimly lit, uncluttered room, but the location need not be soundproof or completely distraction-free, given that the goal is to be able to relax under normal circumstances (McGuigan & Lehrer, 2007). The learner requires a pillow as well as a comfortable place to lie down, such as a couch, a recliner, a cot, or a rug. The learner should also be encouraged to wear comfortable, loose-fitting clothing to subsequent sessions (McGuigan & Lehrer, 2007).

First Session

As described by McGuigan and Lehrer (2007), the clinician begins by explaining the basic functioning of the muscles—as they tense, the fine fibers that comprise them contract and shorten, and when they relax, the fibers lengthen—and its relevance for PMR training: By repeatedly tensing and relaxing a specific set of muscle fibers while attending to the sensations involved, the learner will become better able to pinpoint focal areas of tension and relax it away. The learner should also be advised not to expect instant mastery; PMR is a skill that takes significant time and practice to develop. The duration of a full course of PMR varies depending on the learner's starting point and therapeutic goals; Jacobson's full basic course lasts for 13 weeks and requires at least 1 hour of daily practice (Jacobson, 1964). The learner should be made aware that treatment outcome depends in large part on diligence with the prescribed practice between clinical sessions. Jacobson and others have outlined specific training and practice schedules, but the technique also allows for flexibility in the number and frequency of meetings with the therapist.

At the start of each session, the learner should be encouraged to adopt a frame of mind that is training focused and as free from other concerns as possible during the 1-hour session. The learner begins by lying down with her arms at her sides with her eyes open. After several minutes and without concerted effort, she should gradually allow her eyes to close by simply letting the muscle fibers around the eyes slowly relax and lengthen. The learner lies with eyes closed for a few minutes, then at the therapist's gentle instruction, steadily flexes the left wrist to raise the hand up to be approximately perpendicular to

the resting surface. She holds this position for a minute or two, paying careful attention to the sensations it produces in order to localize the *control signal*, the precise origin point of the muscle contraction. The learner is not told where to seek the control signal (in this case, the dorsal surface of the forearm), and she may be unsure at first what kind of signal or sensation it is. Still, the therapist should not give detailed instruction but should act as a guide through the trial-and-error training process. If the learner misidentifies other tensions as the control signal, she is not corrected, only encouraged to continue searching. The therapist aims to keep the focus on the learner and her independence; she must identify and eliminate (relax away) the control signal herself, which will become easier with practice.

After holding her left hand in the tensed position for a few minutes and attending to the muscle tension, at the therapist's direction the learner allows the hand and wrist muscles to go slack for a few minutes. Rather than purposely moving the hand down, the learner should be encouraged simply to let the tension go, allow the muscles to stop working, or "let the power go off." It may be difficult at first to avoid "trying to relax," and it should be emphasized that relaxation requires no effort in itself; rather, a cessation of prior efforts allows the muscle fibers at the control signal site to lengthen and the hand to fall. For this reason, terminology that denotes effortful behavior like "relaxation exercise" and "relaxation response" is discouraged (McGuigan & Lehrer, 2007). This sequence is repeated two more times during the session. The therapist then ends the meeting by discussing the learner's progress, answering questions, and prescribing a practice schedule for the interval between sessions.

Subsequent Sessions

Later sessions take the same form as the first. With the therapist's guidance, the learner focuses on a single control signal during the hour-long session, repeating and studying the tense-and-relax sequence three times. As training proceeds through the different areas of the body, each region is broken down into smaller muscle groups for study over several days, with each day highlighting a single movement and corresponding control signal. There are minor variations between practitioners in the order in which training progresses; Jacobson's traditional sequence is outlined in Table 15.1. Days 1 through 7 in this table show how the musculature in the left

Table 15.1 Traditional Progressive Muscle Relaxation Practice Sequence

Practice Days	Focal Musculature
7 (days 1–7)	Left arm
Day 1	Left hand bent back
Day 2	Left hand bent forward
Day 3	Relax only
Day 4	Left arm bent at the elbow
Day 5	Left wrist pressed down on books
Day 6	Relax only
Day 7	Entire left arm progressively tensed and relaxed (general, residual tension)
7 (days 8–14)	Right arm
10 (days 15–24)	Left leg
10 (days 25–34)	Right leg
10 (days 35–44)	Trunk
6 (days 45–50)	Neck
12 (days 51–62)	Eye region
9 (days 63–71)	Visualization
19 (days 72–90)	Speech region and speech imagery

Source: After McGuigan, 1991, as adapted from Jacobson, 1964.

arm is studied through a series of small, specific movements.

In sessions focused on generalized or residual tension (see Table 15.1, Day 7), the learner focuses on recognizing and releasing the continuous, low-level muscle contraction throughout a larger region. To study this kind of tension, the learner very gradually stiffens all muscles in this region, in this case the left arm, increasing to a maximum level of muscle contraction over about 15 minutes. The learner holds and observes this tension for roughly 30 to 60 seconds, then very gradually relaxes the whole arm over the remainder of the session. The emphasis on distinguishing localized control signals from generalized tension is a hallmark of Jacobson's method that is not typically included in abbreviated versions of PMR (McGuigan & Lehrer, 2007).

Sessions near the end of the training sequence focus on the especially subtle control signals in the eyes and the speech musculature. The vision- and speech-related components of the program are each followed by a set of sessions training these respective muscle groups to regulate associated cognitive activity. That is, after training to relax the muscles of the eye region, the learner spends 9 days learning to recognize and release similar covert tensions that occur in association with mental imagery. Likewise, after training to relax the speech musculature by purposely moving, tensing, and releasing these muscles, the learner then applies this skill to detect control signals in these muscles that occur during silent, verbal thought. These components of training are considered critical to gaining control of stressful thoughts and emotions.

The goal of PMR is not to eliminate all sources of tension but to become a skilled interpreter of the body's control signals in order to release unwanted tension and stress. When the learner becomes proficient at recognizing and eliminating these signals at will, she can then learn to distinguish the tension's "process," a term for the felt muscle contraction itself, from its "meaning," which refers to the reason for the contraction, such as the thought content associated with the reverberations of specific neuromuscular circuits. If the learner experiences unexpected muscle tension or contractions during training, the first therapeutic priority is for the learner to observe carefully, localize, and describe these sensations. The therapist then guides the learner in considering why those tensions occur where they do, in association with particular kinds of thoughts or feelings. Addressing these issues is not always quick or straightforward; nonetheless, understanding the tension's meaning, perhaps by discovering its link to a particular worry or memory, often facilitates muscle control. Along these same lines, understanding the meaning of muscle tension associated with particular thoughts and emotions is said to provide a mechanism for controlling these mental events. In this view, relaxing the muscles in a neuromuscular circuit where unwanted thoughts or emotions originate stops the circuit's reverberation, which eliminates the thoughts or feelings.

Abbreviated Progressive Muscle Relaxation

As described earlier, classical PMR training is lengthy and requires much practice. Although there is no shortcut to gaining the level of mastery that is possible through a full training program, its briefer version, known as abbreviated progressive muscle relaxation (APMR), has also been found to be beneficial (Bernstein, Carlson, & Schmidt, 2007). The first shortened form of Jacobson's training was developed by the psychiatrist and pioneer of behavior therapy Joseph Wolpe (1958), who took an interest in relaxation as a component of his systematic desensitization approach to anxiety treatment. Over the next decade, other psychologists interested in treating anxiety continued to adapt Jacobson's relaxation methods, shortening them further and providing learners with more overt guidance. These changes, first described and formalized by Gordon Paul (1966) and by Douglas Bernstein and Thomas Borkovec (1973), allowed PMR to be incorporated into a range of behavioral treatments for anxiety.

In practice, APMR proceeds very similarly to classical PMR. After explaining the therapeutic process and rationale, the therapist guides the learner through a series of tense-and-relax cycles focused on particular muscle groups. A key difference in APMR is that, while PMR devotes whole sessions to studying single control signals within major muscle groups, APMR proceeds through a sequence of 16 major muscle groups in each 45-minute session, using shorter tense-and-relax cycles (see Table 15.2). APMR is also more flexible than traditional PMR, so if an individual has trouble with the method of tensing described in a particular APMR program, the therapist is encouraged to work with the learner to devise a more feasible way of tensing and releasing the target muscles (Bernstein, Carlson, & Schmidt, 2007).

Another important difference from traditional PMR methods is that in APMR the learner is generally discouraged from speaking during the relaxation period, since verbal exchanges can distract the learner from his physical sensations, and there is no need to confirm the location of control signals. Before beginning the first session's relaxation training, the therapist and the learner should establish simple signals to guide their progression through the 16 muscle groups. When explaining the method, the therapist should not only describe the tense-and-relax procedure and the muscle sequence to be followed but should also establish with the learner exactly what instructions will be given, what the learner should do in response, and how the learner will signal silently that the target muscles are completely relaxed. For example, the therapist might explain that each instruction will end with the word "now" (e.g., "Tense the muscles in your right hand and forearm by making a tight fist *now*"), and that the word "now" is the learner's

cue to tense or relax those muscles all at once, not gradually. The therapist and the learner should also arrange a comfortable way for the learner to signal that the muscles are fully relaxed without speaking or creating unnecessary muscle tension, such as by lifting the index finger on one hand that is visible to the therapist (Bernstein, Carlson, & Schmidt, 2007). The therapist should briefly work through each of the tense-and-release procedures with the learner before training begins, demonstrating each procedure, observing and coaching the learner as needed, and proceeding in the same order to be used during the session. This guided practice will help ensure that the learner understands the method and put him at ease during relaxation.

Relaxation training begins with the learner reclining comfortably. The therapist asks the learner to focus attention on sensations in the first muscle group, allowing the rest of the body to relax. Using the established instruction, the therapist asks the client to tense the target muscles. They should remain tensed for about 5–7 seconds (or shorter for the muscles of the feet and others that cramp easily), while the therapist suggests ways to focus on the sensations. At the end of the tension interval, the therapist uses the established cue to tell the learner to relax all the muscles completely at once. During the relaxation interval (30 to 40 seconds), the therapist again gently suggests ways of concentrating on the sensations of relaxation in the relevant muscles. In this way, the therapist guides the learner through tensing and relaxing each muscle group twice, allowing a slightly longer relaxation interval of 45 to 60 seconds during the second repetition, before proceeding to the next muscle group. If, after two repetitions with a particular muscle group, the learner has not signaled complete relaxation, the process can be repeated up to four or five times, at which point it is appropriate to try an alternate solution (see Bernstein, Borkovec, & Hazlett-Stevens, 2000).

During the tensing and relaxing intervals, the therapist should use suggestions that help the learner to observe sensory changes (e.g., "Notice what it's like to feel the muscles pulling tight" or "Focus on the feeling in these muscles as they become more relaxed") rather than prescriptive or descriptive statements about what the learner should feel (e.g., "Your muscles are feeling deeply relaxed now"). Using passive suggestions helps show the learner how to become a passive but keen observer of these sensations. It also keeps the focus on the learner's own experience and avoids the possibility

Table 15.2 Abbreviated Progressive Muscle Relaxation Practice Sequence

Muscle Group	Method of Tensing
Dominant hand and forearm	Make a tight fist, allowing upper arm to relax
Dominant upper arm	Press elbow down against chair
Nondominant hand and forearm	Same as dominant
Nondominant upper arm	Same as dominant
Forehead	Raise eyebrows as high as possible
Upper cheeks and nose	Squint eyes, wrinkle nose
Lower face	Clench teeth, pull back corners of mouth
Neck	Counterpose muscles by trying to raise and lower chin simultaneously
Chest, shoulders, upper back	Take a deep breath; hold it and pull shoulder blades together
Abdomen	Counterpose muscles by trying to push stomach out and pull it in simultaneously
Dominant upper leg	Counterpose large muscles on top of leg against two smaller ones underneath (strategies will vary)
Dominant calf	Point toes toward head
Dominant foot	Point toes downward, turn toes in, curl toes gently
Nondominant upper leg	Same as dominant
Nondominant calf	Same as dominant
Nondominant foot	Same as dominant

Source: Bernstein, Carlson, & Schmidt, 2007.

that the therapist's statements will not match what the learner feels—if, for example, he is having trouble relaxing—which can create needless tension (Bernstein, Borkovec, & Hazlett-Stevens, 2000).

At the session's end, one way for the therapist to ease the learner out of the relaxed state is by instructing him to move his feet and legs on the count of 4, hands and arms on 3, head and neck on 2, and to sit up on 1, and then counting backward slowly from 4 to 1. The therapist should then ask open-ended questions to encourage the learner to discuss thoughts and questions about the experience. When the learner has mastered this method of deep relaxation, perhaps after several sessions and regular daily practice, he can move on to progressively shorter relaxation sequences that combine the original 16 muscle groups into 7 groups, then into only 4 groups. Using the same tense-and-relax procedure with these larger muscle groups allows the learner to achieve deep relaxation more quickly. The learner then can move on to releasing tension by systematically, vividly recalling the sensations of muscle relaxation, first while focusing attention on the now-familiar muscle groups in sequence, then by learning to associate the sensations of relaxation with a slow count to 10. By the end of the training, then, the learner should be able to relax thoroughly in the time it takes to focus the mind and make this mental count.

The goal of this comprehensive but less intense training also differs, in part, from that of traditional PMR. Both methods teach similar ways of achieving deep relaxation by systematically lowering autonomic activation. But unlike traditional PMR, APMR focuses on developing the learner's ability to notice and voluntarily release unwanted tension, placing little emphasis if any on achieving automaticity and muscle-mediated control of stressful thoughts.

EMPIRICAL SUPPORT

Several decades of research has provided ample evidence for the benefits of both the traditional and the abbreviated PMR techniques for reducing stress, and for improving a variety of psychiatric and somatoform problems to which stress contributes. Jacobson (e.g., 1938, 1970) documented successful applications of his method for treating nervous hypertension, acute and chronic insomnia, fatigue, cyclothymia, dysthymia, hypochondria, obsessive-compulsive disorder, and several other anxiety problems resembling generalized anxiety disorder or panic (then termed "anxiety neuroses"), as well as essential hypertension, tension headaches, esophageal spasms, several bowel disorders, and convulsive tics.

More recent reviews have bolstered many of Jacobson's findings, consistently supporting the effectiveness of PMR techniques (including APMR) for stress, generalized anxiety, specific anxieties and phobias, hypertension, and tension headaches (Borkovec & Sides, 1979; Carlson & Hoyle, 1993; Hyman, Feldman, Harris, Levin, & Molloy, 1989; King, 1980; Lehrer, 1982; Lehrer & Woolfolk, 1984). Newer studies of PMR have continued to support these conclusions (see Bernstein, Carlson, & Schmidt, 2007), while expanding the list of conditions that PMR can help to improve. In recent years, it has been shown to reduce anxiety and boost well-being for patients with schizophrenia (Vancampfort et al., 2011); reduce chronic pain associated with osteoarthritis (Gay, Philippot, & Luminet, 2002) and cancer (Tatrow & Montgomery, 2006); decrease behavioral problems in Alzheimer's patients (Suhr, Anderson, & Tranel, 1999); and increase adherence to sleep apnea treatment (Wang, He, Wang, Liu, & Tang, 2012); among other benefits.

ISSUES FOR FUTURE RESEARCH

Given the substantial support for PMR's effectiveness, one important area for future research involves finding new ways of deploying the technique, for example, applying it more cost-effectively and combining it with newer therapies that may provide added benefits. Although individual PMR training has been shown to achieve larger effect sizes on average than group sessions (Carlson & Hoyle, 1993), recent work suggests that even a single, large-group training session can significantly reduce anxiety and speed recovery from a brief stress exposure (Rausch, Gramling, & Auerbach, 2006). Extensions of this training model could reduce stress in institutional settings such as workplaces (Hahn, Binnewies, Sonnentag, & Mojza, 2011) and psychiatric facilities (Hall & Long, 2009).

One way in which PMR is being combined with new stress management approaches is its incorporation into computer-supported and computer-delivered therapies. One computer-assisted group treatment for social phobia utilizes palmtop computers to prompt APMR practice and guide clients through the process (Przeworski & Newman, 2004). Palmtop computers and smartphones offer an efficient means of enhancing group PMR therapies with individualized follow-up, which may improve long-term adherence to practice. PMR is also being combined with virtual-reality exposure therapy for phobias (Muhlberger Herrmann,

Wiedemann, Ellgring, & Pauli, 2001) and delivered virtually with immersive video (Mezo, Hall, Duggan, & Noël, 2011).

The period in which evidence supporting PMR's efficacy has accumulated has also seen major advances in psychophysiology and neuroscience, allowing researchers to pursue a more rigorous and detailed account of its mechanisms of action (Conrad & Roth, 2007). These studies often have focused on healthy volunteers, examining physiological correlates of APMR and their possible contributions to stress relief. Findings include evidence of decreases in salivary cortisol (Pawlow & Jones, 2002, 2005); higher salivary concentration and secretion rate of immunoglobulin A, an antibody critical to mucosal immunity (Pawlow & Jones, 2005); and an increased threshold in the nociceptive flexion reflex, a spinal reflex used to study pain processing (Emery, France, Harris, Norman, & VanArsdalen, 2008). At the same time, evidence for its theoretical rationale—particularly pertaining to treatment of anxiety—has been characterized as "mixed at best" (Conrad & Roth, 2007, p. 259). For example, contrary to the assumptions of PMR, patients with panic disorder or generalized anxiety disorder do not consistently show elevated muscle tension and autonomic activation. Because relatively few studies of PMR's effectiveness have included thorough measures of muscle tension, the possibility remains that its effects are largely or entirely cognitive, based on developing a sense of personal control and confidence through the training process. A more precise dismantling of the cognitive and psychophysiological mechanisms of PMR for specific conditions will contribute significantly to the development of a coherent theoretical framework for explaining shared mechanisms of mind-body interventions (Taylor, Goehler, Galper, Innes, & Bourguignon, 2010).

Breathing

BRIEF HISTORY

Western medical and psychological practice tends to regard respiratory changes as signs or symptoms of a health problem, and numerous treatments and therapies have been devised to correct respiratory malfunctions. In contrast, in some areas of the East and particularly in India, breathing techniques have been used for millennia as a means of improving the functioning of many physiological systems as well as for spiritual purposes (Chandra, 1994).

Archaeological evidence suggests that well-developed yogic methods of breath control were used to promote spiritual and physical health as early as 3000 B.C. (Rowland, 1953). The breathing techniques collectively known as *pranayama* incorporate several key features that remain important to various types of yoga practice, which have also been incorporated into some Western cognitive-behavioral stress management therapies (Chandra, 1994). These features include enhancing abdominal or diaphragmatic breathing, and two additional approaches—prolonging exhalation to slow and regularize breathing, and imposing resistance during inhalation and exhalation (described later). Due, in part, to the evidence that purposeful, systematic changes in breathing can affect physiological and psychological arousal, many forms of relaxation training and therapy incorporate controlled breathing techniques. These include progressive relaxation (Bernstein & Borkovec, 1973), autogenics (Luthe, 1969–1973), stress-inoculation training (Meichenbaum, 1977), many forms of yoga practice (Iyengar, 1966), tai chi and qigong (Liao, 1990), and Zen meditation (Kapleau, 1965).

THEORETICAL AND EMPIRICAL BASES

Respiration is the only involuntary vital function that is also subject to direct, intentional control (Ley, 2003). Breathing has pervasive psychophysiological influences, including cardiovascular and neurological effects, so voluntary respiratory control can significantly reduce (or increase) states of physical and psychological tension. Likely because breathing is readily modifiable and has rapid mental and physical effects, it has been ranked as the most popular stress management method (Umezawa, 2001). In this context, it is important to consider the reciprocal relationships between breathing and other body systems: Relaxing slows breathing and lengthens exhalation pauses. Conversely, willfully practicing these respiratory changes often reduces tension. Thus, respiration serves as both an indicator of stress and a potential regulator thereof (van Dixhoorn, 2007).

Several complementary perspectives contribute to the therapist's view of breathing difficulty or dysregulation. The first of these perspectives centers on the primary functions of breathing (van Dixhoorn, 2007). The most common lay understanding focuses on ventilation, the movement of air in and out of the lungs, primarily for the metabolic purposes of gas exchange. Along with its life-sustaining purpose, respiration also serves a necessary, less-recognized role in speech. Consequently, psychosocial factors may cause or exacerbate some kinds of breathing difficulties, and vice versa (De Peuter et al., 2004).

A second perspective focuses on breathing rhythm and mechanics as physiological regulators (van Dixhoorn, 2007). Respiration causes pressure changes that facilitate circulation of blood, lymph, and cerebrospinal fluid, and it is linked to heart rate through oscillatory feedback systems (Hirsch & Bishop, 1981). Parts of the respiratory anatomy affect posture and weight bearing as well as voluntary motor coordination. Additionally, recent evidence suggests that the neural circuits through which perceptual information affects the hypothalamic-pituitary-adrenal axis may simultaneously shape breathing patterns (Abelson, Khan, & Giardino, 2010).

The third perspective, emphasizing breathing as an information source in self-perception, is especially important in breathing therapies (van Dixhoorn, 2007). Internal respiratory feedback can reflect or instill a sense of either unrest or relaxation, linking one's internal state with an appraisal of the immediate environment. Individual variations in sensitivity to this feedback can have significant clinical implications. Among patients with severe asthma, those less attuned to breathing sensations may be more vulnerable to serious attacks (Kikuchi et al., 1994), while less sensitive patients with asthma or chronic obstructive pulmonary disease (COPD) risk delaying self-medication until a breathing problem becomes urgent (Noseda, Schmerber, Prigogine, & Yernault, 1993). Respiratory hypersensitivity is also associated with clinical problems, as patients with panic disorder or hypochondriasis may detect small changes in airway resistance more accurately than do nonpatient controls (Ehlers, 1997). Respiratory sensitivities also influence whether patients report breathing problems and how helpful they find breathing therapies.

CURRENT PRACTICE
Types of Breathing

Chest breathing, or costal breathing, involves movement of the chest wall outward and upward with each draw of breath. This type of breathing, which may be shallower and less regular than other types, is likely to be associated with high-arousal states and is typically more efficient during exercise than at rest (Patel, 1991). *Clavicular breathing* involves maximum-capacity inhalation that completely fills the lungs. It gets its name from the clavicles, or collar bones, which rise slightly at the end of a full inhalation when the tops of the lungs expand.

Clavicular breathing happens only when the body struggles to meet its need for oxygen; it may be seen in patients suffering from chronic bronchitis or asthma (Patel, 1991). *Abdominal breathing*, or diaphragmatic breathing, principally relies on the movements of the diaphragm, a thin, strong muscle sheet that extends across the bottom of the rib cage and separates the thoracic and abdominal cavities. In this type of breathing, which is often used in yoga practice and in relaxation therapies, the diaphragm contracts downward with each breath, the abdominal muscles relax upward, and the lungs expand, drawing in air. During exhalation, the diaphragm relaxes and abdominal muscles contract. Abdominal breathing involves a focus on limiting the upper ribs' movement during each breath and instead pushing out the upper abdominal wall (Chandra, 1994).

No single standard defines the optimal way of breathing. While slow deep breathing is healthy in some conditions and should not cause feelings of dyspnea, this does not imply that it is always, or usually, the best way to breath. Instead, functional breathing is most often variable, changing with little or no effort in response to circumstances (van Dixhoorn, 2007; Ley, 1994). Many of the therapeutic techniques described next aim to promote this responsiveness to visual, auditory, or kinesthetic stimuli. Breathing can also be too irregular, however, as when people with high anxiety alternate between rapid breaths and deep sighs (Wilhelm, Gevirtz, & Roth, 2001). The goal of breathing-focused stress management is to eliminate undue respiratory effort while balancing the emphases on the stability versus the flexibility of the breathing pattern according to the individual's needs.

Finally, although practicing the techniques learned during therapy sessions is extremely important, healthy breathing should happen effortlessly and outside conscious regulation in most circumstances. Therefore, it is equally necessary for the patient to stop practicing and take time to self-observe, with the therapist's guidance, how physical and mental sensations change or persist when conscious regulation of breathing stops. In this respect, therapeutic techniques that involve short periods of controlled breathing followed by relinquishment of control to self-observe one's relaxed mental and physical states resemble the earlier described tense-and-relax cycles of progressive muscle relaxation (van Dixhoorn, 2007). These two types of therapy also take similar approaches to imparting their self-regulatory skills and techniques: In both cases, the therapist seeks to present instructions to the patient in a manner that is "more like an invitation for the system to respond favorably than [as] a dominant influence" (van Dixhoorn, 2007, p. 296).

Breathing Techniques

The technique of *timing breathing* includes several methods of regulating the rate or pace of respiration, typically for the purpose of focusing attention on taking slow, deep breaths. This technique is based on the idea that slowed breathing facilitates relaxation, reduces hyperventilation, or both (van Dixhoorn, 2007). One way of keeping time is to count silently along with each breath, so that the duration of each inhalation and exhalation corresponds to the same rhythmic count with each breathing cycle. For example, counting at a rate that corresponds to comfortable breathing, one might count from 1 to 4 while slowly drawing breath for 4 seconds, and then continue the count from 5 to 8 while smoothly exhaling for 4 seconds. If keeping count is distracting, a count of "1, 1, 1 . . ." can also be used (Benson, 1993). These approaches can also be applied to lengthen inhalation and/or exhalation, by slightly and gradually increasing the count per breath in 1-second (or one-digit) increments, perhaps inhaling for a 1 to 5 (rather than 1 to 4) count, then exhaling from 6 to 10 (rather than 5 to 8) while maintaining the prior pace of the count, and always taking care not to induce labored breathing or discomfort.

Similar methods help lengthen breathing by focusing attention on the exhalation pauses, those transitional moments between the end of an exhalation and the beginning of the next inhalation that emerge during relaxed breathing. Modifying the count to include exhalation pause ("in, 2, 3, out, 2, 3, pause, 2, 3"), or simply maintaining a silent, rhythmic recitation of "in . . . out . . . pause. . . . " in synch with the breathing cycle, can help the patient notice and become accustomed to these points of transition. Another version of this approach that often promotes feelings of calm and control is to focus on both types of transition in the breathing cycle—when the air in the system reverses direction after an exhalation as well as after an inhalation. Though the practice is less common, timing techniques can also be used to encourage faster, shallower breaths to help break a habit of persistent, effortful deep breathing or to demonstrate to patients with medically unwarranted anxieties about airflow that a feared decrease in ventilation is not dangerous (van Dixhoorn, 2007).

When a less direct regulatory approach than the timing method is needed, *linking movement to breathing* can be a helpful strategy, relying on the regulation of movements to regularize breathing indirectly. Rhythmic movements, such as running, walking, and many forms of aerobic exercise, tend to synchronize with breathing. When this kind of concurrence emerges, slowing or speeding up the movement tends to have a similar effect on respiration. Thus, simple rhythmic movements can be used as a mechanism to facilitate changes in breathing patterns without requiring the patient's conscious attention to each breath. Jan van Dixhoorn suggests several movements that tend to become coupled to breathing, which can then be systematically slowed to affect the respiratory rate indirectly, such as "rolling the hands or arms in and out, moving the head up and down, pressing the fingers together and relaxing them, [or] flexing and extending the feet" (2007, p. 299). Walking more slowly than usual also has this effect on breathing, as long as it is not so slow as to become effortful (van Dixhoorn, 2007). If a more direct focus on breathing is desirable (or at least is not contraindicated), breathing cycles can also be paired with the tense-and-release cycles of abbreviated progressive muscle relaxation. Tensing while inhaling is typical, but the reverse pairing of tensing with exhaling is more difficult and therefore can be especially useful for focusing attention on these bodily states (van Dixhoorn, 2007).

Several methods of *monitoring air passage* can also be used to regulate and focus attention on breathing (van Dixhoorn, 2007). Pursed-lips breathing, which involves mouth breathing through the lips while keeping them very gently pressed together, adds resistance to the air and thereby helps to maintain open airways, improving ventilation. Pursed-lips breathing tends to increase tidal volumes and to result in longer exhalation times, so it is important that while using this technique patients inhale slowly and gently, rather than gasping, to maintain a relaxed, focused state. To prevent hyperventilation, this technique should be used for only about 5 to 6 breaths in succession before taking a break and returning to normal breathing through the nose. Another method of monitoring air passage is simply to slow inhalation through the nose. This method poses less risk of hyperventilation than mouth breathing, while maintaining the benefits of increased tidal volumes and greater involvement of the whole body in the slow, steady drawing of breath. The attention-focusing and stress-alleviating potential of this technique can be enhanced by pairing it with imagery. The patient can be guided in imagining the air passing in through the nose and flowing down the throat, into the lungs and chest, and even pervading the rest of the body.

EMPIRICAL SUPPORT

A robust literature developed over several decades shows that voluntary control of breathing can affect physiological and psychological arousal (Ley, 1994). One facet of this research examined direct effects of breathing regulation on psychophysiological measures of experimentally induced arousal. Voluntarily slowed breathing (McCaul, Solomon, & Holmes 1979) and prolonged exhalation relative to inhalation (Cappo & Holmes, 1984) have been associated with lower levels of physiological (e.g., electrodermal response, finger pulse volume) and self-reported arousal. In contrast, hyperventilation has been shown to increase subjective anxiety and its psychophysiological correlates (Thyer, Papsdorf, & Wright, 1984), an effect that may be enhanced in individuals with either high trait anxiety or anxiety sensitivity (Sturges, Goetsch, Ridley, & Whittal, 1998). However, in a more recent study, various breathing instructions tested in a 3-hour session—for example, attending to breathing, or anti-hyperventilation techniques of breathing more slowly, shallowly, or both—had no significant psychophysiological effects. Homeostatic mechanisms counteracted most effects of purposeful control of breathing (Conrad et al., 2007). These authors noted that different instructions, additional practice, and combining instructions with feedback may induce greater physiological changes, and that cognitive training mechanisms underlying breathing-based relaxation also contribute to its efficacy.

Breathing-focused therapies are also incorporated into medical treatment, with the goal of decreasing stress associated with chronic illness (Gilbert, 2003). Given that relaxed, responsive, effortless breathing can have widespread physiological benefits—less upper-body muscle tension, more stable blood chemistry, a more healthful balance of sympathetic–parasympathetic nervous system activation, and improved oxygenation in the lungs—changes in breathing may also improve some medical symptoms (Gilbert, 2003). Many studies investigating this potential have focused on cardiovascular diseases (e.g., essential hypertension, angina, functional chest disorder, and cardiac rehabilitation), as well as COPD, and some therapies appear to be beneficial (see Gilbert, 2003 for a review).

One clinical trial randomly assigned 156 myocardial infarction patients to one of two rehabilitation programs: exercise training alone or exercise plus six sessions of breathing-focused relaxation therapy. Breathing therapy initially was associated with enhanced effects of exercise and improved well-being (van Dixhoorn et al., 1989), and these patients later showed improved return to work and a 50% lower incidence of cardiac medical events (van Dixhoorn & Duivenvoorden, 1999; van Dixhoorn & White, 2005). At 5-year follow-up these patients showed a 31% lower rehospitalization rate than those who rehabilitated with only exercise, offsetting the relaxation therapy costs (van Dixhoorn & Duivenvoorden, 1999).

ISSUES FOR FUTURE RESEARCH

Future research promises to improve the use of breathing therapies for stress by developing increasingly precise ways of measuring respiration outside the laboratory and integrating these measures with other physiological indicators of stress. One such technology operates via personal computer to detect the pace of the user's breathing. The system uses two pairs of small microphones to detect respiratory activity; it eliminates environmental noise from the respiratory signal, and then streams the data to the computer with a latency of less than 5 milliseconds (Leskovsek et al., 2011). The small, noninvasive device requires no external power supply, suggesting it could be incorporated easily into ecologically valid studies of stress or breathing-focused interventions in the workplace, or used to provide feedback during patients' real-world practice of breathing exercises.

Along similar lines, as the use of breathing therapies becomes more common in the context of medical treatment, there is growing interest in the ability to "prescribe" a precise course of breathing exercises that a patient can accurately follow at home. Devices supporting this kind of treatment have existed for decades, but they are becoming much smaller, more cost-effective, and easier for patients to use, and better able to provide physicians and researchers with precise data about patients' treatment adherence and respiratory changes over time (e.g., Gavish, 2010). Other technologies that can help expand the use and understanding of breathing therapies include a wireless, wearable stress monitor that combines heart rate and respiratory information based on spectral density measures (Choi, Ahmed, &

Gutierrez-Osuna, 2012), and a system for measuring mental stress more precisely by distinguishing the influences of breathing on heart rate variability (Choi & Gutierrez-Osuna, 2011). These innovations will not only make gathering data on respiration and stress easier and more precise but will also aid researchers in studying breathing techniques in the naturalistic circumstances where they might be productively applied.

Guided Imagery
BRIEF HISTORY

Therapeutic uses of imagery may seem second nature because people commonly use imagery for psychological benefit—for motivation, escapism, or simply planning activities—without consciously considering its effects (Hatler, 1998). Therapeutic imagery has roots in the earliest psychotherapies, but Freudians typically relied on patients' spontaneous imagery. In contrast, the French psychotherapist Robert Desoille created a technique for directing patients' mental imagery. In his "guided day dream method," developed in the 1920s, the therapist described a series of six narratives or "themes" to the patient (Klapish, 1973; Schoettle, 1980). Each session focused on one theme, which set the patient as the protagonist in an archetypal story thought to facilitate access to unconscious conflicts (e.g., diving into a shipwreck for treasure). The patient elaborated and described this "experience," then the patient and therapist would later discuss the "day dream's" significance. A similar guided affective imagery method, developed by the German psychiatrist Hanscarl Leuner in the late 1940s, involved a series of 10 psychoanalyst-guided visualizations (Leuner, 1969). These scenarios were likewise symbolic but less story-directed to maximize their projective potential. Some of them, like being in a meadow or near a babbling brook, remain popular in relaxation therapies.

Around the same time, the South African psychiatrist Joseph Wolpe (1969) was refining his systematic desensitization treatment for phobias—quite a different enterprise from imagery-driven psychoanalysis, but one that similarly used mental imagery therapeutically. His treatment, which became foundational to behavior therapy, relied on "imaginal exposures" to the phobic stimulus, in which the therapist guided the patient through increasingly frightening imagined encounters with the feared object or situation. Each exposure was coupled with Jacobsonian progressive muscle relaxation to help the patient remain calm. Informed by laboratory research on conditioning, Wolpe based this method on his reciprocal inhibition theory: the idea that because the body cannot be simultaneously relaxed and anxious, patients could face fears by learning to relax during frightening encounters. Though Wolpe used imagery to induce fears, he was a pioneering proponent of its power in treating anxiety. Modern cognitive-behavioral therapies still use imagery as a form of practice for facing anxiety-provoking situations (Ronen, 2011).

THEORETICAL AND EMPIRICAL BASES

Clinical experience has long suggested a close relationship between imagery and emotion, but evidence has been limited and widely dispersed until recently (Hackmann, Bennett-Levy, & Holmes, 2011). Early research showed that people who considered themselves "good" rather than "poor" imagers had stronger psychophysiological responses to highly active or affective (fear, anger) visualizations, and their responses showed more enhancement with training (Miller et al., 1987). These findings were interpreted in support of a bioinformational theory (Lang, 1979), in which recreating or recalling emotional images elicits the same patterns of neural activity as the imagined experiences would (Denis, Mellet, & Kosslyn, 2004; Kosslyn, Ganis, & Thompson, 2001; Lang, Greenwalk, Bradley, & Hamm, 1993). Although findings associating imagery with specific psychophysiological responses are mixed, and some clinical populations have shown different response patterns from controls (see Vianna, Naqvi, Bechara, & Tranel, 2009), imagery's potential for exerting stronger therapeutic emotional change than verbal thought has prompted direct experimental comparisons.

Holmes, Matthews, and colleagues presented participants with verbal descriptions of brief scenarios, each of which began with an emotionally ambiguous premise then resolved in either a neutral or an emotionally charged way (Holmes & Matthews, 2005; Holmes, Mathews, Dalgleish, & Mackintosh, 2006). In each experiment, participants in the verbal condition focused on the meanings of the words describing the scenarios, while those in the imagery condition imagined the scenarios. Between the two, those who imagined the events showed stronger emotional responses (Holmes & Matthews, 2005; Holmes et al., 2006). In another paradigm, participants viewed picture–word pairs in which each word suggested either a negative or a benign interpretation of its associated picture (Holmes, Coughtrey, & Connor, 2008). In one

condition, participants thought of sentences using each picture–word pair; those in the other condition imagined combining each pair (Holmes et al., 2008, p. 401). Again, participants who used imagery showed stronger emotional responses than did those who combined the pairs verbally.

One evolutionary explanation for imagery's emotional power may be relevant to its therapeutic use. Öhman and Mineka (2001) suggested that the neural circuitry supporting fear constitutes an evolved module highly sensitive to perceptual stimuli, such as images, necessary for identifying threats. They proposed that this module operates largely outside conscious control, including regulation by verbal thoughts, because its evolutionary development long predates conscious thought and language (Öhman & Mineka, 2001). In this view, if guided imagery helps patients to replace stress-inducing mental images with calming ones, it may promote relaxation through neural and somatic mechanisms that are less responsive to conscious control.

CURRENT PRACTICE

Guided imagery can be incorporated into a wide variety of therapeutic approaches to stress management, and it has often been studied in combination with other relaxation methods. One reason for its broad use and frequent combination with other techniques is that, to a greater extent than some other relaxation methods (e.g., Jacobson's progressive muscle relaxation training program), the specific content and method of guided imagery can be tailored to suit the individual patient's needs. Another reason is that imagery and relaxation may have reciprocally enhancing effects, so that imagery helps to deepen relaxation, which in turn facilitates immersion in a vivid, imagined scene (Hatler, 1998).

Many practitioners who use guided imagery rely on scripts, which are standardized written scenarios that can be read verbatim or can provide starting points for more improvised guided imagery sessions. Practitioners can acquire them from numerous bookstores and Web sites (also see sample scripts in Hatler, 1998; Tusek & Cwynar, 2000), or they may choose to personalize their scripts, either by revising existing ones for particular patients or problems or creating entirely new scripts. Particularly for less experienced clinicians, using a script can help to ensure that the patient experiences the clinician's guidance during the session as soothing, effortless, and consistent. The scripts themselves can vary from highly individualized to relatively generic, so long as they include cues to help patients elaborate on the evoked mental images with their own most relaxing, personally resonant sensory details. Some clinicians find it useful to create several basic scripts pertaining to the kinds of problems they typically treat and to modify them as needed in their work with individual patients (Hatler, 1998). The scripts can also be provided to the patient for use outside of therapy sessions, either in written form (for use with a close other) or as an audio recording.

During the guided imagery session, the therapist should speak in a soothing, gentle tone that will foster the patient's personal reflections (Hatler, 1998). The script may begin with a brief physical relaxation procedure, such as a form of deep breathing or muscle relaxation, conducted with eyes closed (Tusek & Cwynar, 2000). This process serves as an induction, or a transitional phase, to help the patient enter a different mental state (Battino, 2007). During this time, the patient is encouraged to focus on the present moment and begin letting go of racing thoughts and nagging concerns, instead bringing to mind any images that evoke a sense of peace and restfulness. The patient should remain in a comfortable, relaxed position (seated, reclining, or supine), with eyes closed for the duration of the guided imagery session, in order to focus on the imagined sensations and limit distractions from the physical environment.

An important goal of guided imagery that can inform the clinician's selection or creation of scripts is to help the patient to envision and to experience a special imagined place that serves as a sanctuary from stress and anxiety (Hatler, 1998). For some patients, this place may be a natural environment, while others may prefer a familiar park or a favorite room. Ideally, the patient should choose his own location where he feels completely safe and calm, since a scene chosen by the therapist may have adverse associations for the patient (Hatler, 1998), though some generic locations such as a beach or a meadow may provide a helpful starting point for beginners or patients who have difficulty creating images.

During the session, the therapist's language should reinforce the patient's sense of being protected and at ease in this place, while helping him focus on the soothing sensory qualities of the experience. Rich, absorbing imagery should include not only what the patient sees in this environment but also what he hears, smells, and perhaps tastes, and how these aspects of the experience make him feel. Positive imagery confers stronger emotional benefits

when it is imagined from a first-person perspective rather than a third-person or observer perspective (Holmes et al., 2008); focusing on a variety of sensory experiences may help the patient develop and maintain a first-person perspective that places him within the imagined experience. Additionally, scripts that carefully use repetition and pauses can also help to deepen patients' relaxation and provide opportunities to develop their imagery independently (Hatler, 1998). The general tenor of the script should convey feeling of courage and calm, with a focus on accepting lessons learned from past experiences and moving forward in life with substantial personal capabilities on which to draw (Tusek & Cwynar, 2000). Themes of finding and developing inner resources can support a sense of self-efficacy that contributes to patients' ability to manage daily stress independently through effective self-care (AGI, 2011).

After the person is oriented and comfortable in the imagined place, some scripts may include an encounter with a guide who supports the patient through the imagery experience and can serve as a source of strength and wisdom (Hatler, 1998; Tusek & Cwynar, 2000). The guide can be a loved one, a close friend, a past or present mentor, or even a beloved pet, a favorite animal, or an immaterial spiritual presence. If the script features a guide, it should help to instill a sense of the guide as a trusted companion in the imagined experience or as a watchful, protective presence who can provide help if it is needed. In some cases, patients may discover this kind of supportive, imagined presence on their own, even when they are not explicitly included in the script (Tusek & Cwynar, 2000). The use of imagined guides or protectors is just one means of facilitating the patient's ability to draw on his own inner resources for creative problem-solving and resilience (AGI, 2011). Guided imagery techniques in which patients are encouraged to interact with a guide or with other figures, including symbolic representations, are sometimes called *interactive guided imagery* techniques (Heinschel, 2002). Although this approach has been studied less often than guided imagery that lacks a clear interactive component, the boundary between these types is not always clear, and both appear to have beneficial effects (Heinschel, 2002).

Another common technique for enhancing the guided imagery experience is to combine it with soothing music played in the background at a low to moderate volume (Tusek & Cwynar, 2000). Music has a long history of therapeutic use to reduce stress, anxiety, and pain, as it seems to help distract from negative thoughts and promote a soothing mental escape from pressing concerns (Nilsson, 2008). A recent meta-analysis of music-assisted stress reduction therapies conducted in medical, university, and occupational settings found consistently positive results and noted that "music-assisted verbal suggestion" was one of two procedures producing the largest average effect sizes in stress reduction measures among the 22 studies examined (Pelletier, 2004). For clinicians who wish to incorporate music into the guided imagery experience, this paper also describes the most effective selections for relaxation as typically including "a slower tempo, low pitches. . . . regular rhythmic patterns, no extreme changes in dynamics, and no lyrics" (Pelletier, 2004, p. 209). If the script describes a particular natural setting, such a being on a beach or near a stream, recordings of the sounds of that environment can also enhance the experience (Tusek & Cwynar, 2000), particularly for patients who find it difficult to conjure or maintain vivid mental images.

Finally, it is important to bear in mind that the broadly flexible uses of guided imagery for relaxation and stress management differ significantly from its more restrained and programmatic uses in treating psychological disorders. Imagery is a powerful treatment tool, and different imagery-based techniques have been developed and tested for many specific disorders. Consequently, practitioners must ensure that a particular therapeutic use of guided imagery for stress management is appropriate for the individual patient and is not contraindicated by existing psychopathology (Harding, 1996). Several types of problems that may preclude the use of guided imagery for relaxation include posttraumatic stress disorder or other trauma-related stress, obsessive-compulsive disorder, severe anxiety or phobias, dissociative disorders, and hallucinations or delusions, among others (for additional information, see Arthbhnott, Arbuthnott, & Rossiter, 2001; Courtois, 2001; Harding, 1996).

EMPIRICAL SUPPORT

Relatively little cognitive-behavioral therapy-based research has investigated effects of positive mental imagery (Hackmann, Bennett-Levy, & Holmes, 2011). One review of imagery's uses in symptom management noted five studies in which guided imagery reduced stress in medically healthy individuals (Eller, 1999). Another more recent study of an imagery intervention for people with dysphoria showed that generating positive images in response to picture-word prompts led to mood improvements and related cognitive and behavioral changes that remained evident 24 hours later (Pictet, Coughtrey, Mathews, & Holmes, 2011).

Additional evidence from sports psychology and health psychology has demonstrated guided imagery's value for stress management. Studies of many athletic activities, including basketball, weight lifting, archery, skating, and military parachute jumps, among others, suggest that mental imagery can help athletes reduce anxiety (Jones & Stuth, 1997; Vadoa, Hall, & Moritz, 1997). Researchers have also examined the content of athletes' self-generated imagery and documented links between particular types of imagery, athletes' mental states (e.g., confidence, anxiety), and performance (Jones & Stuth, 1997; Monsma & Overby, 2004; Vadoa, Hall, & Moritz, 1997).

Guided imagery also has a substantial history in medicine, especially as practiced by nurses as an adjuvant therapy to reduce patients' stress (Stephens, 1993a). One transdiagnostic application is its use for pain management across a variety of medical conditions (McCaffery, 1989; Stephens, 1993a). Cognitive mechanisms potentially contributing to this effect include providing distraction, enhancing relaxation, and inducing a state of autohypnosis (Stephens, 1993a); however, like many stress management therapies, its underlying mechanisms are not well understood.

Closely related to its potential contributions to medical symptom management, imagery offers psychological benefits, helping patients manage anxiety and muster the inner resources required to undergo difficult treatments. Many uses of imagery in medical contexts, such as problem reframing, regaining a sense of control in life, facing one's limitations, and developing the strength to make major lifestyle changes (Stephens, 1993b), map clearly onto therapeutic goals of cognitive-behavioral therapists and clients. One study of imagery focused on the intersection of its medical and psychotherapeutic uses involved adding imagery-supported relaxation to prenatal care to reduce maternal stress. Use of a CD-recorded guided imagery intervention for 12 weeks was associated with a significant reduction in the women's state anxiety (Jallo, Bourguignon, Taylor, Ruiz, & Goehler, 2009).

ISSUES FOR FUTURE RESEARCH

The study of positive guided imagery as a technique for relieving stress and promoting relaxation has generated much research (Jones & Stuth, 1997;

Stephens, 1993a, 1993b), but few studies have systematically examined its use in combination with other cognitive-behavioral interventions, making this an important and likely area of future growth (Hackmann, Bennett-Levy, & Holmes, 2011). One productive new avenue of research with likely implications for the use of imagery in stress management is the development of computerized cognitive bias modification (CBM; Hackmann, Bennett-Levy, & Holmes, 2011; Koster, Fox, & MacLeod, 2009). CBM is a computer-based training method designed to help individuals decrease negative biases in information processing and promote more adaptive interpretations. Imagery-based CBM uses a paradigm similar to the earlier described experimental task (Holmes et al., 2006), in which participants heard and envisioned brief descriptions of ambiguous scenarios that then resolved in either a neutral or a positive way. The CBM programs present similarly ambiguous scenarios in repeated trials to help train people with depression to make positive, imagery-supported interpretations more habitually. The investigators suggest that practice with positive-imagery CBM may be most helpful for people who tend to interpret ambiguous everyday situations negatively.

Scientific and Clinical Issues in Cognitive-Behavioral Stress Management
Physiological and Cognitive Mechanisms

The abundance of stress management and relaxation techniques considered "cognitive-behavioral" raises questions about these varied methods' mechanisms of action. Like the refinement of the techniques themselves, the study of their mechanisms has developed within the parallel areas of basic stress science and clinical, efficacy-focused comparisons of treatments for specific stress-related pathologies. Research in both areas was initially framed by a decades-old question: To what extent are the effects of the different techniques mediated by common or modality-specific processes (Lehrer, Carr, Sargunaraj, & Woolfolk, 1994; Smith, Amutio, Anderson, & Aria, 1996)?

This question spurred the development of several theories. First, Benson's (1975) "relaxation response" model suggests that all relaxation techniques have the same complex of generalized physiological effects, resulting in reduced levels of arousal. In contrast, Davidson and Schwartz (1976) proposed a technique-specific model that distinguished between the effects of somatic, cognitive, and behavioral relaxation methods. A third model

then integrated elements of the first two, describing a reduction in physiological activity common to all techniques (consistent with Benson's "relaxation response") on which particular techniques' specific cognitive or somatic effects were then "superimposed" (Schwartz, Davidson, & Goleman, 1978).

Consistent with the third, integrative model, Lehrer and colleagues' extensive meta-analysis of the comparative effectiveness research found both generalized physiological effects of relaxation and technique-specific advantages in many direct treatment-based comparisons (Lehrer et al., 1994). To minimize bias due to methodological differences, they analyzed the *consistency* of significant effects across studies rather than comparing effect sizes. Technique-specific advantages were more likely when the techniques being compared showed a clear contrast between modalities (e.g., PMR versus mantra meditation), and when one of the techniques "directly pinpoint[ed] the system being assessed at outcome" (Lehrer et al., 1994, p. 386). More broadly, findings from many controlled studies of various relaxation techniques' physiological effects (e.g., cardiovascular functioning, glucose tolerance, lipid profiles, and neuroendocrine functioning) are consistent with the general notion that these practices promote a healthy state of dynamic equilibrium (e.g., Gaab et al., 2003; see Taylor et al., 2010 for a review).

Although biological mechanisms for stress management techniques are not well understood, research into the physical and mental workings of both stress and relaxation has implicated some relevant central and peripheral pathways. These approaches often highlight the complex reciprocal connections between the brain, as the "the central mediator and target of stress resiliency and vulnerability processes" and other body systems, which undergo wear and tear in modulating dysregulated threat responses (McEwen & Gianaros, 2011, p. 432).

The neuroscientific study of relaxation has often focused on various meditation techniques. Within this area, findings on the neurocognitive effects of focused attention methods, which combine attentional control (e.g., focusing on breath) and lowered physiological arousal, may help to inform future research into other cognitive-behavioral approaches, including those discussed earlier in this chapter. In this relatively young research area, the heterogeneity in the studied states, control populations, and tasks (Slagter, Davidson, & Lutz, 2011) makes the findings to date difficult to synthesize (see

Cahn & Polich, 2006 for a review). Nonetheless, a number of studies have described potentially beneficial effects of regular focused attention meditation on brain structures involved in sustained attention, as well as on proficient attentional processing abilities (Lutz et al., 2008; Slagter, Davidson, & Lutz, 2011). As research in this area progresses, studies linking the structural and functional changes in the brain that are associated with relaxation practices may provide important insights into their cognitive and physiological mechanisms.

Other researchers have focused on cognitive changes associated with regular use of cognitive-behavioral relaxation techniques, including the development of a common set of skills across techniques as well as technique-specific effects. The common skills theorized to be important to all types of cognitive-behavioral relaxation training include focusing attention (directing and sustaining attention on simple stimuli), passivity (slowing or stopping purposeful, analytic thought), and receptivity (becoming open to unfamiliar subjective states; Smith, 1990). Furthermore, the various focused attention meditation techniques are thought to bolster not only sustained attention but the crucial attention-regulating skills of remaining aware of distractions without losing focus, disengaging from distractions, and returning attention to the object of focus (Slagter, Davidson, & Lutz, 2011). Neuroimaging studies suggest that, with practice, these meditation techniques may produce broad, lasting improvements in sustained attention along with a practice-dependent decrease in the effort required to exert this cognitive control (Slagter, Davidson, & Lutz, 2011).

These and other cognitive changes that may come with relaxation practice help to deepen the experience of relaxation, and they may bring about other therapeutic cognitive effects as well. Over the long term, for example, the learning process and regular practice required to utilize most cognitive-behavioral relaxation techniques may also have implicit effects on the client's values and beliefs (Smith et al., 1996). Because new techniques present clients with challenges that cannot be met successfully through greater striving and pressure, these techniques may provide an opportunity to break stress-increasing mental patterns and to develop healthier approaches to tasks and goals. As Smith and colleagues (1996) describe, training-specific realizations, such as "'relaxation works better if I stop worrying about practicing perfectly' [may] evolve into more encompassing personal philosophies ('I'm an okay person and don't have to be perfect to be accepted')" (p. 65). As a counterpoint to these potentially technique-general cognitive effects, practitioners of the different techniques have described qualitatively distinct relaxation states (e.g., joyful, distant, calm, aware, limp) depending on their preferred technique (Smith et al., 1996). This finding suggests that relaxation-induced psychological changes may follow an integrative model similar to the physiological changes, yielding a combination of generalized and technique-specific effects. As research on the physiological and cognitive substrates of these interventions progresses, it potentially will provide clinicians with increasingly practical guidance for choosing the most suitable techniques, as well as insights about when and whether particular approaches can be productively combined.

Applications in Institutional Settings

Examining the mechanisms of action underlying cognitive-behavioral approaches to stress management necessarily focuses attention on the processes taking place within the minds and bodies of practitioners. As noted earlier in the chapter, however, the development and clinical application of these techniques also has been significantly informed by research into stressful environmental conditions. Much of this work has incorporated Lazarus and colleagues' transactional view of stress, in which stress is caused by the perception of disparities between the environmental demands on an individual and his or her ability to marshal adaptive resources (e.g., Lazarus, 1995). Over the last few decades, many institutions have become more aware of the functional and financial costs of operating as high-stress environments (Pelletier & Lutz, 1990; Weinberg & Cooper, 2011). Consequently, some organizations, including workplaces, and hospitals, have used cognitive-behavioral stress management techniques to address these issues, at the levels of primary stress prevention and secondary interventions for managing stress symptoms (McGregor & Antoni, 2009; McVicar, 2003; Richardson & Rothstein, 2008; van der Hek & Plomp, 1997).

Research into workplace stress management suggests that organization-specific interventions designed by a professional who takes into account feedback from employees at all levels about workplace stressors are especially effective at fostering a positive, collective approach to stress management (Giga, Cooper, & Faragher, 2003). Because an intensive, highly customized approach will not be practical for all workplaces, however, it is important to note that more cost-effective implementation methods can also be helpful. For example, small group interventions teaching several cognitive-behavioral stress management techniques have been shown to be as effective when they are led by paraprofessionals from participating organizations (employees briefly trained by a clinical psychologist) as they are when led by a clinical psychologist (de Jong & Emmelkamp, 2000). This dissemination model, in which paraprofessionals without advanced psychotherapy credentials are trained to administer evidence-based interventions, has been supported empirically in other areas of cognitive-behavioral practice (e.g., Craske et al., 2011). In the workplace, as well as other institutional settings, it could help to reduce the costs and complications of providing supportive, therapeutic interventions for stress.

Whether a workplace custom-designs its stress management program or adopts an existing approach, it will be useful to consider which types of techniques have proven useful in occupational settings. One recent meta-analysis of workplace stress management programs found approaches that allot time to relaxation training during the workday to be less effective on average than interventions that teach adaptive ways of appraising and responding to stressful workplace situations and encourage employees to practice these skills on the job (Richardson & Rothstein, 2008). This finding suggests that teaching employees to cope with job stress effectively as it occurs may be a more suitable workplace goal than helping them to minimize or avoid stressors (Meurs & Perrewé, 2011).

Hospitals can be highly stressful environments for staff and patients alike. Concerns about burnout, shiftwork effects, and understaffing among hospital nurses have led to a number of studies of occupational stress in this population (see Edwards & Burnard, 2003; McVicar, 2003 for reviews). Comparing separate, contemporary literature reviews that focused, respectively, on mental health nurses and nurses in medical hospitals suggests that the sources of nurses' stress in both hospital environments are well characterized, but translating this knowledge into rigorous studies of effective interventions has proven difficult. Notably, most interventions documented in these studies have focused on individual-level changes, which the authors suggest may not be adequate without addressing some key sources of stress at the organizational level. On the other hand, incorporating relaxation

and stress management techniques into patient care has shown some notable benefits for those managing chronic illnesses as well as those undergoing major procedures (Baum, Herberman, & Cohen, 1995; Ludwick-Rosenthal & Neufeld, 1988; Nezu, Nezu, & Xanthopoulos, 2011). One area in which promising in-hospital applications of these techniques have been widely documented is the use of relaxation interventions to manage presurgical stress (reviewed in Johnston, 1993; Powell et al., 2010), which for some patients has been shown to hasten patients' recovery and improve quality of life after surgery.

Conclusions

This overview of muscle relaxation, breathing, and guided imagery illustrates recent developments in cognitive-behavioral approaches to stress management. These and other techniques have generated evidence of efficacy with regard to a number of stress outcomes of importance to a variety of clinical populations. Refinements in technique have been accompanied by adaptations that take advantage of handheld electronic devices and address the need to incorporate stress management into various institutional settings.

References

Abelson, J. L., Khan, S., & Giardino, N. (2010). HPA axis, respiration and the airways in stress—a review in search of intersections. *Biological Psychology, 84*(1), 57–65.

Academy for Guided Imagery (AGI). (2011). *How guided imagery works.* Retrieved March 2012, from http://www.academyforguidedimagery.com/whatisguidedimagery/how-imageryworks/index.html

Almeida, D. M., Stawski, R. S., & Cichy, K. E. (2011). Combining checklist and interview approaches for assessing daily stressors: The Daily Inventory of Stressful Events. In R. J. Contrada & A. Baum (Eds.), *The handbook of stress science: Biology, psychology, and health* (pp. 583–596). New York: Springer.

Anderson, N. B., & Armstead, C. A. (1995). Toward understanding the association of socioeconomic status and health: A new challenge for the biopsychosocial approach. *Psychosomatic Medicine, 23*, 3726–3751.

Anderson, B., Wethington, E., & Kamark, T. W. (2011). Interview assessment of stress exposure. In R. J. Contrada & A. Baum (Eds.), *The handbook of stress science: Biology, psychology, and health* (pp. 565–582). New York: Springer.

Arbuthnott, K. D., Arbuthnott, D. W., & Rossiter, L. (2001). Guided imagery and memory: Implications for psychotherapists. *Journal of Counseling Psychology, 48*(2), 123–132.

Arnsten, A. F. (2009). Stress signaling pathways that impair prefrontal cortex structure and function. *Nature Reviews Neuroscience, 10*(6), 410–422.

Battino, R. (2007). *Guided imagery: Psychotherapy and healing through the mind–body connection.* Carmarthen, Wales: Crown House.

Baum, A. (1987). Social density and perceived control as mediators of crowding stress in high-density residential neighborhoods. *Journal of Personality and Social Psychology, 52*(5), 899–906.

Baum, A., Herberman, H., & Cohen, L. (1995). Managing stress and managing illness: Survival and quality of life in chronic disease. *Journal of Clinical Psychology in Medical Settings, 2*(4), 309–333.

Benson, H. (1975). *The relaxation response.* New York: Morrow.

Benson, H. (1993). The relaxation response. In D. J. Goleman & J. Gurin (Eds.), *Mind body medicine* (pp. 233–257). Yonkers, NY: Consumer Reports Books.

Bernhaut, M., Gelhorn, E., & Rasmussen, A. T. (1953). Experimental contributions to the problem of consciousness. *Journal of Neurophysiology, 16*, 21–35.

Bernstein, D. A., & Borkovec, T. D. (1973). *Progressive relaxation training: A manual for the helping professions.* Champaign, IL: Research Press.

Bernstein, D. A., Borkovec, T. D., & Hazlett-Stevens, H. (2000). *New directions in progressive relaxation training: A guidebook for helping professionals.* Westport, CT: Praeger.

Bernstein, D. A., Carlson, C., & Schmidt, J. E. (2007). Progressive relaxation: Abbreviated methods. In P. M. Lehrer & R. L. Woolfolk (Eds.), *Principles and practice of stress management* (3rd ed. pp. 88–124). New York: Guilford Press.

Berntson, G. G., Cacioppo, J. T., Binkley, P. E., Uchino, B. N., Quigley, K. S., & Fieldstone, A. (1994). Autonomic cardiac control. III. Psychological stress and cardiac response in autonomic space as revealed by pharmacological blockades. *Psychophysiology, 31*, 599–608.

Berntson, G. G., Norman, G. J., Hawkley, L. C., & Cacioppo, J. T. (2008). Cardiac autonomic balance versus cardiac regulatory capacity. *Psychophysiology, 45*(4), 643–652.

Borkovec, T. D., & Sides, J. K. (1979). Critical procedural variables related to the physiological effects of progressive relaxation: A review. *Behaviour Research and Therapy, 17*, 119–125.

Cacioppo, J. T., Tassinary, L. G., & Berntson, G. (Eds.). (2007). *Handbook of psychophysiology* (3rd ed.). New York: Cambridge University Press.

Cahn, B. R., & Polich, J. (2006). Meditation states and traits: EEG, ERP, and neuroimaging studies. *Psychological Bulletin, 132*, 180–211.

Cannon, W. (1929). The sympathetic division of the autonomic system in relation to homeostasis. *Archives of Neurology and Psychiatry, 22*, 284–294.

Cappo, B. M., & Holmes, D. S. (1984). The utility of prolonged respiratory exhalation for reducing physiological and psychological arousal in non-threatening and threatening situations. *Journal of Psychosomatic Research, 28*(4), 265–273.

Carlson, C. R., & Hoyle, R. (1993). Efficacy of abbreviated progressive muscle relaxation training: A quantitative review. *Journal of Consulting and Clinical Psychology, 61*, 1059–1067.

Cerqueira, J. J., Mailliet, F., Almeida, O. F., Jay, T. M., & Sousa, N. (2007). The prefrontal cortex as a key target of the maladaptive response to stress. *Journal of Neuroscience, 27*(11), 2781–2787.

Chandra, F. A. (1994). Respiratory practices in yoga. In B. H. Timmons & R. Ley (Eds.), *Behavioral and psychological approaches to breathing disorders* (pp. 221–232). New York: Plenum Press.

Choi, J., Ahmed, B., & Gutierrez-Osuna, R. (2012). Development and evaluation of an ambulatory stress monitor cased on wearable sensors. *Information Technology in Biomedicine, 16*(2), 279–286.

Choi, J., & Gutierrez-Osuna, R. (2011). Removal of respiratory influences from heart rate variability in stress monitoring. *Sensors Journal, IEEE, 11*(11), 2649–2656.

Cohen, S., Kessler, R. C., & Gordon, L. U. (1997). Strategies for measuring stress in studies of psychiatric and physical disorders. In S. Cohen, R. C. Kessler, & L. U. Gordon (Eds.), *Measuring stress: A guide for health and social scientists* (pp. 3–26). New York: Oxford University Press.

Conrad, A., Müller, A., Doberenz, S., Kim, S., Meuret, A. E., Wollburg, E., & Roth, W. T. (2007). Psychophysiological effects of breathing instructions for stress management. *Applied Psychophysiology and Biofeedback, 32*(2), 89–98.

Conrad, A., & Roth, W. T. (2007). Muscle relaxation therapy for anxiety disorders: It works but how? *Journal of Anxiety Disorders, 21*, 243–264.

Courtois, C. A. (2001). Commentary on "Guided imagery and memory:" Additional considerations. *Journal of Counseling Psychology, 48*(2), 133–135.

Craske, M. G., Stein, M. B., Sullivan, G., Sherbourne, C., Bystritsky, A., Rose, R. D.,…Roy-Byrne, P. (2011). Disorder-specific impact of coordinated anxiety learning and management treatment for anxiety disorders in primary care. *Archives of General Psychiatry, 68*(4), 378–388.

Dantzer, R., O'Connor, J. C., Freund, G. G., Johnson, R. W., & Kelley, K. W. (2008). From inflammation to sickness and depression: When the immune system subjugates the brain. *Nature Reviews Neuroscience, 9*, 46–57.

Davidson, R. J., & Schwartz, G. E. (1976). Psychobiology of relaxation and related states. In D. Mostofsky (Ed.), *Behavior modification and control of physiological activity.* Englewood Cliffs, N J: Prentice-Hall.

De Peuter, S., Van Diest, I., Lemaigre, V., Verleden, G., Demedts, M., & Van den Bergh, O. (2004). Dyspnea: the role of psychological processes. *Clinical Psychology Review, 24*(5), 557–581.

de Jong, G. M., & Emmelkamp, P. M. J. (2000). Implementing a stress management training: Comparative trainer effectiveness. *Journal of Occupational health Psychology, 5*(2), 309–320.

Dedovic, K., D'Aguiar, C., & Pruessner, J. C. (2009). What stress does to your brain: A review of neuroimaging studies. *Canadian Journal of Psychiatry, 54*(1), 6–15.

Denis, M., Mellet, E., & Kosslyn, S. M. (2004). *Neuroimaging of mental imagery.* Hove, UK: Psychology Press.

Edwards, D., & Burnard, P. (2003). A systematic review of stress and stress management interventions for mental health nurses. *Journal of Advanced Nursing, 42*(2), 169–200.

Ehlers, A. (1997). *Perception of heartbeats and airway resistance in hypochondriasis.* Paper presented at the 3rd European Congress of Psychophysiology. Konstanz, Germany. May 29–31.

Eller, L. S. (1999). Guided imagery interventions for symptom management. *Annual Review of Nursing Research, 17*, 57–84.

Emery, C. F., France, C. R., Harris, J., Norman, G., & VanArsdalen, C. (2008). Pain reduction effects of progressive muscle relaxation training on nociceptive flexion reflex threshold in healthy young adults: A randomized trial. *Pain, 138*, 375–379.

Gaab, J., Blättler, N., Menzi, T., Pabst, B., Stoyer, S., & Ehlert, U. (2003). Randomized controlled evaluation of the effects of cognitive–behavioral stress management on cortisol responses to acute stress in healthy subjects. *Psychoneuroendocrinology*, *28*, 767–779.

Gavish, B. (2010). Device-guided breathing in the home setting: Technology, performance and clinical outcomes. *Biological Psychology*, *84*(1), 150–156.

Gay, M-C., Philippot, P., & Luminet, O. (2002). Differential effectiveness of psychological interventions for reducing osteoarthritis pain: A comparison of Erickson hypnosis and Jacobson relaxation. *European Journal of Pain*, *6*, 1–6.

Gelhorn, E. (1958). The physiological basis of neuromuscular relaxation. *Archives of Internal Medicine*, *102*, 392–399.

Gelhorn, E., & Keily, W. F. (1972). Mystical states of consciousness: Neurophysiological and clinical aspects. *Journal of Nervous and Mental Disease*, *154*, 399–405.

Gianaros, P. J., & O. Connor, M-F. (2011). Neuroimaging methods in human stress science. In R. J. Contrada & A. Baum (Eds.), *The handbook of stress science: Biology, psychology, and health* (pp. 543–564). New York: Springer.

Giga, S. I., Cooper, C. L., & Faragher, B. (2003). The development of a framework for a comprehensive approach to stress management interventions at work. *International Journal of Stress Management*, *10*(4), 280–296.

Gilbert, C. (2003). Clinical applications of breathing regulation beyond anxiety management. *Behavior Modification*, *27*(5), 692–709.

Glass, D. C., & Singer, J. E. (1972). *Urban stress: Experiments on noise and social stressors*. New York: Academic Press.

Hackmann, A., Bennett-Levy, J., & Holmes, E. A. (2011). *Oxford guide to imagery in cognitive therapy*. New York: Oxford University Press.

Hahn, V. C., Binnewies, C., Sonnentag, S., & Mojza, E. J. (2011). Learning how to recover from job stress: Effects of a recovery training program on recovery, recovery-related self-efficacy and well-being. *Journal of Occupational Health Psychology*, *16*, 202–216.

Hall, L., & Long, C. G. (2009). Back to basics: Progressive muscle relaxation (PMR) training for women detained in conditions of medium security. *Journal of Forensic Psychiatry and Psychology*, *20*(3), 481–492.

Harding, S. (1996). Relaxation: With or without imagery? *International Journal of Nursing Practice*, *2*, 160–162.

Hatler, C. W. (1998). Using guided imagery in the emergency department. *Journal of Emergency Nursing*, *24*(6), 518–522.

Heinschel, J. A. (2002). A descriptive study of the interactive guided imagery experience. *Journal of Holistic Nursing*, *20*(4), 325–346.

Hirsch, J. A., & Bishop, B. (1981). Respiratory sinus arrhythmia in humans: How breathing pattern modulates heart rate. *American Journal of Physiology: Heart and Circulatory Physiology*, *241*(4), H620–H629.

Holmes, E. A., Coughtrey, A. E., & Connor, A. (2008). Looking at or through rose-tinted glasses? Imagery perspective and positive mood. *Emotion*, *8*(6), 875–879.

Holmes, E. A., & Mathews, A. (2005). Mental imagery and emotion: A special relationship? *Emotion*, *5*(4), 489–497.

Holmes, E. A., Mathews, A., Dalgleish, T., & Mackintosh, B. (2006). Positive interpretation training: Effects of mental imagery versus verbal training on positive mood. *Behavior Therapy*, *37*(3), 237–247.

Hyman, R. B., Feldman, H. R., Harris, R. B., Levin, R. F., & Molloy, G. B. (1989). The effects of relaxation training on clinical symptoms: A meta-analysis. *Nursing Research*, *38*, 216–220.

Iyengar, B. (1966). *Light on yoga*. New York: Schocken.

Jacobson, E. (1938). *Progressive relaxation* (2nd ed.). Chicago: University of Chicago Press.

Jacobson, E. (1964). *Self-operations control: A manual of tension control*. Chicago: National Foundation for Progressive Relaxation.

Jacobson, E. (1970). *Modern treatment of tense patients*. Springfield, IL: Thomas.

Jacobson, E. (1974). *Progressive relaxation* (3rd ed., rev.). Chicago: University of Chicago Press.

Jallo, N., Bourguignon, C., Taylor, A. G., Ruiz, J., & Goehler, L. (2009). The biobehavioral effects of relaxation guided imagery on maternal stress. *Advances in Mind-Body Medicine*, *24*(4), 12–22.

Johnston, M., & Vögele, C. (1993). Benefits of psychological preparation for surgery: A meta-analysis. *Annals of Behavioral Medicine*, *15*(4), 245–256.

Jones, L., & Stuth, G. (1997). The uses of mental imagery in athletics: An overview. *Applied and Preventive Psychology*, *6*(2), 101–115.

Kapleau R. P. (1965). *The three pillars of Zen*. New York: Doubleday.

Kiecolt-Glaser, J. K., & Newton, T. L. (2001). Marriage and health: His and hers. *Psychological Bulletin*, *127*(4), 472–503.

Kikuchi, Y., Okabe, S., Tamura, G., Hida, W., Homma, M., Shirato, K., & Takishima, T. (1994). Chemosensitivity and perception of dyspnea in patients with a history of near-fatal asthma. *New England Journal of Medicine*, *330*(19), 1329–1334.

King, N. J. (1980). Abbreviated progressive muscle relaxation. In M. Hersen, R. M. Eisler, & P. M. Miller (Eds.), *Progress in behavior modification* (pp. 147–182). New York: Academic Press.

Klapish, N. (1973). Introduction to Desoilleṣ methods of "guided day dream." *The Israel Annals of Psychiatry and Related Disciplines*, *11*(4), 330–343.

Kosslyn, S. M., Ganis, G., & Thompson, W. L. (2001). Neural foundations of imagery. *Nature Reviews Neuroscience*, *2*, 635–642.

Koster, E. H., Fox, E., & MacLeod, C. (2009). Introduction to the special section on cognitive bias modification in emotional disorders. *Journal of Abnormal Psychology*, *118*, 1–4.

Lang, P. J. (1979). A bio-informational theory of emotional imagery. *Psychophysiology*, *16*(6), 495–512.

Lang, P. J., Greenwalk, M. K., Bradley, M. M., & Hamm, A. O. (1993). Looking at pictures: Affective, facial, visceral, and behavioral reactions. *Psychophysiology*, *30*, 261–273.

Lazarus, R. S. (1966). *Psychological stress and the coping process*. New York: McGraw-Hill.

Lazarus, R. S. (1995). Psychological stress in the workplace. In R. Crandall & P. L. Perrewe (Eds.), *Occupational stress: A handbook* (pp. 3–14). Boca Raton, FL: CRC Press.

Lazarus, R. S., & Folkman, S. (1984). *Stress, appraisal, and coping*. New York: Springer.

Lehrer, P. M. (1982). How to relax and how not to relax: A re-evaluation of the work of Edmund Jacobson: 1. *Behaviour Research and Therapy*, *20*, 417–428.

Lehrer, P. M., Carr, R., Sargunaraj, D., & Woolfolk, R. L. (1994). Stress management techniques: Are they all equivalent, or do they have specific effects? *Biofeedback and Self-Regulation*, *19*, 353–401.

Lehrer, P. M. & Woolfolk, R. L. (1984). Are stress reduction techniques interchangeable or do they have specific effects?

A review of the comparative empirical literature. In R. L. Woolfolk & P. M. Lehrer (Eds.), *Principles and practice of stress management* (pp. 404–477). New York: Guiliford Press.

Leskovsek, M., Ahlin, D., Cancer, R., Hosta, M., Enova, D., Pusenjak, N., & Bunc, M. (2011). Low latency breathing frequency detection and monitoring on a personal computer. *Journal of Medical Engineering and Technology, 35*(6–7), 322–329.

Leuner, B., & Gould, E. (2010). Structural plasticity and hippocampal function. *Annual Review of Psychology, 61*, 111–140.

Leuner, H. (1969). Guided affective imagery (GAI): A method of intensive psychotherapy. *American Journal of Psychotherapy, 23*(1), 4–22.

Ley, R. (1994). Breathing and the psychology of emotion, cognition, and behavior. In B. H. Timmons & R. Ley (Eds.), *Behavioral and psychological approaches to breathing disorders* (pp. 81–95). New York: Plenum Press.

Ley, R. (2003). Respiratory psychophysiology and the modification of breathing behavior. *Behavior Modification, 27*(5), 603–606.

Liao, W. (1990). *T'ai chi classics*. Boston, MA: Shambhala.

Ludwick-Rosenthal, R., & Neufeld, W. J. (1988). Stress management during noxious medical procedures: An evaluative review of outcome studies. *Psychological Bulletin, 104*(3), 326–342.

Luthe, W. (Ed.). (1969–1973). *Autogenic therapy* (Vols. 1–6). New York: Grune & Stratton.

Lutz, A., Slagter, H. A., Dunne, J. D., & Davidson, R. J. (2008). Attention regulation and monitoring in meditation. *Trends in Cognitive Science, 12*, 163–169.

Marmot, M., & Brunner. E. (2005). Cohort profile: The Whitehall II study. *International Journal of Epidemiology, 34*, 251–256.

McCaffery, M. (1989). *Nursing management of the patient with pain* (3rd ed.). Philadelphia: J. P. Lippincott.

McCaul, K. D., Solomon, S., & Holmes, D. S. (1979). Effects of paced respiration and expectations on physiological and psychological responses to threat. *Journal of Personality and Social Psychology, 37*(4), 564.

McEwen, B. S., & Gianaros, P. J. (2011). Stress- and allostasis-induced brain plasticity. *Annual Review of Medicine, 62*, 431–645.

McGregor, B. A., & Antoni, M. H. (2009). Psychological intervention and health outcomes among women treated for breast cancer: A review of stress pathways and biological mediators. *Brain, Behavior, and Immunity, 23*, 159–166.

McGuigan, F. J. (1978). *Cognitive psychophysiology: Principles of covert behavior*. Englewood Cliffs, NJ: Prentice Hall.

McGuigan, F. J. Culver, V. L., & Kendler, T. S. (1971). Covert behavior as a direct electromyographic measure of mediating responses. *Conditional Reflex, 6*, 145–152.

McGuigan, F. J., & Leherer, P. M. (2007). Progressive relaxation: Origens, principles, and clinical applications. In P. M. Lehrer & R. L. Woolfolk (Eds.) *Principles and practice of stress management* (3rd ed. pp. 57–87). New York: Guilford Press.

McVicar, A. (2003). Workplace stress in nursing: A literature review. *Journal of Advanced Nursing, 44*(6), 633–642.

Meichenbaum, D. (1977). *Cognitive-behavior modification*. New York: Plenum.

Meurs, J. A., & Perrewé, P. L. (2011). Cognitive activation theory of stress: An integrative theoretical approach to work stress. *Journal of Management, 37*(4), 1043–1068.

Mezo, P. G., Hall, J., Duggan, C. M., & Noël, V. A. (2011). An initial comparison of live instruction and immersive video modes of progressive muscle relaxation. *Journal of Technology in Human Services, 29*(3), 212–223.

Miller, G. A., Levin, D. N., Kozak, M. J., Cook, E. W., III, McLean, A., Jr., & Lang, P. J. (1987). Individual differences in imagery and the psychophysiology of emotion. *Cognition and Emotion, 1*(4), 367–390.

Monsma, E. V., & Overby, L. Y. (2004). The relationship between imagery and competitive anxiety in ballet auditions. *Journal of Dance Medicine and Science, 8*(1), 11–18.

Muhlberger, A., Herrmann, M. J., Wiedemann, G. C., Ellgring, H., & Pauli, P. (2001). Repeated exposure of flight phobics to flights in virtual reality. *Behaviour Research Therapy, 39*(9), 1033–1050.

Nezu, A, M., Nezu, C. M., & Xanthopoulos, M. S. (2011). Stress reduction in chronically ill patients. In R. J. Contrada & A. Baum (Eds.), *The handbook of stress science: Biology, psychology, and health* (pp. 475–486). New York: Springer.

Nilsson, U. (2008). The anxiety- and pain-reducing effects of music interventions: A systematic review. *AORN Journal, 87*(4), 780, 782, 785–794, 797–807.

Norris, F. H., Friedman, M. J., & Watson, P. J. (2002). 60,000 disaster victims speak: Part II. Summary and implications of the Disaster Mental Health Research. *Psychiatry: Interpersonal and Biological Processes, 65*(3), 240–260.

Noseda, A., Schmerber, J., Prigogine, T., & Yernault, J. C. (1993). How do patients with either asthma or COPD perceive acute bronchodilation?. *European Respiratory Journal, 6*(5), 636–644.

Öhman, A., & Mineka, S. (2001). Fears, phobias, and preparedness: Toward an evolved module of fear and fear learning. *Psychological Review, 108*(3), 483–522.

Pandey, A., Quick, J. C., Rossi, A. M., Nelson, D. L., & Martin, W. (2011). Stress and the workplace: 10 years of stress science, 1997–2007. In R. J. Contrada & A. Baum (Eds.), *The handbook of stress science: Biology, psychology, and health* (pp. 137–150). New York: Springer.

Patel, C. (1991). *The complete guide to stress management*. New York: Plenum Press.

Paul, G. L. (1966). *Insight versus desensitization in psychotherapy*. Palo Alto, CA: Stanford University Press.

Pawlow, L. A., & Jones, G. A. (2002). The impact of abbreviated progressive muscle relaxation on salivary cortisol. *Biological Psychiatry, 60*(1), 1–16.

Pawlow, L. A., & Jones, G. A. (2005). The impact of abbreviated progressive muscle relaxation on salivary cortisol and salivary immunoglobulin A (sIgA). *Applied Psychophysiology and Biofeedback, 30*(4), 375–387.

Pelletier, C. L. (2004). The effect of music on decreasing arousal due to stress: A meta-analysis. *Journal of Music Therapy, 41*(3), 192–214.

Pelletier, K. R., & Lutz, R. (1990). Healthy people—healthy business: A critical review of stress management programs in the workplace. In J. E. Fielding, A. S. Baum, & S. M. Weiss (Eds.), *Health at work* (pp. 189–204). New York: Psychology Press.

Pictet, A., Coughtrey, A. E., Mathews, A., & Holmes, E. A. (2011). Fishing for happiness: The effects of generating positive imagery on mood and behaviour. *Behaviour Research and Therapy, 49*(12), 885–891.

Porges, S. W. (2009). Stress and parasympathetic control. In G. Fink (Ed.), *Stress science: neuroendocrinology* (pp. 306–312). San Diego, CA: Academic Press.

Powell, R., Bruce, J., Johnston, M., Vogele, C., Scott, N., Shehmar, M., & Roberts, T. (2010). Psychological preparation and postoperative outcomes for adults undergoing surgery under general anaesthesia (Protocol). *Cochrane Database of Systematic Reviews, 8*. doi: 10.1002/14651858.CD008646.

Przeworski, A., & Newman, M. G. (2004). Palmtop computer-assisted group therapy for social phobia. *Journal of Clinical Psychology, 60*(2), 179–188.

Rausch, S. M., Gramling, S. E., & Auerbach, S. M. (2006). Effects of a single session of large-group meditation and progressive muscle relaxation training on stress reduction, reactivity, and recovery. *International Journal of Stress Management, 13*(3), 273–290.

Richardson, K. M., & Rothstein, H. R. (2008). Effects of occupational stress management intervention programs: A meta-analysis. *Journal of Occupational Health Psychology, 13*(1), 69–93.

Ronen, T. (2011). *The positive power of imagery: Harnessing client imagination in CBT and related therapies.* Malden, MA: Wiley-Blackwell.

Roozendaal, B., McEwen, B. S., & Chattarji, S. (2009). Stress, memory and the amygdala. *Nature Reviews Neuroscience, 10*(6), 423–433.

Rowland, B. (1953). *The art and architecture of India.* Pelican history of art. Melbourne: Penguin Books.

Sapolsky, R. (1996). Why stress is bad for your brain. *Science, 273*, 749–750.

Schiffman, S., Stone, A. A., & Hufford, M. R. (2008). Ecological momentary assessment. *Annual Review of Clinical Psychology, 4*, 1–32.

Schoettle, U. C. (1980). Guided imagery—a tool in child psychotherapy. *American Journal of Psychotherapy, 34*(2), 220–227.

Schwartz, G. E., Davidson, R. J., & Goleman, D. T. (1978). Patterning of cognitive and somatic processes in the self-regulation of anxiety: Effects of meditation versus exercise. *Psychosomatic Medicine, 40*, 321–328.

Segerstrom, S. C., & Miller, G. E. (2004). Psychological stress and the human immune system: A meta-analytic study of 30 years of inquiry. *Psychological Bulletin, 130*(4), 610–630.

Selye, H. (1956). *The stress of life.* New York: McGraw-Hill.

Skinner, E. A., Edge, K., Altman, J., & Sherwood, H. (2003). Searching for the structure of coping: A review and critique of category systems for classifying various ways of coping. *Psychological Bulletin, 129*, 216–269.

Slagter, H. A., Davidson, R. J., & Lutz, A. (2011). Mental training as a tool in the neuroscientific study of brain and cognitive plasticity. *Frontiers in Human Neuroscience, 5*(17), 1–12.

Smith, C. A., & Lazarus, R. S. (1993). Appraisal components, core relational themes, and the emotions. *Cognition and Emotion, 7*, 233–269.

Smith, J. C. (1990). *Cognitive behavioral relaxation training: A new system of strategies for treatment and assessment.* New York: Springer.

Smith, J. C., Amutio, A., Anderson, J. P., & Aria, L. A. (1996). Relaxation: Mapping an uncharted world. *Biofeedback and Self-Regulation, 21*(1), 63–90.

Stephens, R. (1993a). Imagery: A strategic intervention to empower clients—Part I–Review of research literature. *Clinical Nurse Specialist, 7*(4), 170–174.

Stephens, R. L. (1993b). Imagery: A strategic intervention to empower clients—Part II–A practical guide. *Clinical Nurse Specialist, 7*(5), 235–240.

Sturges, L. V., Goetsch, V. L., Ridley, J., & Whittal, M. (1998). Anxiety sensitivity and response to hyperventilation challenge: Physiologic arousal, interoceptive acuity, and subjective distress. *Journal of Anxiety Disorders, 12*(2), 103–115.

Suhr, J., Anderson, S., & Tranel, D. (1999). Progressive muscle relaxation in the management of behavioral disturbances in Alzheimer's disease. *Neuropsychological Rehabilitation, 9*(1), 31–44.

Tatrow, K., & Montgomery, G. H. (2006). Cognitive behavioral therapy techniques for distress and pain in breast cancer patients: A meta-analysis. *Journal of Behavioural Medicine, 29*, 17–27.

Taylor, A. G., Goehler, L. E., Galper, D. I., Innes, K. E., & Bourguignon, C. (2010). Top-down and bottom-up mechanisms in mind-body medicine: Development of an integrative framework for psychophysiological research. *Explore (NY), 6*(1), 29–41.

Thyer, B. A., Papsdorf, J. D., & Wright, P. (1984). Physiological and psychological effects of acute intentional hyperventilation. *Behavioral Research and Therapy, 22*(5), 587–590.

Tusek, D. L., & Cwynar, R. E. (2000). Strategies for implementing a guided imagery program to enhance patient experience. *AACN Clinical Issues, 11*(1), 68–76.

Umezawa, A. (2001). Facilitation and inhibition of breathing during changes in emotion. In Y. Haruki, I. Homma, A. Umezawa, & Y. Masaoka (Eds.), *Respiration and emotion* (pp. 139–148). Tokyo: Springer Verlag.

Vadoa, E. A., Hall, C. R., & Moritz, S. E. (1997). The relationship between competitive anxiety and imagery use. *Journal of Applied Sport Psychology, 9*(2), 241–253.

Vancampfort, D., De Hert, M., Knapen, J., Maurissen, K., Raepsaet, J., Deckx, S., … Probst, M. (2011). Effects of progressive muscle relaxation on state anxiety and subjective well-being in people with schizophrenia: A randomized controlled trial. *Clinical Rehabilitation, 25*(6), 567–575.

van der Hek, H., & Plomp, H. N. (1997). Occupational stress management programmes: A practical overview of published effect studies. *Occupational Medicine, 47*(3), 133–141.

van Dixhoorn, J., & Duivenvoorden, H. J. (1999). Effect of relaxation therapy on cardiac events after myocardial infarction: A 5-year follow-up study. *Journal of Cardiopulmonary Rehabilitation, 19*(3), 178–185.

van Dixhoorn, J., Duivenvoorden, H. J., Staal, A., & Pool, J. (1989). Physical training and relaxation therapy in cardiac rehabilitation therapy assessed through a composite criterion for training outcome. *American Heart Journal, 118*(3), 545–552.

van Dixhoorn, J, & White, A. R. (2005). Relaxation therapy for rehabilitation and prevention in ischemic heart disease: A systematic review and meta-analysis. *European Journal of Cardiovascular Prevention and Rehabilitation, 12*, 193–202.

van Dixhoorn, J. J. (2007). Whole-body breathing. In P. M. Leher, R. L. Woolfolk, & W. E. Sime (Eds.), *Principles and practice of stress management* (3rd ed., pp. 291–332). New York: Guiliford Press.

Vianna, E. P. M., Naqvi, N., Bechara, A., & Tranel, D. (2009). Does vivid emotional imagery depend on body signals? *International Journal of Psychophysiology, 72*(1), 46–50.

Wang, W., He, G., Wang, M., Liu, L., & Tang, H. (2012). Effects of patient education and progressive muscle relaxation alone or combined on adherence to continuous positive airway pressure treatment in obstructive sleep apnea patients. *Sleep Breath, 16*(4), 1049–1057.

Weinberg, A., & Cooper, C. (2011). The challenge of stress in modern organizations. In R. J. Contrada & A. Baum (Eds.), *The handbook of stress science: Biology, psychology, and health* (pp. 151–166). New York: Springer.

Wilhelm, F. H., Gevirtz, R., & Roth, W. T. (2001). Respiratory dysregulation in anxiety, functional cardiac, and pain disorders: Assessment, phenomenology, and treatment. *Behavior Modification, 25*(4), 513–545.

Wolpe, J. (1958). *Psychotherapy by reciprocal inhibition.* Palo Alto, CA: Stanford University Press.

Wolpe, J. (1969). *The practice of behavior therapy.* New York: Pergamon Press.

Zapf, D., Dormann, C., & Frese, M. (1996). Longitudinal studies in organizational stress research: A review of the literature with reference to methodological issues. *Journal of Occupational Health Psychology, 1*(2), 145–169.

PART 3

Major Psychological Problems and Populations

Adult Anxiety and Related Disorders

Jacqueline R. Bullis *and* Stefan G. Hofmann

Abstract

Anxiety and related disorders are some of the most common mental disorders. In the absence of treatment, these disorders follow a chronic, persistent course that results in significant distress and functional impairment across various domains of the individual's life. We will present here the contemporary cognitive-behavioral approaches for treating adults with generalized anxiety disorder, obsessive-compulsive disorder, social anxiety disorder, panic disorder, specific phobia, and posttraumatic stress disorder. Following a brief definition of the diagnostic features and possible etiological factors, we discuss for each disorder the specific cognitive-behavioral treatment strategies, their empirical support, and a comparison to other existing psychological or pharmacological treatment approaches. We conclude with a summary of the current status and recommendations for future research.

Key Words: cognitive-behavioral therapy, generalized anxiety disorder, obsessive-compulsive disorder, social anxiety disorder, panic disorder, specific phobias, posttraumatic stress disorder

Introduction

Epidemiological studies suggest that approximately 40 million American adults currently suffer from an anxiety disorder, with a 12-month prevalence rate of 18.1% and a lifetime prevalence rate of 28.8% (Kessler, Berglund, et al., 2005; Kessler, Chiu, Demler, Merikangas, & Walters, 2005). Anxiety disorders are the most commonly diagnosed mental disorder, and frequently occur in the presence of other disorders, including substance use and mood disorders (Grant et al., 2004). They are associated with significant distress and functional impairment in social, occupational, and health-related domains, and result in considerable economic and societal costs each year (Barrera & Norton, 2009; Lepine, 2002).

This chapter will discuss the defining features and conceptualization of the six primary anxiety disorders from a cognitive-behavioral perspective. Treatment implications and empirical support for cognitive-behavioral therapy (CBT) in the treatment of anxiety disorders will also be discussed. A more detailed description of the techniques presented in this chapter can be found in Hofmann (2011).

The American Psychiatric Association recently published the first major revision of the *Diagnostic and Statistical Manual of Mental Disorders* (*DSM*) in 20 years (DSM-5; American Psychiatric Association, 2013). DSM-5 is the product of over a decade of work and reflects many big changes from the previous version of the *DSM* (DSM-IV-TR; American Psychiatric Association, 2000), not least of which include the discontinuation of roman numerals to denote the edition number. The release of DSM-5 has been met with mixed reviews at best, with many critics arguing that there was insufficient evidence for some of the decisions made. The vast majority of changes made in DSM-5 are specific to how diagnoses are assigned and therefore do not necessarily reflect changes to how the disorders are conceptualized in terms of etiological factors or treatment approaches from a CBT perspective. Accordingly, we choose to keep anxiety and related disorders grouped within one chapter while noting any relevant DSM-5 revisions throughout the text.

Generalized Anxiety Disorder
Defining Features

The defining characteristic of generalized anxiety disorder (GAD) is persistent and excessive worry that is difficult to control (American Psychiatric Association, 2000). Worrying involves specific cognitive processes and is not the same as merely anticipating a future event (Hofmann et al., 2005). Worrying is conceptualized as a cognitive avoidance strategy that inhibits the emotional processing of distressing material and thus preserves cognitive-affective fear structures (T. D. Borkovec, Ray, & Stöber, 1998). Individuals with GAD worry about a number of things, including finances, health, family, performance at work or school, foreign affairs, and minor events, such as grocery shopping or scheduling an appointment. These worries are typically exaggerated, excessive, and maladaptive. They are characteristically associated with physiological symptoms, such as muscle tension, irritability, restlessness, feeling keyed up or on edge, being easily fatigued, difficulty concentrating, restless sleep, and difficulty falling or staying asleep. Furthermore, these symptoms are often associated with significant subjective and economic cost. For example, it is estimated that over one-third of individuals with GAD report a minimum of six disability days during the past month (Wittchen, Carter, Pfister, Montgomery, & Kessler, 2000).

Approximately 5.7% of adult Americans suffer from GAD, including nearly twice as many women as men (Kessler, Berglund, et al., 2005; Kessler, Chiu, et al., 2005; Robichaud, Dugas, & Conway, 2003; Wittchen & Hoyer, 2001). GAD tends to develop gradually and has an average age of onset of 31 years, with the majority of individuals developing the disorder between their early 20s and late 40s (Kessler, Berglund, et al., 2005). Earlier age of onset tends to be associated with greater symptom severity, comorbidity, and temperamental vulnerability for developing other emotional disorders (Campbell, Brown, & Grisham, 2003).

CBT Conceptualization
PROBLEM-SOLVING ABILITY AND PROBABILITY OVERESTIMATION

Individuals with GAD report less confidence in their ability to solve problems and a more negative orientation toward their ability to anticipate and respond to real-life problems (Davey, 1994). Individuals with GAD also tend to engage in cognitive errors related to overestimating the probability that a feared event will occur, as well as overestimating the cost of worrying over a future event (Provencher, Freeston, Dugas, & Ladouceur, 2000).

INFORMATION-PROCESSING AND COGNITIVE BIASES

Research using information-processing models suggests that cognitive biases play an important role in the development and maintenance of GAD (Bar-Haim, Lamy, Pergamin, Bakermans-Kranenburg, & van IJzendoorn, 2007). For example, in studies using the emotional Stroop paradigm, individuals with GAD take a longer amount of time to name the color of threatening words than neutral words (Mogg & Bradley, 2005). In addition, individuals with GAD are more likely to interpret ambiguous stimuli as negative or threatening. When asked to listen and then write down homophones with either threatening or neutral spellings (e.g., "sleigh" or "slay"), individuals with GAD wrote down threatening spellings more often than nonanxious controls (Mathews, Richards, & Eysenck, 1989).

METACOGNITION

Theories of metacognition propose that GAD is maintained by both positive and negative beliefs about worry. The metacognitive model of GAD distinguishes two different types of worry: worry about minor matters and events as specified in the DSM-IV, and worry about the worry process itself (Wells, 1999). Positive beliefs about worrying (e.g., beliefs that worrying is adaptive or an effective coping strategy) lead individuals to engage in the first type of worrying, which then activates the second type of worrying about the worry process itself. Contemporary CBT strategies for the treatment of GAD address both types of worry processes.

COGNITIVE AVOIDANCE

Worrying has been described as a cognitive process that largely involves verbal activity and, to a smaller degree, imagery (T. D. Borkovec et al., 1998). Verbalization and imagery each result in different responses, with verbalization of an emotional or feared situation resulting in less cardiovascular arousal than visualization of the situation. For example, in a classic study by Borkovec and Hu (1990), students who were instructed to worry before visualizing giving a speech reported greater subjective anxiety than students who were instructed to relax prior to the visualization task, but demonstrated less physiological arousal. However, in the long term, worrying increases distress and arousal, which is consistent with research suggesting that thought suppression results in greater physiological arousal (Hofmann, Heering, Sawyer, & Asnaani, 2009).

INTOLERANCE OF UNCERTAINTY

It has been suggested that worrying is influenced by an established set of beliefs concerning uncertainty of the world and a dispositional tendency to view ambiguous or uncertain situations as dangerous (Ladouceur, Gosselin, & Dugas, 2000). This intolerance of uncertainty may be viewed as a cognitive vulnerability factor that causes individuals to react to ambiguous situations with extreme worry and anxiety.

Treatment Implications

A number of specific treatment strategies have been developed to target the process and function of worrying and its consequences. These strategies include psychoeducation, cognitive restructuring techniques specifically targeting worrying, meditation and relaxation, as well as exposure and acceptance strategies.

PSYCHOEDUCATION

People with GAD believe that worrying is part of their personality and frequently view their excessive worrying as a positive way of showing concern for loved ones. Some individuals with GAD may view worrying as an adaptive strategy for avoiding negative situations in the future. Therefore, an effective early-treatment strategy is to discuss the function of worrying and address these maladaptive beliefs about worrying by discussing the advantages and emphasizing the disadvantages of worrying.

COGNITIVE RESTRUCTURING

The goal of cognitive restructuring is to initially identify and then to modify the overarching maladaptive beliefs and specific thoughts associated with worrying. For example, the therapist might instruct the patient to record the intensity and context of worry episodes, and to critically examine the function of worrying. The specific beliefs and thoughts are then translated into concrete and testable hypotheses in order to evaluate the validity of them. For example, if the patient believes that

worrying helps prevent bad events from happening, the therapist might explore methods to test the validity of this assumption with the patient.

MEDIATION AND RELAXATION

Worrying is a maladaptive and future-oriented cognitive process. This process can be targeted by enhancing nonjudgmental and present-moment awareness. Meditation, mindfulness practices, and relaxation training can be useful techniques to target worrying about future events by encouraging this nonjudgmental and present-moment awareness. Meditation that employs imagery-focused techniques or enhanced focus on breathing can further help teach patients to mentally distance themselves from unpleasant thoughts and lessen the feelings of autonomic hyperarousal (Roemer, Orsillo, & Salters-Pedneault, 2008).

EXPOSURE AND ACCEPTANCE

As discussed earlier, worrying is conceptualized as a cognitive avoidance strategy that inhibits the emotional processing of distressing material and thus preserves cognitive-affective fear structures (T. D. Borkovec et al., 1998). Therefore, CBT strategies often include exposure procedures that target the worry process. As part of these so-called worry-exposure exercises, the patient may be asked to imagine a worst-case scenario or outcome of an event that is typically associated with the worrying. For example, a patient may report that she worried excessively about not being able to pay her mortgage. In this case, the therapist might ask the patient to imagine the worst-case scenario in which she sees herself as a homeless person alone, without any friends or family members to support her. Instead of suppressing or otherwise avoiding the negative feelings, patients are instructed to accept their feelings of anxiety and focus on the present moment while repeatedly being exposed to this worst-case image.

Empirical Support

CBT is an effective treatment for GAD, producing moderate to large effect sizes that are superior to waitlist controls and nonspecific alternative therapies and similar to pharmacological therapy (T. D. Borkovec & Ruscio, 2001; Mitte, 2005). Whereas gains made during pharmacological therapy often remit when the medication is discontinued, CBT for GAD has been shown to be effective at reducing anxiety in both the short term and the long term (Hofmann & Smits, 2008). At the same time, a substantial proportion of patients still do not respond to CBT and fail to improve even after completing additional treatment sessions (Durham et al., 2004). Future research will need to focus on examining novel and more effective treatment strategies. Acceptance-based and mindfulness meditation strategies might offer such effective interventions, and recent studies have supported the efficacy of these interventions in reducing GAD symptoms when compared to waitlist control conditions (Roemer et al., 2008).

Obsessive-Compulsive Disorder
Defining Features

Obsessive-Compulsive Disorder (OCD) is characterized by the presence of either obsessions or compulsions that are experienced as persistent and relentless (American Psychiatric Association, 2000). Obsessions and compulsions are distressing and time-consuming (e.g., occupy more than an hour a day), and cause significant impairment in occupational or academic performance, day-to-day activities, relationships, and overall quality of life (Markarian et al., 2010). Obsessions are recurrent thoughts, images, or impulses that often feel involuntary, intrusive, and inappropriate. These thoughts or images cause feelings of intense anxiety and distress, and are not related to excessive worry or everyday concerns. People with OCD typically attempt to suppress these thoughts or to counteract them with other thoughts or actions. Obsessions in OCD are very heterogeneous and may involve aggressive thoughts or impulses to self-harm or hurt others, intrusive sexual or religious thoughts, contamination fears, excessive concerns with order and symmetry, or relentless feelings of doubt (McKay et al., 2004; Rasmussen & Eisen, 1992).

Compulsions are repetitive behaviors (e.g., cleaning or decontaminating, repetitive checking, ordering and arranging) or mental rituals (e.g., praying, counting, repeating words or phrases) that are often performed according to strict rules and in response to an obsession. These behaviors and mental rituals are often performed to reduce feelings of anxiety or to prevent a feared outcome (American Psychiatric Association, 2000; Rachman, 2002). For example, someone with OCD may feel driven to arrange food items in the refrigerator in a certain way in order to prevent a loved one's death.

Most individuals with OCD recognize that their obsessions and compulsions are irrational and excessive. However, there is a small subset of people with poor insight who view their persistent thoughts and compulsive acts as logical and reasonable (Ravi Kishore, Samar, Janardhan Reddy, Chandrasekhar, & Thennarasu, 2004). Poor insight is most common among individuals with OCD who endorse obsessive thoughts and impulses related to religion or aggression toward others (Tolin, Abramowitz, Kozak, & Foa, 2001).

OCD is a relatively common psychological disorder, with epidemiological studies reporting lifetime prevalence rates between 1.6% and 2.9% (Kessler, Berglund, et al., 2005; Kolada, Bland, & Newman, 1994). The prevalence rate is slightly higher among women than men, and the average age of onset is earlier for men (21 years of age) than for women (22–24 years of age) (Rasmussen & Eisen, 1992). In the absence of treatment, OCD is a chronic illness that fluctuates in severity throughout the lifespan and rarely remits in entirety.

In DSM-5, OCD was removed from the Anxiety Disorders chapter and moved to a new chapter entitled, "Obsessive-Compulsive and Related Disorders," which follows immediately after Anxiety Disorders to reflect the close relationship between anxiety and obsessive-compulsive spectrum disorders. This new chapter contains the following disorders: OCD, Body Dysmorphic Disorder, Hoarding Disorder (note that hoarding behavior was historically seen as a type of OCD that did not warrant a separate diagnosis), Trichotillomania (i.e., Hair-Pulling Disorder), and Excoriation (Skin-Picking) Disorder. Hoarding disorder was included as a new diagnosis based on data supporting the diagnostic validity and clinical utility of a unique diagnosis (for a review, see Mataix et al., 2010). DSM-5 views obsessive-compulsive and related disorders as defined most principally by repetitive thoughts and behavior (as discussed in greater detail below), which then result in anxious distress.

CBT Conceptualization
DYSFUNCTIONAL BELIEFS

It is normal to experience intrusive or inappropriate thoughts and images that are similar to those reported by individuals with OCD. In fact, over 90% of people in community and analogue samples report the presence of unwanted thoughts, images, or impulses, including urges to harm or attack someone and thoughts of sexually inappropriate acts (Salkovskis & Harrison, 1984). However, people with OCD are not able to dismiss these intrusive thoughts as harmless and instead interpret them as significant and potentially harmful. Studies have shown that individuals with

OCD report an exaggerated sense of responsibility to prevent harm from occurring, and are more apt to overestimate the likelihood of negative or dangerous situations (Frost & Steketee, 2002). Most people view a situation as safe unless there is a sign of danger. In contrast, individuals with OCD generally view a situation as dangerous until they are able confirm its safety (Rachman, 2002). For people with OCD, overestimations of threat are frequently associated with a tendency to place a disproportionate emphasis on widely publicized catastrophes that are highly unlikely to personally affect them (Moritz & Pohl, 2009).

THOUGHT-ACTION FUSION

It is often difficult for individuals with OCD to separate intrusive thoughts about inappropriate content from the consequences of performing an inappropriate action (Shafran, Thordarson, & Rachman, 1996). This phenomenon has been referred to as thought-action fusion (TAF), and is a core characteristic of OCD (Berle & Starcevic, 2005). Thought-action fusion involves two distinct dysfunctional beliefs related to obsessive thoughts and images, including a belief that merely having an inappropriate or unpleasant thought increases the probability that a certain event will occur (Shafran, et al., 1996). In addition, TAF is typically associated with the belief that having an inappropriate or unpleasant thought is equivalent to performing the inappropriate action. More specifically, patients with TAF believe that merely experiencing inappropriate thoughts or images is representative of one's moral character and reflects one's true nature. For example, a person with OCD who experiences an intrusive thought about hitting a pedestrian while driving may believe that it is now more likely that he or she will actually hit a pedestrian, and thinking about hitting a pedestrian is indicative of his or her evil nature. Studies have shown that TAF is associated with religiosity, as well superstitious and magical thinking (Rachman, 1993; Rassin & Koster, 2003).

PERFECTIONISM AND INTOLERANCE OF UNCERTAINTY

In contrast to healthy individuals, individuals with OCD often believe that perfection is an achievable and desirable goal (Wu & Cortesi, 2009). Furthermore, people with OCD may believe that failure to complete an action or task perfectly will result in catastrophic consequences (Frost &

Steketee, 1997). Perfectionism may be measured by an objective, external standard (e.g., writing a letter without any mistakes) or more subjective, internal standards (e.g., opening and closing a door until it feels complete or "right") (Coles, Frost, Heimberg, & Rheaume, 2003). Individuals with OCD who place a heavy emphasis on perfectionism also tend to have a low tolerance for uncertainty (Frost & Steketee, 1997). Even when there is very low probability that a negative event will occur, such as causing a fire by leaving a light on, people with OCD exaggerate this likelihood and experience a great deal of anxiety that frequently manifests itself in compulsive and repetitive checking behaviors (Tolin, Abramowitz, Brigidi, & Foa, 2003).

Treatment Implications

The goals of contemporary CBT approaches for treating OCD are to target dysfunctional beliefs, misappraisal of intrusive thoughts, and overestimation of threat. The specific strategies toward these goals include psychoeducation, cognitive restructuring, attention and situation modification, and exposure and acceptance procedures.

PSYCHOEDUCATION

As discussed earlier, individuals with OCD often show dysfunctional beliefs associated with an inflated sense of personal responsibility for the well-being of others and have maladaptive thought processes that merge thoughts about undesirable behaviors and actual behaviors and their consequences (e.g., thought-action fusion). Accordingly, educating the patient about how these dysfunctional beliefs are maladaptive and contribute to the maintenance of OCD is a critical treatment component.

COGNITIVE RESTRUCTURING

Obsessive thoughts and impulses can be triggered by many stimuli. The goal of cognitive restructuring is to identify and modify cognitions related to the overestimation of threat, as well as catastrophic thinking. It is often helpful for therapists to choose a specific feared outcome and then discuss the sequence of events that would need to occur first in order for the negative outcome to happen. In addition, therapists may ask a patient to rate the probability of each event in the sequence happening, and then calculate and compare the actual probability of a feared outcome occurring to the patient's subjective, overestimated probability.

ATTENTION AND SITUATION MODIFICATION

People with OCD frequently seek out information that is consistent with their obsessive beliefs, which then reinforces their feelings of anxiety and the need to counteract the anxiety by performing compulsive, repetitive acts. Therefore, it is useful for patients to practice directing their attention away from cues or events that trigger their obsessions or provide support for their obsessions. For example, a patient's obsessive thought about contamination might be triggered by public restrooms, and she might spend a great deal of time watching the news for stories about health scares and infectious outbreaks. The therapist can help the patient to resist her urge to engage in checking behaviors and enhance her distress tolerance by accepting her temporary feeling of distress and by replacing her maladaptive behaviors with adaptive responses, such as meditation or physical exercise.

EXPOSURE AND ACCEPTANCE

People with OCD feel driven to perform repetitive behaviors or mental rituals to prevent the occurrence of a specific feared outcome. These compulsive behaviors contribute to the maintenance of the disorder by preventing individuals with OCD from testing whether the feared outcome would actually occur in the absence of the preventative acts. Accordingly, behavioral exposures are an important component of treatment because they allow patients to test specific predictions or hypotheses about engaging in a feared activity without also engaging in safety behaviors or relying on safety signals. In collaboration with the patient, the therapist can construct a fear hierarchy consisting of the patient's least to most feared situations to guide the targets of the exposure exercises. During behavioral exposures, patients often experience progressively more intense feelings of distress and anxiety as they move through more challenging steps of the fear hierarchy. Patients eventually learn to fully experience and accept their feelings of distress and anxiety, which reduces the urge to engage in avoidance behaviors and compulsive acts.

Empirical Support

Studies suggest that CBT is an effective treatment approach and produces a large treatment effect when compared to placebo conditions (Hofmann & Smits, 2008). CBT for the treatment of OCD has demonstrated efficacy in both research studies and outpatient settings, with as many as 80% of patients achieving clinically meaningful reductions in OCD symptoms (Franklin, Abramowitz, Kozak, Levitt, & Foa, 2000). CBT for OCD most often involves a combination of cognitive strategies to target dysfunctional beliefs and behavioral exposure and response prevention (ERP) to target avoidance and compulsive behaviors. A recent study comparing the efficacy of CBT to ERP alone did not find a significant difference in the percentage of patients that achieved a recovered status at posttreatment or at follow-up (Whittal, Thordarson, & McLean, 2005). However, the inclusion of cognitive therapy with ERP protected against attrition during treatment (Vogel, Stiles, & Gotestam, 2004).

Social Anxiety Disorder
Defining Features

Social anxiety disorder (SAD; also referred to as social phobia) is a chronic disorder characterized by excessive anxiety and fear of one or more social or performance situations (American Psychiatric Association, 2000). People with SAD typically avoid these situations due to a fear of negative, and occasionally even positive, evaluation (Weeks, Heimberg, Rodebaugh, & Norton, 2008). If these situations cannot be avoided, patients with SAD endure a great deal of anxiety and distress. Individuals with SAD experience fear and distress that is out of proportion to the actual threat posed by the social situation or the sociocultural context. Typical social situations that are feared or avoided by individuals with SAD include initiating and carrying on conversations, interacting with authority figures, and dating, as well as performance situations that involve speaking, writing, or eating in front of others. In *DSM-IV*, SAD was classified with two subtypes: 1) generalized to reflect individuals who fear most or all social situations, and 2) non-generalized to indicate that the fear is limited to one particular social situation. However, DSM-5 replaced these subtypes with a specifier of "performance only" for when the fear or anxiety is limited to only public speaking or performing. Members of the DSM-5 taskforce felt there to be insufficient evidence supporting the generalized subtype of SAD, namely since individuals with SAD demonstrate a range of social fears (for a review, see Heimberg et al., 2014).

Epidemiological studies report a lifetime prevalence rate of 12.1% and a 12-month prevalence of 6.8%, making SAD the second most commonly diagnosed anxiety disorder following specific phobia (Kessler, Berglund, et al., 2005; Kessler, Chiu, et al., 2005). The average age of onset for SAD is during the teenage years. Individuals with SAD frequently report experiencing extreme shyness, anxiety regarding negative evaluations, school refusal, or separation anxiety as children. In contrast to other anxiety disorders, the prevalence rates for SAD in men and women are roughly the same. In the absence of treatment, SAD follows a chronic, unremitting course, and is associated with substantial disability and functional impairment across interpersonal and occupational domains, often resulting in increased absences from work or school and decreased productivity levels (Katzelnick et al., 2001; Stein & Kean, 2000; Stein, McQuaid, Laffaye, & McCahill, 1999). SAD is additionally associated with high rates of psychiatric comorbidity, with estimates ranging from 56.9% in community samples (Magee, Eaton, Wittchen, McGonagle, & Kessler, 1996) to 83% in clinical samples (Goisman, Goldenberg, Vasile, & Keller, 1995).

CBT Conceptualization

AVOIDANCE

Individuals with SAD engage in a variety of avoidance behaviors, such as avoiding eye contact, or avoiding entering evaluative social and performance situations. Some of these avoidance behaviors are overt and obvious (e.g., canceling a date or job interview or leaving a party); others are subtle (e.g., avoiding eye contact or being overly apologetic) and not immediately evident (e.g., only being able to attend a party if alcohol is served or being aggressive and impolite in interpersonal interactions). Although these avoidance behaviors temporarily reduce anxiety or prevent anxiety from developing, these behaviors are critically important for the maintenance of the problem because they reinforce and maintain social anxiety in the long term by preventing individuals with SAD from testing the outcome and consequences of engaging in the feared situation (Clark & Wells, 1995; Hofmann, 2008; Rapee & Heimberg, 1997).

INFORMATION-PROCESSING AND COGNITIVE BIASES

Individuals with SAD tend to be self-critical and to judge themselves more harshly than they judge other people, as well as more negatively than others judge them (Wallace & Alden, 1991). Research on cognitive and information-processing biases in people with SAD suggests that they preferentially attend to threat-relevant information and environmental cues that indicate negative evaluation

(Heinrichs & Hofmann, 2001). Studies support the vigilance-avoidance model of selective attention (Bögels & Mansell, 2004), suggesting that individuals with SAD are initially hypervigilant to the detection of threatening stimuli and then engage in avoidance to reduce subsequent feelings of anxiety. As a consequence, people with SAD frequently fail to adequately process social stimuli. Furthermore, they are unable to adequately evaluate the outcomes of social situations, preserving the maladaptive beliefs associated with them (Clark & Wells, 1995; Hofmann & Otto, 2008). Finally, post-event processing can cause experiences that were initially positive or pleasant to become viewed as negative and unpleasant (Hofmann, 2007a; Hofmann & Otto, 2008).

Treatment Implications

Effective treatment of SAD involves multiple treatment approaches to target all the components of the cognitive model presented earlier, including poor self-image, overestimation of the likelihood of a feared outcome, and the perceived social cost of a negative outcome.

PSYCHOEDUCATION

Individuals with SAD often believe that social anxiety or intense shyness is part of their personality and cannot be changed through treatment. Psychoeducation prepares patients to actively engage in the treatment process by addressing the misconceptions about SAD and explaining the rationale behind exposure exercises. It is often helpful to discuss the goals of CBT for SAD with the patient in the context of learning objectives over the course of the treatment process.

ATTENTION AND SITUATION MODIFICATION

People with SAD tend to respond to social threats or social situations with hypervigilance to their own behavior and feelings of anxiety, thereby directing attentional resources away from successful performance in social situations. Attention and situation modification teaches individuals with SAD to focus on the present situation instead of the debilitating feelings of anxiety or negative self-image. For example, patients may be instructed to direct their attention to various stimuli when they are in an anxious state, such as their own feelings of anxiety, threat-relevant characteristics of the situation, neutral aspects of the environment, and the task at hand. The goal is for patients to observe how their level of anxiety changes in response to modifying the focus of their attention, and to learn how to stay present in a social situation.

COGNITIVE RESTRUCTURING

People with SAD tend to overestimate the likelihood of a negative outcome in a social situation, as well as the costs of such a negative outcome. Cognitive restructuring involves identifying and then challenging maladaptive thoughts about the probability and cost of negative evaluation, negative attribution bias, and poor self-concept. Challenging and eventually replacing these maladaptive thoughts with more realistic, objective thoughts is an important part of correcting the negative feedback cycle that contributes to the chronic nature of SAD.

EXPOSURE

The most important component for the treatment of SAD is exposing patients to the feared social or performance situation. During an exposure, patients are prevented from engaging in avoidance behaviors, and thus, they must rely on acceptance to cope with their feelings of anxiety. Exposures also provide opportunities for patients to learn how attention and situation modification impacts their level of anxiety by comparing their anxiety ratings (e.g., on a 0–10 scale) before and after the exposure. Exposures using video or audio feedback can help test patients' poor self-concept and false beliefs concerning their presentation in social situations by comparing their predicted presentation to the actual feedback. In vivo exposures, or exposures that involve patients directly confronting the feared situation, allow patients to test assumptions about the likelihood and cost of a negative outcome in a certain social situation. Most often, patients learn that their feared outcome is highly unlikely and will not result in catastrophic consequences.

Empirical Support

The conventional treatment of SAD is conducted in a group setting of five to six patients, and administered in weekly sessions over the course of 12 weeks. Although the treatment of SAD has stimulated a large body of research, cognitive-behavioral group therapy (CBGT) and other treatment approaches have only demonstrated modest efficacy. Randomized controlled trials comparing CBGT to educational support group therapy, waitlist control, pharmacological therapy, and CGBT combined with pharmacological therapy or a placebo pill have reported effect sizes ranging from 0.10 to 0.30, suggesting that there is clearly still room for improvement (Hofmann & Smits, 2008).

Although CBT and exposure therapy provide the best treatment outcome for individuals with SAD, there are still a large number of patients who do not respond to treatment and the majority of patients do not achieve full remission. Future efforts should focus on augmentation strategies for CBT. Recent studies examining the effect of acute administration of d-cycloserine (DCS) prior to exposure exercises has been shown to significantly enhance the efficacy of CBT for SAD (Guastella et al., 2008; Hofmann et al., 2006; Hofmann et al., 2013). In addition, future research should explore potential mediators and moderators of treatment response in order to more precisely target specific maintenance factors.

Panic Disorder
Defining Features

Panic disorder (PD) is characterized by repeated and unexpected panic attacks, which are defined as discrete periods of intense fear and discomfort that develop abruptly and peak within 10 minutes (American Psychiatric Association, 2000). Panic attacks are associated with feelings of choking, dizziness, shortness of breath, nausea or stomach pain, pounding heart, sweating, shakiness, chest pain, numbness, and chills or hot flashes. Panic attacks are also often accompanied by feelings of unreality or detachment, fear of losing control, and fear of dying. After a panic attack, individuals with PD often experience persistent concern related to having another panic attack, worry about the consequences or implications of the panic attack, or a significant change in behavior related to the attacks for at least one month.

It is important to note that panic attacks are not specific to PD; they can occur in many different situations and can be either expected or unexpected. For example, someone with SAD may experience a panic attack when confronted with a stressful social situation, or exposure to blood may trigger a panic attack for someone with OCD and contamination fears. DSM-5 now explicitly recognizes the pervasiveness of panic attacks by introducing a "panic attack" specifier for all anxiety disorders as well as other mental disorders and some medical conditions. However, people with PD experience panic attacks that occur unexpectedly and without any clear triggers.

Historically, individuals who met criteria for a diagnosis for PD and who also reported fear of situations where it would be difficult to escape or to seek help if they were to experience a panic attack or panic-like symptoms (e.g., public transportation, crowds) received a diagnosis of PD with Agoraphobia. In DSM-5, PD and Agoraphobia are no longer linked diagnoses; in another words, individuals who meet the criteria described above would receive two separate diagnoses of PD and Agoraphobia. Although there are some individuals who experience Agoraphobia in the absence of PD, the majority of individuals with Agoraphobia also meet criteria for PD.

Epidemiological studies report a 12-month prevalence rate of 2.7% and a lifetime prevalence rate of 4.7% for PD (Kessler, Berglund, et al., 2005; Kessler, Chiu, et al., 2005). People with PD typically report an age of onset between 21 and 23 years, with more than twice as many women suffering from the disorder as men (Eaton, Kessler, Wittchen, & Magee, 1994). In the absence of treatment, PD follows a chronic course and is associated with high rates of relapse even when symptoms do spontaneously remit.

CBT Conceptualization of the Disorder
FEAR OF BODILY SENSATIONS

Individuals with PD have an intense fear of the physical sensations that accompany anxiety, fear, or panic (McNally, 2002). When people with PD experience the hyperarousal and autonomic activation associated with fear and anxiety, they interpret those sensations as dangerous or harmful. For example, simply climbing a flight of stairs can produce symptoms similar to those experienced during the onset of a panic attack (e.g., shortness of breath and an increase in heart rate). However, someone with PD may interpret these symptoms as indicative of a heart attack or other health-related malady. Therefore, it is not surprising that people with PD tend to avoid exercise like cardiovascular activities more so than people with other anxiety disorders (Jacob, Furman, Durrant, & Turner, 1996).

COGNITIVE BIASES

Individuals with PD possess maladaptive cognitions about the meaning of bodily sensations, and are hypervigilant to the detection of threat and to physical threat in particular (Beck, Stanley, Averill, Baldwin, & Deagle, 1992; Ehlers & Breuer, 1995). The cognitive model of PD asserts that these biases reinforce the salience of threat-relevant cues and are the primary factor that contributes to the maintenance of PD (Clark, 1999). Empirical evaluations of the cognitive model of PD have provided support for the relationship between information-processing biases and PD (Teachman, Smith-Janik, & Saporito, 2007). Automatic associations in memory, interference effects, and interpretation biases were each found to be unique predictors of panic symptoms and independent of one another, suggesting that these cognitive factors may independently contribute to the development and maintenance of PD.

AVOIDANCE

One of the defining features of PD is a fear of experiencing another anxiety attack, which may cause people with PD to either avoid certain situations or behave in a way to prevent the onset of a future panic attack. Individuals with PD frequently engage in agoraphobic avoidance by avoiding situations in which escape would be difficult, or in which they might humiliate themselves during a panic attack. There is a great deal of variability in the degree of agoraphobic avoidance among people with PD, with some individuals confined to their homes for years and others able to maintain relatively normal day-to-day routines (Barlow, 2002).

People with PD often avoid any activities or situations that may produce symptoms that mimic those experienced during a panic attack (e.g., consumption of alcohol or caffeine, sex, horror movies, or exercise), which is referred to as interoceptive avoidance. In addition to avoiding certain behaviors or situations, individuals with PD develop safety behaviors that they believe provide reassurance and protection during a panic attack (Salkovskis, Clark, Hackmann, Wells, & Gelder, 1999). Safety behaviors may include carrying around a lucky charm or talisman, checking for the presence of hospitals in a certain area, wearing a heart rate monitor, or the presence of a particular companion.

Treatment Components

Effective treatment of PD involves multiple treatment approaches to target all the components of the cognitive model presented earlier, including fear of bodily sensations, cognitive biases, and avoidance behaviors (Barlow & Craske, 2006).

PSYCHOEDUCATION

People with PD interpret their physical sensations as dangerous, and continue to believe they are in danger even after receiving confirmation from multiple doctors that they are healthy and in no danger of dying. Accordingly, it is very helpful to explain the nature and adaptive function of panic attacks to patients so they can better understand that the associated symptoms are not dangerous. Once patients learn that panic attacks are part of the body's natural flight-or-fight response that occur in the absence of any real threat or danger, they are less likely to explore medical reasons for their physical symptoms of fear and anxiety.

COGNITIVE RESTRUCTURING

It is a common belief among individuals with PD that it is important to appear strong and in control of one's body at all times, which causes them to become hypervigilant to their bodily sensations. The goal of cognitive restructuring is to identify, challenge, and modify these maladaptive beliefs in addition to those related to misinterpretations of bodily sensations as dangerous. Prior to participating in exposure exercises, it is beneficial for patients to learn that the use of safety or avoidance behaviors does not reduce the anxiety they experience before even entering a feared situation, but instead increases anticipatory anxiety in both current and future situations.

ATTENTION AND SITUATION MODIFICATION

Most people with PD experience unexpected or uncued panic attacks, which results in the perception that the attacks are uncontrollable and unpredictable. However, patients can often identify some patterns when they are instructed to systematically monitor the characteristics of the situation or the timing of panic attacks. In addition, individuals with PD tend to allocate a large amount of their attentional resources toward monitoring their bodily sensations, which can cause hyperarousal in and of itself. When patients learn that focusing on bodily sensations has a counterproductive effect and can even lead to a panic attack, they can exert more control over their symptoms.

EXPOSURE AND ACCEPTANCE

For individuals with PD, panic attacks are often triggered by the experience and misinterpretation of bodily sensations. In order to address avoidance behaviors related to the experience of distressing bodily sensations (e.g., avoiding alcohol or caffeine, exercise, watching scary movies), the therapist must guide patients through exposure to the feared bodily sensations. By asking the patient to breathe through a small straw, spin around in a circle, or hyperventilate, these bodily sensations can be induced. The therapist can also incorporate exposure exercises outside of the office by instructing patients to run on a treadmill or drink a caffeinated beverage.

People with PD who also experience agoraphobia must additionally be exposed to the feared situation or activity. It is important that during exposure to agoraphobic situations, the therapist prevents the patient from engaging in safety behaviors or emotional avoidance strategies. As patients are exposed to fearful situations, the therapist encourages them to accept their feelings of anxiety and may also provide instructions for deep-breathing exercises to help mediate the symptoms of physiological arousal.

Empirical Support

CBT is the most widely researched and empirically supported treatment for PD, and consists of two predominant approaches. Cognitive approaches are often based on Clark's (1986) model of panic and Barlow and Craske's (2006) panic-control treatment (PCT). Both approaches include psychoeducation, cognitive restructuring, interoceptive exposure, and agoraphobic exposure, but PCT emphasizes behavioral exposures as the primary mechanism of change and Clark's cognitive approach views behavioral exposures as secondary to cognitive changes (Barlow & Craske, 1988; Clark, 1986). Studies investigating the efficacy of CBT for PD suggest that 70% to 80% of patients are panic-free after completing treatment (Barlow, Craske, Cerny, & Klosko, 1989).

In a study comparing CBT for PD alone to pharmacological therapy (imipramine) alone, CBT plus imipramine, CBT plus a pill placebo, and the pill placebo alone, both CBT alone and imipramine alone were found to demonstrate limited efficacy at acute outcome (Barlow, Gorman, Shear, & Woods, 2000). Although imipramine produced a higher response at acute outcome, it was associated with high rates of attrition due to adverse effects of the medication, as well as higher rates of relapse at follow-up. The addition of CBT to imipramine did not mitigate the high rate of relapse, and patients who received either CBT alone or with the pill placebo were most likely to maintain treatment gains. These results are consistent with previous studies that suggest that the addition of pharmacological therapy to CBT does not convey any additional benefits to CBT alone (Furukawa, Watanabe, & Churchill, 2006). In addition, mediation analyses of the Barlow et al. (2000) trial suggested that cognitions significantly mediated treatment that involved CBT, but not in treatment that involved imipramine (Hofmann, 2007b).

Studies investigating whether the addition of d-cycloserine (DCS) augments the response to CBT in individuals with PD are producing promising results. In one recent study comparing the addition of CBT plus acute administration of DCS to CBT plus a pill placebo in a double-blind, randomized controlled trial found that 77% of patients in the CBT plus DCS condition achieved clinically significant change status compared to only 33% in the CBT plus pill placebo condition (Otto et al., 2010).

Specific Phobias
Defining Features

Specific phobia is characterized by an intense and persistent fear that is triggered by the presence or anticipation of a specific situation or object (e.g., heights, flying, seeing blood, spiders) (American Psychiatric Association, 2000). When individuals with specific phobia encounter the phobic stimulus, they experience an immediate fear response that frequently manifests as a panic attack. The anxiety and avoidance associated with the feared situation or object results in significant impairment in day-to-day activities, occupational or academic functioning, and relationships.

People with specific phobia experience intense fear or anxiety that is out of proportion to the actual danger posed by the specific object or situation and to the sociocultural context, which then frequently causes them to avoid the situation entirely. Many individuals with specific phobia also experience anxiety over embarrassing themselves in front of others during a panic attack, fainting, or losing control. Symptoms of specific phobia also share many similarities with agoraphobia and panic disorder, which often results in misdiagnosis (Stinson, et al., 2007). Specific phobia is differentiated from agoraphobia and panic disorder by the focus of the fear, with specific phobia characterized by fear of a specific situation and agoraphobia characterized by a fear of being unable to escape or seek help during a panic attack (Barlow, 2002).

DSM-5 classifies specific phobias using five specifiers: 1) animal (e.g., fears of snakes, spiders, insects), natural environment (e.g., fear of stormy weather, heights, being close to water), blood-injection-injury (e.g., fear of needles, seeing blood, surgical procedures), situational (e.g., fear of small places, elevators, airplanes), and an "other" type (e.g., fear of vomiting or choking, loud noises, contracting an illness) (American Psychiatric Association, 2013). It is important to distinguish specific phobia from other anxiety disorders that are also characterized by avoidance and panic attacks. For example, a fear of dirt may be due to an obsession with contamination in someone with obsessive-compulsive disorder, a fear of driving in a car may be the result of a traumatic car accident in someone with posttraumatic stress disorder, and a fear of embarrassing oneself in a social situation may be better accounted for by social anxiety disorder.

According to epidemiological studies, specific phobia has a lifetime prevalence rate of 12.5% and a 12-month prevalence rate of 8.7%, making specific phobia the most common anxiety disorder (Kessler, Berglund, et al., 2005; Kessler, Chiu, et al., 2005). Twice as many women suffer from specific phobia as men, and women also report a greater number of phobias, higher fear ratings, and more animal and situational phobias (Fredrikson, Annas, Fischer, & Wik, 1996). Specific phobia is a chronic disorder and symptomatic episodes tend to persist continuously for an average of 20 years in the absence treatment (Stinson et al., 2007). The onset of specific phobia typically occurs in early childhood, with an average onset of seven years of age (Kessler, Berglund, et al., 2005). Despite the early age of onset, most people with specific phobia do not receive treatment until middle adulthood (average age of first treatment = 31 years) and only 8% of those who seek treatment report receiving treatment specifically for specific phobia (Stinson et al., 2007).

CBT Conceptualization
FEAR ACQUISITION

It has been assumed that specific phobia develops when an association is learned between triggers (e.g., conditioned stimuli) that signal the onset of distress or pain (Mowrer, 1939; Rachman, 1991). However, classical conditioning principles are unable to explain why many individuals with specific phobia cannot recall a traumatic experience at the onset of their phobia, why some people develop phobias after simply hearing about or observing a traumatic conditioning experience, or why many other cases of specific phobia develop in humans (Field, 2006; Rachman, 1991).

The neo-conditioning model emphasizes the role of fear acquisition through information pathways (e.g., a child is taught that spiders are dangerous) and vicarious learning (e.g., a child observes her mother responding fearfully to a spider) (Rachman, 1991). The neo-conditioning model has been supported through animal studies showing that rhesus monkeys display observational learning and will acquire a fear of snakes by watching a video in which other monkeys respond fearfully to snakes (Cook & Mineka, 1990). However, this model does not explain learning that occurs through nonassociative pathways. The nonassociative learning model of fear acquisition proposes that there are a small number of innate fears, which are evolutionarily relevant (e.g., objects that pose a threat to survival), that do not require any form of associative learning to develop (Poulton & Menzies, 2002). There is a great deal of support for nonassociative fear acquisition from animal models of learning, as well as with humans (Cook & Mineka, 1990; Menzies & Parker, 2001). When evaluating empirical support for the conceptualization of specific phobia, it is important to note that the majority of research has been conducted with animal models, which may not translate directly to humans (Hermans, Craske, Mineka, & Lovibond, 2006).

COGNITIVE BIASES

Higher-order cognitive processes play a significant role in fear acquisition and the development of specific phobia, with research suggesting that harm expectancy and perceptions of predictability and controllability are among the most important (Hofmann, 2008). In specific phobia, individuals learn an association between the phobic stimulus and an aversive experience (e.g., panic attack, intense feelings of anxiety), which results in the conclusion that the phobic stimulus is either a direct source of danger or signals a potential threat. The expectation of harm (e.g., dogs are dangerous and will attack me) manifests as behavioral avoidance of the phobic stimulus, as well as intense feelings of distress and anxiety, and consequently reinforces the association between the phobic stimulus and fear.

The inability to predict the onset of a feared situation or object and a lack of control over aversive events each play a causal role in the genesis of anxiety (Barlow, 2002). For individuals with specific phobia, maladaptive cognitions concerning an inability to predict when they will encounter the phobic stimulus results in hypervigilance to threat detection and a tendency to scan their environment for the phobic stimulus or objects that may resemble it. People with specific phobia also believe that they are unable to control their reaction, namely bodily sensations and physical symptoms of anxiety, when they encounter the phobic stimulus (Thorpe & Salkovskis, 1995).

INFORMATION-PROCESSING BIASES

Individuals with specific phobia display an attentional bias toward the detection of relevant phobic stimuli. In both animals and humans, there are certain stimuli that are preferentially activated and particularly susceptible to fear acquisition due to evolutionary relevance (Öhman & Mineka, 2001). Accordingly, attentional biases seem to be more prevalent in people with specific phobias of spiders, snacks, or heights. Attentional biases are often expressed in persistent scanning of the environment for the presence of the phobic stimulus, and result in frequent misinterpretation of a neutral object as the phobic stimulus and subsequent onset of a panic attack or fear response (MacLeod, Rutherford, Campbell, Ebsworthy, & Holker, 2002).

DISGUST SENSITIVITY AND CONTAMINATION FEARS

People with specific phobias of the animal or blood-injection-injury type seem to display a greater sensitivity to stimuli that provoke a disgust response that is unique from their phobic anxiety (Sawchuk, Lohr, Tolin, Lee, & Kleinknecht, 2000). Disgust sensitivity is most common among specific phobia of the spider and blood-injection-injury type, and may manifest as feelings of nausea or aversion (Gross & Levenson, 1993). The disease-avoidance model suggests that these types of specific phobias may be uniquely related to a fear of disease transmission or contamination, and also provides an explanation of why there is a high prevalence of animal phobias for animals that pose minimal harm and are unlikely to physically attack (e.g., insects) (Matchett & Davey, 1991).

Treatment Components

Effective treatment of specific phobia involves multiple treatment approaches to target all the components of the cognitive model presented earlier, including the learned association between the phobic stimulus and fear, cognitive biases, and information-processing biases.

PSYCHOEDUCATION

Specific phobic is associated with a great deal of distress and anxiety, which is frequently amplified by the experience of panic attacks. It is often a significant relief for patients to learn about the nature of specific phobia, as well as to understand how their avoidance behaviors are reinforcing their fear and anxiety. Psychoeducation is also important to prepare patients for treatment by explaining the function of the behavioral exposure exercises and habituation to anxiety.

COGNITIVE RESTRUCTURING

Individuals with specific phobia frequently harbor irrational beliefs about the true degree of danger posed by a phobic stimulus. They also tend to overestimate the probability of encountering the phobic stimulus or feared situation. Cognitive restructuring is a useful tool to address these dysfunctional beliefs by helping the patient to evaluate the accuracy or true probability of each situation. For example, in the case of a patient with a snake phobia and fear of dying from a poisonous snakebite, the therapist may point out the small percentage of snakes that are actually poisonous, as well as the small number of people who actually die from snakebite.

ATTENTION MODIFICATION

As discussed earlier, specific phobia is often associated with an attentional bias toward the detection of the phobic stimulus. This attentional bias toward the detection of threat may have been evolutionarily adaptive in the past, but it interferes with modern life and contributes to the maintenance of specific phobia when it results in hypervigilance (MacLeod et al., 2002). By simply instructing individuals to attend to a threatening stimulus during a computer task, Macleod and colleagues (2002) were able to cause a significant increase in symptoms of anxiety. For the treatment of specific phobia, the therapist may instruct the patient to focus on neutral, nonthreatening environmental stimuli in order to minimize attentional bias toward threat detection.

EXPOSURE AND ACCEPTANCE

Exposure is a critical component of treatment for specific phobia. Before beginning exposure exercises, the therapist must identify the phobic stimulus or situations that trigger the fear response. Once a fear hierarchy has been established, the therapist guides the patient through exposure exercises, beginning with the least fear provoking and gradually progressing through the hierarchy. For example, a patient with a phobia of snakes may begin by viewing photographs of a snake, followed by watching a video of a snake, then handling a realistic rubber snake, and so on and so forth. The therapist should encourage the patient to continue each exposure until the anxiety diminishes or distress tolerance increases, which may require more than one exposure session for a particular step of the fear hierarchy. It is often helpful for the patient to repeat exposures even after they have successfully completed them in order to reinforce the fear extinction process. The therapist must also ensure that the patient is not engaging in any safety or avoidance behaviors during exposure sessions. As patients move through their fear hierarchies, they learn that their feelings of anxiety and distress will naturally diminish over time, and to accept feelings of anxiety without engaging in avoidance or suppression.

Empirical Support

For the treatment of specific phobia, behavioral exposures to the phobic stimulus are the most effective treatment when compared to placebo or active alternative psychotherapeutic approaches (Choy, Fyer, & Lipsitz, 2007; Wolitzky-Taylor, Horowitz, Powers, & Telch, 2008). In a meta-analysis of 33 randomized treatments studies of specific phobia, placebo treatments proved superior to inactive control conditions, which suggests that people with specific phobia may be responsive to placebo treatments (Wolitzky-Taylor et al., 2008). It is noteworthy that behavioral exposures with direct contact with the phobic stimulus produced the most robust effect size at posttreatment. However, it was not significantly different from imaginal exposures or virtual-reality exposures at follow-up. Treatment gains achieved during in vivo exposures are generally maintained for at least one year, but are also associated with high rates of attrition and low ratings of treatment acceptability (Choy et al., 2007).

Systematic desensitization, which emphasizes imaginal exposure to the phobic stimulus while using deep muscle relaxation to suppress anxiety, tends to produce a significant reduction in subjective anxiety but only a minimal effect on phobic avoidance at best (Choy et al., 2007). However, there is some support for treatment specificity among the subtypes of specific phobia. For example, applied muscle tension (e.g., tensing muscles during exposure to the phobic stimulus in order to increase blood pressure and minimize fainting) and tension-only (e.g., without exposure to phobic stimulus) are both superior to in vivo exposures for the treatment of blood phobia (Öst, Fellenius, & Sterner, 1991).

Pharmacological therapy with conventional anxiolytic agents has not demonstrated a therapeutic benefit when administered alone or in combination with CBT. However, there is some support from a pilot investigation of the use of DCS during treatment for acrophobia (e.g., fear of heights) that acute administration of DCS enhances learning during the fear extinction process in a virtual reality exposure (Choy et al., 2007; Ressler et al., 2004).

Posttraumatic Stress Disorder
Defining Features

Posttraumatic stress disorder (PTSD) is unique among anxiety-related disorders in that we are able to identify the trigger, or traumatic event, that serves as a catalyst for the disorder. PTSD is also one of few psychological disorders that require an explicitly defined, identifiable event as an antecedent for its diagnosis. In order to receive a diagnosis of PTSD, an individual must be exposed to actual or threatened death, serious injury, or sexual violence (American Psychiatric Association, 2013). This exposure can occur through direct experience, directly witnessing the event occurring to another person, learning that the event occurred to a close friend or family member, or experiencing repeated or extreme exposure to distressing information related to a traumatic event (e.g., police officers working with victims of sexual assault). Individuals suffering from PTSD continue to reexperience the trauma through persistent, involuntary recollections, flashbacks or feelings of reliving the trauma, recurrent and disturbing dreams, dissociative symptoms, or feelings of intense anxiety and physiological arousal when exposed to objects or bodily sensations associated with the trauma. Individuals with PTSD consistently avoid situations or objects that are associated with the trauma (e.g., thoughts, conversations, places, people, or activities that trigger recollections). They also tend to exhibit less emotional responsiveness (e.g., failure to remember important details of the trauma, decreased interest in important activities, blunted affect, feelings of isolation or detachment, minimal plans for the future). In addition, PTSD is associated with lasting symptoms of hyperarousal, including concentration difficulties, trouble falling asleep or sleeping through the night, moodiness or outbursts of anger, reckless or self-destructive behavior, hypervigilance to threat detection, and an exaggerated startle response.

Epidemiological studies report prevalence rates of 6.8% and 3.6% for lifetime and 12-month diagnoses of PTSD, respectively (Kessler, Berglund, et al., 2005). Although females are less likely to experience a traumatic event, more than three times as many women as men develop PTSD (Kessler, Berglund, et al., 2005; Tolin & Foa, 2006). A meta-analysis of sex differences in PTSD suggests that there are sex-specific risks for exposure to different types of traumatic events, with men more likely to experience or witness trauma related to combat and women more likely to experience sexual assault as adults and children (Tolin & Foa, 2006). However, over half of all men and women experience one or more traumatic events in their lifetime (Kessler, Sonnega, Bromet, Hughes, & Nelson, 1995). Most people who experience a traumatic event exhibit symptoms of PTSD immediately following the trauma, but do not go on to develop PTSD because symptoms remit naturally before the one month duration criterion is met (Gutner, Rizvi, Monson, & Resick, 2006). For example, it is estimated that 80% to 90% of individuals who experience a traumatic event and exhibit symptoms of PTSD immediately after the trauma do not develop PTSD (Kessler et al., 1995). Indeed, PTSD may be best understood as a failure to adapt or effectively cope with the effects of a traumatic event. Meta-analyses exploring risk factors for PTSD support this conceptualization of the disorder, and suggest that factors operating during or after the trauma, such as the use of avoidant coping strategies and low perceived social support, are stronger predictors of PTSD than pretrauma factors (Brewin, Andrews, & Valentine, 2000; Ozer, Best, Lipsey, & Weiss, 2003).

Similarly to OCD, PTSD has been removed from the Anxiety Disorders chapter in DSM-5 and moved to a new chapter entitled, "Trauma- and Stressor-Related Disorders," which includes disorders that require exposure to a stressful or traumatic event as part of the diagnostic criteria.

CBT Conceptualization
MALADAPTIVE COGNITIONS

One of the core components of the classic cognitive theory of emotional disorders is that anxiety is the result of how individuals interpret specific experiences and life events, rather than the event itself. Consistent with this general model, Ehlers and Clark's (2000) suggest that the anxiety experienced by individuals with PTSD is due to errors in cognitive appraisal. People who experience a traumatic event frequently overgeneralize from the specific traumatic event to a variety of other situations, and consequently characterize those situations as dangerous as well. Individuals with PTSD also view themselves or characteristics of their personality as somehow contributing to the traumatic event (e.g., "I am a magnet for disaster" or "This type of thing always happens to me"). In addition, they overestimate the probability that the traumatic event will occur again in the future.

PTSD is associated with a number of distressing and unpleasant symptoms (e.g., involuntary recollections of the trauma, prolonged and constant physiological arousal, sleep difficulties), which are often misinterpreted by individuals with PTSD. Instead of viewing these symptoms as a natural part of the body's response to trauma, they view symptoms as indicative of a permanent change to their mental and physical health. These types of appraisals are maladaptive because they generate negative emotions and frequently lead people with PTSD to employ counterproductive coping strategies (e.g., behavioral avoidance, suppression of emotions or thoughts related to the trauma) that only reinforce the fear structure.

MEMORY OF TRAUMATIC EVENT

Another core component proposed by Ehlers and Clark's (2000) model of PTSD is related to how individuals process and encode the memory of the traumatic event. Autobiographical memories are most often retrieved through higher-order meaning-based retrieval strategies, but can also be triggered by the presence of situational cues associated with the event (Brewin, Dalgleish, & Joseph, 1996). According to Ehlers and Clark, individuals with PTSD do not effectively elaborate the traumatic memory and, thus, it is not successfully integrated into their episodic memory. Consequently, people with PTSD frequently encounter great difficulty during attempts to intentionally recall the traumatic event, but still experience involuntary, distressing recollections of the trauma. In addition, ineffective elaboration prevents the storage of information related to the context of the traumatic memory, which may contribute to the sense of current threat that is attributed to a past event.

BEHAVIORAL AND COGNITIVE AVOIDANCE

In order to cope with the feelings of fear and danger related to the traumatic event and associated symptoms, individuals with PTSD employ cognitive and behavioral strategies (Ehlers & Clark, 2000). They frequently attempt to avoid the experience of intrusive recollections of the trauma by suppressing any thoughts related to the traumatic event, which only increases the frequency of these thoughts. People with PTSD also allocate significant attentional resources toward the detection of threat, which results in heightened autonomic arousal and hypervigilance. Alternatively, some individuals with PTSD will spend a great deal of time ruminating about how the trauma could have been prevented, or how they can seek revenge on the perpetrator of the trauma. Rumination is a cognitive avoidance strategy because it prevents individuals from successfully elaborating and integrating the trauma into autobiographical memory.

Many individuals with PTSD develop a strong reliance on safety behaviors (e.g., behaviors or actions believed to offer protection against future threats). For example, someone who was violently attacked by an intruder in the middle of the night may be unable to fall asleep without a baseball bat next to him in bed. In addition, people with PTSD frequently avoid revisiting the site of the trauma because they mistakenly believe that it will trigger intense anxiety and panic. However, revisiting the location or situation where the trauma took place can help provide additional contextual information, which assists in the construction of a more elaborate trauma memory. Some individuals with PTSD rely on alcohol or other substances to dull the anxiety and associated symptoms.

Treatment Components

Effective treatment of PTSD involves multiple treatment approaches to target all the components of the cognitive model presented earlier, including maladaptive cognitions, memory of the trauma, and behavioral and cognitive avoidance via psychoeducation, cognitive restructuring, stimulus discrimination, and exposure.

PSYCHOEDUCATION

Individuals with PTSD harbor maladaptive and dysfunctional beliefs about both external threats (e.g., characterizing the world as dangerous) and internal threats (e.g., perceiving themselves as unable to deal with the trauma or future threats). The goal of psychoeducation is to educate the patient about the nature of PTSD, and to emphasize that symptoms of PTSD are part of the body's natural response to an abnormal event. It is also important for the patient to learn that coping strategies like safety behaviors or cognitive avoidance are, in fact, producing and maintaining PTSD symptoms.

COGNITIVE RESTRUCTURING

In order to facilitate the contextualization and elaboration of the trauma memory, it is often necessary for the patient to re-experience the trauma by rehearsing distressing details of it with the assistance of the therapist. During this exercise, the patient provides verbal descriptions of the details of trauma, as well as thoughts and feelings related to the trauma.

The therapist is then able to identify and challenge maladaptive cognitions surrounding the traumatic experience (e.g., feelings of being responsible for the trauma, overgeneralization of traumatic event, belief that symptoms of PTSD are permanent). The patient then incorporates the new information and reappraisals into subsequent reliving exercises until a coherent, comprehensive narrative of the trauma is encoded into the patient's memory.

STIMULUS DISCRIMINATION

For individuals with PTSD, intrusive recollections of the trauma and hyperarousal are frequently triggered by situational cues or bodily sensations associated with the traumatic event. It is common among people with PTSD to feel a lack of control over the onset of PTSD symptoms or panic attacks, which increases reliance on maladaptive coping strategies like safety behaviors. The goal of stimulus discrimination is to aid the patient in the identification of internal triggers (e.g., feelings of loneliness, muscle tension, anger) and external triggers (e.g., smell of smoke, certain places, seeing a similar traumatic event in a movie or on the news) that trigger flashbacks of the trauma. The therapist encourages the patient to discuss how these triggers are both similar to and distinct from the situation and sensations experienced during the trauma. The patient then learns to focus his or her attention on these dissimilarities during future encounters with potential internal or external triggers to maximize stimulus discrimination.

EXPOSURE

Avoidance of situations or sensations that are associated with the trauma reinforces and maintains symptoms of PTSD because it prevents the patient from testing maladaptive cognitions about the trauma or modifying the trauma memory. Therefore, exposure to the site of the trauma and associated cues is an important part of contextualizing the trauma as an event that happened in the past. In vivo or behavioral exposures can help a patient who has overgeneralized characteristics of the trauma to other situations to better discriminate between dangerous and relatively innocuous situations. For example, a therapist may instruct a female patient who avoids all public restrooms after she was raped in a rest stop bathroom late at night to engage in exposures that require her to use busy, well-lit public restrooms. When internal triggers are particularly salient (e.g., a man believes that he will lose control or go crazy if exposed to a similar situation), it is often useful for the patient to challenge and disconfirm these negative appraisals through exposure exercises.

Empirical Support

In an empirical investigation of Ehlers and Clark's cognitive model of PTSD, a path analytic examination found both the nature of the trauma memory and cognitions related to the trauma to be unique and independent predictors of PTSD symptom severity (Lancaster, Rodriguez, & Weston, 2011). Accordingly, response to treatment and good outcome are strongly associated with changes in maladaptive cognitions about the trauma, whereas psychiatric comorbidity, trauma history, duration of time since the traumatic event, or type of trauma are not significant predictors of treatment response (Ehlers, Clark, Hackmann, McManus, & Fennell, 2005).

In a meta-analysis of both controlled and uncontrolled studies, psychological therapies (e.g., behavioral therapy, hypnotherapy, dynamic therapy, relaxation training) demonstrated superior efficacy to pharmacological therapies and control conditions, as well as the lowest rates of attrition (van Etten & Taylor, 1998). Cognitive treatments that incorporate repeated exposure to the trauma through imagery or writing exercises and in vivo exposures or a combination of the two can significantly enhance the treatment efficacy (Ehlers et al., 2005). Conversely, a recent meta-analysis by Benish and colleagues (2008) did not find relative differences between the efficacy of psychotherapies, suggesting that all forms of psychotherapy are superior to control conditions and provide comparable treatment gains (Benish, Imel, & Wampold, 2008). However, Ehlers and colleagues (2010) contend that Benish's selection procedures introduced biased results and were methodologically unsound (Ehlers et al., 2010). Further research is necessary to determine whether trauma-focused cognitive therapies are, in fact, more efficacious than psychotherapies that do not incorporate trauma exposure.

Future Directions

Although CBT and exposure therapy provide the best treatment outcome for individuals with anxiety disorders, there are still a large number of patients who do not respond to treatment and many who do not achieve full remission. Support for the acute administration of DCS prior to exposure exercises has been presented throughout the chapter, and future efforts should continue to focus on how we can augment the response to CBT and maximize associative learning during the fear extinction process. Despite sophisticated and heuristically useful models of CBT, very little is known about the mechanism of treatment change. Future studies need to study the hypothesized mediators and moderators in clinical practice. This information would enable future researchers to further improve the existing treatment protocols.

Another urgent area for future development includes the dissemination of CBT. In contrast to pharmacological interventions, there is no specific industry supporting and profiting from the dissemination of CBT. However, CBT is a highly cost-effective family of interventions when considering the enormous economic burden caused by anxiety disorders (Hofmann & Barlow, 1999). Given the high cost-effectiveness of CBT, the United Kingdom (UK) Health Secretary agreed to spend £300 million ($600 million) and train 8,000 new therapists as part of a 6-year program with the goal to provide people with anxiety disorders, as well as depression and other mental disorders, access to CBT. Similarly, the Australian government recommended the provision of CBT in 1996 and introduced a plan to provide better access to these services (Rachman & Wilson, 2008). These efforts are innovative and exemplary, and provide a valuable model of dissemination efforts for other countries, including the United States.

Other notable areas for future research are advancements in technology and computer software, including Internet-based CBT treatments for anxiety disorders. Early interventions have shown efficacy comparable to CBT delivered face-to-face (e.g., Kiropoulos et al., 2008). Another area with great promise includes virtual-reality exposures for treating PTSD and for generating phobic stimuli or situations that are difficult or expensive to reproduce, as well as for patients who are unwilling to engage in behavioral exposures.

Finally, more research is needed to systematically examine the role of emotion regulation in anxiety disorders (Hofmann, Sawyer, Fang, & Asnaani, 2012), and explore promising and alternative interventions, such as mindfulness meditation. Reviews investigating the efficacy of mindfulness-based cognitive therapy (MBCT) suggest a moderate effect size for the treatment of anxiety disorders (Hofmann, Sawyer, Witt, & Oh, 2010), and meta-analytic reviews have found acceptance and commitment therapy (ACT) to be superior to a control condition (Powers, Zum Vorde Sive Vording, & Emmelkamp, 2009). Although there are differences between CBT, MBCT, and ACT with regard to specific treatment strategies, their theoretical approaches to treatment are not incompatible (Hofmann, Sawyer, & Fang, 2010). Future research should focus on whether combining MBCT or ACT with CBT produces an additive effect, or whether treatment response can be enhanced by using a combination of these approaches based on characteristics of each patient.

References

American Psychiatric Association. (2000). *Diagnostic and statistical manual of mental disorders* (4th ed., text rev.). Washington, DC: Author.

Bar-Haim, Y., Lamy, D., Pergamin, L., Bakermans-Kranenburg, M. J., & van IJzendoorn, M. H. (2007). Threat-related attentional bias in anxious and nonanxious individuals: A meta-analytic study. *Psychological Bulletin, 133*, 1–24.

Barlow, D. H. (2002). *Anxiety and its disorders: The nature and treatment of anxiety and panic* (2nd ed.). New York: Guilford.

Barlow, D. H., & Craske, M. G. (1988). *Mastery of your anxiety and panic*. Albany, NY: Graywind Publications.

Barlow, D. H., & Craske, M. G. (2006). *Mastery of your anxiety and panic: Client workbook* (4th ed.). New York: Oxford University Press.

Barlow, D. H., Craske, M. G., Cerny, J. A., & Klosko, J. S. (1989). Behavioral treatment of panic disorder. *Behavior Therapy, 20*, 261–282.

Barlow, D. H., Gorman, J. M., Shear, M. K., & Woods, S. W. (2000). Cognitive-behavioral therapy, imipramine, or their combination for panic disorder: A randomized controlled trial. *JAMA, 283*, 2529–2536.

Barrera, T. L., & Norton, P. J. (2009). Quality of life impairment in generalized anxiety disorder, social phobia, and panic disorder. *Journal of Anxiety Disorders, 23*, 1086–1090.

Beck, J. G., Stanley, M. A., Averill, P. M., Baldwin, L. E., & Deagle, E. A., III. (1992). Attention and memory for threat in panic disorder. *Behaviour Research and Therapy, 30*, 619–629.

Benish, S. G., Imel, Z. E., & Wampold, B. E. (2008). The relative efficacy of bona fide psychotherapies for treating post-traumatic stress disorder: a meta-analysis of direct comparisons. *Clinical Psychology Review, 28*, 746–758.

Berle, D., & Starcevic, V. (2005). Thought-action fusion: review of the literature and future directions. *Clinical Psychology Review, 25*, 263–284.

Bögels, S. M., & Mansell, W. (2004). Attention processes in the maintenance and treatment of social phobia: hypervigilance, avoidance and self-focused attention. *Clinical Psychology Review, 24*, 827–856.

Borkovec, T. D., & Hu, S. (1990). The effect of worry on cardiovascular response to phobic imagery. *Behaviour Research and Therapy, 28*, 69–73.

Borkovec, T. D., Ray, W. J., & Stöber, J. (1998). Worry: A cognitive phenomenon intimately linked to affective, physiological, and interpersonal behavioral processes. *Cognitive Therapy and Research, 22*, 561–576.

Borkovec, T. D., & Ruscio, A. M. (2001). Psychotherapy for generalized anxiety disorder. *Journal of Clinical Psychiatry, 62* Suppl 11, 37–42; discussion 43–35.

Brewin, C. R., Andrews, B., & Valentine, J. D. (2000). Meta-analysis of risk factors for posttraumatic stress disorder in trauma-exposed adults. *Journal of Consulting and Clinical Psychology, 68,* 748–766.

Brewin, C. R., Dalgleish, T., & Joseph, S. (1996). A dual representation theory of posttraumatic stress disorder. *Psychological Review, 103,* 670–686.

Campbell, L. A., Brown, T. A., & Grisham, J. R. (2003). The relevance of age of onset to the psychopathology of generalized anxiety disorder. *Behavior Therapy, 34,* 31–48.

Choy, Y., Fyer, A. J., & Lipsitz, J. D. (2007). Treatment of specific phobia in adults. *Clinical Psychology Review, 27,* 266–286.

Clark, D. M. (1986). A cognitive approach to panic. *Behaviour Research and Therapy, 24,* 461–470.

Clark, D. M. (1999). Anxiety disorders: why they persist and how to treat them. *Behaviour Research and Therapy, 37* Suppl 1, S5–S27.

Clark, D. M., & Wells, A. (1995). A cognitive model of social phobia. In R. G. Heimberg, M. R. Leibowitz, D. A. Hope & F. R. Schneider (Eds.), *Social phobia: Diagnosis, assessment and treatment* (pp. 69–93). New York: Guilford Press.

Coles, M. E., Frost, R. O., Heimberg, R. G., & Rheaume, J. (2003). "Not just right experiences": Perfectionism, obsessive-compulsive features and general psychopathology. *Behaviour Research and Therapy, 41,* 681–700.

Cook, M., & Mineka, S. (1990). Selective associations in the observational conditioning of fear in rhesus monkeys. *Journal of Experimental Psychology: Animal Behavior Processes, 16,* 372–389.

Davey, G. C. (1994). Worrying, social problem-solving abilities, and social problem-solving confidence. *Behaviour Research and Therapy, 32,* 327–330.

Durham, R. C., Fisher, P. L., Dow, M. G. T., Sharp, D., Power, K. G., Swan, J. v., & Morton, R. V. (2004). Cognitive behavior therapy for good and poor prognosis generalized anxiety disorder: A clinical effectiveness study. *Clinical Psychology and Psychotherapy, 11,* 145–157.

Eaton, W. W., Kessler, R. C., Wittchen, H. U., & Magee, W. J. (1994). Panic and panic disorder in the United States. *American Journal of Psychiatry, 151,* 413–420.

Ehlers, A., Bisson, J., Clark, D. M., Creamer, M., Pilling, S., Richards, D.,. . . Yule W. (2010). Do all psychological treatments really work the same in posttraumatic stress disorder? *Clinical Psychology Review, 30,* 269–276.

Ehlers, A., & Breuer, P. (1995). Selective attention to physical threat in subjects with panic attacks and specific phobias. *Journal of Anxiety Disorders, 9,* 11–31.

Ehlers, A., & Clark, D. M. (2000). A cognitive model of posttraumatic stress disorder. *Behaviour Research and Therapy, 38,* 319–345.

Ehlers, A., Clark, D. M., Hackmann, A., McManus, F., & Fennell, M. (2005). Cognitive therapy for post-traumatic stress disorder: development and evaluation. *Behaviour Research and Therapy, 43,* 413–431.

Field, A. P. (2006). Is conditioning a useful framework for understanding the development and treatment of phobias? *Clinical Psychology Review, 26,* 857–875.

Franklin, M. E., Abramowitz, J. S., Kozak, M. J., Levitt, J. T., & Foa, E. B. (2000). Effectiveness of exposure and ritual prevention for obsessive-compulsive disorder: randomized compared with nonrandomized samples. *Journal of Consulting and Clinical Psychology, 68,* 594–602.

Fredrikson, M., Annas, P., Fischer, H., & Wik, G. (1996). Gender and age differences in the prevalence of specific fears and phobias. *Behaviour Research and Therapy, 34,* 33–39.

Frost, R. O., & Steketee, G. (1997). Perfectionism in obsessive-compulsive disorder patients. *Behaviour Research and Therapy, 35,* 291–296.

Frost, R. O., & Steketee, G. (2002). *Cognitive approaches to obsessions and compulsions: Theory, assessment, and treatment.* Oxford, UK: Elsevier.

Furukawa, T. A., Watanabe, N., & Churchill, R. (2006). Psychotherapy plus antidepressant for panic disorder with or without agoraphobia: systematic review. *British Journal of Psychiatry, 188,* 305–312.

Goisman, R. M., Goldenberg, I., Vasile, R. G., & Keller, M. B. (1995). Comorbidity of anxiety disorders in a multicenter anxiety study. *Comprehensive Psychiatry, 36,* 303–311.

Grant, B. F., Stinson, F. S., Dawson, D. A., Chou, S. P., Dufour, M. C., Compton, W.,. . . Kaplan K. (2004). Prevalence and co-occurrence of substance use disorders and independent mood and anxiety disorders: results from the National Epidemiologic Survey on Alcohol and Related Conditions. *Archives of General Psychiatry, 61,* 807–816.

Gross, J. J., & Levenson, R. W. (1993). Emotional suppression: physiology, self-report, and expressive behavior. *Journal of Personality and Social Psychology, 64,* 970–986.

Guastella, A. J., Richardson, R., Lovibond, P. F., Rapee, R. M., Gaston, J. E., Mitchell, P., et al. (2008). A randomized controlled trial of D-cycloserine enhancement of exposure therapy for social anxiety disorder. *Biological Psychiatry, 63,* 544–549.

Gutner, C. A., Rizvi, S. L., Monson, C. M., & Resick, P. A. (2006). Changes in coping strategies, relationship to the perpetrator, and posttraumatic distress in female crime victims. *Journal of Traumatic Stress, 19,* 813–823.

Heimberg R. G., Hofmann, S. G., Liebowitz, M. R., Schneier, F. R., Smits, J. A. J., Stein, M. B., Hinton, D. E., & Craske, M. G. (2014). Social anxiety disorder in DSM-5. *Depression and Anxiety.* doi: 10.1002/da.22231

Heinrichs, N., & Hofmann, S. G. (2001). Information processing in social phobia: a critical review. *Clinical Psychology Review, 21,* 751–770.

Hermans, D., Craske, M. G., Mineka, S., & Lovibond, P. F. (2006). Extinction in human fear conditioning. *Biological Psychiatry, 60,* 361–368.

Hofmann, S. G. (2007a). Cognitive factors that maintain social anxiety disorder: a comprehensive model and its treatment implications. *Cognitive Behaviour Therapy, 36,* 193–209.

Hofmann, S. G. (2007b). Enhancing exposure-based therapy from a translational research perspective. *Behaviour Research and Therapy, 45,* 1987–2001.

Hofmann, S. G. (2008). Cognitive processes during fear acquisition and extinction in animals and humans: implications for exposure therapy of anxiety disorders. *Clinical Psychology Review, 28,* 199–210.

Hofmann, S. G., & Barlow, D. H. (1999). The costs of anxiety disorders: Implications for psychosocial interventions. In N. E. Miller & K. M. Magruder (Eds.), *Cost-Effectiveness of Psychotherapy* (pp. 224–234). New York: Oxford University Press.

Hofmann, S. G., Heering, S., Sawyer, A. T., & Asnaani, A. (2009). How to handle anxiety: The effects of reappraisal, acceptance, and suppression strategies on anxious arousal. *Behaviour Research and Therapy, 47*, 389–394.

Hofmann, S. G., Meuret, A. E., Smits, J. A., Simon, N. M., Pollack, M. H., Eisenmenger, K., (2006). Augmentation of exposure therapy with D-cycloserine for social anxiety disorder. *Archives of General Psychiatry, 63*, 298–304.

Hofmann, S. G., Moscovitch, D. A., Litz, B. T., Kim, H. J., Davis, L. L., & Pizzagalli, D. A. (2005). The worried mind: autonomic and prefrontal activation during worrying. *Emotion, 5*, 464–475.

Hofmann, S. G., & Otto, M. W. (2008). *Cognitive-behavior therapy for social anxiety disorder: Evidence-based and disorder-specific treatment techniques.* New York: Taylor & Francis Group.

Hofmann, S. G., Sawyer, A. T., & Fang, A. (2010). The empirical status of the "new wave" of cognitive behavioral therapy. *Psychiatric Clinics of North America, 33*, 701–710.

Hofmann, S. G., Sawyer, A. T., Fang, A., & Asnaani, A. (2012). Emotion dysregulation model of mood and anxiety disorders. *Depression and Anxiety, 29*, 409–416.

Hofmann, S. G., Sawyer, A. T., Witt, A. A., & Oh, D. (2010). The effect of mindfulness-based therapy on anxiety and depression: A meta-analytic review. *Journal of Consulting and Clinical Psychology, 78*, 169–183.

Hofmann, S. G., & Smits, J. A. (2008). Cognitive-behavioral therapy for adult anxiety disorders: a meta-analysis of randomized placebo-controlled trials. *Journal of Clinical Psychiatry, 69*, 621–632.

Hofmann, S. G., Smits, A. J., Rosenfield, D., Simon, N., Otto, M. W., Meuret, A. E., Marques, L., Fang, A., Tart, C., & Pollack, M. H. (2013). D-cycloserine as an augmentation strategy of cognitive behavioral therapy for social anxiety disorder. *American Journal of Psychiatry, 170*, 751–758.

Jacob, R. G., Furman, J. M., Durrant, J. D., & Turner, S. M. (1996). Panic, agoraphobia, and vestibular dysfunction. *American Journal of Psychiatry, 153*, 503–512.

Katzelnick, D. J., Kobak, K. A., DeLeire, T., Henk, H. J., Greist, J. H., Davidson, J. R., . . . Helstad, C. P. (2001). Impact of generalized social anxiety disorder in managed care. *American Journal of Psychiatry, 158*, 1999–2007.

Kessler, R. C., Berglund, P., Demler, O., Jin, R., Merikangas, K. R., & Walters, E. E. (2005). Lifetime prevalence and age-of-onset distributions of DSM-IV disorders in the National Comorbidity Survey Replication. *Archives of General Psychiatry, 62*, 593–602.

Kessler, R. C., Chiu, W. T., Demler, O., Merikangas, K. R., & Walters, E. E. (2005). Prevalence, severity, and comorbidity of 12-month DSM-IV disorders in the National Comorbidity Survey Replication. *Archives of General Psychiatry, 62*, 617–627.

Kessler, R. C., Sonnega, A., Bromet, E., Hughes, M., & Nelson, C. B. (1995). Posttraumatic stress disorder in the National Comorbidity Survey. *Archives of General Psychiatry, 52*, 1048–1060.

Kiropoulos, L. A., Klein, B., Austin, D. W., Gilson, K., Pier, C., Mitchell, J., &. Ciechomski, L. (2008). Is internet-based CBT for panic disorder and agoraphobia as effective as face-to-face CBT? *Journal of Anxiety Disorders, 22*, 1273–1284.

Kolada, J. L., Bland, R. C., & Newman, S. C. (1994). Epidemiology of psychiatric disorders in Edmonton. Obsessive-compulsive disorder. *Acta Psychiatrica Scandinavica. Supplementum, 376*, 24–35.

Ladouceur, R., Gosselin, P., & Dugas, M. J. (2000). Experimental manipulation of intolerance of uncertainty: a study of a theoretical model of worry. *Behaviour Research and Therapy, 38*, 933–941.

Lancaster, S. L., Rodriguez, B. F., & Weston, R. (2011). Path analytic examination of a cognitive model of PTSD. *Behaviour Research and Therapy, 49*, 194–201.

Lepine, J. P. (2002). The epidemiology of anxiety disorders: prevalence and societal costs. *Journal of Clinical Psychiatry, 63* Suppl 14, 4–8.

MacLeod, C., Rutherford, E., Campbell, L., Ebsworthy, G., & Holker, L. (2002). Selective attention and emotional vulnerability: Assessing the causal basis of their association through the experimental manipulation of attentional bias. *Journal of Abnormal Psychology, 111*, 107–123.

Magee, W. J., Eaton, W. W., Wittchen, H. U., McGonagle, K. A., & Kessler, R. C. (1996). Agoraphobia, simple phobia, and social phobia in the National Comorbidity Survey. *Archives of General Psychiatry, 53*, 159–168.

Markarian, Y., Larson, M. J., Aldea, M. A., Baldwin, S. A., Good, D., Berkeljon, A., . . . McKay, D. (2010). Multiple pathways to functional impairment in obsessive-compulsive disorder. *Clinical Psychology Review, 30*, 78–88.

Mataix-Cols, D., Frost, R. O., Pertusa, A., Clark, L. A., Sacena, S., Leckman, J. F., . . . Wilhem, S. (2010). Hoarding disorder: A new diagnosis for DSM-V? *Depression and Anxiety, 27*, 556–572.

Matchett, G., & Davey, G. C. (1991). A test of a disease-avoidance model of animal phobias. *Behaviour Research and Therapy, 29*, 91–94.

Mathews, A., Richards, A., & Eysenck, M. (1989). Interpretation of homophones related to threat in anxiety states. *Journal of Abnormal Psychology, 98*, 31–34.

McKay, D., Abramowitz, J. S., Calamari, J. E., Kyrios, M., Radomsky, A., Sookman, D., . . . Wilhelm, S. (2004). A critical evaluation of obsessive-compulsive disorder subtypes: Symptoms versus mechanisms. *Clinical Psychology Review, 24*, 283–313.

McNally, R. J. (2002). Anxiety sensitivity and panic disorder. *Biological Psychiatry, 52*, 938–946.

Menzies, R. G., & Parker, L. (2001). The origins of height fear: An evaluation of neoconditioning explanations. *Behaviour Research and Therapy, 39*, 185–199.

Mitte, K. (2005). Meta-analysis of cognitive-behavioral treatments for generalized anxiety disorder: a comparison with pharmacotherapy. *Psychological Bulletin, 131*, 785–795.

Mogg, K., & Bradley, B. P. (2005). Attentional bias in generalized anxiety disorder versus depressive disorder. *Cognitive Therapy and Research, 29*, 29–45.

Moritz, S., & Pohl, R. F. (2009). Biased processing of threat-related information rather than knowledge deficits contributes to overestimation of threat in obsessive-compulsive disorder. *Behavior Modification, 33*, 763–777.

Mowrer, O. H. (1939). A stimulus-response analysis of anxiety and its role as a reinforcing agent. *Psychological Review, 46*, 553–565.

Öhman, A., & Mineka, S. (2001). Fears, phobias, and preparedness: toward an evolved module of fear and fear learning. *Psychological Review, 108*, 483–522.

Öst, L. G., Fellenius, J., & Sterner, U. (1991). Applied tension, exposure in vivo, and tension-only in the treatment of blood phobia. *Behaviour Research and Therapy, 29*, 561–574.

Otto, M. W., Tolin, D. F., Simon, N. M., Pearlson, G. D., Basden, S., Meunier, S. A., . . . Pollack, M. H. (2010). Efficacy of d-cycloserine for enhancing response to cognitive-behavior therapy for panic disorder. *Biological Psychiatry, 67*, 365–370.

Ozer, E. J., Best, S. R., Lipsey, T. L., Weiss, D. S. (2003). Predictors of posttraumatic stress disorder and symptoms in adults: A meta-analysis. *Psychological Bulletin, 129*, 52–73.

Poulton, R., & Menzies, R. G. (2002). Non-associative fear acquisition: A review of the evidence from retrospective and longitudinal research. *Behaviour Research and Therapy, 40*, 127–149.

Powers, M. B., Zum Vorde Sive Vording, M. B., & Emmelkamp, P. M. (2009). Acceptance and commitment therapy: A meta-analytic review. *Psychotherapy and Psychosomatics, 78*, 73–80.

Provencher, M. D., Freeston, M. H., Dugas, M. J., & Ladouceur, R. (2000). Catastrophizing assessment of worry and threat schemata among worriers. *Behavioral and Cognitive Psychotherapy, 28*, 211–224.

Rachman, S. (1991). Neo-conditioning and the classical theory of fear acquisition. *Clinical Psychology Review, 11*, 155–173.

Rachman, S. (1993). Obsessions, responsibility and guilt. *Behaviour Research and Therapy, 31*, 149–154.

Rachman, S. (2002). A cognitive theory of compulsive checking. *Behaviour Research and Therapy, 40*, 625–639.

Rachman, S., & Wilson, G. T. (2008). Expansion in the provision of psychological treatment in the United Kingdom. *Behaviour Research and Therapy, 46*, 293–295.

Rapee, R. M., & Heimberg, R. G. (1997). A cognitive-behavioral model of anxiety in social phobia. *Behaviour Research and Therapy, 35*, 741–756.

Rasmussen, S. A., & Eisen, J. L. (1992). The epidemiology and differential diagnosis of obsessive compulsive disorder. *Journal of Clinical Psychiatry, 53* Suppl, 4–10.

Rassin, E., & Koster, E. (2003). The correlation between thought-action fusion and religiosity in a normal sample. *Behaviour Research and Therapy, 41*, 361–368.

Ravi Kishore, V., Samar, R., Janardhan Reddy, Y. C., Chandrasekhar, C. R., & Thennarasu, K. (2004). Clinical characteristics and treatment response in poor and good insight obsessive-compulsive disorder. *European Psychiatry, 19*, 202–208.

Ressler, K. J., Rothbaum, B. O., Tannenbaum, L., Anderson, P., Graap, K., Zimand, E., . . . Davis, M. (2004). Cognitive enhancers as adjuncts to psychotherapy: use of D-cycloserine in phobic individuals to facilitate extinction of fear. *Archives of General Psychiatry, 61*, 1136–1144.

Robichaud, M., Dugas, M. J., & Conway, M. (2003). Gender differences in worry and associated cognitive-behavioral variables. *Journal of Anxiety Disorders, 17*, 501–516.

Roemer, L., Orsillo, S. M., & Salters-Pedneault, K. (2008). Efficacy of an acceptance-based behavior therapy for generalized anxiety disorder: evaluation in a randomized controlled trial. *Journal of Consulting and Clinical Psychology, 76*, 1083–1089.

Salkovskis, P. M., Clark, D. M., Hackmann, A., Wells, A., & Gelder, M. G. (1999). An experimental investigation of the role of safety-seeking behaviours in the maintenance of panic disorder with agoraphobia. *Behaviour Research and Therapy, 37*, 559–574.

Salkovskis, P. M., & Harrison, J. (1984). Abnormal and normal obsessions—a replication. *Behaviour Research and Therapy, 22*, 549–552.

Sawchuk, C. N., Lohr, J. M., Tolin, D. F., Lee, T. C., & Kleinknecht, R. A. (2000). Disgust sensitivity and contamination fears in spider and blood-injection-injury phobias. *Behaviour Research and Therapy, 38*, 753–762.

Shafran, R., Thordarson, D. S., & Rachman, S. (1996). Thought-action fusion in obsessive compulsive disorder. *Journal of Anxiety Disorders, 10*, 379–391.

Stein, M. B., & Kean, Y. M. (2000). Disability and quality of life in social phobia: epidemiologic findings. *American Journal of Psychiatry, 157*, 1606–1613.

Stein, M. B., McQuaid, J. R., Laffaye, C., & McCahill, M. E. (1999). Social phobia in the primary care medical setting. *Journal of Family Practice, 48*, 514–519.

Stinson, F. S., Dawson, D. A., Patricia Chou, S., Smith, S., Goldstein, R. B., June Ruan, W., . . . (2007). The epidemiology of DSM-IV specific phobia in the USA: results from the National Epidemiologic Survey on Alcohol and Related Conditions. *Psychological Medicine, 37*, 1047–1059.

Teachman, B. A., Smith-Janik, S. B., & Saporito, J. (2007). Information processing biases and panic disorder: Relationships among cognitive and symptom measures. *Behaviour Research and Therapy, 45*, 1791–1811.

Thorpe, S. J., & Salkovskis, P. M. (1995). Phobic beliefs: Do cognitive factors play a role in specific phobias? *Behaviour Research and Therapy, 33*, 805–816.

Tolin, D. F., Abramowitz, J. S., Brigidi, B. D., & Foa, E. B. (2003). Intolerance of uncertainty in obsessive-compulsive disorder. *Journal of Anxiety Disorders, 17*, 233–242.

Tolin, D. F., Abramowitz, J. S., Kozak, M. J., & Foa, E. B. (2001). Fixity of belief, perceptual aberration, and magical ideation in obsessive-compulsive disorder. *Journal of Anxiety Disorders, 15*, 501–510.

Tolin, D. F., & Foa, E. B. (2006). Sex differences in trauma and posttraumatic stress disorder: a quantitative review of 25 years of research. *Psychological Bulletin, 132*, 959–992.

van Etten, M. L., & Taylor, S. (1998). Comparative efficacy of treatments for post-traumatic stress disorder: a meta-analysis. *Clinical Psychology and Psychotherapy, 5*, 126–144.

Vogel, P. A., Stiles, T. C., & Gotestam, K. G. (2004). Adding cognitive therapy elements to exposure therapy for obsessive compulsive disorder: A controlled study. *Behavioural and Cognitive Psychotherapy, 32*, 275–290.

Wallace, S. T., & Alden, L. A. (1991). A comparison of social standards and perceived ability in anxious and nonanxious men. *Cognitive Therapy and Research, 15*, 237–254.

Weeks, J. W., Heimberg, R. G., Rodebaugh, T. L., & Norton, P. J. (2008). Exploring the relationship between fear of positive evaluation and social anxiety. *Journal of Anxiety Disorders, 22*, 386–400.

Wells, A. (1999). A metacognitive model and therapy for generalized anxiety disorder. *Clinical Psychology and Psychotherapy, 6*, 86–95.

Whittal, M. L., Thordarson, D. S., & McLean, P. D. (2005). Treatment of obsessive-compulsive disorder: cognitive behavior therapy vs. exposure and response prevention. *Behaviour Research and Therapy, 43*, 1559–1576.

Wittchen, H. U., Carter, R. M., Pfister, H., Montgomery, S. A., & Kessler, R. C. (2000). Disabilities and quality of life in pure and comorbid generalized anxiety disorder and major depression in a national survey. *International Clinical Psychopharmacology, 15*, 319–328.

Wittchen, H. U., & Hoyer, J. (2001). Generalized anxiety disorder: nature and course. *Journal of Clinical Psychiatry, 62* Suppl 11, 15–19; discussion 20-11.

Wolitzky-Taylor, K. B., Horowitz, J. D., Powers, M. B., & Telch, M. J. (2008). Psychological approaches in the treatment of specific phobias: a meta-analysis. *Clinical Psychology Review, 28*, 1021–1037.

Wu, K. D., & Cortesi, G. T. (2009). Relations between perfectionism and obsessive-compulsive symptoms: examination of specificity among the dimensions. *Journal of Anxiety Disorders, 23*, 393–400.

Adult Mood Disorders: The Case of Major Depressive Disorder

C. Steven Richards

Abstract

Major depressive disorder (MDD) is the most prevalent mood disorder. The 1-year prevalence rate of MDD among adults in the United States is approximately 6.7%. MDD provides an excellent example for examining the efficacy of CBT for adult mood disorders. Cognitive behavior therapy is an evidence-based, psychosocial intervention for MDD. There is substantial research literature on CBT that evaluates the efficacy of CBT for various populations of patients with MDD. Although results are consistently promising, there are a number of important directions for future research. CBT for depression usually has certain components and structure. In addition, the research literature and the extensive clinical experience of experts working in this area lead to some clinical guidelines for practitioners who are using CBT to treat MDD. We conclude with a discussion of future directions for research on CBT for depression.

Key Words: cognitive behavior therapy, major depressive disorder, CBT for depression, CBT components and structure, clinical guidelines

Major Depressive Disorder

Major depressive disorder (MDD) is one of the most common psychiatric disorders in terms of incidence and prevalence. Large-scale epidemiological research conducted in the United States indicates that the 1-year prevalence for MDD among adults is approximately 6.7%, whereas the 1-year prevalence of any mood disorder among adults is approximately 9.5% (Kessler, Chiu, Demler, & Walters, 2005, Table 1, p. 620). Other large-scale epidemiological studies conducted in Europe, Asia, Africa, and South America and elsewhere suggest that the prevalence of MDD is equivalently high in many parts of the world (Gotlib & Hammen, 2009). Therefore, MDD is a very important disorder, and one that provides a useful testing ground for the efficacy of cognitive and behavioral therapies for adult mood disorders. Moreover, CBT for depression has received much more research attention than CBT for other possible mood disorders, such as dysthymic disorder, bipolar disorder,

and depressive disorder not otherwise specified (American Psychiatric Association, 2010; Beck & Dozois, 2011; Craighead et al., 2007; Hollon & Dimidjian, 2009; Young et al., 2008). Hence, for the purposes of this chapter and this book, the case of major depressive disorder is an excellent area to examine the efficacy, strengths, and weaknesses of CBT and associated cognitive and behavioral therapies. The next step, then, is to provide a brief overview of the diagnostic criteria for major depressive disorder.

The two major diagnostic systems presently in use for psychiatric diagnoses are the *Diagnostic and Statistical Manual of Mental Disorders* (American Psychiatric Association, 2013) and the *International Classification of Diseases* (World Health Organization, 1992). These diagnostic systems are usually abbreviated as the *DSM-5* and the *ICD-10*. It should be noted that both of these diagnostic systems regularly go through a massive revision process, based in part on recent research, with the newest editions published in 2013 (*DSM-5*) and to be published in 2015 (*ICD-11*). There is considerable overlap in these two diagnostic systems. We will rely on the *DSM-5* (APA, 2013) for our present discussion. In addition, the diagnostic criteria in *DSM-5*, for major depressive disorder, are virtually identical to those in *DSM-IV* (2000, text revision), with the exception of no longer including an exclusion for "complicated bereavement" (cf. APA, 2013, pp. 160-161*)*. In summary, we will rely on the diagnostic criteria for major depressive disorder, which are spelled out in the *DSM-5* (APA, 2013, pp. 160-161). These criteria are briefly summarized below.

The DSM-5 recognizes 9 symptoms and signs for diagnosing major depressive disorder:

1. Depressed mood.
2. Loss of pleasure (anhedonia).
3. Change in weight or appetite.
4. Sleep disruption.
5. Slow and delayed responses.
6. Tired and fatigued, without a medical reason.
7. Guilty and a sense of worthlessness.
8. Concentration problems.
9. Suicidal thinking, plans, or attempts.

For a diagnosis of major depressive disorder, the patient must exhibit at least 5 of the above 9 symptoms and signs, consistently throughout a 2-week interval. In addition, at least one of the present symptoms must be depressed mood *or* loss of pleasure (anhedonia). Furthermore, the symptoms and signs of depression must be clearly causing distress and interfering with day-to-day functioning. Typically, all these depressive symptoms and signs are assessed via thorough, face-to-face interviews, which may then be supplemented with other assessment modalities such as questionnaires, self-monitoring records, reports from significant others, direct observation of interpersonal interactions when close relationships are involved, and so forth. The assessment portfolio, however, should always include some careful, face-to-face interviewing by the clinician (Gotlib & Hammen, 2009, 2014; Richards & O'Hara, 2014; Richards & Perri, 2002, 2010).

There are a number of rule-outs and alternative diagnostic possibilities, of course, and a complete discussion of these issues is beyond the scope of this chapter (see *DSM-5*, 2013, pp. 160–168). Briefly, however, these rule-outs include the following: not better meeting the diagnostic criteria for another mood disorder, such as dysthymic disorder;

and the depressive symptoms are not directly due to drug effects or medical conditions; moreover, the depressive-symptom profile is not centered on a situation-based adjustment disorder with depressed mood. With this brief overview of the symptom picture in place, we should now discuss the severe disability, extensive comorbidity, and relentless relapse and recurrence that may accompany major depressive disorder.

In addition to having a high prevalence and ubiquitous presence in most of the world, major depressive disorder is frequently listed in the top-10 causes of disability throughout the world, with the exact place dependent on how "disability" is defined and measured (cf. Alexopoulos et al., 2011; American Psychiatric Association, 2010; Gotlib & Hammen, 2009; Kessler et al., 2005; Kocsis & Klein, 1995; Pettit & Joiner, 2006; Richards & Perri, 2002; Young et al., 2008). In some of the lists, major depressive disorder climbs as high as 3 or 4 in the causes of disability, while sharing the top-10 with heart disease, cancer, chronic substance abuse, and so forth. Thus, depression is important, in part, because it is one of the most common causes of disability and disruptions in effective day-to-day functioning.

Another serious feature of major depressive disorder is that it is highly comorbid with a wide array of other psychiatric disorders, chronic health problems, distressed close relationships, and problems at work and home. Depression often goes with other problems. The literature on the depressive-comorbidity issue is so vast that it is far beyond the scope of this chapter or book, but there are numerous recent journal articles and books that attend to the issue of depression and comorbidity (e.g., see APA, 2000 & 2013; Angst et al., 2011; Craske et al., 2011; Curry et al., 2012; Gotlib & Hammen, 2009, 2014; Iverson et al., 2011; Kessler et al., 2011; Kocsis & Klein, 1995; Miklowitz & Craighead, 2007; Pettit & Joiner, 2006; Richards et al., 2013; Richards & O'Hara, 2014; Spitzer, Gibbon, Skodol, Williams, & First, 2002; Steptoe, 2007; Uliaszek et al., 2012; Watson, 2009; WHO, *ICD-10* & *ICD-11*, 1992 & in press). For example, depressive comorbidity with generalized anxiety disorder, cancer and heart disease, and distressed marriage is often over 50% (Richards & O'Hara, 2014; Watson, 2009). In summary, depression is often associated with other problems.

Finally, treatments of depression frequently do not last. Major depressive disorder is often a chronically recurrent disorder, which is highly prone to relapse and recurrence throughout the life span. The "relapse problem" in depression is serious and ubiquitous. Indeed, some investigators have described the relapse problem as one of the most difficult—if not *the* most difficult—challenge that is facing clinicians and their patients who are coping with depression (e.g., Richards & Perri, 2010). Thus, depressive relapse is a big problem. Not surprisingly, therefore, there have been ambitious efforts to describe and understand depressive relapse (and recurrence, e.g., Mueller et al., 1999). There have also been major initiatives to enhance cognitive and behavioral interventions, including CBT and Cognitive Therapy, to reduce and prevent depressive relapse (e.g., see Hans & Hiller, 2013; Hollon et al., 2005; Jarrett, Minhajuddin, Gershenfeld, Friedman, & Thase, 2013; Segal et al., 2010; van Rijsbergen et al., 2013; Young, Klosko, & Weishaar, 2003). Moreover, there has been much collaboration for improving the research methodology to study depressive relapse, and for investigating the associated treatment possibilities (e.g., Craighead et al., 2007; Fullerton et al., 2011; Hofmann et al., 2010; Nezu, 2011; Thoma et al., 2012). Nevertheless, although clear improvement and movement outside the diagnostic range is usually evident within six months of acute treatment with evidence-based interventions, relapse and recurrence is more common than not within the first few years following treatment termination. Therefore, improved long-term outcomes and better research methods to investigate them remain an important challenge for the field.

These concerns for improved research methods, and expanded effectiveness studies under real-world conditions, have also grown regarding other evidence-based, cognitive-behavioral interventions for depression besides CBT and Cognitive Therapy, such as problem-solving therapy (Nezu, Nezu, & D'Zurilla, 2013), interpersonal psychotherapy for depression (Cuijpers et al., 2011), telephone-administered CBT (cf. Joint Task Force for the Development of Telepsychology Guidelines for Psychologists, 2013; Mohr et al., 2011), and computer-assisted interventions for depression (de Graaf et al., 2010; Kiluk et al., 2011). Calls for better methodology, larger studies, and longer follow-ups have also been directed at investigations of the pharmacotherapy treatment of depression with antidepressant medications, with these calls for improvement in the pharmacotherapy of depression coming from both medical professionals and social scientists (e.g., Fournier et al., 2010; Gitlin, 2009; Hollon, Stewart, & Strunk, 2006; Kramer,

2011). We wish to remind readers, however, that despite some limitations in the research literature, CBT treatment of depression remains one of the most researched and one of the best evidence-based interventions available for treating depression (Beck & Dozois, 2011; Craighead et al., 2007; Hollon & Dimidjian, 2009). Moreover, although the relapse problem in depression is far from solved, cognitive and behavioral interventions like CBT and cognitive therapy, and treatment-maintenance trails appear to be among the most promising directions for reducing depressive relapse and recurrence (e.g., Hollon et al., 2005; Jarrett et al., 2013; Segal et al., 2010).

In summary, depression or major depressive disorder (MDD) is highly prevalent; it is important regarding its negative associations, including disability, comorbidity, and relapse; it is sometimes challenging to treat effectively; it is very prone to relapse and recurrence, even after successful acute treatment; and—based on the available research literature—it is amenable to effective treatment with CBT and cognitive therapy, along with some of the other cognitive-behavioral interventions.

Cognitive Behavior Therapy (CBT), Cognitive Therapy, and Other Cognitive-Behavioral Interventions for Depression

In this section on cognitive behavior therapy—or CBT—for depression, along with other cognitive-behavioral approaches, we will briefly discuss the following issues: the cognitive-behavioral model of depression; major components of CBT for depression; CBT case conceptualization and planning; therapeutic alliance in CBT; relapse prevention with CBT; combined and multidisciplinary treatments, plus CBT; follow-up and booster sessions with CBT; prevention of depression via teaching CBT, cognitive therapy and associated skills; and clinical guidelines for practitioners who are using CBT and other cognitive-behavioral interventions for depression.

The Cognitive-Behavioral Model of Depression

The cognitive-behavioral model of depression focuses on dysfunctional thinking styles, negative thought schemas, an array of behavioral and skill deficits, the lowered activity and negative affect that are a central part of the experience of depression, and the relentless risk of relapse and recurrence in a chronic, recurring disorder like depression (or major depressive disorder—MDD). The goals and constraints of this short chapter only allow us to briefly address these issues here. Happily, for the reader interested in extensive and long discussions of these issues, there are many available resources (e.g., Beck & Dozois, 2011; Beck, Rush, Shaw, & Emory, 1979; Clark & Beck, 1999; Elgersma et al., 2013; Goldfried & Davison, 1994; Gotlib & Hammen, 2014; Hollon & Dimidjian, 2009; Persons, Davidson, & Tompkins, 2001; Safran & Segal, 1990; Young et al., 2003; and Young et al., 2008). The emphasis on changing the patient's dysfunctional thinking styles covers several domains of the patient's life.

Therefore, the therapist and the patient collaborate on changing dysfunctional thinking patterns and schemas regarding the patient's personal self, his or her environment, and their future. Depressed patients, of course, may struggle with this change process. This is often slow and hard work. But dysfunctional thinking is at the core of the cognitive-behavioral model of depression.

The cognitive-behavioral model of depression also takes into account behavioral and skill deficits, such as low activity levels, ineffective coping skills, poor interpersonal strategies, and problem-solving strategies that are not efficacious. Moreover, the brutal negative affect, which is often part of the depressive experience, is addressed in the cognitive-behavioral model through a determined effort to help the patient become more behaviorally active, more forward-looking, and more realistically balanced about their prospects for positive experiences in the future. Finally, one way or another, the cognitive-behavioral model acknowledges and accepts the recurring risk of depression, and, therefore, some sort of maintenance phase of therapy or booster sessions are typically built into the model and therapy practice.

Major Components of Cognitive-Behavioral Interventions for Depression

The following discussion borrows heavily from the numerous treatment manuals and discussions of CBT that have already been noted. In addition, we also borrow from some of our own clinical experience of 40-plus years, treating or supervising the treatment of over 1,500 depressed patients.

The major components of cognitive-behavioral interventions for depression are discussed in the following paragraphs.

CBT and cognitive therapy for depression includes *individualized case formulation and treatment planning*. Therefore, each patient's developmental history, current circumstances, cognitive styles, behavioral skills, emotional regulation strategies, and plans for the future are built into their own case formulation and treatment planning. The actual treatment sessions are organized and structured, with this individual patient information serving as guidelines, and with the cognitive-behavioral model of depression serving as formulating principles. The process is collaborative, with a constant attention to the therapeutic alliance and a professional, empathic working relationship. Depressed patients often find therapy difficult. Without a good therapeutic relationship, they find it impossible.

Therefore, CBT and other cognitive-behavioral interventions for depression include *planned, careful, and ongoing attention to the therapeutic alliance*. The research literature supports the importance of this emphasis on the therapeutic alliance for CBT, just as it does for many of the evidence-based psychotherapies (e.g., for relevant reviews and discussions from empirical data, see Aderka, Nickerson, Boe, & Hofmann, 2012; Beck & Dozois, 2011; Craighead et al., 2007; Duncan, Miller, Wampold, & Hubble, 2010; Gotlib & Hammen, 2014; Hollon & Dimidjian, 2009; Karlin et al., 2012; Lewis, Simons, & Kim, 2012; Nezu et al., 2013; Richards & Perri, 2002; Safran & Segal, 1990; Simons et al., 2010; Spitzer et al., 2002; Webb et al., 2012; Weissman, Markowitz, & Klerman, 2007; Young et al., 2003, 2008). CBT and other cognitive-behavioral interventions for depression are enhanced by a warm and gentle interpersonal style. It is also helpful if the clinician shows empathic sensitivity and insight. And, of course, it is helpful if the therapist has a collaborative and respectful professional relationship with their client. It would be difficult to exaggerate the importance of the therapeutic alliance for effective CBT and other cognitive-behavioral interventions for depression.

CBT and other cognitive-behavioral interventions for depression include *structured therapy sessions*. Therefore, the therapist and the patient explore, examine, and "experiment" with the dysfunctional thinking styles, negative schemas, ineffective skills, and low activities levels that are central to the depressive experience. The therapist will gently ask questions about some of this material, sometimes use a gracious "Socratic style" of discussion to enhance patient-therapist collaboration, think out loud, ask for relevant data and examples and role plays, and then discuss it some more. The patient may do some of the same. In the best cases of CBT, and other cognitive-behavioral interventions for depression, the patient and the therapist thereby become a therapy team as they work through the complicated picture of the depressive experience—"I'm bad; my world is bad; and my future is bad." In addition, small exercises of skill training and practice are woven into these sessions, just as they are woven into some of the homework exercises that are discussed next. In addition, almost all contemporary cognitive-behavioral interventions for depression also include some "mindfulness training," to help foster more effective reactions and emotional regulation regarding negative inner experiences, and also negative environmental events and stressors (e.g., see Bieling et al., 2012; Hofmann et al., 2010; Karlin et al., 2012; Nezu et al., 2013; Safran and Segal, 1990; Segal et al., 2010; and Young et al., 2003, 2008).

CBT and other cognitive-behavioral interventions for depression include *homework, practice, thought records, and other data-recording by the patient*. For CBT to work effectively, the patient must do some homework. They need to keep some thought records, particularly regarding their own styles of negative and dysfunctional thinking; "automatic thoughts" that tend to be negative, irrational and unhelpful; and other depressive schemas that are personally relevant. It is also helpful if they self-monitor some crucial behaviors, such as their activity levels and interpersonal experiences. And they need to practice some of the skills, which they learn in therapy, at home, and in the workplace. Then there needs to be more data-recording, which is brought into therapy for simple data analysis and discussion.

CBT and other cognitive-behavioral interventions for depression include *behavioral activation*. Almost always, seriously depressed patients need to become more active. This is typically pursued in a gradual, shaping process that takes the patient's preferences, circumstances, and skills into account. Effective activity scheduling usually requires careful planning, gradual change goals, record keeping, and lots of encouragement for the patient's successive approximations to a more active and reinforcing lifestyle. Moreover, once some progress is made on this goal, behavioral activation can be fun. The positive-affect benefits of behavioral activation are difficult to overemphasize in CBT and other cognitive-behavioral interventions for depression, particularly since loss of pleasure and anhedonia are such central features of the depressive experience.

Furthermore, recent research has produced stunning results regarding the power and importance of behavioral activation—both within CBT and other cognitive-behavioral interventions for depression, and for other psycho-social-behavioral interventions regarding depression (e.g., see the following studies and reviews: Dobson et al., 2008; Driessen et al., 2013; Grant, Huh, Perivoliotis, Stolar, & Beck, 2012; Hollon & Dimidjian, 2009; Hopko et al., 2011; Lincoln et al., 2012; Mata et al., 2012; and Persons et al., 2001). Behavioral activation is very important in CBT for depression. This activation emphasis will effectively complement the cognitive-therapy and skill-enhancement strategies that are always a part of CBT and other cognitive-behavioral interventions for depression.

CBT and other cognitive-behavioral interventions for depression include *attention to negative beliefs and schema change*. Negative beliefs—and complex and harmful schema systems—which are often fed and maintained by dysfunctional thinking styles, are focused on in CBT for depression. This is often difficult work. Therefore, extensive attention to schema change in depressed patients is usually reserved for the later stages of acute treatment with CBT and other cognitive-behavioral interventions. By this point in the therapy process, the patient and the therapist are used to working with each other as an effective team; some symptom reduction has usually occurred; practice with homework, thought records, and changes in dysfunctional thinking are well underway; and some behavioral activation is in progress. Therefore, this is a good point in the therapy process for attention to complex belief systems that are unnecessarily negative—and often very hard to change. In addition, if there are still "cracks" in the therapeutic alliance, then they will show up here. Schema change for long-held, negative belief systems is very important in the CBT and other cognitive-behavioral interventions for depression. It is important to treatment process. It is important to acute-treatment outcome. And it is very important to maintenance and long-term treatment success. Treatment effects often do not last. One of the possible reasons is that acute therapy did not yield schema change and the modification of negative beliefs (cf. studies and reviews by: Bieling et al., 2012; Clark & Beck, 1999; Elgersma et al., 2013; Hollon & Dimidjian, 2009; Karlin et al., 2012; Richards & Perri, 2010; van Rijsbergen et al., 2013; Vittengl et al., 2013; and Young et al., 2003). With a chronic, recurrence-prone disorder such as depression, this issue is very important.

CBT and other cognitive-behavioral interventions for depression include *some follow-up care and maintenance treatment or booster sessions*. The inclusion and necessity of some follow-up care, after acute treatment is completed, dovetails with the typical course/recurrence-proneness of depression and the recent research on relapse prevention (e.g., see studies and reviews by Gotlib & Hammen, 2014; Hollon et al., 2005; Hollon et al., 2006; Jarrett et al., 2013; Richards & Perri, 2010; and Steptoe, 2007). A recent summary of this research literature suggests that the following 10 clinical guidelines, for clinicians and patients, may enhance treatment maintenance and reduce depressive recurrence: (1) individualize treatment; (2) have the patient learn coping skills; (3) incorporate relapse-prevention strategies into acute treatment regimens; (4) consider special populations and diversity issues; (5) monitor chronic health problems; (6) evaluate and treat for comorbid substance abuse; (7) assess and intervene regarding the social environment; (8) follow a team approach, and use a cooperative, multidisciplinary-treatment approach when appropriate; (9) consider the merits of a "continuous-care model" of treatment for chronic and severe cases of depression; (10) evaluate the patient's treatment preferences, and then—when possible—build some of them into the treatment regimen. This is research support for each of these evidence-based, relapse-prevention strategies (Richards & Perri, 2010).

Of course, it would also be wonderfully helpful to prevent depression *in the first place*, in addition to preventing depressive relapses *after* treatment, and there are several promising research programs with this prevention goal (cf. Munoz, Beardslee, & Leykin, 2012; Stice, Rohde, Gau, & Wade, 2010; Tandon, Perry, Mendelson, Kemp, & Leis, 2011). In summary, the relapse problem in depression is *very* important, and it needs to be addressed during and after acute treatment.

Finally, CBT and other cognitive-behavioral interventions for depression *often* include a *combined-intervention* with antidepressant medications as part of the treatment package; and these therapies *sometimes* include a combined intervention with additional evidence-based psychotherapies (often cognitive-behavioral interventions) for depression—such as interpersonal psychotherapy for depression (IPT; cf. Cuijpers et al., 2011; Gotlib & Hammen, 2009, 2014; Uliaszek et al., 2012; Weissman et al., 2007), mindfulness-based CBT for depression (MB-CBT; cf. Hofmann et al.,

2010; Segal et al., 2010), and problem-solving therapy for depression (PST; cf. Alexopoulos et al., 2011; Klein et al., 2011; Nezu et al., 2013). The combination of CBT and pharmacotherapy (antidepressant medications) for treating depression is the most common *combined-treatment* with CBT or other cognitive-behavioral interventions for depression (cf. American Psychiatric Association, 2010; Fullerton et al., 2011; Gitlin, 2009; Gotlib & Hammen, 2009, 2014; Olfson, Blanco, Wang, Laje, & Correll, 2014; and Spitzer et al., 2002). Combinations of CBT with additional psychotherapy approaches, however, will sometimes have considerable merit when there are additional treatment goals that go well beyond the standard CBT and cognitive-behavioral goals (e.g., dramatic improvements in close relationships or better coping strategies for dealing with severe-and-chronic health problems). Moreover, the delivery of CBT and other evidence-based psychotherapies via *group* formats (e.g., Compas et al., 2011; Huntley, Araya, & Salisbury, 2012; Watkins et al., 2011) has promise and practical advantages, just as the *Internet* and *cell-phone delivery* of CBT and other cognitive-behavioral interventions have cost-effectiveness and convenience advantages. These Internet and cell-phone methodologies are discussed further in our "Future Directions" section of this chapter. In summary, CBT does not have to be a monotherapy, and there are often advantages—and evidence-based support—for combining CBT with other well-researched therapies and practical treatment-delivery systems.

Clinical Guidelines

These clinical guidelines for CBT and other cognitive behavioral interventions for major depressive disorder are based on the numerous treatment manuals that were cited earlier in this chapter, comments in the discussion sections of the many randomized controlled trails that have been conducted for CBT (and other cognitive-behavioral interventions) for depression, and our own clinical experience with CBT (and related cognitive and behavioral approaches) over the last 40-plus years. In addition, these guidelines are *aspirational and advisory*, rather than guaranteed and certain. There are many exceptions to individual cases, each patient is unique, and each clinician will use the specific context and their own judgment to inform their practice. Furthermore, these clinical guidelines are generated primarily within the context of face-to-face, individual therapy. Some modifications, obviously, would be necessary for other treatment modalities, such as large-group therapy, cell-phone therapy, and therapy via the Internet. Therefore, these guidelines raise clinical issues to consider in CBT and other cognitive-behavioral interventions for depression, in 1-on-1 in-person therapy, rather than rigid rules that must be followed in all circumstances. The judgment of the clinician, and the perspective of the patient, will often modify these guidelines. Nevertheless, clinical guidelines are usually helpful for practitioners and patients, and, therefore, some are provided here regarding CBT (and other cognitive-behavioral interventions) for depression:

• *Always include a focus on the therapeutic alliance in CBT and other cognitive-behavioral interventions for depression.* This should begin with the first therapy session and continue until the last therapy session. This is hard work. It is stressful. And there will be setbacks. You need a strong therapeutic alliance to make consistent progress and to achieve a positive outcome and follow-up.

• *As part of the initial assessment process, do a thorough case conceptualization within the cognitive and behavioral CBT framework for depression.* Also, include an early assessment for risk factors and co-morbidity. Your treatment plan will follow the individual case conceptualization for each depressed patient, so it is important to conduct this assessment carefully and thoroughly. Moreover, depressed patients should always be immediately evaluated for common risk factors (e.g., suicide) and frequent comorbidities (e.g., other *DSM-5 disorders and associated psychopathology;* chronic health problems; and distressed close relationships).

• *Include planning, structure, and collaborative team work in each of the therapy sessions of cognitive and behavioral CBT for depression.* There is plenty of work to do: (a) gentle discussions and Socratic questioning with the patient; (b) review of homework assignments, self-monitoring records, thought records, and trial "experiments"— where the patient pursues a CBT or other cognitive-behavioral strategy, and collects relevant data on it; (c) discussion of depressive symptoms and signs; and (d) review of progress in areas such as decreasing dysfunctional thinking, increasing behavioral activation, decreasing negative schemas, and increasing effective coping and interpersonal strategies.

• *Include behavioral activation in the process and outcome goals of cognitive and behavioral intervention, such as CBT for depression.*

The recent research literature indicates that behavioral activation is very important—and quite helpful—to depressed patients. Therefore, behavioral activation strategies and goals should be developed early in CBT and other cognitive-behavioral interventions for depression should be pursued throughout the acute treatment protocol and maintained as much as possible during follow-up and maintenance phases of therapy.

• *Include some intensive attention to modifying long-standing, negative schemas—especially during the later stages of acute therapy with cognitive and behavioral interventions, such as CBT for depression.* Once therapy is well underway and progressing positively—in terms of progress on dysfunctional thinking, behavioral activation, problem solving, emotional regulation, health promotion, and interpersonal functioning—then this is a good point in the therapy process to work intensively on modifying some of the depressed patient's long-standing, negative schemas. This is hard to do. Both the clinician and the patient should expect this to be hard work, with occasional frustrations and setbacks. This is very important work, however, and it may reap many benefits regarding a more-effective modification of the dysfunctional thinking patterns in depression, and also regarding the prevention of relapse and recurrence after acute treatment is completed. If the depressive, negative schemas are not effectively modified, then treatment outcome will not usually be as positive, and relapse prevention will rarely be as complete.

• *Expect some setbacks and deal with them assertively during cognitive and behavioral interventions, such as CBT for depression.* The course of depression is not perfectly even. It does not usually get worse in a perfectly linear fashion, and it does not usually get better in a perfectly linear fashion. It is an expected part of the process that the depressed patient will experience some setbacks. The patient and the therapist can effectively cope with these setbacks, however, and the setbacks do provide some "learning opportunities," "problem-solving challenges," and evidence-based "experiments" to better practice the strategies of CBT for depression. Moreover, if the therapeutic alliance is strong and the case conceptualization and session plans are sound, then the patient setbacks can usually be overcome. Finally, this kind of collaborative problem solving and practice with more effective emotional regulation will pay many dividends during long-term follow-up, when the patient will not always be able to rely on help from the therapist and will thereby benefit from "learning to be his or her *own* therapist."

• *Consider the merits of a multi-disciplinary, combined cognitive and behavioral treatmentfor depression.* We particularly recommend considering this combined-treatment strategy when the patient's depression is very chronic and severe, or when it includes dangerous risk factors and extensive comorbidity. A cooperative, collegial, team-player approach for the various clinicians and professionals will be important here. And these more-complex treatment approaches, with several treatment interventions combined together (e.g., CBT and other cognitive-behavioral interventions for depression, plus pharmacotherapy with antidepressant medications) can still be practical—through cost-effective treatment systems such as stepped-care models, Internet and bibliotherapy adjuncts, cell-phone follow-up sessions, and so forth. Major depressive disorder can yield severe disability and dangerous risk. Therefore, it is advantageous to consider the merits of combined-treatment approaches in the more-severe cases of depression.

• *Do some follow-up and maintenance treatment, after the acute-treatment phase of CBT (and other cognitive-behavioral interventions) for depression is completed.* The problem of relapse and recurrence in depression is extremely serious. There is a vast research literature on this issue. Furthermore, there is also extensive research support for the benefits of booster sessions and other forms of follow-up care and long-term maintenance treatment. Acute treatment effects often do not last. Clinicians should plan on follow-up care, implement maintenance treatment with evidence-based strategies, and be prepared to welcome some patients back into intensive acute treatment again if serious depressive relapses and recurrences do occur. In addition, this is another area where modern technology can be helpful, with tools such as follow-up assessments via the Internet and cell-phone calls. Most depressed patients do relapse, so this clinical guideline is *very* important.

Future Directions

There are several future directions regarding CBT and other cognitive-behavioral intervention approaches for treating adult mood disorders.

We will discuss the following important developments: special populations and multicultural issues, comorbidity of adult mood disorders with other disorders, clinical health psychology and behavioral medicine, cell phone and computer/Internet applications, combined and multidisciplinary interventions, and cost-effectiveness issues in managed-care systems or economically challenged environments.

Special Populations and Multicultural Issues

There has been some excellent research regarding CBT and other cognitive-behavioral interventions for mood disorders in special populations, which reflect multicultural issues. More work on this important topic, however, will be helpful. An example of strong work in this area is a study by Watkins and colleagues (2011). This study includes several of the issues in our Future Directions section, including a special population: after screening 1,262 clients, the 299 participants randomized to treatment conditions (Usual Care versus Usual Care + CBT) were diverse in terms of racial/ethnic membership, with 22% African American, 30% Hispanic, 34% White, and 14% of mixed or other racial/ethnic groups. The gender ratio was balanced, with 48% female. Most clients were economically challenged and underserved, with 84% unemployed. In addition, 18% of the clients indicated that they had been arrested in the month before treatment began. The mean age of clients was 36. Moreover, this study also illustrates the comorbidity and behavioral medicine issues for Future Directions, since the participants were receiving residential substance-abuse treatment in addition to having concerns about their co-occurring depression, and the residential treatment and community follow-up programs had a number of behavioral medicine features. Finally, this study exhibits several effectiveness-trial features, or what clinicians sometimes refer to as doing interventions in the "real world."

The CBT intervention for depression was an effective addition to Usual Care. The clients who received the CBT intervention showed a greater reduction in depressive symptoms than those in the Usual Care condition, and measures of their mental health functioning indicated significant improvement toward population averages. In addition, clients in the Usual Care + CBT condition reduced their substance use by more than 50% compared to clients in the Usual Care condition (Watkins et al., 2011). Thus, the CBT intervention was a helpful addition to Usual Care, regarding both depression and substance abuse. This is an impressive result, in a large study, conducted under real-world circumstances.

There are numerous other examples that we could give regarding important research on CBT, other cognitive-behavioral interventions for depression, special populations, and multicultural issues. For example, Le, Perry, and Stuart (2011) have conducted promising research on a CBT preventive intervention for perinatal depression in high-risk, Latina women. There is also important assessment and evaluation research that is ongoing in the depression field, which should impact all evidence-based treatment interventions (e.g., see Gara et al., 2012). This is an important area, and more research is needed (also see: Olfson et al., 2014; Siddique, Chung, Brown, & Miranda, 2012; Tandon et al., 2011).

Comorbidity with Axis I Disorders and Interpersonal Issues

Depression often goes with other problems. Therefore, depressive disorders (and other mood disorders) are often associated with additional psychiatric disorders and associated psychopathology in the *DSM-5* (APA, 2013); depression is also frequently associated with chronic health problems, distressed close relationships, and problems at work (e.g., Angst et al., 2011; Curry et al., 2012; Gotlib & Hammen, 2009, 2014; Kessler et al., 2011; and Richards & O'Hara, 2014). In this section, we will give some recent examples of CBT and other cognitive-behavioral interventions for adult mood disorders, other psychopathology, and close relationship problems. We will save the topic of the comorbidity of depression and chronic health problems for the next section.

Iverson and colleagues (2011) investigated a CBT intervention for reducing both depressive and PTSD symptoms in interpersonal trauma survivors. The participants were a sample of 150 women who were diagnosed with PTSD, including significant depressive symptoms, had experienced interpersonal trauma, and were at a high-risk for intimate partner violence in the future. CBT was effective for reducing the PTSD and depressive symptoms. Furthermore, these improvements were associated with reductions in the probability of intimate partner violence at the 6-month follow-up. This study is a good example of CBT being used to effectively treat several co-occurring disorders, in a high-risk sample, and finding improvements across a wide array of outcomes including the crucial one of intimate partner violence.

McFall and colleagues (2010) conducted a large study comparing an integrated treatment program for PTSD and smoking cessation with usual care. The participants were 943 patients in 10 VA Hospitals, with military-associated PTSD, extensive mood disorder symptoms, other Axis I psychopathology, and a goal of smoking cessation. The intervention included several components of CBT, psycho-education, and pharmacotherapy in a multidisciplinary approach. The treatment program also included a consistent focus on reducing depressive symptoms, since 75% of participating patients had a current or past history of major depressive disorder. On most of the outcome variables, the integrated-treatment program was superior to the usual-care program of separate clinics and treatments for each of the problems (PTSD, depression, smoking cessation, etc.). Moreover, this ambitious study is a reminder that CBT interventions can be easily and effectively combined with other interventions (e.g., psycho-education and pharmacotherapy) in a multidisciplinary context.

Versions of CBT have also been effectively used in contexts in which depression is comorbid with severely distressed close relationships. Of course, with complex relationships and extended families, there are several possible targets in terms of who is (or was or might become) depressed. For instance, Compas et al. (2011) evaluated a CBT intervention for families of depressed parents. In the present report, they conducted 18- and 24-month follow-ups of the parents and their now 11- to 17-year-old children, with the study sample representing 111 families that were randomized to a group, family version of CBT versus a written information comparison intervention. The follow-up results indicated a significantly positive effect for the CBT intervention on depressive and anxiety symptoms and on diagnoses of major depressive disorder for the children, although this effect was stronger at the 18-month follow-up than the 24-month follow-up. The impact of the interventions on parental depression was much more modest. Therefore, this investigation is an example of an effective CBT intervention in the context of families with depressed parents, in terms of protecting high-risk children from developing serious depressive symptoms and major depressive disorder. This style of family research, with variations of CBT that are sculpted to the needs of families, is important and we should see more of it.

Comorbidity with Chronic Health Problems and Diseases

The comorbidity of mood disorders like depression with chronic diseases like cancer and Parkinson's disease is well-established (Andersen, 2002; Freedland & Carney, 2009; Gotlib & Hammen, 2009; Steptoe, 2007). If CBT and other cognitive-behavioral interventions can relieve depressive symptoms and improve associated vulnerabilities such as day-to-day functioning and adherence to medical recommendations in patients with these diseases, then this is a very important result. It appears that CBT can have this result.

For example, a series of studies by Andersen and colleagues (e.g., Brothers, Yang, Strunk, & Andersen, 2011) suggest that CBT and its variations can reduce depressive symptoms and major depressive disorder in cancer patients. In a recent study with 36 cancer survivors (92% female, 89% white, 39% employed, and with primarily breast and gynecological cancers), the investigators used a version of CBT that was molded and revised in previous studies to dovetail closely to the challenges of being a cancer survivor—with a mood disorder (Brothers et al., 2011; see Table 2, p. 256, for a description of the intervention). Although previous studies by this research group had focused more broadly on interventions to reduce cancer stress, the present treatment package included numerous CBT components focused on treating depression. Studies in this area do not always enjoy the huge samples of some CBT studies, and thus the authors used an efficient single group, pre-post design (A "pre-post design" is a standard research design where the participants are only measured pre- and post-treatment). This CBT intervention of 20 individual sessions appears to be effective, with significant improvements in depressive and associated symptoms (e.g., quality of life measures) and with 19 of the 21 patients who completed treatment moving out of the diagnosable range for major depressive disorder (Brothers et al., 2011).

In another recent study of CBT-like interventions for depressed cancer patients, Hopko and colleagues compared versions of CBT that emphasized behavioral activation versus problem-solving therapy (Hopko et al., 2011; see pp. 840–841 for descriptions of the interventions;). These versions of CBT are discussed in detail in the "Major Cognitive and Behavior Therapy Approaches" section of this book. This study involved a randomized controlled trial with 80 participants (100% female, 92% white, 43% employed, & all with breast cancer). The patients were randomly assigned to an 8-session CBT intervention focused on behavioral activation versus an intervention focused on problem-solving therapy. Both interventions were effective at improving depressive symptoms, quality of life, and additional psychological symptoms, with about 75% of the patients showing a clinically relevant improvement on these measures (Hopko et al., 2011). The interventions evidenced similar efficacy at posttreatment. Moreover, these treatment gains were generally maintained at a 12-month follow-up, although the behavioral activation intervention was somewhat more effective than the problem-solving treatment at the follow-up assessment. This important study with a relatively large sample and the merits of randomized-controlled-trial methodology indicates that CBT-like interventions have promise with depressed cancer patients, and that the results at posttreatment and long-term follow-up are not always identical.

As a final example for the section on comorbidity of depression with health problems, we will mention the recent work of Dobkin et al. (2011) on CBT for depressed Parkinson's disease patients. The investigators randomized 80 patients to CBT versus clinical monitoring for the treatment of their depression, during 10 weeks of acute treatment. All patients continued to receive full medical care and pharmacotherapy for their Parkinson's disease. The CBT group showed a clear improvement in their depression, at both posttreatment and the 14-week follow-up. The clinical monitoring group did not. Moreover, 56% of the CBT group responded positively enough during treatment to justify the label of a clear "treatment response" immediately posttreatment, whereas only 8% of the clinical monitoring group showed this much improvement in depressive symptoms. Similarly, 51% of the CBT group maintained this clear improvement at the 14-week follow-up, whereas 0% of the clinical-monitoring group showed this durable a treatment effect for depression. It will be interesting to see extensions and replications of this treatment approach with larger samples, comparison treatment groups (e.g., CBT versus other cognitive-behavioral interventions such as problem-solving therapy or interpersonal psychotherapy for depression), and longer follow-ups. Nevertheless, this study is another indicator that CBT interventions for depression, which are sculpted to meet the specific needs of patients with specific diseases, can be helpful.

Cell Phone and Computer/Internet Applications

Cell phones are virtually ubiquitous for adults in the United States, and in much of the rest of the world. (For instance, public health workers in Haiti, following the recent earthquake there and numerous economic challenges, have found that almost all adults in Haiti have cell phones; Perri, personal communication, August 5, 2011.) Computers and access to the Internet for e-mails and websites are not quite as prevalent as cell phones in the United States, but they are very common. Therefore, practical mediums for communicating with clients, sending information, and doing therapy are afforded by these technological advances of the cell phone and the computer. Moreover, "smart phones" combine both technologies. We will discuss a couple of the recent applications of CBT via the computer and the telephone.

An ambitious example of computerized CBT for depression is the research of de Graaf and colleagues (2010). In this randomized controlled trail, 303 depressed patients were randomized to online computerized CBT, treatment as usual, or combined treatment of online CBT and treatment as usual. How well the treatments worked depended in part on patient characteristics, with outcome assessments conducted at posttreatment and a 12-month follow-up. For example, relatively optimistic patients who used approach-style coping strategies benefited the most from those in the online CBT intervention, and compared favorably with similar patients in treatment as usual. The combined treatment of online CBT plus treatment as usual was more effective than other treatments for the most severely depressed patients, however, who also had the strongest vulnerability characteristics (e.g., severe MDD plus a parental psychiatric history; de Graaf et al., 2010). Therefore, this study indicates that online CBT may be a particularly attractive option for patients with optimistic, approach-styles of coping, whereas online CBT plus treatment as usual may be a more-effective option for severely depressed patients who have numerous vulnerability factors.

An interesting example of CBT delivered via telephone calls, with depressed veterans in the United States, is the work of Mohr and colleagues (2011). As Mohr et al. note, several studies have found telephone versions of CBT to be at least somewhat effective for the treatment of depression. These investigators were interested in extending this approach to a challenging situation, however, which is a group of severely depressed veterans in the VA Health Care System, who, because of their locations, must be treated in rural settings rather than in urban hospitals. In this randomized controlled trail, 85 depressed patients—in rural environments—were randomized to a telephone version of CBT versus treatment as usual (at satellite outpatient clinics). The patients in the telephone-administered CBT condition received 16 sessions of CBT over 20 weeks, whereas the treatment-as-usual patients received their usual care for the same time interval via the community clinics. Outcome assessments were conducted posttreatment and at a 6-month follow-up. The results indicated that the telephone-administered CBT was *not* effective in this sample of depressed veterans, compared to treatment as usual. The negative outcome surprised the investigators, considering that their own and others' previous research with telephone CBT for depression had often yielded positive results. They speculate that telephone-administered CBT, without complementary and treatment-as-usual interventions added to it, may not be sufficient for treating severe depression in some rural situations. This may particularly be the case when the participants are vulnerable to depressive risk factors and refractory to treatment. It is possible that their sample of veterans, who were all diagnosed with MDD and significant impairment, fit this high-risk category (Mohr et al., 2011).

More research on this topic is needed (also see the APA guidelines for telepsychology; Joint Task Force for the Development of Telepsychology Guidelines for Psychologists, December, 2013). Adult mood disorders are highly prevalent, they usually cause significant impairment, and many people live in rural areas. Therefore, we need to develop practical and effective interventions for these clients, and telephone-administered and computer-assisted versions of CBT (and other cognitive-behavioral interventions for depression) would seem to be practical options. In addition, although the studies discussed in this section are methodologically strong, not all studies on this topic enjoy these elegant methodologies, and research design should be a careful consideration in future work (cf. Kiluk et al., 2011).

Combined Cognitive Behavioral and Multidisciplinary Interventions

Combined and multidisciplinary interventions for mood disorders—and indeed, for many other disorders also—are receiving more attention and support from the professional community in recent years, with review articles and book chapters frequently discussing the potential merits of these approaches (e.g., Gotlib & Hammen, 2009, 2014; Nathan & Gorman, 2007; Thase & Jindal, 2004). Furthermore, there is a rapidly expanding empirical literature on these approaches with mood disorders. We will give a couple of examples here.

Segal and his colleagues (Segal et al., 2010) conducted an interesting study where they compared a relapse-prevention phase of (1) mono-therapy with antidepressant medication to (2) a mindfulness version of CBT (following pharmacotherapy), or to (3) placebo, for preventing relapse in patients with recurrent depression. Thus, 84 patients in remission, after 8 months of acute treatment with pharmacotherapy, were randomized to maintenance pharmacotherapy or mindfulness CBT (via 8 weekly group sessions) or placebo, and then evaluated during 18 months of follow-up. The investigators' findings indicated that the relapse-prevention effects of mindfulness CBT were similar to maintenance pharmacotherapy (Segal et al., 2010). These maintenance interventions appeared to be particularly helpful (73% reduction in the relapse hazard) for patients who had not achieved a stable remission at the end of acute treatment. In summary, this study included combined treatments and a multidisciplinary treatment team, and the relapse-prevention results for mindfulness CBT were as favorable as those for the most common maintenance intervention with mood disorders, which is long-term pharmacotherapy.

Another interesting example of combined and multidisciplinary treatments is a randomized controlled trial by Craske and her colleagues (Craske et al., 2011). In this large study with 1,004 patients, a combination of CBT and pharmacotherapy was compared to usual care (medication, and brief counseling in some cases) for patients for whom the principal diagnosis was an anxiety disorder, but up to 88% of the patients in the diagnostic groups *also had comorbid major depressive disorder* (the range of depressive disorders was 53% to 88% across the anxiety-disorder groups). The version of CBT that was implemented in this study included 8 treatment modules, and it was tailored to the circumstances of primary-care patients with anxiety disorders, but also reflected the complexity that most patients had comorbid disorders such as depression and chronic medical conditions (see pp. 380-381 for a description of the treatments). The combined intervention of CBT and pharmacotherapy was more effective than usual care, through 18 months of follow-up

assessment, but the advantage in effectiveness decreased as the extent of patients' comorbidity increased (Craske et al., 2011). This investigation is another illustration of the attractiveness of combined interventions, with CBT and pharmacotherapy, in real-world settings that include a diverse array of practitioners and disciplines. Furthermore, this trend toward combined and multidisciplinary interventions that include CBT (and other cognitive-behavioral interventions) is evident in recent treatment programs for many types of psychopathology beyond the mood and anxiety disorders. For example, Grant and his colleagues have recently demonstrated effectiveness for a CBT intervention that is focused on cognitive-therapy components from Aaron Beck's treatment model (Beck & Dozois, 2011), plus standard pharmacotherapy, in patients with schizophrenia (Grant et al., 2012; also see: Lincoln et al., 2012). In summary, we think *combined and multidisciplinary interventions* that include CBT and other cognitive-behavioral interventions have an auspicious future for treating numerous types of psychopathology, including the mood disorders.

Cost-Effectiveness Issues

The public media and the professional forums in the United States (and most other countries) frequently discuss the issue of cost effectiveness. Interventions need to be cost effective. The more cost-effective treatments are, the better. This includes CBT for mood disorders. Therefore, we will discuss a few recent studies in which cost-effectiveness issues, and associated variables, are among the primary concerns that were investigated.

Simons and her colleagues (Simons et al., 2010) investigated the effectiveness of brief training in CBT for depression, regarding a group of experienced therapists working in a community mental health center. The training intervention entailed a 2-day workshop, and then phone consultations with expert CBT therapists during the next year. The workshop included didactic, written, audio-visual, role-play, and interactive instructional methods. The 16, one-hour group phone consultations over the following year were focused on questions about CBT, not on supervision of specific cases. A total of 12 therapists who were novices regarding CBT, but experienced therapists with an average of 21 years of work in the field, participated in the study. In addition, 116 depressed clients participated in the study, with the clients receiving either CBT or treatment as usual (TAU). We should note that the clients were not randomly assigned to the two treatment groups, which is a significant methodological limitation of this study. The results suggested that therapists demonstrated significant improvement in CBT skills, and these skills were maintained at the 12-month follow-up. Both treatments led to significant decreases in depressive symptoms, CBT led to significantly more decreases in depressive symptoms than TAU, and CBT lead to decreases in anxiety symptoms whereas TAU did not (Simons et al., 2010). Therefore, this study indicates that CBT skills can be efficiently taught to therapists in real-world, primary-care settings like a large community mental health center. Additional research in this area will be interesting, including further investigations of alternative delivery mediums regarding the CBT training for therapists, such as extensive audio-visual presentations, computer-assisted training via the Internet, more-extensive use of cell-phone consultations, and so forth. An important aspect of cost-effectiveness for CBT is training the therapists. This study illustrates that a brief training-and-consultation program for experienced therapists can be effective.

Some of the stronger research investigations and review articles that have cost-effectiveness implications regarding CBT for mood disorders may mix-and-match a wide range of issues, only some of which are relevant to CBT and cost-effectiveness. For example, a 10-year study of quality of care for depression in Florida Medicaid enrollees ($N = 42,975$) found that cost is going up (29%), quality is going down (especially regarding follow-up care), and the major factor regarding increased costs is the increased use of pharmacotherapy—both for antidepressants and antipsychotics (Fullerton et al., 2011). The use of psychotherapy for this sample of patients actually decreased during the assessment period—56% to 37%—but there was little attention paid in this particular study to different types of psychotherapy, such as CBT versus the many alternatives. There are a number of studies involving CBT for adolescent depression that have cost-effectiveness implications, but this chapter is focused on adult mood disorders. Nevertheless, it is worth mentioning that several studies have suggested that CBT may have attractive cost-effectiveness implications for preventing and treating adolescent depression, both as a monotherapy and as a combined therapy with antidepressant medications (e.g., Curry et al., 2012; Stice et al., 2010). Moreover, variations of CBT have been extended to other age groups with

positive outcomes and cost-effective results, such as problem-solving therapy (PST) for older adults with depression and executive dysfunction (e.g., Alexopoulos et al., 2011). CBT and PST interventions for depression in older adults are also an attractive treatment option because these older patients are frequently resistant to pharmacotherapy for their mood disorders. Finally, there are a number of discussion articles that are relevant to cost-effectiveness issues, and associated methodological issues, regarding CBT, other cognitive-behavioral interventions, and their variations (e.g., Aderka et al., 2012; American Psychiatric Association, 2010; Hofmann et al., 2010; Nezu, 2011; Olfson et al., 2014; Thoma et al., 2012).

Cost-effectiveness is important. CBT and other cognitive-behavioral interventions for depression, such as major depressive disorder, appear to be relatively cost-effective compared to many of the older psychotherapy and pharmacotherapy options, but improvements and extensions regarding this issue are needed (e.g., see Gotlib & Hammen, 2009, 2014; Nathan & Gorman, 2007; Webb et al., 2012). For example, strong research regarding relapse prevention is ongoing, with some very promising results in some studies, but more work on this important issues is needed (e.g., see Bieling et al., 2012). Regarding the most severe-and-chronic cases of depression, combined interventions with CBT (and other cognitive-behavioral interventions) and pharmacotherapy appear to be common and practical (e.g., see Gitlin, 2009; Hollon & Dimidjian, 2009; Thase & Jindal, 2004). CBT and additional cognitive-behavioral interventions for some of the other adult mood disorders besides depression (MDD), such as bipolar disorder, are usually combined with pharmacotherapy in a multidisciplinary treatment context (cf. relevant discussions by Miklowitz & Craighead, 2007; Olfson et al., 2014). We predict that this topic of cost-effectiveness will receive *increased attention* in the future.

Conclusions

Major depressive disorder is highly prevalent, seriously debilitating, and potentially treatable with CBT and other cognitive-behavioral interventions. A large body of research indicates that CBT is an efficacious treatment for MDD. CBT for depression includes a standard content and structure, which entails a data-based case conceptualization; the development of a strong therapeutic alliance; a collaborative team effort to reducing the depressed patient's dysfunctional thinking; assertive implementation of behavioral activation for the patient; extensive homework and in-session discussions regarding the goal of reducing the patient's long-standing negative schemas; and careful attention, planning, and skill-development regarding relapse prevention and maintenance treatment during a follow-up phase. Based on the research literature and the clinical experience of numerous experts in this area, we recommended some clinical guidelines for practitioners who are using CBT (and other cognitive-behavioral interventions) to treat their depressed patients. There are a number of future research directions regarding CBT for depression, including more investigations with diverse populations; research on depressive comorbidity; studies of technological advancements in treatment delivery, such as interventions via cell phones and the Internet; further research on combined and multidisciplinary interventions; and additional studies on cost-effectiveness issues, which would include further attention to reducing depressive relapse and recurrence. This is an exciting and important area. CBT for depression is efficacious. More research needs to be done, however, and depression remains an important and disabling type of psychopathology, which is difficult to treat with complete effectiveness and full maintenance of long-term positive results.

References

Aderka, I. M., Nickerson, A., Boe, H. J., & Hofmann, S. G. (2012). Sudden gains during psychological treatments of anxiety and depression: A meta-analysis. *Journal of Consulting and Clinical Psychology, 80*, 93–101.

Alexopoulos, G. S., Raue, P. J., Kiosses, D. N., Mackin, R. S., Kanellopoulos, D., McCulloch, C., & Arean, P. A. (2011). Problem-solving therapy and supportive therapy in older adults with major depression and executive dysfunction: Effect on disability. *Archives of General Psychiatry, 68*, 33–41.

American Psychiatric Association. (2000). *Diagnostic and statistical manual of mental disorders* (4th ed., text revision, *DSM-IV*). Washington, DC: Author.

American Psychiatric Association. (2010). *Practice guideline for the treatment of patients with major depressive disorder* (3rd ed.). Washington, DC: Author.

American Psychiatric Association. (2013). *Diagnostic and statistical manual of mental disorders* (5th ed., *DSM-5*). Washington, DC: Author.

Andersen, B. L. (2002). Biobehavioral outcomes following psychological interventions for cancer patients. *Journal of Consulting and Clinical Psychology, 70*, 590–610.

Angst, J., Azorin, J. M., Bowden, C. L., Perugi, G., Vieta, E., Gamma, A., & Young, A. H. (2011). Prevalence and characteristics of undiagnosed bipolar disorders in patients with a major depressive episode: The BRIDGE Study. *Archives of General Psychiatry, 68*, 791–799.

Beck, A. T., & Dozois, D. J. (2011). Cognitive therapy: Current status and future directions. *Annual Review of Medicine, 62*, 397–409.

Beck, A. T., Rush, A. J., Shaw, B. F., & Emery, G. (1979). *Cognitive therapy of depression*. New York: Guilford Press.

Bieling, P. J., Hawley, L. L., Bloch, R. T., Corcoran, K. M., Levitan, R. D., Young, L. T., . . . Segal, Z. V. (2012). Treatment-specific changes in decentering following mindfulness-based cognitive therapy versus antidepressant medication or placebo for prevention of depressive relapse. *Journal of Consulting and Clinical Psychology, 80*, 365–372.

Brothers, B. M., Yang, H. C., Strunk, D. R., & Andersen, B. L. (2011). Cancer patients with major depressive disorder: Testing a biobehavioral/cognitive behavior intervention. *Journal of Consulting and Clinical Psychology, 79*, 253–260.

Clark, D. A., & Beck, A. T. (1999). *Scientific foundations of cognitive theory and therapy of depression*. New York, NY: Wiley.

Compas, B. E., Forehand, R., Thigpen, J. C., Keller, G., Hardcastle, E. J., Cole, D. A., . . . Roberts, L. (2011). Family group cognitive-behavioral preventive intervention for families of depressed parents: 18- and 24-month outcomes. *Journal of Consulting and Clinical Psychology, 79*, 488–499.

Craighead, W. E., Sheets, E. S., Brosse, A. L., & Ilardi, S. S. (2007). Psychosocial treatments for major depressive disorder. In P. E. Nathan & J. M. Gorman (Eds.), *A guide to treatments that work* (3rd ed., pp. 289–307). New York, NY: Oxford University Press.

Craske, M. G., Stein, M. B., Sullivan, G., Sherbourne, C., Bystritsky, A., Rose, R. D., . . . Roy-Byrne, P. (2011). Disorder-specific impact of coordinated anxiety learning and management treatment for anxiety disorders in primary care. *Archives of General Psychiatry, 68*, 378–388.

Cuijpers, P., Geraedts, A. S., van Oppen, P., Andersson, G., Markowitz, J. C., & van Straten, A. (2011). Interpersonal psychotherapy for depression: A meta-analysis. *American Journal of Psychiatry, 168*, 581–592.

Curry, J., Silva, S., Rohde, P., Ginsburg, G., Kennard, B., Kratochvil, C., . . . March, J. (2012). Onset of alcohol or substance use disorders following treatment for adolescent depression. *Journal of Consulting and Clinical Psychology, 80*, 299–312.

de Graaf, L. E., Hollon, S. D., & Huibers, M. J. H. (2010). Predicting outcome in computerized cognitive behavioral therapy for depression in primary care: A randomized trial. *Journal of Consulting and Clinical Psychology, 78*, 184–189.

Dobkin, R. D., Menza, M., Allen, L. A., Gara, M. A., Mark, M. H., Tiu, J., . . . Friedman, J. (2011). Cognitive-behavioral therapy for depression in Parkinson's Disease: A randomized, controlled trial. *American Journal of Psychiatry, 168*, 1066–1074.

Dobson, K. S., Hollon, S. D., Dimidjian, S., Schmaling, K. B., Kohlenberg, R. J., Gallop, R. J., . . . Jacobson, N. S. (2008). Randomized trial of behavioral activation, cognitive therapy, and antidepressant medication in the prevention of relapse and recurrence in major depression. *Journal of Consulting and Clinical Psychology, 76*, 468–477.

Driessen, E., Van, H. L., Don, F. J., Peen, J., Kool, S., Westra, D., . . . Dekker, J. J. M. (2013). The efficacy of cognitive-behavioral therapy and psychodynamic therapy in the outpatient treatment of major depression: A randomized clinical trial. *American Journal of Psychiatry, 170*, 1041–1050.

Duncan, B. L., Miller, S. D., Wampold, B. E., & Hubble, M. A. (Eds.). (2010). *The heart and soul of change* (2nd ed.). Washington, DC: American Psychological Association.

Elgersma, H. J., Glashouwer, K. A., Bockting, C. L. H., Penninx, B. W. J. H., & de Jong, P. J. (2013). Hidden scars in depression? Implicit and explicit self-associations following recurrent depressive episodes. *Journal of Abnormal Psychology, 122,* 951–960.

Fournier, J. C., DeRubeis, R. J., Hollon, S. D., Dimidjian, S., Amsterdam, J. D., Shelton, R. C., & Fawcett, J. (2010). Antidepressant drug effects and depression severity: A patient-level meta-analysis. *Journal of the American Medical Association, 303,* 47–53.

Freedland, K. E., & Carney, R. M. (2009). Depression and medical illness. In I. H. Gotlib & C. L. Hammen (Eds.), *Handbook of depression* (2nd ed., pp. 113–141). New York, NY: Guilford Press.

Fullerton, C. A., Busch, A. B., Normand, S. L. T., McGuire, T. G., & Epstein, A. M. (2011). Ten-year trends in quality of care and spending for depression: 1996 through 2005. *Archives of General Psychiatry, 68,* 1218–1226.

Gara, M. A., Vega, W. A., Arndt, S., Escamilla, M., Fleck, D. E., Lawson, W. B., . . . Strakowski, S. M. (2012). Influence of patient race and ethnicity on clinical assessment in patients with affective disorders. *Archives of General Psychiatry, 69,* 593–600.

Gitlin, M. J. (2009). Pharmacotherapy and other somatic treatments for depression. In I. H. Gotlib & C. L. Hammen (Eds.), *Handbook of depression* (2nd ed., pp. 554–585). New York, NY: Guilford Press.

Goldfried, M. R., & Davison, G. C. (1994). *Clinical behavior therapy* (2nd ed.). New York, NY: Wiley.

Gotlib, I. H., & Hammen, C. L. (Eds.). (2009). *Handbook of depression* (2nd ed.). New York, NY: Guilford Press.

Gotlib, I. H., & Hammen, C. L. (Eds.). (2014). *Handbook of depression* (3rd ed.). New York, NY: Guilford Press.

Grant, P. M., Huh, G. A., Perivoliotis, D., Stolar, N. M., & Beck, A. T. (2012). Randomized trial to evaluate the efficacy of cognitive therapy for low-functioning patients with schizophrenia. *Archives of General Psychiatry, 69,* 121–127.

Hans, E., & Hiller, W. (2013). Effectiveness of and dropout from outpatient cognitive behavioral therapy for adult unipolar depression: A meta-analysis of nonrandomized effectiveness studies. *Journal of Consulting and Clinical Psychology, 81,* 75–88.

Hofmann, S. G., Sawyer, A. T., Witt, A. A., & Oh, D. (2010). The effect of mindfulness-based therapy on anxiety and depression: A meta-analytic review. *Journal of Consulting and Clinical Psychology, 78,* 169–183.

Hollon, S. D., DeRubeis, R. J., Shelton, R. C., Amsterdam, J. D., Salomon, R. M., O'Reardon, J. P., . . . Gallop, R. (2005). Prevention of relapse following cognitive therapy versus medications in moderate to severe depression. *Archives of General Psychiatry, 62,* 417–422.

Hollon, S. D., & Dimidjian, S. (2009). Cognitive and behavioral treatment of depression. In I. H. Gotlib & C. L. Hammen (Eds.), *Handbook of depression* (2nd ed., pp. 586–603). New York, NY: Guilford Press.

Hollon, S. D., Stewart, M. O., & Strunk, D. (2006). Cognitive behavior therapy has enduring effects in the treatment of depression and anxiety. *Annual Review of Psychology, 57,* 285–315.

Hopko, D. R., Armento, M. E. A., Robertson, S. M. C., Ryba, M. M., Carvalho, J. P., Colman, L. K., . . . Lejuez, C. W. (2011). Brief behavioral activation and problem-solving therapy for depressed breast cancer patients: Randomized trial. *Journal of Consulting and Clinical Psychology, 79,* 834–849.

Huntley, A. L., Araya, R., & Salisbury, C. (2012). Group psychological therapies for depression in the community: Systematic review and meta-analysis. *British Journal of Psychiatry, 200,* 184–190.

Iverson, K. M., Gradus, J. L., Resick, P. A., Suvak, M. K., Smith, K. F., & Monson, C. M. (2011). Cognitive-behavioral therapy for PTSD and depression symptoms reduces risk for future intimate partner violence among interpersonal trauma survivors. *Journal of Consulting and Clinical Psychology, 79,* 193–202.

Jarrett, R. B, Minhajuddin, A., Gershenfeld, H., Friedman, E. S., & Thase, M. E. (2013). Preventing depressive relapse and recurrence in higher-risk cognitive therapy responders: A randomized trial of continuation phase cognitive therapy, fluoxetine, or matched pill placebo. *JAMA—Psychiatry, 70,* 1152–1160.

Joint Task Force for the Development of Telepsychology Guidelines for Psychologists, American Psychological Association. (2013, December). Guidelines for the practice of telepsychology, *American Psychologist, 68,* 791–800.

Karlin, B. E., Brown, G. K., Trockel, M., Cunning, D., Zeiss, A. M., & Taylor, C. B. (2012). National dissemination of cognitive behavioral therapy for depression in the Department of Veterans Affairs Health Care System: Therapist and patient-level outcomes. *Journal of Consulting and Clinical Psychology, 80,* 707–718.

Kessler, R. C., Chiu, W. T., Demler, O., & Walters, E. E. (2005). Prevalence, severity, and comorbidity of 12-month DSM-IV disorders in the National Comorbidity Survey Replication. *Archives of General Psychiatry, 62,* 617–627.

Kessler, R. C., Ormel, J., Petukhova, M., McLaughlin, K. A., Green, J. G., Russo, L. J., . . . Ustun, T. B. (2011). Development of lifetime comorbidity in the World Health Organization world mental health surveys. *Archives of General Psychiatry, 68,* 90–100.

Kiluk, B. D., Sugarman, D. E., Nich, C., Gibbons, C. J., Martino, S., Rounsaville, B. J., & Carroll, K. M. (2011). A methodological analysis of randomized clinical trials of computer-assisted therapies for psychiatric disorders; Toward improved standards for an emerging field. *American Journal of Psychiatry, 168,* 790–799.

Klein, D. N., Leon, A. C., Li, C., D'Zurilla, T. J., Black, S. R., Vivian, D., . . . Kocsis, J. H. (2011). Social problem solving and depressive symptoms over time: A randomized clinical trial of cognitive-behavioral analysis system of psychotherapy, brief supportive psychotherapy, and pharmacotherapy. *Journal of Consulting and Clinical Psychology, 79,* 342–352.

Kocsis, J. H., & Klein, D. N. (Eds.). (1995). *Diagnosis and treatment of chronic depression.* New York, NY: Guilford Press.

Kramer, P. D. (2011). In defense of antidepressants. *The New York Times,* p. SR1, New York edition. Le, H. N., Perry, D. F., & Stuart, E. A. (2011). Randomized controlled trial of a preventive intervention for perinatal depression in high-risk Latinas. *Journal of Consulting and Clinical Psychology, 79,* 135–141.

Lewis, C. C., Simons, A. D., & Kim, H. K. (2012). The role of early symptom trajectories and pretreatment variables in predicting treatment response to cognitive behavioral therapy. *Journal of Consulting and Clinical Psychology, 80,* 525–534.

Lincoln, T. M., Ziegler, M., Mehl, S., Kesting, M.-L., Lullmann, E., Westermann, S., & Rief, W. (2012). Moving from efficacy to effectiveness in cognitive behavioral therapy for psychosis: A randomized clinical practice trial. *Journal of Consulting and Clinical Psychology, 80,* 674–686.

Mata, J., Thompson, R. J., Jaeggi, S. M., Buschkuehl, M., Jonides, J., & Gotlib, I. H. (2012). Walk on the bright side: Physical activity and affect in major depressive disorder. *Journal of Abnormal Psychology, 121,* 297–308.

McFall, M., Saxon, A. J., Malte, C. A., Chow, B., Bailey, S., Baker, D. G.,…Lavori, P. W. (2010). Integrating tobacco cessation into mental health care for posttraumatic stress disorder: A randomized controlled trial. *JAMA, 304,* 2485–2493.

Miklowitz, D. J., & Craighead, W. E. (2007). Psychosocial treatments for bipolar disorder. In P. E. Nathan & J. M. Gorman (Eds.), *A guide to treatments that work* (3rd ed., pp. 309–322). New York, NY: Oxford University Press.

Mohr, D. C., Carmody, T., Erickson, L., Jin, L., & Leader, J. (2011). Telephone-administered cognitive behavioral therapy for veterans served by community-based outpatient clinics. *Journal of Consulting and Clinical Psychology, 79,* 261–265.

Mueller, T. I., Leon, A. C., Keller, M. B., Solomon, D. A., Endicott, J., Coryell, W.,…Maser, J. D. (1999). Recurrence after recovery from major depressive disorder during 15 years of observational follow-up. *American Journal of Psychiatry, 156,* 1000–1006.

Munoz, R. F., Beardslee, W. R., & Leykin, Y. (2012). Major depression can be prevented. *American Psychologist, 67,* 285–295.

Nathan, P. E., & Gorman, J. M. (Eds.). (2007). *A guide to treatments that work* (3rd ed.). New York, NY: Oxford University Press.

Nezu, A. M. (2011). Editorial. *Journal of Consulting and Clinical Psychology, 79,* 1–5.

Nezu, A. M., Nezu, C. M., & D'Zurilla, T. J. (2013). *Problem-solving therapy: A treatment manual.* New York, NY: Springer.

Olfson, M., Blanco, C., Wang, S., Laje, G., & Correll, C. U. (2014). National trends in the mental health care of children, adolescents, and adults by office-based physicians. *JAMA—Psychiatry, 71,* 81–90.

Perri, M. G. (2011, August 5). *Personal communication* with M. G. Perri, College of Public Health and Health Professions, Health Sciences Center, University of Florida, Gainesville, FL.

Persons, J. B., Davidson, J., & Tompkins, M. A. (2001). *Essential components of cognitive-behavior therapy for depression.* Washington, DC: American Psychological Association.

Pettit, J. W., & Joiner, T. E. (2006). *Chronic depression.* Washington, DC: American Psychological Association.

Richards, C. S., Cohen, L. M., Morrell, H. E. R., Watson, N. L., & Low, B. E. (2013). Treating depressed and anxious smokers in smoking cessation programs. *Journal of Consulting and Clinical Psychology, 81,* 263–273.

Richards, C. S., & O'Hara, M. W. (Eds.). (2014). *The Oxford handbook of depression and comorbidity.* New York, NY: Oxford University Press.

Richards, C. S., & Perri, M. G. (2002). *Depression.* Thousand Oaks, CA: Sage.

Richards, C. S., & Perri, M. G. (Eds.). (2010). *Relapse prevention for depression.* Washington, DC: American Psychological Association.

Safran, J. D., & Segal, Z. V. (1990). *Interpersonal process in cognitive therapy.* New York, NY: Basic Books.

Segal, Z. V., Bieling, P., Young, T., MacQueen, G., Cooke, R., Martin, L.,…Levitan, R. D. (2010). Antidepressant monotherapy vs sequential pharmacotherapy and mindfulness-based cognitive therapy, or placebo, for relapse prophylaxis in recurrent depression. *Archives of General Psychiatry, 67,* 1256–1264.

Siddique, J., Chung, J. Y., Brown, C. H., & Miranda, J. (2012). Comparative effectiveness of medication versus cognitive-behavioral therapy in a randomized controlled trial of low—income young minority women with depression. *Journal of Consulting and Clinical Psychology, 80,* 995–1006.

Simons, A. D., Padesky, C. A., Montemarano, J., Lewis, C. C., Murakami, J., Lamb, K.,…Beck, A. T. (2010). Training and dissemination of cognitive behavior therapy for depression in adults: A preliminary examination of therapist competence and client outcomes. *Journal of Consulting and Clinical Psychology, 78,* 751–756.

Spitzer, R. L., Gibbon, M., Skodol, A. E., Williams, J. B. W., & First, M. B. (Eds.). (2002). *DSM-IV-TR Casebook.* Washington, DC: American Psychiatric Publishing.

Steptoe, A. (Ed.). (2007). *Depression and physical illness.* New York, NY: Cambridge University Press.

Stice, E., Rohde, P., Gau, J. M., & Wade, E. (2010). Efficacy trial of a brief cognitive-behavioral depression prevention program for high-risk adolescents: Effects at 1- and 2-year follow-up. *Journal of Consulting and Clinical Psychology, 78,* 856–867.

Tandon, S. D., Perry, D. F., Mendelson, T., Kemp, K., & Leis, J. A. (2011). Preventing perinatal depression in low-income home visiting clients: A randomized controlled trial. *Journal of Consulting and Clinical Psychology, 79,* 707–712.

Thase, M. E., & Jindal, R. D. (2004). Combining psychotherapy and psychopharmacology for treatment of mental disorders. In M. J. Lambert (Ed.), *Bergin and Garfield's handbook of psychotherapy and behavior change* (5th ed., pp. 743–766). New York, NY: John Wiley & Sons, Inc.

Thoma, N. C., McKay, D., Gerber, A. J., Milrod, B. L., Edwards, A. R., & Kocsis, J. H. (2012). A quality-based review of randomized controlled trials of cognitive-behavioral therapy for depression: An assessment and metaregression. *American Journal of Psychiatry, 169,* 22–30.

Uliaszek, A. A., Zinbarg, R. E., Mineka, S., Craske, M. G., Griffith, J. W., Sutton, J. M.,…Hammen, C. (2012). A longitudinal examination of stress generation in depressive and anxiety disorders. *Journal of Abnormal Psychology, 121,* 4–15.

van Rijsbergen, G. D., Bockting, C. L. H., Burger, H., Spinhoven, P., Koeter, M. W. J., Ruhe, H. G.,…Schene, A. H. (2013). Mood reactivity rather than cognitive reactivity is predictive of depressive relapse: A randomized study with 5.5-year follow-up. *Journal of Consulting and Clinical Psycholohy, 81,* 508–517.

Vittengl, J. R., Clark, L. A., Thase, M. E., & Jarrett, R. B. (2013). Nomothetic and idiographic symptom change trajectories in acute-phase cognitive therapy for recurrent depression. *Journal of Consulting and Clinical Psychology, 81,* 615–626.

Watkins, K. E., Hunter, S. B., Hepner, K. A., Paddock, S. M., de la Cruz, E., Zhou, A. J., & Gilmore, J. (2011). An effectiveness trial of group cognitive behavioral therapy for patients with persistent depressive symptoms in substance abuse treatment. *Archives of General Psychiatry, 68*, 577–584.

Watson, D. (2009). Differentiating the mood and anxiety disorders: A quadripartite model. *Annual Review of Clinical Psychology, 5*, 221–247.

Webb, C. A., DeRubeis, R. J., Dimidjian, S., Hollon, S. D., Amsterdam, J. D., & Shelton, R. C. (2012). Predictors of patient cognitive therapy skills and symptom change in two randomized clinical trials: The role of therapist adherence and the therapeutic alliance. *Journal of Consulting and Clinical Psychology, 80*, 373–381.

Weissman, M. M., Markowitz, J. C., & Klerman, G. L. (2007). *Clinician's quick guide to interpersonal psychotherapy.* New York, NY: Oxford University Press.

World Health Organization (WHO). (1992). *International classification of diseases* (10th revision, *ICD-10*). Geneva, Switzerland: Author.

World Health Organization (WHO). (in preparation, 2015). *International classification of diseases* (11th revision, *ICD-11*). Geneva, Switzerland: Author.

Young, J. E., Klosko, J. S., & Weishaar, M. E. (2003). *Schema therapy: A practitioner's guide.* New York, NY: Guilford Press.

Young, J. E., Rygh, J. L., Weinberger, A. D., & Beck, A. T. (2008). Cognitive therapy for depression. In D. H. Barlow (Ed.), *Clinical handbook of psychological disorders* (4th ed., pp. 250–305). New York, NY: Guilford Press.

Cognitive-Behavioral Interventions in Psychosis

Elizabeth Kuipers, Suzanne Jolley, *and* Juliana Onwumere

Abstract

This chapter focuses on cognitive-behavioral interventions for people with psychosis, including individual and family interventions. It examines the key components of each intervention, the underlying models, and the evidence base related to outcomes. The chapter first considers individual cognitive-behavioral therapy and cognitive models of psychosis before turning to family interventions, with particular emphasis on the importance of informal caregiving relationships, positive communication styles, facilitated information sharing, improved problem-solving skills, and emotional processing. It concludes by outlining future directions for cognitive-behavioral interventions for people with psychosis.

Key Words: psychosis, evidence base, cognitive-behavioral therapy, cognitive models, individual interventions, family interventions, caregiving, communication styles, information sharing, problem solving

Psychotic disorders are complex and heterogeneous. The hallmark symptoms of psychosis are the positive symptoms of hallucinations: sensory experiences in the absence of a corresponding external stimulus; delusions, which are strong beliefs that seem unfounded or irrational to others; and thought disorder, which is cognitive disorganization apparent in an individual's thinking and often his or her speech (e.g., World Health Organization [WHO], 1992). Negative symptoms of psychosis include lack of motivation; affective blunting; and difficulty initiating movement, speech, or thought (e.g., Foussias et al., 2014). Affective disturbance may arise as a precursor to, alongside, or as a reaction to psychotic illness (Freeman & Garety, 2003; Krabbendam & van Os, 2005). Rates of trauma and adverse life events, particularly interpersonal and victimization events, are high (e.g., Bebbington et al., 2011). Social or occupational impairment is common, and the high cost of care, alongside increased physical health needs, elevated rates of suicide, excess mortality, and social exclusion contribute to the substantial personal impact and societal cost of schizophrenia (Chang et al., 2011; Kennedy, Altar, Taylor, Degtiar, & Hornberger, 2014; Killaspy, Mas-Expósito, Marston, & King, 2014; Mangalore & Knapp, 2007; Robinson et al., 2010; Saha, Chant, & McGrath, 2007), rendering it a globally recognized burdensome condition (Whiteford et al., 2013). The adverse impact, however, is rarely limited to the service user alone; relatives and close others will also be affected (Andrews, Knapp, McCrone, Parsonage, & Trachtenberg, 2012).

Traditionally, medications are the cornerstone of mental health treatments for people with psychosis and the first-line intervention, improving symptoms for up to 60% of individuals (National Institute for Health and Care Excellence [NICE], 2014). However, over the last 20 years, cognitive-behavioral approaches for individuals, for families when there is close contact with an individual with psychosis, and, most recently, for caregivers (NICE, 2014) have become increasingly well-established components of routine care. The most recent United

Kingdom government recommendations advocate these interventions across the life span, including young people under the age of 18 years, as a preventative measure for those who may be at risk of developing psychosis, at first episode and for persisting difficulties, during any period of crisis or recurrence, and irrespective of comorbid substance misuse (NICE, 2009, 2011, 2013, 2014). The interventions are cost-effective by virtue of reducing the number of days spent in psychiatric hospital, at best delivering a cost saving of between £2,000 and £4,000 per course of therapy (Knapp et al., 2014). International recommendations are similar (Dixon et al., 2010; Gaebel, Weinmann, Sartorius, Rutz, & McIntyre, 2005; Kreyenbuhl, 2010), but access remains limited, due to common factors of the prioritization of other interventions and limited investment in mental health care generally, and therapy specifically (e.g., Haddock et al., 2014; The Schizophrenia Commission, 2012). The current global drive, consequently, is the refinement of intervention protocols that hold the promise of easier implementation and wider dissemination to improve access in front-line services (WHO, 2013).

In this chapter we present an overview of cognitive-behavioral interventions, focusing first upon individual interventions for people with psychosis and then on family interventions. For each, we discuss underlying models and the key components of intervention, together with a critical review of the evidence relating to outcomes, the latest developments, and future directions.

Individual Cognitive-Behavioral Therapy for People with Psychosis
Cognitive Models of Psychosis

Psychosis is considered by many to represent the epitome of abnormal psychological functioning, and recognizing abnormality or "illness" in oneself through increasing "insight" is still held to be key to recovery in many mental health settings. However, it is increasingly well accepted that psychosis can be considered to lie on a continuum with normal experience, whereby increasing disability is associated with the persistence and the distressing or adversely impacting nature of psychotic-like experiences, occurring in the context of a complex and heterogeneous biopsychosocial vulnerability (e.g., Linscott & van Os, 2013). Recent reviews indicate prevalence rates of frank psychotic symptoms of up to 20% in the general population, with up to two thirds endorsing similar content in questionnaire measures (van Os, Linscott, Myin-Germeys,

Delespaul, & Krabbendam, 2009). Van Os and colleagues have proposed a continuum of proneness and persistence from psychosis at the extreme, through psychotic-like symptom states, decreasing in severity until presentations merge imperceptibly with common everyday experiences.

The continuum concept underpins cognitive models of psychosis (e.g., Garety, Bebbington, Fowler, Freeman, & Kuipers, 2007; Garety, Kuipers, Fowler, Freeman, & Bebbington, 2001). Just as cognitive models of anxiety and depression draw on normal experiences of low mood and fear, so models of psychosis emphasize the normality both of the experiences that are characteristic of psychosis and of the social, emotional, and cognitive mechanisms that lead to their development and maintenance. Psychosis is therefore currently understood as the end result of a multifactorial interplay of biopsychosocial processes, which will be different for each individual.

Individual Cognitive-Behavioral Interventions for Psychosis: Key Components
Background

Cognitive-behavioral therapies for people with psychosis draw on these models, together with knowledge of the difficulties facing people with psychosis, to adapt Beckian approaches to working with emotional problems (e.g., Beck, Rush, Shaw, & Emery, 1979). A wide range of cognitive, behavioral, and self-management strategies may be employed to promote new learning and change, with an emphasis on facilitating between-session work. Strategies target the key factors implicated in an individualized formulation of the development, maintenance, and recurrence of psychosis. Particular attention is paid to the therapeutic relationship and engagement skills, with a collaborative and goal-focused stance, and a normalizing approach to the experiences of psychosis. The overarching aim is to reduce adverse impact and promote movement toward the individual's valued life goals and recovery. The large number of available treatment manuals and self-help guides (e.g., Fowler, Garety, & Kuipers, 1995; Freeman, Freeman, & Garety, 2006; Gumley & Schwannauer, 2006; Meaden, Keen, Aston, Barton, & Bucci, 2012; Morrison, Renton, French, & Bentall, 2008) tend to emphasize these common components of cognitive-behavioral therapy for psychosis (CBTp), summarized in a Delphi study by Morrison and Barratt (2010). The evidence suggests a longer duration of treatment (16 sessions or more, over at least 6 months) confers greater benefits, although this may vary in early intervention services (NICE, 2009, 2014).

ESTABLISHING A FOCUS OF THERAPY

Identifying a specific and achievable goal is particularly important in CBTp, as people with psychosis have often had distressing unusual experiences over many years, with a long history of adversity. It can be tempting therapeutically to try to assess all these experiences, but this risks insufficient focus on active change methods, given the often time-limited nature of the intervention. Assessing and formulating which initially targets the key obstacles to goal attainment also promotes better engagement because it facilitates assessment-formulation-intervention links that emphasize movement toward personally valued outcomes.

ENGAGEMENT

Attachment problems and negative beliefs about the self and others, arising from difficult interpersonal histories, are very common in psychosis and impede the formation of a trusting therapeutic relationship (e.g., Berry, Barrowclough, & Wearden, 2008; Berry, Wearden, Barrowclough, Oakland, & Bradley 2012; Fowler et al., 2006, 2012). Persecutory ideation can extend to the therapeutic relationship, and therapist behaviors (even a cough, hand movements, or welcoming smiles) may be interpreted otherwise and perceived as threatening (Lawlor, Hall, & Ellett, 2014). Safety behaviors to avoid threat can limit the person's attendance, and voices may warn against engagement or distract the person during therapy. Ongoing unusual experiences, disorganization, negative symptoms, working memory problems, and poorly regulated affect can also impair communication and make the process of engaging with the therapist and the therapeutic approach feel aversive, rather than supportive. Strongly held beliefs often center on an external cause for the presenting problems (e.g., the police or neighbors), placing the onus on therapists to provide a rationale for how therapy may help that is acceptable to each individual. Service users may be particularly sensitive to any sign that their problems will not be taken seriously, and at face value, because of frequent experiences of being disbelieved and of feeling socially devalued and disempowered.

CBTp incorporates a range of techniques for addressing these difficulties. Supervision often involves careful thought about how best to frame the intervention so that service users can appreciate, within their current belief system, how therapy could help them to achieve valued life goals. For example, a person whose beliefs center on neighbors repeatedly breaking into his home and interfering with his belongings, who ideally wants the therapist to help to move his neighbors, or have them brought to justice, may find that intrusions from neighbors are more or less disruptive on different days depending on what else has happened or his own mood or focus of attention. This person may also find certain responses more or less helpful. Drawing on normative models of belief formation and change (e.g., Evans, Over, & Manktelow, 1993), therapists are careful to make "helpfulness" the aim of interventions, rather than necessarily identifying what is right or wrong, "logical" or "just." Therapists need to fit their language, pace, and emotional tone to that of the service user; they are warm, transparent, and genuinely keen for the person to engage.

Therapists try to compensate for any difficulties in attention, concentration, and motivation by being flexible with times, lengths, and locations of meetings, and by summarizing, repeating, and reminding (to help with memory problems), without being intrusive or patronizing. Empathy often needs to be clearly and explicitly expressed (e.g., "That sounds really scary"; "It seems like that was an awful time for you"), as service users may not easily pick up, or may misinterpret, the usual, more subtle indicators of empathy, such as head nodding and concerned looks. Therapists adopt an explicitly tentative and "one down" stance, of being ready to learn from the service user about what the difficulties are and to puzzle together over what might be helpful. Strategies are offered for the service user's consideration, or to try out, carefully weighing the possible benefits against the potential for unintended adverse effects (for example, checking out whether a change in a belief or behavior would feel better *before* questioning it, thereby avoiding accidentally increasing distress by creating aversive uncertainty and confusion). Therapists also take responsibility for the smooth running of the session, apologizing for any rifts, which are not uncommon early in therapy (e.g., *"I'm* sorry—I didn't mean to be unhelpful" or *"I'm* not explaining this very well"), while promoting the service user's ownership of positive changes (e.g., "Sounds like you've come up with a really good way of tackling that"). Therapy most usually occurs alongside medication and with the support of a community mental health team, as many service users have significant social care needs or high levels of risk to themselves or others. However, recent studies suggest efficacy as a stand-alone intervention for those preferring not to take medication (Morrison et al., 2014). With the service user's consent, it can be helpful to involve family members or keyworkers, and it is sometimes possible to use cognitive-behavioral therapy principles in the wider setting even if the service user himself is not able to engage (e.g., Meaden & Hacker, 2011).

STRUCTURING THE SESSION

Much of the usual cognitive-behavioral therapy session structure and content requires adaptation to the specific problems of psychosis. Collaborative agenda-setting may require extra bridging to bring to mind previous sessions, goals, and progress to date. Eliciting in-session feedback includes explicit sensitivity to signs of distressing psychotic experiences or other changes in mental state (e.g., asking directly if voices or other unusual perceptions are occurring, or if the person has noticed or remembered something untoward). Explicit feedback on the therapeutic relationship and interaction is usually sought (e.g., "How has it felt talking about this with me today?" "How do you feel about how I have reacted to what you've said?" "How do the plans we've made sound to you?"). Sensitivity is often needed in identifying key cognitions, as the associated affect may feel particularly destabilizing and aversive for people with psychosis (e.g., "It feels like there may be something especially upsetting about that—how would it be to ask you a little more about it—it may give us some more ideas about what would help?"). Homework may need more troubleshooting, reminders, or more involvement from supportive others, but should be set, as it is associated with better outcomes irrespective of completion (e.g., Glaser, Kazantzis, Deane, & Oades, 2000; Mueser et al., 2008).

CHANGE PROCESSES

As in cognitive-behavioral therapy for other disorders, CBTp concentrates on identifying and modifying key appraisals, associated emotions, and behavioral reactions, but with the inclusion of unusual experiences as an additional trigger. Monitoring forms and diaries may need to be modified to reduce burden, or be completed in vivo, by going into trigger situations together or from memory in session. The emphasis is usually on identifying patterns of better and worse times and building up coping in the early stages and moving to reappraisal and schema work in the later stages. Care may be needed over the term used for cognitions; service users may prefer to talk about "knowing" or "being sure" rather than "thinking." In general, the aim is to reduce the pervasiveness of the external, personal, and threatening interpretations characteristic of psychosis and to create room for maneuver: a change from "the neighbors come into my house all the time, with completely malign intent, and there is nothing I can do about it ever" to considering that sometimes, even if on a very small number of occasions, events may not be due to the deliberate and personal actions of the neighbors, and may be managed, can have substantial clinical implications.

For voices, appraisals of identity, intention, power, control, and perceived rank are prioritized (e.g., Birchwood et al., 2014; Trower et al., 2004). Thinking style may be particularly important in working with delusions, attributional biases, a tendency to jump to conclusions, overcertainty, and difficulty identifying acceptable alternatives that have all been shown to contribute to belief maintenance (e.g., Garety & Freeman, 2013). Other important maintaining factors are attentional biases, deriving from preoccupation, often with the threatening nature of experiences, as well as thinking biases and styles associated with affective disorders (e.g., worry and anxiety, negative memories, and rumination with low mood; e.g., Freeman & Garety, 2014); for instance, those who had received CBTp showed a reduced reaction to threat in a functional magnetic resonance imaging (fMRI) study compared to matched controls (Kumari et al., 2011). Previous traumatic experiences and adversity shape both processing style and schematic beliefs, as well as affect regulation, and psychotic experiences are often either directly or indirectly associated. This makes reprocessing and schema work important, with an emerging evidence base for a range of trauma-focused interventions (e.g., Croes et al., 2014; Ison, Medoro, Keen, & Kuipers, 2014; Mueser et al., 2008; van den Berg et al., 2015). There have also been recent advances in approaches for negative symptoms, building experiences of, and beliefs about the potential for, success, alongside self-compassion (e.g., Grant, Huh, Perivoliotis, Stolar, & Beck, 2011; Johnson et al., 2011; Staring, Ter Huurne, & van der Gaag, 2013). This is in addition to more remedial approaches to (re)learning social cognitive skills, such as theory of mind, emotion recognition, and interpersonal interactions (e.g., Velligan et al., 2014).

Evidence Base

Meta-analytic evidence suggests that CBTp results in small but reliable improvements compared to treatment as usual, with no evidence of publication bias (e.g., Jauhar et al., 2014; Wykes, Steel, Everitt, & Tarrier, 2008). Several studies suggest good translation into routine services (e.g., Jolley et al., 2014a; Peters et al., 2010) and persistence of, or increased, effects at follow-up (e.g., Sarin, Wallin, & Widerlöv, 2011). The most recent meta-analyses support the preventative impact of CBTp as a way of reducing transition to psychosis for those presenting with an at-risk mental state (e.g., van der Gaag et al., 2013). Evidence for cost-effectiveness is good, reducing bed days, even by intervening at very first onset or before (McCrone et al., 2013). Few studies to date have compared cognitive-behavioral therapy to another active intervention: Those that do suggest equal impact but are of poor quality (Jones, Hacker, Cormac, Meaden, & Irving, 2012; Lynch et al., 2010). Effects appear to be stronger for hallucinations than delusions, perhaps because of the heterogeneity of presentation in delusions, and strongest for those with persisting symptoms (Burns, Erickson, & Brenner, 2014; Thomas et al., 2014; Turner, van der Gaag, Karyotaki, & Cuijpers, 2014). The majority of trials have evaluated heterogeneous multifactorial interventions, including work on affect, coping, appraisals of psychotic symptoms, schematic beliefs, and relapse, with scope to tailor the precise content of therapy to suit an individual's presentation (e.g., Garety et al., 2008). This is necessary in trials of cognitive-behavioral therapy for "psychosis," as the range of potential therapy targets is broad, but it provides little information on the important question of "what works for whom." "Third-wave" cognitive therapies, such as acceptance and commitment therapy (ACT) are an exception to this, as they target specific processes for intervention in order to change a person's relationship with her mental events, and consequently their impact on functioning (e.g., White et al., 2011). Evidence to date is promising, and the interventions appear to be deliverable in a brief, group format, which should further reduce costs (Morris, Johns, & Oliver, 2013; Ost, 2014). Another alternative is to select participants with a specific difficulty and target therapy on a particular maintenance mechanism. A developing evidence base suggests efficacy both in changing the targeted mechanism and in reducing problematic symptomatology, with good effect sizes reported for the impact of reasoning interventions on delusions (Garety et al., 2011,

2014); of changing voice appraisals to reduce compliance with command hallucinations (Birchwood et al., 2014; Trower et al., 2004); and of modifying a range of emotional and self-management processes, including worry, on paranoia (Freeman et al., 2011; Freeman & Garety, 2014; Freeman et al. 2015). However, trauma and dual-diagnosis interventions have tended to show mixed results, perhaps because there remains a lack of mechanistic clarity in selecting for these difficulties (Barrowclough et al., 2014; Jackson et al., 2009).

Future Directions

A key advantage of targeted interventions is that they tend to be deliverable over fewer sessions and to be easier to manualize as a disseminable protocol; therefore, they lend themselves to training and workforce development initiatives (e.g., Waller et al., 2014). Pilot studies suggest that such initiatives are feasible and helpful (Waller, Freeman, Jolley, Dunn, & Garety, 2011; Waller et al., 2013a, 2013b). Group interventions may improve cost-effectiveness in delivery, as a number of participants can receive intervention at the same time, and confer additional benefits of normalizing, validating, and providing a supportive social context (Lecomte, Leclerc, Wykes, Nicole, & Abdel, 2014). Computer-assisted, Internet, or telephone delivery may also confer cost advantages with comparable outcomes to face-to-face interventions (e.g., Gottlieb, Romeo, Penn, Mueser, & Chiko, 2013; Hartley et al., 2014). Identifying the key mechanisms of change can inform the refinement of therapies: This work is in its infancy, but developing (e.g., Freeman et al., 2013a, 2014; Garety et al., 2013). Further, identifying those most likely to benefit from therapy and those requiring a different or adapted approach may improve effects. Recent studies have highlighted how an individual's beliefs about her difficulties influence both engagement and outcome (Freeman et al., 2013b; Marcus et al., 2014) and the characteristics both of service users (higher functioning, better insight, e.g., Lincoln et al., 2014) and therapists (better rapport, setting homework, higher competence e.g., Jung, Wiesjahn, Rief, & Lincoln, 2014; Miles, Peters, & Kuipers, 2007; Steel, Tarrier, Stahl, & Wykes, 2012) associated with better outcomes and higher user satisfaction. Other important areas of development include therapies for specific groups, such as children and adolescents (e.g., Browning, Corrigall, Garety, Emsley, & Jolley, 2013; Maddox et al., 2013), people with learning disabilities (e.g.,

Oathamshaw et al., 2011), people with histories of aggression (Haddock et al., 2009), and older adults (Granholm, Holden, Link, McQuaid, & Jeste, 2013), as well as consideration of psychotic symptoms occurring in the context of other psychiatric disorders, where they are associated with persisting difficulties and treatment failures, suggesting specific targeting may be beneficial (van Os & Murray, 2013). Given the focus on workforce development and implementation, the identification of core competences and tools for measuring competence (e.g., Fowler, Rollinson, & French, 2011), together with evaluations of training (e.g., Jolley et al., 2012, 2013), are particularly pertinent areas of development. The United Kingdom extension of the Increasing Access to Psychological Therapies initiative to people with severe mental illness, including psychosis, has afforded the opportunity to develop a competency framework (Roth & Pilling, 2013) and pilot models of service delivery (e.g., Jolley et al., 2014a), with plans for the development of national curricula to inform a national rollout in progress (http://www.iapt.nhs.uk/smi-/).

Cognitive-Behavioral Family Interventions for People with Psychosis

The importance of informal caregiving relationships on service user outcomes is emphasized in cognitive models of caregiving (e.g., Kuipers, Onwumere, & Bebbington, 2010) and psychosis (e.g., Garety et al., 2007).

Many relatives take on the responsibility and caregiving role for service users with psychosis. Thus, informal caregiving relationships can make an important contribution to the illness course and outcomes (Bebbington & Kuipers, 1994). During onset and periods of crisis, caregivers will often play a pivotal role in securing the input of relevant services, particularly at a time when symptoms and formal diagnosis are unclear (Bergner et al., 2008; Fridgen et al., 2013; Morgan et al., 2006).

Engagement with services, treatment gains, and service user symptomatology can be significantly better when service users have informal caregiving relationships (Garety et al., 2008; Jolley et al., 2014b; Stowkowy, Addington, Liu, Hollowell, & Addington, 2012). Moreover, support from informal caregivers has been linked to reduced levels of relapse and inpatient admissions (Norman et al., 2005) and improved mortality risk in first episode (Reininghaus et al., 2014).

Impact of Care

Relapse rates in psychosis can be high, particularly during the early illness phase (Alvarez-Jimenez et al., 2012; Hui et al., 2014; Robinson et al., 1999). The caregiver role can therefore be a long-term undertaking. As part of this role, caregivers will often undertake a wide range of duties to support their relative, including advocating for services; dispensing medications and monitoring their effects; helping with self-care, daily living, and budgeting skills; and providing a supportive environment in which to recover.

Unfortunately, the role can impact negatively on caregiver well-being, which is frequently described as caregiver burden. This is a global phenomenon, reported in diverse populations, including those from the Middle East, Asia, Europe, and Africa (Awad & Voruganti, 2008; C4C Survey, 2014; Igberase, Morakinyo, Lawani, James, & Omoaregba, 2012; Karanci & Inandilar, 2002; Ostman & Hansson, 2004; Tang, Leung, & Lam, 2008; Ukpong, 2006) and across different caregiver-type relationships such as spouses, parents (Jungbauer & Angermeyer, 2002; Seeman, 2012), and siblings (Bowman, Alvarez-Jimenez, Wade, McGorry, & Howie, 2014).

We already know that higher rates of common mental disorders are found in caregivers (Phillips et al., 2009), particularly for those providing a greater number of caregiving duties each week (Smith et al., 2014; Stansfeld et al., 2014). In psychosis, several studies confirm high rates of stress and affective disturbance in caregivers. Approximately 30%–40% of caregivers will report clinical depression (e.g., Dyck, Short, & Vitaliano, 1999). Reports of distress are known to endure over the course of the illness (Brown & Birtwistle, 1998) but can peak during difficult periods such as an inpatient admission and initial onset (Boydell et al., 2014; Boye & Malt, 2002; Jansen, Gleeson, & Cotton, 2015; Martens & Addington, 2001). Research evidence confirms that caregivers report experiencing a broad range of negative emotional reactions, including feelings of loss, stigma, worry, guilt, fear, and anger (Kuipers et al., 2010; McCann, Lubman, & Clark, 2011). Reports of trauma have been reported by caregivers (Barton & Jackson, 2008; Hanzawa et al., 2013; Kingston, 2012; Loughland et al., 2009), and many have found themselves the targets of service user aggression (Belli et al., 2010; Kjellin & Ostman, 2005; Loughland et al., 2009; Onwumere et al., 2014). Psychosis caregivers can report burnout and exhaustion from their role (Cuijpers & Stam, 2000), even during the early illness phases (Onwumere et al., 2015) and at equivalent levels to those observed in paid psychiatric staff (Angermeyer, Bull, Bernert, Dietrich, & Kopf, 2006).

The strategies used by caregivers to cope with their situation and access support have important implications for their well-being (Jansen et al., 2015). Caregivers characteristically employ a broad range of strategies to cope with the challenges of their role (e.g., denial, optimism, problem solving, religion; Cotton et al., 2013). Though debate continues in the wider literature about what is considered the most adaptive strategies, the pattern of evidence confirms that avoidant styles of coping (e.g., trying not to think about it; hoping problems will go away) yield poorer results in terms of reports of caregiver distress (Cotton et al., 2013; Onwumere et al., 2011). Caregivers, similar to their relatives they provide care for, can also find themselves socially isolated, particularly when compared to caregivers from other long-term challenging conditions (Magliano, Fiorillo, Malangone, De Rosa, & Maj, 2006). Moreover, caregivers who report greater levels of social isolation also report higher levels of distress and burden (Magliano et al., 2002).

THE CAREGIVING RELATIONSHIP: LINKS WITH SERVICE USER AND CAREGIVER OUTCOMES

For several decades, the quality of the caregiving relationship has been studied using the expressed emotion (EE) framework. Using recorded speech samples from caregivers, EE provides a quantitative assessment of the caregiving relationship. It is argued that this rating provides a "snapshot" of typical exchanges and communication patterns in the family (Miklowitz, Goldstein, Falloon, & Doane, 1984; Scazufca & Kuipers, 1997). Specifically, EE reflects the degree of criticism, hostility, emotional overinvolvement (EOI), and positivity caregivers express toward the service user, which typically develops as an initial response to psychosis onset (McFarlane & Cook, 2007). Ratings of EE are most reliably measured during a semistructured interview (i.e., Camberwell Family Interview, Brown & Rutter, 1966; Vaughn & Leff, 1976) and can fluctuate over time (Moller-Leimkuhler & Jandi, 2011).

High EE relationships reflect elevated levels of criticism and/or hostility and/or EOI and predict poorer service user outcomes in psychosis and across a range of other health conditions (Finnegan

et al., 2014; Hooley, 2007; Wearden, Tarrier, Barrowclough, Zastowny, & Rahill, 2000). In psychosis, high EE predicts more than twice the relapse or hospital admission rates recorded in low EE families (50.1% versus 21.1%) (Bebbington & Kuipers, 1994; Butzlaff & Hooley, 1998). Criticism, the most frequent rating, is identified as being particularly predictive of poorer service user outcomes (Cechnicki, Bielanska, Hanuszkiewicz, & Daren, 2013).

The importance of high EE relationships lies not only with its predictive links to poorer service user outcomes across many samples but with its association with key beliefs caregivers report about the service user and illness. To illustrate, caregivers reporting high levels of EE (criticism) are more likely to apportion blame and responsibility to the service user for their problems and fail to appraise their symptoms and behavior as forming part of a recognized illness. For example, high EE criticism caregivers may be more likely to attribute negative symptoms as being the result of "laziness" in their relative (Barrowclough & Hooley, 2003; Hooley & Campbell, 2002). In addition, high EE critical caregivers are more likely to engage in behaviors designed to directly change and control the service user's behavior compared to low EE caregivers (Vasconelos, Wearden, & Barrowclough, 2013). Even at first episode, they are likely to believe in the benefits of criticism as a method to effect behavior change (McNab, Haslam, & Burnett, 2007). Finally, high levels of criticism are linked to caregivers with a reduced understanding of psychosis and more pessimistic illness beliefs in terms of its course, timeline, and impact (Bentsen et al., 1998; Lobban, Barrowclough, & Jones, 2005, 2006).

In contrast, high EE (EOI) caregivers tend to apportion blame to themselves (rather than the service user) and perceive their relative as having very little control over the illness experience (Peterson & Docherty, 2004). Consequently, high EOI caregivers tend to actively assume greater control of events and undertake additional tasks, including service user self-care in some instances. EOI has been identified as a longitudinal predictor of burden (Alvarez-Jimenez et al., 2010) and of poorer mental health in caregivers (Breitborde, Lopez, & Kopelowicz, 2010). In contrast, low EOI caregivers tend to attribute more positive events to their relatives (Grice et al., 2009).

In high EE relationships, differences between service users and caregivers in how they conceptualize the illness, for example, in terms of illness impact and consequences, appear more evident (Lobban et al., 2006), and such differences have been linked to affective disturbance in both groups (Kuipers et al., 2007). Styles of communication can also vary depending on EE ratings. High EE caregivers, compared to low EE peers, are more likely to be rated as less effective listeners given their tendency to talk more (Kuipers et al., 1983; Wuerker, Long, Haas, & Bellack, 2002) and convey their thoughts in a less clear manner (Kymalainen, Weisman, Rosales, & Armesto, 2006). In comparison, low EE caregivers demonstrate better skills in being able to extricate themselves from potentially difficult situations before they escalate and defuse situations (Rosenfarb, Goldstein, Mintz, & Nuechterlein, 1995; Simoneau, Miklowitz, & Saleem, 1998).

Running parallel to the body of the evidence on caregiver EE and outcomes has been the more recent focus on service user perceptions of caregiver criticism. Service users with psychosis are able to accurately perceive negative and critical emotions from caregivers (Onwumere et al., 2009; Renshaw, 2008; Tomlinson, Onwumere, & Kuipers, 2014), which can also be predictive of their outcomes (Tompson et al., 1995). Thus, there is evidence that poor relationships in psychosis are important markers for poor outcomes via their impact on both service user and caregiver appraisals (Kuipers et al., 2010).

POSITIVE CAREGIVING PROCESSES

Positive processes also have a role to play in caregiving relationships in psychosis, even alongside negative ones (Bauer, Koepke, Sterzinger, & Spiessl, 2012; Kulhara, Kate, Grover, & Nehra, 2012) Positive experiences have been linked to optimistic beliefs about treatment (Onwumere et al., 2008), greater social support (Boydell et al., 2014), and greater metacognitive skills in carers (Jansen et al., 2014).

Links between positive family relationships and optimal service user outcomes in psychosis are increasingly noted (Bebbington & Kuipers, 1994; Ierago et al., 2010; Lee, Barrowclough, & Lobban, 2014; Tienari et al., 2004). The impact of positive caregiving processes can vary across different cultural groups (Breitborde, Lopez, Wickens, Jenkins, & Karno, 2007; Lopez et al., 2004). Some of the earlier studies (e.g., Bertrando et al., 1992) reported that caregiver warmth was linked to significantly fewer relapses in service users from low and high EE households. More recent investigations, using first-episode groups, similarly observed significantly fewer relapses over a 12-month period when caregivers were rated with more warmth or when service users perceived greater warmth from caregivers (Lee, McKeith, Mosimann, Ghosh-Nodyal, & Thomas, 2013). In prodromal groups, improved service user symptomatology, including social functioning, were linked to caregiver warmth and expression of positive comments (O'Brien et al., 2006).

SUMMARY

Individuals with psychosis can be socially isolated, but many will have contact with informal caregivers who are often close relatives such parents or partners. Informal caregiving relationships make an important contribution to service user outcomes in psychosis. Difficulties in the caregiving relationship can impact negatively on both caregiver and service user outcomes. Reassuringly, positive caregiving processes also impact on service user outcomes, even in the context of negative caregiving relationships.

Family Interventions in Psychosis: Key Components

BACKGROUND

The development of family interventions for psychosis (FIp) was initially prompted by the published links between poorer service user outcomes in psychosis and familial settings (e.g., Brown & Rutter, 1966) and more recently supported by data on the impact of care (Kuipers & Bebbington, 2005) and caregiver attributions about service user symptoms and behaviors (Barrowclough & Hooley, 2003; Vasconcelos, Weardon and Barrowclough 2013).

The current NICE UK guidance for adults with Psychosis and Schizophrenia (2014) recommends the provision of evidence-based family interventions, as an adjunct to routine treatment packages, to families of service users with psychosis who are in close contact for a minimum of 10 sessions delivered over the course of 3 to 12 months.

There are a small number of evidence-based treatment manuals (e.g., Addington & Burnett, 2004; Barrowclough & Tarrier, 1992; Falloon, Boyd, & McGill, 1984; Kuipers, Leff, & Lam, 2002). The manuals differ depending on the emphasis given to where sessions are held, if the service user is included in sessions, and whether sessions are offered as part of a group intervention or with individual families. However, the commonalities of the treatment manuals predominately relate to a stress-vulnerability framework for understanding the development and course of psychosis, an emphasis on present-day (here and now) problem solving, with an explicit focus on reducing risk of future relapse, improving family relationships, adaptive coping styles, and recovery outcomes.

All family interventions are based on therapists adopting a nonblaming stance and positive attitudes toward families. The Kuipers et al. (2002) treatment manual is designed to improve service user and caregiver outcomes via facilitating cognitive and behavioral changes linked to a small range of key therapeutic activities. Some of the primary activities include establishing shared goals between family members; information sharing between caregiver and service user (psychoeducation); emotional processing and stress management; and enhancing problem-solving skills and positive communication styles. The interventions are provided by two therapists and, where possible, will be offered in the family home as a deliberate means to facilitate engagement. Home-based sessions also ensure that difficulties of the illness (e.g., negative symptoms, poor motivation, and isolation) do not, by themselves, serve as barriers to accessing the intervention.

COMMUNICATION

Given the impact of negative communication styles on measures of service user affect and functioning (Finnegan et al., 2014), and the challenges that can be imposed by psychosis during family interactions, supporting positive communication styles between family members is a key therapeutic activity in FIp. Optimal communication styles also facilitate the implementation of additional FIp therapeutic activities, such as problem solving and psychoeducation (Onwumere & Kuipers, 2009). Communication styles that are emphasized include family members talking directly to each other instead of about one another. This serves a number of purposes. First, direct speech can help to minimize negative exchanges and support family members to give more immediate attention to the content and tone of their comments. Direct speech also minimizes the potential for negative comments (e.g., "He is so selfish"; "She is so careless"), replicating negative verbal hallucinations where service users are left feeling isolated, victimized, or humiliated (e.g., Birchwood et al., 2000). Family members are also asked by therapists to talk one person at a time. This is designed to ensure that all family members (and therapists) are able to hear what is being said, including the important exchanges of warmth and positive comments between family members, which will often go unheard when several people talk at once. A final key communication strategy is

that therapists ensure that talking time is divided equally among all family members. Thus, the typical 60-minute session is not dominated by one individual (service user or caregiver), which reduces the likelihood of family members disengaging within a session and subsequently from the intervention altogether.

INFORMATION SHARING

Facilitated information sharing between family members about the subjective experience and impact of psychosis plays a central role in improving understanding between family members, dispelling myths and inaccuracies, and facilitating cognitive reappraisals about psychosis. Psychoeducation facilitates a move toward fewer person-blaming appraisals and a family-based adaptive approach to coping. The psychoeducation process offers a framework for discussions around relevant topic areas, including diagnosis, symptoms, causal models, treatments, and recovery strategies. All family members are seen by therapists as experts in their experiences and are supported in sharing these experiences with one another. Consequently, family members are supported to provide their own views and comment on the feedback from fellow family members and therapists. Information-sharing sessions are not conceived as, or delivered as, "teaching" sessions. If completed well, the process is interactive, questions are answered, and discussions can offer a new way to appraise experiences and effective coping.

PROBLEM SOLVING

Improving skills in solving and responding to the everyday problems commonly reported in families where a relative has psychosis (e.g., managing housework, shopping, daily living activities) forms an important component for FIp. We know that improved problem-solving skills in service users are positively linked to better social functioning and to caregivers reporting greater warmth. Similarly, caregiver problem-solving skills are linked to positive caregiving processes (O'Brien et al., 2009). Interventions are based on adopting a simple and generic approach to problem solving where families are supported to focus on one problem at a time; to specify in exact terms the nature of the problem to be solved; and to negotiate solutions between all family members. As part of their problem-solving strategies and skill acquisition, families are encouraged to make relevant changes and implement the negotiated solutions outside of sessions. The in-between session work serves as a helpful vehicle for facilitating learning and adaptive coping. Therapists have a facilitative role to play in working toward a common goal, supporting efforts to try things differently and reinforcing positive change.

EMOTIONAL PROCESSING

Given the negative emotional impact of psychosis for service users and relatives, families are supported to address their emotional upset (e.g., grief, loss, anger, fear) through different strategies such as active listening, normalization of affective and behavioral reactions, and positive reframing (Kuipers et al., 2002). Relatives are also encouraged to attend support groups and to make contact with other relatives to widen their social networks and access to adaptive coping strategies (Mentis et al., 2014).

Evidence Base

The efficacy of family interventions is well documented (NICE, 2009; Pharoah, Mari, Rathbone, & Wong, 2010). The largest meta-analyses to date, drawn from a Cochrane review of 53 randomized controlled studies in settings across Europe, North America, and Asia, confirmed significantly reduced levels of relapse and readmission in psychosis and reductions in EE (Pharoah et al., 2010). The fixed effect relative risk (RR) for reduced relapse rates was 0.55 (95% CI 0.5–0.6); for reduced hospitals admissions it was 0.78 (95% CI 0.6–1.0); and for medication compliance it was 0.60 (95% CI 0.5–0.7) (Pharoah et al., 2010). Family interventions are also cost-effective (Christenson, Crane, Bell, Beer & Hillin, 2014; Mihalopoulos, Magnus, Carter, & Vos, 2004; NICE Schizophrenia Update, 2009).

Longer length interventions have proved more efficacious compared to brief interventions (Mari & Streiner, 1994; Pfammatter et al., 2006; Pitschel-Walz, Leucht, Bauml, Kissling, & Engel, 2001). For example, interventions lasting more than 3 months and over nine sessions yielded larger effect sizes (Cuijpers et al., 1999; Pitschel-Walz, Leucht, Bauml, Kissling, & Engel, 2004). Nevertheless, results taken from a recent Cochrane review of brief family interventions (of five sessions or fewer), based on four randomized studies, offer some preliminary evidence that brief interventions may help with improvements in family members' understanding of the service user (Okpokoro, Adams, & Sampson, 2014).

Comparatively fewer studies have been undertaken in the early illness phase compared to longer term psychosis groups despite the evidence that service users are more likely to be embedded in close familial networks at this stage (Fisher et al., 2008). Where studies have been undertaken, most have published outcomes on FIp provision delivered as a component within an early intervention program alongside other psychosocial interventions (Grawe, Falloon, Widen, & Skogvoll, 2006). The earlier studies tended to provide mixed findings on efficacy; for example, Leavey et al. (2004), in a study of 106 first-episode caregivers, compared a seven-session family intervention to standard care. Results highlighted no significant differences in service user outcomes of inpatient days or caregiver levels of satisfaction. Linszen et al. (1996) evaluated the impact of family interventions following completion of individual psychosocial interventions. No significant benefit on rates of service user relapse was identified using a protocol of 18 sessions of behavioral family intervention delivered over 12 months. However, subsequent data from a 5-year follow-up indicated reductions to inpatient admission times for those who received the family interventions (Lenior, Dingemans, Linszen, de Haan, & Schene, 2001).

As part of a meta-analyses of family interventions in early psychosis, based on three published trials of family interventions (N = 288), the authors observed significantly reduced relapse and hospital admission rates for those completing FIp compared to standard care (Bird et al., 2010). Recent developments offer preliminary findings on the efficacy of applying family interventions to psychosis prodrome groups (O'Brien et al., 2014). For example, data from a randomized trial confirmed the superiority of an 18-session intervention in clinical high-risk populations when compared to standard care or brief psychoeducational intervention. The results indicated significant decreases in conflictual behaviors, irritability, anger, and criticism, and improved constructive communication styles in family members following family participation in family interventions (O'Brien et al., 2014).

Though fewer investigations have focused on recording the impact of family interventions on caregiver outcomes, we know they can have a positive impact on caregivers, too (Lobban et al., 2013; Pharoah et al., 2010). Reductions in caregiver burden (Cuijpers et al., 1999; Giron et al., 2010; Tomas et al., 2012), increases to positive caregiving appraisals (Gleeson et al., 2010), and readiness to continue providing care have also been noted as positive outcomes for caregivers (Berglund, Vahlne, & Edman, 2003; Giron et al., 2010). The most recent meta-analysis of interventions for psychosis caregivers themselves showed improved outcomes after psychoeducation and support (Yesufu-Udechuku et al., 2015).

To date, there remains a lack of investigations outlining the mechanism via which FIp exert their positive outcomes for service users and caregivers. The work from Giron et al. (2014) suggests that reductions in caregiver attempts to take control of their relative and an increase in empathy toward service users mediated positive effects of family interventions. Qualitative feedback from service users and relatives highlights a better understanding of the illness, recognition of early indicators of relapse, improved communication styles between family members, improved problem solving, improved activity and functioning, and better support for caregivers as key treatment factors (Budd & Hughes, 1997; Gregory, 2009; Nilsen, Frich, Friis, Norheim, & Rossberg, 2014).

Future Directions

Future developments in assessing the impact of FIp include Web-based interventions (Rotondi et al., 2010); applications with different cultural groups (Asmal, Mall, Emsley, Chiliza, & Swartz, 2014); peer-based (Duckworth & Halpern, 2014) and triaged family interventions, which offer increasing levels of intervention, from information, crisis meetings and family work, only if family distress continues (Cohen et al., 2008).

Despite treatment guidelines, access to and provision of family interventions for psychosis remain low (Berry & Haddock, 2008; Dixon et al., 2001; Glynn, 2012; Haddock et al., 2014). Issues identified as barriers include difficulties engaging service users and relatives, reluctance from staff to offer help outside of the service users' immediate needs, and limited understanding from staff about what role FIp can have in optimizing outcomes. Some families, for example, may not perceive a need for support, or they may have concerns about the function and consequences of the intervention. In addition, organizational difficulties (e.g., high caseloads and limited time) alongside a lack of training and supervision opportunities for staff are emphasized (Fadden, 2006; Kuipers, 2010; Onwumere et al., 2013; Prytys, Garety, Jolley, Onwumere, & Craig, 2011). Although evidence exists confirming the effectiveness and cost-effectiveness of family interventions in routine services (e.g., Kelly & Newstead,

2004; NICE, 2009), the transfer of research findings to routine delivery remains problematic.

Conclusions

Cognitive-behavioral interventions for individuals with psychosis, families in close contact, and caregivers have a consistent evidence base for both clinical and cost-effectiveness, with an emerging evidence base for the mechanisms of change that will allow more specific targeting of therapy. The latter is at present better developed for individual CBTp interventions. Nevertheless, implementation remains limited internationally, with particular obstacles to the delivery of family interventions, despite a superior evidence base for both clinical and economic gains. The further development of therapies and the workforce to promote cost-effective and equitable delivery, particularly in the early stages of psychosis, is a current global priority.

References

Addington, J., & Burnett, P. (2004). Working with families in the early stages of psychosis. In J. F. M. Gleeson & P. D. McGorry (Eds.), *Psychological interventions for early psychosis.* Chichester, UK: Wiley.

Alvarez-Jimenez, M., Gleeson, J. F., Cotton, S. M., Wade, D., Crisp, K., Yap, M. B. H., & McGorry, P. D. (2010). Differential predictors of critical comments and emotional over-involvement in first-episode psychosis. *Psychological Medicine, 40,* 63–72. doi: 10.1017/S0033291708004765

Alvarez-Jimenez, M., Priede, A., Hetrick, S. E., Bendall, S., Killackey, E., Parker, A. G., ... Gleeson, J. F. (2012). Risk factors for relapse following treatment for first episode psychosis: A systematic review and meta-analysis of longitudinal studies. *Schizophrenia Research, 139*(1–3), 116–128.

Andrews, A., Knapp, M., McCrone, P., Parsonage, M., & Trachtenberg, M. (2012). *Effective interventions in schizophrenia the economic case: A report prepared for the Schizophrenia Commission.* London: Rethink Mental Illness.

Angermeyer, M. C., Bull, N., Bernert, S., Dietrich, S., & Kopf, A. (2006). Burnout of caregivers: A comparison between partners of psychiatric patients and nurses. *Archives of Psychiatric Nursing, 20*(4), 158–165. doi: 10.1016/j.apnu.2005.12.004

Asmal, L., Mall, S., Emsley, R., Chiliza, B., & Swartz, L. (2014). Towards a treatment model for family therapy for schizophrenia in an urban African setting: Results from a qualitative study. *International Journal of Social Psychiatry, 60*(4), 315–320. doi: 10.1177/0020764013488569

Awad, A. G., & Voruganti, L. N. (2008). The burden of schizophrenia on caregivers: A review. *Pharmacoeconomics, 26*(2), 149–162.

Barrowclough, C., & Hooley, J. M. (2003). Attributions and expressed emotion: A review. *Clinical Psychology Review, 23*(6), 849–880.

Barrowclough, C., Marshall, M., Gregg, L., Fitzsimmons, M., Tomenson, B., Warburton, J., & Lobban, F. (2014). A phase-specific psychological therapy for people with problematic cannabis use following a first episode of psychosis: A randomized controlled trial. *Psychological Medicine, 44*(13), 2749–2761. doi: 10.1017/S0033291714000208

Barrowclough, C. T., & Tarrier, N. (1992). *Families of schizophrenic patients: Cognitive behavioural intervention.* Cheltenham, UK: Stanley Thornes.

Barton, K., & Jackson, C. (2008). Reducing symptoms of trauma among carers of people with psychosis: Pilot study examining the impact of writing about caregiving experiences. *Australian and New Zealand Journal of Psychiatry, 42*(8), 693–701. doi: 10.1080/00048670802203434

Bauer, R., Koepke, F., Sterzinger, L., & Spiessl, H. (2012). Burden, rewards, and coping–the ups and downs of caregivers of people with mental illness. *Journal of Nervous and Mental Disease, 200*(11), 928–934. doi: 10.1097/NMD.0b013e31827189b1

Bebbington, P., & Kuipers, L. (1994). The predictive utility of expressed emotion in schizophrenia: An aggregate analysis. *Psychological Medicine, 24*(3), 707–718.

Bebbington, P. E., Jonas, S., Brugha, T., Meltzer, H., Jenkins, R., Cooper, C., . . . McManus, S. (2011). Child sexual abuse reported by an English national sample: Characteristics and demography. *Social Psychiatry and Psychiatric Epidemiology, 46*(3), 255–262.

Beck, A. T., Rush, A. J., Shaw, B. F., & Emery, G. (1979). *Cognitive therapy of depression.* New York: Guilford Press.

Belli, H., Ozcetin, A., Ertem, U., Tuyluoglu, E., Namli, M., Bayik, Y., & Simsek, D. (2010). Perpetrators of homicide with schizophrenia: Sociodemographic characteristics and clinical factors in the eastern region of Turkey. *Comprehensive Psychiatry, 51*(2), 135–141. doi: 10.1016/j.comppsych.2009.03.006

Bentsen, H., Munkvold, O. G., Notland, T. H., Boye, B., Oskarsson, K. H., Uren, G., . . . Malt, U. F. (1998). Relatives' emotional warmth towards patients with schizophrenia or related psychoses: Demographic and clinical predictors. *Acta Psychiatrica Scandinavica, 97*(1), 86–92.

Berglund, N., Vahlne, J. O., & Edman, A. (2003). Family intervention in schizophrenia–impact on family burden and attitude. *Social Psychiatry and Psychiatric Epidemiology, 38*(3), 116–121. doi: 10.1007/s00127-003-0615-6

Bergner, E., Leiner, A. S., Carter, T., Franz, L., Thompson, N. J., & Compton, M. T. (2008). The period of untreated psychosis before treatment initiation: A qualitative study of family members' perspectives. *Comprehensive Psychiatry, 49*(6), 530–536. doi: 10.1016/j.comppsych.2008.02.010

Berry, K., & Haddock, G. (2008). The implementation of the NICE guidelines for schizophrenia: Barriers to the implementation of psychological interventions and recommendations for the future. *Journal of Psychology and Psychotherapy, 81*(Pt 4), 419–436. doi: 10.1348/147608308X329540

Berry, K., Barrowclough, C., & Wearden, A. (2008). Attachment theory: A framework for understanding symptoms and interpersonal relationships in psychosis. *Behaviour Research and Therapy, 46*(12), 1275–1282.

Berry, K., Wearden, A., Barrowclough, C., Oakland, L., & Bradley, J. (2012). An investigation of adult attachment and the nature of relationships with voices. *British Journal of Clinical Psychology, 51*(3), 280–291. doi: 10.1111/j.2044-8260.2011.02027.x

Bertrando, P., Beltz, J., Bressi, C., Clerici, M., Farma, T., Invernizzi, G., & Cazzullo, C. L. (1992). Expressed emotion and schizophrenia in Italy. A study of an urban population. *British Journal of Psychiatry, 161*, 223–229.

Birchwood, M., Meaden, A., Trower, P., Gilbert, P., & Plaistow, J. (2000). The power and omnipotence of voices: Subordination and entrapment by voices and significant others. *Psychological Medicine, 30*(2), 337–344.

Birchwood, M., Michail, M., Meaden, A., Tarrier, N., Lewis, S., Wykes, T., . . . Peters, E. (2014). Cognitive behaviour therapy to prevent harmful compliance with command hallucinations (COMMAND): A randomised controlled trial. *Lancet Psychiatry, 1*(1), 23–33. doi: 10.1016/S2215-0366(14)70247-0

Bird, V., Premkumar, P., Kendall, T., Whittington, C., Mitchell, J., & Kuipers, E. (2010). Early intervention services, cognitive-behavioural therapy and family intervention in early psychosis: Systematic review. *British Journal of Psychiatry, 197*(5), 350–356. doi: 10.1192/bjp.bp.109.074526

Bowman, S., Alvarez-Jimenez, M., Wade, D., McGorry, P., & Howie, L. (2014). Forgotten family members: The importance of siblings in early psychosis. *Early Intervention in Psychiatry, 8*(3), 269–275. doi: 10.1111/eip.12068

Boydell, J., Onwumere, J., Dutta, R., Bhavsar, V., Hill, N., Morgan, C., . . . Fearon, P. (2014). Caregiving in first-episode psychosis: Social characteristics associated with perceived "burden" and associations with compulsory treatment. *Early Intervention in Psychiatry, 8*(2), 122–129. doi: 10.1111/eip.12041

Boye, B., & Malt, U. F. (2002). Stress response symptoms in relatives of acutely admitted psychotic patients: A pilot study. *Nordic Journal of Psychiatry, 56*(4), 253–260. doi: 10.1080/08039480260242732

Breitborde, N. J. K., Lopez, S. R., & Kopelowicz, A. (2010). Expressed emotion and health outcomes among Mexican-Americans with schizophrenia and their caregiving relatives. *Journal of Nervous and Mental Disease, 198*, 105–109.

Breitborde, N. J., Lopez, S. R., Wickens, T. D., Jenkins, J. H., & Karno, M. (2007). Toward specifying the nature of the relationship between expressed emotion and schizophrenic relapse: The utility of curvilinear models. *International Journal of Methods in Psychiatric Research, 16*(1), 1–10.

Brown, G. W., & Rutter, M. (1966). The measurement of family activities and relationships: A methodological study. *Human Relations, 19*(3), 241–263. doi: 10.1177/001872676601900301

Brown, S., & Birtwistle, J. (1998). People with schizophrenia and their families. Fifteen-year outcome. *British Journal of Psychiatry, 173*, 139–144.

Browning, S., Corrigall, R., Garety, P., Emsley, R., & Jolley, S. (2013). Psychological interventions for adolescent psychosis: A pilot controlled trial in routine care. *European Psychiatry, 28*(7), 423–426.

Budd, R. J., & Hughes, I. C. T. (1997). What do relatives of people with schizophrenia find helpful about family intervention? *Schizophrenia Bulletin, 23*(2), 341–347.

Burns, A. M., Erickson, D. H., & Brenner, C. A. (2014). Cognitive-behavioral therapy for medication-resistant psychosis: A meta-analytic review. *Psychiatric Services,* doi: 10.1176/appi.ps.201300213

Butzlaff, R. L., & Hooley, J. M. (1998). Expressed emotion and psychiatric relapse: A meta-analysis. *Archives of General Psychiatry, 55*(6), 547–552.

Caring for Carers (C4C) survey, LUCAS Centre for Care Research, September 2014.

Cechnicki, A., Bielanska, A., Hanuszkiewicz, I., & Daren, A. (2013). The predictive validity of expressed emotions (EE) in schizophrenia. A 20-year prospective study. *Journal of Psychiatric Research, 47*(2), 208–214. doi: 10.1016/j.jpsychires.2012.10.004

Chang, C-K., Hayes, R. D., Perera, G., Broadbent, M. T. M., Fernandes, A. C., Lee, W. E., . . . Stewart, R. (2011). Life expectancy at birth for people with serious mental illness and other major disorders from a secondary mental health care case register in London. *PLoS ONE, 6*(5), e19590. doi: 10.1371/journal.pone.0019590

Christenson, J. D., Crane, D. R., Bell, K. M., Beer, A. R., & Hillin, H. H. (2014). Family intervention and health care costs for Kansas medicaid patients with schizophrenia. *Journal of Marital and Family Therapy, 40*(3), 272–286. doi: 10.1111/jmft.12021

Cohen, S. P., Christo, P. J., Wang, S., Chen, L., Stojanovic, M. P., Shields, C. H., & Mao, J. (2008). The effect of opioid dose and treatment duration on the perception of a painful standardized clinical stimulus. *Regional Anesthesia and Pain Medicine, 33*(3), 199–206. doi: 10.1016/j.rapm.2007.10.009

Cotton, S. M., McCann, T. V., Gleeson, J. F., Crisp, K., Murphy, B. P., & Lubman, D. I. (2013). Coping strategies in carers of young people with a first episode of psychosis. *Schizophrenia Research, 146*(1–3), 118–124. doi: 10.1016/j.schres.2013.02.008

Croes, C. F., van Grunsven, R., Staring, A. B., van den Berg, D. P., de Jongh, A., & van der Gaag, M. (2014). [Imagery in psychosis: EMDR as a new intervention in the treatment of delusions and auditory hallucinations]. *Tijdschr Psychiatr, 56*(9), 568–576.

Cuijpers, P. (1999). The effects of family intervention on relatives' burden: A meta analysis. *Journal of Mental Health, 8,* 275–285.

Cuijpers, P., & Stam, H. (2000). Burnout among relatives of psychiatric patients attending psychoeducational support groups. *Psychiatric Services, 51*(3), 375–379. doi: 10.1176/appi.ps.51.3.375

Dixon, L., McFarlane, W. R., Lefley, H., Lucksted, A., Cohen, M., Falloon, I., & Sondheimer, D. (2001). Evidence-based practices for services to families of people with psychiatric disabilities. *Psychiatric Services, 52,* 903–910.

Dixon, L. B., Dickerson, F., Bellack, A. S., Bennett, M., Dickinson, D., Goldberg, R. W., . . . Kreyenbuhl, J. (2010). The 2009 Schizophrenia PORT psychosocial treatment recommendations and summary statements. *Schizophrenia Bulletin, 36,* 48–70.

Duckworth, K., & Halpern, L. (2014). Peer support and peer-led family support for persons living with schizophrenia. *Current Opinion in Psychiatry, 27*(3), 216–221. doi: 10.1097/YCO.0000000000000051

Dyck, D. G., Short, R., & Vitaliano, P. P. (1999). Predictors of burden and infectious illness in schizophrenia caregivers. *Psychosomatic Medicine, 61*(4), 411–419.

Evans, J. S., Over, D. E., & Manktelow, K. I., (1993). Reasoning, decision making and rationality. *Cognition, 49*(1–2), 165–187.

Fadden, G. (2006). Training and disseminating family interventions for schizophrenia: Developing family intervention skills with multi-disciplinary groups. *Journal of Family Therapy, 28*(1), 23–38. doi: 10.1111/j.1467-6427.2006.00335.x

Falloon, I. R. H., Boyd, J. L., & McGill, C. W. (1984). *Family care of schizophrenia.* New York: Guildford Press.

Finnegan, D., Onwumere, J., Green, C., Freeman, D., Garety, P. & Kuipers, E. (2014). Negative communication in psychosis: Understanding pathways to poorer patient outcomes. *Journal of Nervous and Mental Disease, 202*(11), 829–832. doi: 10.1097/NMD.0000000000000204

Fisher, H., Theodore, K., Power, P., Chisholm, B., Fuller, J., Marlowe, K., & Johnson, S. (2008). Routine evaluation in first episode psychosis services: Feasibility and results from the MiData project. *Social Psychiatry and Psychiatric Epidemiology, 43*(12), 960–967. doi: 10.1007/s00127-008-0386-1

Foussias, G., Siddiqui, I., Fervaha, G., Agid, O., & Remington G. (2014). Dissecting negative symptoms in schizophrenia: Opportunities for translation into new treatments. *Journal of Psychopharmacology,* pii: 0269881114562092. [Epub ahead of print]

Fowler, D., Freeman, D., Smith, B., Kuipers, E., Bebbington, P., Bashforth, H., . . . Garety, P. (2006). The Brief Core Schema Scales (BCSS): Psychometric properties and associations with paranoia and grandiosity in non-clinical and psychosis samples. *Psychological Medicine, 36*(6), 749–759.

Fowler, D., Garety, P., & Kuipers, E. (1995). *Cognitive behaviour therapy for psychosis: theory and practice.* Chichester, UK: John Wiley and Sons.

Fowler, D., Rollinson, R., & French, P. (2011). Adherence and competence assessment in studies of CBT for psychosis: Current status and future directions. *Epidemiology and Psychiatric Sciences, 20,* 121–126.

Fowler, D. J., Hodgkins, P., Garety, D., Freeman, E., Kuipers, G., Dunn, B., . . . Bebbington, P. E. (2012). Negative cognition, depressed mood, and paranoia: A longitudinal pathway analysis using structural equation modeling. *Schizophrenia Bulletin, 38*(5), 1063–1073. doi: 10.1093/schbul/sbr019

Freeman, D. (2011). Improving cognitive treatments for delusions. *Schizophrenia Research, 132*(2–3), 135–139.

Freeman, D., Dunn, G., Fowler, D., Bebbington, P., Kuipers, E., Emsley, R., . . . Garety, P. (2013a). Current paranoid thinking in patients with delusions: the presence of cognitive-affective biases. *Schizophrenia Bulletin, 39*(6), 1281–1287. doi: 10.1093/schbul/sbs145

Freeman, D., Dunn, G., Garety, P., Weinman, J., Kuipers, E., Fowler, D., . . . Bebbington, P. (2013b). Patients' beliefs about the causes, persistence and control of psychotic experiences predict take-up of effective cognitive behaviour therapy for psychosis. *Psychological Medicine, 43*(2), 269–277. doi: 10.1017/S0033291712001225

Freeman, D., Emsley, R., Dunn, G., Fowler, D., Bebbington, P., Kuipers, E., . . . Garety, P. (2014). The stress of the street for patients with persecutory delusions: A test of the symptomatic and psychological effects of going outside into a busy urban area. *Schizophrenia Bulletin,* pii: sbu173 [Epub ahead of print]

Freeman, D., Freeman, J., & Garety, P. (2006). *Overcoming paranoid and suspicious thoughts.* London: Constable Robinson.

Freeman, D., & Garety, P. (2014). Advances in understanding and treating persecutory delusions: A review. *Social Psychiatry and Psychiatric Epidemiology, 49*(8), 1179–1189. doi: 10.1007/s00127-014-0928-7

Freeman, D., & Garety, P. A. (2003). Connecting neurosis and psychosis: The direct influence of emotion on delusions and hallucinations. *Behaviour Research and Therapy*, *41*, 923–947.

Freeman D, Dunn G, Startup H, Pugh K, Cordwell J, Mander H,. . .. Kingdon, D. (2015). An explanatory randomised controlled trial testing the effects of cognitive behaviour therapy for worry on persecutory delusions in psychosis: the Worry Intervention Trial (WIT). *Lancet Psychiatry*, *2*, 305–313.

Fridgen, G. J., Aston, J., Gschwandtner, U., Pflueger, M., Zimmermann, R., Studerus, E., . . . Riecher-Rossler, A. (2013). Help-seeking and pathways to care in the early stages of psychosis. *Social Psychiatry and Psychiatric Epidemiology*, *48*(7), 1033–1043. doi: 10.1007/s00127-012-0628-0

Gaebel, W., Weinmann, S., Sartorius, N., Rutz, W., & McIntyre, J. S. (2005). Schizophrenia practice guidelines: International survey and comparison. *British Journal of Psychiatry*, *187*, 248–255.

Garety, P. A., Bebbington, P., Fowler, D., Freeman, D., & Kuipers, E. (2007). Implications for neurobiological research of cognitive models of psychosis: A theoretical paper. *Psychological Medicine*, *37*(10), 1377–1391. doi: 10.1017/S003329170700013X

Garety, P. A., Fowler, D. G., Freeman, D., Bebbington, P., Dunn, G., & Kuipers, E. (2008). Cognitive–behavioural therapy and family intervention for relapse prevention and symptom reduction in psychosis: Randomised controlled trial. *British Journal of Psychiatry*, *192*(6), 412–423. doi: 10.1192/bjp.bp.107.043570

Garety, P. A., & Freeman, D. (2013). The past and future of delusions research: From the inexplicable to the treatable. *British Journal of Psychiatry*, *203*, 327–333.

Garety, P. A., Freeman, D., Jolley, S., Ross, K., Waller, H., & Dunn, G. (2011). Jumping to conclusions: The psychology of delusional reasoning. *Advances in Psychiatric Treatment*, *17*, 332–339.

Garety, P. A., Gittins, M., Jolley, S., Bebbington, P., Dunn, G., Kuipers, E., . . . Freeman, D. (2013). Differences in cognitive and emotional processes between persecutory and grandiose delusions. *Schizophrenia Bulletin*, *39*, 629–639.

Garety, P. A., Kuipers, E., Fowler, D., Freeman, D., & Bebbington, P. E. (2001). A cognitive model of the positive symptoms of psychosis. *Psychological Medicine*, *31*, 189–195.

Garety, P. A., Waller, H., Emsley, R., Jolley, S., Kuipers, E., Bebbington, P., . . . Freeman, D. (2014). Cognitive mechanisms of change in delusions: An experimental investigation targeting reasoning to effect change in paranoia. *Schizophrenia Bulletin*, *41*(2), 400–410.

Giron, M., Fernandez-Yanez, A., Mana-Alvarenga, S., Molina-Habas, A., Nolasco, A., & Gomez-Beneyto, M. (2010). Efficacy and effectiveness of individual family intervention on social and clinical functioning and family burden in severe schizophrenia: A 2-year randomized controlled study. *Psychological Medicine*, *40*(1), 73–84. doi: 10.1017/S0033291709006126

Giron, M., Nova-Fernandez, F., Mana-Alvarenga, S., Nolasco, A., Molina-Habas, A., Fernandez-Yanez, A., . . . Gomez-Beneyto, M. (2014). How does family intervention improve the outcome of people with schizophrenia? *Social Psychiatry and Psychiatric Epidemiology*, *50*(3), 379–387. doi: 10.1007/s00127-014-0942-9

Glaser, N., Kazantzis, N., Deane, F., & Oades, L. (2000). Critical issues in using homework assignments within cognitive-behavioral therapy for schizophrenia. *Journal of Rational-Emotive and Cognitive-Behavior Therapy*, *18*, 247–261.

Gleeson, J. F., Cotton, S. M., Alvarez-Jimenez, M., Wade, D., Crisp, K., Newman, B., . . . McGorry, P. D. (2010). Family outcomes from a randomized control trial of relapse prevention therapy in first-episode psychosis. *Journal of Clinical Psychiatry*, *71*(4), 475–483. doi: 10.4088/JCP.08m04672yel

Glynn, S. M. (2012). Family interventions in schizophrenia: Promise and pitfalls over 30 years. *Current Psychiatry Reports*, *14*(3), 237–243. doi: 10.1007/s11920-012-0265-z

Gottlieb, J. D., Romeo, K. H., Penn, D. L., Mueser, K. T., & Chiko, B. P. (2013). Web-based cognitive-behavioral therapy for auditory hallucinations in persons with psychosis: A pilot study. *Schizophrenia Research*, *145*(1–3), 82–87. doi: 10.1016/j.schres.2013.01.002

Granholm, E., Holden, J., Link, P. C., McQuaid, J. R., & Jeste, D. V. (2013). Randomized controlled trial of cognitive behavioral social skills training for older consumers with schizophrenia: Defeatist performance attitudes and functional outcome. *American Journal of Geriatric Psychiatry*, *21*(3), 251–262. doi: 10.1016/j.jagp.2012.10.014

Grant, P. M., Huh, G. A., Perivoliotis, D., Stolar, N. M., & Beck, A. T. (2011). Randomized trial to evaluate the efficacy of cognitive therapy for low-functioning patients with schizophrenia. *Archives of General Psychiatry*, *69*, 121–127.

Grawe, R. W., Falloon, I. R., Widen, J. H., & Skogvoll, E. (2006). Two years of continued early treatment for recent-onset schizophrenia: A randomised controlled study. *Acta Psychiatrica Scandinavica*, *114*(5), 328–336. doi: 10.1111/j.1600-0447.2006.00799.x

Gregory, M. (2009). Why are family interventions important? A family member perspective. In F. Lobban & C. Barrowclough (Eds.), *A casebook of family interventions in psychosis* (pp. 3–19). London: Wiley.

Grice, S. J., Kuipers, E., Bebbington, P., Dunn, G., Fowler, D., Freeman, D., & Garety, P. (2009). Carers' attributions about positive events in psychosis relate to expressed emotion. *Behaviour Research and Therapy*, *47*(9), 783–789.

Gumley, A. I., & Schwannauer, M. (2006). Staying well after psychosis: A cognitive interpersonal approach to recovery and relapse prevention. Chichester, UK: Wiley.

Haddock, G., Barrowclough, C., Shaw, J. J., Dunn, G., Novaco, R. W., & Tarrier, N. (2009). Cognitive-behavioural therapy v. social activity therapy for people with psychosis and a history of violence: Randomised controlled trial. *British Journal of Psychiatry*, *194*, 152–157.

Haddock, G., Eisner, E., Boone, C., Davies, G., Coogan, C., & Barrowclough, C. (2014). An investigation of the implementation of NICE-recommended CBT interventions for people with schizophrenia. *Journal of Mental Health*, *23*(4), 162–165. doi: 10.3109/09638237.2013.869571

Hanzawa, S., Bae, J. K., Bae, Y. J., Chae, M. H., Tanaka, H., Nakane, H., . . . Nakane, Y. (2013). Psychological impact on caregivers traumatized by the violent behavior of a family member with schizophrenia. *Asian Journal of Psychiatry*, *6*(1), 46–51. doi: 10.1016/j.ajp.2012.08.009

Hartley, S., Scarratt, P., Bucci, S., Kelly, J., Mulligan, J., Neil, S. T., . . . Haddock, G. (2014). Assessing therapist adherence to recovery-focused cognitive behavioural therapy for psychosis delivered by telephone with support from a self-help guide: psychometric evaluations of a new fidelity scale. ROSTA. Alliance important again. *Behavioural and Cognitive Psychotherapy*, 42(4), 435–451.

Hooley, J. M. (2007). Expressed emotion and relapse of psychopathology. *Annual Review of Clinical Psychology*, 3, 329–352. doi: 10.1146/annurev.clinpsy.2.022305.095236

Hooley, J. M., & Campbell, C. (2002). Control and controllability: Beliefs and behaviour in high and low expressed emotion relatives. *Psychological Medicine*, 32(6), 1091–1099.

Hui, C. L., Chang, W. C., Chan, S. K., Lee, E. H., Tam, W. W., Lai, D. C., & Chen, E. Y. (2014). Early intervention and evaluation for adult-onset psychosis: The JCEP study rationale and design. *Early Intervention in Psychiatry*, 8(3), 261–268. doi: 10.1111/eip.12034

Ierago, L., Malsol, C., Singeo, T., Kishigawa, Y., Blailes, F., Ord, L., & Ngiralmau, H. (2010). Adoption, family relations and psychotic symptoms among Palauan adolescents who are genetically at risk for developing schizophrenia. *Social Psychiatry and Psychiatric Epidemiology*, 45(12), 1105–1114. doi: 10.1007/s00127-009-0154-x

Igberase, O. O., Morakinyo, O., Lawani, A. O., James, B. O., & Omoaregba, J. O. (2012). Burden of care among relatives of patients with schizophrenia in midwestern Nigeria. *International Journal of Social Psychiatry*, 58(2), 131–137. doi: 10.1177/0020764010387544

Ison, R., Medoro, L., Keen, N., & Kuipers, E. (2014). The use of rescripting imagery for people with psychosis who hear voices. *Behavioural and Cognitive Psychotherapy*, 42(2), 129–142.

Jackson, C., Trower, P., Reid, I., Smith, J., Hall, M., Townend, M., Barton, K., & Birchwood, M. (2009). Improving psychological adjustment following a first episode of psychosis: A randomised controlled trial of cognitive therapy to reduce post psychotic trauma symptoms. *Behaviour Research and Therapy*, 47, 454–462.

Jansen, J. E., Gleeson, J., & Cotton, S. (2015). Towards a better understanding of caregiver distress in early psychosis: A systematic review of the psychological factors involved. *Clinical Psychology Review*, 35, 55–66.

Jansen, J. E., Lysaker, P. H., Harder, S., Haahr, U. H., Lyse, H. G., Pedersen, M. B., & Simonsen, E. (2014). Positive and negative caregiver experiences in first-episode psychosis: Emotional overinvolvement, wellbeing and metacognition. *Psychology and Psychotherapy*, 87(3), 298–310. doi: 10.1111/papt.12014

Jauhar, S., McKenna, P. J., Radua, J., Fung, E., Salvador, R., & Laws, K. R. (2014). Cognitive behavioural therapy for the symptoms of schizophrenia: Systematic review and meta-analysis with examination of potential bias. *British Journal of Psychiatry*, 204, 20–29.

Johnson, D. P., Penn, D. L., Fredrickson, B. L., Kring, A. M., Meyer, P. S., Catalino, L. I., & Brantley, M. (2011). A pilot study of loving-kindness meditation for the negative symptoms of schizophrenia. *Schizophrenia Research*, 129, 137–140.

Jolley, S., Ferner, H., Bebbington, P., Garety, P., Dunn, G., Freeman, D., . . . Kuipers, E. (2014b). Delusional belief flexibility and informal caregiving relationships in psychosis: A potential cognitive route for the protective effect of social support. *Epidemiology and Psychiatric Sciences*, 23(4), 389–397.

Jolley, S., Garety, P., Peters, E., Fornells-Ambrojo, M., Onwumere, J., Harris, V., . . . Johns, L. (2014a). Opportunities and challenges in Improving Access to Psychological Therapies for people with Severe Mental Illness (IAPT-SMI): Evaluating the first operational year of the South London and Maudsley (SLaM) demonstration site for psychosis. *Behaviour Research and Therapy*, 64C, 24–30. doi: 10.1016/j

Jolley, S., Onwumere, J., Bissoli, S., Bhayani, P., Singh, G., Kuipers, E., . . . Garety, P. (2013). A pilot evaluation of therapist training in cognitive therapy for psychosis: therapy quality and clinical outcomes. *Behavioural and Cognitive Psychotherapy*, 23, 1–12.

Jolley, S., Onwumere, J., Kuipers, E., Craig, T., Moriarty, A., & Garety, P. (2012). Increasing access to psychological therapies for people with psychosis: Predictors of successful training. *Behaviour Research and Therapy*, 50, 457–462.

Jones, C., Hacker, D., Cormac, I., Meaden, A., & Irving, C. B. (2012). Cognitive behaviour therapy versus other psychosocial treatments for schizophrenia (Review). *Cochrane Database of Systematic Reviews*, 4, CD008712.

Jung, E., Wiesjahn, M., Rief, W., & Lincoln, T. M. (2014). Perceived therapist genuineness predicts therapeutic alliance in cognitive behavioural therapy for psychosis. *British Journal of Clinical Psychology*, 54(1), 34–48. doi: 10.1111/bjc.12059

Jungbauer, J., & Angermeyer, M. C. (2002). Living with a schizophrenic patient: A comparative study of burden as it affects parents and spouses. *Psychiatry*, 65(2), 110–123.

Karanci, A. N., & Inandilar, H. (2002). Predictors of components of expressed emotion in major caregivers of Turkish patients with schizophrenia. *Social Psychiatry and Psychiatric Epidemiology*, 37(2), 80–88.

Kelly, M. & Newstead, L. (2004). Family intervention in routine practice: it is possible! *Journal of Psychiatric and Mental Health Nursing*, 11, 64–72.

Kennedy, J. L., Altar, C. A., Taylor, D. L., Degtiar, I., & Hornberger, J. C. (2014). The social and economic burden of treatment-resistant schizophrenia: A systematic literature review. *International Clinical Psychopharmacology*, 29(2), 63–76. doi: 10.1097/YIC.0b013e32836508e6

Killaspy, H., Mas-Expósito, L., Marston, L., & King, M. (2014). Ten year outcomes of participants in the REACT (Randomised Evaluation of Assertive Community Treatment in North London) study. *BMC Psychiatry*, 14, 296. doi: 10.1186/s12888-014-0296-6

Kingston, C. (2012). *Understanding posttraumatic stress symptoms in carers of people with psychosis: A cross-sectional study*. Department of Clinical Psychology, King's College, London.

Kjellin, L., & Ostman, M. (2005). Relatives of psychiatric inpatients–do physical violence and suicide attempts of patients influence family burden and participation in care? *Nordic Journal of Psychiatry*, 59(1), 7–11. doi: 10.1080/08039480510018850

Knapp, M., Andrew, A., McDaid, D., Iemmi, V., McCrone, P., Park, A., . . . Shepherd, G. (2014). *Investing in recovery: Making the business case for effective interventions for people with schizophrenia and psychosis*. PSSRU, The London School of Economics and Political Science, and Centre for Mental Health, London.

Krabbendam, L., & van Os, J. (2005). Affective processes in the onset and persistence of psychosis. *European Archives of Psychiatry and Clinical Neuroscience*, 255, 185–189.

Kreyenbuhl, J., Buchanan, R. W., Dickerson, F. B., & Dixon, L. B. (2010). The Schizophrenia Patient Outcomes Research Team (PORT): updated treatment recommendations 2009.

Schizophrenia Bulletin, 36(1), 94–103. doi: 10.1093/schbul/sbp130

Kuipers, E. (2010). Time for a separate service caregiver service? *Journal of Mental Health, 19*(5), 401–404.

Kuipers, E., & Bebbington, P. (2005). Research on burden and coping strategies in families of people with mental disorders: Problems and perspectives. In J. L. N. Sartorius, J. J. L'opez-Ibor, M. Maj & A. Okasha (Eds.), Families and mental disorders: From burden to empowerment (pp. 217–234). London: Wiley.

Kuipers, E., Garety, P., Dunn, G., Bebbington, P., Fowler, D., & Freeman, D. (2002). CBT for psychosis. *British Journal of Psychiatry, 181*, 534; author reply 534.

Kuipers, E., Leff, J., & Lam, D. (2002). Family work for schizophrenia: A practical guide (2nd ed.). London: Gaskell.

Kuipers, E., Onwumere, J., & Bebbington, P. (2010). Cognitive model of caregiving in psychosis. *British Journal of Psychiatry, 196*(4), 259–265. doi: 10.1192/bjp.bp.109.070466

Kuipers, E., Watson, P., Onwumere, J., Bebbington, P., Dunn, G., Weinman, J., & Garety, P. (2007). Discrepant illness perceptions, affect and expressed emotion in people with psychosis and their carers. *Social Psychiatry and Psychiatric Epidemiology, 42*(4), 277–283. doi: 10.1007/s00127-007-0165-4

Kuipers, L., Sturgeon, D., Berkowitz, R., & Leff, J. (1983). Characteristics of expressed emotion: Its relationship to speech and looking in schizophrenic patients and their relatives. *British Journal of Clinical Psychology, 22* (Pt 4), 257–264.

Kulhara, P., Kate, N., Grover, S., & Nehra, R. (2012). Positive aspects of caregiving in schizophrenia: A review. *World Journal of Psychiatry, 22*(2), 43–48.

Kumari, V., Fannon, D., Peters, E. R., Ffytche, D. H., Sumich, A. L., Premkumar, P., & Kuipers, E. (2011). Neural changes following cognitive behaviour therapy for psychosis: A longitudinal fMRI study. *Brain, 134*, 2396–2407.

Kymalainen, J. A., Weisman, A. G., Rosales, G. A., & Armesto, J. C. (2006). Ethnicity, expressed emotion, and communication deviance in family members of patients with schizophrenia. *Journal of Nervous and Mental Disease, 194*(6), 391–396. doi: 10.1097/01.nmd.0000221171.42027.5a

Lawlor, C., Hall, K., & Ellett, L. (2014). Paranoia in the therapeutic relationship in cognitive behavioural therapy for psychosis. *Behavioural and Cognitive Psychotherapy,* doi: 10.1017/S1352465814000071 [Epub ahead of print]

Leavey, G., Gulamhussein, S., Papadopoulos, C., Johnson-Sabine, E., Blizard, B., & King, M. (2004). A randomized controlled trial of a brief intervention for families of patients with a first episode of psychosis. *Psychological Medicine, 34*(3), 423–431.

Lecomte, T., Leclerc, C., Wykes, T., Nicole, L., & Abdel, B. A. (2014). Understanding process in group cognitive behaviour therapy for psychosis. *Psychology and Psychotherapy,* doi: 10.1111/papt.12039 [Epub ahead of print]

Lee, D. R., McKeith, I., Mosimann, U., Ghosh-Nodyal, A., & Thomas, A. J. (2013). Examining carer stress in dementia: The role of subtype diagnosis and neuropsychiatric symptoms. *International Journal of Geriatric Psychiatry, 28*(2), 135–141. doi: 10.1002/gps.3799

Lee, G., Barrowclough, C., & Lobban, F. (2014). Positive affect in the family environment protects against relapse in first-episode psychosis. *Social Psychiatry and Psychiatric Epidemiology, 49*(3), 367–376. doi: 10.1007/s00127-013-0768-x

Lenior, M. E., Dingemans, P. M., Linszen, D. H., de Haan, L., & Schene, A. H. (2001). Social functioning and the course of early-onset schizophrenia: Five-year follow-up of a psychosocial intervention. *British Journal of Psychiatry, 179*, 53–58.

Lincoln, T. M., Rief, W., Westermann, S., Ziegler, M., Kesting, M. L., Heibach, E., & Mehl, S. (2014). Who stays, who benefits? Predicting dropout and change in cognitive behaviour therapy for psychosis. *Psychiatry Research, 216*(2), 198–205.

Linscott, R. J., & van Os, J. (2013). An updated and conservative systematic review and meta-analysis of epidemiological evidence on psychotic experiences in children and adults: On the pathway from proneness to persistence to dimensional expression across mental disorders. *Psychological Medicine, 43*(6), 1133–1149. doi: 10.1017/S0033291712001626

Linszen, D., Dingemans, P., Van der Does, J. W., Nugter, A., Scholte, P., Lenior, R., & Goldstein, M. J. (1996). Treatment, expressed emotion and relapse in recent onset schizophrenic disorders. *Psychological Medicine, 26*(2), 333–342.

Lobban, F., Barrowclough, C., & Jones, S. (2005). Assessing cognitive representations of mental health problems. II. The illness perception questionnaire for schizophrenia: Relatives' version. *British Journal of Clinical Psychology, 44*, 163–179.

Lobban, F., Barrowclough, C., & Jones, S. (2006). Does expressed emotion need to be understood within a more systemic framework? An examination of discrepancies in appraisals between patients diagnosed with schizophrenia and their relatives. *Social Psychiatry and Psychiatric Epidemiology, 41*(1), 50–55. doi: 10.1007/s00127-005-0993-z

Lobban, F., Glentworth, D., Chapman, L., Wainwright, L., Postlethwaite, A., Dunn, G., Pinfold, V., . . . Haddock, G. (2013). Feasibility of a supported self-management intervention for relatives of people with recent-onset psychosis: REACT study. *British Journal of Psychiatry, 203*(5), 366–372. doi: 10.1192/bjp.bp.112.113613

Lopez, S. R., Nelson, H. K., Polo, A. J., Jenkins, J. H., Karno, M., Vaughn, C., & Snyder, K. S. (2004). Ethnicity, expressed emotion, attributions, and course of schizophrenia: Family warmth matters. *Journal of Abnormal Psychology, 113*(3), 428–439. doi: 10.1037/0021-843X.113.3.428

Loughland, C. M., Lawrence, G., Allen, J., Hunter, M., Lewin, T. J., Oud, N. E., & Carr, V. J. (2009). Aggression and trauma experiences among carer-relatives of people with psychosis. *Social Psychiatry and Psychiatric Epidemiology, 44*(12), 1031–1040. doi: 10.1007/s00127-009-0025-5

Lynch. D., Laws, K. R., & McKenna, P. J. (2010). Cognitive behavioural therapy for major psychiatric disorder: does it really work? A meta-analytical review of well-controlled trials. *Psychological Medicine, 40*(1), 9–24.

Maddox, L., Jolley, S., Laurens, K., Hirsch, C., Hodgins, S., Browning, S., . . . Kuipers, E. (2013). Cognitive behavioural therapy for unusual experiences in children: A case series. *Behavioural and Cognitive Psychotherapy, 41*, 344–58.

Magliano, L., Fiorillo, A., Malangone, C., De Rosa, C., & Maj, M. (2006). Social network in long-term diseases: A comparative study in relatives of persons with schizophrenia and physical illnesses versus a sample from the general population. *Social Science and Medicine, 62*(6), 1392–1402.

Magliano, L., Marasco, C., Fiorillo, A., Malangone, C., Guarneri, M., & Maj, M. (2002). The impact of professional and social network support on the burden of families of patients with schizophrenia in Italy. *Acta Psychiatrica Scandinavica, 106*(4), 291–298.

Mangalore, R., & Knapp, M. (2007). Cost of schizophrenia in England. *Journal of Mental Health Policy and Economics*, *10*, 23–41.

Marcus, E., Garety, P., Weinman, J., Emsley, R., Dunn, G., Bebbington, P., . . . Jolley, S. (2014). A pilot validation of a modified Illness Perceptions Questionnaire designed to predict response to cognitive therapy for psychosis. *Journal of Behavior Therapy and Experimental Psychiatry*, *45*(4), 459–466.

Mari, J. J., & Streiner, D. L. (1994). An overview of family interventions and relapse on schizophrenia: Meta-analysis of research findings. *Psychological Medicine*, *24*(3), 565–578.

Martens, L., & Addington, J. (2001). The psychological well-being of family members of individuals with schizophrenia. *Social Psychiatry and Psychiatric Epidemiology*, *36*(3), 128–133.

McCann, T. V., Lubman, D. I., & Clark, E. (2011). First-time primary caregivers' experience of caring for young adults with first-episode psychosis. *Schizophrenia Bulletin*, *37*(2), 381–388. doi: 10.1093/schbul/sbp085

McCrone, P., Singh, S. P., Knapp, M., Smith, J., Clark, M., Shiers, D., & Tiffin, P. A. (2013). The economic impact of early intervention in psychosis services for children and adolescents. *Early Intervention in Psychiatry*, *7*(4), 368–373.

McFarlane, W. R., & Cook, W. L. (2007). Family expressed emotion prior to onset of psychosis. *Family Process*, *46*(2), 185–197.

McNab, C., Haslam, N., & Burnett, P. (2007). Expressed emotion, attributions, utility beliefs, and distress in parents of young people with first episode psychosis. *Psychiatry Research*, *151*(1–2), 97–106. doi: 10.1016/j.psychres.2006.08.004

Meaden, A., & Hacker, D. (2011). *Problematic and risk behaviours in psychosis: A shared formulation approach*. Hove, UK: Routledge.

Meaden, A., Keen, N., Aston, R., Barton, K., & Bucci, S. (2012). *Cognitive therapy for command hallucinations: An advanced practical companion*. Hove, UK: Routledge.

Mentis, M., Messinis, L., Kotrotsiou, E., Angelopoulos, N. V., Marneras, C., Papathanasopoulos, P., & Dardiotis, E. (2014). Efficacy of a support group intervention on psychopathological characteristics among caregivers of psychotic patients. *International Journal of Social Psychiatry*. doi: 10.1177/0020764014547075 [Epub ahead of print]

Mihalopoulos, C., Magnus, A., Carter, R., & Vos, T. (2004). Assessing cost-effectiveness in mental health: Family interventions for schizophrenia and related conditions. *Australian and New Zealand Journal of Psychiatry*, *38*, 511–519.

Miklowitz, D. J., Goldstein, M. J., Falloon, I. R., & Doane, J. A. (1984). Interactional corelates of expressed emotion in the families of schizophrenics. *British Journal of Psychiatry*, *144*, 482–487.

Miles, H., Peters, E., & Kuipers, E. (2007). Service-user satisfaction with CBT for psychosis. *Behavioural and Cognitive Psychotherapy*, *35*, 109–116.

Moller-Leimkuhler, A. M., & Madger, F. (2011). Personality factors and mental health outcome in caregivers of first hospitalized schizophrenic and depressed patients: 2-year follow-up results. *European Archives of Psychiatry and Clinical Neuroscience*, *261*(3), 165–172. doi: 10.1007/s00406-010-0155-5

Morgan, C., Abdul-Al, R., Lappin, J. M., Jones, P., Fearon, P., Leese, M., . . . Murray, R. (2006). Clinical and social determinants of duration of untreated psychosis in the AESOP first-episode psychosis study. *British Journal of Psychiatry*, *189*, 446–452. doi: 10.1192/bjp.bp.106.021303

Morris, E. M. J., Johns, L. C., & Oliver, J. E. (2013). *Acceptance and commitment therapy and mindfulness for psychosis*. London: Wiley Blackwell.

Morrison, A. P., & Barratt, S. (2010). What are the components of CBT for psychosis? A Delphi study. *Schizophrenia Bulletin*, *36*(1), 136–142. doi: 10.1093/schbul/sbp118

Morrison, A. P., Renton, J. C., French, P., Bentall, R. P. (2008). *Think you're crazy? Think again: A cognitive therapy resource book*. London: Routledge.

Morrison, A. P., Turkington, D., Pyle, M., Spencer, H., Brabban, A., Dunn, G., . . . Hutton, P. (2014). Cognitive therapy for people with schizophrenia spectrum disorders not taking antipsychotic drugs: A single-blind randomised controlled trial. *Lancet*, *383*(9926), 1395–1403. doi: 10.1016/S0140-6736(13)62246-1

Mueser, K. T., Rosenberg, S. D., Xie, H., Jankowski, M. K., Bolton, E. E., Lu, W., . . . Wolfe, R. (2008). A randomized controlled trial of cognitive-behavioral treatment for post-traumatic stress disorder in severe mental illness. *Journal of Consulting and Clinical Psychology*, *76*, 259–271.

NICE. (2009). Schizophrenia- core interventions in the treatment and management of schizophrenia in adults in primary and secondary. Clinical guideline 82. London: National Institute for Health and Care Excellence.

NICE. (2011). Psychosis with coexisting substance misuse. Assessment and management in adults and young people. Clinical guideline 120. London: National Institute for Health and Care Excellence.

NICE. (2013). *Psychosis and schizophrenia in children and young people (CG155)*. London: National Institute for Health & Care Excellence.

NICE. (2014). Psychosis and schizophrenia: Treatment and management. Clinical guideline 178. London: National Institute of Health and Care Excellence.

Nilsen, L., Frich, J. C., Friis, S., Norheim, I., & Rossberg, J. I. (2014). Participants' perceived benefits of family intervention following a first episode of psychosis: A qualitative study. *Early Intervention in Psychiatry*, doi: 10.1111/eip.12153 [Epub ahead of print]

Norman, R. M. G., Malla, A. K., Manchanda, R., Harricharan, R., Takhar, J., & Northcott, S. (2005). Social support and three-year symptom and admission outcomes for first episode psychosis. *Schizophrenia Research*, *80*, 227–234.

Oathamshaw, S., Barrowcliff, A. & Haddock, G. (2011). CBT for people with intellectual disabilities and psychosis. In J. Taylor, W. Lindsay, R. Hastings, & C. Hatton (Eds.), *Psychological therapies for adults with intellectual disabilities* (pp. 157–172). Oxford: Wiley.

O'Brien, M. P., Gordon, J. L., Bearden, C. E., Lopez, S. R., Kopelowicz, A., & Cannon, T. D. (2006). Positive family environment predicts improvement in symptoms and social functioning among adolescents at imminent risk for onset of psychosis. *Schizophrenia Research*, *81*(2–3), 269–275. doi: 10.1016/j.schres.2005.10.005

O'Brien, M. P., Miklowitz, D. J., Candan, K. A., Marshall, C., Domingues, I., Walsh, B. C., & Cannon, T. D. (2014). A randomized trial of family focused therapy with populations at clinical high risk for psychosis: Effects on interactional behavior. *Journal of Consulting and Clinical Psychology*, *82*(1), 90–101. doi: 10.1037/a0034667

O'Brien, M. P., Zingberg, J. L., Ho, L., Rudd, A., Kopelowicz, A., Daley, M., . . . Cannon, T. D. (2009). Family problem solving interactions and 6-month symptomatic and functional outcomes in youth at ultra-high risk for psychosis and with recent onset psychotic symptoms: A longitudinal study. *Schizophrenia Research, 107*, 198–205.

Okpokoro, U., Adams, C. E., & Sampson, S. (2014). Family intervention (brief) for schizophrenia (Review). *Cochrane Database of Systematic Reviews* (3). doi: 10.1002/14651858. CD009802.pub2

Onwumere, J., Chung, A., Boddington, S., Little, A., & Kuipers, E. (2013). Older adults with psychosis: A case for family interventions. *Psychosis, 6*(2), 181–183. doi: 10.1080/1752 2439.2013.774436

Onwumere, J., Grice, S., Garety, P., Bebbington, P., Dunn, G., Freeman, D., . . . Kuipers, E. (2014). Caregiver reports of patient-initiated violence in psychosis. *Canadian Journal of Psychiatry, 59*(7), 376–384.

Onwumere, J., Kuipers, E., Bebbington, P., Dunn, G., Fowler, D., Freeman, D., . . . Garety, P. (2008). Care-giving and illness beliefs in the course of psychotic illness. *Canadian Journal of Psychiatry, 53*(7), 460–468.

Onwumere, J., Kuipers, E., Bebbington, P., Dunn, G., Freeman, D., Fowler, D., & Garety, P. (2009). Patient perceptions of caregiver criticism in psychosis: Links with patient and caregiver functioning. *Journal of Nervous and Mental Disease, 197*(2), 85–91. doi: 10.1097/NMD.0b013e3181960e57

Onwumere, J., Kuipers, E., Bebbington, P., Dunn, G., Freeman, D., Fowler, D., & Garety, P. (2011). Coping styles in carers of people with recent and long-term psychosis. *Journal of Nervous and Mental Disease, 199*(6), 423–424. doi: 10.1097/ NMD.0b013e31821ccb07

Onwumere, J., Lotey, G., Schulz, J., James, G., Afsharzadegan, R., Harvey, R., . . . Raune D. (2015). Burnout in early course psychosis caregivers: The role of illness beliefs and coping styles. *Early Intervention in Psychiatry, 59*(7), 376–384.

Onwumere, J., & Kuipers, E. (2009). Family Communication in Psychosis. In K. Bryan (Ed.), Communication in Healthcare (pp. 333–362). Germany: Peter Lang.

Ost, L. G. (2014). The efficacy of acceptance and commitment therapy: An updated systematic review and meta-analysis. *Behaviour Research and Therapy, 61*, 105–121.

Ostman, M., & Hansson, L. (2004). Appraisal of caregiving, burden and psychological distress in relatives of psychiatric inpatients. *European Psychiatry, 19*(7), 402–407. doi: 10.1016/j. eurpsy.2004.06.030

Peters, E., Landau, S., McCrone, P., Cooke, M., Fisher, P., Steel, C., . . . Kuipers, E. (2010). A randomised controlled trial of cognitive behaviour therapy for psychosis in a routine clinical service. *Acta Psychiatrica Scandinavica, 122*(4), 302–318. doi: 10.1111/J.1600-0447.2010.01572.X

Peterson, E. C., & Docherty, N. M. (2004). Expressed emotion, attribution, and control in parents of schizophrenic patients. *Psychiatry, 67*(2), 197–207. doi: 10.1521/ psyc.67.2.197.35959

Pfammatter, M., Junghan, U. M., & Brenner, H. D. (2006). Efficacy of psychological therapy in schizophrenia: Conclusions from meta-analyses. *Schizophrenia Bulletin, 32*(Suppl 1), S64–S80. doi: 10.1093/schbul/sbl030

Pharoah, F., Mari, J., Rathbone, J., & Wong, W. (2010). Family intervention for schizophrenia. *Cochrane Database of Systematic Reviews, 12*, CD000088. doi: 10.1002/14651858. CD000088.pub2

Phillips, A. C., Gallagher, S., Hunt, K., Der, G., & Carroll, D. (2009). Symptoms of depression in non-routine

caregivers: The role of caregiver strain and burden. *British Journal of Clinical Psychology, 48*, 335–346.

Pitschel-Walz, G., Leucht, S., Bauml, J., Kissling, W., & Engel, R. R. (2001). The effect of family interventions on relapse and rehospitalization in schizophrenia–a meta-analysis. *Schizophrenia Bulletin, 27*(1), 73–92.

Pitschel-Walz, G., Leucht, S., Bauml, J., Kissling, W., & Engel, R. R., (2004). The effect of family interventions on relapse and rehospitalisation in schizophrenia: A meta-analysis. *Journal of Lifelong Learning in Psychiatry, Winter II*(1), 78–94.

Prytys, M., Garety, P. A., Jolley, S., Onwumere, J., & Craig, T. (2011). Implementing the NICE guideline for schizophrenia recommendations for psychological therapies: A qualitative analysis of the attitudes of CMHT staff. *Clinical Psychology and Psychotherapy, 18*(1), 48–59.

Reininghaus, U., Dutta, R., Dazzan, P., Doody, G. A., Fearon, P., Lappin, J., & Jones, P. B. (2014). Mortality in schizophrenia and other psychoses: A 10-year follow-up of the SOP First-Episode Cohort. *Schizophrenia Bulletin, 41*(3), 665–673. doi: 10.1093/schbul/sbu138

Renshaw, K. D. (2008). The predictive, convergent, and discriminant validity of perceived criticism: A review. *Clinical Psychology Review, 28*(3), 521–534. doi: 10.1016/j. cpr.2007.09.002

Robinson, D., Woerner, M. G., Alvir, J. M., Bilder, R., Goldman, R., Geisler, S., & Lieberman, J. A. (1999). Predictors of relapse following response from a first episode of schizophrenia or schizoaffective disorder. *Archives of General Psychiatry, 56*(3), 241–247. doi: 10.1001/archpsyc.56.3.241

Robinson, J., Harris, M. G., Harrigan, S. M., Henry, L. P., Farrelly, S., Prosser, A., . . . McGorry, P. D. (2010). Suicide attempt in first-episode psychosis: A 7.4 year follow-up study. *Schizophrenia Research, 116*, 1–8.

Rosenfarb, I. S., Goldstein, M. J., Mintz, J., & Nuechterlein, K. H. (1995). Expressed emotion and subclinical psychopathology observable within the transactions between schizophrenic-patients and their family members. *Journal of Abnormal Psychology, 104*(2), 259–267. doi: 10.1037/0 021–843x.104.2.259

Roth, A. D., & Pilling, S. (2013). *A competence framework for psychological interventions with people with psychosis and bipolar disorder.* University College London, Centre for Outcomes Research & Effectiveness.

Rotondi, A. J., Anderson, C. M., Haas, G. L., Eack, S. M., Spring, M. B., Ganguli, R., . . . Rosenstock, J. (2010). Web-based psychoeducational intervention for persons with schizophrenia and their supporters: One-year outcomes. *Psychiatric Services, 61*(11), 1099–1105. doi: 10.1176/appi.ps.61.11.1099

Saha, S., Chant, D., & McGrath, J. (2007). A systematic review of mortality in schizophrenia: Is the differential mortality gap worsening over time? *Archives of General Psychiatry, 64*, 1123–1131.

Sarin, F., Wallin, L., & Widerlöv, B. (2011). Cognitive behavior therapy for schizophrenia: A meta-analytical review of randomized controlled trials. *Nordic Journal of Psychiatry, 65*, 162–174.

Scazufca, M., & Kuipers, E. (1997). The impact on women who care for those with schizophrenia. *Psychiatric Bulletin, 22*, 1–3.

Seeman, M. V. (2012). Bad, burdened or ill? Characterizing the spouses of women with schizophrenia. *International Journal of Social Psychiatry, 59*(8), 805–810. doi: 10.1177/0020764012456818

Simoneau, T., Miklowitz, D. J., & Saleem, R. (1998). Expressed emotion and interactional patterns in the families of bipolar patients. *Journal of Abnormal Psychology, 107*(3), 497–507.

Smith, L., Onwumere, J., Craig, T., McManus, S., Bebbington, P., & Kuipers, E. (2014). Mental and physical illness in caregivers: Results from an English national survey sample 2007. *British Journal of Psychiatry, 205*(3), 197–203.

Stansfeld, S., Smuk, M., Onwumere, J., Clark, C., Pike, C., McManus, S., & Bebbington, P. (2014). Stressors and common mental disorder in informal carers–An analysis of the English Adult Psychiatric Morbidity Survey 2007. *Social Science and Medicine, 120*, 190–198. doi: 10.1016/j.socscimed.2014.09.025

Staring, A. B., Ter Huurne, M. A., & van der Gaag, M. (2013). Cognitive behavioral therapy for negative symptoms (CBT-n) in psychotic disorders: A pilot study. *Journal of Behavior Therapy and Experimental Psychiatry, 44*(3), 300–306. doi: 10.1016/j.jbtep.2013.01.004

Steel, C., Tarrier, N., Stahl, D., & Wykes, T. (2012). Cognitive behaviour therapy for psychosis: The impact of therapist training and supervision. *Psychotherapy and Psychosomatics, 81*(3), 194–195.

Stowkowy, J., Addington, D., Liu, L., Hollowell, B., & Addington, J. (2012). Predictors of disengagement from treatment in an early psychosis program. *Schizophrenia Research, 136*(1–3), 7–12. doi: 10.1016/j.schres.2012.01.027

Tang, V. W., Leung, S. K., & Lam, L. C. (2008). Clinical correlates of the caregiving experience for Chinese caregivers of patients with schizophrenia. *Social Psychiatry and Psychiatric Epidemiology, 43*(9), 720–726. doi: 10.1007/s00127-008-0357-6

The Schizophrenia Commission. (2012). *The abandoned illness: A report from the Schizophrenia Commission.* London: Rethink Mental Illness.

Thomas, N., Hayward, M., Peters, E., van der Gaag, M., Bentall, R. P., Jenner, J., . . . McCarthy-Jones, S. (2014). Psychological therapies for auditory hallucinations (voices): Current status and key directions for future research. *Schizophrenia Bulletin, 40*(Suppl 4), S202–S212. doi: 10.1093/schbul/sbu037

Tienari, P., Wynne, L. C., Sorri, A., Lahti, I., Laksy, K., Moring, J., & Wahlberg, K. E. (2004). Genotype-environment interaction in schizophrenia-spectrum disorder. Long-term follow-up study of Finnish adoptees. *British Journal of Psychiatry, 184*, 216–222.

Tomas, E. P., Hurtado, G., Noguer, S., Domenech, C., Garcia, M., Lopez, N., & Gallo, P. (2012). Effectiveness of family work interventions on schizophrenia: Evidence from a multicentre study in Catalonia. *International Journal of Social Psychiatry, 58*(6), 587–595. doi: 10.1177/0020764011415595

Tomlinson, E., Onwumere, J., & Kuipers, E. (2014). Distress and negative experiences of the caregiving relationship in early psychosis: Does social cognition play a role? *Early Intervention in Psychiatry, 8*(3), 253–260. doi: 10.1111/eip.12040

Tompson, M. C., Goldstein, M. J., Lebell, M. B., Mintz, L. I., Marder, S. R., & Mintz, J. (1995). Schizophrenic-patients perceptions of their relatives' attitudes. *Psychiatry Research, 57*(2), 155–167.

Trower, P., Birchwood, M., Meaden, A., Byrne, S., Nelson, A., & Ross, K. (2004). Cognitive therapy for command hallucinations: Randomised controlled trial. *British Journal of Psychiatry, 184*(4), 312–320.

Turner, D. T, van der Gaag, M., Karyotaki, E., & Cuijpers, P. (2014). Psychological interventions for psychosis: A meta-analysis of comparative outcome studies. *American Journal of Psychiatry, 171*(5), 523–538. doi: 10.1176/appi.ajp.2013.13081159

Ukpong, D. I. (2006). Demographic factors and clinical correlates of burden and distress in relatives of service users experiencing schizophrenia: A study from south-western Nigeria. *International Journal Mental Health Nursing, 15*(1), 54–59. doi: 10.1111/j.1447-0349.2006.00403.x

van den Berg, D. P, de Bont, P. A, van der Vleugel, B. M, de Roos, C., de Jongh, A., Van Minnen, A., & van der Gaag, M. (2015). Prolonged exposure vs eye movement desensitization and reprocessing vs waiting list for posttraumatic stress disorder in patients with a psychotic disorder: A randomized clinical trial. *JAMA Psychiatry, 72*(3), 259–267. doi: 10.1001/jamapsychiatry.2014.2637

van der Gaag, M., Smit, F., Bechdolf, A., French, P., Linszen, D. H., Yung, A. R., . . . Cuijpers, P. (2013). Preventing a first episode of psychosis: Meta-analysis of randomized controlled prevention trials of 12 month and longer-term follow-ups. *Schizophr Research, 149*(1–3), 56–62. doi: 10.1016/j.schres.2013.07.004

van Os, J., Linscott, R. J., Myin-Germeys, I., Delespaul, P., & Krabbendam, L. (2009). A systematic review and meta-analysis of the psychosis-continuum: Evidence for a psychosis- proneness-persistence-impairment model of psychotic disorder. *Psychological Medicine, 39*, 179–195.

van Os, J., & Murray, R. M. (2013). Can we identify and treat "schizophrenia light" to prevent true psychotic illness? *British Medical Journal, 18*, 346:f304. doi: 10.1136/bmj.f304

Vasconcelos, E. S. D., Wearden, A., & Barrowclough, C. (2013). Expressed emotion, types of behavioural control and controllability attributions in relatives of people with recent-onset psychosis. *Social Psychiatry and Psychiatric Epidemiology, 48*(9), 1377–1388. doi: 10.1007/s00127-013-0659-1

Vaughn, C., & Leff, J. (1976). The measurement of expressed emotion in the families of psychiatric patients. *British Journal of Social and Clinical Psychology, 15*(2), 157–165.

Velligan, D. I., Tai, S., Roberts, D. L., Maples-Aguilar, N., Brown, M., Mintz, J., & Turkington, D. (2014). A randomized controlled trial comparing cognitive behavior therapy, cognitive adaptation training, their combination and treatment as usual in chronic schizophrenia. *Schizophrenia Bulletin, 41*(3), 597–603.

Waller, H., Craig, T., Landau, S., Fornells-Ambrojo, M., Hassanali, N., Iredale, C., . . . Garety, P. (2014). The effects of a brief CBT intervention, delivered by frontline mental health staff, to promote recovery in people with psychosis and comorbid anxiety or depression (the GOALS study): Study protocol for a randomized controlled trial. *Trials, 15*, 255. doi: 10.1186/1745-6215-15-255

Waller, H., Freeman, D., Jolley, S., Dunn, G., & Garety, P. (2011). Targeting reasoning biases in delusions: A pilot study of the Maudsley Review Training Programme for individuals with persistent, high conviction delusions. *Journal of Behavior Therapy and Experimental Psychiatry, 42*, 414–421.

Waller, H., Garety, P. A., Jolley, S., Fornells-Ambrojo, M., Kuipers, E., Onwumere, J., . . . Craig, T. (2013a). Low intensity cognitive behavioural therapy for psychosis: a pilot study. *Journal of Behavioural Therapy and Experimental Psychiatry, 44*(1), 98–104. doi: 10.1016/j.jbtep.2012.07.013

Waller, H., Garety, P., Jolley, S., Fornells-Ambrojo, M., Kuipers, E., Onwumere, J.,...Craig, T. (2013b). Training frontline mental health staff to deliver "low intensity" psychological therapy for psychosis: A qualitative analysis of therapist and service user views on the therapy and its future implementation. *Behavioural and Cognitive Psychotherapy*, *23*, 1–16.

Wearden, A. J., Tarrier, N., Barrowclough, C., Zastowny, T. R., & Rahill, A. A. (2000). A review of expressed emotion research in health care. *Clinical Psychology Review*, *20*(5), 633–666.

White, R., Gumley, A., McTaggart, J., Rattrie, L., McConville, D., Cleare, S., & Mitchell, G. (2011). A feasibility study of acceptance and commitment therapy for emotional dysfunction following psychosis. *Behavioral Research and Therapy*, *49*, 901–907.

Whiteford, H. A., Degenhardt, L., Rehm, J., Baxter, A. J., Ferrari, A. J., Erskine, H. E.,...Vos, T. (2013). Global burden of disease attributable to mental and substance use disorders: Findings from the Global Burden of Disease Study 2010. *Lancet*, *382*(9904), 1575–1586. doi: 10.1016/s0140-6736(13)61611-6

World Health Organization. (1992). *The ICD–10 classification of mental and behavioural disorders: Clinical description and diagnostic guidelines*. Geneva: WHO.

World Health Organization. (2013). *Mental health action plan 2013–2020*. Geneva: WHO.

Wuerker, A. K., Long, J. D., Haas, G. L., & Bellack, A. S. (2002). Interpersonal control, expressed emotion, and change in symptoms in families of persons with schizophrenia. *Schizophrenia Research*, *58*(2–3), 281–292.

Wykes, T., Steel, C., Everitt, B., & Tarrier, N. (2008). Cognitive behaviour therapy for schizophrenia: Effect sizes, clinical models, and methodological rigor. *Schizophrenia Bulletin*, *34*, 523–537.

Yesufu-Udechuku, A., Harrison, B., Mayo-Wilson, E., Young, N., Woodhams, P., Shiers, D., Kendall, T. (2015). Interventions to improve the experience of caring for people with severe mental illness: systematic review and meta-analysis. *British Journal of Psychiatry*, *206*(4), 268–274.

Cognitive-Behavioral Therapies in Older Adult Populations

Michelle M. Braun, Bradley E. Karlin, *and* Antonette Zeiss

Abstract

Cognitive-behavioral therapies have a strong history of effectiveness in treating mental and behavioral health conditions and improving quality of life in adults 65 years of age and older. As the provision of mental health treatment has increasingly shifted from specialty mental health settings to medical and long-term care settings, cognitive and behavioral therapies have been more widely utilized in the context of comorbid medical disorders and have contributed to improved clinical outcomes. Innovative models of service delivery by video, telephone, and to rural populations have provided additional evidence of their flexibility and value. Quality of life for our growing older adult population may be enhanced through improved detection of mental and behavioral health conditions and expanded awareness of the effectiveness of cognitive and behavioral therapies.

Key Words: older adults, cognitive-behavioral therapy, geropsychology, psychotherapy, CBT, effectiveness

The effectiveness of various cognitive-behavioral therapies in treating mental and behavioral health conditions and improving quality of life in older adults is well established (Barrowclough et al, 2001; Scogin, Welsh, Hanson, Stump, & Coates, 2005). This chapter provides an overview of the effectiveness of these techniques across various mental and behavioral health conditions, comorbid chronic medical conditions, and comorbid cognitive disorders, with the goal of summarizing the broad applicability of cognitive-behavioral approaches with older adults. Although there are multiple forms of cognitive-behavioral therapies, this chapter primarily reviews the effectiveness of an integrated cognitive-behavioral intervention, which we will refer to as CBT.

Additionally, CBT is the most widely studied type of cognitive-behavioral therapy in older adults. Readers are encouraged to refer to other chapters of this handbook to obtain additional details about other cognitive-behavioral approaches that are briefly summarized in the current chapter, including problem-solving therapy (PST), relaxation training, and behavioral activation. In an effort to highlight the breadth and flexibility of CBT, we identify multiple modalities and formats of CBT delivery (e.g., groups, telephone, clinical video teleconferencing), comparisons between CBT and other types of treatment (medication, other psychotherapies), and various settings for CBT delivery (e.g., community, medical, long-term care). When possible, meta-analytic and review studies are included to enhance the strength of conclusions in a given topic area. Also included is a case study highlighting the use of CBT in an older adult with depression. The chapter concludes with a focus on integrating cognitive-behavioral therapies into our changing health care system and suggestions for future research.

Prevalence of Mental Disorders in Older Adults

Our burgeoning older adult population is poised to create exponentially increased demands for mental health care. In 2009, adults aged 65 years and older represented 12.9% of the United States population (39.6 million people, or one in every eight Americans). By 2030, older adults are estimated to represent 19% of the population (72.1 million people, or more than twice their number in 2000; Administration on Aging, 2010). Approximately 16% of the older adult population meets criteria for a mental disorder (not including dementia), which is likely to increase dramatically as the older adult population grows (Jeste et al., 1999). In a recent review of the prevalence of mental disorders in community-dwelling older adults, anxiety disorders were reported to be most prevalent (7.0% of the population, including 4.7% phobia, 2.3% social phobia, 1.2% generalized anxiety disorder, 0.7% panic disorder, 0.4% posttraumatic stress disorder [PTSD], and 0.4% agoraphobia), with mood disorders second most prevalent (2.6% of the population, including 2.3% major depression, 0.5% dysthymia, 0.2% bipolar disorder) (Gum, King-Kallimanis, & Kohn, 2009). These rates are similar to other estimates based on national survey data (e.g., Karlin, Duffy, & Gleaves, 2008). Although the prevalence of mental disorders is consistently higher in younger adults, clinically significant psychiatric symptoms that are subthreshold for a diagnosis occur more frequently in older adults, and symptoms are more likely to be persistent, to be chronic, and to co-occur with physical and pain conditions (Gum, King-Kallimanis, & Kohn, 2009). In addition, unique factors may impact the detection of mental disorders in older adults. For example, although the prevalence of anxiety disorders is lower in older adults than younger adults, assessment of anxiety in older adults is limited, and anxiety disorders may be masked by comorbid depression, medical illnesses, and cognitive decline (Wolitzky-Taylor, Castriotta, Lenze, Stanley, & Craske, 2010).

CBT in Older Adults: General Considerations

We define integrated CBT as an action-oriented psychotherapy based on empirically supported theories of psychopathology that involves recognizing and changing maladaptive thoughts and behaviors to decrease symptoms of mental illness and enhance quality of life. The primary goal of CBT is to help individuals identify, challenge, and alter negative or extreme thought patterns that contribute to, maintain, and/or exacerbate psychological symptoms. Behavioral techniques are also incorporated, including but not limited to activity scheduling, assertiveness training, and problem solving for depressive disorders; and relaxation training and exposure techniques for anxiety disorders (Scogin et al., 2005). CBT is effective in treating a variety of mental health disorders in older adults, with most research to date focusing on the treatment of depression (Ayers et al, 2007; Dick-Siskin, 2002; Gallagher-Thompson & Thompson, 1996; Satre, Knight, & David, 2006; Sorocco & Lauderdale, 2011; Zeiss & Steffen, 1996a). CBT is also effective in treating anxiety disorders (Barrowclough et al., 2001; Stanley et al., 2003), behavioral challenges in dementia (Burgio & Fisher, 2000; Gatz et al., 1998; Teri, Huda, Gibbons, Young, & van Leynseele, 2005), late-life insomnia (Morin, Colecchi, Stone, Sood, & Brink, 1999; Vitiello, Rybarczyk, Von Korff, & Stepanski, 2009), pain (Jackson, O'Malley, & Kroenke, 2006), and anxiety and depression in a variety of comorbid medical conditions. CBT is equally effective in treating older and younger adults (Payne & Marcus, 2008; Walker & Clarke, 2001) and is effective across a variety of settings, including primary care, hospice and palliative care, and home-based care (as reviewed in Sorocco & Lauderdale, 2011). In addition, CBT has enduring effects that reduce the risk of recurring depression and anxiety (Hollon, Stewart, & Strunk, 2006; Stanley et al., 2003).

There are several methods for tailoring CBT techniques to maximize effectiveness with older adults. Research and clinical reports have revealed that relatively minor adaptations to accommodate age-related changes in information processing, sensory abilities, learning style, and memory are helpful (Karlin, 2011; Laidlaw & McAlpine, 2008; Zeiss & Steffen, 1996a, 1996b). In addition, a focus on religion and/or spirituality may be useful with many older adults (Hodge & Bonifas, 2010; Paukert et al., 2009; Stanley et al., 2011). Integration of issues related to sexuality, including lesbian, gay, bisexual, and transgender considerations, may also help to maximize outcomes for many older adults—a finding that can be counterintuitive, given the stereotypical desexualized concepts of older adults (Kimmel, Rose, & David, 2006).

The expanding ethnic diversity of our older adult population makes cultural considerations in psychotherapy increasingly important (Lau & Kinoshita, 2006). In 2003, 83% of older adults in the United States were non-Hispanic White, 8% were non-Hispanic Black, 6% were Hispanic, and 3% were Asian. However, by 2030, it is projected that 72% of older adults will be non-Hispanic White; 11% will be Hispanic; 10% will be Black; and 5% will be Asian (Centers for Disease Control and Prevention, 2007). These changing demographics will require greater attention to issues of ethnic diversity in order to enhance CBT effectiveness. Socioeconomic status is another important element of diversity that may require tailored techniques for therapy and outreach. For example, although research has shown that low-income older adults with depression benefit from increased access to psychosocial services, either alone or when combined with cognitive-behavioral group therapy (Areán et al., 2005), low-income older adults are less likely to access such services. As such, potential special needs of this population are not well understood.

CBT and Mental Health Disorders in Older Adults
CBT for Depression

CBT with older adults has been most widely studied in the treatment of depression, with significant research supporting its effectiveness (e.g., Areán, 2004; Mackin & Arean, 2005; Moss & Scogin, 2008; Qualls & Knight, 2006; Scogin et al., 2005), including CBT in the treatment of poststroke depression (Laidlaw, 2008) and CBT offered in group formats (DeVries & Coon, 2002; Krishna et al., 2011). CBT provides specific benefits as compared to "talking control" conditions (Serfaty et al., 2009; Serfaty, Csipke, Haworth, Murad, & King, 2011) and in the treatment of residual depressive symptoms after pharmacotherapy (Scogin et al., 2001).

Effectiveness of CBT as a function of depression severity has been examined as a potential modifier of treatment outcome. For example, in a study of mild to moderate depression in older adults, although all treatments resulted in substantial improvement (CBT, medication/desipramine, and combined CBT/desipramine), the CBT-only and combined groups showed similar levels of improvement, with combined therapies shown to be most effective in severe depression, particularly when desipramine was at or above recommended dosage levels (Thompson, Coon, Gallagher-Thompson, Sommer, & Koin, 2001). In a placebo-controlled trial of treatment for moderate to severe depression, DeRubeis et al. (2005) showed that cognitive therapy was as effective as medications for the initial treatment of moderate to severe major depression, but that the degree

of effectiveness might depend on a high level of therapist expertise.

Other effective cognitive-behavioral therapies for the treatment of depression in older adults include problem-solving therapy (PST) and behavioral activation (Fiske, Wetherell, & Gatz, 2009; Scogin et al., 2005; Yon & Scogin, 2009). In PST, older adults learn to approach problems actively and to view problem solving as a coping strategy. Skills in some forms of PST that have been used with older adults include learning to define problems more effectively, formulating alternative solutions to problems, examining the consequences of each solution, and evaluating the outcomes of solutions after implementation (Scogin et al., 2005). Behavioral activation involves encouraging individuals to become more active, often through the use of activity-scheduling exercises that increase contact with positive environmental reinforcers (Bottonari, Roberts, Thomas, & Read, 2008; Kanter, Busch, & Rusch, 2009). As noted earlier, other chapters in the current volume provide additional details on these therapies.

The use of CBT techniques and the common issues that arise in treating depression in older adults might best be illustrated with the following case example.

Mrs. P—Depressed and "Useless"

Mrs. P is an 82-year-old African American female with a history of osteoarthritis, diabetes, chronic generalized anxiety disorder, and mild cognitive impairment (MCI) (amnestic multiple-domain subtype, with deficits in memory and semantic naming). She was widowed 5 years ago and has lived with her son and three grandchildren since then. At a recent check-up with her primary care physician, family members reported that she had been quieter and more somber over the past few months, a notable shift from her fun-loving personality. She also stopped driving 3 months ago, reportedly due to visual difficulties. Her family reports frustration because she does not ask for assistance with transportation and says she would be "burdening" them to do so. They have also noticed that she sits in her room and stares out the window more frequently since her last grandchild was born about 3 months ago.

During an initial interview with Mrs. P, she became tearful, noting that her family members "have lives of their own" and that she feels "useless." She reported that she spent her early years as a caretaker for her siblings and later became a nurse.

She felt that "the best times" of her life were when she raised five children with her beloved husband, Harold. She reported that she has been a "worrywart" since her teenage years, and that working helped to keep her mind on other things. She felt depressed after her children moved out of the home 30 years ago, with increased depression after her retirement 20 years ago and the death of her husband 5 years ago. She reported feeling "glad at first" when she moved in with her son and his family 5 years ago, but since then she has felt increasingly "left out" of the family, especially since her last grandchild was born 3 months ago. She reported several symptoms, including increased crying, increased sleeping, decreased appetite, difficulty concentrating, and feeling depressed on most days over the past 3 months. Upon further questioning, she reported that she voluntarily stopped driving because it was difficult for her to see at night, and because she felt that her diagnosis of MCI implied that she should no longer be driving ("I stopped it myself"). Review of her medical records suggested that her MCI was quite mild, that her diabetes and osteoarthritis were generally under control, and that her visual difficulties were due to cataracts. Further discussion with Mrs. P revealed that she had been informed about her cataracts several years ago and had since forgotten why she was having visual problems. A risk assessment revealed that she was not suicidal and had no history of suicide attempts or ideation.

Consistent with the clinical approach to CBT described in Karlin (2011), the following steps were taken in structuring CBT with Mrs. P:

1. *Case conceptualization, with integration of age-related factors that may impact symptoms.* Mrs. P appears to be suffering from depression that was exacerbated by several factors, including a perceived shift in her role as family caregiver, decreased self-worth since discontinuing driving, and increased isolation from her family due to feeling "useless." Mrs. P's interpretation of these experiences, as well as her assumptions (e.g., that she had to discontinue driving due to MCI and visual problems) may be a focus of CBT. Case conceptualization was modified throughout treatment based on new information.

2. *Motivation enhancement and treatment socialization.* Mrs. P's feelings and experiences were validated, and she was informed that working with her therapist on "exercises" that examined her thoughts and her behaviors might help her feel better. She and her therapist discussed her motivation for treatment, and she indicated that she would be willing to do "anything" to feel better, even though she did not have much energy. She was informed that she might feel an increase in her energy if she committed to participating in at least a few sessions. She agreed to "partner" with her therapist and reevaluate her progress with her therapist after six sessions. She and her therapist agreed that initial goals for therapy would include an improvement in her mood (as measured by the Geriatric Depression Scale [GDS]; Yesavage et al., 1983) and 25% increased time spent out of her room with her family. She was in agreement with informing her family about this plan.

3. *Integrate behavioral components.* She first completed an activity-monitoring log, which revealed that she spent 12 hours in her room daily and 12 hours watching television in the living room of her son's home. The following week she agreed to engage in activity scheduling, spending increased time with her new grandchild (three times weekly for 30 minutes). With the permission of her physician, she returned to daytime driving and agreed to drive to a hair appointment weekly and lunch once per week with her daughter.

4. *Integrate cognitive components.* During her third week of therapy, she reported decreased depression, which she attributed to "getting around more." She agreed to learn more about how her thoughts might be impacting her mood. Her therapist helped her to identify her most prominent automatic thought (AT) ("I will never be able to do anything anymore"). This AT typically occurred when she was by herself and not interacting with her family. Over the next few sessions, as she continued her activity scheduling, Mrs. P and her therapist examined the evidence for her AT and uncovered a related core belief ("I'm useless"), which they focused on over the next few sessions.

5. *Outcome.* After 12 weekly sessions, and gradual normalization of her GDS scores, Mrs. P reported feeling much happier. After five additional sessions, Mrs. P reported that she was feeling significantly better and agreed to terminate therapy.

CBT for Anxiety

CBT for the treatment of anxiety in older adults involves the use of anxiety-reduction strategies, including cognitive techniques (e.g., cognitive restructuring, worry-behavior prevention, active problem solving) and behavioral exercises (e.g., progressive muscle relaxation, diaphragmatic breathing, interoceptive exposure, activity structuring, in vivo exposure, and sleep hygiene) (Gorenstein, Papp, & Kleber, 1999).

Recent reviews show that CBT and relaxation training (RT) are effective in treating anxiety in older adults. For example, in a review of randomized, controlled trials, RT was effective in treating subjective anxiety symptoms, whereas CBT was effective in treating generalized anxiety disorder (GAD) and miscellaneous anxiety syndromes, including panic disorder (Wetherell, Sorrell, Thorp, & Patterson, 2005). A review of 17 studies in older adults with GAD or mixed anxiety disorders showed that CBT had the most consistent support, with RT judged to be an efficacious, relatively low-cost intervention (Ayers, Sorrell, Thorp, & Wetherell, 2007). Although a meta-analysis of 19 studies showed no additive value of CBT beyond relaxation training, it was noted that direct comparison was compromised by differences in control groups (Thorp et al., 2009). CBT has also been shown to be effective in treating GAD in older adults in primary care settings (Brenes, Wagener, & Stanley, 2008).

Studies comparing CBT to nonbehavioral therapies have generally shown superior effectiveness of CBT. For example, Barrowclough et al. (2001) found that although older adults treated with CBT and supportive counseling (SC) both showed improvement on anxiety measures following treatment, the CBT group had lower self-ratings of anxiety and depression. Over the follow-up period, the CBT group maintained improvement and had significantly greater improvement than the SC group on anxiety and depression measures, and treatment response for anxiety was also superior. In a study of older adults receiving an anxiolytic medication taper, adjunctive CBT (versus medication taper alone) correlated with significantly reduced psychological symptoms, even 6 months posttreatment (Gorenstein et al., 2005). In addition, a randomized clinical trial of CBT in primary care showed greater improvement in worry severity, depressive symptoms, and general mental health for older patients with GAD as compared to a supportive telephone intervention (Stanley et al., 2009).

GAD has been frequently studied in older adults, with some studies correlating symptom variables with treatment response. One study determined that age of onset is an important modifier of GAD symptoms, especially given that most older adults report onset of symptoms in childhood or adolescence, and earlier-onset symptoms are more likely to be associated with pathological worry and a more severe course than later-onset symptoms (which were more often associated with role disability; Le Roux, Gatz, & Wetherell, 2005). The timeline for symptom reduction may also be an important modifier. For example, in a study of older adults with GAD treated in a multispecialty health organization, early symptom reduction (after 1 month of CBT) predicted symptom improvement after treatment (3 months) and posttreatment (15 months), suggesting that early response or lack of response to treatment should be investigated as a prognostic factor in older adults (Bradford et al., 2011). Modifiers for treatment response in group therapy for GAD included better homework adherence, higher baseline GAD severity, comorbid psychiatric diagnosis, and at-home practice of techniques (Wetherell et al., 2005b).

CBT for Other Mental Health Conditions in Older Adults

In addition to evidence of effectiveness in treating depression and anxiety, CBT has been shown to be effective in treating bipolar disorder (Nguyen, Truong, Marquett, & Reiser, 2007), suicidality (Coon, DeVries, & Gallagher-Thompson, 2004), and alcohol abuse (Dupree, Schonfeld, Dearborn-Harshman, & Lynn, 2008). In addition, a review of 34 randomized controlled trials involving 3,922 patients showed that CBT was the best established and most effective treatment for somatoform disorders (Kroenke, 2007). CBT has also been shown to be effective in treating symptoms of schizophrenia (Granholm, Gottlieb, McQuaid, & McClure, 2006), and a CBT-based conceptual model for the treatment of visual hallucinations has been proposed (Collerton & Dudley, 2004).

CBT in Medical Populations

Given that 80% of older adults have one chronic health condition and 50% have two (Centers for Disease Control and Prevention, 2011a), it is important to note that cognitive-behavioral therapies have been shown to be effective in treating depression and anxiety in the context of common chronic medical conditions, including coronary artery disease, diabetes, arthritis, and insomnia. In addition, extensive evidence supports the efficacy of CBT in treating symptoms that may be either directly due to various medical conditions or due to the psychological impact of such medical conditions.

CBT for Insomnia

As reviewed in Rybarczyk et al. (2005), older and younger adults showed similar benefit from CBT for insomnia (CBT-I), and multicomponent CBT-I approaches (combining sleep restriction, stimulus control, relaxation training, and sleep hygiene) yielded effect sizes 20% greater than single-component treatments. In a review of effective treatments for insomnia in older adults, only multicomponent CBT-I and sleep restriction–sleep compression therapy met criteria for evidence-based therapies, with insufficient evidence to consider cognitive therapy, relaxation therapy, and sleep hygiene education as stand-alone interventions (McCurry, Logsdon, Teri, & Vitiello, 2007). The positive effects from CBT-I were shown to generalize beyond improvement in insomnia, often positively impacting physical functioning, emotional role limitation, and mental health over 6 months (Dixon, Morgan, Mathers, Thompson, & Tomeny, 2006).

Although many older adults prefer CBT to sleep medication (Stone, Booth, & Lichstein, 2008), a review on the management of chronic insomnia found an underutilization of nonpharmacologic approaches such as CBT-I (Bain, 2006), which may relate in part to limited professional training in CBT-I (Manber et al., 2012). Treatment of insomnia is particularly important for broader psychological wellness, given that older adults with persistent insomnia are at greater risk for the development of depression (Perlis et al., 2006).

CBT has also been shown effective in treating insomnia in older adults with comorbid medical disorders. For example, in a study examining the use of CBT-I in treating primary and comorbid insomnia in older adults with osteoarthritis or coronary artery disease, self-help CBT for insomnia showed good potential to serve as a first-line, cost-effective treatment, with maintenance of results for 81% of treatment responders after 1-year follow-up (Rybarczyk, Mack, Harris, & Stepanski, 2011). Rybarczyk et al. (2005) also showed that CBT resulted in notable improvements on 8 out of 10 self-report sleep measures in older adults with comorbid osteoarthritis, coronary artery disease, or pulmonary disease, with similar outcomes regardless of the type of chronic disease. In addition, a recent large-scale implementation of CBT-I with older Veterans revealed large improvements in insomnia, depression, and quality of life in routine treatment settings, with effects equivalent to those observed with younger patients (Karlin, Trockel, Spira, Taylor, & Manber, 2015). Guidelines for utilizing CBT to treat insomnia are available (Stone, Booth, & Lichstein, 2008) and might be modified based on specific protocols that are used in certain subpopulations of older adults.

CBT for Arthritis

CBT has been shown to be helpful in managing the mood and functional issues related to arthritis. For example, in older adults with osteoarthritis and comorbid depression, CBT, coupled with integrated depression care management and exercise therapy, was associated with reduced depressive symptoms (Yohannes & Caton, 2010). In a study of individuals with early rheumatoid arthritis, CBT resulted in significant reductions in fatigue, depression, and helplessness at posttreatment and 6-month follow-up (Evers, Kraaimaat, van Riel, & deJong, 2002).

CBT for Cardiac Conditions

As reviewed in Clabby and Howarth (2007), several studies have shown that older adults with congestive heart failure (CHF) are likely to have comorbid depression, and that CBT can effectively treat CHF-related depression, alone or in combination with a disease management program to improve physical health. In a review examining the effectiveness of several nonpharmacologic approaches in treating depression in coronary heart disease (CHD)—including CBT, interpersonal therapy (IPT), aerobic exercise, St. John's wort (SJW), essential fatty acids (EFAs), S-Adenosylmethionine (SAMe), acupuncture, and chromium picolinate (CP)—CBT and IPT were shown to be most effective (Lett, Davidson, & Blumenthal, 2005). Treatment of depression with CBT has also been shown to reduce heart rate and thus may have a beneficial effect on a known risk factor for mortality in depressed patients with CHD (Carney et al., 2000). In a clinical trial of individuals with a history of acute myocardial infarction (MI), successful treatment of depression varied as a function of CBT homework completion, and not antidepressant use (Cowan et al., 2008).

CBT for Diabetes

The prevalence of depressive disorder in older adults with type 2 diabetes is significantly higher than in nondiabetic older adults (Shehatah, Rabie, & Al-Shahry, 2010), especially in individuals with poor glycemic control. A study by Gonzalez and colleagues (2010) found that individuals participating in a 10–12 session CBT team intervention exhibited decreased depression and improved diabetes self-care and glycemic control. CBT has also been shown effective in improving self-management in patients with poorly controlled type 1 diabetes, resulting in increased blood glucose testing and decreased hypoglycemia, distress, anxiety, and depression (Amsberg et al., 2009).

CBT for Other Medical Issues

CBT has been shown to be more effective than antidepressants in treating a variety of pain syndromes, including irritable bowel syndrome, chronic back pain, headache, fibromyalgia, chronic fatigue syndrome, tinnitus, menopausal symptoms, chronic facial pain, noncardiac chest pain, interstitial cystitis, and chronic pelvic pain (Jackson, O'Malley, & Kroenke, 2006). In individuals with chronic obstructive pulmonary disease (COPD), a 2-hour CBT group intervention resulted in reduced anxiety and depression (Kunik et al., 2001). For individuals with heart failure and COPD, a modular CBT approach was successful in treating depression and anxiety (Cully, Paukert, Falco, & Stanley, 2009). In addition, a recent review of randomized controlled trials evaluating psychological treatment in individuals with spinal cord injury (SCI) found that CBT was effective in treating depression, anxiety, and adjustment issues (Mehta et al., 2011).

CBT for Older Adults with Cognitive Disorders

As reviewed in Dreer, Copeland, and Cheavens (2011), several studies have shown promising results when CBT is modified to account for neurocognitive weaknesses identified through neuropsychological testing. In particular, performance on measures of executive functioning (EF) (measures of judgment, problem solving, mental flexibility, and self-monitoring) is valuable to incorporate, given that some older adults with EF deficits and anxiety symptoms showed decreased benefit from CBT (Mohlman & Gorman, 2005), and older adults who received CBT with concomitant executive skills training for GAD showed greater improvement in executive skills and worry than older adults who received CBT without executive skills training (Mohlman, 2008).

Several studies have shown that older adults with a variety of cognitive disorders benefit from CBT. For example, individuals with mild cognitive impairment (MCI) who participated in CBT group therapy with their spouses reported increased acceptance of MCI, and spouses showed increased awareness of memory and behavioral issues (Banningh et al.,

2008). For individuals with early-stage dementia, CBT is helpful in developing coping strategies and reducing distress (Kasl-Godley & Gatz, 2000), and, in an innovative study utilizing CBT and Tai Chi, depression was decreased and balance was improved (Burgener, Yang, & Gilbert, 2008). CBT can also be successfully modified to treat GAD in dementia (Kraus et al., 2008) and to decrease depression in Alzheimer's disease when used with behavioral treatments including pleasant event scheduling and caregiver problem solving (Teri, Logsdon, Uomoto, & McCurry, 1997; Walker, 2004). CBT, coupled with a cognitive enhancement intervention, has also been shown effective in treating anxiety, memory problems, and attention problems in Parkinson's disease (Mohlman et al., 2010). In addition, CBT has been shown to be helpful when treating individuals in long-term care with chronic pain and comorbid physical or cognitive impairments (Glifford, Cipher, Roper, Snow, & Molinari 2008). A model for providing CBT to individuals with dementia is provided by Snow, Powers, and Liles (2006).

Cognitive correlates of CBT treatment response in older adults with anxiety have also been identified. For example, older adults with lower "fluid intelligence" (i.e., ability to perceive and adapt to novel situations) exhibited less benefit from supportive counseling, but good response to CBT regardless of fluid intelligence level (Doubleday, King, & Papageorgiou, 2002). Another study found that older adults with GAD and poor performance on the Mini-Mental Status Examination (MMSE) Working Memory index exhibited increased baseline anxiety and depression, and baseline performance differences on the MMSE Orientation domain predicted outcome 6 months after CBT intervention (Caudle et al., 2007).

Challenging behaviors such as agitation, aggression, and wandering are more common as dementia progresses and are often stressful for caregivers. Behavioral interventions have been increasingly studied, especially given significant concerns about increased mortality risk and limited efficacy associated with the use of antipsychotic medications in dementia (Huybrechts et al., 2012; Kales et al., 2009). Behavioral interventions for dementia-related behaviors include but are not limited to functional analysis of behaviors, promoting engagement in pleasant activities, communication training, and individualized behavioral reinforcement strategies. In a review of 162 studies that utilized psychological interventions to manage challenging neuropsychiatric symptoms in dementia, only behavioral management strategies and staff/caregiver education showed lasting effectiveness (Livingston, Johnston, Katona, Paton, & Lyketsos, 2005). Individualized behavioral interventions also are more successful than those that are not individualized (Livingston et al., 2005).

One interdisciplinary behavioral approach to managing challenging dementia-related behaviors is STAR (Staff Training in Assisted Living Residences; Teri, Huda, Gibbons, Young, & van Leynseele, 2005). STAR is a multicomponent intervention designed for professional caregivers that focuses on behavior modification strategies, increasing pleasant events, and promoting effective communication with and maintaining realistic expectations of individuals with dementia. STAR has recently been adapted as part of a pilot implementation initiative in the Veterans Health Administration (VHA). This intervention, known as STAR-VA, has been implemented in 17 VA community living centers (CLCs; formerly known as "nursing home care units") (Karlin et al., 2011). Clinical outcome data demonstrate significant reductions in the frequency and severity of challenging behaviors, depression, and anxiety (Karel, Teri, McConnell, Visnic, & Karlin, in press; Karlin, Visnic, McGee, & Teri, L., 2014).

In addition to providing behavioral techniques for professional caregivers, CBT is effective in decreasing depression and stress for family caregivers (Coon, Shurgot, Gillispie, Cardenas, & Gallagher-Thompson, 2005; Gallagher-Thompson, Gray, Dupart, Jimenez, & Thompson, 2008), and even telephone CBT interventions can effectively help caregivers attain specific goals related to improving their caregiving experience (Wilz, Schinköthe, & Soellner, 2011).

CBT across Settings

As previously highlighted, CBT has been paired with various medical interventions to treat depression and anxiety in the context of comorbid medical issues, and it has been effectively used in long-term care settings to manage challenging behaviors and neuropsychiatric symptoms in dementia. In addition, cognitive and behavioral therapies are used in specialty mental health settings, outpatient settings, hospice and palliative care, home-based environments, cognitive rehabilitation, and throughout various settings in the VA health care system (as reviewed in Sorocco & Lauderdale, 2011). Similarly, a consensus study of community-based treatment for depression concluded that individual CBT was

the most effective treatment modality (Steinman et al., 2006).

Other delivery models with growing empirical support include home-based CBT for insomnia (Rybarczyk, Lopez, Benson, Alsten, & Stepanski. 2002), depression (Maxfield & Segal, 2008), and anxiety (Diefenbach, Tolin, & Meunier, 2008); treatment of depression in community and extended-care settings (Thompson & Gallagher-Thompson, 1997); CBT-I via clinical video teleconferencing to treat insomnia (Rybarczyk, Lopez, Schelble, & Stepanski, 2005); and home-based CBT to treat psychological symptoms and improve quality of life in primarily rural, African American, low-resource, physically frail older adults (Scogin et al., 2007). In long-term care settings, the GIST model (Group, Individual, and Staff Therapy) has been shown to be effective in treating depression, with participants reporting high subjective ratings of treatment satisfaction (Hyer & Hilton, 2006). A multitheoretical model for treating depression, focusing on growth, adaptability, and change, may be particularly helpful in the nursing home environment (Duffy & Karlin, 2006).

Limited Utilization of CBT

Despite the wealth of data supporting the effectiveness of CBT for various mental disorders and in various settings, CBT and other psychological interventions are underutilized in the older adult population, and older adults are three times less likely to receive mental health treatment than younger adults (Karlin, Duffy, & Gleaves, 2008). Although older adults often fail to recognize a need for mental health care (Karlin et al., 2008), underidentification of mental health disorders by professionals has also been noted. For example, older adults typically seek treatment for mental health concerns from a primary care physician, and many primary care physicians report both a lack of confidence in diagnosing mental health disorders and an expectation that depression is normative in older adults and therefore not an appropriate target for treatment (Jeste et al., 1999). Recent data support this finding, suggesting that primary care physicians are less successful in detecting depression in older than younger adults (Mitchell, Rao, & Vaze, 2010), and that anxiety symptoms are not documented in the medical records of many older adults (Calleo et al., 2009).

Identification of mental health issues is important not only for psychological treatment but also because some disorders, such as depression, serve as risk factors for future medical conditions. For example, one study showed that working-age adults (ages 50–62 years) with depression at baseline were at significantly higher risk to develop diabetes, heart problems, and arthritis during 12-year follow-up (Karakus & Patton, 2011). In addition, a 15-year longitudinal study found that late-life depression was a risk factor for the development of dementia (Li et al., 2011).

A long-recognized solution to the underdetection of mental health issues in primary care is the integration of mental health care and primary care services (Coleman & Patrick, 1976), which was formally recommended by the World Health Organization in 2001, and in the United States health care reform bill (i.e., Patient Protection and Affordability Care Act). Promising research shows that integration of services can help to improve care (Fiske, Wetherell, & Gatz, 2009; Speer & Schneider, 2003), especially when older adults are connected to clinicians trained in evidence-based therapies (Gatz, 2007). Although various approaches for integration have been proposed (Thielke, Vannoy, & Unutzer, 2007), a "blended" approach, incorporating evidence-based approaches of care management and colocated/collaborative care that has been implemented in primary care settings throughout VHA, has proven particularly successful (Post, Metzger, Dumas, & Lemann, 2010; Zeiss & Karlin, 2008).

New changes in Medicare reimbursement for outpatient mental health treatment may help to support the increased use of CBT and other psychological treatments by older adults over the coming years (Karlin & Humphries, 2007). For example, although Medicare previously reimbursed mental health treatment at a rate of 50% (while reimbursing ambulatory medical services at 80%), in 2008, Congress enacted the Medicare Improvements for Patients and Providers Act, which eliminated the disparity in Medicare mental health care coverage through a phased process that has now been fully implemented.

A multicomponent approach to improving mental health outcomes for older adults might involve both systems-level changes to improve detection, access, and reimbursement; and interventions targeted at the individual level (e.g., patient education). For example, patient receptivity to psychotherapy might be increased by focusing on related physical, financial, cognitive, emotional, educational, and attitudinal issues. In addition, receptivity to therapy might be increased with expanded options for service provision, including the use of in-home psychotherapy, telephone sessions, support groups, strong community outreach, and liaisons with other professionals (Yang & Jackson, 1998).

Conclusion

CBT is effective in treating anxiety, depression, and other mental and behavioral health issues in older adults, with or without comorbid medical and neurocognitive conditions, and across a variety of settings. Despite the evidence for effectiveness and the growing need for psychological treatments in the older adult population, barriers to accessing CBT still exist. A continued focus on enhanced awareness and access, including integrating mental health services into primary care settings, educating health care providers and consumers about the benefits of CBT, development of innovative methods for service delivery, and influencing health care policy, is likely to increase the demand for CBT and enhance the quality of life and functioning for a greater number of older adults.

Future Directions

The effectiveness of CBT in older adults might be enhanced through additional research into variables associated with improved clinical outcomes. Randomized controlled trials are especially encouraged, given that they are most likely to influence health care policy. Continued investigations into the importance of culture (DeVries & Coon, 2002); modifications to CBT as a function of cognitive abilities (Dreer, Copeland, & Cheavens, 2011); early identification of symptoms; improved tools to assess symptoms and measure outcomes; and personalization of treatments (Beck, 2008) might be particularly helpful. Expanded integration of mental health treatment into primary care settings (Stanley et al, 2009) and the development of additional strategies to bundle CBT with medical interventions is highly recommended. This is especially important given that several national organizations—including VHA, the American Psychological Association (APA), the National Institutes of Health, and the National Institute of Mental Health—support the integration of mental health treatment into primary care (APA, 2010).

Expanding upon innovations to treat depression in community-dwelling older adults is also encouraged (Centers for Disease Control and Prevention, 2011b). In addition, improving access to CBT by increasing the availability of specialty training (Pachana, Knight, Karel, & Beck, 2008) and demonstrating cost-effectiveness are highly recommended. Prevention of mental health disorders—focusing broadly on avoiding a first onset of illness, a recurrence in late life, or a relapse following treatment (Fiske, Wetherell, & Gatz, 2009)—is another vital area for additional study (Steinman et al., 2006), especially given that identification and modification of risk factors can decrease future symptoms of mental illness (Cole, 2008; Hsu et al., 2010; Konnert & Stelmach, 2009).

References

Administration on Aging, US Department of Health and Human Services. (2010). *A profile of older Americans.* Retrieved December 2011, from http://www.aoa.gov/Aging_Statistics/Profile/2010/docs/2010profile.pdf

American Psychological Association. (2010). APA health reform matrix: Key provisions by APA priority. Retrieved December 2011, from http://www.apa.org/about/gr/issues/health-care/health-reform-matrix.pdf

Amsberg, S., Anderbro, T., Wredling, R., Lisspers, J., Lins, P., Adamson, U., & Johansson, U. B. (2009). A cognitive behavior therapy-based intervention among poorly controlled adult type 1 diabetes patients—A randomized controlled trial. *Patient Education and Counseling, 771,* 72–80.

Areán, P. A. (2004). Psychosocial treatments for depression in the elderly. *Primary Psychiatry, 11*(5), 48–53.

Areán, P. A., Gum, A., McCulloch, C. E., Bostrom, A., Gallagher-Thompson, D., & Thompson, L. (2005). Treatment of depression in low-income older adults. *Psychology and Aging, 20,* 601–609.

Ayers, C. R., Sorrell, J. T., Thorp, S. R., & Wetherell, J. L. (2007). Evidence-based psychological treatments for late-life anxiety. *Psychology and Aging, 22*(1), 8–17.

Bain, K. T. (2006). Management of chronic insomnia in elderly persons. *American Journal of Geriatric Pharmacotherapy, 4,* 168–192.

Banningh, L. W. A. J., Kessels, R. P. C., Nijmegen, R., Rikkert, M. G. M. O., Geleijns-Lanting, C. E., & Kraaimaat, F. W. (2008). A cognitive behavioural group therapy for patients diagnosed with mild cognitive impairment and their significant others: Feasibility and preliminary results. *Clinical Rehabilitation, 22,* 731–740.

Barrowclough, C., King, P., Colville, J., Russell, E., Burns, A., & Tarrier, N. (2001). A randomized trial of the effectiveness of cognitive-behavioral therapy and supportive counseling for anxiety symptoms in older adults. *Journal of Consulting and Clinical Psychology, 69,* 756–762.

Beck, J. G. (2008). Treating generalized anxiety in a community setting. In D. Gallagher-Thompson, A. M. Steffen, & L. W. Thompson (Eds.), *Handbook of behavioral and cognitive therapies with older adults* (pp. 18–32). New York: Springer Science.

Bottonari, K. A., Roberts, J. E., Thomas, S. N., & Read, J. P. (2008). Stop thinking and start doing: Switching from cognitive therapy to behavioral activation in a case of chronic treatment-resistant depression. *Cognitive and Behavioral Practice, 15,* 376–386.

Bradford, A., Cully, J., Rhoades, H., Kunik, M. Kraus-Schuman, C., Wilson, N., & Stanley, M. (2011). Early response to psychotherapy and long-term change in worry symptoms in older adults with generalized anxiety disorder. *American Journal of Geriatric Psychiatry, 19,* 347–356.

Brenes, G. A., & Wagener, P., & Stanley, M. A. (2008). Treatment of late-life generalized anxiety disorder in primary care settings. In D. Gallagher-Thompson, A. M. Steffen, & L. W. Thompson (Eds.), *Handbook of behavioral and cognitive therapies with older adults* (pp. 33–47). New York: Springer Science.

Burgener, S. C., Yang, Y., & Gilbert, R., (2008). The effects of a multimodal intervention on outcomes of persons with early-stage dementia. *American Journal of Alzheimer's Disease and Other Dementias, 23,* 382–394.

Burgio, L. D., & Fisher, S. E. (2000). Application of psychosocial interventions for treating behavioral and psychological symptoms of dementia. *International Psychgeriatrics, 12,* 351–358.

Calleo, J., Stanley, M. A., Greisinger, A., Wehmanen, O., Johnson, M., Novy, D.,...Kunik, M. (2009). Generalized anxiety disorder in older medical patients: Diagnostic recognition, mental health management and service utilization. *Journal of Clinical Psychology in Medical Settings, 16,* 178–185.

Carney, R. M., Freedland, K. E., Stein, P. K., Skala, J. A., Hoffman, P., & Jaffe, A. S. (2000). Change in heart rate variability during treatment for depression in patients with coronary heart disease. *Psychosomatic Medicine, 62,* 639–647.

Caudle, D. D., Senior, A. C., Wetherell, J. L., Rhoades, H. M., Beck, J. G., Kunik, M. E.,...Stanley, M. A. (2007). Cognitive errors, symptom severity, and response to cognitive behavior therapy in older adults with generalized anxiety disorder. *American Journal of Geriatric Psychiatry, 15,* 680–689.

Centers for Disease Control and Prevention. (2007). *The state of aging and health in America, 2007.* Retrieved on December 2011, from http://www.cdc.gov/aging/pdf/saha_2007.pdf

Centers for Disease Control and Prevention. (2011a). *Healthy aging.* Retrieved June 2012, from http://www.cdc.gov/chronicdisease/resources/publications/aag/aging.htm

Centers for Disease Control and Prevention. (2011b). *Evidence-based programs for treatment of depression in community-dwelling older adults.* Retrieved December 2011, from http://apps.nccd.cdc.gov/MAHA/EBPrograms.aspx

Clabby, J., & Howarth, D. (2007). Managing CHF and depression in an elderly patient: Being open to collaborative care. *Families, Systems, and Health, 25,* 457–464.

Cole, M. G. (2008). Brief interventions to prevent depression in older subjects: A systematic review of feasibility and effectiveness. *Psychiatric Clinics of North America, 28,* 785–803.

Coleman, J. V., & Patrick, D. L. (1976). Integrating mental health services into primary medical care. *Medical Care, 14,* 654–661.

Collerton, D., & Dudley, R. (2004). A cognitive behavioural framework for the treatment of distressing visual hallucinations in older people. *Behavioural and Cognitive Psychotherapy, 32,* 443–455.

Coon, D. W., DeVries, H. M., & Gallagher-Thompson, D. (2004). Cognitive behavioral therapy with suicidal older adults. *Behavioural and Cognitive Psychotherapy, 32,* 481–493.

Coon, D. W., Shurgot, G. R., Gillispie, Z., Cardenas, V., & Gallagher-Thompson, D. (2005). Cognitive-behavioral group interventions. In G. O. Gabbard, J. S. Beck, & J. Homes (Eds.), *Oxford textbook of psychotherapy* (pp. 45–55). New York: Oxford University Press.

Cowan, M. J., Freedland, K. E., Burg, M. M., Saab, P. G., Youngblood, M. E., Cornell, C. E.,...ENRICHD Investigators. (2008). Predictors of treatment response for depression and inadequate social support—The ENRICHD randomized clinical trial. *Psychotherapy and Psychosomatics*, 77(1), 27–37.

Cully, J. A., Paukert, A., Falco, J., & Stanley, M. (2009). Cognitive-behavioral therapy: Innovations for cardiopulmonary patients with depression and anxiety. *Cognitive and Behavioral Practice*, 16, 394–407.

DeRubeis, R. J., Hollon, S. D., Amsterdam, J. D., Shelton, R. C., Young, P. R., Salomon, R. M.,... Gallop, R. (2005). Cognitive therapy vs medications in the treatment of moderate to severe depression. *Archives of General Psychiatry*, 62, 409–416.

DeVries, H. M., & Coon, D. W. (2002). Cognitive/behavioral group therapy with older adults. In F. W. Kaslow & T. Patterson (Eds.), *Comprehensive handbook of psychotherapy: Cognitive-behavioral approaches* (Vol. 2, pp. 547–567). Hoboken, NJ: Wiley.

Dick-Siskin, L. P. (2002). Cognitive-behavioral therapy with older adults. *Behavior Therapist*, 25(1), 3–6.

Diefenbach, G. J., Tolin, D. F., & Meunier, S. A. (2008). Extending cognitive-behavioral therapy for late-life anxiety to home care: Program development and case examples. *Behavior Modification*, 32, 595–610.

Dixon, S., Morgan, K., Mathers, N., Thompson, J., & Tomeny, M. (2006). Impact of cognitive behavior therapy on health-related quality of life among adult hypnotic users with chronic insomnia. *Behavioral Sleep Medicine*, 4, 71–84.

Doubleday, E. K., King, P., & Papageorgiou, C. (2002). Relationship between fluid intelligence and ability to benefit from cognitive-behavioural therapy in older adults: A preliminary investigation. *British Journal of Clinical Psychology*, 41, 423–428.

Dreer, L. E., Copeland, J. N., & Cheavens, J. S. (2011). Integrating neuropsychological functioning into cognitive behavioral therapy: Implications for older adults. In K. H. Sorocco & S. Lauderdale (Eds.), *Cognitive behavior therapy with older adults: Innovations across care settings* (pp. 317–365). New York: Springer.

Duffy, M., & Karlin, B. E. (2006). Treating depression in nursing homes: Beyond the medical model. In L. Hyer & R. Intrieri (Eds.), *Geropsychological interventions in long-term care* (pp. 109–135). New York: Springer.

Dupree, L. W., Schonfeld, L., Dearborn-Harshman, K. O., & Lynn, N. (2008). A relapse prevention model for older alcohol abusers. In D. Gallagher-Thompson, A. M. Steffen, & L. W. Thompson (Eds.), *Handbook of behavioral and cognitive therapies with older adults* (pp. 61–75). New York: Springer Science.

Evers, A. W. M., Kraaimaat, F. W., van Riel, L. C. M., & deJong, A. J. L. (2002). Tailored cognitive-behavioral therapy in early rheumatoid arthritis for patients at risk: A randomized controlled trial. *Pain*, 100(1–2), 141–153.

Fiske, A., Wetherell, J. L., & Gatz, M. (2009). Depression in older adults. *Annual Review of Clinical Psychology*, 5, 363–389.

Gallagher-Thompson, D., Gray, H., Dupart, T., Jimenez, D., & Thompson, L. W. (2008). Effectiveness of cognitive/behavioral small group intervention for reduction of depression and stress in non-Hispanic White and Hispanic/Latino women dementia family caregivers: Outcomes and mediators of change. *Journal of Rational-Emotive and Cognitive Behavior Therapy*, 26, 286–303.

Gallagher-Thompson, D., & Thompson, L. (1996). Applying cognitive-behavioral therapy to the psychological problems of later life. In S. H. Zarit & B. Knight (Eds.), *A guide to psychotherapy and aging: Effective clinical interventions in a life-stage context* (pp. 61–82). Washington, DC: American Psychological Association.

Gatz, M. (2007). Commentary on evidence-based psychological treatments for older adults. *Psychology and Aging*, 22(1), 52–55.

Gatz, M., Fiske, A., Fox, L. S., Kaskie, B., Kasl-Godley, J. E., McCallum, T. J., & Wetherell, J. L. (1998). Empirically validated psychological treatments for older adults. *Journal of Mental Health and Aging*, 4, 9–46.

Glifford, P. A., Cipher, D. J., Roper, K. D., Snow, A. L., & Molinari, V. (2008). Cognitive-behavioral pain management interventions for long-term care residents with physical and cognitive disabilities. In D. Gallagher-Thompson, A. M. Steffen, & L. W. Thompson (Eds.), *Handbook of behavioral and cognitive therapies with older adults* (pp. 76–101). New York: Springer Science.

Gonzalez, J. S., McCarl, L. A., Wexler, D. A., Cagliero, E., Delahanty, L., Soper, T. D.,... Safren, S. A. (2010). Cognitive-behavioral therapy for adherence and depression (CBT-AD) in type 2 diabetes. *Journal of Cognitive Psychotherapy*, 24, 329–343.

Gorenstein, E. E., Kleber, M. S., Mohlman, J., DeJesus, M., Gorman, J. M., & Papp, L. A. (2005). Cognitive-behavioral therapy for management of anxiety and medication taper in older adults. *American Journal of Geriatric Psychiatry*, 13, 901–909.

Gorenstein, E. E., Papp, L. A., & Kleber, M. S. (1999). Cognitive-behavioral treatment of anxiety in later life. *Cognitive and Behavioral Practice*, 6, 305–319.

Granholm, E., Gottlieb, J. D., McQuaid, J. R., & McClure, F. S. (2006). Therapeutic factors contributing to change in cognitive-behavioral group therapy for older persons with schizophrenia. *Journal of Contemporary Psychotherapy*, 36(1), 31–41.

Gum, A. M., King-Kallimanis, B., & Kohn, R. (2009). Prevalence of mood, anxiety, and substance-abuse disorders for older Americans in the national comorbidity survey-replication. *American Journal of Geriatric Psychiatry*, 17, 769–781.

Hodge, D. R., & Bonifas, R. P. (2010). Using spiritually modified cognitive behavioral therapy to help clients wrestling with depression: A promising intervention for some older adults. *Social Thought: Journal of Religion and Spirituality in Social Work*, 29, 185–206.

Hollon, S. D., Stewart, M. O., & Strunk, D. (2006). Enduring effects for cognitive behavior therapy in the treatment of depression and anxiety. *Annual Review of Psychology*, 57, 285–315.

Hsu, C. T., Weng, C. Y., Kuo, C. S., Lin, C., Jong, M., Kuo, S. Y., & Chen, P. F. (2010). Effects of a cognitive-behavioral group program for community-dwelling elderly with minor depression. *International Journal of Geriatric Psychiatry*, 25, 654–655.

Huybrechts, K. F., Schneeweiss, S., Gerhard, T., Olfson, M., Avorn, J., Levin, R.,... Crystal, S. (2012). Comparative safety of antipsychotic medications in nursing home residents. *Journal of the American Geriatrics Society*, 60, 420–429.

Hyer, L., & Hilton, N., (2006). Group, individual, and staff therapy: An efficient and effective cognitive behavioral therapy in long-term care. *American Journal of Alzheimer's Disease and Other Dementias, 23,* 528–539.

Jackson, J. L., O'Malley, P. G., & Kroenke, K. (2006). Antidepressants and cognitive-behavioral therapy for symptom syndromes. *CNS Spectrums, 11,* 212–222.

Jeste, D. V., Alexopoulos, G. S., Bartels, S. J., Cummings, J. L., Gallo, J. J., Gottlieb, G. L., . . . Lebowitz, B. D. (1999). Consensus statement on the upcoming crisis in geriatric mental health: Research agenda for the next 2 decades. *Archives of General Psychiatry, 56,* 848–853.

Kales, H. C., Valenstein, M., Kim, H. M., McCarthy, J. F., Ganoczy, D., Cunningham, F., & Blow, F. C. (2009). Mortality risk in patients with dementia treated with antipsychotics versus other psychiatric medications. *American Journal of Psychiatry, 164,* 1568–1576.

Kanter, J., Busch, A. M., & Rusch, L. C. (2009). *Behavioral activation: distinctive features.* New York: Routledge.

Karakus, M. C., & Patton, L. C. (2011). Depression and the onset of chronic illness in older adults: A 12-year prospective study. *Journal of Behavioral Health Services and Research, 38,* 373–382.

Karel, M. J., Teri, L., McConnell, E., Visnic, & Karlin, B. E. (in press). Effectiveness of a psychosocial intervention for managing challenging behaviors among veterans with dementia: Outcomes from the expanded implementation of STAR-VA. *The Gerontologist.*

Karlin, B. E. (2011). Cognitive behavioral therapy with older adults. In K. H. Sorocco & S. Lauderdale (Eds.), *Cognitive behavior therapy with older adults: Innovations across care settings* (pp. 1–28). New York: Springer.

Karlin, B. E., Duffy, M., & Gleaves, D. H. (2008). Patterns and predictors of mental health service use and mental illness among older and younger adults in the United States. *Psychological Services, 5,* 275–294.

Karlin, B. E., & Humphries, K. (2007). Improving medicare coverage of psychological services for older Americans. *American Psychologist, 62,* 637–649.

Karlin, B. E., Teri, L, McGee, J. S., Sutherland, E., Asghar-Ali, A., Crocker, S. M., . . . Drexler, M. (2011). *STAR-VA: Manual for community living center mental health providers.* Washington, DC: US Department of Veterans Affairs.

Karlin, B. E., Trockel, M., Spira, A., Taylor, C. B., & Manber, R. (2015). National evaluation of the effectiveness of Cognitive Behavioral Therapy for insomnia among older versus younger Veterans. *International Journal of Geriatric Psychiatry, 30,* 308–315.

Karlin, B. E., Visnic, S., McGee, J. S., & Teri, L. (2014). Results from the multi-site implementation of STAR-VA— A multi-component psychosocial intervention for managing challenging dementia-related behaviors of Veterans. *Psychological Services, 11,* 200–208.

Kasl-Godley, J., & Gatz, M. (2000). Psychosocial interventions for individuals with dementia: An integration of theory, therapy, and a clinical understanding of dementia. *Clinical Psychology Review, 20,* 755–782.

Kimmel, D., Rose, T., & David, S. (Eds.). (2006). *Lesbian, gay, bisexual, and transgender aging: Research and clinical perspectives.* New York: Columbia University Press.

Konnert, C., & Stelmach, L. (2009). The prevention of depression in nursing home residents: A randomized clinical trial of cognitive-behavioral therapy. *Aging and Mental Health, 13,* 288–299.

Kraus, C. A., Seignourel, P., Snow, A. L., Wilson, N. L., Kunik, M. E., Schulz, P. E., & Stanley, M. A. (2008).

Cognitive-behavioral treatment for anxiety in patients with dementia: Two case studies. *Journal of Psychiatric Practice, 14,* 186–192.

Krishna, M., Jauhari, A., Lepping, P., Turner, J., Crossley, D., & Krishnamoorthy, A. (2011). Is group psychotherapy effective in older adults with depression? A systematic review. *International Journal of Geriatric Psychiatry, 26,* 331–340.

Kroenke, K. (2007). Efficacy of treatment for somatoform disorders: A review of randomized controlled trials. *Psychosomatic Medicine, 69,* 881–888.

Kunik, M. E., Braun, U., Stanley, M. A., Wristers, K., Molinari, V., Stoebner, D., Orengo, C. A. (2001). One session cognitive behavioural therapy for elderly patients with chronic obstructive pulmonary disease. *Psychological Medicine, 31,* 717–723.

Laidlaw, K. (2008). Post-stroke depression and CBT with older people. In D. Gallagher-Thompson, A. M. Steffen, & L. W. Thompson (Eds.), *Handbook of behavioral and cognitive therapies with older adults* (pp. 223–248). New York: Springer Science.

Laidlaw, K., & McAlpine, S. (2008). Cognitive behaviour therapy: How is it different with older people? *Journal of Rational-Emotive and Cognitive Behavior Therapy, 26,* 250–262.

Lau, A. W., & Kinoshita, L. M. (2006). Cognitive-behavioral therapy with culturally diverse older adults. In P. A. Hays & G. Y. Iwamasa (Eds.), *Culturally responsive cognitive-behavioral therapy: Assessment, practice, and supervision* (pp. 179–197). Washington, DC: American Psychological Association.

Le Roux, H., Gatz, M., & Wetherell, J. L. (2005). Age at onset of generalized anxiety disorder in older adults. *American Journal of Geriatric Psychiatry, 13,* 23–30.

Lett, H. S., Davidson, J., & Blumenthal, J. A. (2005). Nonpharmacologic treatments for depression in patients with coronary heart disease. *Psychosomatic Medicine, 67,* S58–S62.

Li, G., Wang, L. Y., Shofer, J. B., Thompson, M. L., Peskind, E. R., McCormick, W., . . . Larson, E. B. (2011). Temporal relationship between depression and dementia: Findings from a large community-based 15-year follow-up study. *Archives of General Psychiatry, 68,* 970–977.

Livingston, G., Johnston, K., Katona, C., Paton, J., & Lyketsos, C. G., (2005). Systematic review of psychological approaches to the management of neuropsychiatric symptoms of dementia. *American Journal of Psychiatry, 162,* 1996–2021.

Mackin, R. S., & Areán, P. A. (2005). Evidence-based psychotherapeutic interventions for geriatric depression. *Psychiatric Clinics of North America, 28,* 805–820.

Manber, R., Carney, C., Edinger, J., Epstein, D., Friedman, L., Haynes, P. L., . . . Trockel, M. (2012). Dissemination of CBTI to the non-sleep specialist: Protocol development and training issues. *Journal of Clinical Sleep Medicine, 8,* 209–218.

Maxfield, M., & Segal, D. L. (2008). Psychotherapy in non-traditional settings: A case of in-home cognitive-behavioral therapy with a depressed older adult. *Clinical Case Studies, 7,* 154–166.

McCurry, S. M., Logsdon, R. G., Teri, L., & Vitiello, M. V. (2007). Evidence-based psychological treatments for insomnia in older adults. *Psychology and Aging, 22*(1), 18–27.

Mehta, S., Orenczuk, S., Hansen, K. T., Aubut, J. L., Hitzig, S. L., Legassic, M., . . . Spinal Cord Injury Rehabilitation Evidence Research Team. (2011). An evidence-based review of the effectiveness of cognitive behavioral therapy for psychosocial issues post-spinal cord injury. *Rehabilitation Psychology, 56,* 15–25.

Mitchell A. J., Rao S., & Vaze, A. (2010). Do primary care physicians have particular difficulty identifying late-life depression? A meta-analysis stratified by age. *Psychotherapy and Psychosomatics, 79,* 285–294.

Mohlman, J. (2008). More power to the executive? A preliminary test of CBT plus executive skills training for treatment of late-life GAD. *Cognitive and Behavioral Practice, 15,* 306–316.

Mohlman, J., & Gorman, J. M. (2005). The role of executive functioning in CBT: A pilot study with older adults. *Behaviour Research and Therapy, 43,* 447–465.

Mohlman, J., Reel, D. H., Chazin, D., Ong, D., Georgescu, B., Tiu, J., & Dobkin, R. D. (2010). A novel approach to treating anxiety and enhancing executive skills in an older adult with Parkinson's disease. *Clinical Case Studies, 9*(1), 74–90.

Morin, C. M., Colecchi, C., Stone, J., Sood, R., & Brink, D. (1999). Behavioral and pharmacological therapies for late-life insomnia. *Journal of the American Medical Association, 281,* 991–999.

Moss, K. S., & Scogin, F. R. (2008). Behavioral and cognitive treatments for geriatric depression: An evidence-based perspective. In D. Gallagher-Thompson, A. M. Steffen, & L. W. Thompson (Eds.), *Handbook of behavioral and cognitive therapies with older adults* (pp. 1–17). New York: Springer Science.

Nguyen, T., Truong, D., Marquett, R., & Reiser, R. (2007). Response to group-based cognitive behavioral therapy for older adults with bipolar disorder. *Clinical Gerontologist, 30,* 103–110.

Pachana, N. A., Knight, B., Karel, M. J., & Beck, J. S. (2008). Training of geriatric mental health providers in CBT interventions for older adults. In D. Gallagher-Thompson, A. M. Steffen, & L. W. Thompson (Eds.), *Handbook of behavioral and cognitive therapies with older adults* (pp. 295–308). New York: Springer Science.

Paukert, A. L., Phillips, L., Cully, J. A., Loboprabhu, S. M., Lomax, J. W., & Stanley, M. A. (2009). Integration of religion into cognitive-behavioral therapy for geriatric anxiety and depression. *Journal of Psychiatric Practice, 15,* 103–112.

Payne, K. T., & Marcus, D. K. (2008). The efficacy of group psychotherapy for older adult clients: A meta-analysis. *Theory, Research, and Practice, 12,* 268–278.

Perlis, M. L., Smith, L. J., Lyness, J. M., Matteson, S. R., Pigeon, W. R., Jungquist, C. R., & Tu, X. (2006). Insomnia as a risk factor for onset of depression in the elderly. *Behavioral Sleep Medicine, 4,* 104–113.

Post, E. P., Metzger, M., Dumas, P., & Lemann, L. (2010). Integrating mental health into primary care within the Veterans Health Administration. *Families, Systems and Health, 28,* 83–90.

Qualls, S. H., & Knight, B. G. (2006). *Psychotherapy for depression in older adults.* Hoboken, NJ: Wiley.

Rybarczyk, B., Lopez, M., Benson, R., Alsten, C., & Stepanski, E. (2002). Efficacy of two behavioral treatment programs for comorbid geriatric insomnia. *Psychology and Aging, 17,* 288–298.

Rybarczyk, B., Lopez, M., Schelble, K., & Stepanski, E. (2005). Home-based video CBT for comorbid geriatric insomnia: A pilot study using secondary data analyses. *Behavioral Sleep Medicine, 3,* 158–175.

Rybarczyk, B., Mack, L., Harris, J. H., & Stepanski, E. (2011). Testing two types of self-help CBT-I for insomnia in older adults with arthritis or coronary artery disease. *Rehabilitation Psychology, 56,* 257–266.

Rybarczyk, B., Stepanski, E., Fogg, L., Lopez, M., Barry, P., & Davis, A. (2005). A placebo-controlled test of cognitive-behavioral therapy for comorbid insomnia in older adults. *Journal of Consulting and Clinical Psychology, 73,* 1164–1174.

Satre, D. D., Knight, B. G., & David, S. (2006). Cognitive-behavioral interventions with older adults: Integrating clinical and gerontological research. *Professional Psychology: Research and Practice, 37,* 489–498.

Scogin, F., Morthland, M., Kaufman, A., Burgio, L., Chaplin, W., & Kong, G. (2007). Improving quality of life in diverse rural older adults: A randomized trial of a psychological treatment. *Psychology and Aging, 22,* 657–665.

Scogin, F., Shackelford, J., Rohen, N., Stump, J., Floyd, M., McKendree-Smith, N., & Jamison, C. (2001). Residual geriatric depression symptoms: A place for psychotherapy. *Journal of Clinical Geropsychology, 7,* 271–283.

Scogin, F., Welsh, D., Hanson, A., Stump, J., & Coates, A. (2005). Evidence-based psychotherapies for depression in older adults. *Clinical Psychology: Science and Practice, 12,* 222–237.

Serfaty, M., Csipke, E., Haworth, D., Murad, S., & King, M. (2011). A talking control for use in evaluating the effectiveness of cognitive-behavioral therapy. *Behaviour Research and Therapy, 49,* 433–440.

Serfaty, M. A., Haworth, D., Blanchard, M., Buszewicz, M., Murad, S., & King, M. (2009). Clinical effectiveness of individual cognitive behavioral therapy for depressed older people in primary care: A randomized controlled trial. *Archives of General Psychiatry, 66,* 1332–1340.

Shehatah, A., Rabie, M. A., & Al-Shahry, A (2010). Prevalence and correlates of depressive disorders in elderly with type 2 diabetes in primary health care settings. *Journal of Affective Disorders, 123,* 197–201.

Snow, L. A., Powers, D., & Liles, D. (2006). Cognitive-behavioral therapy for long-term care patients with dementia. In L. Hyer & R. Intrieri (Eds.), *Geropsychological interventions in long-term care* (pp. 265–293). New York: Springer.

Sorocco, K., & Lauderdale, S. (Eds.). (2011). *Cognitive behavior therapy with older adults: Innovations across care settings.* Pittsburgh, PA: Pittsburgh State University.

Speer, D. C., & Schneider, M. G. (2003). Mental health needs of older adults and primary care: Opportunity for interdisciplinary geriatric team practice. *Clinical Psychology: Science and Practice, 10*(1), 85–101.

Stanley, M. A., Beck, J. G., Novy, D. M., Averill, P. M., Swann, A. C., Diefenbach, G. J., & Hopko, D. R. (2003). Cognitive-behavioral treatment of late-life generalized anxiety disorder. *Journal of Consulting and Clinical Psychology, 71,* 309–319.

Stanley, M.A., Bush, A.L., Camp, M.E., Jameson, J.P., Phillips, L.L., Barber, C. R., . . . Cully, J. A. (2011). Older adults' preferences for religion/spirituality in treatment for anxiety and depression. *Aging and Mental Health, 15,* 334–343.

Stanley, M. A., Wilson, N. L., Novy, D. M., Rhoades, H. M. Wagener, P. D., Greisinger, J., . . . Kunik, M. E. (2009). Cognitive behavior therapy for generalized anxiety disorder among older adults in primary care: A randomized clinical trial. *Journal of the American Medical Association, 301,* 1460–1467.

Steinman, L. E., Frederick, J. T., Prohaska, T., Satariano, W. A., Dornberg-Lee, S., Graub, P. B., . . . Late Life Depression Special Interest Project (SIP) Panelists. (2006). Recommendations for treating depression in community-based older adults. *American Journal of Preventive Medicine, 33*, 175–181.

Stone, K. C., Booth, A. K., & Lichstein, K. L. (2008). Cognitive-behavior therapy for late-life insomnia. In D. Gallagher-Thompson, A. M. Steffen, & L. W. Thompson (Eds.), *Handbook of behavioral and cognitive therapies with older adults* (pp. 48–60). New York: Springer Science.

Teri, L., Huda, P., Gibbons, L., Young, H., & van Leynseele, J. (2005). STAR: A dementia-specific training program for staff in assisted living residences. *Gerontologist, 45*, 686–693.

Teri, L., Logsdon, R. G., Uomoto, J., & McCurry, S. M. (1997). Behavioral treatment of depression in dementia patients: A controlled clinical trial. *Journals of Gerontology: Series B: Psychological Sciences and Social Sciences, 52B*(4), P159–P166.

Thielke, S., Vannoy, S., & Unutzer, J. (2007). Integrating mental health and primary care. *Primary Care: Clinics in Office Practice, 34*, 571–592.

Thompson, L. W., Coon, D. W., Gallagher-Thompson, D., Sommer, B. R., & Koin, D. (2001). Comparison of desipramine and cognitive/behavioral therapy in the treatment of elderly outpatients with mild-to-moderate depression. *American Journal of Geriatric Psychiatry, 9*, 225–240.

Thompson, L. W., & Gallagher-Thompson, D. (1997). Psychotherapeutic interventions with older adults in outpatient and extended care settings. In R. L. Rubinstein & M. P. Lawton (Eds.), *Depression in long term and residential care: Advances in research and treatment* (pp. 169–184). New York: Springer.

Thorp, S. R., Ayers, C. R., Nuevo, R., Stoddard, J. A., Sorrell, J. T., & Wetherell, J. L. (2009). Meta-analysis comparing different behavioral treatments for late-life anxiety. *American Journal of Geriatric Psychiatry, 17*, 105–115.

Vitiello, M. V., Rybarczyk, B., Von Korff, M., & Stepanski, E. J., (2009). Cognitive behavioral therapy for insomnia improves sleep and decreases pain in older adults with co-morbid insomnia and osteoarthritis. *Journal of Clinical Sleep Medicine, 15*, 355–362.

Walker, D. A. (2004). Cognitive behavioural therapy for depression in a person with Alzheimer's dementia. *Behavioural and Cognitive Psychotherapy, 32*, 495–500.

Walker, D. A., & Clarke, M. (2001). Cognitive behavioural psychotherapy: A comparison between younger and older adults in two inner city mental health teams. *Aging and Mental Health, 5*, 197–199.

Wetherell, J. L, Hopko, D. R., Averill, P. M., Beck, J. G., Craske, M. G., Gatz, M., . . . Stanley, M. A. (2005b). Cognitive-behavioral therapy for late-life generalized anxiety disorder: Who gets better? *Behavior Therapy, 36*, 147–156.

Wetherell, J. L., Sorrell, J. T., Thorp, S. R., & Patterson, T. L. (2005). Psychological interventions for late-life anxiety: A review and early lessons from the CALM Study. *Journal of Geriatric Psychiatry and Neurology, 18*, 72–82.

Wilz, G., Schinköthe, D., & Soellner, R. (2011). Goal attainment and treatment compliance in a cognitive-behavioral telephone intervention for family caregivers of persons with dementia. *GeroPsych: The Journal of Gerontopsychology and Geriatric Psychiatry, 24*, 115–125.

Wolitzky-Taylor, J. B., Castriotta, N., Lenze, E. J., Stanley, M. A., & Craske, M. G. (2010). Anxiety disorders in older adults: A comprehensive review. *Depression and Anxiety, 27*, 190–211.

World Health Organization. (2001). *The world health report, 2001: Mental health: new understanding, new hope.* Retrieved on December 2011, from http://www.who.int/whr/2001/en/whr01_en.pdf

Yang, J. A., & Jackson, C. L. (1998). Overcoming obstacles in providing mental health treatment to older adults: Getting in the door. *Psychotherapy: Theory, Research, Practice, Training, 35*, 498–505.

Yesavage, J. A., Brink, T. L., Rose, T. L., Lum, O., Huang, V., Adey, M. B., & Leirer, V. O. (1983). Development and validation of a geriatric depression rating scale: A preliminary report. *Journal of Psychiatric Research, 17*, 37–49.

Yohannes, A. M., & Caton, S. (2010). Management of depression in older people with osteoarthritis: A systematic review. *Aging and Mental Health, 14*, 637–651.

Yon, A., & Scogin, F., (2009). Behavioral activation as a treatment for geriatric depression. *Clinical Gerontologist: The Journal of Aging and Mental Health, 32*, 91–103.

Zeiss, A., & Karlin, B. (2008). Integrating mental health and primary care services in the Department of Veterans Affairs health care system. *Journal of Clinical Psychology in Medical Settings, 15*, 73–78.

Zeiss, A., & Steffen, A. (1996a). Behavioral and cognitive-behavioral treatments: An overview of social learning. In S. H. Zarit & B. G Knight (Eds.), *A guide to psychotherapy and aging: Effective clinical interventions in a life-stage context* (pp. 35–60). Washington, DC: American Psychological Association.

Zeiss, A., & Steffen, A. (1996b). Treatment issues with elderly clients. *Cognitive and Behavioral Practice, 3*, 371–389.

Treating Children and Adolescents

Philip C. Kendall, Jeremy S. Peterman, Marianne A. Villabø, Matthew Mychailyszyn, *and* Kelly A. O'Neil Rodriguez

Abstract

Advances in the development of cognitive-behavioral therapy (CBT) and the findings from outcome research with youth are noted. CBT has empirical support for treating a variety of childhood and adolescents disorders (e.g. anxiety, OCD, depression, disruptive behavior disorders). This chapter begins by defining empirically supported and evidence-based treatment and reviewing its history, and considers the developmental context that guides the adaptation of CBT for youth. We overview common CBT components, and we discuss the implementation of CBT for specific childhood disorders. The chapter concludes by discussing the dissemination of evidence-based treatment, school-based interventions, brief CBT, computer-assisted CBT, and transdiagnostic approaches.

Key Words: cognitive-behavioral therapy, childhood disorders, adolescents, psychopathology, outcomes, treatment response

The history of psychology is laced with a focus on the provision of optimal possible care to those in need. In the seminal meta-analysis, Smith and Glass (1977) summarized the findings to date and claimed that their results provided convincing evidence of the efficacy of psychological treatment. In retrospect, the promising findings may have merely opened the door to an expanded era characterized by both an endorsement of empirical support and the debate as to what constitutes the most optimal approach to care. In the interim, there emerged numerous examples of the development and implementation of interventions that do and do not truly lead to substantive improvement (e.g., Lynam et al., 1999)—or, in especially troubling instances, can lead to unfavorable outcomes (see Lilienfeld, Fowler, Lohr, & Lynn, 2005).

There has been a major effort to develop an agreed-upon set of standards to evaluate the efficacy of services being provided. These laudatory efforts have led to an evolution in the terminology applied to psychological treatments and to the studies that evaluate them. In 1993, the board of the Division of Clinical Psychology (12) of the American Psychological Association (APA) adopted policies regarding "empirically validated treatments" that had been developed by the Task Force on Promotion and Dissemination of Psychological Procedures and published the report in 1995. Acknowledging the arbitrary nature of determining the sufficiency of evidence required for treatment efficacy, the Task Force proposed that psychological therapies be grouped into the following categories with corresponding definitions: "Well established treatments" are those supported either by (a) two or more quality group design studies, conducted by different investigators that have demonstrated efficacy by being superior to a pill placebo, psychological placebo, or another treatment and/or being found to produce equivalent outcomes to a previously established treatment using studies with sufficient statistical power, or (b) a large series of single-case design studies that have demonstrated efficacy while using good experimental designs and by comparing the intervention to another treatment; additionally, studies must have clearly specified the characteristics of client samples used and had treatment implementation guided by manuals. "Probably efficacious treatments" are identified by (a) the presence of at least two studies demonstrating that the treatment is more effective than a waiting-list control group, (b) at least two studies otherwise meeting the well-established treatment criteria but with both having been conducted by the same investigator, or only one good study demonstrating effectiveness by established criteria, (c) two or more quality studies that demonstrate effectiveness but are flawed by the heterogeneity of the client samples, or (d) a series of single-case design studies otherwise meeting the well-established treatment criteria but that is not yet large enough to be deemed well established. Finally, "experimental treatments" are those that have not yet garnered enough sound data to be deemed at least probably efficacious.

A succeeding Task Force on Psychological Interventions was charged with providing ongoing review of the treatment literature to identify psychosocial treatment approaches meeting the criteria. Chambless and colleagues (1996) provided an update to the 1995 Task Force report, providing a preliminary list of therapies that qualify for the various levels of empirical support. It was footnoted that the term "validation" may lead to the mistaken conclusion that research on a treatment is complete. In various reports, the term "empirically supported treatments" (ESTs) was proposed and has emerged as a preferred language to present the nature of the topic and emphasize the ongoing evaluation of treatment efficacy through research (Kendall, 1998).

"ESTs" has increasingly been relied upon in narrative descriptions of the evolving project. In a separate effort, Chambless and Hollon (1998) proposed distinct criteria for "ESTs". The framework of classification advocates that studies be identified as "efficacious," "possibly efficacious," or "efficacious and specific," with detailed guidelines provided for evaluating the strength of the methodology of the study.

In 2000, the APA approved a set of criteria for evaluating treatment guidelines (APA, 2002). As contrasted with practice guidelines, treatment guidelines were described as providing "specific recommendations about treatments to be offered to patients" and as being "patient directed or patient focused as opposed to practitioner focused"

(p. 1052). The report revolves around features of "treatment efficacy" as the "systematic and scientific evaluation of whether a treatment works" as well as on "clinical utility" as "the applicability, feasibility, and usefulness of the intervention in the local or specific setting where it is to be offered" (p. 1053). In this way, the APA put forth a system to assist in the assessment of the guidelines and the shaping of clinical services.

A recent development in the evolving terminology is the emergence of "evidence-based practice in psychology" (EBPP). In a continued expansion of the APA efforts, evidence-based practice (APA, 2006) seeks to integrate science and practice in terms of psychological assessment, conceptualization, and intervention. The Task Force defines EBPP as "the integration of the best available research with clinical expertise in the context of patient characteristics, culture, and preferences" (p. 273).

Within this context, cognitive-behavioral therapies (CBT) collectively emerge as EST that qualifies for evidence-based treatment (EBT). Although it is beyond the present scope to review the following extensive research that provides empirical support for a variety of versions of CBT with youth, two examples illustrate the broad-reaching esteem that CBT now holds as a first-line treatment of choice for a number of mental health disorders. In 2007, the government of Great Britain made a commitment of £170 million to the Increasing Access to Psychological Therapies (IAPT) program that is devoted to providing training in CBT to thousands of health care providers across Great Britain. In New York State, the Evidence Based Treatment Dissemination Center (EBTDC) is focused on providing training and consultation in CBT for youth with internalizing and externalizing mental health problems (Gleacher et al., 2011). The New York example fits within the larger picture of how a growing number of states in the United States are heeding the exhortations from federal leadership and national policymakers to increase the reliance on evidence-based services for youth and families.

Developmentally Informed Differentiations in Treatment

To be optimally effective, CBT for children and adolescents is implemented with consideration of developmental factors. To illustrate, consider several factors that differentiate CBT with youth from CBT with adults: (a) the entry into treatment; (b) the mode of therapy delivery; (c) the client's level of cognitive, emotional, and social understanding; (d) the role of parents; and (e) the role of the therapist. Each factor is discussed next, along with related recommendations for therapists conducting CBT with youth.

Entry into Therapy

Unlike adult clients, children and adolescents rarely initiate psychological services for themselves. Rather, parents, pediatricians, or teachers are typical referral sources for youth. This distinction is important. Children and adolescents may not be eager or willing to discuss their problems with the therapist or to be involved in sessions. Accordingly, it is important that the therapist working with youth creates a pleasant experience so that youth are willing to return for future sessions. Rapport-building activities may include playing get-to-know-you games, taking a tour of the clinic or office area, and engaging in activities of the child's choice, such as drawing or playing board games.

Age-Appropriate Delivery

Play activities can be an age-appropriate and effective way to facilitate the implementation of CBT for youth. Fun activities foster a collaborative relationship between client and therapist, and they can boost the learning of therapy content. Play activities allow the therapist to observe the child's expectations and beliefs, and they can be used to introduce coping skills that promote adaptive behavior. Fun activities may include art projects, role plays, songs, board games, and computer time. For example, within the *Coping Cat* program for child anxiety disorders, therapists engage in a "Body Drawing" art activity that helps youth identify somatic anxiety.

Level of Cognitive, Emotional, and Social Development

Not all youth are comparably mature, so the implementation of any treatment, including CBT with youth, requires that the therapist be aware of cognitive, emotional, and social development. For example, children may not understand a type of cognitive restructuring used with adults: a refutation of a personal style might be taken as punitive rather than explorative. Children may not have the cognitive maturity or vocabulary to distinguish rational and irrational thoughts, but they can label thoughts as "helpful or not helpful" or "scary or coping thoughts." Probabilities may be difficult, but children can understand that certain events have a "small" or "big" chance of

happening, and they can be coached to gather evidence or "clues" about the possibility of their feared outcome occurring.

Therapists working with children benefit from awareness of typical psychosocial development and recognition of a child's delayed or impaired social functioning. Youth face different social issues at different points in their development, and these issues may influence treatment. For example, academic performance and peer relationships take on increased importance during adolescence. For teens, social issues can be folded into CBT as they relate to treatment goals.

Role of Parents

For several reasons, including the fact that children and adolescents are not fully independent, it is critical to consider the role of parents when treating youth. Parents can serve as consultants (e.g., provide information about symptoms and impairment), collaborators (e.g., bring youth to treatment, assist with implementation of therapy techniques), or co-clients in the treatment itself (Kendall, 2012).

The benefits of including parents in CBT for youth with behavioral and emotional problems can vary depending on the specific problem and the child's age. Younger children may benefit more when parents are involved from the beginning, whereas adolescents may accrue more gains when parents are not regularly included in treatment. Some treatments for disruptive behavior problems involve parent training as a core component of treatment and thus require parental involvement (e.g., Kazdin, 2005). On the other hand, CBT for child anxiety can be implemented in a child-focused format and, with adolescents, less parental involvement. However, research examining the benefit of including parents in CBT for child anxiety has produced mixed findings (e.g., Barmish & Kendall, 2005), and it is complicated by varying types of parental involvement. Research is needed to examine the ideal involvement of parents in CBT for the different childhood disorders.

Therapist's Role and Expectations

When working with children and adolescents, the CBT therapist fills multiple roles, including diagnostician, consultant, and educator (Kendall, 2012). As diagnostician, the therapist uses multimethod, multi-informant assessment of the child's symptomatology and functioning in multiple domains to create a case conceptualization. As a consultant, the CBT therapist works with the client and family to share perspectives and select treatment goals. As an educator, the CBT therapist provides information about the disorder and the likely course of treatment. It can be helpful to view the therapist's role as that of a *coach* for the youth (Kendall, 2012). The coaching analogy helps communicate that the therapist will provide information, provide opportunities to learn, teach coping skills, and provide opportunities to practice the use of coping skills in real situations.

Common Components in CBT for Youth

Many of the central components of CBT for children and adolescents do not differ greatly from those applied with adults (Kendall, 1993). Models of learning, such as operant conditioning and social learning theory, underlie many of the CBT strategies that treat both adults and children (March & Morris, 2004). Although many of the core strategies remain the same, the use of visual aids, fun activities, and metaphors help make the concepts more accessible for children. In the following section we discuss several CBT strategies, including problem solving, affective education, relaxation, cognitive restructuring, modeling and role playing, and behavioral contingencies. Please note, however, that these strategies are not isolated but are interconnected and build upon one another. For example, affective education cues the child to use relaxation techniques, and cognitive restructuring promotes engagement in behavioral tasks (Kendall et al., 1992).

Problem Solving

With early roots in behavioral therapy (D'Zurilla & Goldfried, 1971), problem solving is a procedure in which one generates solutions to a dilemma and systematically determines the most effective response. Core problem-solving strategies for children are consistent with planful problem-solving skills that are used with adults (Nezu, Nezu, & D'Zurilla, 2013; Nezu, Nezu, & Perri, 1990). Children are introduced to a series of steps that they refer to when they identify a problem. The problem-solving steps are frequently made into an acronym to help children remember them. For example, a treatment for youths with aggression called *Keeping Your Cool* uses the acronym SPEAR (Nelson & Finch, 2008). The SPEAR sequence consists of the following: Stop: what's the problem (understanding the situation), Plan: what can I do (generating solutions), Evaluate: what is the best solution (choosing a plan of action),

Act: try it out, React: did it work (self-evaluation). Other treatments use variations of the same fundamental problem-solving steps and tailor them to a specific disorder. Initially the therapist helps the child generate solutions and process the outcome of selected strategies. As children repeat the problem-solving process and apply it to a variety of situations, they learn to better resolve future problems (Gosch, Flannery-Schroeder, Mauro, & Compton, 2006).

Problem solving has been incorporated into treatments targeting a variety of childhood mental health problems. Children with aggression tend to believe that their aggressive behavior is instrumental to achieve a desired goal (Lochman & Dodge, 1994). An important part of problem solving for this population is to help them recognize the advantages and disadvantages for each potential plan of action and to choose one with a reasonable outcome (Lochman, Powell, Boxmeyer, & Jimenez-Camargo, 2011). Problem solving is a balanced approach that acknowledges the potential benefits for an unproductive or impractical solution, as well as the benefits of a more appropriate solution. In problem solving, the therapist validates the child's experience while also showing that problems can have several potential solutions. Treatments for aggressive children focus on developing nonaggressive strategies to express anger and alternative means to achieve a desired goal (Lochman, Powell, Whidby, & Fitzgerald, 2012).

Problem solving has been used with impulsive children (Kendall, Padever, & Zupan, 1980). The components resemble those from other CBT protocols with the addition of a step to maintain focused attention. For depressed children, problem solving (Stark et al., 2012) may require added attention to negative affect and thoughts that may be an obstacle for depressed youth. Children are encouraged to do something pleasurable to improve mood and to facilitate problem solving. Therapists may also need to pay special attention when depressive youth disqualify positive outcomes after a problem-solving strategy has been used effectively. Across target problems, unorthodox strategies are welcomed when brainstorming potential solutions. Deriving silly solutions to problems can add humor to the setting and highlight the sensibility of other solutions.

Affective Education

Affective education helps the child recognize, differentiate, and express emotion. Affective education has several parts and is implemented to be consistent with the presenting problem and stage of treatment. For example, often early in CBT, clinicians normalize the child's experience of certain emotions. For example, an anxious child would be told that anxiety is a normal emotion experienced by everyone (including adults). When it is too intense or too frequent, then it requires "dialing down." The therapist may even share instances in which he or she has experienced anxiety. Children are also taught to distinguish among emotional states (Davis & Boster, 1992). In the *Coping Cat* program children with anxiety disorders create feelings dictionaries (Kendall, 2012). The therapist and child cut out pictures of people from magazines and label their emotions based on facial expressions. Another option would be to play "feelings charades" in which the therapist and child alternate acting out and guessing various emotions.

Affective education includes learning how to identify physiological cues of emotional distress or arousal. Recognition of low-level emotional distress can then signal the child to use problem solving. To raise physiological awareness, youth with anxiety may draw a picture of their body and highlight the parts that are active when anxious (e.g., butterflies in their stomach or sweat on their palms). Youth or therapists can create a "feelings thermometer" to represent the range of a particular emotion. The thermometer is a visual aid for children to better comprehend the varying intensity of negative emotions (Lochman et al., 2011). For example, when children with depression reach a particular threshold on their "mood thermometer," they are encouraged to do something they enjoy (Stark et al., 2012). The thermometer can help reveal common triggers that elicit a particular negative emotion, and the mere construction of the thermometer can provide an opportunity for rapport building. Younger children often enjoy the task of decorating and personalizing their feelings thermometer.

Relaxation

Relaxation training has a long history in the treatment of some mental health problems (e.g., Jacobson, 1938) and has been incorporated within some protocols to treat children (e.g., Koeppen, 1974). Children are taught to use relaxation as a means to reduce and/or cope with stress. Debate exists regarding the precise mechanism accounting for the effects of relaxation, with some researchers arguing that the process helps children regulate emotional and physiological responses to negative life events (Gosch et al., 2006), while others theorize that its effects are due to cognitive changes such as increased self-efficacy and control (Conrad & Roth, 2007). There is also controversy regarding the necessity of relaxation training within some CBT protocol for children. Some research on treatment of anxiety suggests that CBT remains effective even after the removal of relaxation training (Rapee, 2000). However, other results suggest that relaxation training may be as effective as other treatment components (Goldfried & Trier, 1974; Kahn, Kehle, Jenson, & Clark, 1990). Although its centrality has been questioned, relaxation continues to be a feature in CBT programs targeting a variety of disorders in children (Crawley, Podell, Beidas, Braswell, & Kendall, 2010).

A common form of relaxation treatment is progressive muscle relaxation (PMR). In PMR children learn to systematically tense and relax muscle groups, moving from head to toe. A child might be instructed to clench his fist as tightly as he can, count to ten, and then slowly relax the muscle while counting back to one (March & Mulle, 1998; Ollendick & Cerny, 1981). The use of metaphors, such as "squeezing lemons" when tightening a fist and "going into a shell" when tensing shoulders, helps make it fun and understandable for youth. The robot-ragdoll exercise is another method to highlight the distinction between tense and relaxed states (Kendall & Braswell, 1993). First, therapists and children pretend to be robots by stiffening their limbs and walking about. Afterward they act as ragdolls by slumping in a chair and relaxing their arms, legs, and neck.

Relaxation training often includes diaphragmic breathing exercises. Children are taught to breathe deeply and slowly from their diaphragm rather than take quick and shallow breaths from their chest. For example, children can rest one hand on their diaphragm and feel it move up and down as they breathe into their mouth and exhale from their nose. The therapist discusses physiological changes that occur during diaphragmic breathing. Again, the use of metaphors such as "let your stomach inflate like a balloon" can be helpful. Unlike PMR, children can engage in diaphragmic breathing without others easily noticing (Gosch et al., 2006). Therapists can make CDs of relaxation exercises that children can personalize and use to practice at home.

Cognitive Restructuring (Changing Self-Talk)

According to Beck (1976), dysfunctional and distorted thoughts mediate the relationship between stressful life events and psychopathology. Within depression, cognitive distortions refer to negative misperceptions about oneself, the world, or the future. Children with a variety of disorders display distorting thinking (Crick & Dodge, 1994; Kendall, 1993; Rudolph & Clark, 2001), and there are data to suggest that the content of the negative thoughts reflects the specific psychopathology. For example, core cognitive features in depression include attribution of positive events to external, unstable, and specific causes (Curry & Craighead, 1990). Externalizing disorders, on the other hand, are associated with distorted processing of ambiguous situations, seeing them as hostile (Lansford et al., 2006) and potentially requiring retaliation. Cognitive restructuring refers to the process of helping youth to see alternate views and change distorted thinking. Additionally, cognitive restructuring involves identifying distorted beliefs and negative thoughts, connecting thoughts to feelings and behaviors, challenging the validity of the thoughts and beliefs with evidence, and developing new and helpful patterns of thinking. This strategy is modified depending on the age and presenting problem of the child.

Children learn to recognize some of their unfounded negative thoughts early in cognitive restructuring. In one exercise children are presented with various cartoons of people in ambiguous situations. Children fill in a blank thought bubble above the character's head to express the thoughts (Kendall & Hedtke, 2006a). After identifying the thoughts of others, the therapist can inquire about what is in the child's own thought bubble. For homework, children keep a journal, record their thoughts, and note the situation and their accompanying emotion. This self-monitoring exercise helps children become aware of the link between thoughts, feelings, and behaviors. The therapist can also take time to identify a situation from the child's life; write down thoughts, feelings, and behaviors; and review how the three components are interconnected. Integrating the mood thermometer into the discussion of thoughts (self-talk) is another way to show that emotions and thoughts influence one another.

After identifying maladaptive self-talk, children move on to challenging their thoughts/beliefs and eventually developing coping thoughts. Children can become "thought detectives" who objectively evaluate the validity of self-talk. The therapist and child examine maladaptive thoughts and ask, "What is the evidence for that?" or "What's another way of looking at it?" The latter question can be helpful for aggressive children who misinterpret ambiguous social cues as having hostile intent. "Decatastrophizing" refers to when the therapist asks, "If a feared or nonpreferred outcome happens or if your thought is true, so what?" By exploring the worst-case consequences of some thoughts, the child learns that he or she can very likely cope with the situation. A child learns to identify "thinking traps." Thinking traps, adapted from Beck's cognitive errors for adults (Beck, 1995), include mind reading (knowing what others are thinking), fortune telling (being certain about an ambiguous future event), and black-and-white thinking (dichotomizing things on a continuum), among others. Finally, therapists and children collaborate to develop coping thoughts. An aggressive child might try, "It may have been an accident; I won't get angry until I learn more," or an anxious child might think, "I tried it a few times, and did OK, so I may do OK when I try it again."

Although not a formal component of cognitive restructuring, several CBT protocols "externalize" the disorder. The idea is for the child to realize that his or her symptoms do not define who he or she is but represent something to be managed or addressed. "Externalizing" reduces self-blame and distances the child from negative thoughts. A treatment for depression externalizes the collective symptoms into "the muck monster" (Stark, Schnoebelen, et al., 2005; Stark, Simpson, et al., 2005). The child draws a picture of the monster and can direct his or her coping statements at it. In treating obsessive-compulsive disorder (OCD), children name their symptoms (e.g., "stupid thing"), and a treatment goal is to reclaim control by "bossing back OCD" (March & Mulle, 1998).

Modeling and Role Playing

Modeling, a form of observational learning, allows a child to acquire a new skill by viewing the behavior of others (despite no explicit reinforcement; Benjamin et al., 2011). Modeling exemplifies social learning theory in that individuals learn through observation in addition to direct experience (Bandura, 1969). Several types of modeling exist including covert, filmed, live, and participant-guided modeling. Covert modeling strategies have the child imagine the therapist or another model coping with a difficult situation.

Children can visualize a model, such as a cartoon character, superhero, or celebrity in addition to the therapist (Kendall, Chu, Pimentel, & Choudhury, 2012). In filmed modeling, children watch a video of a model engaging in the problem scenario. Live modeling involves the therapist demonstrating a behavior for a child. For example, the therapist may approach a feared stimulus while verbalizing coping statements. In some protocols same-aged peers proficient in a particular behavior serve as live models (Beidel, Turner, & Morris, 2000). In guided modeling the therapist interacts with the child as they navigate the situation. Research has found that participant-guided modeling is an effective treatment for reducing avoidance (Barrios & O'Dell, 1998).

Role plays provide a safe environment in which to practice new skills. In a role play the therapist and child typically act out a scenario in which the child faces a challenge and uses problem-solving and coping skills. Role plays simulate real-life situations. They do not provide the real-life consequences, but they do provide therapist feedback. For example, the therapist could pretend to be the child's friend who is experiencing negative thoughts (Deblinger & Heflin, 1996). The child's task is to be a good friend and help the friend to challenge the negative thoughts. With practice and feedback, the child can internalize the skills and challenge his or her own thoughts.

Behavioral Contingencies

Behavioral contingencies include positive reinforcement, punishment, shaping, and extinction. Contingency management strategies help to promote targeted behavior and encourage treatment compliance. Often, the initial reinforcers are tangible, whereas later in treatment they are social or self-reward. It is important that rewards reflect the developmental level of the child. For example, younger children may require concrete and frequent rewards (Crawley et al., 2010). However, rewards do not necessarily have to be large or material. Getting to be the person who chooses the meal for a family dinner, earning computer time, or spending time alone with a parent can all be effective rewards. In addition, therapists can print Certificates of Achievement (as in the *Coping Cat* program) to increase self-esteem and motivation after the child successfully completes a task (March & Mulle, 1998). The certificate provides an opportunity for children to brag about their accomplishments to others, which in turn is reinforcing. Separate

from the specific reinforcer, it is important that the reward be contingent and meaningful to the child.

In many of the CBT programs for youth, parents play a role and are taught how to use behavioral contingencies. Parents are taught to be consistent in their implementation and, depending on the age of the child, may be encouraged to set up a sticker chart or other system to track the child's progress. Effort and partial success are always rewarded, particularly in children who have perfectionistic tendencies.

Applications with Specific Childhood Disorders

Despite the many common elements in CBT, it is not uniform in its application. Treatments are developed for specific disorders with differential use of strategies consistent with the research data on the nature of each disorder. In this section we describe some disorder-focused applications of CBT and related research findings.

Anxiety Disorders

The experience of anxiety or fear, such as being afraid of the dark or being mildly distressed when separated from a parent, is part of normal development for most children. As children get older, anxiety and worries about appearances and peer relationships are common. However, excessive anxiety can cause distress and interfere with the youth's daily activities at home or school and with peer or family relationships. Youth with anxiety disorders view the world as a disproportionately dangerous place and tend to avoid situations that make them anxious.

CBT for anxiety disorders in youth targets the somatic (arousal), cognitive (self-talk), and behavioral (avoidance) aspects of anxiety. Treatments typically include psychoeducation, somatic management skills, cognitive restructuring, and gradual exposure to feared situations. The *Coping Cat* program (Kendall & Hedtke, 2006a, 2006b) is representative of CBT, and variations of the program have been developed to include group (Mendlowitz et al., 1999), family (Howard, Chu, Krain, Marrs-Garcia, & Kendall, 2000), group school-based (Masia-Warner, Nangle, Hansen, & David, 2006), and computer-assisted treatments (Kendall & Khanna, 2008). The *Coping Cat* is tailored toward children aged 7–14 years with a principal diagnosis of separation anxiety disorder, social phobia, or generalized anxiety disorder, addressing the basic similarities among them. In the

16-session child-focused program, youths learn to recognize somatic reactions to anxiety (e.g., sweating, stomach aches, rapid heartbeat, dizziness) and apply cognitive and relaxation skills to manage their symptoms. Cognitive restructuring focuses on identifying and challenging anxious self-talk and applying coping-focused thinking. After acquiring these skills, treatment focuses on gradual and planned exposure tasks—exposure to feared stimuli and situations. During the exposure tasks the youth practices applying the skills taught in the earlier sessions in actual anxiety-provoking situations. Parents typically attend weekly check-ins and there are two parent-only sessions. The *Coping Cat* program has been evaluated in several randomized controlled trials (RCTs) and found to effectively reduce anxiety in youth (e.g., Kendall, 1994; Kendall et al., 1997; Kendall, Hudson, Gosch, Flannery-Schroeder, & Suveg, 2008; Walkup et al., 2008).

Other CBT interventions for child anxiety have also been developed and evaluated. Albano and DiBartolo (2007) group CBT is for socially anxious adolescents, and includes strategies such as cognitive restructuring to identify and change cognitive distortions that maintain anxiety, social skills training, and problem solving. Some applications of CBT for child anxiety have added parent and/or family involvement (e.g., Barrett, Dadds, & Rapee, 1996; Cobham, Dadds, & Spence, 1998; Wood, Piacentini, Southam-Gerow, Chu, & Sigman, 2006) but the incremental effect of adding parental involvement has yet to be clearly demonstrated (Barmish & Kendall, 2005; Breinholst, Esbjørn, Reinholdt-Dunne, & Stallard, 2012). Not surprisingly, given the reported efficacy of CBT for child anxiety, treatment programs based on CBT are being developed for other anxiety-related conditions. New research is examining the treatment of selective mutism: a challenging condition associated with severe social anxiety and involving consistent lack of speech in important social situations despite being able to speak in familiar settings. Initial favorable results have been reported (Oerbeck, Johansen, Lundahl, & Kristensen, 2012; Reuther, Davis, Moore, & Matson, 2011), but more outcome evaluation research is needed.

The literature identifies CBT as an EBT for anxiety disorders in youth (Seligman & Ollendick, 2011). CBT is considered a "well-established" treatment for youth anxiety, and its efficacy has been demonstrated in a number of studies (for a review, see Ollendick & King, 2012; Silverman, Pina, & Viswesvaran, 2008). The largest treatment trial to date (Walkup et al., 2008) evaluated outcomes for 488 youth aged 7–17 years with an anxiety disorder who were treated either with CBT (i.e., the age-appropriate *Coping Cat*), medication (i.e., sertraline), their combination, or a pill placebo. Of the youth receiving CBT, 60% were found to have "very much" or "much improved" outcomes after treatment compared to 55% receiving medication only. The combination treatment resulted in the best outcome, with 80% favorable responders. Efforts to better understand the mechanisms of change within CBT for child anxiety endorse the exposure tasks as a critical component and suggest that changed self-talk is a key to change. Kendall and Treadwell (2007; Treadwell & Kendall, 1996) found that changes in children's anxious, but not positive or depressed, self-talk mediated treatment-produced gains. Those youth who reduced their negative anxious self-talk were the youth who showed the beneficial gains. Although most youth benefit, across ages, ethnicities, gender, and principal disorder, having social phobia and some added depression has been associated with less favorable outcomes (Crawley, Beidas, Benjamin, Martin, & Kendall, 2008; Ginsburg et al., 2011). Ginsburg and colleagues (2011) found that low severity of anxiety, absence of a comorbid internalizing disorder, and absence of social phobia were associated with higher remission. Despite the favorable outcomes for 50%–72% of youth receiving CBT, many continue to experience some residual symptoms. Further work is needed to address treatment partial responders and nonresponders.

Obsessive-Compulsive Disorder

Evidence supports the use of CBT with exposure and response prevention (ERP) for youth obsessive-compulsive disorder (OCD), both alone or in combination with medication (Kircanski, Peris, & Piacentini, 2011; Watson & Rees, 2008). CBT is considered as the initial treatment of choice for mild to moderate OCD in children and adolescents based on the literature and expert consensus of efficacy, safety, and durability of response (AACAP, 2012; Barrett, Farrell, Pina, Peris, & Piacentini, 2008). For severe OCD, medication is often prescribed along with CBT.

A behavioral model of OCD considers obsessions as intrusive, unwanted thoughts, images, or impulses that cause distress or anxiety. Compulsions, either as overt behavior or cognition, serve to reduce these negative feelings (Albano, March, & Piacentini, 1999). Compulsions reduce obsession-triggered distress and are thus negatively reinforced. The more compulsions reduce the child's anxiety, the more powerful they become. In more cognitive models, beliefs are considered influential (Kiracinski et al., 2011). Treatments for OCD, such as March and Mulle (1998), apply gradual exposure according to a hierarchy of OCD symptoms while preventing the child from carrying out compulsive rituals. The symptom hierarchy provides a guide for designing individual exposure tasks as well as the sequence for implementation. A goal of ERP is to teach the youth that, via repeated exposures, the obsession-triggered anxiety will dissipate and that the feared consequences of not ritualizing will not happen (Barrett et al., 2008). Even if total extinction of the anxiety does not occur, the youth learns to tolerate the distress during ERP. Cognitive interventions are also a part of treatment. The youth learns to recognize that the intrusive thoughts are part of OCD and to reevaluate the likelihood of feared consequences. During the psychoeducation phase the therapist educates the youth and his or her family about OCD within a cognitive-behavioral framework. Inclusion of the family at this stage can be important as family factors play a role in OCD treatment. In many families with a child with OCD both parents and siblings many participate or accommodate rituals on a daily basis (e.g., by providing clean towels and soap for hand washing, taking over chores the child is unable to carry out). A family-based CBT intervention has been found to effectively reduce OCD severity and impairment as well as parent-reported involvement in symptoms (e.g., Piacentini et al., 2011).

Using meta-analysis, Watson and Rees (2008) reported on five RCTs of CBT in children with OCD and found a large effect size. Findings from the Pediatric OCD Treatment Study (POTS) suggest that greater OCD severity and related functional impairment, more comorbid externalizing symptoms, and higher levels of family accommodation were associated with poorer treatment outcome (Garcia et al., 2010). When there is a family history of OCD, the authors recommend combining CBT with medication (an SSRI).

Depression

Depressed youth are characterized by feelings of sadness, a sense of being unlovable, and a negative belief about the future. In accordance with a behavioral model, depression is associated with behavioral inactivity and social behavior resulting in low rates of positive reinforcement. In treatment, behavioral activation and social skills training seek to stimulate behavior that will elicit positive environmental consequences. Cognitive models underscore that automatic negative thoughts underlie depression and are associated with depressed persons interpreting ambiguous situations in a pessimistic and negative way (Beck, Rush, Shaw, & Emery, 1979). In accordance, cognitive components of treatment target negative self-talk. CBT is the most widely researched psychological therapy for treating depression in youth. In a recent review of evidence-based psychotherapies for youth depression, David-Ferdon and Kaslow (2008) concluded that CBT meet the criteria for a "well-established" treatment. Group-based programs are considered well-established treatments for treating depression in youth, with or without a parent component, whereas individually delivered treatments for adolescents are rated as probably efficacious. Studies of younger children typically focus on school-based interventions for children with elevated symptoms of depression. In contrast, studies of adolescent samples focus more on youth meeting criteria for a depressive disorder.

The *ACTION* program (Stark, Schnoebelen, et al., 2005; Stark, Simpson, et al., 2005) was developed as a CBT treatment for depressed girls, although it can be adapted for use with boys, applying the same core techniques. *ACTION* is a group-based intervention for youth aged 9–13 years typically implemented in schools with 20 group meetings and two individual sessions over 11 weeks. Youth learn coping skills to manage the stress and emotions they experience and to recognize problems and apply problem-solving skills. Behavioral activation is accomplished through scheduling of pleasant activities. Interactions with the therapist and with peers are used to change maladaptive beliefs and build beliefs that they are lovable and worthy. The parent component for *ACTION* provides parents with information to reinforce the skills the girls learn in their sessions and to create a supportive and positive home environment. In anevaluation of *ACTION* (Stark, Streusand, Krumholz, & Patel, 2010), 159 girls aged 9–13 years with depressive disorders were treated with CBT alone or CBT plus a parent component. More than 80% of the girls no longer met criteria for a depressive disorder at the end of treatment. The girls in the CBT-alone treatment showed a more positive sense of self and future at the end of treatment compared to girls whose parents also participated. Parent training participants reported greater family cohesiveness and improved communication at posttreatment. At 1-year follow-up, 73% of CBT-only youth and 84% of the CBT-plus-parent youth maintained their improvement.

A modular treatment of adolescent depression, *Adolescent Coping with Depression* (CWDA; Clarke, Lewinsohn, & Hops, 1990) has been evaluated. Each module targets specific problem areas that may be experienced by the teen. Cognitive skills target depressogenic patterns of thinking and seek to increase positive thinking. Behavioral modules aim to reduce social withdrawal and impaired interpersonal interactions. The downward spiral of thoughts and behavior is turned upward by stimulating more positive interactions and positive thinking. To address conflicts with others, CWDA includes training in problem solving, communication, and negotiating skills. Several studies document the efficacy of CWDA in alleviating symptoms of depression in youths aged 13–17 years (Clarke et al., 1999; Lewinsohn, Clarke, Hops, & Andrew, 1990; Rohde, Clarke, Mace, Jorgensen, & Seeley, 2004). However, CWDA was comparable to treatment as usual (therapy and/or medication) for depressed offspring of depressed parents (Clarke et al., 2002). Based on a meta-analysis of seven studies of CWDA, the observed average effect size was in the low to medium range (Cuijpers, Muñoz, Clarke, & Lewinsohn, 2009). Although a parent companion group course has been developed (Lewinsohn, Rohde, Hops, & Clarke, 1991), research suggests that there is little incremental benefit to adding a parent course (Lewinsohn et al., 1990). Another study found that supplementing the original program with booster sessions did not reduce the rate of recurrence (Clarke et al., 1999). Kaufman and colleagues (Kaufman, Rohde, Seeley, Clarke, & Stice, 2005) examined possible mediators of treatment and observed that reducing negative thinking (similar to the Kendall & Treadwell findings for anxiety) may be a mechanism through which CBT reduces depressive symptoms.

The relative efficacy of CBT for depression in adolescents was evaluated in a large study of depressed youth aged 12 to 17 years (March et al., 2004). The study compared the effects of fluoxetine, CBT, and their combination. The 12-week CBT treatment was a combination of strategies that included psychoeducation, goal setting, mood monitoring, behavioral activation, and cognitive restructuring. The results indicated that the short-term effect of CBT was no better than placebo in reducing symptoms, whereas response rates for medication alone

and the combination of CBT and medication were greater (March et al., 2004). In contrast, the longer term results suggested that medication may produce more rapid effects, whereas CBT may take a little longer before a positive treatment response is observed. The efficacy of CBT was comparable to that of medication by weeks 18–24 and to combination therapy by weeks 30–36 (TADS, 2007). At 9 months follow-up there were no differences in response rates between the treatment conditions, with all showing a favorable effect. Interestingly, suicidal ideation decreased with treatment, but greater reduction in suicidal ideation was found when treatment included CBT, either alone or with medication. As the authors postulated, CBT may protect against treatment-emergent suicidal events in patients taking fluoxetine (TADS, 2007).

Depression can be episodic, so relapse prevention becomes an important treatment concern. Youth with residual symptoms at the end of treatment are at greater risk of relapse (Emslie et al., 2008; Kennard et al., 2009), and some youth do not maintain their remission over time, emphasizing the need for therapists to monitor clients even after they have reached remission status (Kennard et al., 2009). Adolescent girls who have recovered from their depression have a relatively high risk of recurrence (Curry et al., 2011). Of particular interest, adding CBT to medication was successful at reducing the risk of relapse in youth responding to medications (Kennard et al., 2008). On the other hand, Clarke and colleagues (1999), studying a preventive intervention, found that booster sessions did not reduce recurrence rates during a 2-year follow-up.

CBT has been deemed a "well-established" treatment for youth depression. However, the proportion of unsuccessfully treated youth is high in some of the studies, and there is need for more studies and improved interventions. In particular, more knowledge is needed about potential moderators of the effectiveness of treatment and which specific components of CBT are especially effective.

Aggression and Disruptive Behavior Disorders

Aggression is a pattern of interpersonal behavior that is injurious or destructive to others or to objects (Bandura, 1973). Aggressive behavior problems are among the most common causes of referrals to mental health services for youth (Steiner & Remsing, 2007). Children showing high levels of aggressive behavior are typically diagnosed with oppositional defiant disorder (ODD) or conduct disorder (CD), and comorbidity with other disorders is high.

The social-cognitive model is the CBT framework for understanding aggression in youth. According to the social-cognitive model, the emotional and physiological reaction of an aggressive child to a distressing event is due to the child's misperceptions and inaccurate appraisal of the event rather than the event itself (Crick & Dodge, 1994). Aggressive youth typically misattribute hostile intentions to others (Lochman & Dodge, 1994) in an ambiguous conflict situation with their peers or others, thereby justifying retaliation (Lochman, Powell, Whidby, & Fitzgerald, 2012). Distorted perceptions, misattributions of intentionality, overreliance on nonverbal solutions, and underreliance on verbal solutions are targeted in CBT for aggressive youth (Lochman, Powell, Whidby, & Fitzgerald, 2012).

Multiple studies have evaluated CBT for aggression, and meta-analyses have found CBT to be effective for aggressive and externalizing behavior problems in youth with medium effect sizes (Robinson, Smith, Miller, & Brownell, 1999; Sukhodolsky, Kassinove, & Gorman, 2004). Several specific ESTs for aggression in youth have been identified (see Eyberg, Nelson, & Boggs, 2008; Pardini & Lochman, 2006). Although there are some differences between the various programs, there are many common factors, giving clinicians a firm theoretical and empirical foundation when working with aggressive youth and their families. Parenting processes have been linked to aggression in children (Jaffe, Caspi, Moffitt, & Taylor, 2004) and parent training components are common in CBT for youth aggression. Parenting components typically focus on teaching parents how to reinforce and shape prosocial, nonaggressive behavior. Parents are also taught how to communicate in a firm but flexible manner, and how to use selective ignoring and time-outs to reduce aggressive behavior. In the child programs, children are often taught skills such as emotion awareness, perspective taking, problem solving, and goal setting.

Problem-solving skills training (PSST) and parent management training (PMT; Kazdin, 2005) are treatment programs originally developed for inpatient care for children ages 5–12 years and their families, but they have been extended for use in outpatient settings. Children are typically referred for oppositional, aggressive, and antisocial behavior and usually meet criteria for CD or ODD. PSST consists of 12 weekly sessions with the child (may be supplemented with additional sessions if required). A central component of treatment is teaching problem solving to develop and apply prosocial solutions to interpersonal problems, with an emphasis on situations that the child actually encounters in his or her life. The therapist and child practice problem solving through role plays before the child applies the behavior at home as part of homework assignments. Rewards systems, contingent social reinforcement, and modeling are also part of the program. PMT also consists of 12 sessions with the possibility to add further sessions when necessary. The parent program teaches parents skills that they apply with the child at home. In the child sessions, skills are practiced in session, modeled by the therapist, and rehearsed in role plays. Parents are also taught how to use positive reinforcements to increase prosocial behavior as well as effective applications of time-out and ignoring to reduce aggressive behavior. Typically, the treatment is not implemented so much in therapy sessions as it is carried out by the parents and children at home. A number of studies (see Kazdin, 2010) have reported positive effects of PSST and PMT alone or in combination with both inpatient and outpatient samples of youth. Both PSST and PMT have been reported to be effective in reducing oppositional and aggressive behavior and increasing prosocial behavior in youth compared to control conditions, and effects have held up at 1-year follow-up (Kazdin, Esveldt-Dawson, French, &Unis, 1987a, 1987b; Kazdin, Siegel, & Bass, 1992). The combination of problem-solving training with the child and the parent management training has resulted in greater improvements than using one of the treatments alone, moving more children from clinical to normal levels of functioning. Children with cognitive deficits and severe impairment have also benefited significantly from the treatment (Kazdin & Crowley, 1997), and case complexity and comorbidity did not result in poorer treatment outcomes (Kazdin & Whitley, 2006).

CBT interventions have been adapted for group implementation and developed for use in schools. Results indicate that the programs have been effective in reducing delinquent behavior and preventing substance use. The *Anger Coping* (Larson & Lochman, 2002) and *Coping Power* programs (Lochman, Wells, & Lenhart, 2008; Wells, Lochman, & Lenhart, 2008) target social-cognitive problems characteristic of aggressive children using a group format for fourth through sixth graders. These CBT programs have been successfully implemented in school and clinical settings (Lochman,

Boxmeyer, Powell, Barry, & Pardini, 2010). The programs include training in problem-solving skills, recognition of physiological cues of arousal, goal setting, and use of calming self-talk in conflict situations. The *Coping Power Program*, an extension of the *Anger Coping Program*, includes a 16-session parent component in addition to the 34 child sessions that are usually implemented over 16 to 18 weeks. Parents learn to use behavior management skills and social learning procedures as ways of managing the child's behavior at home. Evaluations of the programs have found that participant children had lower rates of aggressive behavior as per parent report and independent observer ratings of classroom behavior (Lochman, Burch, Curry, & Lampron, 1984; Lochman, Lampron, Gemmer, Harris, & Wyckoff, 1989). At 3-year follow-up, children who had participated in the program showed lower rates of substance use and had maintained their increases in self-esteem and problem-solving skills compared to an untreated group (Lochman, 1992). In other reports, youth who received the *Coping Power Program* showed lower rates of delinquent behavior, parent-rated drug use, and teacher-rated externalizing behavior (Lochman, Boxmeyer, Powell, Roth, & Windle, 2006; Lochman & Wells, 2004). Adapted for use with samples of youth diagnosed with ODD or CD, youth treated with the *Coping Power Program* were found to have greater reductions in overt aggression relative to a treatment as usual group (Van de Wiel, Matthys, Cohen-Kettenis, & van Engeland, 2003).

Attention-Deficit/Hyperactivity Disorder

Youth diagnosed with attention-deficit/hyperactivity disorder (ADHD) show levels of inattention, impulsivity, or hyperactivity that exceed age appropriate levels. Given the association between ADHD and poor self-regulation and cognitive deficits, one might consider CBT a suitable approach to treating ADHD. However, problem-solving and cognitive self-instructional methods, while helpful, may not be sufficiently powerful to influence the full symptomology or course of ADHD, and the use of cognitive interventions alone is not considered to be empirically supported (Miller & Hinshaw, 2012). One possible explanation for this may be that cognitive therapies are better suited for changing cognitive *distortions* rather than *deficiencies* in cognitive strategies (see Kendall & MacDonald, 1993). More traditional behavioral interventions form the foundation of effective psychosocial intervention for this condition and, in combination with

stimulant medication, are recommended as the first line of treatment for youth with ADHD (Pelham & Fabiano, 2008). The evidence base for the short-term benefits of behavioral parent training, behavioral classroom management, and intensive peer-focused behavioral interventions in recreational settings (e.g., summer programs) indicate that these interventions improve the functioning of children with ADHD and such behavioral interventions have been considered "well established" (Fabiano et al., 2009; Pelham & Fabiano, 2008). Behavioral interventions teach skills to parents, teachers, and youth in real-life settings that overcome some of the important functional impairments seen in patients with ADHD in areas such as peer relationships, school functioning, and parenting. In contrast to traditional clinic-based social skills groups, recent treatment studies have targeted peer relationships and functioning in recreational settings conducted in summer programs. These are typically intensive programs with daily activities involving brief segments of social skills training and coached group play concurrent with contingency management systems and home rewards from parents (Pelham, Fabiano, Gnagy, Greiner, & Hoza, 2005). Summer treatment programs have been included in comprehensive treatment approaches to ADHD (e.g., MTA Cooperative Group, 1999a).

The Multimodal Treatment Study of Children with Attention-Deficit/Hyperactivity Disorder (MTA Cooperative Group, 1999a) was a randomized trial comparing the effects of medication management, behavior modification, and their combination and usual community practice. Medication management was found to have the greatest impact on the core symptoms of ADHD, while combination therapy and behavioral intervention showed positive effect on coexisting issues such as oppositional/defiant symptoms, internalizing symptoms, and parent–child relationship Behavioral intervention without medication outperformed community care only for those children who had comorbid anxiety symptoms (MTA Cooperative Group, 1999b). This study indicates that medication or combination therapy may be superior to behavioral intervention alone for ADHD and supports recommendations for a two-pronged treatment approach for ADHD. The advantages of combination therapy and medication management were still evident at a 2-year follow-up (MTA Cooperative Group, 2004). However, participants in the medication-only condition received higher dose levels than youth in the combination group. This may suggest that the combination of medication and behavioral intervention may permit lower medication requirements over time.

Special Issues
Transportability of Interventions

Our brief historical overview introduced the notion of and criteria for "efficacy," or "demonstrations that a treatment is beneficial for patients or clients in well-controlled treatment studies" (Chambless & Hollon, 1998, p. 3). Important questions remain, however, regarding the potential for empirically supported interventions to be successful when implemented in community and private settings, where they are delivered by a variety of individuals (Owens & Murphy, 2004) and where training and supervision may be less focused.

Such questions revolve around issues of transportability——the degree to which EBTs work when implemented in community contexts (Schoenwald & Hoagwood, 2001). Over 15 years ago the *Journal of Consulting and Clinical Psychology* devoted a special issue to an examination of "how findings from carefully controlled studies of efficacious psychosocial interventions for children can be transported into naturalistic studies of the effectiveness of services" (Hoagwood, Hibbs, Brent, & Jensen, 1995, p. 683). Transportability has been discussed at multiple levels, for instance, surfacing in the Surgeon General's Conference on Children's Mental Health, which promoted increased reliance on the use of "scientifically proven" mental health services (U.S. Public Health Service, 2000). Indeed, the issue remains before us today. Ginsburg and colleagues (2008) point out that the challenges that continue to confront psychology regard successful dissemination of empirically supported intervention strategies to community treatment settings—especially those serving youth from diverse racial and ethnic backgrounds. The difficulty, however, may be found in the gap between research and service clinics (Weisz, Donenberg, Han, & Weiss, 1995).

The achievement of transportability thus requires a "bridging of the gap," which has also been referred to as "translating science into practice" (Chorpita, 2003). This entails a move from "efficacy" to "effectiveness" (Mufson, Dorta, Olfson, Weissman, & Hoagwood, 2004; Schoenwald & Hoagwood, 2001) or from "research therapy" to "clinic therapy" (Weisz et al., 1995) studies. The former (in each case) is often characterized by clinicians with in-depth training in the use of manualized treatments and the goal of testing the intervention. On the other hand, the latter seeks to evaluate applications of such efficacious treatments in community settings that commonly lack resources.

A consequence of limited resources may be lower adherence to treatment fidelity and a corresponding drop in treatment effects (e.g., Henggeler, Melton, Brondino, Scherer, & Hanley, 1997). Thus, a critical future goal is to address the issues raised by articles included in the special section of the *Journal of Consulting and Clinical Psychology*, which discussed how such a goal might be realized (Weisz et al., 1995), the implications of transportability (Henggeler, Schoenwald, & Pickrel, 1995), and the use of manual-based treatment (Kendall & Southam-Gerow, 1995), the latter of which should always be done with "flexibility" (Kendall & Beidas, 2007).

Although transporting efficacious treatments may incur expenses, the investment is worthwhile when compared to providing ineffective services (Henggeler et al., 1997). Successfully doing so will yield what Schoenwald and Hoagwood (2001) refer to as "street-ready" interventions—ones that can be applied in representative settings and systems. To achieve such an end, being guided by empirical support for the efficacy of treatment is required in order to effectively implement broader applications in needed community settings.

The School Setting

The dissemination and implementation of ESTs would be markedly enhanced by their inclusion within school systems—a favorable change from the manner in which mental health services are traditionally provided to youth (Evans & Weist, 2004). Challenges exist with regard to schools' acceptance of a greater role in children's mental health (Owens & Murphy, 2004; Pincus & Friedman, 2004; Weisz et al., 1995), and difficult questions remain unanswered. For instance, Owens and Murphy (2004) asked: How effective are these treatments when delivered to diverse populations by mental health professionals in community settings who struggle with the added burdens of higher caseloads and fewer resources? Schools represent such a community setting.

The link between children's mental health and academic success would seemingly provide a natural avenue for collaborative efforts among professionals in psychology and education (Mufson, Dorta, Olfson, Weissman, & Hoagwood, 2004), as research has demonstrated the deleterious effects of psychopathology on children and adolescents' school functioning (Ialongo et al., 1993, 1994; Mychailyszyn, Mendez, & Kendall, 2010). However, developing and sustaining working relationships can be difficult because schools may be wary of having researchers on-site for their studies. Additionally, research may be stymied when parents and/or school administrations have negative perceptions of research.

According to some, a particularly problematic obstacle for school-based mental health interventions will be getting teachers "on board" (Pincus & Friedman, 2004). Although other school personnel might carry the burden, teachers are often asked to play an active part in the delivery of school-based interventions, with related tasks including identification of eligible participants, completion of research measures, and perhaps even implementation of the program itself within class time. These tasks require considerable training, reflecting a time commitment that competes with an already demanding schedule (Owens & Murphy, 2004). Combined with the possibility that children may need to spend time out of the classroom to participate in the intervention, it is somewhat understandable that teachers may not be enthusiastic about involvement in school-based research. It may be that state or other government agencies will need to assign funds and staff to schools for the implementation and evaluation of empirically supported programs for children's mental health.

Conclusions and Future Directions

Cognitive-behavioral therapy has substantial empirical support for the treatment of many, but not all, psychological disorders of youth. Therapists conducting CBT with children and adolescents attend to a number of factors that differentiate the treatment of children from that of adults, including the entry into therapy; mode of delivery; level of cognitive, emotional, and social development; and the role of parents. Although CBT applications for specific disorders vary in the use of specific treatment strategies, there are several strategies common to CBT, including affective education, cognitive restructuring, problem solving, modeling and role play, behavioral contingencies, and exposure and behavioral activation. There have been advances and encouraging findings, but there are important directions for future research. Suggested future directions include brief CBT, computer-assisted CBT, and transdiagnostic CBT approaches.

Brief CBT

Many CBT protocols for psychological disorders in youth are built on 16–20 sessions of therapy (e.g., 16 sessions in *Coping Cat*, Kendall & Hedtke, 2006a; 20 sessions in *ACTION*, Stark et al., 2007). There are many reasons that shorter protocols (e.g., 8–10 sessions) may be desirable for dissemination and implementation in practice. For example, it may be easier to implement brief CBT treatments in community settings because shorter treatments would be less costly and each trained therapist could treat more youth. Although caution is needed not to assume that quality CBT can be accomplished "quickly," research is needed to explore whether CBT approaches for various childhood disorders can be delivered in more brief formats while at the same time maintaining an acceptable level of efficacy. For example, regarding the treatment of childhood anxiety disorders, a brief version (8 sessions) of the *Coping Cat* program was found to be acceptable and beneficial in a pilot study (Crawley et al., 2013). Further investigation is needed to examine the relative efficacy of brief CBT and CBT for child anxiety.

Computer-Assisted CBT

Computers offer a novel format for CBT with youth. There are numerous potential advantages of computer-assisted CBT, including increased access to mental health services for underserved populations, standardization of treatment content and delivery, and cost-effectiveness (Hofmann, 1999). Initial investigations have found support for computer-assisted CBT for child anxiety. For example, Spence and colleagues (2006) compared group CBT, group CBT with half of the sessions delivered via the Internet, and a waitlist condition for 7- to 14-year-old youth diagnosed with an anxiety disorder. Both treatment conditions demonstrated significantly greater improvement at posttreatment compared to the waitlist condition, and diagnostic recovery rates did not differ across treatment conditions. Treatment satisfaction also did not differ across the two active treatments. Similarly, March and colleagues (2009) compared the *BRAVE-ONLINE* program, an Internet-delivered CBT program with minimal therapist support, to a waitlist control and reported positive effects of the program. Cunningham and colleagues (2009), in a small pilot study, reported beneficial effects for the *Cool Teens CD-ROM* for youth anxiety. More recently, Kendall and Khanna (2008a, 2008b) developed *Camp Cope-a-Lot: The Coping Cat DVD* for youth ages 7–13 years with anxiety. The Camp Cope-a-Lot (CCAL) program is a computer-assisted CBT based on the *Coping Cat* program. Half of the 12 sessions—the exposure task sessions—are overseen by a therapist, or "coach." Feasibility and acceptability of the CCAL was favorable and an RCT (Khanna & Kendall, 2010) comparing CCAL, CBT, and an education, support, and attention (ESA) control condition indicated higher diagnostic recovery rates in the CCAL and CBT conditions compared to the ESA condition. Improvement rates did not differ between the two active conditions.

To recap, several investigations report support for the use of computer-assisted CBT for childhood anxiety. Additional work is justified to expand the use of computer-assisted CBT to other childhood disorders and to examine the relative efficacy of these novel treatments to traditional CBT for childhood psychological disorders.

Transdiagnostic CBT

Although originally conceived as a more broad-based approach to treating psychological disorders, CBT has typically been viewed as a disorder-specific approach in recent decades, in part due to external pressures (Mansell, Harvey, Watkins, & Shafran, 2009). Disorder-specific treatment protocols have been developed for a variety of psychological disorders in youth. Transdiagnostic treatment approaches target multiple disorders within a single treatment, and they have been proposed as complements to disorder-specific treatments (Mansell et al., 2009). Transdiagnostic treatments could be made available to youth with comorbid diagnoses. Although a number of different definitions of transdiagnostic treatments have been offered, one proposal states that a transdiagnostic model is a treatment that is flexible enough to simultaneously address multiple problems at a time using principles and strategies that target transdiagnostic mechanisms of change (Kendall et al., 2012). For instance, targets of change within transdiagnostic CBT for youth may include disturbances in cognitive processing, emotion regulation, and problem solving.

Anxiety and depressive disorders are diagnostic classes that may fit transdiagnostic CBT because they are highly comorbid in youth (Angold, Costello, & Erkanli, 1999), share symptoms and etiological factors (Axelson & Birmaher, 2001), and have similar treatment structures, strategies, and response rates (Kendall et al., 2008; Stark,

Streusand, Arora, & Patel, 2012). Efforts to develop transdiagnostic CBT treatments for anxiety and depressive disorders are under way among several research groups (e.g., Chu, Colognori, Weissman, & Bannon, 2009; Ehrenreich, Goldstein, Wright, & Barlow, 2009; Ehrenreich-May & Bilek, 2012; Kendall, Stark, Martinsen, Rodrigues, & Arora, 2013; Weersing, Gonzalez, Campo, & Lucas, 2008). Efforts notwithstanding, proper outcome evaluation is required to examine the efficacy of transdiagnostic CBT and to evaluate their relative efficacy compared to disorder-specific treatments. Future research is also needed to identify other areas where transdiagnostic approaches may be developed and evaluated.

References

American Academy of Child & Adolescent Psychiatry. (2012). Practice parameter for the assessment and treatment of children and adolescents with obsessive-compulsive disorder. *Journal of the American Academy of Child and Adolescent Psychiatry, 51,* 98–113.

American Psychological Association. (2002). Criteria for evaluating treatment guidelines. *American Psychologist, 57,* 1052–1059.

American Psychological Association. (2006). Evidence-based practice in psychology. *American Psychologist, 61,* 271–285.

Albano, A. M., & DiBartolo, P. M. (2007). *Cognitive behavioral therapy for social phobia in adolescents: Stand up, speak out therapist guide.* New York, NY: Oxford University Press.

Albano, A. M., March, J. S., & Piacentini, J. (1999). Cognitive behavioral treatment of obsessive-compulsive disorder. In R. T. Ammerman (Ed.), *Handbook of prescriptive treatments for children and adolescents* (pp. 193–213). Boston, MA: Allyn & Bacon.

Angold, A., Costello, E. J., & Erkanli, A. (1999). Comorbidity. *Journal of Child Psychology and Psychiatry, 40,* 57–87.

Axelson, D. A., & Birmaher, B. (2001). Relation between anxiety and depressive disorders in childhood and adolescence. *Depression and Anxiety, 14,* 67–78.

Bandura, A. (1969). *Principles of behavior modification.* New York, NY: Holt, Rinehart & Winston.

Bandura, A. (1973). *Aggression: A social learning analysis.* Englewood Cliffs, NJ: Prentice-Hall.

Barmish, A. J., & Kendall, P. C. (2005). Should parents be co-clients in cognitive-behavioral therapy for anxious youth? *Journal of Clinical Child and Adolescent Psychology, 34,* 569–581.

Barrett, P. M., Dadds, M. R., & Rapee, R. M. (1996). Family treatment of childhood anxiety: A controlled trial. *Journal of Consulting and Clinical Psychology, 64,* 333–342. doi:10.1037/0022-006X.64.2.333

Barrett, P. M., Farrell, L., Pina, A. A., Peris, T. S., & Piacentini, J. (2008). Evidence-based psychosocial treatments for child and adolescent obsessive-compulsive disorder. *Journal of Clinical Child and Adolescent Psychology, 37,* 131–155.

Barrios, B. A., & O'Dell, S. L. (1998). Fears and anxieties. In E. J. Mash & R. A. Barkley (Eds.), *Treatment of childhood disorders* (2nd ed., pp. 249–337). New York, NY: Guilford Press.

Beck, A. (1976). *Cognitive therapy and the emotional disorders*. New York, NY: International Universities Press.

Beck, A. (1995). *Cognitive therapy: Basics and beyond*. New York, NY: Guilford Press.

Beck, A. T., Rush, A. J., Shaw, B. F., & Emery, G. (1979). *Cognitive therapy of depression*. New York, NY: Guilford Press.

Beidel, D. C., Turner, S. M., & Morris, T. L. (2000). Behavioral treatment of childhood social phobia. *Journal of Consulting and Clinical Psychology, 68*(6), 1072–1080.

Benjamin, C. L., Puleo, C. M., Settipani, C. A., Brodman, D. M., Edmunds, J. M., Cummings, C. M., & Kendall, P. C. (2011). History of cognitive-behavioral therapy in youth. *Child and Adolescent Psychiatric Clinics of North America, 20*(2), 179–189.

Breinholst, S., Esbjørn, B. H., Reinholdt-Dunne, M. L., & Stallard, P. (2012). CBT for the treatment of child anxiety disorders: A review of why parental involvement has not enhanced outcomes. *Journal of Anxiety Disorders, 26*(3), 416–424.

Chambless, D. L., & Hollon, S. D. (1998). Defining empirically supported treatments. *Journal of Consulting and Clinical Psychology, 66*, 7–18.

Chambless, D. L., Sanderson, W. C., Shoham, V., Bennett Johnson, S., Pope, K. S., Crits-Christoph, P., ... & McCurry, S. (1996). An update on empirically validated therapies. *Clinical Psychologist, 49*, 5–18.

Chorpita, B. F. (2003). The frontier of evidence-based practice. In A. E. Kazdin & J. R. Weisz (Eds.), *Evidence-based psycho-therapies for children and adolescents* (pp. 42–59). New York, NY: Guildford Press.

Chu, B. C., Colognori, D., Weissman, A. S., & Bannon, K. (2009). An initial description and pilot of group behavioral activation therapy for anxious and depressed youth. *Cognitive and Behavioral Practice, 16*, 408–419.

Clarke, G. N., Hornbrook, M., Lynch, F., Polen, M., Gale, J., O'Connor, E., ... Debar, L. (2002). Group cognitive-behavioral therapy for depressed adolescent offspring of depressed parents in a health maintenance organization. *Journal of the American Academy of Child and Adolescent Psychiatry, 41*, 305–313

Clarke, G. N., Lewinsohn, P. M., & Hops, H. (1990). *Instructor's manual for the adolescent coping with depression course*. Portland, OR: Kaiser Permanente Center for Health Research.

Clarke, G. N., Rohde, P., Lewinsohn, P. M., Hops, H., & Seeley, J. R. (1999). Cognitive-behavioral treatment of adolescent depression: Efficacy of acute group treatment and booster sessions. *Journal of the American Academy of Child and Adolescent Psychiatry, 38*, 272–279.

Cobham, V. E., Dadds, M. R., & Spence, S. H. (1998). The role of parental anxiety in the treatment of childhood anxiety. *Journal of Consulting and Clinical Psychology, 66*, 893–905. doi:10.1037/0022-006X.66.6.893

Conrad, A., & Roth, W. T. (2007). Muscle relaxation therapy for anxiety disorders: It works but how? *Journal of Anxiety Disorders, 21*(3), 243–264.

Crawley, S. A., Beidas, R. S., Benjamin, C. L., Martin, E., & Kendall, P. C. (2008). Treating socially phobic youth with CBT: Differential outcomes and treatment considerations. *Behavioural and Cognitive Psychotherapy, 36*, 379–389.

Crawley, S. A., Kendall, P. C., Benjamin, C. L., Brodman, D. M., Wei, C., Beidas, R. S., ... Mauro, C. (2013). Brief cognitive-behavioral therapy for anxious youth: Feasibility and initial outcomes. *Cognitive and Behavioral Practice, 20*, 123–133. doi:10.1016/j.cbpra.2012.07.003

Crawley, S. A., Podell, J. L., Beidas, R. S., Braswell, L., & Kendall, P. C. (2010). Cognitive-behavioral therapy with youth. In K. S. Dobson (Ed.), *Handbook of cognitive-behavioral therapies* (3rd ed., pp. 375–410). New York, NY: Guilford Press.

Crick, N. R., & Dodge, K. A. (1994). A review and reformulation of social information- processing mechanisms in children's social adjustment. *Psychological Bulletin, 115*(1), 74–101.

Cuijpers, P., Muñoz, R. F., Clarke, G. N., & Lewinsohn, P. M. (2009). Psychoeducational treatment and prevention of depression: The "coping with depression" course thirty years later. *Clinical Psychology Review, 29*, 449–458.

Cunningham, M. J., Wuthrich, V. M., Rapee, R. M., Lyneham, H. J., Schniering, C. A., & Hudson, J. L. (2009). The Cool Teens CD-ROM for anxiety disorders in adolescents. *European Child and Adolescent Psychiatry, 18*, 125–129.

Curry, J. F., & Craighead, W. (1990). Attributional style in clinically depressed and conduct disordered adolescents. *Journal of Consulting and Clinical Psychology, 58*(1), 109–115.

Curry, J., Silva. S., Rohde, P., Ginsburg, G., Kratochvil, C., Simons, A., ... March, J. (2011). Recovery and recurrence following treatment for adolescent major depression. *Archives of General Psychiatry, 68*, 263–270.

David-Ferdon, C., & Kaslow, N. J. (2008). Evidence-based psychosocial treatments for child and adolescent depression. *Journal of Clinical Child and Adolescent Psychology, 37*, 62–104.

Davis, D., & Boster, L. (1992). Cognitive-behavioral-expressive interventions with aggressive and resistant youths. *Child Welfare: Journal of Policy, Practice, and Program, 71*(6), 557–573.

Deblinger, E., & Heflin, A. H. (1996). *Treating sexually abused children and their nonoffending parents: A cognitive behavioral approach*. Thousand Oaks, CA: Sage.

D'Zurilla, T. J., & Goldfried, M. R. (1971). Problem solving and behavior modification. *Journal of Abnormal Psychology, 78*(1), 107–126.

Ehrenreich, J. T., Goldstein, C. R., Wright, L. R., & Barlow, D. H. (2009). Development of a unified protocol for the treatment of emotional disorders in youth. *Child and Family Behavior Therapy, 31*, 20–37.

Ehrenreich-May, J., & Bilek, E. L. (2012). The development of a transdiagnostic, cognitive behavioral group intervention for childhood anxiety disorders and co-occurring depression symptoms. *Cognitive and Behavioral Practice, 19*, 41–55.

Emslie, G, J., Kennard, B. D., Mayes, T. L., Nightingale-Teresi, J., Carmody, T., Hughes, C. W., ... Rintelmann, J. W. (2008). Fluoxetine versus placebo in preventing relapse of major depression in children and adolescents. *American Journal of Psychiatry, 165*, 459–467.

Evans, S. W., & Weist, M. D. (2004). Implementing Empirically Supported Treatments in the Schools: What Are We Asking? *Clinical Child and Family Psychology Review, 7*, 263–267. doi:10.1007/s10567-004-6090-0

Eyberg, S. M., Nelson, M. M., & Boggs, S. R. (2008). Evidence-based psychosocial treatments for children and adolescents with disruptive behavior. *Journal of Clinical Child and Adolescent Psychology, 37*, 215–237.

Fabiano, G. A., Pelham, W. E., Coles, E. K., Gnagy, E. M., Chronis-Tuscano, A., & O'Connor, B. (2009). A meta-analysis of behavioral treatments for attention- deficit/

hyperactivity disorder. *Clinical Psychology Review, 29*, 129–140.

Garcia, A. M., Sapyta, J. J., Moore, P. S., Freeman, J. B., Franklin, M. E., March, J. S., & Foe, E. B. (2010). Predictors and moderators of treatment outcome in the Pediatric Obsessive Compulsive Treatment Study (POTS I). *Journal of the American Academy of Child and Adolescent Psychiatry, 49*, 1024–1033.

Ginsburg, G. S., Becker, K. D., Kingery, J. N., & Nichols, T. (2008). Transporting CBT for childhood anxiety disorders into inner-city school-based mental health clinics. *Cognitive and Behavioral Practice, 15*, 148–158.

Ginsburg, G. S., Kendall, P. C., Sakolsky, D., Compton, S. N., Piacentini, J., Albano, A. M., ... March, J. (2011). Remission after acute treatment in children and adolescents with anxiety disorders: Findings from the CAMS. *Journal of Consulting and Clinical Psychology, 79*, 806–813. doi:10.1037/a0025933

Gleacher, A. A., Nadeem, E., Joy, A. J., Whited, A. L., Albano, A. M., Radigan, M., ... Eaton, K. (2011). Statewide CBT training for clinicians and supervisors treating youth: The New York State evidence based treatment dissemination center. *Journal of Emotional and Behavioral Disorders, 19*, 182–192.

Goldfried, M. R., & Trier, C. S. (1974). Effectiveness of relaxation as an active coping skill. *Journal of Abnormal Psychology, 83*(4), 348–355.

Gosch, E. A., Flannery-Schroeder, E., Mauro, C. F., & Compton, S. N. (2006). Principles of cognitive-behavioral therapy for anxiety disorders in children. *Journal of Cognitive Psychotherapy, 20*(3), 247–292.

Henggeler, S. W., Melton, G. B., Brondino, M. J., Scherer, D. G., & Hanley, J. H. (1997). Multisystemic therapy with violent and chronic juvenile offenders and their families: The role of treatment fidelity in successful dissemination. *Journal of Consulting and Clinical Psychology, 65*, 821–833.

Henggeler, S. W., Schoenwald, S. K., & Pickrel, S. G. (1995). Multisystemic therapy: Bridging the gap between university- and community-based treatment. *Journal of Consulting and Clinical Psychology, 63*, 709–717. doi:10.1037/0022-006X.63.5.709

Hoagwood, K., Hibbs, E., Brent, D., & Jensen, P. (1995). Introduction to the special section: Efficacy and effectiveness in studies of child and adolescent psychotherapy. *Journal of Consulting and Clinical Psychology, 63*, 683–687.

Hofmann, S. (Ed.). (1999). Innovations in cognitive behavioral treatments of anxiety disorders: Of treatments and technologies [Special Series]. *Cognitive and Behavioral Practice, 6*, 221–270.

Howard, B., Chu, B. C., Krain, A. L., Marrs-Garcia, A. L., & Kendall P. C. (2000). Cognitive-behavioral therapy for anxious children: Therapist manual, second addition. Workbook publishing. Ardmore, PA.

Ialongo, N., Edelsohn, G., Werthamer-Larsson, L., Crockett, L., & Kellam, S. (1994). The significance of self-reported anxious symptoms in first-grade children. *Journal of Abnormal Child Psychology, 22*, 441–455. doi:10.1007/BF02168084

Ialongo, N. S., Horn, W. F., Pascoe, J. M., Greenberg, G., Packard, T., Lopez, M., ... Puttler, L. (1993). The effects of a multimodal intervention with attention-deficit hyperactivity disorder children: A 9-month follow-up. *Journal of the American Academy of Child and Adolescent Psychiatry, 32*, 182–189. doi:10.1097/00004583-199301000-00026

Jacobson, E. (1938). *Progressive relaxation* (2nd ed.). Chicago, IL: University of Chicago Press.

Jaffe, S. R., Caspi, A., Moffitt, T. E., & Taylor, A., (2004). Physical maltreatment victim to antisocial child: Evidence of an environmentally mediated process. *Journal of Abnormal Psychology, 113*, 44–55.

Kahn, J. S., Kehle, T. J., Jenson, W. R., & Clark, E. (1990). Comparison of cognitive-behavioral, relaxation, and self-modeling interventions for depression among middle-school students. *School Psychology Review, 19*(2), 196–211.

Kaufman, N. K., Rohde, P., Seeley, J. R., Clarke, G. N., & Stice, E. (2005). Potential mediators of cognitive-behavioral therapy for adolescents with comorbid major depression and conduct disorder. *Journal of Consulting and Clinical Psychology, 73*, 38–46.

Kazdin, A. E. (2005). *Parent management training: Treatment for oppositional, aggressive, and antisocial behavior in children and adolescents*. New York, NY: Oxford University Press.

Kazdin, A. E. (2010). Problem-solving skills training and parent management training for oppositional defiant disorder and conduct disorder. In J. R. Weisz & A. E. Kazdin (Eds.), *Evidence-based psychotherapies for children and adolescents* (2nd ed., pp. 211–227). New York, NY: Guilford Press.

Kazdin, A. E., & Crowley, M. (1997). Moderators of treatment outcome in cognitively based treatment of antisocial behavior. *Cognitive Therapy and Research, 21*, 185–207.

Kazdin, A. E., Esveldt-Dawson, K., French, N. H., & Unis, A. S. (1987a). The effects of parent management training and problem-solving skills training combined in the treatment of antisocial child behavior. *Journal of the American Academy of Child and Adolescent Psychiatry, 26*, 416–424.

Kazdin, A. E., Esveldt-Dawson, K., French, N. H., & Unis, A. S. (1987b). Problem-solving skills training and relationship therapy in the treatment of antisocial child behavior. *Journal of Consulting and Clinical Psychology, 55*, 76–85.

Kazdin, A. E., Siegel, T., & Bass, D. (1992). Cognitive problem-solving skills training and parent management training in the treatment of antisocial behavior in children. *Journal of Consulting and Clinical Psychology, 60*, 733–747.

Kazdin, A. E., & Whitley, M. K. (2006). Comorbidity, case complexity, and effects of evidence-based treatment for children referred for disruptive behavior. *Journal of Consulting and Clinical Psychology, 74*, 455–467.

Kendall, P. C. (2012). Guiding theory for therapy with children and adolescents. In P. C. Kendall (Ed.), *Child and adolescent therapy: Cognitive-behavioral procedures* (4th ed., pp. 1–24) New York, NY: Guilford Press.

Kendall, P. C. (1993). Cognitive-behavioral therapies with youth: Guiding theory, current status, and emerging developments. *Journal of Consulting and Clinical Psychology, 61*, 235–247.

Kendall, P. C. (1994). Treating anxiety disorders in children: Results of a randomized clinical trial. *Journal of Consulting and Clinical Psychology, 62*, 100–110.

Kendall, P. C. (1993). Cognitive-behavioral therapies with youth: Guiding theory, current status, and emerging developments. *Journal of Consulting and Clinical Psychology, 61*, 235–247.

Kendall, P. C. (1998). Empirically supported psychological therapies. *Journal of Consulting and Clinical Psychology, 66*, 3–7.

Kendall, P. C., & Beidas, R. (2007). Smoothing the trail for dissemination of evidence-based practices for youth: Flexibility within fidelity. *Professional Psychology: Research and Practice*, *38*, 13–20.

Kendall, P. C., & Braswell, L. (1993). *Cognitive behavioral therapy for impulsive children* (2nd ed.). New York, NY: Guilford Press.

Kendall, P. C., Chansky, T. E., Kane, M. T., Kim, R., Kortlander, E., Ronan, K. R.,…Siqueland, L. (1992). *Anxiety disorders in youth: Cognitive-behavioral interventions*. Needham Heights, MA: Allyn & Bacon.

Kendall, P. C., Chu, B., Pimentel, S., & Choudhury, M. (2012). Treating anxiety disorders in youth. In P. C. Kendall (Ed.), *Child and adolescent therapy: Cognitive-behavioral procedures* (4th ed., pp. 143–189) New York, NY: Guilford Press.

Kendall, P. C., Flannery-Schroeder, E., Panichelli-Mindel, S. M., Southam-Gerow, M., Henin, A., & Warman, M. (1997). Therapy for youths with anxiety disorders: A second randomized clinical trial. *Journal of Consulting and Clinical Psychology*, *65*, 366–380.

Kendall, P. C., & Hedtke, K. (2006a). *Coping Cat workbook* (2nd ed.). Ardmore, PA: Workbook Publishing.

Kendall, P. C., & Hedtke, K. (2006b). *Cognitive-behavioral therapy for anxious children: Therapist manual* (3rd ed.). Ardmore, PA: Workbook Publishing.

Kendall, P. C., Hudson, J. L., Gosch, E., Flannery-Schroeder, E., & Suveg, C. (2008). Cognitive-behavioral therapy for anxiety disordered youth: A randomized clinical trial evaluating child and family modalities. *Journal of Consulting and Clinical Psychology, 76*, 282–297.

Kendall, P. C., & Khanna, M. S. (2008a). *Camp Cope-A-Lot: The Coping Cat CD ROM*. Ardrmore, PA: Workbook Publishing.

Kendall, P. C., & Khanna, M. S. (2008b). *Coach's manual for Camp Cope-A-Lot: The Coping Cat CD ROM*. Ardmore, PA: Workbook Publishing.

Kendall, P. C., & MacDonald, J. P. (1993). Cognition in the psychopathology of youth and implications for treatments. In K. S. Dobson & P. C. Kendall (Eds.), *Psychopathology and cognition* (pp. 387–427). San Diego, CA: Academic Press.

Kendall, P. C., Padever, W., & Zupan, B. (1980). *Developing self-control in children: A manual of cognitive-behavioral strategies*. Minneapolis: University of Minnesota.

Kendall, P. C., Stark, K., Martinsen, K., Rodrigues, K., & Arora, P. (2013). *Group leader manual for EMOTION: "Coping kids" managing anxiety and depression*. Ardmore, PA: Workbook Publishing.

Kendall, P. C.(2012). Treating anxiety disorders in youth. In P. C. Kendall (Ed.). *Child and adolescent therapy: Cognitive-behavioral procedures* (4th ed., pp. 143–189) New York, NY: Guilford Press.

Kendall, P. C., & Treadwell, K. H. (2007). The role of self-statements as a mediator in treatment for youth with anxiety disorders. *Journal of Consulting and Clinical Psychology*, *75*, 380–389. doi:10.1037/0022-006X.75.3.380

Khanna, M. S., & Kendall, P. C. (2008). Computer-assisted CBT for child anxiety: The coping cat CD-ROM. *Cognitive and Behavioral Practice*, *15*, 159–165. doi:10.1016/j.cbpra.2008.02.002

Khanna, M., & Kendall, P. C. (2010). Computer-assisted cognitive-behavioral therapy for child anxiety: Results of a randomized clinical trial. *Journal of Consulting and Clinical Psychology*, *78*, 737–745.

Kendall, P. C., & Southam-Gerow, M. A. (1995). Issues in the transportability of treatment: The case of anxiety disorders

in youths. *Journal of Consulting and Clinical Psychology*, *63*, 702–708. doi:10.1037/0022-006X.63.5.702

Kennard, B. D., Emslie, G. J., Mayes, T. L., Nightingale-Teresi, J., Nakonezny, P. A., Hughes, J. L.,…Jarrett, R. B. (2008). Cognitive-behavioral therapy to prevent relaps in pediatric responders to pharmacotherapy for major depressive disorder. *Journal of the American Academy of Child and Adolescent Psychiatry*, *47*, 1395–1404.

Kennard, B. D., Silva, S. G., Tonev, S., Rohde, P., Hughes, J. L., Vitiello, B.,…March, J. (2009). Remission and recovery in the treatment for adolescents with depression study (TADS): Acute and long-term outcomes. *Journal of the American Academy of Child and Adolescent Psychiatry*, *48*, 186–195.

Kircanski, K., Peris, T. S., & Piacentini, J. C. (2011). Cognitive-behavioral therapy for obsessive-compulsive disorder in children and adolescents. *Child and Adolescent Psychiatric Clinics of North-America*, *20*, 239–254.

Koeppen, A. S. (1974). Relaxation training for children. *Elementary School Guidance and Counseling*, *9*, 14–26.

Lansford, J. E., Malone, P. S., Dodge, K. A., Crozier, J. C., Pettit, G. S., & Bates, J. E. (2006). A 12-year prospective study of patterns of social information processing problems and externalizing behaviors. *Journal of Abnormal Child Psychology*, *34*(5), 715–724.

Larson, J., & Lochman, J. E. (2002). *Helping school children cope with anger: A cognitive- behavioral intervention*. New York, NY: Guilford Press.

Lewinsohn, P. M., Clarke, G., N., Hops, H., & Andrews, J. A. (1990). Cognitive-behavioral treatment for depressed adolescents. *Behavior Therapy*, *21*, 385–401.

Lewinsohn, P. M., Rohde, P., Hops, H., & Clarke, G. N. (1991). *Leader's manual for parent groups: Adolescent coping with depression*. Eugene, OR: Casalia Press.

Lilienfeld, S. O., Fowler, K. A., Lohr, J. M., & Lynn, S. J. (2005). Pseudoscience, nonscience, and nonsense in clinical psychology: Dangers and eemedies. In R. H. Wright & N. A. Cummings (Eds.), *Destructive trends in mental health: The well-intentioned path to harm* (pp. 187–218). New York, NY: Routledge.

Lochman, J. E. (1992). Cognitive-behavioral interventions with aggressive boys: Three-year follow-up and preventive effects. *Journal of Consulting and Clinical Psychology*, *60*, 426–432.

Lochman, J. E., Boxmeyer, C. L., Powell, N. P., Barry, T. D., & Pardini, D. A. (2010). Anger control training for aggressive youths. In J. R. Weisz & A. E. Kazdin (Eds.), *Evidence-based psychotherapies for children and adolescents* (2nd ed., pp. 227–243). New York, NY: Guilford Press.

Lochman, J. E., Boxmeyer, C. L., Powell, N. P., Roth, D., & Windle, M. (2006). Masked intervention effects: Analytic methods for addressing low dosage of intervention. *New Directions for Evaluations*, *110*, 19–32.

Lochman, J. E., Burch, P. P., Curry, J. F., & Lampron, L. B. (1984). Treatment and generalizations of cognitive-behavioral and goal setting interventions with aggressive boys. *Journal of Consulting and Clinical Psychology*, *52*, 915–916.

Lochman, J. E., & Dodge, K. A. (1994) Social-cognitive processes of severely violent, moderately aggressive and nonaggressive boys. *Journal of Consulting Clinical Psychology*, *62*, 366–374.

Lochman, J. E., Lampron, L. B., Gemmer, T. C., Harris, S. R., & Wyckoff, G. M. (1989). Teacher consultation and cognitive-behavioral interventions with aggressive boys. *Psychology in the Schools, 26,* 179–188.

Lochman, J. E., Powell, N. P., Boxmeyer, C. L., & Jimenez-Camargo, L. (2011). Cognitive- behavioral therapy for externalizing disorders in children and adolescents. *Child and Adolescent Psychiatric Clinics of North America, 20*(2), 305–318.

Lochman, J., Powell, N., Whidby, J., & Fitzgerald, D. (2012). Aggressive children: Cognitive-behavioral assessment and treatment. In P. C. Kendall (Ed.), *Child and adolescent therapy: Cognitive-behavioral procedures* (4th ed., pp. 27–60) New York, NY: Guilford Press.

Lochman, J. E., & Wells, K. C. (2004). The Coping Power Program for preadolescent aggressive boys and their parents: Outcome effects at the one-year follow-up. *Behavior Therapy, 34,* 493–515.

Lochman, J. E., Wells, K. C., & Lenhart, L. (2008). *Coping Power: Child group facilitators' guide.* New York, NY: Guilford Press.

Lynam, D. R., Milich, R., Zimmerman, R., Novak, S. P., Logan, T. K., Martin, C., … Clayton, R. (1999). Project DARE: No effects at 10-year follow-up. *Journal of Consulting and Clinical Psychology, 67,* 590–593.

Mansell, W., Harvey, A., Watkins, E., & Shafran, R. (2009). Conceptual foundations of the transdiagnostic approach to CBT. *Journal of Cognitive Psychotherapy, 23,* 6–19.

March, J., Silva, S., Petrycki, S., Curry, J., Wells, K., Fairbank, J., & Severe, J. (2004). Fluoxetine, cognitive-behavioral therapy, and their combination for adolescents with depression: Treatment for adolescent depression study (TADS) randomized controlled trial. *Journal of the American Medical Association, 292,* 807–820.

March, J. S., & Morris, M. L. (2004). *Anxiety disorders in children and adolescents* (2nd ed.). New York, NY: Guildford Press

March, J. S., & Mulle, K. (1998). *How I ran OCD off my land: A guide to cognitive behavioral psychotherapy for children and adolescents with obsessive-compulsive disorder.* New York, NY: Guilford Press

March, S., Spence, S. H., & Donovan, C. L. (2009). The efficacy of an internet-based cognitive-behavioral therapy intervention for child anxiety disorders. *Journal of Pediatric Psychology, 34,* 474–487.

Masia-Warner, C., Nangle, D. W., & Hansen, D. J. (2006). Bringing Evidence-Based Child Mental Health Services to the Schools: General Issues and Specific Populations. *Education and Treatment of Children, 29,* 165–172.

Mendlowitz, S. L., Manassis, K., Bradley, S., Scapillato, D., Miezitis, S., & Shaw, B. F. (1999). Cognitive-Behavioral group treatments in childhood anxiety disorders: The role of parental involvement. *Journal of the American Academy of Child and Adolescent Psychiatry, 38,* 1223–1229.

Miller, M., & Hinshaw, S. P. (2012). Attention-Deficit/Hyperactivity Disorder. In P. C. Kendall (Ed.), *Child and adolescent therapy* (4th ed., pp. 61–91). New York, NY: Guilford Press.

MTA Cooperative Group. (1999a). 14-month randomized clinical trial of treatment strategies for attention-deficit/hyperactivity disorder. *Archives of General Psychiatry, 56,* 1073–1086.

MTA Cooperative Group. (1999b). Moderators and mediators of treatment response for children with attention-deficit/hyperactivity disorder: the multimodal treatment study of children with ADHD. *Archives of General Psychiatry, 56,* 1088–1096.

MTA Cooperative Group. (2004). National Institute of Mental Health Multimodal Treatment Study of ADHD Follow-up: 24-month outcomes of treatment strategies for attention- deficit/hyperactivity disorder. *Pediatrics, 113,* 754–761.

Mufson, L. H., Dorta, K. P., Olfson, M., Weissman, M. M., & Hoagwood, K. (2004). Effectiveness research: Transporting interpersonal psychotherapy for depressed adolescents (IPT-A) from the lab to school-based health clinics. *Clinical Child and Family Psychology Review, 7,* 251–261.

Mychailyszyn, M. P., Mendez, J. L., & Kendall, P. C. (2010). School functioning in youth with and without anxiety disorders: Comparisons by diagnosis and comorbidity. *School Psychology Review, 39,* 106–121.

Nelson, W., & Finch, A. (2008). *Keeping your cool: The anger management workbook* (2nd ed., Parts 1 & 2). Ardmore, PA: Workbook Publishing.

Nezu, A. M., Nezu, C. M., & D'Zurilla, T. J. (2013). *Problem-solving therapy: A treatment manual.* New York, NY: Springer.

Nezu, A. M., Nezu, C. M., & Perri, M. G. (1990). Psychotherapy for adults within a problem solving framework: Focus on depression. *Journal of Cognitive Psychotherapy, 4,* 247–256.

Oerbeck, B., Johansen, J., Lundahl, K., & Kristensen, H. (2012). Selective mutism: A home-and kindergarten-based intervention for children 3-5 years: A pilot study. *Clinical Child Psychology and Psychiatry, 17*(3), 370–383.

Ollendick, T. H., & Cerny, J. A. (1981). *Clinical behavior therapy with children.* New York, NY: Plenum Press.

Ollendick, T. H., & King, N. J. (2012). Evidence-based treatments for children and adolescents: Issues and commentary. In P. C. Kendall (Ed.), *Child and adolescent therapy* (4th ed., pp. 499–519). New York, NY: Guilford Press

Owens, J. S., & Murphy, C. E. (2004). Effectiveness research in the context of school-based mental health. *Clinical Child and Family Psychology Review, 7,* 195–209.

Pardini, D. A., & Lochman, J. (2006). Treatments for oppositional defiant disorder. In M. A. Reinecke, F. M. Dattilio, & A. Freeman (Eds.), *Cognitive therapy with children and adolescents* (2nd ed., pp. 43–69) New York, NY: Guilford Press.

Pelham, W. E., & Fabiano, G. A. (2008). Evidence-based psychosocial treatments for attention-deficit/hyperactivity disorder. *Journal of Clinical Child and Adolescent Psychology, 37,* 184–214.

Pelham, W. E., Fabiano, G. A., Gnagy, E. M., Greiner, A. R., & Hoza, B (2005). The role of summer treatment programs in the context of comprehensive treatment for ADHD. In E. Hibbs & P. Jensen (Eds.), *Psychosocial treatments for child and adolescent disorders: Empirically based strategies for clinical practice* (pp. 377–410). Washington, DC: APA Press.

Piacentini, J., Bergman, R. L., Chang, S., Lanley, A., Peris, T., Woods, J. J., & McCracken, J. (2011). Controlled comparison of family cognitive behavioral therapy and psychoeducation/relaxation training for child obsessive-compulsive disorder. *Journal of the American Academy of Child and Adolescent Psychiatry, 50,* 1149–1161.

Pincus, D. B., & Friedman, A. G. (2004). Improving children's coping with everyday stress: Transporting treatment interventions to the school setting. *Clinical Child and Family Psychology Review, 7*(4), 223–240.

Rapee, R. M. (2000). Group treatment of children with anxiety disorders: Outcomes and predictors of treatment response. *Australian Journal of Psychology, 52,* 125–130.

Reuther, E. T., Davis, T. E., Moore, B. N., & Matson, J. L. (2011). Treating selective mutism using modular CBT for child anxiety: A case study. *Journal of Clinical Child & Adolescent Psychology, 40*, 156–63

Robinson, T. R., Smith, S. W., Miller, M. D., & Brownell, M. T. (1999). Cognitive behavior modification of hyperactivity-impulsivity and aggression: A meta-analysis of school- based studies. *Journal of Educational Psychology, 91*, 195–203.

Rohde, P., Clarke, G. N., Mace, D. E., Jorgensen, J. S., & Seeley, J. R. (2004). An efficacy/effectiveness study of cognitive-behavioral treatment for adolescents with comorbid major depression and conduct disorder. *Journal of the American Academy of Child Psychiatry, 43*, 660–668.

Rudolph, K. D., & Clark, A. G. (2001). Conceptions of relationships in children with depressive and aggressive symptoms: Social-cognitive distortion or reality? *Journal of Abnormal Child Psychology, 29*(1), 41–56.

Schoenwald, S. K., & Hoagwood, K. (2001). Effectiveness, transportability, and dissemination of interventions: What matters when? *Psychiatric Services, 52*, 1190–1197. doi:10.1176/appi.ps.52.9.1190

Seligman, L. D., & Ollendick, T. H. (2011). Cognitive-behavioral therapy for anxiety disorders in youth. *Child and Adolescent Psychiatric Clinics of North America, 20*, 217–238.

Silverman, W. K., Pina, A. A., & Viswesvaran, C. (2008). Evidence-based psychosocial treatments for phobic and anxiety disorders in children and adolescents. *Journal of Clinical Child and Adolescent Psychology, 37*, 105–130.

Smith, M. L., & Glass, G. V. (1977). Meta-analysis of psychotherapy outcome studies. *American Psychologist, 32*, 752–760.

Spence, S. H., Holmes, J., March, S., & Lipp, O. (2006). The BRAVE internet program for children aged 7–12 years from the University of Queensland: The feasibility and outcome of clinic plus internet delivery of cognitive-behavioural therapy for childhood anxiety. *Journal of Consulting and Clinical Psychology, 74*, 614–621.

Stark, K. D., Hargrave, J., Sander, J, Custer, G., Schnnoebelen, S., & Simpson, J. (2012). Treatment of childhood depression: The ACTION treatment program. In P. C. Kendall (Ed.), *Child and adolescent therapy: Cognitive-behavioral procedures* (4th ed.). New York, NY: Guilford Press.

Stark, K. D., Schnoebelen, S., Simpson, J., Hargrave, J., Molnar, J., & Glenn, R. (2005). *Treating depressed children: Therapist manual for ACTION.* Ardmore, PA: Workbook Publishing.

Stark, K. D., Simpson, J., Schnoebelen, S., Glenn, R., Hargrave, J., & Molnar, J. (2005). *ACTION workbook.* Ardmore, PA: Workbook Publishing.

Stark, K. D., Simpson, J., Schnoebelen, S., Hargrave, J., Molnar, J., & Glen, R. (2007). *Treating depressed youth: Therapist manual for 'ACTION.'* Ardmore, PA: Workbook Publishing.

Stark, K. D., Streusand, W., Arora, P., & Patel, P. (2012). Childhood depression: The ACTION treatment program. In P. C. Kendall (Ed). *Child and adolescent therapy: Cognitive-behavioral procedures* (4th ed., pp. 190–233) New York, NY: Guilford Press.

Stark, K. D., Streusand, W., Krumholz, L. S., & Patel, P. (2010). Cognitive-behavioral therapy for depression: The ACTION treatment program for girls. In J. R. Weisz & A. E. Kazdin (Eds.), *Evidence-based psychotherapies for children and adolescents* (pp. 93–109). New York, NY: Guilford Press.

Steiner, H., & Remsing, L. (2007). Practice parameter for the assessment and treatment of children and adolescents with oppositional defiant disorder. *Journal of the American Academy of Child and Adolescent Psychiatry, 46*, 126–141.

Sukhodolsky, D. G., Kassinove, H., & Gorman, B. S. (2004) Cognitive-behavioral therapy for anger in children and adolescents: a meta-analysis. *Aggression and Violent Behaviour, 9*, 247–269.

TADS. (2007). The treatment for adolescents with depression study (TADS): Long-term effectiveness and safety outcomes. *Archives of General Psychiatry, 64*(10), 1132–1144.

Task Force on Promotion and Dissemination of Psychological Procedures. (1995). Training in and dissemination of empirically-validated psychological treatments. *Clinical Psychologist, 48*(1), 3–23.

Treadwell, K. R. H., & Kendall, P. C. (1996). Self-talk in anxiety-disordered youth: States-of- mind, content specificity, and treatment outcome. *Journal of Consulting and Clinical Psychology, 64*, 941–950.

US Public Health Service (2000). *Report on the surgeon general's conference on children's mental health: A national action agenda.* Washington, DC: US Government Printing Office.

van de Wiel, N. M. H., Matthys, W., Cohen-Kettenis, P. T., & van Engeland, H. (2003). Application of the Utrecht Coping Power Program and care as usual to children with disruptive behavior disorders: A comparative study of cost and course of treatment. *Behavior Therapy, 34*, 421–436.

Walkup, J. T., Albano, A. M., Piacentini, J., Birmaher, B., Compton, S. N., Sherrill, J. T., … Kendall, P. C. (2008). Cognitive behavioral therapy, sertraline, or a combination in childhood anxiety. *The New England Journal of Medicine, 359*, 2753–2766. doi:10.1056/NEJMoa0804633

Watson, H. J., & Rees, C. S. (2008). Meta-analysis of randomized, controlled treatment trials for pediatric obsessive-compulsive disorder. *Journal of Child Psychology and Psychiatry, 49*, 489–498.

Weersing, V. R., Gonzalez, A., Campo, J. V., & Lucas, A. N. (2008). Brief behavioral therapy for pediatric anxiety and depression: Piloting an integrated treatment approach. *Cognitive and Behavioral Practice, 15*, 126–139.

Weisz, J. R., Donenberg, G. R., Han, S. S., & Weiss, B. (1995). Bridging the gap between laboratory and clinic in child and adolescent psychotherapy. *Journal of Consulting and Clinical Psychology, 63*, 688–701.

Wood, J. J., Piacentini, J. C., Southam-Gerow, M., Chu, B. C., & Sigman, M. (2006). Family Cognitive Behavioral Therapy for Child Anxiety Disorders. *Journal of the American Academy of Child & Adolescent Psychiatry, 45*, 314–321. doi:10.1097/01.chi.0000196425.88341.b0

Couple Therapy

Kristina Coop Gordon, Katie Wischkaemper, *and* Lee J. Dixon

Abstract

This chapter provides a broad view of the history of cognitive and behavioral couples therapy. First, the authors explore the conceptualization of a healthy relationship and establish a theoretical foundation for cognitive and behavioral couple therapy. Next, the chapter describes the major empirically supported treatments within the cognitive behavioral arena such as traditional behavioral couples therapy, cognitive-behavioral couples therapy, and integrative behavioral couples therapy. Then, the chapter highlights techniques that address a variety of specific issues that couples may face such as intimate partner violence and a host of individual disorders commonly treated within a dyadic framework including depression, chronic illness, and alcohol abuse. Subsequent sections outline the need for replication and cost-effectiveness studies as well as tailoring treatments to meet the specific needs of couples. Finally, the chapter concludes with a discussion about unifying principles common to effective couples treatments demonstrating shared themes across treatment modalities.

Key Words: couple therapy, marital therapy, healthy relationship, cognitive and behavioral couples therapy, empirically supported

One of the leading reasons that people seek any type of professional assistance is because they are experiencing relationship difficulties (i.e., divorce, marital strains, marital separation, and troubles with members of the opposite sex; Swindle, Heller, Pescosolido, & Kikuzawa, 2000). Recent data indicate that in the United States there was exactly half the number of divorces per 1,000 inhabitants as there were marriages, suggesting that roughly half of all marriages will end in divorce (Tejada-Vera & Sutton, 2010). Although this statistic itself may seem daunting, it also might understate the amount of distress that couples experience, as many couples that do not seek divorce also experience distress (Baucom, Epstein, Rankin, & Burnett, 1996). At the same time, research suggests that only 10% of married couples seek professional help for their problems (Johnson et al., 2002). However, for those who do seek help, the outcome of receiving couple therapy is usually positive (Pinsof, Wynne, & Hambright, 1996).

Conceptualization of a Healthy Relationship

The primary goal of couple therapy is almost always to improve the health of an intimate relationship, which is usually defined as romantic in nature and shared between two individuals. Although couple therapy is most often sought out by heterosexual married couples, there are many types of couples for whom therapy can be beneficial (e.g., cohabitating, premarital, gay, lesbian; Martell, Safren, & Prince, 2004; Wetchler, 2011). Just as there are many types of couples that present for therapy, there are also myriad reasons that they decide to seek out professional help. The most common reasons for which couples seek therapy are difficulties with communication and a lack of emotional affection (Doss, Simpson, & Christensen, 2004; Whisman, Dixon, & Johnson, 1997). However, couples also have reported other reasons for seeking therapy, including deciding whether to divorce or separate, sexual/affection difficulties, improving the relationship, and infidelity (Doss et al., 2004). Adding even more complexity to couples' reasons for receiving therapy, Doss and his colleagues found that within couples spouses often give differing reasons for seeking therapy.

Regardless of the couple's reason for seeking help, because the primary goal of couple therapy is the health of the relationship, it is important to understand what differentiates a well-functioning couple from one that is dysfunctional. From a primarily behavioral perspective, a relationship is viewed as rewarding to the partners if it increases their desire to remain with each other in the future. Therefore, for a relationship to remain rewarding, there should be more qualities of the relationship that reinforce the partners to stay together than there are qualities that act as punishers (see Atkins, Dimidjian, & Christensen, 2003). However, it is important to note that inherent in this view is the notion that reinforcers and punishers within a relationship are not necessarily "good" or "bad"; they simply either increase or decrease the chance of a given behavior and can vary both within and between individuals. In order to understand the health of a couple, it is essential for therapists to have a functional understanding of partners' behaviors. This assessment is carried out by completing a functional analysis, which reveals the contingencies of a given behavior and thus guides how the treatment should be targeted. Atkins and colleagues (2003) point out that although the behavioral theory of relationships is quite simple, in practice it is often very difficult to understand these contingencies because the instrumental functions of behavior, as well as the classical conditioning of emotional responses of which partners are consciously aware, can be complex.

With regard to cognitive-behavioral couple therapy (CBCT), traditionally, the cognitive-behavioral conceptualization of a healthy couple is one in which both partners are contributing to form an effective partnership in which (a) decisions are reached and problems are resolved effectively, (b) there is a sense of intimacy and caring, (c) partners communicate constructively, and (d) they participate in activities as a couple that they both find to be mutually rewarding.

Extending beyond this traditional conceptualization, Baucom, Epstein, and LaTaillade (2002) have suggested that in order to best understand couple functioning, the CBCT therapist should not solely focus on the couple as the unit of analysis, but examine the relationship "within the context of the individual partners, the couple, and the couple's environment..." (p. 29). They add that a healthy relationship contributes to the well-being and personal growth of each of the individuals that form the couple and that the relationship should be responsive to each partner's individual needs on both a day-to-day basis and in the long-term (e.g., spending time alone and with friends without one's partner being present). Furthermore, a healthy couple has a symbiotic relationship with their physical and social environment that is beneficial to the couple, each individual, and their community.

A healthy couple also is able to adapt over time to both normative and non-normative circumstances that involve the individual partners, the couple, and the environment in which they live (Baucom, Epstein, LaTaillade, & Kirby, 2008). For example, a healthy couple should adapt to changes that most couples experience, such as the addition of children or career changes, as well as changes that happen less frequently, such as the loss of one's home to a natural disaster. In other words, as the world within and around a couple changes, a healthy relationship is able to meet the challenges inherent in such changes. In contrast, a couple that is less healthy is not as capable of adapting to these types of changes and is more likely to experience both personal and interpersonal distress as a result. Thus, depending upon the health of the relationship, it can both buffer against and exacerbate the difficulties experienced when new stressors present themselves.

As was mentioned earlier, the two primary reasons that many couples seek therapy are communication difficulties and difficulties related to emotional affect (Doss et al., 2004). It is not surprising that difficulties in these areas would act as catalysts for couples to seek therapy given the relational risks that are associated with each of these domains. A review of longitudinal marital research found that both poor communication and the expression of negative affect were primary predictors of poor relationship functioning over time (Karney & Bradbury, 1995). Based on their thorough review of literature regarding communication skills, Baucom and Epstein (1990) suggested that there are three general characteristics of communications skills that repeatedly predict whether a couple is distressed. The first characteristic is the amount that is communicated. Healthy couples tend to simply communicate more information than those who are unhealthy, and are more equipped to clearly communicate emotions, wishes, and needs. The second characteristic is the specificity and clarity of the communication. For example, unhealthy couples tend to communicate how they feel in very general terms, such as, "I was upset," as opposed to, "I feel like you ignored my feelings and it made me feel lonely." The third characteristic is whether a couple's communication decreases or escalates marital conflict and distress. For example, healthy couples tend to speak to each other in ways that do not cause the other partner to become angrier or more defensive. Instead, they communicate information in a manner that is less blaming and more tactful.

Although poor communication can be detrimental to the health of a romantic relationship, it is important to note that simply improving partners' communication skills may not have as beneficial an impact as is desired. Indeed, Baucom and his colleagues (2002) posited that often partners' unmet fundamental needs, such as the needs for intimacy, affiliation, and autonomy, influence the manner in which they communicate with one another, and that the responses that are exhibited are relationally corrosive. The distress that is associated with these unmet needs is termed "primary distress," whereas "secondary distress" occurs as a result of one's reaction to the unmet needs. For example, a wife who desires more emotional intimacy may communicate this need in a way that is perceived as demanding by her husband, who in turn might react with a rejecting or negative response, ultimately undermining the relationship. In this case, it may not be that the wife lacks the necessary skills to communicate her needs effectively, but that the husband's response to the unfulfilled need is problematic. Thus, Baucom et al. (2002) suggest that CBCT therapists attend to both the communication patterns that are exhibited within the relationship and the themes and underlying emotional issues that may be contributing to these negative patterns of communication.

Theoretical Foundation and Basic Treatment Components

Both CBCT and its predecessor, Traditional Behavioral Couples Therapy (TBCT), have their roots in two very influential theories that are both expansions of basic learning theory: social exchange theory and social learning theory. These broad, systemic theories attempt to explain how people interact with each other and are related in a number of ways. Because these theories pay particular attention to understanding and describing dyadic functioning, most TBCT and CBCT treatments draw heavily from a basic notion shared by both theories: the

behaviors exhibited in dyadic romantic relationships are multiply determined and reciprocal.

In concordance with social exchange theory, a CBT or CBCT therapist does not view behavioral interactions between partners as coincidental; instead, they are guided by each partner's best, most cost-effective efforts to resolve presenting problems (Thibaut & Kelley, 1959). It is understood that even when the responses made by members of a dyad appear to be relationally destructive, they are believed by the partner to be the most rewarding, or less punishing, of his or her available response options. According to social exchange theory, whether an outcome of an interpersonal interaction is rewarding is solely based on one's intrapersonal perception of the outcome. Although social learning theory also describes dyadic relationships as being driven by an attempt to increase the rewards and reduce the costs that are associated with the relationship, its approach is more interpersonal (Bradbury & Karney, 2010; Thibaut & Kelley, 1959). In other words, in social exchange theory, the rewards and costs are viewed in terms of individual perspectives, whereas, within social learning theory, the rewards and costs are the actual behaviors that are exhibited in dyadic behavioral exchanges. According to social learning theory, a partner's behaviors in the presence of the other may be viewed as either rewarding or punishing, which will lead to either a rewarding or punishing response, which will then be responded to. The behaviors that are exchanged can be either positive or negative, with the accrual of positive interactions leading to greater relationship satisfaction and the accrual of negative interactions having the opposite effect (e.g., Weiss, Hops, & Patterson, 1973). In turn, greater satisfaction leads to more positive exchanges, and lower satisfaction leads to more negative exchanges, and so on and so forth. In other words, the relationship between these exchanges and relationship partners' relationship satisfaction is cyclical in nature. For example, partner 1 might ignore partner 2's request to take out the garbage. This response could make partner 2 frustrated, which could lead to nagging partner 1 to fulfill the original request. This nagging, in turn, could be interpreted as punishing by partner 1, who might then respond with an angry outburst. Over time, a large number of these kinds of negative interactions can lead to lowered relationship satisfaction, which would most likely result in more negative behaviors. Conversely, responding quickly to the request to take out the trash would most likely be seen as a rewarding behavior, which could prompt the requesting partner to respond with a rewarding behavior such as expressing gratitude. This type of interaction could lead to greater relationship satisfaction in both partners, along with more rewarding behavioral interactions.

Consequently, the goal of changing the response patterns of individuals must include increasing the rewards gained from responding to one's partner in a more constructive manner, reducing the costs associated with this response, and working to alter the contingencies within the dyadic system that elicit a particular response pattern. For example, behavioral couple therapists attempt to alter a couple's unbalanced cost-benefit ratios by using behavior-exchange procedures to increase positive experiences between the partners; an example of this technique would be "caring days" (Stuart, 1980), in which each partner agrees to enact on particular days positive behaviors requested by his or her partner.

Another technique used by traditional behavioral couple therapists to increase positive experiences is to coach couples in creating behavioral contracts, in which each person agrees to behave in specific ways desired by the partner during a specific trial period of time, such as the following week. These contracts can be set up as *quid pro quo* (where the partners' responses are contingent on the other person also following through on his or her side of the agreement) or as "good faith" agreements (in which each person agrees to engage in the positive behaviors desired by the partner, even if the partner does not reciprocate), the latter approach being the preferred one by most TBCT therapists at the present time. Consistent with their behavioral approach, behavior therapists also teach couples specific skills for expressing thoughts and feelings, active empathic listening, and problem-solving. Bolstering problem-solving skills may not seem challenging for couples at first glance, yet an often overlooked obstacle in mastering problem-solving is failure to arrive at a mutual agreement of how the problem is defined. Even after an adequate definition is agreed on, working with both partners can be complicated when the basic skills are translated from safe, "easy" topics, like how the towels are folded, to more emotionally provoking problems, like reinforcing parenting tactics. The classic training manuals by Jacobson and Margolin (1979) and Stuart (1980) provide more complete details on these interventions; however, these models have been largely eclipsed by the newer generations of behavioral couple therapy.

There are many components of CBCT that are similar to TBCT, particularly its use of interventions such as communication skills training for expressing thoughts and feelings, actively listening and responding constructively, problem-solving, and attention to increasing positive couple behaviors to provide more pleasure in the relationship. However, CBCT treatments extend beyond focusing solely on the behaviors that couples exhibit, understanding that once the contingencies of a situation are altered via these new behaviors, significant changes in cognition and affect within the dyadic system are expected to follow, and that these cognitive changes sometimes require additional attention. Thus, although cognitive-behavioral treatments tend to incorporate many behavioral interventions, they also place a greater emphasis on having partners better understand their interactions, in an attempt to more directly intervene in problematic cognitions (e.g., Baucom & Epstein, 1990).

Common techniques to assess partners' cognitions concerning their relationships are self-report questionnaires, interviews, and observation of a couple's behavioral interactions in which the partners spontaneously verbalize their thoughts about each other or exhibit emotional and behavioral reactions to particular types of situations (e.g., becomes angry whenever the partner disagrees with him or her). The therapist then explores how the partners are interpreting their interactions with each other and what meanings they are attaching to behaviors (e.g., "When she interrupts me, it means she doesn't respect me"). During this exploration, the therapist is careful to use nondirective, open-ended questions to reduce the likelihood of shaping the client's reported experience according to the therapist's own beliefs or views of the situation. Once the relevant cognitions have been uncovered, examples of standard cognitive restructuring strategies would be: (a) helping an individual to generate alternative attributions for a partner's negative behavior, (b) asking an individual to conduct daily "experiments" to assess the accuracy of a negative perception concerning his or her partner (e.g., that the partner always disagrees with requests for help), and (c) costs and benefits of expecting one's relationship to live up to an extreme standard.

As the therapist engages in the more "behavioral" communication-skills training, the changes effected as the couples engage in more positive, skillful interactions can alter how the partners perceive each other. For example, if a wife observes her husband struggling to inhibit his tendency to interrupt and communicate more effectively, this observation might challenge her view that he does not care about her or the relationship. Consequently, she may soften toward him and strive to become less attacking in her own communication. The CBCT therapist is alert to these changes and draws couples' attention to them during the session as a means to reinforce these alterations.

Moreover, as mentioned by Gordon, Dixon, Willett, and Hughes (2009), as the field of couple therapy advances, the newer generations of CBCT treatments have expanded to attend to more developmental issues and to more directly elicit and affect emotional experiences. For example, with regard to family of origin issues, schema-focused couple therapy has as a central focus on how ingrained belief systems about self, partner, and relationships in general (a.k.a., schemata) developed over long periods of time and usually within the family of origin which can play a crucial role in understanding couple distress (e.g., Dattilio, 2006; Whisman & Uebelacker, 2007). These therapies believe that exploring individuals' experiences in their family of origin is critical to unlocking couples' current enmeshment in rigid, negative interactions. Consequently, a key intervention in this group of therapies is to conduct a developmental exploration with each partner regarding their earlier relational experiences in their families of origin. These explorations tend to be targeted toward issues that are currently problematic for the couples; for example, if the couple is having difficulties regarding how they express affection for one another, these explorations look carefully at how affection was shown in their families of origin in hopes of uncovering for the partners what beliefs and "rules" they developed about this issue from watching their parents' modeling of this behavior.

With regard to eliciting and affecting emotional experiences, Epstein and Baucom's (2002) enhanced cognitive-behavioral therapy for couples strongly emphasizes the importance of emotion in impacting relationship functioning. This approach recognizes that some partners have difficulties with experiencing and addressing negative and/or positive emotions; thus therapists treating clients from this perspective are likely to provide interventions that are aimed at accessing emotions that are minimized and avoided. For example, with those clients who are avoiding uncomfortable emotions, the therapist would use questions, reflections, and interpretations that would help them express their emotions to their partners. Conversely, cognitive and behavioral techniques would be used to prevent clients from dwelling on negative emotions and assist them in expressing emotions at a level that is more adaptive.

At least four investigations found cognitive restructuring effective in altering dysfunctional cognitions and improving relationship health (Emmelkamp et al., 1988; Epstein, Pretzer, & Fleming, 1982; Huber & Milstein, 1985). The technique of interest in these studies involved the therapist guiding the couple in exploring several cognitive processes, namely the variables of selective attention, causal attributions, expectancies, relationship assumptions, and relationship standards (Baucom, Epstein, Sayers, & Sher, 1989). However, the cognitive restructuring treatments were no more effective than the traditional behavioral and communication-skills training with which they were compared. This finding also held true when Baucom, Sayers, and Sher (1990) supplemented TBCT with both sessions of cognitive restructuring and emotional expressiveness training. In a more recent case study, Dattilio (2005) describes the cognitive restructuring process in depth and suggests that restructuring couples' cognitive schemas is inherent to all therapeutic modalities.

Both TBCT and CBCT share the assumption that the couple therapist's role is part educator and part coach, as he or she interrupts destructive interactions during therapy sessions, educates the couple about the impact of cognitions and behavior on relationship satisfaction, increases the partners' awareness of their own behavioral patterns, and teaches them how to use specific relational skills. Typically, the therapist provides concrete instructions about how to use a skill, models the desired behavior, coaches the partners as they rehearse the skills in the therapy office, provides feedback on communication processes, and helps the couple plan how and when they will apply the skills at home.

In general, behavioral and cognitive-behavioral psychologists tend to approach therapy in a collaborative manner; for example, they arrive at the specific formulations, goals, and procedures of treatment through open discussions with their clients. Clients are usually given homework assignments that are jointly generated out of the work accomplished in their sessions, and the following session usually begins with a review of the homework to see what the couple learned from the experience and to "trouble-shoot" any problems that they had in carrying it out. The emphasis is on teaching couples a number of skills that they can apply on their own. Thus, therapy does not necessarily end when the clients are "problem-free"; rather, the therapy ends when they are judged to have the ability to use their new skills and understandings to arrive at their own solutions to their problems. Consequently the task of the couples therapist is to provide a great deal of modeling and shaping during the early part of treatment, and then remove those supports gradually until the couple can move forward on their own.

However, despite these many fundamental similarities, each behavioral and cognitive-behavioral approach to couple therapy has its own unique perspective on the mechanisms of change in therapy, and, similarly, each has its own unique interventions and contributions to the field. Below, we outline several of the major approaches to TBCT and CBCT treatments and their empirical support.

Overview of Empirically Supported Behavioral and Cognitive-Behavioral Treatments

Traditional Behavioral Couple Therapy

Originally known as Behavioral Marital Therapy (BMT), Traditional Behavioral Couple Therapy (TBCT) is a therapeutic treatment designed for distressed couples. As described earlier, this treatment is grounded in social learning and social exchange theory, combining problem solving and communication skills training with behavioral contracting within a relational context (Baucom, Shoham, Mueser, Daiuto, & Stickle, 1998). This treatment has been rigorously studied and is an established empirically supported treatment (Chambless & Hollon, 1998), as well as a meta-analytically supported treatment (Shadish & Baldwin, 2003), for couple distress. Outcome studies, reviews, and meta-analyses over the last 25 years have found TBCT to be superior to no-treatment groups in improving relationship distress in seriously and chronically distressed couples (Baucom & Lester, 1986; Baucom, et al., 1998; Christensen, Atkins, Baucom, & Yi, 2010; Dunn & Schwebel, 1995; Hahlweg & Markman, 1988; Johnson & Lebow, 2000; Shadish & Baldwin, 2003).

Despite TBCT's historical findings of positive results, a substantial minority of couples showed no improvement in marital satisfaction and almost two-thirds of the couples remained somewhat maritally distressed after receiving TBCT when treatment outcome data were re-analyzed (Jacobson et al., 1984). Also, longer-term follow-ups have demonstrated that the effects of TBCT may not remain as strong several years after treatment (Snyder, Wills, & Grady-Fletcher, 1991). Given the limitations of TBCT, researchers began exploring different

techniques that could enhance the effectiveness of traditional couples therapy. Ideas ranged from integrating theoretically based techniques from cognitive psychology to adding affective change strategies into the primarily behavioral treatment.

Cognitive Behavioral Couple Therapy

Early forms of CBCT, referred to as "enhanced behavioral marital therapy" in the literature, emerged during this refinement process (Baucom & Lester, 1986). The enhancement initially consisted of adding sessions focused on couples' cognitions about the relationship based on the theory used to develop similar techniques within individual therapy. For example, Ellis (1981) proposed three unrealistic beliefs that are characteristic of all intrapersonal and relational dysfunction: (1) all significant others must show love and approval; (2) one must prove competence, adequacy, and achievement; and (3) significant others and life events should always live up to expectations and desires. Upon further examination of intimate relationships, similar extreme and unrealistic beliefs held by partners about their relationship predicted marital discord (Epstein & Eidelson, 1981). These beliefs included: (1) partner conflict indicates a poor relationship; (2) partners should be able to mind read; and (3) positive change within partners and the relationship is impossible. Because identifying and modifying such unrealistic beliefs and cognitive reframing were explored by researchers on an individual basis, these techniques were proposed for application in couple therapy based on correlational findings between marital satisfaction and irrational relationship beliefs (Epstein, 1982; Epstein & Eidelson, 1981). Along these lines, Margolin and Weiss (1978) reported on the relative effectiveness of three common procedures used in marital therapy: behavior modification only, behavior and attitude modification combined, and nonspecific therapeutic tools. Results showed decreases in negative relationship behavior for all three groups, but overall the behavioral-attitudinal group demonstrated greater improvement in marital satisfaction when compared to the other groups. However, since only four sessions were used and the treatment was provided by trained undergraduate students, conclusions from this study were severely limited.

Huber and Milstein (1985) added to the early effort of CBCT efficacy research with a study of 17 couples randomly assigned to one of two groups: cognitive-restructuring treatment or waiting list. They found that couples receiving six sessions of treatment that focused on modifying unrealistic relationship beliefs showed statistically significant improvement in marital satisfaction, beliefs about therapeutic assessment, and desire to improve the relationship from pretreatment to post-treatment measurements compared to a no-treatment group. These results offered support for the effectiveness of cognitive techniques to increase partners' expectations of couple therapy and enhance baseline relationship satisfaction (Huber & Milstein, 1985). The implications of these early studies were critical in introducing the idea that creating a positive collaborative set and combining cognitive tools with behavior change strategies when treating distressed couples could be beneficial.

At this stage in the development of CBCT, many behavioral couple therapists had long recognized the importance of couples' cognitions and emotions in relationship functioning, but their point of entry for intervention remained first and foremost on the couples' behavior. In an effort to improve the delivery of TBCT to distressed couples, Baucom and Lester (1986) were the first to compare the effects of TBCT alone with a cognitive-behavioral version of couple therapy which they called "enhanced behavioral marital therapy" in a controlled outcome study with 24 maritally distressed couples. This study met the need for more rigorous testing of cognitive factors added to behavioral couples therapy. TBCT alone consisted of 12 sessions focused on communication and problem-solving skills training and quid pro quo contracting, whereas enhanced TBCT consisted of six sessions of cognitive restructuring followed by six sessions focused on the behavioral-therapy skills mentioned earlier. Both treatment groups, TBCT alone and enhanced TBCT, showed statistically more improvement in marital adjustment than the waiting-list group, but neither treatment was superior to the other. These findings echo the overriding results across TBCT studies. Although this particular design included limitations such as small sample size, early stage in the development of the content of the cognitive-behavioral sessions, and failure to match couples with treatment components, it constituted an important stepping stone in the empirical testing of cognitive-behavioral treatments with distressed couples.

Emmelkamp and colleagues (1988) evaluated the mediating effects of cognitive processes within CBCT by randomly assigning 32 severely distressed couples to one of two treatment groups: behavioral therapy or cognitive therapy. The behavioral-treatment group focused primarily on communication-skills training as practiced in TBCT, and the cognitive therapy followed a format based on Ellis (1964) and Beck (1980) that focused on training couples to analyze faulty attributions and irrational expectations and replace them with more realistic beliefs. Results indicated that cognitive restructuring was as effective as communication-skills training, but there was little evidence that changes in cognitive processes mediated the effects of cognitive therapy. In fact, this study suggested that changes in irrational relationship beliefs occurred regardless of the treatment received (Emmelkamp, et al., 1988). Although this study lacked the level of attention to research design and methodology provided by Baucom and Lester (1986), it raised more questions about the contribution of cognitive factors to TBCT and motivated additional research in the field.

A few years later, Baucom, Sayers, and Sher (1990) completed one of the most rigorous outcome investigations of CBCT to date. They randomly assigned 60 couples to one of five groups: (1) TBCT alone, (2) cognitive restructuring (CR) combined with TBCT, (3) emotional expressiveness training (EET) combined with TBCT, (4) cognitive restructuring (CR) and emotional expressiveness training (EET) combined with TBCT, and (5) wait-list control. Manuals were developed and used by three master's level therapists to conduct treatment. The treatment groups were formatted in the following manner. The first group received TBCT alone: six weeks of problem-solving and communication-skills training followed by 6 weeks of quid pro quo contracting. The second group received CR + TBCT: six sessions of CR and six sessions devoted to an abbreviated TBCT (session 1–3 focused on attributions; sessions 4–5 focused on relationship standards; session 6 focused on integration of concepts; sessions 7–9 focused on problem-solving and communication-skills training; and sessions 10–12 focused on contracting). The third group received TBCT + EET: six weeks TBCT followed by sessions 7–9 focusing on expressing emotions and responding empathically, session 10 focusing on mode switching and alternating speakers, and sessions 11–12 focused on practicing EET skills. Finally, the fourth group received CR + TBCT + EET: three weeks of CR covering the same issues but having less time for couples to practice, six weeks of TBCT, then three weeks of EET with a discussion of aforementioned skills but with less time for couples to practice.

For both husbands and wives, findings indicated that all active treatment groups showed greater improvement in marital adjustment than the wait-list control group, and adding cognitive and/or affective components to TBCT did not result in more effective treatment outcome than TBCT presented alone (Baucom, Sayers, & Sher, 1990). The authors suggested that future studies include implementing research efforts aimed at integrating cognitive components into existing behavioral frameworks, matching couples to specific interventions rather than random assignment, investigating differences made by various lengths of treatment, and activating treatment paradigms outside of university training clinics and research institutions.

In further pursuit of determining the efficacy of CBCT, Halford, Sanders, and Behrens (1993) compared the effects of a treatment based on Jacobson and Margolin's (1979) description of behavioral marital therapy to a treatment based on adding cognitive restructuring as developed and implemented by Baucom and Lester (1986). They implemented procedures to test the generalization of couple therapy across settings by coding couples' interactions that had been recorded both at the treatment location and in participants' homes. As in previous outcome studies, no evidence was found to support the superiority of an enhanced version of TBCT. Both treatments conducted in this study significantly reduced negative behavior, cognitions, and affect in participating couples. Encouragingly though, both treatment groups resulted in generalization of therapeutic effects in both the treatment and home settings.

The consistent pattern of results across this series of studies indicates that specific interventions may not necessarily produce specific effects as once assumed. In sum, TBCT, a treatment designed to target behavioral modification within a relationship, appears to be related to change in cognition and affect surrounding the relationship despite its distinct focus. Thus, the possibility emerges that couples intervention may be effective on a more systematic level, instigating broader changes within dyads rather than acting on relationship components (such as behaviors or cognitions) in isolation.

Integrative Behavioral Couple Therapy

In response to the limitations of TBCT and CBCT, particularly the disappointing deterioration of long-term treatment gains, Jacobson and Christensen (1996) developed an alternative treatment, namely, integrative behavioral couple therapy (IBCT). Integrative behavioral couple therapy builds on the theories behind TBCT and CBCT and attempts to improve the long-term sustainability of couple therapy. A unique characteristic of IBCT is its strong emphasis on the emotional context between partners and promoting change through natural contingencies. Integrative behavioral couple therapy strives to assist couples in achieving greater acceptance for situations in which behavior change is not possible while increasing intimacy during such interactions. This therapy assumes that all couples face genuine incompatibilities that are unlikely to change (e.g., personality traits, differing worldviews, or desires to have children). Thus, the emotional responses to such irreconcilable differences are as important as the behavioral exchanges between the partners.

In practice, IBCT balances behavior exchange procedures such as problem-solving and communication skills with a desire to stimulate emotional acceptance. For example, instead of teaching communication skills as the one and only way to communicate, IBCT therapists help partners process natural reactions to each other's comments, thereby allowing personal responses, or natural contingencies, to impact and shape each other's behavior. Therefore, the therapeutic focus in this treatment rests more heavily on fostering an environment that allows for emotional acceptance of the differences within the couple and less so on identifying and monitoring specific behavior change. Developers of this model hypothesized IBCT would bring about more durable change for severely distressed couples (Christensen et al., 2004).

As a brief example of the differences between IBCT and the previously explored methods of therapy, imagine the use of the word *never* during an interchange between partners. Within the TBCT framework, a partner stating "*you never* take out the trash" would be treated as a communication error, something that the partner should not do. Thus, the couple might be instructed by the therapist to practice a more correct way to communicate their message without using extremes like "always" and "never." According to the conceptualization of CBCT, the use of such words indicates the occurrence of a cognitive distortion known as black and white thinking. The therapist may guide a partner through finding exceptions in the other partner's behavior, thus increasing tolerance for accepting the grayer areas of reality. For instance, the therapist could ask the speaking partner to remember the last time they saw their partner taking out the trash, and in the future, compliment their partner when the trash is taken out.

Alternatively, the IBCT approach to this scenario is to catch an occurrence in vivo or discuss a recent incident. The therapist might pay special attention to ask about what is going on internally for both partners as they discuss the problem. For example, the therapist might ask "What is going on for you right now as you make this statement toward your partner?" This question is asked to uncover understandable reasons for each partner's reactions during the conflict. For example, the first partner might discuss how having to make the request multiple times makes her feel disrespected and unimportant to her partner, which leads her to express her request with an angry tone. In turn, the other partner might experience the initial request as demanding and insensitive to the other tasks in which that partner is currently engaging, but because she doesn't believe her partner will listen to her request to do it later, she chooses to ignore the request to avoid conflict, which in turn creates more frustration and conflict. The therapist also helps the couple to identify how these interactions reflect recurring patterns in their relationship and by naming the patterns they are able to externalize the problem and join together around it by understanding and often empathizing with each other's responses. In noticing the pattern and then helping them to choose different responses, the couple has the opportunity to change their experiences of each other. These new experiences create a more lasting shift in the couple's communication patterns over time as a result of new contingency-shaped behavior rather than rule-governed behavior (Christensen, 2011).

In the largest clinical trial of couple therapy to date with one of the most distressed and also diverse samples of couples, Christensen and colleagues (2004) began to follow 134 moderately to severely distressed couples and collected outcome data for 5 years after treatment completion (Christensen et al., 2010). The couples were randomly assigned to either TBCT or IBCT and experienced up to 26 sessions of couple therapy. Upon treatment completion, results revealed significant pre- to post-treatment effect sizes on marital satisfaction. At the 2-year follow-up, IBCT demonstrated statistically significant superiority over TBCT (Christensen, Atkins, Yi, Baucom, & George, 2006). After the 5-year follow-up, TBCT and IBCT with a highly distressed sample both demonstrated substantial effect sizes in marital satisfaction, as compared to before treatment. Since the post-treatment and

long-term outcomes of this study were equal to or superior to most other random clinical trials of couple therapy, these findings provide encouragement to couple researchers and practitioners alike regarding the efficacy of this new approach to treatment.

Techniques for Intimate Partner Aggression or Violence

Another branch of the literature discusses CBCT techniques as applied to couples experiencing psychological or physical aggression and intimate partner violence. O'Leary, Heyman, and Neidig (1999) examined the effects of Physical Aggression Couples Treatment (PACT), which integrates CBCT-based techniques and is delivered to groups of couples experiencing psychological and physical aggression, but not severe violence, from wife abuse in a longitudinal study. Results of this study showed that separating men and women into different treatment groups versus couple-based treatment was equally effective in reducing violence, increasing husbands' taking responsibility for aggression, and improving wives' depression levels. However, husbands who received aggression-specific couple therapy improved more on marital adjustment levels than husbands who were treated separately from wives.

A more recent study questions the appropriateness and effectiveness of conjoint approaches in treating intimate partner violence (LaTaillade, Epstein, & Werlinich, 2006). The authors argue that conjoint approaches in the treatment of intimate partner violence are appropriate as long as couples have not experienced battering of severe violence and have a desire to remain in and work on their relationship during treatment. A pilot study with couples considered appropriate for conjoint treatment compared a CBCT treatment to treatment as usual, and no differences were found in posttreatment levels of all forms of psychological aggression between the two treatment modalities (Epstein et al., 2005). The pilot study also found that the CBCT treatment produced a significant increase in relationship satisfaction for husbands but only a trending increase for wives on self-report measures. Observational data of the participating couples indicated a significant decrease in negative communication in both males and females in the CBCT group compared to no change in treatment as usual couples. Although this treatment has not been subjected to further empirical study, these early findings suggest that cognitive-behavioral interventions when applied in a couples context can be instrumental in decreasing negative communication linked to intimate partner violence, decreasing psychological and physical aggression, and improving relationship satisfaction.

Couple Techniques for Individual Disorders

Although targeted to assist distressed couples, recent research efforts on CBCT have shifted their focus in recent years in response to the availability of research funding. Federal government funding policies in the United States have encouraged a movement toward research focused on individual psychological disorders as described in the Diagnostic and Statistical Manual of the American Psychiatric Association by limiting funding for clinical trials comparing different types of more generalized couple therapy (Lebow, Chambers, Christensen, & Johnson, 2012). Unfortunately, the *DSM* does not recognize couple distress as a disorder, and reallocation of research funding has made large-scale empirical examination of CBCT and other couple treatments extremely difficult to pursue over the last decade. However, this newly directed focus has instigated promising findings for the effectiveness of couple treatments in situations in which one partner has been diagnosed with specific Axis I disorders. Techniques from couple and family therapy have been implemented to study the treatment of schizophrenia, bipolar disorder, alcohol abuse, mood disorders, anxiety disorders, chronic illness, and anorexia in one partner.

Schizophrenia and Bipolar Disorder

Behavioral family therapy (BFT) promotes efficient family functioning and upholds the principle that significant change for an individual with a psychological disorder is only possible when the immediate social system is able to make changes in their behavioral patterns (Falloon, 2003). Behavioral family therapy works to apply theoretical concepts such as social-learning theory in families by using techniques similar to those found in TBCT, such as building more effective communication patterns and addressing problem solving. Behavioral family therapy is the most researched treatment intervention for schizophrenia and bipolar disorder since symptoms of each disorder place tremendous strain on family members and partners. Falloon, Boyd, & McGill (1984) produced one of the first detailed manuals for conducting BFT with families impacted by schizophrenia, and building on this progress, another group published a manual describing applying BFT to other severe mental illnesses like bipolar disorder (Mueser & Glynn, 1999). A later review of 14 randomized controlled trials found statistically significant support for the effectiveness of family interventions versus medication and case management alone using outcome variables of psychotic episodes, deaths, hospital admissions, and serious noncompliance or withdrawal from interventions (Falloon, Held, Coverdale, Roncone, & Laidlaw, 1999).

Alcohol Abuse

TBCT also has been shown to be efficacious when treating individuals with alcohol abuse problems. Generally, TBCT for alcohol abuse consists of 15–20 outpatient sessions with both partners over a period of five to six months. O'Farrell and colleagues (1993) found that participants receiving TBCT and relapse prevention (n= 30) had a statistically significantly higher percent of abstinent days than participants in an attention-placebo group (n= 29). Another meta-analysis concluded that TBCT results in better outcomes than more traditional individual-based treatments for married or cohabitating individuals seeking treatment for alcohol or drug dependence (Powers, Vedel, & Emmelkamp, 2008). A more recent study comparing alcohol behavioral couple therapy and alcohol behavioral individual therapy for women with alcohol use disorders reveals that women in the behavioral couples treatment group had more abstinent days and less days of heavy drinking than women in the individual therapy (McCrady, Epstein, Cook, Jensen, & Hildebrandt, 2009). Overall, TBCT demonstrates promising results when working with couples impacted by alcohol abuse.

Depression

Regarding the treatment of an individual with clinical depression via couple therapy, Barbato and D'Avanzo (2008) conducted a meta-analysis of 8 controlled trials. The literature suggests that there is no difference in depressive symptomatology between those treated with couple therapy and individual psychotherapy; however, relationship distress significantly decreased in those who received couple therapy. The authors suggest that improving the quality of relationship for depressed individuals may play a mediating role in ameliorating their depressive symptoms, but also state that this hypothesis has not been adequately tested. With cognitive and behavioral couple therapy specifically, two studies have found that TBCT is as effective as individual cognitive therapy when treating a depressed partner (Jacobson, Dobson, Fruzzetti, Schmaling, &

Salusky, 1991; O'Leary & Beach, 1990). A more recent clinical trial demonstrates TBCT interventions for a depressed partner are effective for relationally distressed couples (Gupta, Coyne, & Beach, 2003). Specific interventions emphasize behavior exchange, training in communication and problem-solving skills, and cognitive techniques such as cognitive reframing and directing attention to positive change. Beach & Gupta (2003) outline specific clinical guidelines for working with a depressed partner in a couple-therapy context.

Anxiety Disorders

Anxiety disorders can disrupt patterns of relationship interaction, increase number of arguments, restrict pleasant activities, and limit the acknowledgment of the needs of the partner who is not anxious (Baucom, Stanton, & Epstein, 2003). Cognitive and behavioral techniques to treat anxiety disorders in a couple-therapy setting include exposure and response prevention, cognitive restructuring, and relaxation training. Empirical studies have shown that partner-assisted exposure treatment for obsessive-compulsive disorder is at least as effective as individual treatment and an alternative for individuals with this disorder who desire treatment (Emmelkamp, de Hann, & Hoodguim, 1990; Emmelkamp & de Lange, 1983).

Agoraphobia is another anxiety-related disorder that has received attention from couple-therapy researchers. After nearly 50 years of debating whether to include partners in the treatment of agoraphobia and, more recently, how to utilize partners in the treatment process, the empirical findings are limited. However, a review by Daiuto, Baucom, Epstein, and Dutton (1998) provides recommendations on assessing relationship quality in these couples and treating the marital relationship based on extant literature. The authors report that the findings suggest more effective partner involvement occurs during interventions focused on changing the couples' interaction patterns:

> Whereas exposure therapy is likely the active therapeutic ingredient in terms of producing an immediate decrease in phobic symptoms, additional interventions aimed at fostering positive, direct, and constructive dialogues between the partners may serve to enhance the effectiveness of exposure by promoting the maintenance of treatment gains at follow-up.... (Daiuto, Baucom, Epstein, & Dutton, 1998, p. 17)

Eating Disorders

Eating disorders pose unique challenges for couples. Therefore, based on the efficacy of CBCT and the importance of relationships in anorexia nervosa, a couple-based cognitive-behavioral intervention for adult anorexia nervosa was developed by Bulik, Baucom, Kirby, and Pisetsky (2011). Uniting Couples in the treatment of Anorexia Nervosa (UCAN) posits that the disorder occurs in an interpersonal context and helps partners approach the disorder as a team. Currently, UCAN is undergoing empirical evaluation in a clinical trial, and an endeavor to modify the treatment specifically for Latino populations is underway.

Chronic Illness

Chronic illnesses confront couples with a variety of obstacles including new information to fit into existing cognitive structures and often vast changes to current patterns of behavior. As Berg & Upchurch (2007) describe in their developmental-contextual model of couples coping with chronic illness, dyadic coping may be different depending on the stage of life in which a diagnosis is received. These authors also highlight the range of issues that affect couples engaged in this coping process including both broad sociocultural factors (e.g., gender and culture) and more narrow proximal factors (e.g., relationship quality and demands of the specific chronic illness).

Whereas the difficulties imposed by chronic illness vary, research findings demonstrate that the quality of marital relationships can affect feelings, thoughts, self-care behavior, and ways of coping with illness and physiological changes (Kiecolt-Glaser & Newton, 2001). In addition, research has shown that modifying health behavior is more effective when a partner jointly participates in the lifestyle changes (Tucker & Mueller, 2000). Specifically, including spouses in medically necessary behavioral changes brings more opportunity for maintaining meaningful behavior change in the targeted patients for patients attempting to reduce their risk for heart problems (Sher & Baucom, 2001). Along these lines, numerous studies have shown that persons whose partners supported their efforts to quit smoking were more likely to quit and maintain abstinence (e.g., Cohen & Lichtenstein, 1990). Furthermore, results from a recent pilot study comparing cognitive-behavioral couples-based relationship enhancement to treatment-as-usual for women with breast cancer suggest that both men and women improve on individual measures and relationship functioning when they receive relationship enhancement as an adjunct to medical treatment (Baucom et al. 2009).

In a randomly assigned trial of partner-assisted coping with chronic, osteoarthritic knee pain, Keefe, Caldwell, Baucom, & Salley (1996) implemented cognitive and behavioral pain-coping skills (e.g. relaxation, imagery, distraction techniques, activity pacing, goal setting, and cognitive restructuring) with the partner-assisted condition. Patients and partners received training in communication skills, behavioral rehearsal, problem solving, joint practice, and maintenance training. Results indicated that the partner-assisted condition had the best outcomes, and that the couples who demonstrated increased marital adjustment also had lower levels of physical and psychological disability and pain behavior at the one-year follow-up.

Future Directions

Empirical findings in the cognitive and behavioral therapy literature consistently demonstrate that TBCT is an effective treatment for relationship distress and a variety of other individual disorders. Research on IBCT has shown encouraging findings using this type of treatment with couples, especially severely and chronically distressed couples. CBCT is another effective treatment in changing cognitions about relationships and behaviors within a couple and treating individual psychopathology within a couples context; however, findings also consistently show that CBCT is not significantly more effective than TBCT. Since Jacobson, et al. (1984) demonstrated that 35–40% of couples changed from the distressed to nondistressed range of marital adjustment after receiving TBCT, further research on these specific types of cognitive and behavioral couples therapies is warranted to improve the outcomes for couples seeking therapy. Although a significant amount of work already has been conducted on behavioral and cognitive couple therapy, the field still could be considered as in its early stages. The gaps in the literature give new researchers in this area of study plenty of room to expand on existing work by addressing topics likely to be of great utility to clinicians. Below, we describe a few of the potential directions for further research and exploration.

Replication and Cost-effectiveness Studies

One of the most obvious future directions is the need for replication and further validation for existing cognitive and behavior couple therapies. As of the last formal review by the APA Task Force on Empirically Supported Treatments (Baucom et al., 1998), only one treatment, TBCT, had met the necessary requirement of validation in two separate laboratories. Since that time, little has changed (Lebow et al., in press; Snyder, Castellani, & Whisman, 2006) and few additional randomized controlled trials for couple distress have been conducted; the few studies that have occurred primarily focus on targeting individual disorders within a conjoint format. As suggested earlier, the NIH is currently less open to funding studies that are not directly connected to *DSM* diagnoses (Lebow, et al., 2012). Consequently, the field sorely lacks replication studies, and this creates a large gap in the overall body of literature on couple treatments.

In addition to applying couple therapy to more fundable individual disorders, another mechanism to reduce this gap might be for couple researchers and therapists to make a better case to policy makers and granting agencies for the cost-effectiveness of couple treatments in order to increase their motivation to fund this area of research. Some evidence indicates that couple-based treatments result in significant savings over time; for example, individuals receiving services from a health-maintenance organization who also engaged in marital and family therapy reduced their use of health care services by 21.5% (Law & Crane, 2000). Cordova and colleagues report similar findings (Cordova et al., 2005). Along these lines, O'Farrell and colleagues (1995) demonstrated that adding a BMT module as an adjunctive treatment for substance abuse yielded decreases in both health care and legal costs following treatment, and that the cost savings resulting from these decreases were significantly greater than the costs of providing adjunctive marital treatment.

Estimates of the cost of systematically assessing for couple distress and providing empirically supported treatments as part of a government or health-insurer process indicate that the costs of screening and providing treatment would far offset the costs of divorce or the increased health-care expenses associated with divorce (Caldwell, Wooley, & Caldwell, 2007); further, Bray and Jouriles (1995) suggest that, given that the average length of couple therapy is 10 sessions, and the average cost is $60–$100, the average costs of $600–$1,000 for couple therapy is still far below the long-term costs of divorce and continuing couple distress. Still more research is needed to determine the actual cost-effectiveness to both couples and to government and civic organizations of providing couple therapy services; for those researchers who are seeking to answer this call, Mackinnon (2005) provides an excellent road map for conducting this type of research.

Tailoring Treatments to Couples' Developmental Stages and Individual Differences

The concept of matching individuals to types of treatment has a complicated history in the treatment of individual disorders and rarely has this effort yielded clear guidelines as to which treatments are better for which individual characteristics. However, another form of matching might be more applicable to couple therapy per se. There are identifiable developmental stages across the life of the relationship (e.g., Carstensen, Graff, Levenson, & Gottman,, 1996; Lawrence, Eldridge, & Christensen, 1998), and each of these stages present specific challenges for couple functioning. For example, the transition to parenthood requires different adjustments within the couple compared to the aging process, which often brings with it greater physical challenges and changing relational roles. Consequently, researchers and therapists might benefit by developing treatments that are tailored to these specific challenges to aid couples in negotiating these difficult transitions; unfortunately, very few of these types of treatment exist. Of the ones that do exist, more interventions are targeted toward earlier stages in a relationship, such as premarital interventions (e.g., Stanley, Blumberg, & Markman, 1999) or the transition to parenthood (e.g., Schulz, Cowan, & Cowan, 2006). Currently, we are aware of no empirical research conducted on behavioral or cognitive couple therapies targeted toward older adults dealing with transitions into retirement or physical declines.

Furthermore, as with much of the psychotherapy literature, couple therapy is lacking in validation with diverse samples. Kelly (2005) provided an overview of how empirically validated couple therapies, including TBCT, CBCT, and IBCT, might accommodate diversity issues; however, in general, these approaches have not been specifically empirically validated with differing ethnic and cultural populations, as well as sexual orientations, and diversity within the initial validation studies for these treatments has been limited. Strikingly, one study that examined ethnicity as a moderator of treatment efficacy for a stand-alone TBCT treatment for drug use found that this treatment was less effective for Black couples than for White or Latino couples (Epstein et al., 2007), underlining the great need to examine these treatments in diverse populations rather than applying them without consideration for variations within cultures. Furthermore, the field could benefit from studying other individual differences that might impact response to treatment such as personality characteristics, family of origin histories, and blended families.

Process and Mechanism of Change Studies

Another gap in the research on behavioral and cognitive couple therapies is in the area of process research and identification of mechanisms of change. Although both cognitions and affect appear to change over the course of behavioral and cognitive couple therapy, these changes do not consistently mediate therapeutic improvements, nor do they appear to be specific to types of therapy; couples demonstrated changes in cognition and behavior regardless of whether they received traditional behavioral therapy or cognitive-behavioral couple therapy (e.g., Snyder et al., 2006). Whereas it is apparent that both TBCT and CBCT are effective at reducing couple distress, the primary mechanisms underlying this change are still not known. Furthermore, findings seem to suggest that they are equally effective in producing change, but it is unclear whether the important change processes might be due to broader systemic changes rather than changes that are particular to each treatment, or whether each treatment effects a mechanistic change that is particular to that approach and yet are equally effective at reducing marital distress.

Two notable exceptions are studies conducted on IBCT. Potential change mechanisms have been examined comparing IBCT and TBCT using hierarchical linear modeling and task analysis, and these approaches seem to yield more promising findings regarding change mechanisms (Doss, Thum, Sevier, Atkins, & Christensen, 2005). Specifically, both approaches increase emotional acceptance and also communication from pretreatment to post-treatment; however, gains were larger in acceptance for IBCT and larger for positive communication for TBCT, suggesting that these treatments might target certain change mechanisms differentially. Furthermore, task analysis suggests that couples in IBCT become more detached and emotionally vulnerable when discussing problems over the course of treatment, and that these changes predict changes in relationship satisfaction (Cordova, Jacobson, & Christensen, 1998). More research along these lines is needed, and Heatherington and colleagues (Heatherington, Friedlander, & Greenberg, 2005) provide an excellent review on conducting this type of research for those who wish to address this problem.

The Ivory Tower and Beyond

Finally, Bray and Jouriles noted in their 1995 review of marital therapy that a major shortcoming of the literature was the failure to demonstrate how well these empirically supported therapies fared outside university settings; furthermore, in their meta-analysis of couple therapies, Shadish and Baldwin (2003) found that couple-therapy-outcome research tended to occur in conditions that were less generalizable than treatment-outcome research for other problems. Sadly, more than a decade and a half after Bray and Jouriles' review, the same state of affairs exists. There is very little true effectiveness research conducted on couple therapy; it is still unclear how well these treatments generalize to the average couple who enters into treatment, particularly in community mental health settings. However, the little existing research on behavioral and cognitive couple therapies is somewhat encouraging; for example, a recent study examining the effectiveness of couple therapy in a community setting in Germany indicated that these treatments can be successfully transported and alleviate both couple distress and individual depression (Klann, Hahlweg, Baucom, & Kroger, 2011).

Not only has the field, in general, failed to move its findings out of the ivory tower to demonstrate their effectiveness, it also appears that practitioners in general have little interest in seeking out these treatments and practicing from an empirically manualized format. Marriage and family therapy researchers note that the practice-research gap appears to be widening and, as outcome studies become more specified and controlled, clinicians are becoming simultaneously more eclectic and integrative rather than specified (Norcross, Karpiak, & Santoro, 2005; Pinsof & Wynne, 2000). Accordingly, more recent treatment models for couple therapy are emerging that parallel this integrative movement. IBCT can be considered an example of this change; similarly, Snyder has integrated cognitive and behavioral strategies with his more psychodynamic Insight-Oriented Marital Therapy (Snyder et al., 1991) to create a more integrative, yet structured model of treatment called Affective Reconstructive Marital Therapy (Snyder & Mitchell, 2008). Similarly, Whisman and Uebelacker (2007) and Dattilio (2006) also proposed a model of couple

therapy based on Young's Schema Therapy, which is integrative in its approach. Unfortunately, none of these new approaches have empirical support other than the support for the treatments on which these new combinations are based.

An additional approach to narrowing the practice-research gap that is receiving greater support in both the general psychotherapy literature and, more recently, in the couple therapy literature is the concept of overarching principles across treatments (Sexton et al., 2011). Several models of unifying protocols exist in the treatments for mood disorders (e.g., Beutler, 2003; Ellard, Fairholme, Boisseau, Farchione, & Barlow, 2010), and these models are currently being applied to existing couple therapies. There are two versions of this approach, the first of which is the more prevalent idea regarding "common factors" in treatment. The common-factors perspective stems from the oft-cited findings that few empirically supported treatments can be consistently demonstrated as superior to other empirically supported treatments. Consequently, proponents of the common factors model suggest that these therapies' efficacy rests more in the elements they share in common rather than in the specific models themselves (e.g., Sprenkle & Blow, 2004). These shared or common factors include the therapeutic alliance, client factors, therapist factors, and the instillation of "hope" (Blow & Sprenkle, 2001). The extreme version of the common-factors approach suggests that treatments have their effects solely through these elements and that the models themselves mean little (e.g., Wampold, 2001). On the other hand, more moderate approaches hold that specific-treatment models might offer additional benefits beyond their common factors and that some treatments might eventually be proven to be more effective for certain problems or types of couples than others (Sprenkle & Blow, 2004).

Unifying principle theories also examine empirically supported treatment models for similarities across treatments; however, they are looking for specific factors in the treatments that might be considered part of the same class of interventions. Similar to models proposed for mood-disorder treatment (Beutler, 2003; Ellard et al., 2010), the major couple therapies can be viewed as all tapping into identifiable and similar principles of change. Five unifying principles of change in couple therapy have been suggested: (1) altering views of the relationship, (2) modifying dysfunctional interactional behavior, (3) eliciting avoided private behavior, (4) improving communication, and (5) promoting strengths (Benson, McGinn, & Christensen, 2012). It is hypothesized that all successful couple-therapy models tap into these unifying principles.

The APA Division 43 Task Force on Empirically Supported Couple and Family Therapies (Sexton et al., 2011) suggests that identifying such unifying principles might allow treatment-outcome researchers to develop more treatments built around these identified common principles, which, in turn, might make it easier for the field to coalesce around these treatments and simpler for clinicians to learn new treatment models. The task force also suggested that in identifying these common principles, the baby should not be thrown out with the bathwater. It is likely that treatment models provide structure for where, when, and how these overarching principles should be accessed and utilized. Consequently, it is possible that the future of our field lies in identifying common treatment factors, common treatment principles, and specific treatment models that can organize and direct therapists in their use of these common factors and approaches.

References

Atkins, D. C., Dimidjian, S., & Christensen, A. (2003). Behavioral couple therapy: Past, present, and future. In T. L. Sexton, G. Weeks, & M. Robbins (Eds.), *Handbook of family therapy: Theory, research, and practice* (pp. 281–302). New York: Brunner-Routledge.

Barbato, A., & D'Avanzo, B. (2008). Efficacy of couple therapy as a treatment for depression: A meta-analysis. *Psychiatric Quarterly, 79*(2), 121–132.

Baucom, D. H., & Epstein, N. (1990). *Cognitive-behavioral marital therapy* (p. 482). Philadelphia, PA, US: Brunner/Mazel.

Baucom, D. H., Epstein, N., & LaTaillade, J. J. (2002). Cognitive-behavioral couple therapy. In A. S. Gurman & N. S. Jacobson (Eds.), *Clinical handbook of couple therapy* (3rd ed., pp. 26–58). New York: Guilford.

Baucom, D. H., Epstein, N. B., LaTaillade, J. J., & Kirby, J. S. (2008). Cognitive behavioral couple therapy. In A. S. Gurman (Ed.), *Clinical handbook of couple therapy* (3rd ed., pp. 31–72). New York: Guilford Press.

Baucom, D. H., Epstein, N., Rankin, L. A., & Burnett, C. K. (1996). Assessing relationship standards: The inventory of specific relationship standards. *Journal of Family Psychology, 10*, 72–88.

Baucom, D. H., Epstein, N., Sayers, S., & Sher, T. G. (1989). The role of cognitions in marital relationships: Definitional, methodological, and conceptual issues. *Journal of Consulting and Clinical Psychology, 57*, 31-38.

Baucom, D. H., & Lester, G. W. (1986). The usefulness of cognitive restructuring as an adjunct to behavioral marital therapy. *Behavior Therapy, 17*(4), 385–403. doi: 10.1016/s0005-7894(86)80070-3

Baucom, D. H., Porter, L. S., Kirby, J. S., Gremore, T. M., Wiesenthal, N., Aldridge, W.,...Keefe, F. J. (2009). A couple-based intervention for female breast cancer. *Psycho Oncology, 18*(3), 276–283. doi: 10.1002/pon.1395

Baucom, D. H., Sayers, S. L., & Sher, T. G. (1990). Supplementing behavioral marital therapy with cognitive restructuring and emotional expressiveness training: An outcome investigation. *Journal of Consulting and Clinical Psychology, 58*(5), 636–645. doi: 10.1037/0022-006x.58.5.636

Baucom, D. H., Shoham, V., Mueser, K. T., Daiuto, A. D., & Stickle, T. R. (1998). Empirically supported couple and family interventions for marital distress and adult mental health problems. *Journal of Consulting and Clinical Psychology, 66*(1), 53–88. doi: 10.1037/0022-006x.66.1.53

Baucom, D. H., Stanton, S., & Epstein, N. B. (2003). Anxiety disorders. In D. Snyder & M. Whisman (Eds.), *Treating difficult couples: Helping clients with coexisting mental and relationship disorders.* (pp. 57–87). New York: Guilford Press.

Beach, S. R. H., & Gupta, M. (2003). Depression. (pp. 88–113) Guilford Press, New York, NY. Retrieved from http://search.proquest.com/docview/620274392?accountid=14766

Beck, A. T. (1980). *Cognitive aspects of marital interactions.* Paper presented at the 14th AABT Conference, New York.

Benson, L., McGinn, M., & Christensen, A. (2012). Common principles of couple therapy. *Behavior Therapy.*

Berg, C. A., & Upchurch, R. (2007). A developmental-contextual model of couples coping with chronic illness across the adult life span. *Psychological Bulletin, 133*(6), 920–954. doi: 10.1037/0033-2909.133.6.920

Beutler, L. E. (2003). David and Goliath: When empirical and clinical standards of practice meet. *American Psychologist, 55*, 997–1007.

Blow, A. J., & Sprenkle, D. H. (2001). Common factors across theories of marriage and family therapy: A modified delphi study. *Journal of Marital and Family Therapy, 27*(3), 385–401. doi:http://dx.doi.org/10.1111/j.1752-0606.2001.tb00333.x

Bradbury, T. N., & Karney, B. R. (2010). *Intimate relationships.* New York: Norton.

Bray, J. H., & Jouriles, E. N. (1995). Treatment of marital conflict and prevention of divorce. *Journal of Marital and Family Therapy, 21*, 461–473.

Bulik, C. M., Baucom, D. H., Kirby, J. S., & Pisetsky, E. (2011). Uniting Couples (in the treatment of) Anorexia Nervosa (UCAN). *International Journal of Eating Disorders, 44*(1), 19–28. doi: 10.1002/eat.20790

Caldwell, B. E., Woolley, S. R., & Caldwell, S. J. (2007). Preliminary estimates of cost-effectiveness for marital therapy. *Journal of Marital and Family Therapy, 33*, 392–405.

Carstensen L. L, Graff, J., Levenson, R. W., & Gottman, J. M. (1996). Affect in intimate relationships: The developmental course of marriage. In Magai, C., & McFadden, S. H. (Eds.), *Handbook of emotion, adult development, and aging* (pp. 227–247). San Diego: Academic Press.

Chambless, D. L., & Hollon, S. D. (1998). Defining empirically supported therapies. *Journal of Consulting and Clinical Psychology, 66*(1), 7–18. doi: 10.1037/0022-006x.66.1.7

Christensen, A. (2011). Acceptance and change in couple therapy: Integrative behavioral couple therapy. [PowerPoint slides]. Retrieved from Association for Behavioral and Cognitive Therapies Workshop, Toronto, Canada.

Christensen, A., Atkins, D. C., Berns, S., Wheeler, J., Baucom, D. H. & Simpson, L. E. (2004). Traditional versus integrative behavioral couple therapy for significantly and chronically distressed married couples. *Journal of Consulting and Clinical Psychology, 72*(2), 176–191.

Christensen, A., Atkins, D. C., Yi, J., Baucom, D. H., & George, W. H. (2006). Couple and individual adjustment for 2 years following a randomized clinical trial comparing traditional versus integrative behavioral couple therapy. *Journal of Consulting and Clinical Psychology, 74*(6), 1180–1191.

Christensen, A., Atkins, D. C., Baucom, B., & Yi, J. (2010). Marital status and satisfaction five years following a randomized clinical trial comparing traditional versus integrative behavioral couple therapy. *Journal of Consulting and Clinical Psychology, 78*(2), 225–235. doi: 10.1037/a0018132

Cohen, S., & Lichtenstein, E. (1990). Partner behaviors that support quitting smoking. *Journal of Consulting and Clinical Psychology, 58*(3), 304–309.

Cordova, J. V., Jacobson, N. S., & Christensen, A. (1998). Acceptance versus change interventions in behavior therapy: impact on couples' in-session communication. *Journal of Marital and Family Therapy, 24*, 437–455.

Cordova, J. V., Scott, R. L., Dorian, M., Mirgain, S., Yaeger, D., & Groot, A. (2005). The marriage checkup: A motivational interviewing approach to the promotion of marital health with couples at-risk for relationship deterioration. *Behavior Therapy, 36*, 301–310.

Daiuto, A. D., Baucom, D. H., Epstein, N., & Dutton, S. S. (1998). The application of behavioral couples therapy to the assessment and treatment of agoraphobia: Implications of empirical research. *Clinical Psychology Review, 18*(6), 663–687.

Dattilio, F. M. (2005). The critical component of cognitive restructuring in couples therapy: A case study. *ANZJFT Australian and New Zealand Journal of Family Therapy, 26*(2), 73–78.

Dattilio, F. M. (2006). Restructuring schemata from family of origin in couple therapy. *Journal of Cognitive Psychotherapy. Special Issue: Cognitive-Behavioral Assessment and Treatment of Couples, 20*, 359–373.

Doss, B. D., Simpson, L. E., & Christensen, A. (2004). Why do couples seek marital therapy? *Professional Psychology: Research and Practice, 35*, 608–614.

Doss, B. D., Thum, Y. M., Sevier, M, Atkins, D. C., & Christensen, A. (2005). Improving relationships: mechanisms of change in couple therapy. *Journal of Consulting and Clinical Psychology, 73*, 624–633.

Dunn, R. L., & Schwebel, A. I. (1995). Meta-analytic review of marital therapy outcome research. *Journal of Family Psychology, 9*(1), 58–68. doi: 10.1037/0893-3200.9.1.58

Ellard, K. K., Fairholme, C. P., Boisseau, C. L., Farchione, T. J., & Barlow, D. H. (2010). Unified protocol for the transdiagnostic treatment of emotional disorders: Protocol development and initial outcome data, *Cognitive and Behavioral Practice, 17*, 88–101.

Ellis, A. (1964). *The nature of disturbed marital interactions.* Paper presented at the American Psychological Association Convention, Los Angeles.

Ellis, A. (1981). *Ideas to make you disturbed.* New York: Institute for Rational-Emotive Therapy.

Emmelkamp, P. M. G., de Hann, E., & Hoodguin, C. A. L. (1990). Marital adjustment and obsessive-compulsive disorder. *British Journal of Psychiatry, 156* 55–60.

Emmelkamp, P. M. G., van Linden van den Heuvell, C., Rüphan, M., Sanderman, R., Scholing, A., & Stroink, F. (1988). Cognitive and behavioral interventions: A comparative evaluation with clinically distressed couples. *Journal of Family Psychology, 1*(4), 365–377. doi: 10.1037/h0080472

Emmelkamp, P. M. G., & de Lange, I. (1983). Spouse involvement in the treatment of obsessive-compulsive patients. *Behavioural Research and Therapy, 25*, 407–429.

Epstein, N. (1982). Cognitive therapy with couples. *American Journal of Family Therapy, 10*(1), 5–16. doi: 10.1080/01926188208250432

Epstein, N., & Eidelson, R. J. (1981). Unrealistic beliefs of clinical couples: Their relationship to expectations, goals and satisfaction. *American Journal of Family Therapy, 9*(4), 13–22. doi: 10.1080/01926188108250420

Epstein, N., Pretzer, J. L., & Fleming, B. (1982, November). *Cognitive therapy and communication training: Comparisons of effects with distressed couples.* Paper present at the annual meeting of the Association of Advancement of Behavior Therapy, Los Angeles.

Epstein, N. B., & Baucom, D. H. (2002). *Enhanced cognitive-behavioral therapy for couples: A contextual approach*: American Psychological Association.

Epstein, N. B., Werlinich, C. A., LaTaillade, J. J., Hoskins, L. H., Dezfulian, T., & Kursch, M. K. (2005). *Couple therapy for domestic abuse: A cognitive-behavioral approach.* Institute presented at the annual convention of the American Association for Marriage and Family Therapy, Kansas City, MO.

Epstein, E. E., McCrady, B. S., Morgain, T. J., Cook, S. M., Kugler, G., & Ziedonis, D. (2007). Couples treatment for drug-dependent males: Preliminary efficacy of a stand-alone outpatient model. *Addictive Disorders & Their Treatment, 6*, 21–37.

Falloon, I. R. (2003). Behavioral family therapy. In G. P. Sholevar (Ed.), *Textbook of family and couples therapy: Clinical applications* (pp. 147–172). Washington, DC: American Psychiatric Publishing.

Falloon, I. R., Boyd, J. L., & McGill, C. W. (1984). *Family care of schizophrenia: A problem-solving approach to the treatment of mental illness.* New York: Guilford Press.

Falloon, I. R., Held, T., Coverdale, J. H., Roncone, R., Laidlaw, T. M. (1999). Family interventions for schizophrenia: A review of long-term benefits of international studies. *Psychiatric Rehabilitation Skills. Special Issue: Integration of Assessment with Intervention for Psychiatric Rehabilitation, 3*(2), 268–290.

Gordon, K. C., Dixon, L. J., Willett, J. M., & Hughes, F. M. (2009). Behavioral and cognitive-behavioral therapies. In J. H. Bray & M. Stanton (Eds.), *The Wiley-Blackwell Handbook of Family Psychology* (pp. 226–239). Oxford, England: Wiley Blackwell Publishing.

Gupta, M., Coyne, J. C., & Beach, S. R. H. (2003). Couples treatment for major depression: Critique of the literature and suggestions for some different directions. *Journal of Family Therapy, 25*(4), 317–346. doi: 10.1111/1467–6427.00253

Hahlweg, K., & Markman, H. J. (1988). Effectiveness of behavioral marital therapy: Empirical status of behavioral techniques in preventing and alleviating marital distress. *Journal of Consulting and Clinical Psychology, 56*(3), 440–447. doi: 10.1037/0022-006x.56.3.440

Halford, W. K., Sanders, M. R., & Behrens, B. C. (1993). A comparison of the generalization of behavioral marital therapy and enhanced behavioral marital therapy. *Journal of Consulting and Clinical Psychology, 61*(1), 51–60. doi: 10.1037/0022-006x.61.1.51

Heatherington, L., Friedlander, M. L., & Greenberg, L. (2005). Change process research in couple and family therapy: Methodological challenges and opportunities. *Journal of Family Psychology*, 19(1), 18–27. doi:10.1037/0893-3200.19.1.18

Huber, C. H., & Milstein, B. (1985). Cognitive restructuring and a collaborative set in couples' work. *The American Journal of Family Therapy*, 13(2), 17–27.

Jacobson, N. S., & Christensen, A. (1996). *Integrative couple therapy*. New York: Norton.

Jacobson, N. S., Follette, W. C., Revenstorf, D., Hahlweg, K., Baucom, D. H., & Margolin, G. (1984). Variability in outcome and clinical significance of behavioral marital therapy: A reanalysis of outcome data. *Journal of Consulting and Clinical Psychology*, 52(4), 497–504. doi: 10.1037/0022-006x.52.4.497

Jacobson, N. S., & Margolin, G. (1979). *Marital therapy: Strategies based on social learning and behavior exchange principles*. New York: Guilford Press.

Jacobson, N. S., Dobson, K., Fruzzetti, A. E., Schmaling, K. B., & Salusky, S. (1991). Marital therapy as a treatment for depression. *Journal of Consulting and Clinical Psychology*, 59(4), 547–557. doi: 10.1037/0022-006x.59.4.547

Johnson, S., & Lebow, J. (2000). The "coming of age" of couple therapy: A decade review. *Journal of Marital and Family Therapy*, 26(1), 23–38. doi: 10.1111/j.1752-0606.2000.tb00273.x

Johnson, C. A., Stanley, S. M., Glenn, N. D., Amato, P. A., Nock, S. L., Markman, H. J., & Dion, M. R. (2002). *Marriage in Oklahoma: 2001 baseline statewide survey on marriage and divorce (S02096 OKDHS)*. Oklahoma City: Oklahoma Department of Human Services.

Karney, B. R. & Bradbury, T. N. (1995) The longitudinal course of marital quality and stability: A review of theory, method, and research. *Psychological Bulletin*, 118, 3–34.

Keefe, F. J., Caldwell, D. S., Baucom, D., & Salley, A. (1996). Spouse-assisted coping skills training in the management of osteoarthritic knee pain. *Arthritis Care and Research*, 9(4), 279–291. doi:10.1002/1529-0131(199608)9:4<279::AID-ANR1790090413>3.0.CO;2–6

Kelly, S. (2005). Enhancing behavioral couple therapy: Addressing the therapeutic alliance, hope, and diversity. *Cognitive and Behavioral Practice*, 12, 102–112.

Kiecolt-Glaser, J. K., & Newton, T. L. (2001). Marriage and health: His and hers. *Psychological Bulletin*, 127(4), 472–503. doi: 10.1037/0033-2909.127.4.472

Klann, N., Hahlweg, K., Baucom, D. H., & Kroeger, C. (2011). The effectiveness of couple therapy in Germany: A replication study. *Journal of Marital and Family Therapy*, 37, 200–208.

LaTaillade, J. J., Epstein, N. B., & Werlinich, C. A. (2006). Conjoint treatment of intimate partner violence: A cognitive behavioral approach. *Journal of Cognitive Psychotherapy. Special Issue: Cognitive behavioral assessment and treatment of couples*, 20(4), 393–410. doi: 10.1891/jcpiq-v20i4a005

Law, D. D., & Crane, R. D. (2000). The influence of marital and family therapy on health care utilization in a health-maintenance organization. *Journal of Marital and Family Therapy*, 26, 281–291.

Lawrence, E. E., Eldridge, K. A., & Christensen, A. (1998). The enhancement of traditional behavioral couples therapy: Consideration of individual factors and dyadic development. *Clinical Psychology Review*, 18, 745–764.

Lebow, J. L., Chambers, A., Christensen, A., & Johnson, S. M. (2012). Marital distress. In D. Sprenkle & R. Chenail (Eds.), *Effectiveness research in marriage and family therapy*. Washington, DC: AAMFT.

Lebow, J. L., Chambers, A. L., Christensen, A., & Johnson, S. M. (2012). Research on the treatment of couple distress. *Journal of Marital and Family Therapy*, 38(1), 145–168. doi:http://dx.doi.org/10.1111/j.1752-0606.2011.00249.x

Mackinnon, D. P. (2005). Economic evaluation methodology for family therapy outcome research. In Sprenkle, D. H., & Piercy, F. P. (Eds.). *Research methods in family therapy* (2nd ed., pp. 339–367). New York: Guilford Press.

Margolin, G., & Weiss, R. L. (1978). Comparative evaluation of therapeutic components associated with behavioral marital treatments. *Journal of Consulting and Clinical Psychology*, 46(6), 1476–1486. doi: 10.1037/0022-006X.46.6.1476

Martell, C. R., Safren, S. A., & Prince, S. E. (2004). *Cognitive-behavioral therapies with lesbian, gay, and bisexual clients*. New York: Guildford Press.

McCrady, B. S., Epstein, E. E., Cook, S., Jensen, N., & Hildebrandt, T. (2009). A randomized trial of individual and couple behavioral alcohol treatment for women. *Journal of Consulting and Clinical Psychology*, 77(2), 243–256. doi: 10.1037/a0014686

Mueser, K. T., & Glynn, S. M. (1999). *Behavioral family therapy for psychiatric disorders*. Oakland, CA: New Harbinger.

Norcross, J. C., Karpiak, C. P., & Santoro, S. O. (2005). Clinical psychologists across the years: The division of clinical psychology from 1960 to 2003. *Journal of Clinical Psychology*, 61 1467–1483.

O'Farrell, T. J., Choquette, K. A., Cutter, H. S., Brown, E. D., & McCourt, W. F. (1993). Behavioral marital therapy with and without additional couples relapse prevention sessions for alcoholics and their wives. *Journal of Studies on Alcohol*, 54(6), 652–666. Retrieved from http://search.proquest.com/docview/618445826?accountid=14766

O'Farrell, T. J., Choquette, K. A., Cutter, H. S. G., Floyd, F. J., Bayog, R., Brown, E. D.,...Denault, P. (1996). Cost-benefit and cost-effectiveness analyses of behavioral marital therapy as an addition to outpatient alcoholism treatment. *Journal of Substance Abuse*, 8(2), 145–166. Retrieved from http://search.proquest.com/docview/618876915?accountid=14766

O'Leary, K. D., Heyman, R. E., & Neidig, P. H. (1999). Treatment of wife abuse: A comparison of gender-specific and conjoint approaches. *Behavior Therapy*, 30(3), 475–505. doi: 10.1016/s0005-7894(99)80021–5

O'Leary, K. D., & Beach, S. R. (1990). Marital therapy: A viable treatment for depression and marital discord. *The American Journal of Psychiatry*, 147(2), 183–186.

Pinsof, W. M., Wynne, L. C., & Hambright, A. B. (1996). The outcomes of couple and family therapy: Findings, conclusions, and recommendations. *Psychotherapy*, 33, 321–331.

Pinsof, W. M., & Wynne, L. C. (2000). Toward progress research: Closing the gap between family therapy practice and research. *Journal of Marital and Family Therapy*, 26, 1–8.

Powers, M. B., Vedel, E., & Emmelkamp, P. M. G. (2008). Behavioral couples therapy (BCT) for alcohol and drug use disorders: A meta-analysis. *Clinical Psychology Review*, 28(6), 952–962. doi: 10.1016/j.cpr.2008.02.002

Schulz, M. S., Cowan, C. P., & Cowan, P. A. (2006). Promoting healthy beginnings: A randomized controlled trial of a preventive intervention to preserve marital quality during the transition to parenthood. *Journal of Consulting and Clinical Psychology*, *74*, 20–31.

Sexton, T. L., Gordon, K. C., Gurman, A. S., Lebow, J. L., Holtzworth-Monroe, A., & Johnson, S. M. (2011). Recommendations from the Division 43: Family Psychology Task Force on Evaluating Evidence-Based Treatments in Couple and Family Psychology. *Family Process.*

Shadish, W. R., & Baldwin, S. A. (2003). Meta-analysis of MFT interventions. *Journal of Marital and Family Therapy*, *29*(4), 547–570. doi: 10.1111/j.1752-0606.2003.tb01694.x

Sher, T. G., & Baucom, D. H. (2001). Mending a broken heart: A couples approach to cardiac risk reduction. *Applied & Preventive Psychology*, *10*(2), 125–133.

Snyder, D. K., & Mitchell, A. E. (2008). Affective-reconstructive couple therapy: A pluralistic, developmental approach. In Gurman, A. S. (Ed.), *Clinical handbook of couple therapy* (4th ed., pp. 353–382). New York: Guilford Press.

Snyder, D. K., Castellani, A. M., & Whisman, M. A. (2006). Current status and future directions in couple therapy. *Annual Review of Psychology*, *57*, 317–344.

Snyder, D. K., Wills, R. M., & Grady-Fletcher, A. (1991). Long-term effectiveness of behavioral versus insight-oriented marital therapy: A 4-year follow-up study. *Journal of Consulting and Clinical Psychology*, *59*(1), 138–141. doi: 10.1037/0022-006x.59.1.138

Sprenkle, D. H., & Blow, A. J. (2004). Common factors and our sacred models. *Journal of Marital and Family Therapy*, *30*, 113–129.

Stanley, S. M., Blumberg, S. L., & Markman, H. J. (1999). Helping couples fight for their marriages: The PREP approach. In Berger, R., & Hannah, M. T. (Eds.), *Preventive approaches in couples therapy* (pp. 279–303). Philadelphia: Brunner/Mazel.

Stuart, R. B. (1980). *Helping couples change: A social learning approach to marital therapy.* Champaign, IL: Research Press.

Swindle, R. Jr., Heller, K., Pescosolido, B., & Kikuzawa, S. (2000). Responses to nervous breakdowns in America over a 40-year period. *American Psychologist*, *55*, 740–749.

Tejada-Vera, B., & Sutton, P. D. (2010). Births, marriages, divorces, and deaths: Provisional data for 2009. *National Vital Statistics Reports*, *58*(25).

Thibaut, J. W., & Kelley, H. H. (1959). *The social psychology of groups.* New York: Wiley.

Tucker, J. S., & Mueller, J. S. (2000). Spouses' social control of health behaviors: Use and effectiveness of specific strategies. *Personality and Social Psychology Bulletin*, *26*(9), 1120–1130. doi: 10.1177/01461672002611008

Wampold, B. E. (2001). *The great psychotherapy debate: Models, methods, and findings* Lawrence Erlbaum Associates Publishers, Mahwah, NJ. Retrieved from http://search.proquest.com/docview/619566790?accountid=14766

Weiss, R. L., Hops, H., & Patterson, G. R. (1973). A framework for conceptualizing marital conflict: A technology for altering it, some data for evaluating it. In L. D. Handy, & E. L. Mash (Eds.), *Behavior change: Methodology concepts and practice* (pp. 309–342). Champaign, IL: Research Press.

Wetchler, J. L. (Ed.). (2011). *Handbook of clinical issues in couple therapy (2nd ed.).* New York: Routledge.

Whisman, M. A., Dixon, A. E., & Johnson, B. (1997). Therapists' perspectives of couple problems and treatment issues in couple therapy. *Journal of Family Psychology*, *11*, 361–366.

Whisman, M. A., & Uebelacker, L. A. (2007). Maladaptive schemas and core beliefs in treatment and research with couples. In D. J. Stein, J. E. Young, L. P. Riso, & P. L. du Toit (Eds.), *Cognitive schemas and core beliefs in psychological problems: A scientist-practitioner guide* (pp. 199–220). Washington, DC: American Psychological Association.

Intellectual Disability

James K. Luiselli

Abstract

Applied behavior analysis (ABA) is an intervention philosophy and methodology for treating challenging behaviors of children and adults who have intellectual disability. This chapter reviews functional behavioral assessment and functional analysis as initial steps in formulating an intervention plan for serious problems such as self-injury, aggression, property destruction, and stereotypy. The conceptual basis and the process of matching hypothesized behavior-function with consequence control and antecedent control intervention procedures are described. The chapter also details selective cognitive-behavioral therapy and self-management training options. A concluding section discusses several intervention enhancement tactics. Throughout the chapter the emphasis is on evidence-based and empirically supported intervention procedures that can be profitably adopted by care providers within school, home, day-habilitation, and community settings.

Key Words: intellectual disability, applied behavior analysis, functional behavioral assessment, functional analysis, self-management training

People with intellectual disability (intellectual developmental disorder) (ID) have deficits in general mental abilities and adaptive functioning with onset during the developmental period (American Psychiatric Association, 2013; Harris, 2005). The cognitive challenges associated with ID affect abstract thinking, problem solving, reasoning, and academic learning. Intellectual functioning is usually measured through standardized, norm-referenced testing—a score that is two or more standard deviations below the population mean is indicative of ID. Concerning adaptive abilities, the key diagnostic criteria are "failure to meet developmental and sociocultural standards for personal independence and social responsibility" (American Psychiatric Association, 2013, p. 33). Deficits in adaptive functioning are further delineated into conceptual (e.g., language, reading, memory), social (e.g., awareness of emotions, communication skills, establishing friendships), and practical

(e.g., self-control, money management, vocational responsibility) domains. Several methods are used to measure adaptive functioning, including informant-based assessment protocols, observation, clinical evaluation, and whenever possible, interview with the person. On the basis of adaptive functioning within the conceptual, social, and practical domains, severity of ID is classified as mild, moderate, severe, or profound.

People with ID also demonstrate challenging behaviors that can be self-harming, health-threatening, environmentally disruptive, and socially stigmatizing (Luiselli, 2012). Common examples of these problems are self-injury, aggression, property destruction, and stereotypy. To a large extent these and similar behaviors are the result of a person having limited skills for interacting successfully with her or his surroundings. In fact, teaching adaptive and compensatory skills is a critical component of intervention planning that targets challenging behaviors.

Over four decades ago Baer, Wolf, and Risley (1968) published a seminal article that defined the then-emerging discipline of applied behavior analysis (ABA). In the year 2014, ABA represents an evidence-based and empirically supported approach to behavioral intervention for people with ID (Luiselli, 2011b; Matson, 2009). Indeed, the basis of this chapter is ABA applications, highlighting several dominant themes and contemporary "best practices." However, as an introductory précis, it is instructive to briefly consider the characteristics of ABA that Baer et al. (1968) emphasized and are true in the present day. First, the "applied" in ABA has to do with "real-world" issues and concerns that extend beyond the experimental laboratory. Reflecting prose of years past, Baer et al. (1968) wrote, "In behavioral application, the behavior, stimuli, and/or organism under study are chosen because of their importance to man and society, rather than their importance to theory" (p. 92). Concerning "behavior," the key element is that "Applied research is eminently pragmatic; it asks how it is possible to get an individual to do something effectively" (p. 93). Thus, directly observing and measuring people behaving is integral to ABA. Finally, "analysis" means demonstrating lawful changes in behavior by manipulating independent variables in the context of single-case experimental designs (Barlow, Nock, & Hersen, 2008; Kazdin, 2011). Citing a popular quote by Baer et al. (1968), "An experimenter has achieved an analysis of behavior when he can exercise control over it" (p. 94).

Baer et al. (1968) also alerted the professional community to other key features of ABA. They used the term "technical" to refer to operationally defined procedures or, "behavioral applications," which practitioners can implement reliably to produce (replicate) the same results. Furthermore, procedures should be conceptually sound by virtue of being derived from established learning principles (Cooper, Heron, & Heward, 2007). And the procedures must be "effective" because they produce results that are practical and socially important. Finally, behavior change should ideally generalize to nonintervention settings and be durable over time.

This chapter focuses on ABA among people with ID, emphasizing intervention for decreasing challenging behaviors. I define challenging behaviors according to several criteria. First, some behaviors cause tissue damage and internal injury: striking face and head with hands, biting skin, slamming body into objects, and poking eyes. Other behaviors, such as aggression, pose a risk to care providers. Environmentally destructive behaviors include destroying property and throwing objects. Sometimes all or some of these behaviors occur simultaneously or in rapid succession. Beyond the dire physical effects, these and similar behaviors are socially stigmatizing, may prevent a person from participating in normative life experiences, and almost always interfere with educational and habilitation training efforts.

In order to adequately capture the evolution of ABA philosophy and methodology, I organized the chapter according to topics that are central to current-day practice and research. The first section describes functional behavioral assessment (hereafter, FBA) and functional analysis (hereafter, FA) methodologies. Next, I present examples of function-based intervention for challenging behaviors frequently addressed in clinical and applied research, one section dealing with consequence-control procedures and another section dealing with antecedent-control procedures. Although traditional cognitive-behavioral therapy (CBT) approaches have been examined less frequently within the ID population, the chapter has a section about CBT and self-management training options. I conclude by highlighting several intervention enhancement tactics when formulating and implementing behavior support plans.

Functional Behavioral Assessment and Functional Analysis

Intervention plans for challenging behaviors are most effective when they are function based—that is, the procedures are "matched" to controlling variables (Matson & Minshawi, 2007). It is important to realize, however, that this orientation was not always the case with ABA. I have noted previously, for example, that the "first generation" of behavioral intervention in ID during the 1960s and 1970s was devoted to establishing a technology of procedures that targeted specific challenging behaviors without regard to motivational influences or systematically assessing conditions that set the occasion for and maintained these behaviors (Luiselli, 2004). As highlighted in this section, the eventual emergence of FBA and FA improved dramatically our understanding of the environmental determinants of challenging behavior, the process of case formulation, and the selection of person-specific intervention procedures.

Concerning the role of reinforcement in establishing function, behavior analysts emphasize three behavior–environment relationships. *Social positive reinforcement* is defined as pleasurable social (e.g., attention) or tangible (e.g., access to preferred objects) consequences. *Social negative reinforcement* operates when behavior terminates an unpleasant situation. The third category, *automatic reinforcement*, represents nonsocial consequences such as sensory stimulation that the behavior itself produces. Conducting FBA and FA is intended to isolate these sources of reinforcement and, in turn, design an intervention plan for the corresponding challenging behaviors.

Functional Behavioral Assessment

FBA is the process of correlating environmental events with challenging behaviors. One approach toward FBA relies on *indirect* methods based principally on the subjective reports of care providers. Instruments such as the *Motivation Assessment Scale (MAS)* (Durand & Crimmins, 1988), the *Functional Analysis Screening Tool (FAST)* (Iwata, 1995), and the *Questions About Behavior Function (QABF)* (Matson & Vollmer, 1995) are informant surveys that target social and nonsocial contingencies responsible for challenging behaviors. Cut-off scores derived from the surveys are used to endorse one or more sources of control (e.g., attention, tangible, escape, automatic).

The *Functional Assessment Interview (FAI)* (O'Neill, Horner, Albin, Sprague, Storey, & Newton, 1997) is another informant-driven protocol. During an interview conducted by a responsible professional, the informant is asked questions about antecedent and consequence events often associated with occurrence and nonoccurrence of challenging behaviors. The *FAI* examines a variety of ecological events (e.g., medical status, sleep patterns, mealtime routines) and interpersonal contacts, thereby producing a comprehensive formulation that guides intervention planning.

Descriptive methods are a second type of FBA, characterized by direct observation of a person under naturalistic conditions. Bijou, Peterson, and Ault (1968) pioneered this approach with their presentation of antecedent-behavior-consequence (A-B-C) data collection. For a child who has challenging behaviors, an observer would watch her or him participate in a variety of activities, noting particular events that immediately precede (antecedents) and follow (consequences) the behaviors (Luiselli, 2006). The resulting data then are evaluated to determine whether specific situations reliably predict the challenging behaviors. In doing so, hypotheses about behavior can be inferred.

More recently, Martens, DiGennaro, Reed, Szczech, and Rosenthal (2008) described a contingency space analysis (CSA) of direct observational data. In a CSA, conditional probabilities are computed from sequential recordings of behaviors and the corresponding contingent consequences. As a type of FBA, the CSA quantifies the probability of specified consequences (e.g., attention and escape) following the occurrence and nonoccurrence of challenging behaviors. I refer the reader to Reed, Luiselli, Morizio, and Child (2010) for a clinical example of CSA applied to a child with ID who had chronic and high-frequency self-injurious behavior.

To be addressed later in the chapter, antecedent events can set the occasion for challenging behaviors through established stimulus control (Luiselli, 2008). Touchette, MacDonald, and Langer (1985) presented a *scatter-plot* analysis as a first step toward confirming stimulus control over challenging behaviors. The recording protocol requires a care provider to indicate if the behaviors did not occur, occurred one time, or occurred two times or more during successive 30-minute intervals within the day. Of course, the intervals can be shorter or longer depending on the prevailing conditions and exigencies. By reviewing data over several days, "Problem behavior may be correlated with a time of day, the presence or absence of certain people, a social setting, a class of activities, a contingency of reinforcement, a physical environment, and combinations of these and other variables" (Touchette et al., 1985, p. 345). Accordingly, intervention can proceed by modifying one or more of these behavior–environment relationships.

Both indirect and descriptive FBA have the advantage of being easily administered by practitioners. From a clinical perspective, it is important to gather information from individuals who are knowledgeable about the person and to document objectively how often challenging behaviors occur and under what conditions. Typically, both assessment methods are performed together, for example, obtaining informant impressions about behavior function followed by direct observation and data collection. To reiterate, FBA enables one to form a working hypothesis (e.g., "The child's aggression appears to be escape motivated.") but not a confirmatory "cause and effect" relationship (see Reed & Azulay, 2011 for practical guidance in conducting FBA).

Functional Analysis

In contrast to FBA, an FA measures challenging behaviors during experimentally manipulated conditions. In the seminal publication on this topic, Iwata, Dorsey, Slifer, Bauman, and Richman (1994) constructed conditions to represent social positive reinforcement, social negative reinforcement, and automatic reinforcement functions. Iwata et al. (1994) studied nine children who had ID and self-injurious behavior (SIB) during daily 15-minute sessions with each session featuring a condition linked to one of four functions:

Social Disapproval. A therapist sat in a room and allowed the child access to toys. The therapist sat away from the child, reading a book or magazine. When the child displayed SIB, the therapist disapproved by stating, "Don't do that, you're going to hurt yourself." This condition provided social attention contingent on SIB.

Academic Demand. A therapist sat in a room with the child and presented her or him with instructional tasks that were difficult to complete. When the child displayed SIB, the therapist removed the task, turned away for 30 seconds, and then resumed instruction. This condition provided escape from demands contingent on SIB.

Unstructured Play. A therapist sat in a room and allowed the child access to toys. There were no consequences for SIB. Instead, the therapist presented the child with social praise and brief physical contact (hand on shoulder) every 30 seconds without SIB. "This condition served as a control procedure for the presence of an experimenter, the availability of potentially stimulating materials, the absence of demands, the delivery of social approval for appropriate behavior, and the lack of approval for self-injury" (Iwata et al., 1994, p. 203).

Alone. The child was present in the room without the therapist or access to toys or other potentially stimulating materials. This condition tested for automatic (sensory) reinforcement as a source of control over SIB.

Iwata et al. (1994) found that for six of the nine children, higher frequencies of SIB were associated with a specific experimental condition. When the data from an FA are graphed, the response differentiation among conditions isolates controlling variables. Although Iwata et al. (1994) concentrated on SIB, FA methodology has been applied to other challenging behaviors of children and adults who have ID and other neurodevelopmental disorders (Hanley, Iwata, & McCord, 2003).

The advantages of FA notwithstanding, the methodology requires greater sophistication than a typical FBA. Another concern is the "ecological validity" of an FA, namely that it is conducted under simulated (analog) conditions that are removed from the natural environment. Hanley et al. (2003) concluded that there has been "Systematic growth in the use of functional analysis methodology as a primary method of behavior assessment and, more generally, as a means of studying environment-behavior relations" (p. 178). Furthermore, many FAs have been performed in applied settings such as schools, and it appears that the time commitment is no greater than that required for an FBA (Iwata et al., 2000). Care providers, in fact, can be taught the skills to independently conduct an FA (Moore & Fisher, 2007; Moore et al., 2002; Stokes & Luiselli, 2008). In summary, FA methodologies continue to be refined and adapted to clinical constraints, and they represent the experimental standard when targeting challenging behaviors (Hanley, 2010).

Before describing function-based intervention, I would like to emphasize that a single challenging behavior can have multiple functions. That is, a child with ID might display attention-maintained self-injury when playing with peers and escape motivated self-injury during instructional activities with a teacher. Also, behavior function can change over time. For example, self-injury in an adult with ID could have started because of a medical condition but subsequently been maintained through social reinforcement. Accordingly, intervention plans must conform to context-specific variables which usually have to do with multiple and/or changing functions on challenging behaviors.

Function-Based Consequence Intervention

The following section describes function-based intervention for attention-maintained, escape-motivated, and automatically reinforced challenging behaviors from a consequence control perspective. Consequence control is established by manipulating behavior-contingent events, intended to either increase desirable behaviors or decrease challenging behaviors. Figure 22.1 shows four behavior-contingent consequence relationships for achieving intervention objectives. Presenting a pleasurable consequence that increases behavior is *positive reinforcement.* Contingent removal of an undesirable consequence, *negative reinforcement,* also has the objective of increasing behavior. Conversely,

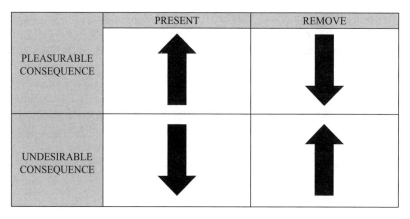

	PRESENT	REMOVE
PLEASURABLE CONSEQUENCE	⬆	⬇
UNDESIRABLE CONSEQUENCE	⬇	⬆

Figure 22.1 Consequence effects on behavior (increase or decrease) by presenting and removing pleasurable and undesirable consequences.

contingently removing a pleasurable consequence (*time-out*) and contingently presenting an undesirable consequence (*punishment*) serve to decrease behavior.

Because it is not possible to adequately represent the vast behavioral intervention research literature in ID, I selected self-injury, aggression, stereotypy, and noncompliance to illustrate procedures that have been effective within the three behavior-function categories. In some instance, the participants in this research had cognitive impairments but were not diagnosed with ID. I included these studies because they aptly depict particular intervention procedures that are applicable to people who have ID.

Attention-Maintained Challenging Behaviors

Attention-maintained challenging behaviors are those reinforced by social attention and access to tangible objects. One function-based intervention in such cases is differential reinforcement (DR) in which (a) a pleasurable stimulus (e.g., praise, approval, food, toy) is delivered when a child or adult does not demonstrate challenging behaviors and (b) the pleasurable stimulus is withheld when the behaviors occur (*extinction*). Differential reinforcement is a relatively straightforward procedure that can be implemented in several ways. With the *differential reinforcement of other behavior (DRO)*, a care provider gives the person a pleasurable stimulus when she or he does not display challenging behaviors for a specified amount of time. Another alternative is the *differential reinforcement of alternative behavior (DRA)* in which the pleasurable stimulus follows behaviors that are physically incompatible with the challenging behaviors. A third option, the *differential reinforcement of low rate behavior (DRL)*, provides a pleasurable stimulus when challenging behaviors do not exceed a predetermined criterion. DRO, DRA, and DRL procedures sometimes are effective when they are applied isolation, but more commonly, when combined with antecedent control manipulations and other behavior-contingent consequences (Kern & Kokina, 2008).

Presenting reinforcement on a noncontingent or fixed-time (FT) schedule can also reduce and eliminate attention-maintained challenging behaviors (Carr & LeBlanc, 2006). Note that noncontingent reinforcement (NCR), in fact, is a misnomer because reinforcement, by definition, is a contingent event that increases behavior (Skinner, 1948). However, NCR has become the conventional terminology accepted by behavior analysts. In one of the first evaluations of NCR, Vollmer, Iwata, Zarcone, Smith, and Mazaleski (1993) treated attention-maintained self-injury of three adults who had ID. The NCR intervention had a therapist provide brief social attention to the adults every few seconds on an FT schedule whether or not they displayed self-injury. Over successive days, the FT schedule was increased gradually to a terminal criterion of 5 minutes. The results of this study were that NCR was as effective as DRO in reducing each adult's self-injury to near-zero frequency.

In a study that addressed several attention-maintained challenging behaviors (aggression, self-injury, disruption) in 5-year-old female quadruplets diagnosed with PDD and ID, Hagopian, Fisher, and Legacy (1994) evaluated two NCR interventions. Following a baseline phase, a therapist presented social attention to the children on an FT 10-second schedule ("dense" schedule condition), then on an FT 5-minute schedule ("lean" schedule condition). The "dense" schedule of reinforcement was associated with the largest decrease in challenging behaviors, suggesting that at the onset of NCR intervention, the FT schedule should be near continuous. Hagopian et al. (1994) eventually were able to fade the delivery of social attention so that by conclusion of the study, a near-zero rate of problem behaviors was maintained by an FT-5 minute schedule.

NCR is relatively easy to implement because it is not behavior dependent. That is, presentation of reinforcement is based on the passage of time and not the occurrence of challenging behaviors as is customary with DR procedures. NCR also maximizes a person's exposure to reinforcement (Vollmer et al., 1993). As a decelerative intervention, it appears that NCR operates by reducing a person's motivation to perform challenging behaviors because delivering pleasurable stimuli noncontingently serves as an *abolishing operation (AO)* (Friman & Hawkins, 2006).

Functional communication training (FCT), initially reported by Carr and Durand (1985), is another intervention procedure that has been effective with attention-maintained challenging behaviors (Durand & Carr, 1991; Peterson et al., 2005). The basis of FCT is teaching a child or adult to use language as a substitute for challenging behaviors. For example, a child who has learned that aggression produces adult attention might be taught to ask, "Am I doing good work?" or "Can I talk to you?" instead of hitting the care provider. Similarly, challenging behaviors that have been reinforced by contingent access to tangibles would be approached by having the child make requests for preferred objects (e.g., "I want to play with that toy"). Because many people with ID do not acquire speech, research in the area of alternative and augmentative communication (AAC) has shown that FCT can be successful by teaching a child or adult to activate vocal output communication aids (Sigafoos, Arthur, & O'Reilly, 2003) and to make requests with visual materials such as the Picture Exchange Communication System (PECS) (Charlop-Christy, Carpenter, Le, LeBlanc, & Kellet, 2002). Thus, FCT appears to be a versatile procedure that can be adapted to more than one behavior function and more than one communication training modality.

Escape-Motivated Challenging Behaviors

Challenging behaviors that result in a person escaping a nonpreferred situation are maintained by social negative reinforcement. One consequence intervention is to prevent escape, otherwise known as *escape extinction* (Carr, Newsom, & Binkoff, 1980), by prompting a person to perform alternative behavior, blocking the challenging behaviors, or restraining movement. Notably, although escape extinction procedures properly address behavior function, they are not easy to implement, may provoke other challenging behaviors, and necessitate at least initially, negative physical contact between the child or adult and the intervening care provider. Therefore, it is desirable to consider other less invasive procedures.

Functional communication training (FCT), described earlier, can be formulated for escape-motivated challenging behaviors by teaching a child or adult to request a "break" from nonpreferred situations (e.g., "Can we stop now?"). Break requests usually are honored continuously and then faded gradually. To illustrate, a child or adult accustomed to taking a break every time the request is made might be required to complete several tasks or participate in instruction for a longer duration before time away from tasks and instruction are permitted. Johnson, McComas, Thompson, and Symons (2004) evaluated FCT with an 11-year-old boy who had autism and displayed aggression (hitting, kicking, pinching, biting, pulling hair) toward his mother and infant brother. An FA conducted in the boy's home revealed that aggression was negatively reinforced by his mother picking up the infant brother and leaving the room. Aggression was reduced to a near-zero rate by teaching the boy to request separation from his mother and brother. Interestingly, the positive effect from FCT was more pronounced when the mother frequently prompted the boy to make requests.

Noncompliant behavior is frequently escape motivated in function—a person learns that nonpreferred directions and instructions are withdrawn when she or he "refuses" to carry them out or demonstrates challenging behaviors that effectively terminate an interaction. In Peyton, Lindauer, and Richman (2005), a 10-year-old girl with autism displayed vocal behavior involving a refusal to comply with requests (e.g., "I won't do it"). An FA suggested that noncompliance was reinforced by escaping task demands. One intervention evaluation showed that noncompliant vocal behavior persisted whether demands were or were not accompanied by removal of task materials. When the manner of prompting the girl included a nondirective request (e.g., "I wonder where the — is") instead of a direct request (e.g., "Show me the —"), noncompliance quickly extinguished. Therefore, for this child, it was how requests were presented and not demands per se that occasioned the noncompliant behavior.

Automatically Reinforced Challenging Behaviors

Stereotypy and self-injury are the automatically reinforced challenging behaviors represented most frequently in the ABA intervention literature. Concerning stereotypy, the defining characteristic is motor and vocal behaviors that are repetitive and invariant, for example, rocking the body rhythmically, flapping hands in front of the eyes, tapping objects with fingers, and repeating sounds, words, and phrases. The automatic reinforcement produced by these and similar behaviors stems from visual, auditory, and proprioceptive sensory stimulation. Self-injury also occurs as repetitive responses that mimic stereotypy but, additionally, can cause tissue damage and bodily harm.

Reinforcing the nonoccurrence of stereotypy and self-injury through DRO has been effective (Cowdery, Iwata, & Pace, 1990; Luiselli, Helfen, Colozzi, Donellon, & Pemberton, 1978; Repp & Deitz, 1974), but in most cases, the required interval of nonresponding must be low duration and it can be difficult identifying and programming stimuli that compete with automatic sensory pleasurable consequences. An alternative is NCR in which stimuli, ideally matched to the preferred stimulation that stereotypy and self-injury produce, are presented on a fixed-time (FT) or variable-time (VT) schedule (Goh et al., 1995; Piazza, Adelinis, Hanley, Goh, & Delia, 2000; Simmons, Smith, & Kliethermes, 2003; Vollmer, Marcus, & LeBlanc, 1994).

Studies have shown that combining DRO and NCR with stereotypy-contingent and self-injury-contingent consequences may be needed as intervention. Early research on *overcorrection* found that stereotypy and self-injury could be reduced by having a child or adult perform opposite-behavior movements in rapid sequence (Foxx & Azrin, 1973). More recently, *response blocking* has been implemented successfully for different motor stereotypies (e.g., hand and object mouthing) and self-injurious behaviors (Hagopian & Adelinis, 2001; Lerman, Kelley, Vorndran, & Van Camp, 2003; Luiselli, 1992a; Reid, Parsons, Phillips, & Green, 1993). With response blocking, a care provider manually interrupts a child or adult from completing stereotypy and self-injury. But like similar physical intervention procedures, overcorrection and response blocking have the disadvantages of being labor intensive and possibly provoking other challenging behaviors (e.g., aggression) (Fisher, Lindauer, Alterson, & Thompson, 1998).

Although fitting more with an antecedent intervention approach (described below), other procedures for automatically reinforced stereotypy and self-injury are (a) enriching the physical environment to occasion incompatible behaviors (Ahearn, Clark, DeBar, & Florentino, 2005; Lindberg, Iwata, & Kahng, 1999; Ringdahl, Vollmer, Marcus, & Roane, 1997), (b) modifying materials so that stereotypy and self-injury do not produce reinforcing sensory stimulation (Rincover, Cook, Peoples, & Packard, 1979), and (c) having a person wear clothing or a piece of equipment (e.g., gloves) which eliminates the source of automatic reinforcement (Luiselli, 1988; Luiselli & Waldstein, 1994; Rincover & Devany, 1982; Tang, Patterson, & Kennedy, 2003). It should be noted that in some cases, clothing and equipment have been applied to *mechanically restrain* a child or adult from engaging in stereotypy and self-injury (Luiselli, 1992b; Oliver, Hall, Hales, Murphy, & Watts, 1998; Zhou, Goff, & Iwata, 2000). Unfortunately, mechanical restraint limits purposeful movement and can have health complications, making equipment fading a necessary component of an intervention plan (Moore, Fisher, & Pennington, 2004; Wallace, Iwata, Zhou, & Goff, 1999).

Finally, Thompson, Fisher, Piazza, and Kuhn (1998) found that hitting, kicking, pinching, and scratching by a 7-year-old boy diagnosed with PDD were attention maintained, while a separate topography of aggression, "grinding" his chin against a person's body, was automatically reinforced by tactile stimulation. Intervention for the attention-maintained aggression consisted of FCT and social extinction. The procedures implemented to reduce automatically reinforced aggression included response blocking and giving the child access to alternative forms of chin stimulation. This study is instructive because it shows how multiple aggressive responses can have different sources of operant control, including automatic reinforcement, which require separate function-based intervention plans.

Function-Based Antecedent Intervention

Defined broadly, antecedent intervention manipulates conditions and implements procedures to *prevent* challenging behaviors. Thus, instead of waiting for a child to display aggression and having someone apply a controlling consequence, an antecedent approach strives to eliminate the probability that aggression is encountered. Among several benefits, antecedent intervention is particularly advantageous for seriously challenging behaviors. To illustrate, therapeutic restraint (protective holding) might be indicated as a behavior support plan consequence for self-injury, aggression, and other high-risk problems (Harris, 1996; Luiselli, 2009, 2011c). However, it is always desirable to minimize intervention procedures that require a care provider to make physical contact with a child or adult when they are agitated and distressed. Also, challenging behaviors are frequently situation specific, meaning that they occur under certain environmental conditions and not others. Often, these conditions can be modified by changing distinct antecedent features, the result being permanent elimination of the challenging behaviors. And as noted previously, care providers may judge antecedent intervention as being more acceptable than "reactive" (consequence) methods. Note, though, that antecedent procedures are rarely incorporated as a sole component of intervention but typically are applied in concert with one or more consequence strategies (Ricciardi, 2006).

The conceptual framework for antecedent intervention is that both people and the physical environment can acquire *stimulus control* over behavior. For example, if a teacher is consistently positive during interactions with students, they may be more likely to approach the teacher, follow her instructions, and participate in activities. Conversely, if a teacher is harsh and rarely positive, students may avoid her and respond less favorably during instruction. Similarly, children and adults may be uncomfortable within, avoid, or seek to escape settings where they had negative experiences. Common examples in this regard are receiving treatment at a hospital or dental clinic where physically invasive procedures are encountered (O'Callaghan, Allen, Powell, & Salama, 2006).

Stimulus control occurs through the pairing of "antecedents" (people, places, objects) with positive and negative consequences. A *discriminative stimulus*, or Sd, is defined as a stimulus that has been associated with positive reinforcement. Relative to antecedent intervention, the principle of discriminative stimulus control allows for various manipulations to induce behavior change. Consider again the teacher who has positive stimulus control with her students. She could conduct instruction simultaneously with less effective staff in order to "transfer" stimulus control to them. Once control is achieved, the teacher could remove herself gradually so that staff eventually is solely responsible for instruction.

A stimulus control approach to intervention also can be applied to environments. In the case of a child or adult who becomes agitated within a medical setting, the intervention might concentrate on teaching her or him to tolerate the earliest steps in a graduated "approach" sequence (Cavalari, DuBard, Luiselli, & Birtwell, 2013; Grider, Luiselli, & Turcotte-Shamski, 2012; Luiselli, 2011a; Ricciardi, Luiselli, & Cammere, 2006). Using the dental distress example, this sequence could start by having the person sit calmly and quietly in a dentist's office. The next steps might be the person interacting briefly with the dentist in the reception area, walking into the dental suite, sitting in the dentist's chair, and so on until she or he is about to receive treatment compliantly. Again, this example illustrates how an emphasis on stimulus control qualifies as antecedent intervention.

Changing a person's *motivation* to respond is another antecedent manipulation. Behavior analysts explain motivation with reference to the concept of an *establishing operation* (EO). As defined by Michael (1993), an EO is "an environmental event, operation, or stimulus condition that affects an organism by momentarily altering (a) the reinforcing effectiveness of other events and (b) the frequency of occurrence of that part of the organism's repertoire to those events as consequences" (p. 192). So conceived, an EO influences responding first by increasing the value (or potency) of consequences that have functioned as positive reinforcement and second, by evoking behaviors that were previously reinforced. As exemplified by a child who receives food as positive reinforcement for correct learning responses, her or his motivation to respond accurately should be greater in instructional sessions that are scheduled before instead of after the lunch meal (Zhou, Iwata, & Shore, 2002). This effect is predicted because being hungry (a state of deprivation) increases the enjoyment of food consumption and, contemporaneously, the behaviors that produce food.

Food is a primary, or tangible, consequence but the concept of an EO extends to other events. With a child or adult who experiences long periods without social contact, subsequent peer or adult attention may be highly reinforcing. The same result is apparent if the child or adult enjoys sensory stimulation but has not had access to toys, music, television, or motor activities. Keep in mind that deprivation states relative to tangible, social, and sensory stimuli strengthen motivation, but the resulting increase in "stimuli-contacting" behavior could be appropriate or inappropriate. As an example, consider that increasing a student's motivation to consume food may lead to better performance in a classroom where food is used as positive reinforcement but also an unacceptable behavior such as food stealing.

The concept of an EO extends to *biological* influences and health conditions as well (Kennedy & Becker, 2006). In one study, Kennedy and Meyer (1996) found that the challenging behaviors of three students during instruction were most frequent when one student had allergy symptoms and two students had reduced hours of sleep the night before. When the students were allergy-free and had slept more soundly, challenging behaviors were less frequent. A similar relationship has been reported with conditions such as constipation (Carr & Smith, 1995), otitis media (Luiselli, Cochran, & Huber, 2005; O'Reilly, 1997), and premenstrual syndrome (Carr, Smith, Giacin, Whelan, & Pancari, 2003). From a clinical perspective, care providers should consider a range of preventive and ameliorative health care treatments combined with evidence-based behavior supports.

Michael (1993) also proposed the term "abolishing operation" for events that *reduce* the effectiveness of consequences that were reinforcing and the frequency of behavior that has been reinforced. More recently, Friman and Hawkins (2006) suggested "disestablishing operation," or DO, to explain the same concept. Whereas deprivation is the critical element with an EO, satiation is linked to an abolishing/disestablishing operation. So for a child or adult who demonstrates challenging behaviors reinforced by adult attention, giving her or him more frequent and noncontingent praise and approval could be therapeutic because the motivation to behave inappropriately is lessened. Or challenging behaviors that are maintained by sensory consequences could be reduced by allowing the child or adult scheduled access to acceptable objects that produce the same or similar preferred stimulation.

In summary, this conceptual framework for antecedent intervention includes discriminative stimulus control and motivational operations (EO and DO). Acknowledging that an Sd and EO/DO are defined in relation to positive reinforcement, the distinction is that an Sd signals the availability of reinforcement, whereas an EO/DO determines the relative strength (effectiveness) of reinforcement.

My colleagues and I have evaluated several approaches to antecedent intervention with children and adults who have ID. One case, reported by Carlson, Luiselli, Slyman, and Markowski (2008), featured *choice making* as an intervention to reduce public disrobing and associated urinary incontinence displayed by a 13-year-old girl with autism and a 5-year-old boy with PDD-NOS. Functional behavioral assessment suggested that the children removed and urinated on their clothing because the customary consequence was to have them change into "preferred" apparel. The resulting intervention plan provided each child with daily, scheduled choice opportunities to change into alternative clothes presented by staff at their schools. Compared to a baseline phase, the choice-making intervention eliminated public disrobing and urinary incontinence by both children. This study identified the challenging behaviors as having a tangible-eliciting function and by giving the children acceptable choices to change their clothes, the procedure served as an abolishing operation that lessened their motivation to disrobe.

It is not unusual to implement several antecedent intervention procedures simultaneously. In Butler and Luiselli (2007), we combined *instructional fading* (Zarcone et al., 1993) and *noncontingent escape* (NCE) (Kodak, Miltenberger, & Romaniuk, 2003; Vollmer, Marcus, & Ringdahl, 1995) with a 13-year-old girl who had autism and escape-motivated self-injury, aggression, and tantrum outbursts. The NCE component of intervention allowed the girl a brief break from an instructional session starting at a fixed-time 20-second schedule (FT-20s) and advanced in 10- to 30-second increments whenever the challenging behaviors were recorded during 20% or less in a session. With instructional fading, requests initially were eliminated during sessions and thereafter, increased by two per session when challenging behaviors were recorded during 20% or less in a session. This multicomponent intervention plan successfully eliminated challenging behaviors, NCE was increased to a fixed-time 300-second schedule (FT-300s), and by the final session, the girl was responding correctly to one instructional request approximately every 20 seconds. Other instruction-focused antecedent intervention procedures for escape-motivated challenging behaviors have manipulated task preferences, duration, and difficulty (Dunlap, Kern-Dunlap, Clarke, & Robbins, 1991; Foster-Johnson, Ferno, & Dunlap, 1994; Kennedy, Itkoken, & Lindquist, 1995).

Luiselli, Ricciardi, Schmidt, and Tarr (2004) described an antecedent intervention evaluation with a 6-year-old boy who had autism and oral-motor stereotypy characterized by repetitive saliva play in which he placed his fingers in his mouth, rubbed together his saliva-coated fingers, and drooled saliva onto his chin. This study began with an FA that was conducted each day at the boy's school and confirmed that saliva play was maintained by oral-digital stimulation. The question that we posed was whether saliva play could be decreased by allowing the boy continuous access to alternative and competing sensory stimulation, either chewing gum or mouthing a hygienic "chew object"? Both types of stimulation were compared with a baseline (nonintervention) condition in a multielement experimental design. Saliva play persisted when the boy chewed gum but never occurred when he could access the "chew object." In a similar study, Ladd, Luiselli, and Baker (2009) decreased self-injurious finger picking in a 9-year-old girl with autism by giving her continuous access to preferred stimuli that she could manipulate with her hands. One interpretation of these findings is that to be optimally effective, antecedent intervention for stereotypy and self-injury through continuous access to sensory stimulation must include stimuli that are equally or more reinforcing than the stimulation that maintains the challenging behaviors.

Finally, Haley, Heick, and Luiselli (2010) conducted research with an 8-year-old boy who had autism and vocal stereotypy defined as "audible vocalizing of non-contextual and non-functional speech that included repetitive sounds, singing, humming, and phrases unrelated to the activity in progress" (p. 313). We evaluated intervention with the boy in his school classroom, under baseline (no intervention) conditions and during antecedent intervention phases that compared (1) presenting a cue card with the word "Quiet" (signifying that vocal stereotypy should not occur) and (2) presenting a visual card with the words "Okay to speak out" (signifying that vocal stereotypy could occur). The boy was first exposed to the cue cards during discrimination training sessions that preceded the intervention evaluation. We found that the presence of the "quiet" visual cue reduced vocal stereotypy from levels recorded during baseline and when the "okay to speak out" visual cue was present. Of clinical importance, the same results were documented when intervention was extended to a school setting outside of the boy's classroom.

CBT and Self-Management Training

Few studies have evaluated conventional CBT with people who have ID. However, there is some evidence that cognitive mediation plays a role in symptom presentation within this population (Nezu, Nezu, Rothenberg, DelliCarpini, & Groag, 1995). Focusing on clinical intervention, Nezu, Nezu, and Arean (1991) reported promising effects from assertiveness and problem-solving training with individuals who had mild ID. In a group comparison design, Sofronoff, Attwood, and Hinton (2005) explored CBT with children diagnosed with Asperger's disorder. Some of the children received a brief CBT intervention, some children received the same intervention combined with parent training, and some children formed a wait-list control group. Both intervention groups had significant decreases in parent-reported anxiety symptoms. Among children and adults with ID and other neurodevelopmental disorders, there are case reports of modified CBT being effective for obsessive-compulsive disorder (Pence, Aldea, Sulkowski, & Storch, 2011; Storch et al., 2011) and panic disorder (Hurley, 2007). The adapted CBT protocols in these cases (a) simplified written and spoken language, (b) incorporated visual cues, (c) relied on less sophisticated cognitive techniques, (d) made liberal use of contingency management "rewards," and (e) enlisted parents as therapy supports. Though promising, these CBT applications must be qualified because the research lacked experimental rigor and the intervention methods, though clinically justified, were so highly individualized that is difficult to generalize the findings to other people with the same disorders.

Dialectical behavior therapy (DBT) encompasses many CBT methods and several years ago, Lew, Matta, Tripp-Tebo, and Watts (2006) proposed a DBT model for adults with ID and comorbid psychiatric problems. Their rationale was that many people with ID have the same clinical presentation as typically developing individuals that have benefited from DBT. To best fit a pilot sample of eight adults (25–61 years old), Lew et al. (2006) modified the constituent "modes of therapy" in DBT, namely individual counseling, group skills training, coaching in crisis, supportive environmental treatment, and collaborative consultation (Linehan, 1993). As one example, skills training with groups emphasized hands-on experiences through music, pictures, and movies. Diary cards, a staple of DBT, were simplified and included graphic cues for nonreaders. Language, too, was altered from the standard DBT framework. Lew et al. (2006) reported outcome data for an 18-month evaluation period, but there was not sufficient experimental control to conclude about the therapeutic effects of DBT. Whether DBT is a viable modality for people with ID awaits further study.

Self-management training might be considered a variant of CBT because there is a mutually desired goal that children and adults learn to behave successfully without relying exclusively on external supports. Dixon and McKeel (2011) commented about self-management training in this way:

> Typical behavior management approaches require the caregiver to arrange learning opportunities, prompt and encourage positive (or reduction of negative) behaviors, and deliver appropriate consequences for task completion. When self-management is implemented, these caregiver responsibilities are transferred to the learner—that is, the learner now seeks out the conditions under which a behavior is to occur, responds within the current repertoire, and then self-reinforces appropriate behavior. The role of the caregiver is altered from managing contingencies to supporting successful implementation of the self-management system. Over time, both caregiver supervision and self-management programs can be faded so that naturalistic contingencies sustain the behavior of interest. (p. 111)

The preceding definition illustrates that self-management training combines several procedures (Shogren, Lang, Machalicek, Rispoli, and O'Reilly, 2011). With *self-monitoring* a person is taught to observe and accurately record her or his behavior. *Self-evaluation* has a person rate her or his behavior according to some relevant dimension (e.g., "acceptable" or "unacceptable"). Through *self-reinforcement* a person makes available or accesses pleasurable consequences when she or he achieves criteria specified in an intervention plan. It is likely that these three components contribute in different ways to the clinical effects produced with self-management training. That is, self-monitoring alone can promote behavior change independent of self-evaluation and self-reinforcement. Relative to self-evaluation, the corresponding valence (e.g., rating "positive" behaviors or "negative"

behaviors) can influence responding regardless of how self-monitoring was performed.

Koegel and Koegel (1990) sought to reduce vocal and motor stereotypy of four children with autism through self-management training that was initially conducted in a clinic setting. Therapists first taught the children to discriminate their stereotypic behaviors from appropriate, alternative behaviors. In the next phase of training, the children learned to place a check mark on a recording form immediately following timed intervals in which they did not display stereotypy. The intervals started at a low duration, increased gradually, and were cued by the chronograph alarm on a watch. Check marks were exchanged for preferred food items and toys that had been selected for each child. The final phase of self-management training had the therapists fade their instructional prompts, which were ultimately eliminated. A multiple baseline design evaluation showed that self-management training reduced stereotypy among all of the children. These clinic-based findings were also replicated when training was extended to novel community settings.

How does self-management training compare to other behavioral interventions? Shogren et al. (2011) reported that self-management was as effective as a teacher-implemented program for improving classroom behaviors (staying in seat, following directions) and academic engagement of two children with Asperger's disorder. Following a baseline phase, teachers presented tokens ("smiley faces") to the students following activities in which they complied with three classroom rules that were represented by drawings on a daily data sheet. Accumulated tokens could be exchanged for edible treats. Self-management training was virtually identical to these conditions except that "instead of one of the teachers marking down how well they did during each activity, the students would mark down how well they did with the marker that was on their data collection sheet" (p. 91). The positive effects of both the teacher implemented token program and self-management training endured 8 weeks post intervention. Social validity assessment revealed that the teachers preferred self-management because it was easier to apply and focused on student responsibility.

Drawing from the sparse CBT and self-management training literature with children and adults who have neurodevelopmental disorders, including ID, it appears that regardless of clinical objectives, procedures must be adapted to a person's learning challenges. Where applicable, cognitive-mediated strategies can facilitate generalization of skills acquired during therapy and training and, as noted, reduce reliance on external supports. To date, there are no absolute prerequisite abilities that would predict success from CBT and self-management training, notwithstanding that a child or adult should be able to understand basic directions, communicate effectively, follow task sequences (e.g., complete a self-monitoring recording form), and transfer skills to settings with reduced supervision. Absent these and related abilities, it is unlikely that CBT and self-management training would be indicated for people with severe-profound ID or those with co-occurring sensory, motor, and communication impairments (unspecified intellectual disability).

Conclusion

With nearly 50 years of experimental and clinical research, ABA is a dominant methodology in the field of ID. When considering function-based consequence and antecedent intervention, there are several tactics for enhancing ABA implementation and promoting desirable outcomes. As presented in this concluding section, they include stimulus preference assessment, intervention integrity, programming for generalization and maintenance, and social validity.

Stimulus Preference Assessment

Positive reinforcement is the basis of differential reinforcement and skill-building procedures. Hence, stimuli that will function as reinforcers must be identified. It is possible to select preferences by observing a child or adult participating in free-choice activities. Or questions about preferences can be posed to care providers. Unfortunately, these subjectively derived selections may not be supported empirically (Fisher, Piazza, Bowman, & Amari, 1996). Instead, preferences are best identified through formal assessment in which (a) a person is presented with different stimuli and choice options, (b) contact with selected stimuli are measured, and (c) preferences are rank-ordered on a high-to-low continuum. It is expected that high-preference stimuli will function as reinforcement more effectively than low-preference stimuli.

Behavior analysts have evaluated several methods for conducting stimulus preference assessment (DeLeon & Iwata, 1996; Fisher et al., 1992; Pace, Ivancic, Edwards, Iwata, & Page, 1985). With *single-stimulus preference assessment* a child or adult is presented with one stimulus such as a food item

or an object (e.g., toy, game, book). The percentage of food items consumed per opportunity and the duration of time engaged with objects would be measured, respectively. By contrast, *paired-stimulus assessment* offers the child or adult an option between two simultaneously presented choices. Rank-ordered preferences are then determined by calculating a selection percentage from the number of times each stimulus was available. Finally, with *multiple-stimulus assessment*, all stimuli are presented at the same time and each selected stimulus is either removed (multiple stimuli without replacement) or returned (multiple stimuli with replacement) during subsequent presentations.

It should be noted that even with stimulus preference assessment, high-ranked preferences may not always function as effective reinforcement. As such, additional assessment that incorporates novel stimuli may have to be conducted. Another finding with clinical implications is that identified high-preference stimuli can, and often do, change over time. Therefore, stimulus preference assessment should not be a one-time exercise but should be repeated routinely to ensure that high-quality reinforcers are always incorporated in a behavior support plan.

Intervention Integrity

Care providers such as classroom teachers, direct-support staff, and parents are usually responsible for implementing behavioral intervention with children and adults who have ID. Most behavior support plans include more than one procedure, and care providers must record occurrences of the intervention target behaviors. If the intervention and measurement procedures are not applied accurately, outcome evaluation is compromised. That is, a planned intervention could be judged to be ineffective based solely on poor implementation.

Intervention integrity assessment is the process of documenting that care providers implement instructional and behavior support procedures as specified in a written plan. DiGennaro Reed and Codding (2011) described how such assessment is usually performed. First, the steps within a plan are listed sequentially on a recording form. A clinician or consultant watches a care provider implementing the plan, scoring performance of each step as "implemented correctly," "implemented incorrectly," or "no opportunity to observe." Following observation the clinician or consultant reviews each plan step with the care provider during a brief 1:1 interaction. Using performance feedback (Codding,

Feinberg, Dunn, & Pace, 2005), the clinician or consultant praises the steps that were implemented correctly and reviews the steps that were implemented incorrectly. The review of incorrect steps might include practicing them a few times and answering questions to clarify procedural inconsistencies. It has been found that performance feedback initially is most effective when it is initiated immediately following observation. Contingent on performance improvement, it is possible to gradually reduce the frequency of feedback interactions. In addition to verbal feedback, a clinician or consultant can also inform the care provider by referencing a written summary sheet or graph (Hagermoser Sanetti, Luiselli, & Handler, 2007). Video modeling, in which a care provider views a highly competent performer implementing steps correctly, is yet another medium for providing feedback.

Low intervention integrity can sometimes improve through regularly scheduled performance feedback sessions, as outlined earlier. If integrity remains poor despite ongoing feedback, the clinician or consultant can intensify training with the care provider by having more rigorous practice sessions. Or simplifying the instructional or behavior support plan combined with feedback can increase intervention integrity to an acceptable level. Recently, Strohmeier, Mule, and Luiselli (2014) found that special education service providers had definitive preferences for methods to improve intervention integrity, namely receiving performance feedback, completing online training modules, avoiding supervisory meetings, and earning a financial "reward."

Generalization and Maintenance

In a seminal publication, Stokes and Baer (1977) admonished behavior analysts that generalization must be programmed rather than expected or lamented. They acknowledged the all-too-often observation that positive effects of intervention do not automatically transfer to novel (untreated) behaviors, settings, and people. For example, reducing or eliminating a child's self-injury does not guarantee the same result for co-occurring aggression. Similarly, successful intervention outcome with an adult at a day-habilitation setting may not occur in that person's home. Desirable intervention effects may also be specific to care providers who implemented the respective procedures with a child or adult but absent in the presence of people who do not have the same learning history with them.

Response, setting, and stimulus generalization are, of course, valued clinically and for this reason, there are several procedures that can and should be implemented. First, intervene in all relevant settings by having multiple care providers apply procedures. A second strategy is to target all challenging behaviors with a function-based intervention plan. From a skills perspective, it is desirable to teach responses that will contact "natural" sources of reinforcement such as praise and acknowledgment. Care providers should also be instructed in how to gradually withdraw intervention procedures to approximate the conditions found in nonintervention settings. I add that teaching self-regulation competencies to a child or adult can facilitate generalization, which has implications for further research about self-management training and CBT applications. A more detailed conceptual analysis and description of generalization programming strategies can be found in Ghezzi and Bishop (2008).

In rare cases, positive clinical change may persist without further intervention. However, like generalization, maintenance typically must be strategically programmed. Unfortunately, few studies have reported long-term maintenance outcomes, in part, because most applied settings do not have the resources available to conduct extended measurement months and years after planned intervention. One approach to support maintenance is gradually withdrawing procedures compromising an intervention plan following an extended period with low- to no-frequency challenging behaviors. Ideally, challenging behaviors should be brought under the control of natural contingencies that a person likely will encounter following intervention. In this regard, switching from tangible (primary) to social (secondary) reinforcement and from a continuous to intermittent reinforcement schedule is advised. Because most intervention plans initially demand close and continuous supervision by one or more care providers, relevant maintenance-facilitating strategies are to (a) withdraw supervision for brief periods that are increased slowly, (b) provide supervision on an unpredictable schedule, and (c) remove supervision while simultaneously transferring stimulus control to an alternative source such as an inanimate object. Lastly, because complete suppression of challenging behaviors is unusual in clinical practice, care providers in maintenance settings are likely to encounter the behaviors even if the frequency has been greatly reduced or the behaviors seemingly have been eliminated. As it pertains to maintenance then, clinicians and consultants should ensure that care providers are provided "maintenance plans," especially for individuals who may be unfamiliar with former intervention or have never witnessed the child or adult demonstrate the targeted challenging behaviors.

Social Validity

Social validity refers to the acceptability or viability of intervention objectives, procedures, and outcome (Schwartz & Baer, 1991; Wolf, 1978). The purpose of social validity assessment is to survey the consumers of behavioral intervention to determine whether the goals were important and relevant to desired lifestyle change, whether the procedures were acceptable, and whether the results were meaningful. Direct consumers are the clients themselves and their care providers. Indirect consumers would be community members, school principals, program administrators, and the like. Through social validity assessment, behavior clinicians and consultants are able to examine factors that lead to better intervention integrity, resonate positively with the people responsible for intervention, and promote acceptance by the public at large.

Social validity assessment methods include interviews, surveys, and questionnaires. Typically, several statements or questions are posed, such as "The behavior support plan for John helped him complete more instructional tasks" or "I found the intervention procedures for Mary easy to implement." Using a Likert-type scale, consumers respond to each statement or question by selecting a number ranking, for example, 1: I strongly disagree, 2: I disagree, 3: I have no opinion, 4: I somewhat agree, or 5: I strongly agree. Average scores for each item comprising the social validity assessment are calculated, making it possible to quantify an overall measure of acceptability and satisfaction. Following the advice of Schwartz and Baer (1991), it is best if social validity assessment includes observable behaviors that correlate with program approval.

Expert validation is another focus of social validity assessment. The usual method is for a clinician or consultant to have several experienced colleagues review the procedures and objectives of an intervention plan before implementation. Expert validation puts eyes on the technical aspects of proposed intervention by professionals who are knowledgeable about standards of practice and can advise on many matters that could influence outcome.

Future Directions

Future directions for ABA practice and research include comparing the effects of different intervention methods and evaluating variations of established procedures. Care provider training should also be emphasized: what types of instruction work best, are time efficient, and yield durable results? Certain intervention approaches such as teaching self-management deserve more attention given the need to expose people with ID to natural settings that may be unable to provide intensive supports. Concerning CBT, more research is clearly needed to expand its utility and treatment effectiveness whether as a primary therapeutic approach or in conjunction with other learning-based methods. Finally, clinicians and behavior specialists must continue to inquire about the efficacy of ABA and CBT not only for treating isolated challenging behaviors but also for improving a person's happiness, well-being, and quality of life.

References

Ahearn, W. H., Clark, K. M., DeBar, R., & Florentino, C. (2005). On the role of preference in response competition. *Journal of Applied Behavior Analysis, 38*, 247–250.

American Psychiatric Association. (2013). *Diagnostic and statistical manual of mental disorders* (5th ed). Washington, DC: Author.

Baer, D. M., Wolf, M. M., & Risley, T. R. (1968). Some current dimensions of applied behavior analysis. *Journal of Applied Behavior Analysis, 1*, 1–14.

Barlow, D. H., Nock, M. K., & Hersen, M. (2008). *Single-case experimental designs: Strategies for studying behavior change* (3rd ed.). Boston: Allyn & Bacon.

Bijou, S. W., Peterson, R. F., & Ault, M. H. (1968). A method to integrate descriptive and experimental field studies at the level of data and empirical concepts. *Journal of Applied Behavior Analysis, 1*, 175–191.

Butler, L. R., & Luiselli, J. K. (2007). Escape maintained problem behavior in a child with autism: Antecedent functional analysis and intervention evaluation of noncontingent escape (NCE) and instructional fading. *Journal of Positive Behavior Interventions, 9*, 195–202.

Carlson, J. I., Luiselli, J. K., Slyman, A., & Markowski, A. (2008). Choice-making as intervention for public disrobing in children with developmental disabilities. *Journal of Positive Behavior Interventions, 10*, 86–90.

Carr, E. G., & Durand, V. M. (1985). Reducing behavior problems through functional communication training. *Journal of Applied Behavior Analysis, 18*, 111–126.

Carr, E. G., Newsom, C. D., & Binkoff, J. A. (1980). Escape as a factor in the aggressive behavior of two retarded children. *Journal of Applied Behavior Analysis, 13*, 101–117.

Carr, E. G., & Smith, C. E. (1995). Biological setting events for self-injury. *Mental Retardation and Developmental Disabilities Research Reviews, 1*, 94–98.

Carr, E. G., Smith, C. E., Giacin, T. A., Whelan, B. M., & Pancari, J. (2003). Menstrual discomfort as a biological setting event for severe problem behavior: Assessment and intervention. *American Journal on Mental Retardation, 108,* 117–133.

Carr, J. E., & LeBlanc, L. A. (2006). Noncontingent reinforcement as antecedent behavior support. In J. K. Luiselli (Ed.), *Antecedent control: Innovative approaches to behavior support* (pp. 147–164). Baltimore, MD: Paul H. Brookes.

Cavalari, R. N. S., DuBard, M., Luiselli, J. K., & Birtwell, K. (2013). Teaching an adolescent with autism to tolerate routine medical examination: Effects of compliance training through graduated exposure and positive reinforcement. *Clinical Practice in Pediatric Psychology, 1,* 121–218.

Charlop-Christy, M. H., Carpenter, M., Le, L., LeBlanc, L. A., & Kellet, K. (2002). Using the Picture Exchange Communication System (PECS) with children with autism: Assessment of PECS acquisition, speech, social-communication behavior, and problem behavior. *Journal of Applied Behavior Analysis, 35,* 213–231.

Codding, R. S., Feinberg, A., Dunn, E. K., & Pace, G. M. (2005). Effects of immediate performance feedback in implementation of behavior support plans. *Journal of Applied Behavior Analysis, 38,* 205–219.

Cooper, J. O., Heron, T. E., & Heward, W. L. (2007). *Applied behavior analysis* (2nd ed.). Upper Saddle River, NJ: Pearson.

Cowdery, G. E., Iwata, B. A., & Pace, G. M. (1990). Effects and side effects of DRO as treatment for self-injurious behavior. *Journal of Applied Behavior Analysis, 23,* 497–506.

DeLeon, I. G., & Iwata, B. A. (1996). Evaluation of a multiple-stimulus presentation format for assessing reinforcer preferences. *Journal of Applied Behavior Analysis, 29,* 519–533.

DiGennaro Reed, F., & Codding, R. S. (2011). Intervention integrity assessment. In J. K. Luiselli (Ed.), *Teaching and behavior support for children and adults with autism spectrum disorder: A practitioner's guide* (pp. 38–47). New York: Oxford University Press.

Dixon, M. R., & McKeel, A. N. (2011). Self-management. In J. K. Luiselli (Ed.), *Teaching and behavior support for children and adults with autism spectrum disorder: A practitioner's guide* (pp. 111–116.). New York: Oxford University Press.

Dunlap, G., Kern-Dunlap, L., Clarke, S., & Robbins, F. R. (1991). Functional assessment, curricular revision, and severe problem behavior. *Journal of Applied Behavior Analysis, 24,* 387–397.

Durand, V. M., & Carr, E. G. (1991). Functional communication training to reduce challenging behavior: Maintenance and application in new settings. *Journal of Applied Behavior Analysis, 24,* 251–264.

Durand, V. M., & Crimmins, D. B. (1988). Identifying the variables maintaining self-injurious behavior. *Journal of Autism and Developmental Disorders, 18,* 99–117.

Fisher, W. W., Lindauer, S. E., Alterson, C. J., & Thompson, R. H. (1998). Assessment and treatment of destructive behavior maintained by stereotypic object manipulation. *Journal of Applied Behavior Analysis, 31,* 513–527.

Fisher, W. W., Piazza, C. C., Bowman, L. G., & Amari, A. (1996). Integrating caregiver report with a systematic choice assessment to enhance reinforcer identification. *American Journal on Mental Retardation, 101,* 15–25.

Fisher, W. W., Piazza, C. C., Bowman, L. G., Hagopian, L. P., Owens, L. C., & Slevin, I. (1992). A comparison of two approaches for identifying reinforcers for persons with severe and profound disabilities. *Journal of Applied Behavior Analysis, 25,* 491–498.

Foster-Johnson, L., Ferro, J., & Dunlap, G. (1994). Preferred curricular activities and reduced problem behaviors in students with intellectual disabilities. *Journal of Applied Behavior Analysis, 27,* 493–504.

Foxx, R. M., & Azrin, N. H. (1973). The elimination of autistic self-stimulatory behavior by overcorrection. *Journal of Applied Behavior Analysis, 6,* 1–14.

Friman, P. C., & Hawkins, R. O. (2006). Contribution of establishing operations to antecedent intervention. In J. K. Luiselli (Ed.), *Antecedent control: Innovative approaches to behavior support* (pp. 31–52). Baltimore, MD: Paul H. Brookes.

Ghezzi, P. M., & Bishop, M. R. (2008). Generalized behavior change in young children with autism. In J. K. Luiselli, D. C. Russo, W. P. Christian, & S. M. Wilczynski (Eds.), *Effective practices for children with autism: Educational and behavior support interventions that work* (pp. 137–158). New York: Oxford University Press.

Goh, H., Iwata, B. A., Shore, B. A., DeLeon, I. G., Lerman, D. C., Ulrich, S. M., & Smith, R. G. (1995). An analysis of the reinforcing properties of hand mouthing. *Journal of Applied Behavior Analysis, 28,* 269–283.

Grider, B., Luiselli, J. K., & Turcotte-Shamski, W. (2012). Graduated exposure, positive reinforcement, and stimulus distraction in a compliance-with-blood draw intervention for an adult with autism. *Clinical Case Studies, 11,* 253–260.

Hagermoser Sanetti, L., Luiselli, J. K., & Handler, M. W. (2007). Effects of verbal and graphic performance feedback on behavior support plan implementation in a public elementary school. *Behavior Modification, 31,* 454–465.

Hagopian, L. P., & Adelinis, J. D. (2001). Response blocking with and without redirection for the treatment of pica. *Journal of Applied Behavior Analysis, 34,* 527–530.

Hagopian, L. P., Fisher, W. W., & Legacy, S. M. (1994). Schedule effects of noncontingent reinforcement on attention-maintained destructive behavior in identical quadruplets. *Journal of Applied Behavior Analysis, 27,* 317–325.

Haley, J. L., Heick, P. F., & Luiselli, J. K. (2010). Use of an antecedent intervention to decrease vocal stereotypy of a student with autism in the general education classroom. *Child & Family Behavior Therapy, 32,* 311–321.

Hanley, G. P. (2010). Functional assessment of problem behavior: Dispelling myths, overcoming implementation obstacles, and developing new lore. *Behavior Analysis in Practice, 5,* 54–72.

Hanley, G. P., Iwata, B. A., & McCord, B. E. (2003). Functional analysis of problem behavior: A review. *Journal of Applied Behavior Analysis, 36,* 147–185.

Harris, J. (1996). Physical restraint procedures for managing challenging behaviors presented by mentally retarded adults and children. *Research in Developmental Disabilities, 17,* 99–134.

Harris, J. C. (2005). *Intellectual disability: Understanding its development, causes, classification, and treatment.* New York: Oxford University Press.

Hurley, A. D. (2007). A case of panic disorder treated with cognitive behavioral therapy. *Mental Health Aspects of Developmental Disabilities, 10,* 25–30.

Iwata, B. A. (1995). *Functional analysis screening tool (FAST).* Gainesville: University of Florida.

Iwata, B. A., Dorsey, M. F., Slifer, K. J., Bauman, K. E., & Richman, G. S. (1994). Toward a functional analysis of self-injury. *Journal of Applied Behavior Analysis, 27,* 197–209.

(Reprinted from *Analysis and Intervention in Developmental Disabilities, 2,* 3–20, 1982).

Iwata, B. A., Wallace, M. D., Kahng, S., Lindeberg, J. S., Roscoe, E. M., Conners, J., . . . Worsdell, A. S. (2000). Skill acquisition in the implementation of functional analysis methodology. *Journal of Applied Behavior Analysis, 33,* 181–194.

Johnson, L., McComas, J., Thompson, A., & Symons, F. J. (2004). Obtained versus programmed reinforcement: Practical considerations in the treatment of escape-reinforced aggression. *Journal of Applied Behavior Analysis, 37,* 239–242.

Kazdin, A. E. (2011). *Single-case research designs: Methods for clinical and applied settings* (2nd ed.). New York: Oxford University Press.

Kennedy, C. H., & Becker, A. (2006). Health conditions in antecedent assessment and intervention of problem behavior. In J. K. Luiselli (Ed.), *Antecedent control: Innovative approaches to behavior support* (pp. 73–97). Baltimore, MD: Paul H. Brookes.

Kennedy, C. H., Itkonen, T., & Lindquist, K. (1995). Comparing interspersed requests and social comments as antecedents for increasing student compliance. *Journal of Applied Behavior Analysis, 29,* 97–98.

Kennedy, C. H., & Meyer, K. A. (1996). Sleep deprivation, allergy symptoms, and negatively reinforced problem behavior. *Journal of Applied Behavior Analysis, 29,* 133–135.

Kern, L., & Kokina, A. (2008). Using positive reinforcement to decrease challenging behavior. In J. K. Luiselli, D. C. Russo, W. P. Christian, & S. M. Wilczynski (Eds.), *Effective practices for children with autism: Educational and behavior support interventions that work* (pp. 413–432). New York: Oxford University Press.

Kodak, T., Miltenberger, R. G., & Romaniuk, C. (2003). The effects of differential negative reinforcement of other behavior and noncontingent escape on compliance. *Journal of Applied Behavior Analysis, 36,* 379–382.

Koegel, R. L., & Koegel, L. K. (1990). Extended reductions in stereotypic behavior of students with autism through a self-management treatment package. *Journal of Applied Behavior Analysis, 23,* 119–127.

Ladd, M. V., Luiselli, J. K., & Baker, L. (2009). Continuous access to competing stimulation as intervention for self-injurious skin picking in a child with autism. *Child and Family Behavior Therapy, 31,* 54–60.

Lerman, D. C., Kelley, M. E., Vorndran, C. M., & Van Camp, C. M. (2003). Collateral effects of response blocking during the treatment of stereotypic behavior. *Journal of Applied Behavior Analysis, 36,* 119–123.

Lew, M., Matta, C., Tripp-Tebo, C., & Watts, D. (2006). Dialectical behavior therapy (DBT) for individuals with intellectual disabilities: A program description. *Mental Health Aspects of Developmental Disabilities, 9,* 1–12.

Lindberg, J. S., Iwata, B. A., & Kahng, S. W. (1999). On the relation between object manipulation and stereotypic self-injurious behavior. *Journal of Applied Behavior Analysis, 32,* 51–62.

Linehan, M. M. (1993). *Cognitive-behavioral treatment of borderline personality disorder.* New York: The Guilford Press.

Luiselli, J. K. (1988). Comparative analysis of sensory extinction treatments for self-injury. *Education and Treatment of Children, 11,* 149–156.

Luiselli, J. K. (1992a). Assessment and treatment of self-injury in a deaf-blind child. *Journal of Developmental and Physical Disorders, 4,* 219–226.

Luiselli, J. K. (1992b). Protective equipment. In J. K. Luiselli, J. L. Matson, & N. N. Singh (Eds.), *Analysis, assessment and treatment of self-injury* (pp. 235–268). New York: Springer-Verlag.

Luiselli, J. K. (2004). Behavior support and intervention: Current issues and practices in developmental disabilities. In J. L. Matson, R. B. Laud, & M. L. Matson (Eds.), *Behavior modification for persons with developmental disabilities: Treatments and supports* (pp. 33–54). Kingston, NY: NADD.

Luiselli, J. K. (2006). *Antecedent assessment and intervention: Supporting children and adults with developmental disabilities in community settings.* Baltimore, MD: Paul H. Brookes.

Luiselli, J. K. (2008). Antecedent (preventive) intervention. In J. K. Luiselli, D. C. Russo, W. P. Christian, & S. Wilczynski. *Effective practices for children with autism: Educational and behavior support interventions that work* (pp. 393–412). New York: Oxford University Press.

Luiselli, J. K. (2009). Physical restraint of people with intellectual disability: A review of implementation reduction and elimination procedures. *Journal of Applied Research in Intellectual Disability, 22,* 126–134.

Luiselli, J. K. (2011a). Fears and phobias. In J. K. Luiselli (Ed.), *Teaching and behavior support for children and adults with autism spectrum disorder: A practitioner's guide* (pp. 159–164). New York: Oxford University Press.

Luiselli, J. K. (Ed.). (2011b). *Teaching and behavior support for children and adults with autism spectrum disorder: A practitioner's guide.* New York: Oxford University Press.

Luiselli, J. K. (2011c). Therapeutic implementation of physical restraint. In J. K. Luiselli (Ed.), *Handbook of high-risk challenging behaviors in intellectual and developmental disabilities* (pp. 243–256). Baltimore, MD: Paul H. Brookes.

Luiselli, J. K. (Ed.). (2012). *Handbook of high-risk challenging behaviors in intellectual and developmental disabilities.* Baltimore, MD: Paul H. Brookes.

Luiselli, J. K., Cochran, M. L., & Huber, S. A. (2005). Effects of otitis media on a child with autism receiving behavioral intervention for self-injury. *Child and Family Behavior Therapy, 27,* 51–56.

Luiselli, J. K., Helfen, C. S., Colozzi, G., Donellon, S., & Pemberton, B. (1978). Controlling self-inflicted biting of a retarded child by the differential reinforcement of other behavior. *Psychological Reports, 42,* 435–438.

Luiselli, J. K., Ricciardi, J. N., Schmidt, S., & Tarr, M. (2004). Brief functional analysis and intervention evaluation for treatment of saliva-play. *Child and Family Behavior Therapy, 26,* 53–61.

Luiselli, J. K., & Waldstein, N. (1994). Evaluation of restraint-elimination interventions for students with multiple disabilities in a pediatric nursing-care setting. *Behavior Modification, 18,* 352–365.

Martens, B. K., DiGennaro, F. D., Reed, D. D., Szczech, F. M., & Rosenthal, B. D. (2008). Contingency space analysis: An alternative method for identifying contingent relations from observational data. *Journal of Applied Behavior Analysis, 41,* 69–81.

Matson, J. L. (Ed.). (2009). *Applied behavior analysis for children with autism spectrum disorders.* New York: Springer.

Matson, J. L., & Minshawi, N. F. (2007). Functional assessment of challenging behavior: Toward a strategy for applied settings. *Research in Developmental Disabilities, 28,* 353–361.

Matson, J. L., & Vollmer, T. R. (1995). *User's guide: Questions about behavioral function (QABF).* Baton Rouge, LA: Scientific Publishers.

Michael, J. (1993). Establishing operations. *Behavior Analyst, 16*, 191–206.

Moore, J. W., Edwards, R. P., Sterling-Turner, H. E., Riley, J., DuBard, M., & McGeorge, A. (2002). Teacher acquisition of functional analysis methodology. *Journal of Applied Behavior Analysis, 35*, 73–77.

Moore, J. M., & Fisher, W. W. (2007). The effects of videotape modeling on staff acquisition of functional analysis methodology. *Journal of Applied Behavior Analysis, 40*, 197–202.

Moore, J. W., Fisher, W. W., & Pennington, A. (2004). Systematic application and removal of protective equipment in the assessment of multiple topographies of self-injury. *Journal of Applied Behavior Analysis, 37*, 73–77.

Nezu, C. M., Nezu, A. M., & Arean, P. (1991). Assertiveness and problem-solving training for mildly mentally retarded persons with dual diagnoses. *Research in Developmental Disabilities, 12*, 371–386.

Nezu, C. M., Nezu, A. M., Rothenberg, J. L., DelliCarpini, L., & Groag, I. (1995). Depression in adults with mild mental retardation: Are cognitive variables involved? *Cognitive Therapy and Research, 19*, 227–239.

O'Callaghan, P. M., Allen, K. D., Powell, S., & Salama, F. (2006). The efficacy of noncontingent escape for decreasing children's disruptive behavior during restorative dental treatment. *Journal of Applied Behavior Analysis, 39*, 161–171.

Oliver, C., Hall, S., Hales, J., Murphy, G., & Watts, D. (1998). The treatment of self-injurious behavior by the systematic fading of restraints: Effects on self-injury, self-restraint, adaptive behavior, and behavioral correlates of affect. *Research in Developmental Disabilities, 19*, 143–165.

O'Neill, R. E., Horner, R. H., Albin, R. W., Sprague, J. R., Storey, K., & Newton, J. S. (1997). *Functional assessment and program development for problem behavior: A practical handbook.* Pacific Grove, CA: Brookes/Cole.

O'Reilly, M. F. (1997). Functional analysis of episodic self-injury correlated with recurrent otitis media. *Journal of Applied Behavior Analysis, 30*, 165–167.

Pace, G. M., Ivancic, M. T., Edwards, G. L., Iwata, B. A., & Page, T. J. (1985). Assessment of stimulus preference assessment and reinforcer value with profoundly retarded individuals. *Journal of Applied Behavior Analysis, 18*, 249–255.

Pence, S. L., Aldea, M. A., Sulkowski, M. L., & Storch, E. A. (2011). Cognitive behavioral therapy in adults with obsessive-compulsive disorder and borderline intellectual functioning: A case series of three patients. *Journal of Developmental and Physical Disabilities, 23*, 71–85.

Peterson, S. M., Caniglia, C., Royster, A. J., Macfarlane, E., Plowman, K., Baird, S. J., & Wu, N. (2005). Blending functional communication training and choice making to improve task engagement and decrease problem behavior. *Educational Psychology, 25*, 257–274.

Peyton, R., Lindauer, S. E., & Richman, D. M. (2005). The effects of directive and nondirective prompts on noncompliant vocal behavior exhibited by a child with autism. *Journal of Applied Behavior Analysis, 38*, 251–255.

Piazza, C. C., Adelinis, J. D., Hanley, G. P., Goh, H. L., & Delia, M. D. (2000). An evaluation of the effects of matched stimuli on behaviors maintained by automatic reinforcement. *Journal of Applied Behavior Analysis, 33*, 13–27.

Reed, D. D., & Azulay, R. L. (2011). Functional behavioral assessment (FBA). In J. K. Luiselli (Ed.), *Teaching and behavior support for children and adults with autism spectrum disorder: A practitioner's guide* (pp. 13–21). New York: Oxford University Press.

Reed, D. D., Luiselli, J. K., Morizio, L. C., & Child, S. N. (2010). Sequential modification and the identification of instructional components occasioning self-injurious behavior. *Child & Family Behavior Therapy, 32*, 1–16.

Reid, D. H., Parsons, M. B., Phillips, J. F., & Green, C. W. (1993). Reduction of self-injurious hand mouthing using response blocking. *Journal of Applied Behavior Analysis, 26*, 139–140.

Repp, A. C., & Deitz, S. M. (1974). Reducing aggressive and self-injurious behavior of institutionalized retarded children through reinforcement of other behaviors. *Journal of Applied Behavior Analysis, 7*, 313–325.

Ricciardi, J. N. (2006). Combining antecedent and consequence procedures in multicomponent behavior support plans: A guide to writing plans with functional efficacy. In J. K. Luiselli (Ed.), *Antecedent control: Innovative approaches to behavior support* (pp. 227–245). *Baltimore, MD: Brookes.*

Ricciardi, J. N., Luiselli, J. K., & Cammare, M. (2006). Shaping approach responses as intervention for specific phobia in a child with autism. *Journal of Applied Behavior Analysis, 39*, 445–448.

Rincover, A., Cook, A. R., Peoples, A., & Packard, D. (1979). Sensory extinction and sensory reinforcement principles for programming multiple adaptive behavior change. *Journal of Applied Behavior Analysis, 12*, 221–233.

Rincover, A., & Devany, J. (1982). The application of sensory extinction to self-injury. *Analysis and Intervention in Developmental Disabilities, 2*, 67–82.

Ringdahl, J. E., Vollmer, T. R., Marcus, B. A., & Roane, H. S. (1997). An analogue evaluation of environmental enrichment: The role of stimulus preference. *Journal of Applied Behavior Analysis, 30*, 203–216.

Schwartz, I. S., & Baer, D. M. (1991). Social validity assessments: Is current practice state of the art? *Journal of Applied Behavior Analysis, 24*, 189–204.

Shogren, K. A., Lang, R., Machalicek, W., Rispoli, M. J., & O'Reilly, M. (2011). Self- versus teacher management of behavior for elementary school students with Asperger syndrome: Impact on classroom behavior. *Journal of Positive Behavior Interventions, 13*, 87–96.

Sigafoos, J., Arthur, M., & O'Reilly, M. F. (2003). Effects of speech output on maintenance of requesting and frequency of vocalizations in three children with developmental disabilities. *Augmentative and Alternative Communication, 19*, 37–47.

Simmons, J. N., Smith, R. G., & Kliethermes, L. (2003). A multiple-schedule evaluation of immediate and subsequent effects of fixed-time food presentation on automatically maintained mouthing. *Journal of Applied Behavior Analysis, 36*, 541–544.

Skinner, B. F. (1948). "Superstition" in the pigeon. *Journal of Experimental Psychology, 38*, 168–172.

Sofronoff, K., Attwood, T., & Hinton, C. (2005). A cognitive behaviour therapy intervention for anxiety in children with Asperger's syndrome. *Good Autism Practice, 3*, 2–8.

Stokes, T. F., & Baer, D. M. (1977). An implicit technology of generalization. *Journal of Applied Behavior Analysis, 10*, 349–367.

Stokes, J. V., & Luiselli, J. K. (2008). In-home parent training of functional analysis skills. *International Journal of Behavioral Consultation and Therapy, 4*, 259–263.

Storch, E. A., Rahman, O., Morgan, J., Brauer, L., Miller, J., & Murphy, T. K. (2011). Case series of behavioral psychotherapy for obsessive-compulsive symptoms in youth with Prader-Willi syndrome. *Journal of Developmental and Physical Disabilities, 23,* 359–368.

Strohmeier, C., Mule, C., & Luiselli, J. K. (2014). Social validity assessment of training methods to improve treatment integrity of special education service providers. *Behavior Analysis in Practice, 7,* 15–20.

Tang, J., Patterson, T. G., & Kennedy, C. H. (2003). Identifying specific sensory modalities maintaining the stereotypy of students with multiple profound disabilities. *Research in Developmental Disabilities, 24,* 433–451.

Thompson, R. H., Fisher, W. W., Piazza, C. C., & Kuhn, D. E. (1998). The evaluation and treatment of aggression maintained by attention and automatic reinforcement. *Journal of Applied Behavior Analysis, 31,* 103–116.

Touchette, P. E., MacDonald, R. F., & Langer, S. N. (1985). A scatter plot for identifying stimulus control of problem behavior. *Journal of Applied Behavior Analysis, 18,* 343–351.

Vollmer, T. R., Iwata, B. A., Zarcone, J. R., Smith, R. G., & Mazaleski, J. L. (1993). The role of attention in the treatment of attention-maintained self-injurious behavior: Noncontingent reinforcement and differential reinforcement of other behavior. *Journal of Applied Behavior Analysis, 26,* 9–21.

Vollmer, T. R., Marcus, B. A., & LeBlanc, L. A. (1994). Treatment of self-injury and hand mouthing following inconclusive functional analyses. *Journal of Applied Behavior Analysis, 27,* 331–344.

Vollmer, T. R., Marcus, B. A., & Ringdahl, J. E. (1995). Noncontingent escape as treatment for self-injurious behavior maintained by negative reinforcement. *Journal of Applied Behavior Analysis, 28,* 15–26.

Wallace, M. D., Iwata, B. A., Zhou, L., & Goff, G. A. (1999). Rapid assessment of the effects of restraint on self-injury and adaptive behavior. *Journal of Applied Behavior Analysis, 32,* 525–528.

Wolf, M. M. (1978). Social validity: The case for subjective measurement or how applied behavior analysis is finding its heart. *Journal of Applied Behavior Analysis, 11,* 203–214.

Zarcone, J. R., Iwata, B. A., Vollmer, T. A., Jagtiani, S., Smith, R. G., & Mazaleski, J. L. (1993). Extinction of self-injurious escape behavior with and without instructional fading. *Journal of Applied Behavior Analysis, 26,* 353–360.

Zhou, L., Goff, G. A., & Iwata, B. A. (2000). Effects of increased response effort on self-injury and object manipulation as competing response. *Journal of Applied Behavior Analysis, 33,* 29–40.

Zhou, L., Iwata, B. A., & Shore, B. A. (2002). Reinforcing efficacy of food on performance during pre- and post-meal sessions. *Journal of Applied Behavior Analysis, 35,* 411–414.

Delivery, Evaluation, and Future Directions for Cognitive-Behavioral Treatments of Obesity

Gareth R. Dutton *and* Michael G. Perri

Abstract

Cognitive-behavioral treatment for weight management involves the application of cognitive and behavioral principles and techniques, including self-monitoring, goal setting, problem solving, and cognitive restructuring, to modify eating behaviors and physical activity. Treatment is based on the principles of classical conditioning, operant conditioning, and social cognitive theory. Treatment is most commonly offered in weekly group sessions lasting up to 6 months. Reduction of 8%-10% of initial body weight is typical, which is associated with clinically meaningful improvements in several chronic conditions. Weight regain is common following treatment, although about 20% of participants achieve long-term success. The provision of extended care contacts following initial treatment significantly improves weight loss maintenance. While efficacy trials document the significant outcomes of behavioral interventions, additional research examining the effectiveness and dissemination of these treatments into applied real-world settings is needed. Additional research focused on young adults, older adults, and at-risk groups (e.g., racial minorities) is also warranted.

Key Words: overweight, obesity, weight loss, behavioral treatment, lifestyle intervention, efficacy, effectiveness

Introduction
Definition of Obesity

Overweight and obesity can be defined or measured in several ways, although body mass index (BMI) is the most common method for establishing weight status in epidemiological surveys as well as clinical assessments (National Heart, Lung, and Blood Institute [NHLBI], 1998). BMI is calculated by dividing one's weight (in kilograms) by one's height (in meters) squared (i.e., BMI = kg/m^2). Based on this calculation, normal weight is defined as a BMI between 18.5 and 24.9 kg/m^2. Overweight status is defined as a BMI of 25.0-29.9 kg/m^2, while obesity is defined as a BMI ≥ 30 kg/m^2. The category of obesity can be further divided by levels of severity, including Class 1 (30.0-34.9 kg/m^2), Class 2 (35.0-39.9 kg/m^2), and Class 3 obesity (≥40.0 kg/m^2).

Prevalence of Obesity

Recent epidemiological data indicate that more than two thirds (68.5%) of adults in the United States are overweight (i.e., ≥25 kg/m^2). Further, the prevalence of obesity (i.e., BMI ≥30 kg/m^2) is nearly 35% (Ogden, Carroll, Kit, & Flegal, 2014). Certain groups, including ethnic minorities, are at even greater risk. For instance, 33% of White women are obese compared to approximately 44% of Mexican American women and 57% of Black women (Ogden et al., 2014). Additional risk factors for excess weight include lower socioeconomic status, less education, and older age (Flegal, Carroll, Kit, & Ogden, 2012; Valdez & Williamson, 2002). Excess weight among US children and adolescents has increased in recent years as well, with current estimates

419

indicating that approximately 32% are overweight or obese (Ogden, Carroll, Kit, & Flegal, 2012; Ogden et al., 2014). However, there are encouraging indications that the prevalence of obesity among younger children (aged <5 years) has decreased based on recent estimates (Ogden et al., 2014).

Consequences of Obesity

There are a number of chronic and costly medical conditions associated with excess body weight. Overweight and obese individuals are at increased risk of hypertension, hyperlipidemia, type 2 diabetes, stroke, osteoarthritis, certain types of cancers, and sleep apnea (Field, Barnoya, & Colditz, 2002; NHLBI, 1998). Higher BMI is associated with increased depressive symptoms, diminished physical functioning, and reduced quality of life as well (Coakley et al., 1998; Fine et al., 1999; Petry, Barry, Pietrzak, & Wagner, 2008; Zhao et al., 2009). Obesity is related to increased overall mortality, which is primarily due to deaths from cardiovascular disease, certain types of cancers, and diabetes/kidney diseases (Flegal, Graubard, Williamson, & Gail, 2007). Not surprisingly, health care expenditures are significantly higher among overweight and obese individuals (Bell, Zimmerman, Arterburn, & Maciejewski, 2011). Based on 2006 estimates, obesity-related health care costs were $86 billion annually (Finkelstein, Trogdon, Cohen, & Dietz, 2009). At the individual level, this corresponded to $1,429 more in annual medical spending for obese patients as compared to normal-weight patients (Finkelstein et al., 2009).

Overview of Treatment Approaches

Given the prevalence as well as the consequences of obesity, the development and dissemination of effective weight loss treatments are imperative. Obesity treatment options can be broadly categorized into one of three approaches, including (1) pharmacotherapy; (2) surgical intervention; and (3) cognitive-behavioral, or lifestyle, interventions. While each approach has merits and limitations, behavioral interventions have been the most commonly employed treatment method and have a large amount of data supporting their utility. Also, it is generally accepted that other types of obesity treatment, including surgery and medications, include some components of cognitive-behavioral treatment as well. While a detailed description of nonbehavioral approaches is beyond the scope of this work, a brief summary of pharmacological and surgical interventions is provided later. Also, Table 23.1 provides a summary of treatment options, including behavioral treatment, pharmacotherapy, and surgery, appropriate for different levels of overweight and obesity.

Nonbehavioral Approaches to Weight Management
Pharmacotherapy

There are a few options for the pharmacological treatment of obesity. Orlistat, a lipase inhibitor that reduces the intestine's absorption of dietary fat, is one medication currently approved for weight management (Fujioka & Lee, 2007; Powell, Apovian, & Aronne, 2011). There are also a handful of appetite suppressants, including phentermine, that are approved for weight loss, although these are only recommended for short-term use (i.e., less than

Table 23.1 Weight Management Treatment Options Based on Weight Status

Weight Category	BMI Range (kg/m²)	Behavioral/ Lifestyle	Pharmacotherapy	Surgery
Overweight	25.0–29.9	√	√ (with presence of weight-related comorbidity and BMI >27)	
Class 1 Obesity	30.0–34.9	√	√	
Class 2 Obesity	35.0–39.9	√	√	√ (with presence of weight-related comorbidity)
Class 3 Obesity	>40	√	√	√

3 months) due to potential adverse cardiovascular effects and the potential for drug tolerance (Fujioka & Lee, 2007; Powell et al., 2011). There are other medications, such as metformin (indicated for the treatment of type 2 diabetes), bupropion (indicated for the treatment of depression), and topiramate (indicated for the treatment of epilepsy and migraine headaches), which previously have been used off-label for weight management as well (Fujioka & Lee, 2007; LeBlanc, O'Connor, Whitlock, Patnode, & Kapka, 2011). However, two new medications were recently approved for the treatment of obesity, including lorcaserin (Smith et al., 2010) and a combination of phentermine/topiramate (Allison et al., 2011; Garvey et al., 2012).

Bariatric Surgery

There are a few surgical options available for the treatment of obesity, although bariatric surgery is currently reserved for patients with a BMI >40 kg/m^2 or those with a BMI >35 kg/m^2 who are also diagnosed with one or more weight-related comorbidities, such as type 2 diabetes or sleep apnea (National Institutes of Health [NIH], 1992). The most common bariatric procedures include Roux-en-Y gastric bypass and adjustable gastric banding (Vetter, Dumon, & Williams, 2011). Gastric bypass involves creating a small gastric pouch from a portion of the stomach. This gastric pouch is surgically disconnected from the remaining section of the stomach and reconnected further down the intestinal tract, resulting in food bypassing 95% of the stomach. With gastric banding, an inflatable silicone band is placed around a portion of the stomach to create a small gastric pouch, and the band's diameter can be adjusted depending on the amount of weight loss achieved and side effects experienced (Vetter et al., 2011). Bariatric surgery can produce significant weight loss that is greater than weight loss achieved with other methods, although surgery is associated with greater risk and potential complications, including infection, embolism, and gastrointestinal leaks (Colquitt, Picot, Loveman, & Clegg, 2009; Vetter et al., 2011).

Cognitive-Behavioral Conceptualization of Obesity

Cognitive-behavioral treatment for obesity targets clients' eating habits, physical activity, and thought patterns. Cognitive-behavioral approaches to weight management are largely based on theories of classical conditioning and operant conditioning (Ferster, Nurnberger, & Levitt, 1962; Foster, Makris, & Bailer, 2005; Stuart, 1967; Wadden & Foster, 2000). From the perspective of classical conditioning, eating behaviors co-occur within the context of other activities, situations, and locations, and these pairings become associated through repeated experience. The association is strengthened with repeated pairings, and these antecedents become powerful triggers for eating behaviors. In fact, eating is often associated with a number of triggers, which highlights the importance of understanding the "behavior chain" that ultimately leads to undesirable eating and activity habits. A primary goal of treatment is to help clients identify these triggers in order to break associations and replace them with healthier, alternative responses.

Principles of operant conditioning are also important in the treatment of obesity. In this paradigm, the likelihood of adopting and maintaining behaviors can be increased or decreased depending on the positive or negative consequences of those behaviors. For eating behaviors and physical activity, the short-term consequences of unhealthy eating and inactivity tend to be positive (e.g., enjoyable taste of high-calorie food) despite the potentially negative, long-term consequences of these behaviors (e.g., excess weight gain, development of weight-related medical conditions, weight-based social stigma). This contrast in the valence of short- and long-term consequences of health behaviors can make modifying these behaviors particularly challenging. Therefore, behavioral treatment aims to help clients identify and employ short-term reinforcement of the adoption of healthy eating and activity behaviors in order to facilitate successful behavior change. Self-monitoring of eating and activity behaviors (described in more detail later) is also useful in helping clients identify antecedents and consequences that facilitate or hinder adoption of these behavioral goals.

The more recent generation of cognitive-behavioral protocols for obesity treatment has extended beyond the application of classical and operant conditioning to include constructs from social cognitive theory (Bandura, 1986) as well. Thus, addressing issues of social support and social context, identifying personalized motivational factors, enhancing problem-solving skills, and bolstering self-efficacy for behavior change have become important components of treatment. Similarly, treatment does not focus only on the modification of overt eating and activity behaviors; it includes the identification and modification of maladaptive or irrational cognitions related to food, weight loss, and one's ability to successfully navigate behavioral changes as well.

Similar to other dietary approaches to weight management, cognitive-behavioral treatment subscribes to the basic principle that excess weight results from consuming more energy through food than is expended through basic physiological functioning, daily activities, and exercise. Because this energy surplus results in weight gain, individuals are directed to decrease their energy intake (i.e., caloric and fat intake) while increasing their energy expenditure through physical activity. Although this energy balance equation is simple on a theoretical level, implementation of these lifestyle changes is less straightforward. Modification of dietary and physical activity behaviors occurs within the complexities of social and familial networks, cultural attitudes and practices, and other environmental constraints. Brownell and others have described a "toxic environment," which refers to social, environmental, organizational, and technological forces that encourage intake of high-fat, high-sugar foods while discouraging energy expenditure through increasingly sedentary lifestyles (Horgen & Brownel, 1998). In addition, genetic, metabolic, hormonal, and other biological factors clearly influence weight status and one's ability to lose weight (Cummings et al., 2002; Wadden, Foster, Letizia, & Mullen, 1990; Wren et al., 2001). Indeed, these biological factors predispose certain individuals to develop obesity and may determine the actual

weight range that can be achieved by those attempting weight loss (Foster et al., 2005).

While acknowledging these biological and environmental factors impacting weight, cognitive-behavioral treatment incorporates a variety of evidence-based strategies to help clients develop and refine a set of skills that lead to healthier diets, physical activity, and cognitions. Wadden and Foster (2000) summarized three guiding principles of cognitive-behavioral treatments for obesity. First, treatment is goal directed, and there is an emphasis on creating goals that are specific, measurable, and realistic. Second, treatment is process oriented and actively involves the client. More specifically, treatment is focused on building and practicing skills that allow individuals to achieve specified goals. When goals are not attained, active problem-solving skills are employed to develop new strategies to address barriers (Foster et al., 2005). Finally, treatment is focused on incremental, short-term, and cumulative changes in behavior (Wadden & Foster, 2000). Figure 23.1 illustrates how these overarching principles of cognitive-behavioral treatment can be put into practice with clients.

Components of Cognitive-Behavioral Treatment
Self-Monitoring

Similar to cognitive-behavioral interventions targeting other psychological and physical conditions, a fundamental component of obesity

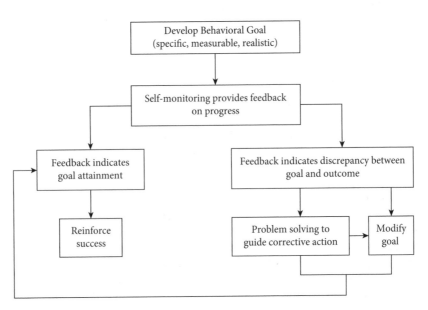

Figure 23.1 Process-oriented and goal-directed activities in cognitive-behavioral treatment.

treatment includes self-monitoring. At a minimum, self-monitoring involves daily recordings of food intake, including caloric/fat values of food consumed and time of meals and snacks. Clients are initially instructed to monitor, but not change, their eating patterns. Participants may also be encouraged to monitor other aspects of their dietary intake, such as location or situation of consumption as well as mood or cognitions experienced at the time. This additional information can be useful to help clients identify triggers and high-risk situations for eating and/or overeating. Self-monitoring of physical activity (i.e., minutes per day or step counts) is also useful to track physical activity levels and goal attainment.

Nutrition and Exercise Education

A necessary component of treatment, particularly in the first few sessions, includes education on appropriate levels of nutritional intake, with a particular focus on kilocalories and fat grams consumed. To achieve this goal, clients are taught how to weigh and measure foods so that accurate estimates can be recorded and appropriate portion sizes are achieved. Clients learn how to accurately read and interpret food labels in order to make appropriate and informed food selections. They also receive information about how to modify recipes and make food substitutions to reduce caloric and fat intake. While the focus is on caloric and fat intake, clients also receive information on the recommended levels of other nutrients, including fiber, protein, and calcium, in order to achieve a balanced and healthy diet. These efforts also help clients discover foods that increase satiety in order to prevent overeating during and between meals.

In addition to nutritional counseling, clients are taught about various forms of physical activity and how much energy is expended with different types of activity. Both programmed exercise (e.g., cycling, aerobic classes) as well as lifestyle modifications (e.g., taking the stairs rather than the elevator) are reviewed and encouraged. Moderate-intensity activities, such as brisk walking, are most commonly recommended. Clients learn about appropriate methods for warming up, cooling down, and stretching in order to reduce injury. While nutritional and activity education is a necessary component of treatment, this involves more than direct provision of information. Rather, health education is incorporated into an interactive process of helping clients set behavioral targets, provide corrective feedback, and encourage reinforcement of behavioral modification.

Behavior Modification and Goal Setting

Once clients are taught to accurately measure and record dietary intake and physical activity, they are then encouraged to reduce their caloric/fat intake in order to achieve an energy deficit for weight loss. Typically, clients are instructed to consume 1,200-1,600 kcal/day, although the exact goal may depend on the individual's baseline weight and activity level (NHLBI, 1998). As caloric intake is reduced, it is important that clients also monitor proteins, carbohydrates, and fats to ensure they are consuming appropriate and balanced amounts of each macronutrient. Although the precise proportions of nutrient intake may depend on the specifics of the program as well as individualized needs of the client, recommended ranges of energy intake include 45%-65% for carbohydrates, 10%-35% for protein, and 20%-35% for fats (US Department of Agriculture & US Department of Health and Human Services, 2010). In particular, adequate protein intake is important to avoid excess loss of muscle mass during weight loss treatment.

As for physical activity, a goal of at least 30 minutes of moderate-intensity activity on at least 5 days per week (i.e., 150 minutes/week) is typical of behavioral programs (NHLBI, 1998; Wadden, Butryn, & Byrne, 2004), which is consistent with current physical activity guidelines (US Department of Health and Human Services, 2008). National guidelines further recommend that increasing levels of aerobic activity to 300 minutes/week and incorporating muscle-strengthening exercises have additional health benefits as well (US Department of Health and Human Services, 2008). Gradual changes in activity levels are advised, and goals are tailored to the baseline activity levels, activity preferences, and physical limitations of clients. Also, evidence suggests that multiple short bouts of activity (i.e., 10-minute periods) are comparably effective to a single, long bout of activity (Jakicic, Wing, Butler, & Robertson, 1995; Jakicic, Winters, Lang, & Wing, 1999).

In addition to the dietary and physical activity goals prescribed to clients, participants are taught how to set other goals during treatment. As mentioned previously, behavioral therapy is goal oriented, so it is important that clients set goals that are specific and measurable (e.g., "consume three servings of vegetables per day" rather than "eat healthier foods"). After such goals have been established, clients should explore factors that will promote goal attainment while identifying factors that may impede successful implementation and outcomes (Foster et al., 2005). Clients are typically encouraged to formulate one or more weekly goals to work on between treatment sessions.

Problem Solving

Closely related to goal setting, problem-solving skills training is another foundational component of cognitive-behavioral obesity treatment. To cope more effectively with treatment barriers and setbacks, problem-solving therapy is designed to target both "motivational" deficits (i.e., negative affective and cognitive responses) as well as behavioral skills deficits (Nezu, Nezu, & Perri, 2006). A defined problem-solving model is employed, which includes the following five steps: (1) problem orientation, (2) problem definition, (3) generation of alternative solutions, (4) decision making to identify the best solution, and (5) implementation and evaluation of selected solution (Murawski et al., 2009; Perri et al., 2001). Effective problem-solving skills have been associated with initial weight loss (Murawski et al., 2009) as well as successful weight loss maintenance (Perri et al., 2001).

Stimulus Control

Stimulus control refers to modification of one's environment to increase the likelihood of engaging in behaviors that promote weight loss while discouraging circumstances that interfere with treatment success (Berkel, Poston, Reeves, & Foreyt, 2005). For instance, clients may be encouraged to keep healthy, low-calorie snacks with them to avoid unplanned eating episodes and decisions to consume "fast food" or similar high-calorie snacks. Another example of stimulus control would be having clients keep a gym bag with comfortable clothes and sneakers in their car to promote walking during their lunch break or at the end of the workday.

Social Support

Therapists as well as peers (for treatment delivered in groups) can serve as important sources of social support for clients attempting weight loss. In addition, cognitive-behavioral interventions encourage clients to identify and enlist additional sources of support from family members, coworkers, friends, and others who may be able to offer emotional encouragement and assistance in meeting program goals (e.g., providing child care while one goes to the gym). Clients are also taught how to use effective communication strategies to deal with unsupportive or "difficult" individuals and high-risk social situations. Treatment sessions can include opportunities to role-play various social situations in order to practice and refine clients' skills in building social support and improving assertive communication. Studies with clinical and community samples have illustrated the important role that social support and social influences/norms can play on individuals' intentions to lose weight as well as weight loss success (Gorin et al., 2005; Leahey, Crowther, & Ciesla, 2011; Wing & Jeffery, 1999).

Cognitive Restructuring

Clients are taught to recognize, challenge, and modify irrational thoughts that contribute to negative mood states and counterproductive health behaviors. Common maladaptive thought patterns, such as dichotomous (all-or-none) thinking, "should" or "must" statements, fortune telling, and catastrophizing, are reviewed and discussed in the context of their impact on eating and activity behaviors. In this way, cognitive therapy for obesity is very similar to the rationale, approach, and strategies employed in the treatment of depressive and anxiety disorders (Beck, 1976). Cognitive restructuring can be particularly useful for improving behavioral and affective responses to setbacks or slips encountered during weight loss efforts (Wadden & Foster, 2000). This technique can also be useful for clients who engage in overly critical and punitive self-talk in order to enhance self-efficacy and self-esteem (Berkel et al., 2005).

Relapse Prevention

Based on the relapse prevention framework (Brownell, Marlatt, Lichtenstein, & Wilson, 1986), clients are taught to distinguish between a lapse (isolated slip back into previously unhealthy behavior) and a relapse (a consistent return to previous behavior). Once this distinction is clear, therapists stress the importance of problem solving, cognitive restructuring, stimulus control, and other strategies to ensure that a lapse does not lead to a full-blown relapse. Related to this, it is helpful to frame the causes of setbacks as a lack of planning or skills rather than a lack of motivation or "willpower" (Foster et al., 2005). Reframing lapses as learning opportunities to develop more effective coping skills (rather than "failures") can lead to problem solving for future situations instead of rumination on past behaviors. Although it is not productive for clients to become overly critical of themselves following lapses, it is important that they take responsibility for their actions and identify aspects of their own behavior that can be targeted for modification.

Other Treatment Topics

In addition to the strategies summarized previously, weight loss interventions often cover other cognitive-behavioral techniques or topics, including stress management and body image disturbance. While these topics are not specific to obesity or weight loss, both can be important contributors to the success (or difficulties) experienced by program participants. As with other stress management protocols, clients are taught appropriate coping methods to deal with stress, such as time management/prioritizing, seeking social support, and maintaining physical activity. In session, participants may be guided through relaxation techniques such as progressive muscle relaxation, diaphragmatic breathing, and visual imagery. Sessions addressing body image dissatisfaction rely heavily upon cognitive therapy to target and modify critical and negative thoughts and attitudes about one's body shape and size (Cash, 1994). Graded body exposure exercises (i.e., viewing oneself in a mirror while engaging in cognitive restructuring and relaxation strategies) may be encouraged in order to desensitize individuals to anxiety or discomfort experienced from viewing their own body (Rosen, Reiter, & Orosan, 1995).

There also has been recent interest in incorporating mindfulness-based approaches into behavioral weight loss interventions. Mindfulness, which is conceptualized as a nonjudgmental and present-focused attention to one's physical sensations, thoughts, and emotional experiences (Godsey, 2013), can be targeted through a variety of techniques such as meditation and mindful eating exercises. Mindful eating involves the use of mindful meditation applied to the experience of food intake, including a heightened awareness of the sensory, cognitive, and affective components of eating (Miller, Kristeller, Headings, & Nagaraja, 2014). The goal is to reduce eating in response to emotions or external cues as well as episodes of overeating. A recent literature review highlights the potential efficacy of mindfulness-based approaches for improving eating behaviors and reducing weight, although much of the research to date is limited by small samples, brief follow-up, and non-randomized designs (O'Reilly, Cook, Spruijt-Metz, & Black, 2014).

Structure of Treatment
Frequency and Duration of Treatment

Behavioral obesity interventions typically include 4-6 months of weekly sessions (i.e., 16-24 contacts). A recent trial indicated that a moderate dose of 16 initial weekly contacts (followed by 16 extended care contacts) achieved weight reductions comparable to a higher dose of 24 initial weekly contacts (followed by 24 extended care contacts) (Perri et al., 2014). Both of these conditions resulted in significantly greater weight loss than a low-dose condition of eight initial visits plus eight extended care contacts. Importantly, the moderate-intensity intervention was more cost-effective than the high-intensity version (Perri et al., 2014).

Most weight loss occurs during the first 6 months of treatment, and extending weekly treatment contacts beyond this point does not significantly enhance initial losses (Wing, 2002). While extending initial treatment beyond the 6-month window has limited utility for greater weight loss, extended treatment can dramatically improve maintenance of treatment effects. Therefore, the initial 16-24 weekly sessions may be followed by additional extended care maintenance sessions designed to promote weight loss maintenance and prevent weight regain. The schedule of extended care sessions can vary, but most typically these occur on a biweekly or monthly basis, although the interval between contacts may be extended over time. This maintenance phase may last anywhere from 6 to 12 months, and this type of continued treatment contact is one of the most effective ways to improve long-term outcomes (Perri et al., 1987; Perri, Nezu, Patti, & McCann, 1989).

Organization of Treatment Sessions

Sessions typically begin with measuring and recording participants' weight. While this weight will be kept by the interventionist in the client's clinic record, it is also provided to the client for his or her feedback and self-monitoring. Even in group-based treatments, weights are measured individually and in private prior to the start of the group session. Interventionists also review clients' food and activity records from the previous week and provide reinforcement and corrective feedback as appropriate.

After client(s) have been weighed and self-monitoring records reviewed, treatment sessions can be generally divided into three segments. First, the therapist and client(s) review progress during the past week, including successes achieved as well as challenges or setbacks encountered during the week. During this initial phase of the session, time is spent reviewing problem-solving skills employed to address specific challenges in order to achieve goals set by the client. The session then includes coverage of the week's new content or topic, which often includes a combination of didactic presentation and in-group discussions and activities relevant to the topic (e.g., snack tasting, identification of food triggers). Finally, the remaining time is spent planning and setting goals for the coming week. These goals generally pertain to the topic covered in the session (e.g., increasing fiber intake, identifying sources of positive social support, challenging and restructuring negative cognitions). These obesity treatment sessions typically last from 60 to 90 minutes (Wadden et al., 2004).

Method of Treatment Delivery

GROUP VERSUS INDIVIDUAL TREATMENT

Most commonly, these interventions are delivered in group formats, with typical group sizes ranging from 10 to 20 participants. While there is no definitive recommendation for the ideal group size, a recent trial indicated that treatment delivered in small groups of approximately 12 participants resulted in greater weight loss and treatment adherence than larger groups of approximately 30 participants (Dutton et al., 2014). While the same content can be delivered individually, there is some indication that group-based programs are more effective than one-on-one treatment (Renjilian et al., 2001). In addition to being more efficient for clinicians and organizations, group-based treatment may be more helpful to participants, as it provides opportunities for them to receive additional support, empathy, role modeling of healthy choices, and a dose of healthy competition (Hayaki & Brownell, 1996; Latner, Stunkard, Wilson, & Jackson, 2006; Wadden et al., 2004; Wadden & Osei, 2002).

ALTERNATIVE METHODS OF DELIVERY

While behavioral obesity treatment is most commonly delivered in person, alternative methods of delivery have been explored, including Internet- and telephone-based treatments. For instance, researchers have examined the effects of providing behavioral weight loss programs via the Internet (Harvey-Berino, Pintauro, & Gold, 2002; Tate, Jackvony, & Wing, 2003; Tate, Wing, & Winett, 2001). Internet-based approaches have been applied to weight loss maintenance as well (Svetkey et al., 2008; Wing, Tate, Gorin, Raynor, & Fava, 2006). Internet-based interventions commonly include weekly lessons provided by therapists via e-mail, and participants similarly submit self-monitoring records electronically for review and feedback (Tate et al., 2001). These interventions may also include

online discussion groups and video segments (Harvey-Berino et al., 2002). Recent technological advancements, including personal digital assistants (PDAs) and smartphones, have expanded opportunities to utilize handheld electronic equipment to complement existing behavioral interventions to facilitate self-monitoring and overcome barriers to behavior change (Duncan et al., 2011). Similarly, telephone-based interventions include behavioral counseling and support provided through regular (typically weekly or biweekly) telephone contacts between the therapist and client (Hellerstedt & Jeffery, 1997; Jeffery, Sherwood, et al., 2003; Perri et al., 2008).

One unique study examined the effects of a telephone-based weight loss intervention while also addressing the issue of individual versus group treatment (Befort, Donnelly, Sullivan, Ellerbeck, & Perri, 2010). In this study, obese women received a behavioral weight loss program by telephone either individually with a therapist or via conference call (i.e., a therapist and group of participants). Results of this pilot project indicated that women in the telephone conference-call condition lost significantly more weight than women receiving one-on-one telephone counseling (Befort et al., 2010), again underscoring the potential benefits of group-based treatments.

Whether delivered to individuals or groups, there are several potential benefits of Internet- and telephone-based programs. First, many individuals seeking information about weight loss already access the Internet to obtain this knowledge (Berkel et al., 2005), making this a logical venue for the delivery of accurate and evidence-based dietary and activity recommendations. Second, Internet- and telephone-based programs may decrease participants' burden of attending weekly in-person sessions over an extended period of time. Also, face-to-face treatment (delivered individually or in groups) may not be available to many overweight and obese individuals who would otherwise benefit from treatment. Therefore, Internet- and telephone-based interventions may be more accessible to the population and have greater reach in addressing the public health crisis of obesity.

Overall, research suggests that interventions delivered by phone or Internet can produce clinically meaningful weight loss that differs significantly from control conditions, at least in the short term (Jeffery, Sherwood, et al., 2003; Tate et al., 2001, 2003). However, these alternative approaches have not always been superior to control conditions

(Hellerstedt & Jeffery, 1997), particularly in longer term follow-up (Sherwood et al., 2006). Also, weight loss achieved with some alternative approaches, including Internet-based treatments, tend to be more modest than outcomes observed with in-person interventions (Dutton, Laitner, & Perri, 2014). Direct comparisons have demonstrated that face-to-face delivery methods yield significantly greater weight loss than Web-based approaches (Harvey-Berino et al., 2002; Svetkey et al., 2008; Wadden et al., 2004; Wing et al., 2006). In contrast to Internet-based interventions, telephone-based programs appear to achieve weight reductions similar in magnitude to face-to-face treatment (Dutton et al., 2014; Perri et al., 2008). Other trials are planned to further evaluate the efficacy of telephone-based treatment for weight loss maintenance (Sherwood et al., 2011).

Effects of Treatment
Efficacy, Effectiveness, and Dissemination

Before summarizing the outcomes literature on obesity interventions, it is important to distinguish between studies of efficacy, effectiveness, and dissemination. Most of what is known about obesity treatment outcomes is based on findings from efficacy clinical trials, which are designed to determine the outcomes of a program when executed under well-controlled or "ideal" circumstances (Simons-Morton et al., 2010). These circumstances are evidenced by some of the following typical characteristics of an efficacy trial: (1) highly screened and motivated participants, (2) provision of incentives to maximize participants' adherence and retention, (3) state-of-the-art treatment protocols delivered by experienced and well-trained interventionists, and (4) resource-intensive environments that are often affiliated with specialty clinics of academic medical centers.

In contrast, effectiveness studies are designed to determine the effectiveness of an intervention in real-world circumstances (Simons-Morton et al., 2010). Studies of effectiveness generally take programs shown to be efficacious in prior controlled trials and modify these for delivery in other community, clinical, and educational settings. Therefore, these are designed to be more practical for use in applied settings, which typically have fewer resources to provide for interventionists (e.g., training, supervision) as well as program participants (e.g., incentives, feedback). Effectiveness trials generally have less stringent inclusion criteria for participants. These studies also must consider issues

of resource allocation, particularly given potential limited reimbursement or coverage for services rendered. While less research has focused on treatment effectiveness as compared to efficacy, there are growing efforts to examine the feasibility and outcomes of weight management programs delivered in applied clinical and community settings (Appel et al., 2011; Perri et al., 2008; Wadden et al., 2011).

Finally, dissemination research focuses on the most appropriate and efficient methods for translating efficacious and effective interventions in order to make them more broadly available to overweight and obese members of the general population who would benefit from these services (Simons-Morton et al., 2010). Of these three general categories of obesity treatment outcomes research, this latter area of dissemination is the least developed. Future research on the dissemination and implementation of weight management programs is vitally important in order to adequately address obesity prevention and treatment from a public health perspective.

Initial Weight Loss

As mentioned previously, there is a robust treatment literature supporting the efficacy of cognitive-behavioral interventions for weight loss. Reviews of cognitive-behavioral weight loss interventions indicate weight losses of nearly 10 kg, or 8%-10% reductions in body weight (Foster et al., 2005; Institute of Medicine, 1995; Wadden et al., 2004; Wing, 2002; Wing & Phelan, 2005). These weight loss amounts have been achieved during treatments averaging 4-6 months in duration (Foster et al., 2005; Wadden et al., 2004; Wing, 2002). This translates to weight loss of 0.5-1.0 kg per week during the primary treatment phase, which is a typical goal of behavioral weight loss programs (Berkel et al., 2005).

An important question surrounding the treatment effects of cognitive-behavioral interventions involves the relative contribution of dietary modification and increased physical activity to successful weight management. This research suggests that weight loss achieved through physical activity alone is quite modest (Wing, 1999). While the addition of physical activity to a program targeting dietary modification results in some improvements in weight loss relative to dietary changes alone, this difference often is not significant (Wadden & Foster, 2000; Wing, 1999). Thus, it is generally concluded that behavioral interventions should target diet as well as exercise, but inclusion of dietary modification is crucial to maximize treatment effects. Other predictors of weight loss success include regular self-monitoring of food intake and physical activity. In fact, self-monitoring is the most important behavioral strategy associated with successful weight management (Baker & Kirschenbaum, 1993; Perri et al., 2008; Streit, Stevens, Stevens, & Rossner, 1991). For instance, Perri et al. (2008) demonstrated that completion of self-monitoring records mediated the treatment effects of the behavioral weight management program.

Long-Term Weight Loss

The Institute of Medicine (1995) has defined long-term "success" in weight loss treatment as losing at least 5% of one's initial body weight and keeping this weight off for at least one year. Recent clinical guidelines from the American Heart Association and National Institutes of Health (Jensen et al., 2013) also recommend a goal of 5%-10% weight reduction. Maintaining these losses for 1 year or longer is a common defining feature of successful weight loss maintenance (e.g., McGuire, Wing, & Hill, 1999a). The rationale for these goals is that this amount of weight loss is associated with clinically meaningful improvements in numerous weight-related health outcomes.

Although behavioral interventions promote initial weight loss, keeping the weight off and achieving long-term success prove to be more challenging. Without additional or ongoing contact, weight loss program participants typically regain about one half of their lost weight within a year after treatment, and many have regained nearly all of the weight within 5 years after treatment (Institute of Medicine, 1995; Perri, 2002). Weight regain is most pronounced during the first year following treatment (Kramer, Jeffery, Forster, & Snell, 1989; Wadden et al., 2004). However, the recently completed Look AHEAD weight loss trial provided ongoing behavioral treatment for 8+ years, representing one of the most extensive periods of follow-up available (Wadden et al., 2014). These results demonstrated that behavioral interventions can achieve successful long-term weight loss maintenance with intensive, comprehensive, and ongoing contact, as participants maintained more than half of their initial losses 8 years after initiating treatment (Perri, 2014; Wadden et al., 2014).

There are multiple factors contributing to the difficulties of successful weight loss maintenance. From a physiological perspective, compensatory metabolic changes occur in response to weight loss. Such changes include reductions in resting energy expenditure (Wadden et al., 1990) as well as increases in ghrelin levels, which serve to increase appetite and food intake (Cummings et al., 2002; Wren et al., 2001). In combination, these biological changes make weight loss more difficult to maintain. There are also psychosocial factors at work in the process of weight regain. Following treatment, individuals are confronted with an environment and numerous high-risk situations involving the availability of energy-dense foods (Perri & Corsica, 2002; Wadden et al., 2004). In addition, weight maintenance (i.e., keeping one's weight stable) is inherently less reinforcing than actual weight loss, so the balance between perceived costs/benefits for maintaining weight tends to change over time for many individuals.

Despite the difficulties associated with weight loss maintenance, approximately 20% of weight loss program participants succeed with long-term weight loss (McGuire, Wing, Klem, Lang, & Hill, 1999b; Wing & Phelan, 2005). Data from the National Weight Control Registry (NWCR), which includes a database of individuals who have lost ≥30 lb and kept it off for 1 year or longer, have been particularly helpful in identifying characteristics and behaviors associated with long-term success. One of the best predictors of successful weight loss maintenance is engagement in regular physical activity (Klem, Wing, McGuire, Seagle, & Hill, 1997). In fact, at least 1 hour of moderate-intensity activity (e.g., walking) each day may be necessary to promote weight loss maintenance (Wing & Phelan, 2005), and as much as 75-90 minutes per day may be advisable (Jeffery, Wing, Sherwood, & Tate, 2003; Klem et al., 1997).

Not surprisingly, successful maintainers report continuation of healthy eating habits as well. On average, female registry participants reported consuming less than 1,300 calories/day, and men reported consuming approximately 1,700 calories/day (Klem et al., 1997). However, Wing and Phelan (2005) suggest these may represent underestimates and actual values may be closer to 1,800 calories/day. Successful maintainers also report limiting their fat intake and their frequency of dining out, particularly limiting consumption of fast food meals (Klem et al., 1997; Wing & Phelan, 2005). Interestingly, weight maintainers report eating breakfast on a regular basis (Wyatt et al., 2002), and they eat slightly more frequently (i.e., snacks) than overweight individuals who have not achieved weight loss (Bachman, Phelan, Wing, & Raynor, 2011).

Other behavioral and psychological factors have been associated with weight loss maintenance. For instance, self-monitoring of body weight and food intake are both important for successful weight loss maintenance. Frequent and consistent (i.e., >3 days/week) dietary self-monitoring is associated with successful long-term weight management (Peterson et al., 2014). In regard to monitoring body weight, most individuals in the NWCR weigh themselves at least weekly, and many weigh daily (Klem et al., 1997; Wing & Phelan, 2005). Lower levels of depressive symptoms and low dietary disinhibition (periodic loss of control over eating) have also been associated with better outcomes (McGuire et al., 1999b).

As mentioned previously, extending therapist-client contacts beyond the initial 4-6 months of treatment is very effective for improving weight loss maintenance. For instance, Perri et al. (1988) demonstrated that 1 year of biweekly maintenance sessions resulted in participants maintaining 13.0 kg of their 13.2 kg posttreatment losses (98% maintenance) compared to maintenance of 5.7 kg of 10.8 kg losses among controls (53% maintenance). In general, the duration of behavioral weight loss interventions has been extended over the past few decades, which has resulted in greater weight losses achieved by these programs (Wadden et al., 2004).

Effects on Weight-Related Comorbidities

Given the weight loss success achieved with cognitive-behavioral interventions, such programs also are effective in improving other weight-related clinical outcomes. For instance, modest weight losses (even less than 4%) have been associated with significant and substantial reductions in the incidence of hypertension and diabetes (Knowler et al., 2002; Pan, Yang, Li, & Liu, 1997; Trials of Hypertension Prevention Collaborative Research Group, 1997; Tuomilehto et al., 2001; Whelton et al., 1998). Results from the Diabetes Prevention Program, a behavioral weight loss program targeting diet and physical activity, demonstrated a 58% reduction in diabetes risk with modest initial weight losses of approximately 7 kg (Knowler et al., 2002). Modest weight loss is also associated with improvements in cholesterol, triglycerides, insulin level, and glycated hemoglobin in both general and disease-specific samples (Gregg & Williamson, 2002). Even with the weight regain that commonly occurs following treatment, long-term health benefits may remain (Knowler et al., 2002; Wadden et al., 2004).

The recently concluded Look AHEAD trial evaluated the impact of weight loss on the prevention of cardiovascular disease among overweight and obese individuals with type 2 diabetes, a group at elevated risk of cardiovascular complications associated with their diabetes. While the intervention did not reduce risk for cardiovascular events (e.g., death due to cardiovascular causes, nonfatal myocardial infarction) (The Look AHEAD Research Group, 2013), weight loss treatment was associated with a wide array of other significant benefits, including improvements in blood pressure, triglyceride levels, HDL cholesterol, glycemic control, physical functioning, physical fitness, mobility, sleep apnea, quality of life, and depression (Foster et al., 2009; Look AHEAD Research Group, 2007; 2010; 2013; Perri, 2014; Rejeski et al., 2012; Rubin et al., 2014; Williamson et al., 2009; Wing et al., 2011).

Treatment with Special Populations

Most of the weight loss trials conducted to date have focused on middle-aged adults and often included predominantly White samples. However, growing attention has been paid to other populations, and the status of this research with other age groups and ethnic minorities deserves special attention.

Children and Adolescents

As mentioned previously, approximately 32% of US children and adolescents are overweight or obese (Ogden et al., 2014). Behavioral weight management programs for children and adolescents share many of the same treatment components as those outlined for overweight and obese adults. However, some distinctions should be highlighted. First, the goals of treatment with children and adolescents may vary depending on the age of the child as well as the severity of obesity. Weight loss may be desirable for older children and adolescents, particularly when they are above the 95th percentile for their age-specific BMI (Wilfley, Vannucci, & White, 2010). When working with younger children as well as adolescents with less severe levels of excess weight, weight gain prevention may be indicated rather than weight loss (Wilfley et al., 2010).

Regardless of which treatment goal is indicated, a family-based program involving children and their parents or other caregivers is the most common approach to behavioral weight management interventions with pediatric populations (Epstein, Myers, Raynor, & Saelens, 1998). Parental and family involvement is particularly important given the role they play in children's activity routine and food selections (Wilfley et al., 2010). Similar to the outcomes literature with adults, there are a robust number of trials indicating the efficacy of cognitive-behavioral interventions for pediatric obesity (Oude Luttikhuis et al., 2009). One meta-analysis indicated that behavioral interventions result in an average decrease of 8.9% in percentage overweight, which differed significantly from control conditions (Wilfley et al., 2007).

Young Adults

Evidence indicates that weight gain over the life span is most pronounced in early adulthood (Lewis et al., 2000; Williamson, Kahn, Remington, & Anda, 1990). This suggests that early adulthood (i.e., early to mid-20s) may be an appropriate and effective time to target obesity prevention and weight management interventions. Unfortunately, previous intervention research has typically overlooked this at-risk population. However, there are several ongoing clinical trials that will examine the effects of behavioral and environmental approaches to weight control in young adults employing novel technologies, such as social networking and other Internet and communication-based technologies. This collaborative group of trials, known as the Early Adult Reduction of Weight through Lifestyle Intervention (EARLY) trials funded by the NIH, will provide needed information on the implementation of behavioral weight loss efforts targeting this age group (National Institutes of Health [NIH], 2010).

Older Adults

The benefit of weight loss relative to potential risks for overweight and obese older adults has been a topic of some controversy. In fact, being overweight (but not obese) may be protective against mobility limitations for older adults (Marsh et al., 2011). Further, overweight status may be associated with reduced mortality risk relative to normal weight BMIs in this population (Auyeung et al., 2010; Marsh et al., 2011). Regarding weight loss efforts, intentional weight loss by overweight, older adults was associated with increased risk of subsequent mobility limitations (Lee et al., 2005). This could be because older adults are at greater risk of losing lean mass during weight loss, and this reduction in lean mass is not fully recovered even with subsequent weight regain (Lee et al., 2005).

While the relationship between overweight and health outcomes is less clear, obesity appears to confer significant health risks for older adults (Koster et al., 2008). Also, some researchers have observed benefits of weight loss for obese, older adults. For instance, Rejeski et al. (2011) reported that weight loss was an integral component for improving mobility among obese, older adults. In this behavioral trial, an intervention incorporating weight loss in addition to physical activity achieved significantly greater and sustained improvements in mobility as compared to a lifestyle intervention focused on physical activity only.

Ethnic Minorities and Other At-Risk Groups

Given the higher prevalence of obesity and weight-related comorbidities among racial/ethnic minorities (Flegal et al., 2012), understanding the effects of treatment for these groups is clearly warranted. When compared to Caucasians participating in weight loss treatment, some studies have concluded that African Americans (and African American women in particular) lose less weight initially and lose weight more slowly (Kumanyika, 2002; West, Elaine Prewitt, Bursac, & Felix, 2008). Consistent with this conclusion, recent findings from the Weight Loss Maintenance trial indicated that African American participants lost significantly less weight during the initial phase of treatment (Svetkey et al., 2011).

However, examination of long-term outcomes may provide a different perspective, as weight change during the extended, maintenance phase of this trial did not differ by race (Svetkey et al., 2011). Rickel et al. (2011) also found that African American women lost less initial weight than Caucasians in a behavioral weight loss trial, but African Americans demonstrated better weight loss maintenance during extended follow-up, even in the absence of ongoing therapeutic support. Additional research is needed to understand the differential trajectory of weight loss for Caucasian and minority participants as well as possible sociocultural, socioeconomic, or environmental factors that may influence short-term and long-term treatment responses.

Another underserved and high-risk group includes individuals living in rural areas. Similar to the racial disparities observed for obesity, rates of obesity are higher in rural settings as compared to urban settings (Jackson, Doescher, Jerant, & Hart, 2005). Yet residents of rural communities have limited access to appropriate treatment resources and experience other environmental barriers to care (Phillips & McLeroy, 2004). While interventions targeting rural populations are limited, initial findings are very promising on the effectiveness of obesity treatment for women (Perri et al., 2008), children (Janicke et al., 2008), and older adults (Rejeski et al., 2011) living in rural settings.

Conclusions

Given the high prevalence of overweight and obesity, it is imperative that effective interventions are developed and delivered to address this public health crisis. Cognitive-behavioral treatment for obesity is one of the most commonly used approaches to weight management and is generally considered the first choice in treatment for the majority of clients. Cognitive-behavioral treatment includes a variety of evidence-based techniques targeting dietary and activity modifications, including self-monitoring, problem solving, stimulus control, social support, cognitive restructuring, stress management, and relapse prevention. Cognitive-behavioral interventions for obesity have demonstrated statistically significant and clinically meaningful weight loss outcomes and reduction in risk for weight-related comorbidities such as diabetes and cardiovascular disease. Although treatment is associated with

significant reductions in body weight and improved health, a remaining challenge for many is sustaining this weight loss after the termination of treatment.

Future Directions

There are a number of important areas of future investigation that may inform the delivery of cognitive-behavioral weight loss interventions and strengthen our understanding of program outcomes. First, most of the conclusions regarding treatment outcomes are based on randomized controlled trials conducted in specialized clinics affiliated with academic medical centers. These interventions rely on well-trained and experienced therapists and often include substantial eligibility restrictions for participants. Therefore, more work on dissemination and implementation of these interventions in applied clinical and community settings is needed, particularly if there is going to be a meaningful, evidence-based public health effort to address these conditions.

On a related front, there is a need to explore the most appropriate treatment approach and the effects of these approaches among different patient populations. For example, the development of alternative delivery methods (e.g., telephone-, Internet-based

Table 23.2 Future Research Directions for Specific Populations

Population	Examples of Research Topics
Children and adolescents	• Effectiveness trials and dissemination research to examine treatment effects in typical, real-world conditions • Methods to promote weight loss maintenance • Most appropriate and efficient levels of inclusion of parents and children in family-based treatments
Young adults	• Among normal-weight adults, interventions targeting weight gain prevention and increased physical activity • Among overweight/obese adults, interventions targeting weight loss and increased physical activity • Use of alternative and innovative methods of treatment delivery (e.g., social media)
Adults	• Effectiveness trials and dissemination research to examine treatment effects in typical, real-world conditions • Methods to promote weight loss maintenance • Most appropriate levels of treatment contacts • Obesity management among clients with psychiatric comorbidities
Older adults	• Importance of weight loss for preserving mobility and other age-related outcomes • Balance of benefits/risks of weight loss for older adults
Racial/ethnic minorities	• Treatment response, including weight loss trajectories (initial and long-term weight change) • Impact of cultural tailoring of treatment (compared with standard treatment protocols) • Methods to promote recruitment and retention in treatment

treatment) as well as the increased usage of communication technologies (e.g., smartphones, social media) raises the issue of whether an age by treatment modality interaction impacts the effectiveness of these treatments. The need to examine weight management techniques among young adults is an emerging area of research as well as understanding potential differences in the weight loss patterns of racial and ethnic minorities participating in treatment. Table 23.2 summarizes some of the emerging research questions specific to different demographic groups.

Another important practical consideration for behavioral obesity interventions involves the most appropriate methods for delivering these programs. While these programs typically involve 4-6 months of weekly group sessions, this frequency and duration of contact may not be feasible in certain settings or with particular populations. Also, groups most commonly include 10-20 participants, but there is little research (e.g., Dutton et al., 2014) to indicate whether treatment could be conducted more efficiently with larger numbers of participants and still achieve meaningful results. There is also limited research (e.g., Perri et al., 2014) to identify the minimum number of sessions required to achieve clinically meaningful weight loss. Both topics are relevant for balancing treatment outcomes with practical considerations for implementation. Similarly, therapists with advanced training in cognitive-behavioral treatment may not be available in certain settings or programs, and research exploring the feasibility of using interventionists with limited specialized training may be informative.

Another area for future work involves examination of the delivery of obesity treatment in the context of comorbid psychological conditions. In particular, the relationship between obesity and depression and the impact of this comorbidity on treatment is needed. While a significant proportion of overweight and obese clients also suffer from depression (Petry et al., 2008; Zhao et al., 2009), these individuals traditionally have been excluded from weight loss trials and weight management programs, as it was assumed that depressive symptoms would interfere with obesity treatment engagement, adherence, and outcomes. Indeed, the presence of depressive symptoms has been associated with poorer weight loss outcomes (Linde et al., 2004) and greater likelihood of weight regain following treatment (McGuire et al., 1999b). However, a recent study demonstrated no significant difference in weight loss or program attendance for depressed and nondepressed women participating in a cognitive-behavioral intervention (Ludman et al., 2010). Additional work examining the impact of comorbid depression on obesity treatment is needed, and this research may point toward modified interventions that concurrently address both conditions (Linde et al., 2011).

Perhaps one of the most urgent and challenging areas of inquiry involves the problem of weight loss maintenance. As mentioned previously, cognitive-behavioral treatments are quite effective in inducing initial weight loss, although treatment is followed by significant weight regain for the majority of participants. Innovative strategies to prevent weight regain and sustain clients' motivation for continued engagement in lifestyle modification is warranted. Because a significant minority of weight loss participants achieve weight loss maintenance, continued examination of biological, behavioral, and psychological factors that contribute to this long-term success is also important.

References

Allison, D. B., Gadde, K. M., Garvey, W. T., Peterson, C. A., Schwiers, M. L., Najarian, T., … Day, W. W. (2011). Controlled-release phentermine/topiramate in severely obese adults: A randomized controlled trial (EQUIP). *Obesity*, *20*(2), 330–342.

Appel, L. J., Clark, J. M., Yeh, H. C., Wang, N. Y., Coughlin, J. W., Daumit, G., & Brancati, F. L. (2011). Comparative effectiveness of weight-loss interventions in clinical practice. *New England Journal of Medicine*, *365*(21), 1959–1968.

Auyeung, T. W., Lee, J. S., Leung, J., Kwok, T., Leung, P. C., & Woo, J. (2010). Survival in older men may benefit from being slightly overweight and centrally obese—A 5-year follow-up study in 4,000 older adults using DXA. *Journals of Gerontology. Series A, Biological Sciences and Medical Sciences*, *65*(1), 99–104.

Bachman, J. L., Phelan, S., Wing, R. R., & Raynor, H. A. (2011). Eating frequency is higher in weight loss maintainers and normal-weight individuals than in overweight individuals. *Journal of the Amercian Dietetic Association*, *111*(11), 1730–1734.

Baker, R. C., & Kirschenbaum, D. S. (1993). Self-monitoring may be necessary for successful weight control. *Journal of Behavior Therapy and Experimental Psychiatry*, *24*, 377–394.

Bandura, A. (1986). *Social foundations of thought and action: A social cognitive theory.* Englewood Cliffs, NJ: Prentice Hall.

Beck, A. T. (1976). *Cognitive therapy and the emotional disorders.* New York, NY: Int. Univ Press.

Befort, C. A., Donnelly, J. E., Sullivan, D. K., Ellerbeck, E. F., & Perri, M. G. (2010). Group versus individual phone-based obesity treatment for rural women. *Eating Behaviors*, *11*(1), 11–17.

Bell, J. F., Zimmerman, F. J., Arterburn, D. E., & Maciejewski, M. L. (2011). Health-care expenditures of overweight and obese males and females in the medical expenditures panel survey by age cohort. *Obesity (Silver Spring)*, *19*(1), 228–232.

Berkel, L. A., Poston, W. S., Reeves, R. S., & Foreyt, J. P. (2005). Behavioral interventions for obesity. *Journal of American Dietetic Association, 105*(5 Suppl 1), S35–S43.

Brownell, K. D., Marlatt, G. A., Lichtenstein, E., & Wilson, G. T. (1986). Understanding and preventing relapse. *American Psychologist, 41*(7), 765–782.

Cash, T. F. (1994). Body-image attitudes: Evaluation, investment, and affect. *Perceptual and Motor Skills, 78*(3 Pt 2), 1168–1170.

Coakley, E. H., Kawachi, I., Manson, J. E., Speizer, F. E., Willet, W. C., & Colditz, G. A. (1998). Lower levels of physical functioning are associated with higher body weight among middle-aged and older women. *International Journal of Obesity and Related Metabolic Disorders, 22*(10), 958–965.

Colquitt, J. L., Picot, J., Loveman, E., & Clegg, A. J. (2009). Surgery for obesity. *Cochrane Database of Systematic Reviews,* (2), CD003641.

Cummings, D. E., Weigle, D. S., Frayo, R. S., Breen, P. A., Ma, M. K., Dellinger, E. P., & Purnell, J. Q. (2002). Plasma ghrelin levels after diet-induced weight loss or gastric bypass surgery. *New England Journal of Medicine, 346*, 1623–1630.

Duncan, J. M., Janke, E. A., Kozak, A. T., Roehrig, M., Russell, S. W., McFadden, H. G.,... Spring, B. (2011). PDA+: A Personal Digital Assistant for Obesity Treatment—An RCT testing the use of technology to enhance weight loss treatment for veterans. *BioMed Central Psychiatry, 11*, 223.

Dutton, G. R., Laitner, M. H., & Perri, M. G. (2014). Lifestyle interventions for cardiovascular disease risk reduction: A systematic review of the effects of diet composition, food provision, and treatment modality on weight loss. *Current Atherosclerosis Reports, 16*(10), 442. Epub ahead of print.

Dutton, G. R., Nackers, L. M., Dubyak, P. J., Rushing, N. C., Huynh, T. T., Tan, F.,... Perri, M. G. (2014). A randomized trial comparing weight loss treatment delivered in large versus small groups. *International Journal of Behavioral Nutrition and Physical Activity, 11*, 123. Epub ahead of print.

Epstein, L. H., Myers, M. D., Raynor, H. A., & Saelens, B. E. (1998). Treatment of pediatric obesity. *Pediatrics, 101*(3 Pt 2), 554–570.

Ferster, C. B., Nurnberger, J. I., & Levitt, E. B. (1962). The control of eating. *Journal of Mathematics, 1*, 87–109.

Field, A. E., Barnoya, J., & Colditz, G. A. (2002). Epidemiology and health and economic consequences of obesity. In T. A. Wadden & A. J. Stunkard (Eds.), *Handbook of obesity treatment* (pp. 3–18). New York, NY: Guilford Press.

Fine, J. T., Colditz, G. A., Coakley, E. H., Moseley, G., Manson, J. E., Willett, W. C., & Kawachi, I. (1999). A prospective study of weight change and health-related quality of life in women. *Journal of the American Medical Association, 282*(22), 2136–2142.

Finkelstein, E. A., Trogdon, J. G., Cohen, J. W., & Dietz, W. (2009). Annual medical spending attributable to obesity: Payer-and service-specific estimates. *Health Affairs (Millwood), 28*(5), w822–w831.

Flegal, K. M., Carroll, M. D., Kit, B. K., & Ogden, C. L. (2012). Prevalence of obesity and trends in the distribution of body mass index among US adults, 1999-2010. *Journal of the American Medical Association, 307*(5), 491–497.

Flegal, K. M., Graubard, B. I., Williamson, D. F., & Gail, M. H. (2007). Cause-specific excess deaths associated with underweight, overweight, and obesity. *Journal of the American Medical Association, 298*(17), 2028–2037.

Foster, G. D., Borradaile, K. E., Sanders, M. H., Millmann, R., Zammit, G., Newman, A. B.,... Kuna, S. T. (2009). A randomized study on the effect of weight loss on obstructive sleep apnea among obese patients with type 2 diabetes. *Archives of Internal Medicine, 169*(17), 1619–1626.

Foster, G. D., Makris, A. P., & Bailer, B. A. (2005). Behavioral treatment of obesity. *American Journal of Clinical Nutrition, 82*(Suppl 1), 230S–235S.

Fujioka, K., & Lee, M. W. (2007). Pharmacologic treatment options for obesity: Current and potential medications. *Nutrition in Clinical Practice, 22*(1), 50–54.

Garvey, W. T., Ryan, D. H., Look, M., Gadde, K. M., Allison, D. B., Peterson, C. A.,... Bowden, C. H. (2012). Two-year sustained weight loss and metabolic benefits with controlled-release phentermine/topiramate in obese and overweight adults (SEQUEL): A randomized, placebo-controlled, phase 3 extension study. *American Journal of Clinical Nutrition, 95*, 297–308.

Godsey, J. (2013). The role of mindfulness based interventions in the treatment of obesity and eating disorders: An integrative review. *Complimentary Therapies in Medicine, 21*, 430–439.

Gorin, A., Phelan, S., Tate, D., Sherwood, N., Jeffery, R., & Wing, R. (2005). Involving support partners in obesity treatment. *Journal of Consulting and Clinical Psychology, 73*(2), 341–343.

Gregg, E. W., & Williamson, D. F. (2002). The relationship of intertional weight loss to disease incidence and mortality. In T. A. Wadden & A. J. Stunkard (Eds.), *Handbook of obesity treatment* (pp. 125–143). New York, NY: Guilford Press.

Harvey-Berino, J., Pintauro, S. J., & Gold, E. C. (2002). The feasibility of using Internet support for the maintenance of weight loss. *Behavior Modification, 26*(1), 103–116.

Hayaki, J., & Brownell, K. D. (1996). Behaviour change in practice: group approaches. *International Journal of Obesity and Related Metabolic Disorders, 20*(Suppl 1), S27–S30.

Hellerstedt, W. L., & Jeffery, R. W. (1997). The effects of a telephone-based intervention on weight loss. *American Journal of Health Promotion, 11*(3), 177–182.

Horgen, K. B., & Brownel, K. D. (1998). Policy change as a means for reducing the prevalence and impact of alcoholism, smoking, and obesity. In M. W. R. & H. N. (Eds.), *Treating addictive behaviors* (2nd ed., pp. 105–118). New York, NY: Plenum Press.

Institute of Medicine. (1995). *Weighing the options: Criteria for evaluating weight-management programs.* Washington, DC: National Academy of Sciences.

Jackson, J. E., Doescher, M. P., Jerant, A. F., & Hart, L. G. (2005). A national study of obesity prevalence and trends by type of rural county. *Journal of Rural Health, 21*(2), 140–148.

Jakicic, J. M., Wing, R. R., Butler, B. A., & Robertson, R. J. (1995). Prescribing exercise in multiple short bouts versus one continuous bout: Effects on adherence, cardiorespiratory fitness, and weight loss in overweight women. *International Journal of Obesity and Related Metabolic Disorders, 19*(12), 893–901.

Jakicic, J. M., Winters, C., Lang, W., & Wing, R. R. (1999). Effects of intermittent exercise and use of home exercise equipment on adherence, weight loss, and fitness in overweight women: A randomized trial. *Journal of the American Medical Association, 282*(16), 1554–1560.

Janicke, D. M., Sallinen, B. J., Perri, M. G., Lutes, L. D., Huerta, M., Silverstein, J. H., & Brumback, B. (2008). Comparison of parent-only vs family-based interventions for overweight children in underserved rural settings: Outcomes from project STORY. *Archives of Pediatrics and Adolescent Medicine*, *162*(12), 1119–1125.

Jeffery, R. W., Sherwood, N. E., Brelje, K., Pronk, N. P., Boyle, R., Boucher, J. L., & Hase, K. (2003). Mail and phone interventions for weight loss in a managed-care setting: Weigh-To-Be one-year outcomes. *International Journal of Obesity and Related Metabolic Disorders, 27*(12), 1584–1592.

Jeffery, R. W., Wing, R. R., Sherwood, N. E., & Tate, D. F. (2003). Physical activity and weight loss: Does prescribing higher physical activity goals improve outcome? *American Journal of Clinical Nutrition, 78*(4), 684–689.

Jensen, M. D., Ryan, D. H., Apovian, C. M., Ard, J. D., Comuzzie, A. G., Donato, K. A.,. . . Yanovski, S. Z. (2013). AHA/ACC/TOS guideline for the management of overweight and obesity in adults: A report of the American College of Cardiology/American Heart Association Task Force on Practice Guidelines and The Obesity Society. *Journal of the American College of Cardiology, 63*, 2985–3023.

Klem, M. L., Wing, R. R., McGuire, M. T., Seagle, H. M., & Hill, J. O. (1997). A descriptive study of individuals successful at long-term maintenance of substantial weight loss. *American Journal of Clinical Nutrition, 66*(2), 239–246.

Knowler, W. C., Barrett-Connor, E., Fowler, S. E., Hamman, R. F., Lachin, J. M., Walker, E. A.,. . . Nathan, D. M. (2002). Reduction in the incidence of type 2 diabetes with lifestyle intervention or metformin. *New England Journal of Medicine, 346*(6), 393–403.

Koster, A., Patel, K. V., Visser, M., van Eijk, J. T., Kanaya, A. M., de Rekeneire, N.,. . . Harris, T. B. (2008). Joint effects of adiposity and physical activity on incident mobility limitation in older adults. *Journal of the American Geriatrics Society, 56*(4), 636–643.

Kramer, F. M., Jeffery, R. W., Forster, J. L., & Snell, M. K. (1989). Long-term follow-up of behavioral treatment for obesity: Patterns of weight regain among men and women. *International Journal of Obesity (Lond), 13*(2), 123–136.

Kumanyika, S. (2002). Obesity treatment in minorities. In T. A. Wadden & A. J. Stunkard (Eds.), *Handbook of obesity treatment* (pp. 416–446). New York, NY: Guilford Press.

Latner, J. D., Stunkard, A. J., Wilson, G. T., & Jackson, M. L. (2006). The perceived effectiveness of continuing care and group support in the long-term self-help treatment of obesity. *Obesity (Silver Spring), 14*(3), 464–471.

Leahey, T. M., Crowther, J. H., & Ciesla, J. A. (2011). An ecological momentary assessment of the effects of weight and shape social comparisons on women with eating pathology, high body dissatisfaction, and low body dissatisfaction. *Behavior Therapy, 42*(2), 197–210.

LeBlanc, E. S., O'Connor, E., Whitlock, E. P., Patnode, C. D., & Kapka, T. (2011). Effectiveness of primary care-relevant treatments for obesity in adults: A systematic evidence review for the US Preventive Services Task Force. *Annals of Internal Medicine, 155*(7), 434–447.

Lee, J. S., Kritchevsky, S. B., Tylavsky, F., Harris, T., Simonsick, E. M., Rubin, S. M., & Newman, A. B. (2005). Weight change, weight change intention, and the incidence of mobility limitation in well-functioning community-dwelling older adults. *Journals of Gerontology. Series A, Biological Sciences and Medical Sciences, 60*(8), 1007–1012.

Lewis, C. E., Jacobs, D. R., Jr., McCreath, H., Kiefe, C. I., Schreiner, P. J., Smith, D. E., & Williams, O. D. (2000). Weight gain continues in the 1990s: 10-year trends in weight and overweight from the CARDIA study. Coronary Artery Risk Development in Young Adults. *American Journal of Epidemiology, 151*(12), 1172–1181.

Linde, J. A., Jeffery, R. W., Levy, R. L., Sherwood, N. E., Utter, J., Pronk, N. P., & Boyle, R. G. (2004). Binge eating disorder, weight control self-efficacy, and depression in overweight men and women. *International Journal of Obesity and Related Metabolic Disorders, 28*(3), 418–425.

Linde, J. A., Simon, G. E., Ludman, E. J., Ichikawa, L. E., Operskalski, B. H., Arterburn, D.,. . . Jeffrey, R. W. (2011). A randomized controlled trial of behavioral weight loss treatment versus combined weight loss/depression treatment among women with comorbid obesity and depression. *Annals of Behavioral Medicine, 41*(1), 119–130.

Look AHEAD Research Group. (2007). Reduction in weight and cardiovascular disease risk factors in individuals with type 2 diabetes: One-year results of the Look AHEAD trial. *Diabetes Care, 30*(6), 1374–1383.

Look AHEAD Research Group. (2010). Long-term effects of a lifestyle intervention on weight and cardiovascular risk factors in individuals with type 2 diabetes mellitus. *Archives of Internal Medicine, 170*(17), 1566–1575.

Look AHEAD Research Group. (2013). Cardiovascular effects of intensive lifestyle intervention in type 2 diabetes. *New England Journal of Medicine, 369*(2), 145–154.

Ludman, E. J., Russo, J. E., Katon, W. J., Simon, G. E., Williams, L. H., Lin, E. H.,. . . Young, B. A. (2010). How does change in depressive symptomatology influence weight change in patients with diabetes? Observational results from the Pathways longitudinal cohort. *Journal of Gerontology. Series A, Biological Sciences and Medical Sciences, 65*(1), 93–98.

Marsh, A. P., Rejeski, W. J., Espeland, M. A., Miller, M. E., Church, T. S., Fielding, R. A.,. . . Pahor, M. (2011). Muscle strength and BMI as predictors of major mobility disability in the Lifestyle Interventions and Independence for Elders pilot (LIFE-P). *Journals of Gerontology. Series A, Biological Sciences and Medical Sciences, 66*(12), 1376–1383.

McGuire, M. T., Wing, R. R., & Hill, J. O. (1999a). The prevalence of weight loss maintenance among American adults. *International Journal of Obesity and Related Metabolic Disorders, 23*(12), 1314–1319.

McGuire, M. T., Wing, R. R., Klem, M. L., Lang, W., & Hill, J. O. (1999b). What predicts weight regain in a group of successful weight losers? *Journal of Consulting and Clinical Psychology, 67*(2), 177–185.

Miller, C. K., Kristeller, J. L., Headings, A., & Nagaraja, H. (2014). Comparison of a mindful eating intervention to a diabetes self-management intervention among adults with type 2 diabetes: A randomized controlled trial. *Health Education and Behavior, 41*(2), 145–154.

Murawski, M. E., Milsom, V. A., Ross, K. M., Rickel, K. A., DeBraganza, N., Gibbons, L. M., & Perri, M. G. (2009). Problem solving, treatment adherence, and weight-loss outcome among women participating in lifestyle treatment for obesity. *Eating Behaviors, 10*(3), 146–151.

National Heart Lung Blood Institute. (1998). *Clinical guidelines on the identification, evaluation, and treatment of overweight and obesity in adults: The evidence report.* Bethesda, MD: NHLBI.

National Institute of Health. (1992). Gastrointestinal surgery for severe obesity (National Institutes of Health Consensus Development Conference Statement). *American Journal of Clinical Nutrition, 55*, 615S–619S.

National Institutes of Health. (2010). *Trials use technology to help young adults achieve healthy weights*. Bethesda, MD: NHLBI Communications Office.

Nezu, A. M., Nezu, C. M., & Perri, M. G. (2006). Problem solving to promote treatment adherence. In W. T. O'Donohue & E. R. Levensky (Eds.), *Promoting treatment adherence: A practical handbook for health care providers* (pp. 135–148). Thousand Oaks, CA: Sage.

Ogden, C. L., Carroll, M. D., Kit, B. K., & Flegal, K. M. (2012). Prevalence of obesity and trends in body mass index among US children and adolescents, 1999-2010. *Journal of the American Medical Association, 307*(5), 483–490.

Ogden, C. L., Carroll, M. D., Kit, B. K., & Flegal, K. M (2014). Prevalence of childhood and adult obesity in the United States, 2011-2012. *Journal of the American Medical Association, 311*(8), 806–814.

O'Reilly, G. A., Cook, L., Spruijt-Metz, D., & Black, D. S. (2014). Mindfulness-based interventions for obesity-related eating behaviours: A literature review. *Obesity Reviews, 15*, 453–461.

Oude Luttikhuis, H., Baur, L., Jansen, H., Shrewsbury, V. A., O'Malley, C., Stolk, R. P., & Summerbell, C. D. (2009). Interventions for treating obesity in children. *Cochrane Database of Systematic Reviews*, (1), CD001872.

Pan, X. R., Yang, W. Y., Li, G. W., & Liu, J. (1997). Prevalence of diabetes and its risk factors in China, 1994. National Diabetes Prevention and Control Cooperative Group. *Diabetes Care, 20*(11), 1664–1669.

Perri, M. G. (2002). Improving maintenance in behavioral treatment. In C. C. Fairburn & K. D. Brownell (Eds.), *Eating disorders and obesity treatment* (2nd ed., pp. 593–598). New York, NY: Guilford Press.

Perri, M. G. (2014). Effects of behavioral treatment on long-term weight loss: Lessons learned from the look AHEAD trial. *Obesity, 22*(1), 3–4.

Perri, M. G., & Corsica, J. A. (2002). Improving the maintenance of weight lost in behavioral treatment of obesity. In T. A. Wadden & A. J. Stunkard (Eds.), *Handbook of obesity treatment* (pp. 267–282). New York, NY: Guilford Press.

Perri, M. G., Limacher, M. C., Durning, P. E., Janicke, D. M., Lutes, L. D., Bobroff, L. B., … Martin, A. D. (2008). Extended-care programs for weight management in rural communities: The treatment of obesity in underserved rural settings (TOURS) randomized trial. *Archives of Internal Medicine, 168*(21), 2347–2354.

Perri, M. G., Limacher, M. C., von Castel-Roberts, K., Daniels, M. J., Durning, P. E., Janicke, D. M., … Martin, A. D. (2014). Comparative effectiveness of three doses of weight loss counseling: Two-year findings from the Rural LITE Trial. *Obesity, 22*(11), 2293–2300.

Perri, M. G., McAdoo, W. G., McAllister, D. A., Lauer, J. B., Jordan, R. C., Yancey, D. Z., & Nezu, A. M. (1987). Effects of peer support and therapist contact on long-term weight loss. *Journal of Consulting and Clinical Psychology, 55*(4), 615–617.

Perri, M. G., McAllister, D. A., Gange, J. J., Jordan, R. C., McAdoo, G., & Nezu, A. M. (1988). Effects of four maintenance programs on the long-term management of obesity. *Journal of Consulting and Clinical Psychology, 56*(4), 529–534.

Perri, M. G., Nezu, A. M., McKelvey, W. F., Shermer, R. L., Renjilian, D. A., & Viegener, B. J. (2001). Relapse prevention training and problem-solving therapy in the long-term management of obesity. *Journal of Consulting and Clinical Psychology, 69*(4), 722–726.

Perri, M. G., Nezu, A. M., Patti, E. T., & McCann, K. L. (1989). Effect of length of treatment on weight loss. *Journal of Consulting and Clinical Psychology, 57*(3), 450–452.

Peterson, N. D., Middleton, K. R., Nackers, L. M., Medina, K. E., Milsom, V. A., & Perri, M. G. (2014). Dietary self-monitoring and long-term success with weight management. *Obesity, 22*(9), 1962–1967.

Petry, N. M., Barry, D., Pietrzak, R. H., & Wagner, J. A. (2008). Overweight and obesity are associated with psychiatric disorders: Results from the National Epidemiologic Survey on Alcohol and Related Conditions. *Psychosomatic Medicine, 70*(3), 288–297.

Phillips, C. D., & McLeroy, K. R. (2004). Health in rural America: Remembering the importance of place. *American Journal of Public Health, 94*(10), 1661–1663.

Powell, A. G., Apovian, C. M., & Aronne, L. J. (2011). New drug targets for the treatment of obesity. *Clinical Pharmacology and Therapeutics, 90*(1), 40–51.

Rejeski, W. J., Brubaker, P. H., Goff, D. C., Jr., Bearon, L. B., McClelland, J. W., Perri, M. G., & Ambrosius, W. T. (2011). Translating weight loss and physical activity programs into the community to preserve mobility in older, obese adults in poor cardiovascular health. *Archives of Internal Medicine, 171*(10), 880–886.

Rejeski, W. J., Ip, E. H., Bertoni, A. G., Bray, G. A., Evans, G., Gregg, E. W., & Zhang, Q. (2012). Lifestyle change and mobility in obese adults with type 2 diabetes. *New England Journal of Medicine, 366*(13), 1209–1217.

Renjilian, D. A., Perri, M. G., Nezu, A. M., McKelvey, W. F., Shermer, R. L., & Anton, S. D. (2001). Individual versus group therapy for obesity: Effects of matching participants to their treatment preferences. *Journal of Consulting and Clinical Psychology, 69*(4), 717–721.

Rickel, K. A., Milsom, V. A., Ross, K. M., Hoover, V. J., Peterson, N. D., & Perri, M. G. (2011). Differential response of African American and Caucasian women to extended-care programs for obesity management. *Ethnicity and Disease, 21*(2), 170–175.

Rosen, J. C., Reiter, J., & Orosan, P. (1995). Cognitive-behavioral body image therapy for body dysmorphic disorder. *Journal of Consulting and Clinical Psychology, 63*(2), 263–269.

Rubin, R., Wadden, T. A., Bahnson, J. L., Blackburn, G. L., Brancati, F. L., Bray, G. A., … Zhang, P. (2014). Impact of intensive lifestyle intervention on depression and health-related quality of life in type 2 diabetes: The Look AHEAD trial. *Diabetes Care, 37*(6), 1544–1553.

Sherwood, N. E., Crain, A. L., Martinson, B. C., Hayes, M. G., Anderson, J. D., Clausen, J. M., … Jeffrey, R. W. (2011). Keep it off: A phone-based intervention for long-term weight-loss maintenance. *Contemporary Clinical Trials, 32*(4), 551–560.

Sherwood, N. E., Jeffery, R. W., Pronk, N. P., Boucher, J. L., Hanson, A., Boyle, R., … Chen, V. (2006). Mail and phone interventions for weight loss in a managed-care setting: Weigh-to-be 2-year outcomes. *International Journal of Obesity (Lond), 30*(10), 1565–1573.

Simons-Morton, D. G., Donato, K., Loria, C. M., Pratt, C. A., Ershow, A. G., Morrissette, M. A., … Obarzanek, E. (2010). Obesity research and programs at the National Heart, Lung, and Blood Institute. *Journal of the American College of Cardiology, 55*(9), 917–920.

Smith, S. R., Weissman, N. J., Anderson, C. M., Sanchez, M., Chuang, E., Stubbe, S., ... Shanahan, W. R. (2010). Multicenter, placebo-controlled trial of lorcaserin for weight management. *New England Journal of Medicine, 363*(3), 245–256.

Streit, K. J., Stevens, N. H., Stevens, V. J., & Rossner, J. (1991). Food records: A predictor and modifier of weight change in a long-term weight loss program. *Journal of American Dietetic Association, 91*(2), 213–216.

Stuart, R. B. (1967). Behavioral control of overeating. *Behavioural Research and Therapy, 5*, 357–365.

Svetkey, L. P., Ard, J. D., Stevens, V. J., Loria, C. M., Young, D. Y., Hollis, J. F., ... Vollmer, W. M. (2011). Predictors of long-term weight loss in adults with modest initial weight loss, by sex and race. *Obesity (Silver Spring), 20*(9), 1820–1828.

Svetkey, L. P., Stevens, V. J., Brantley, P. J., Appel, L. J., Hollis, J. F., Loria, C. M., ... Aicher, K. (2008). Comparison of strategies for sustaining weight loss: The weight loss maintenance randomized controlled trial. *Journal of the American Medical Association, 299*(10), 1139–1148.

Tate, D. F., Jackvony, E. H., & Wing, R. R. (2003). Effects of Internet behavioral counseling on weight loss in adults at risk for type 2 diabetes: A randomized trial. *Journal of the American Medical Association, 289*(14), 1833–1836.

Tate, D. F., Wing, R. R., & Winett, R. A. (2001). Using Internet technology to deliver a behavioral weight loss program. *Journal of the American Medical Association, 285*(9), 1172–1177.

Trials of Hypertension Prevention Collaborative Research Group. (1997). Effects of weight loss and sodium reduction intervention on blood pressure and hypertension incidence in overweight people with high-normal blood pressure. The trials of hypertension prevention, phase II. The trials of Hypertension Prevention Collaborative Research Group. *Archives of Internal Medicine, 157*, 657–667.

Tuomilehto, J., Lindstrom, J., Eriksson, J. G., Valle, T. T., Hamalainen, H., Ilanne-Parikka, P., ... Uusitupa, M. (2001). Prevention of type 2 diabetes mellitus by changes in lifestyle among subjects with impaired glucose tolerance. *New England Journal of Medicine, 344*(18), 1343–1350.

US Department of Agriculture & US Department of Health and Human Services. (2010). *Dietary guidelines for Americans 2010* (7th ed.). Washington, DC: US Government Printing Office.

US Department of Health and Human Services. (2008). *Physical activity guidelines for Americans*. Retrieved March 2012, from http://www.health.gov/paguidelines/

Valdez, R., & Williamson, D. F. (2002). Prevalence and demographics of obesity. In C. G. Fairburn & K. D. Brownell (Eds.), *Eating disorders and obesity treatment* (pp. 417–421). New York, NY: Guilford Press.

Vetter, M. L., Dumon, K. R., & Williams, N. N. (2011). Surgical treatments for obesity. *Psychiatric Clinics of North American, 34*(4), 881–893.

Wadden, T. A., Bantle, J. P., Blackburn, G., Bolin, P., Brancati, F. L., Bray, G. A., ... Yanovski, S. Y. (2014). Eight-year weight losses with an intensive lifestyle intervention: The Look AHEAD study. *Obesity, 22*(1), 5–13.

Wadden, T. A., Butryn, M. L., & Byrne, K. J. (2004). Efficacy of lifestyle modification for long-term weight control. *Obesity Reviews, 12*(Suppl), 151S–162S.

Wadden, T. A., & Foster, G. D. (2000). Behavioral treatment of obesity. *Medical Clinics of North America, 84*(2), 441–461, vii.

Wadden, T. A., Foster, G. D., Letizia, K. A., & Mullen, J. L. (1990). Long-term effects of dieting on resting metabolic rate in obese outpatients. *Journal of the American Medical Association, 264*(6), 707–711.

Wadden, T. A., & Osei, E. S. (2002). The treatment of obesity: An overview. In T. A. Wadden & A. J. Stunkard (Eds.), *Handbook of obesity treatment* (pp. 229–248). New York, NY: Guilford Press.

Wadden, T. A., Volger, S., Sarwer, D. B., Vetter, M. L., Tsai, A. G., Berkowitz, R. I., ... Moore, R. H. (2011). A two-year randomized trial of obesity treatment in primary care practice. *New England Journal of Medicine, 365*(21), 1969–1979.

West, D. S., Elaine Prewitt, T., Bursac, Z., & Felix, H. C. (2008). Weight loss of black, white, and Hispanic men and women in the Diabetes Prevention Program. *Obesity (Silver Spring), 16*(6), 1413–1420.

Whelton, P. K., Appel, L. J., Espeland, M. A., Applegate, W. B., Ettinger, W. H., Jr., Kostis, J. B., ... Cutler, J. A. (1998). Sodium reduction and weight loss in the treatment of hypertension in older persons: a randomized controlled trial of nonpharmacologic interventions in the elderly (TONE). TONE Collaborative Research Group. *Journal of the American Medical Association, 279*(11), 839–846.

Wilfley, D. E., Tibbs, T. L., Van Buren, D. J., Reach, K. P., Walker, M. S., & Epstein, L. H. (2007). Lifestyle interventions in the treatment of childhood overweight: A meta-analytic review of randomized controlled trials. *Health Psychology, 26*(5), 521–532.

Wilfley, D. E., Vannucci, A., & White, E. K. (2010). Early intervention of eating- and weight-related problems. *Journal of Clinical Psychology in Medical Settings, 17*(4), 285–300.

Williamson, D. F., Kahn, H. S., Remington, P. L., & Anda, R. F. (1990). The 10-year incidence of overweight and major weight gain in US adults. *Archives of Internal Medicine, 150*(3), 665–672.

Williamson, D. A., Rejeski, J., Lang, W., Van Dorsten, B., Fabricatore, A. N., & Toledo, K. (2009). Impact of a weight management program on health-related quality of life in overweight adults with type 2 diabetes. *Archives of Internal Medicine, 169*(2), 163–171.

Wing, R. R. (1999). Physical activity in the treatment of adult overweight and obesity: Current evidence and research issues. *Medicine and Science in Sports and Exercise, 31*, S547–S552.

Wing, R. R. (2002). Behavioral weight control. In T. A. Wadden & A. J. Stunkard (Eds.), *Handbook of obesity treatment* (pp. 301–316). New York, NY: Guilford Press.

Wing, R. R., & Jeffery, R. W. (1999). Benefits of recruiting participants with friends and increasing social support for weight loss and maintenance. *Journal of Consulting and Clinical Psychology, 67*(1), 132–138.

Wing, R. R., Lang, W., Wadden, T. A., Safford, M., Knowler, W. C., Bertoni, A. G., ... Wagenknecht, L. (2011). Benefits of modest weight loss in improving cardiovascular risk factors in overweight and obese individuals with type 2 diabetes. *Diabetes Care, 34*(7), 1481–1486.

Wing, R. R., & Phelan, S. (2005). Long-term weight loss maintenance. *American Journal of Clinical Nutrition, 82*(1 Suppl), 222S–225S.

Wing, R. R., Tate, D. F., Gorin, A. A., Raynor, H. A., & Fava, J. L. (2006). A self-regulation program for maintenance of weight loss. *New England Journal of Medicine, 355*(15), 1563–1571.

Wren, A. M., Seal, L. J., Cohen, M. A., Brynes, A. E., Frost, G. S., Murphy, K. G., ... Bloom, S. R. (2001). Ghrelin enhances appetite and increases food intake in humans. *Journal of Clinical Endocrinology and Metabolism, 86*(12), 5992.

Wyatt, H. R., Grunwald, G. K., Mosca, C. L., Klem, M. L., Wing, R. R., & Hill, J. O. (2002). Long-term weight loss and breakfast in subjects in the National Weight Control Registry. *Obesity Reviews, 10*(2), 78–82.

Zhao, G., Ford, E. S., Dhingra, S., Li, C., Strine, T. W., & Mokdad, A. H. (2009). Depression and anxiety among US adults: Associations with body mass index. *International Journal of Obesity (Lond), 33*(2), 257–266.

Personality Disorders

Mary McMurran *and* Mike J. Crawford

Abstract

Personality disorders are common problems that place a significant burden on the individual, his or her family and friends, and society in general. There are effective treatments based on cognitive and behavioral theories. Most treatment evaluations relate to borderline personality disorder, and treatments for other personality disorders need to be developed. High-intensity, multidimensional, and comprehensive interventions are effective, but limited resources mean that few people have access to these treatments. Attention needs to be paid to developing alternative services, including good clinical management and service user support groups, and briefer interventions. Taking steps to promote engagement with treatments is an important consideration.

Key Words: personality disorder, cognitive and behavioral theories, cognitive and behavioral therapies, clinical guidelines, treatment engagement

Personality Disorders

Personality disorders (PDs) are adult psychiatric conditions described in the American Psychiatric Association's *Diagnostic and Statistical Manual of Mental Disorders* (*DSM*) and the World Health Organization's *International Classification of Diseases (ICD), Classification of Mental and Behavioural Disorders* (World Health Organization, 1992). The fourth edition of *DSM* (*DSM-IV-TR*; American Psychiatric Association, 2000) defines personality disorder as "an enduring pattern of inner experience and behavior that deviates markedly from the expectations of the individual's culture, is pervasive and inflexible, has an onset in adolescence or early adulthood, is stable over time, and leads to distress or impairment" (p. 685). This problematic pattern is manifested in two or more of the following areas: (1) cognition (i.e., ways of perceiving and interpreting self, other people, and events), (2) affectivity (i.e., the range, intensity, lability, and appropriateness of emotional response), (3) interpersonal functioning, and (4) impulse control. The key features of personality disorder are that the person's troubling or troublesome behavior and experiences are persistent, pervasive, and problematic.

In *DSM-IV-TR*, PDs are grouped in three clusters: Cluster A: odd or eccentric (paranoid, schizoid, and schizotypal); Cluster B: dramatic or flamboyant (antisocial, borderline, histrionic, and narcissistic); and Cluster C: anxious or fearful (avoidant, dependent, and obsessive-compulsive). The main features of the *DSM-IV* PDs are listed in Table 24.1.

Diagnosis

Personality disorders as a distinct diagnostic entity first appeared in *DSM-III* (American Psychiatric Association, 1980), placed on a separate axis (Axis II) that distinguished them from clinical syndromes (Axis I). Conceptual problems with PD diagnoses have been aired ever since their conception, including their atheoretical origins, major disconnect with "normal" personality theories and research, lack of comprehensiveness, poor validity, and poor reliability (Lenzenwenger

Table 24.1 *DSM-IV* personality disorders

Cluster A

Paranoid

Distrust and suspiciousness of others, indicated by four or more of the following: (a) unfounded suspicions that others are exploiting, harming or deceiving him or her; (b) preoccupation with unjustified doubts about others' loyalty or trustworthiness; (c) reluctance to confide in others for unwarranted fear that information will be maliciously used against him or her; (d) reading hidden demeaning or threatening meaning into benign remarks or events; (e) persistent bearing of grudges; (f) readiness to perceive attacks on his or her character or reputation that are not apparent to others and quickness to react angrily; (g) recurrent unjustified suspiciousness about the faithfulness of spouse or sexual partner.

Schizoid

Detachment from social relationships a restricted range of expression of emotions in interpersonal situations, indicated by four or more of the following: (a) does not desire or enjoy close relationships, including being part of a family; (b) prefers solitary activities; (c) has little interest in having sex with another person; (d) takes pleasure in few, if any, activities; (e) lacks close friends; (f) appears indifferent to the praise or criticism of others; (g) shows emotional coldness, detachment, or flattened affectivity.

Schizotypal

Social and interpersonal deficits marked by acute discomfort with close relationships, along with cognitive or perceptual distortions and eccentricities of behavior, indicated by five or more of the following: (a) ideas of reference; (b) odd beliefs or magical thinking that is inconsistent with subcultural norms and which influences behavior; (c) unusual perceptual experiences; (d) odd thinking and speech; (e) suspiciousness or paranoid ideas; (f) inappropriate or constricted affect; (g) odd, eccentric or peculiar behavior; (h) lack of close friends; (i) persistent and excessive social anxiety associated with paranoid fears rather than negative judgments about self.

Cluster B

Antisocial

The presence of Conduct Disorder with onset before age 15 years AND, in adulthood, a pervasive pattern of disregard for and violation of the rights of others evident since at least age 15 years, indicated by three or more of the following: (a) failure to abide by the law, as indicated by repeatedly behaving in ways that are grounds for arrest; (b) deceitfulness; (c) impulsivity or failure to plan ahead; (d) irritability and aggressiveness; (e) reckless disregard for the safety of self or others; (f) consistent irresponsibility, as indicated by repeated failure to sustain work and honor financial obligations; (g) lack of remorse.

Borderline

Pervasive instability of interpersonal relationships, self-image, and affects, and marked impulsivity, indicated by five or more of the following: (a) frantic efforts to avoid real or imagined abandonment; (b) unstable and intense interpersonal relationships; (c) unstable sense of self; (d) impulsivity in at least two areas that are potentially self-damaging (e.g., sex, substance abuse); (e) recurrent suicidal behavior or self-mutilation; (f) affective instability; (g) chronic feelings of emptiness; (h) inappropriate, intense anger; (i) transient stress-related paranoid ideation or severe dissociative symptoms.

Histrionic

Excessive emotionality and attention seeking, indicated by five or more of the following: (a) discomfort in situations in which he or she is not the center of attention; (b) inappropriate sexually seductive or provocative behavior in interactions with others; (c) rapidly shifting and shallow expression of emotions; (d) use of physical appearance to draw attention to self; (e) speech is excessively impressionistic and lacking in detail; (f) self-dramatization, theatricality, and exaggerated expression of emotion; (g) suggestibility; (h) considers relationships to be more intimate than they are.

(continued)

Table 24.1 Continued

Narcissistic

Grandiosity, need for admiration and lack of empathy, indicated by five or more of the following: (a) grandiose sense of self-importance; (b) preoccupation with fantasies of unlimited success, power, brilliance, beauty, or ideal love; (c) belief that he or she is special and unique and can only be understood by or associate with other special or high-status people; (d) requires excessive admiration; (e) has a sense of entitlement; (f) is interpersonally exploitative; (g) lacks empathy; (h) is often envious of others or believes others are envious of him or her; (i) shows arrogant behaviors or attitudes.

Cluster C

Avoidant

Social inhibition, feelings of inadequacy and hypersensitivity to negative evaluation, indicated by four or more of the following: (a) avoidance of occupations that involve significant interpersonal contact for fear of criticism, disapproval or rejection; (b) unwillingness to get involved with people unless certain of being liked; (c) shows restraint in intimate relationships for fear of being shamed or ridiculed; (d) preoccupation with being criticized or rejected in social situations; (e) feels inhibited in new interpersonal situations because of feelings of inadequacy; (f) views self as socially inept, personally unappealing or inferior to others; (g) reluctance to take personal risks or engage in new activities because they may prove embarrassing.

Dependent

An excessive need to be taken care of that leads to submissive and clinging behavior and fears of separation, indicated by five or more of the following: (a) difficulty making everyday decisions without an excessive amount of advice and reassurance from others; (b) needs others to assume responsibility for most major areas of his or her life; (c) has difficulty expressing disagreement with others because of unrealistic fears of loss of support or approval; (d) has difficulty initiating projects or doing things on his or her own because of lack of self-confidence; (e) goes to excessive lengths to obtain nurturance and support; (f) feels uncomfortable or helpless when alone because of fears of being unable to care for himself or herself; (g) urgently seeks another relationship when a close relationship ends; (h) is unrealistically preoccupied with fears of being left to take care of himself or herself.

Obsessive-compulsive

Preoccupation with orderliness, perfectionism, and mental and interpersonal control at the expense of flexibility, openness and efficiency, indicated by four or more of the following: (a) preoccupation with details, rules, lists, order, and schedules, to the extent that the main point of the activity is lost; (b) perfectionism that interferes with task completion; (c) excessive devotion to work and productivity to the exclusion of leisure activities and friendships; (d) overconscientious, scrupulous and inflexible about matters of morality, ethics or values; (e) unable to discard worn-out or worthless objects; (f) reluctance to delegate tasks or work with others unless others submit to his or her way of doing things; (g) miserly with money and saving money for future catastrophes; (h) rigid and stubborn.

Personality disorder not otherwise specified

There is a disorder of personality functioning but the criteria for any one specific personality disorder are not met. There may be features of more than one specific personality disorder that together cause distress or impairment, or a personality disorder not included in the classification is considered important (e.g., depressive personality disorder or passive-aggressive personality disorder).

& Clarkin, 2005). Although research has mitigated some of these problems over the years, most notably improving diagnostic reliability through the development of structured clinical assessment schedules, dissatisfaction with PD diagnoses has not disappeared.

Revisions of *DSM-IV* and *ICD-10* address problems with the validity, reliability, and utility of PD diagnoses. In 2013, after much controversy (Livesley, 2013), the fifth version of *DSM* was published (American Psychiatric Association, 2013). In this version, the 10 personality disorders of *DSM-IV-TR* are retained, but there is an optional hybrid model aimed at furthering research. In this, personality disorders are characterized not only by impairments in personality functioning (identity problems or problems in interpersonal functioning) but also by the presence of pathological personality traits (negative affectivity, detachment, antagonism, disinhibition, and psychoticism). *DSM-5* directs clinicians to assess the level of impairment (little, some, moderate, severe, or extreme) in relation to six specific PD types (antisocial, avoidant, borderline, narcissistic, obsessive-compulsive, and schizotypal) with the option for diagnosis of a PD that is trait specified (Skodol, 2011). This hybrid model is not without its critics, who have commented that proposed classification is unnecessarily complex, incoherent, and inconsistent, and that the typal and dimensional models are probably incompatible and certainly not well integrated (Frances, 2012). *ICD-11* is set to take a different course, retaining five PDs (schizotypal, avoidant, antisocial, borderline, and obsessive-compulsive) and classifying them by severity (no PD; PD difficulty; PD disorder; complex PD; severe PD; Tyrer et al., 2011). Again, this model has its critics, who are not convinced that the five types map onto models of normal personality or that the severity scale is a valid one (Gunderson & Zanarini, 2011). The landscape of PD looks set to change, and this will have an impact on how the results of new and existing research are interpreted and applied. However, since research based on the new criteria set forth in *DSM-5* is not yet mainstream, in this chapter, earlier definitions of personality disorder will be used.

Prevalence

Estimates of the prevalence of PD in general populations vary from 4.4% in the United Kingdom (Coid, Yang, Tyrer, Roberts, & Ullrich, 2006), 9.0% in one U.S. sample (Samuels et al., 2002) and 11.9% in another U.S. sample (Lenzenweger, Lane, Loranger, & Kessler, 2007), to 13.4% in a Norwegian sample (Torgerson, Kringlen, & Kramer, 2001). These differences in prevalence may reflect the use of different versions of the *DSM* or *ICD*, variations in the sensitivity of the diagnostic tests used, differences in how the data were analyzed, or genuine differences between cultures in the prevalence of personality disorders. Nonetheless, to put PD prevalence rates into perspective, the lifetime prevalences in the general population for other major mental disorders are: 0.87% for schizophrenia, 0.24% for bipolar I disorder, and 0.35% for major depressive disorder with psychotic features (Perälä et al., 2007). PDs are, therefore, a highly prevalent disorder.

Comorbidity

There is considerable comorbidity of PDs both with other PDs and with major mental disorders. In Coid et al.'s (2006) sample of people with PD, 53% had one disorder, 22% had two disorders, 11% had three disorders, and 14% had four or more disorders, and the average number of PDs was 1.92. PDs also frequently co-occur with Axis I disorders, although, for the most part, the co-occurrence follows base rates (McGlashan et al., 2000). Most people with PD seek help for their Axis I disorders rather than their PD (Coid et al., 2006). This suggests that people with PD will be present in mental health services generally, not just in dedicated PD services. When PD occurs in association with an Axis 1 disorder, this generally has further negative impact upon the individual's functioning (Newton-Howes, Tyrer, & Weaver, 2008) and treatment outcome (Mennin & Heimberg, 2000; Newton-Howes, Tyrer, & Johnston, 2006; Reich, 2003). There is, therefore, a need to treat PD in conjunction with the treatment of other mental disorders.

The Impact of Personality Disorders

The case for treating people diagnosed with PD rests on the impact of PD on the individual, on other people, and on society generally. PDs are associated with significantly increased rates of premature mortality (Fok et al., 2012). This may be because people with PDs commonly engage in health-compromising behaviors, such as substance abuse (Coid et al., 2006; Verheul, van den Brink, & Hartgers, 1995). Compared with people with no disorder, those with PDs suffer more general health problems (Noren et al., 2007), use health-care services more (Powers & Oltmanns, 2012), and the costs of treating people with PD in primary care is about double that of people without PD (Rendu, Moran, Patel, Knapp, & Mann, 2002). Central to PD is interpersonal and social dysfunction and how this prevents the satisfactory achievement of life tasks (Livesley & Lang, 2005; Nur, Tyrer, Merson, & Johnson, 2004; Seivewright, Tyrer & Johnson, 2004; Skodol et al., 2005). PD is associated with financial difficulties and problems maintaining jobs (Noren et al., 2007), marital dissatisfaction and intimate partner violence (South, Turkheimer, & Oltmanns, 2008), crime (Johnson et al., 2000), and poor quality of life (Soeteman, Verheul, & Busschbach, 2008). Although PD can remit, social-functioning problems tend to persist over time (Gunderson, Stout, et al., 2011). These matters make a strong case for treating people with PD.

We now turn to an understanding of PD within a cognitive and behavioral framework.

Theories of Personality Disorder

Diagnostic categories fulfill the function of organizing clinical phenomena into groups for clinical and scientific purposes; however, although they describe PDs, they do not explain these disorders (Millon, Meagher, & Grossman, 2001). Theories of PD are essential to guide scientific enquiry by formulating testable models of the etiology of PD, the processes of developing a disorder, its course over the life span, and hence to provide a rational basis on which to design treatments (Lenzenweger & Clarkin, 2005). There are different levels of exploration and explanation, from biological, through psychological, to societal, and within each level there are different theories of functioning. Although theories at all levels have a contribution to make to our understanding of PD, the focus here is on cognitive and behavioral theories.

Cognitive and behavioral theories in general recognize that the individual is born with a constellation of dispositions or basic traits, relating to affect, activity, and attention, which have biological bases. Reciprocal interactions between the individual with a unique set of traits and his or her social environment across the lifespan produce the adult with a particular personality profile. Personality traits are behavioral patterns that may have once had survival value, but when they are no longer adaptive, and if they are inflexible and persistent, they may be detrimental to well-being and, thereby, constitute a disorder. There are a number of specific cognitive and behavioral theories of PD, some of which explain particular PDs and others that explain PDs more generally.

Cognitive Theory

The focus in cognitive theories is on the individual's core beliefs or basic schemas that activate affective responses and behavioral strategies (Beck & Freeman, 1990). Cognitive theories of PD are based on the notion that an individual's emotional and behavioral responses to a situation are determined by systematic errors, biases, and distortions in how that person perceives and interprets events (Pretzer & Beck, 2005).

Beck and colleagues focus on *basic or core beliefs* that are linked with overt behavior strategies (Beck & Freeman, 1990). For example, narcissistic PD is characterized by the basic belief "I am special" and the overt behavior is self-aggrandizement; dependent PD is characterized by the basic belief "I am helpless"

and the overt behavior is attachment; and paranoid PD is characterized by the basic belief "People are potential adversaries" and the overt behavior is wariness. These beliefs formed the basis of the Personality Belief Questionnaire (PBQ; Beck & Beck, 1991), a 126-item self-report questionnaire that aims to assess respondents' personality beliefs. Beck et al. (2001) found that people with avoidant, dependent, obsessive-compulsive, narcissistic, and paranoid PDs scored significantly higher on the relevant PD subscale of the PBQ than did those with no disorder or other PDs, supporting the association between certain personality beliefs and corresponding PDs. There is no specific borderline scale in the PBQ, since this disorder was seen as more variable in presentation and less specific in content than other disorders (Beck & Freeman, 1990); nonetheless, items that discriminate borderline PD have been identified and a score for borderline beliefs may be calculated (Butler, Brown, Beck, & Grisham, 2002). Bhar, Brown, and Beck (2008) found that this subscale consisted of three factors—dependency, distrust, and protection (i.e., the need to take pre-emptive action to prevent rejection)—which were associated with depressive psychopathology. McMurran and Christopher (2008) found that antisocial beliefs as measured by the PBQ did not discriminate men with antisocial PD from those without, but that the avoidant and paranoid scales did. The PBQ avoidant scale items focus upon fear of criticism, failure, intimacy, and rejection, and the PBQ paranoid scale items cover expectations that others are untrustworthy, duplicitous, and intend to exploit and harm. The PBQ antisocial scale may be tapping primary psychopathy, which is related to selfishness and callousness, whereas secondary psychopathy is actually related to other basic beliefs. Blackburn (2009) suggested that both groups of psychopaths might be behaviorally alike but that primary psychopaths respond aggressively when their perceived high status is threatened, whereas secondary psychopaths respond aggressively to threat because of anxiety and emotional vulnerability. These variations have relevance for cognitive theory and therapy with different subtypes of psychopath.

Schema Theory

A schema approach to PD was developed by Young (1990). Schemas are mental representations of an individual's social knowledge and experience. When triggered, schemas guide affective and behavioral responses in the present. Some schemas may lead to maladaptive responses, and, according to

Young, those of particular importance for PD are *early maladaptive schemas*. An early maladaptive schema is defined as "a broad, pervasive theme or pattern, comprised of memories, emotions, cognitions, and bodily sensations, regarding oneself and one's relationships with others, developed during childhood or adolescence, elaborated throughout one's lifetime, and dysfunctional to a significant degree" (Young, Klosko, & Weishaar, 2003, p. 7). Many maladaptive schemas are built from adverse childhood experiences, such as abuse or neglect, but also from other types of damaging experiences, such as overprotection. They share the common feature of stemming from one or more unmet core emotional needs. As before, the child's innate temperament has a role to play in the interactions that lead to the formation of schemas.

Young lists 18 schemas in five categories, these categories being: (1) *Disconnection and rejection*, which includes fear of abandonment, feeling unlovable and disconnected from other people, and the expectation that others will hurt or neglect one; (2) *Impaired autonomy and performance*, which includes feelings of inadequacy, excessive emotional involvement with others, and fear of imminent harm or illness; (3) *Impaired limits*, which includes entitlement beliefs and difficulty tolerating frustration; (4) *Other directedness,* which includes excessively meeting the needs of others at one's own expense and emphasis on gaining others' approval; and (5) *Over-vigilance and inhibition,* which includes excessive negativity and pessimism, excessive inhibition of spontaneous action, feeling, or communication; perfectionism; and punitiveness. Associated with schemas are specific maladaptive coping responses, which vary both between people and within any one person depending on circumstances. Responses fall into three basic coping styles—overcompensation, avoidance, and surrender. Overcompensation is where individuals act as if the opposite of the schema were true, for example by conveying oneself to be of some importance when the schema is actually one of feeling worthless. Avoidance is where steps are taken to prevent the schema being activated, either by avoiding risky situations such as intimate relationships, or by blotting out thoughts and feelings using drink, drugs, or excessive activity. Surrender is where the schemas are allowed to trigger the maladaptive response learned in childhood, and maladaptive behavior repeats itself. Schemas are assessed using versions of the Young Schema Questionnaire (YSQ; see www.schematherapy.com). These schemas have

been validated through factor analyses of YSQ items, and correlations with *DSM* personality traits have been evidenced (Hoffart et al., 2005; Jovev & Jackson, 2004; Petrocelli, Glaser, Calhoun, & Campbell, 2001).

Emotion Dysregulation Theory

The predominant theory of dysregulation is Linehan's (1993) theory of borderline PD. She argues that the *DSM-IV* diagnostic criteria may be organized into five areas of dysregulation: (1) emotional, (2) cognitive, (3) behavioral, (4) self, and (5) interpersonal. Linehan (1993) positioned emotional dysregulation central to borderline PD, noting its occurrence in people with high emotional reactivity, strong experienced emotional intensity, and a lack of skills for managing strong emotions. Dysregulation in other areas occurs as a consequence of emotional dysregulation or as maladaptive attempts to regulate problematic emotions.

A hyperbolic temperament, which is highly heritable, interacts with adverse experiences (e.g., abuse or neglect) across the lifespan to produce an adult who responds to triggering events with the behaviors that are symptomatic of borderline PD (Zanarini & Frankenburg, 2007). One particularly pertinent type of adverse experience is an invalidating environment, in which an individual's experiences (emotions and thoughts) and behaviors are judged as inappropriate, unimportant, or unacceptable and are punished or disregarded (Robins, Ivanoff, & Linehan, 2001). This may lead to an escalation of emotional responses in order to get the required attention and recognition, with a resultant pattern of extremes of emotional inhibition and emotional expression.

Research into emotion dysregulation and borderline PD indicates that this is indeed a core feature (Cheavens, Strunk, & Chriki, 2012; Glenn, & Klonsky, 2009; Reeves, James, Pizzarello, & Taylor, 2010). People with borderline PD have high baseline emotional intensity (Kuo & Linehan, 2009), and evidence low tolerance for emotional distress (Gratz, Rosenthal, Tull, Lejeuz, & Gunderson, 2006), although invalidation may not be central to the development of emotional deregulation (Reeves et al., 2010).

Attachment Theory

PD is considered by many to be essentially a problem in relating to others; therefore, attachment theory provides a useful framework of understanding PD. Originating with Bowlby (1969), the theory states that attachments are formed in infancy between infant and caregiver, that these bonds develop over childhood with experiences of social interactions, and childhood bonds provide a model for adult attachments. Bartholomew and Horowitz (1991) have identified two underlying dimensions and four styles of adult attachment. The underlying dimensions are (1) how one views oneself, a positive view being an internalized sense of self-worth and a negative view being low self-worth and a need for external validation in relationships; and (2) how one views others, a positive view being the expectation that others will be available and supportive and a negative view being that others are untrustworthy and rejecting. Different positions on these dimensions produce four attachment prototypes: (1) *secure attachment* (positive self-model, positive other model), in which individuals are self-confident, warm, and friendly toward others, have close friendships, and appraise intimate relationships realistically; (2) *fearful attachment* (negative self-model, negative other model), in which individuals avoid intimacy for fear of rejection; (3) *preoccupied attachment* (negative self-model, positive other model), in which individuals idolize others, and are needing of attention, excessively emotionally expressive, and highly dependent in relationships; (4) *Dismissing attachment* (positive self-model, negative other model), which is characterized by superficial friendships and low-intimacy relationships.

Empirical studies have shown associations between attachment styles and PD. Investigations using the Bartholomew and Horowitz (1991) model show that dependent, histrionic, and borderline PDs are associated with a preoccupied style (Patrick, Hobson, Castle, Hobson, & Maughan, 1994; Timmerman & Emmelkamp, 2006; West, Rose, & Sheldon-Keller, 1994); antisocial PD and psychopathy are associated with a dismissing style (Frodi, Dernevik, Sepa, Philipson, & Bragesjö, 2001; Rosenstein & Horowitz, 1996; Timmerman & Emmelkamp, 2006); and Cluster A PDs are associated with a fearful style (Timmerman & Emmelkamp, 2006). Other research has identified latent dimensions of avoidance and anxiety in attachments, with avoidance associated with avoidant, paranoid, schizotypal, and schizoid PDs, and anxiety associated with dependent and borderline PDs (Fossati et al., 2003). Clearly, different attachment styles are a feature of certain PDs.

Interpersonal Theory

Interpersonal theories have their origins with Sullivan (1953) and Leary (1957), who viewed PDs as maladaptive patterns of social interaction and communication. Individuals are born with "integrating tendencies" that support mutual cooperation with the goal of satisfying the basic and higher-order needs that are necessary for survival and well-being. From infancy, complex patterns of relating are developed and internalized, and the outcomes of these patterns of interaction shape the person's concept of self. PD is when maladaptive relational strategies develop and persist, and their outcomes lead to a dysfunctional conception of self (Pincus, 2005). Pincus pointed out that it is not just actual interactions that have an effect, but that mental representations of interpersonal functioning occur in memories and fantasies and these internal experiences are also important influences.

Several authors have developed versions of the *interpersonal circumplex* or *interpersonal circle*, a means of assessing interpersonal behaviors and interpersonal style. Originally constructed by Leary (1957) around two orthogonal dimensions of power or control (dominant-submissive) and affiliation (hostile-friendly), the interpersonal circle was later developed by others (Benjamin, 1974; Blackburn 1998; Kiesler, 1983; Wiggins, 1982). These circles show blends of the dimensions in segments, although the boundaries of these segments are not rigid, and there are positions within segments that describe the level of the dimension described by the segment—normal behavior is placed near the center of the circle and extreme and inflexible behavior nearer the perimeter. The principle of complementarity in interpersonal theory is that particular behaviors and styles of interacting evoke reciprocal responses from the other person, for instance dominance evokes submission and friendliness evokes friendliness.

A number of measures have been constructed to assess interpersonal behaviors and styles, and these confirm the validity of the interpersonal circle (Acton & Revelle, 2002; Monsen, von der Lippe, Havik, Halvorsen, & Eilersten 2007). Additionally, there is some evidence that PDs map onto the circumplex, positioned as one might expect in relation to vectors of control and affiliation (Birtchnell & Shine, 2000; Pukrop, Sass, & Steinmeyer, 2000).

Social Problem Solving Theory

McMurran and colleagues (McMurran, Duggan, Christopher, & Huband, 2007; McMurran, Egan, & Duggan, 2005) proposed a model in which the concept of social problem solving is central to PD. Assuming that innate traits are the developmental start-point for behavioral patterns, they postulated that certain personality traits limit and bias information processing, interfering with the acquisition of good social problem solving skills and consequently leading to dysfunctional ways of operating in everyday life. Interpersonal dysfunction causes stress, experienced affectively in a number of ways including anxiety, depression, and anger, which further impairs problem-solving abilities and may also lead to problematic stress-relieving behaviors, such as substance use, which still further impair social problem-solving abilities and also potentially create additional interpersonal problems. Persistent dysfunction leads to a negative approach to life's problems and the development of maladaptive self-schemas that have a further deleterious effect on information processing and social problem solving.

People diagnosed with personality disorders have been identified as poorer on a test of social problem solving (the Social Problem Solving Inventory-Revised; D'Zurilla, Nezu, & Maydeu-Olivares, 2002) compared to samples of mature students and offenders (Hayward, McMurran, & Sellen, 2008; Huband, McMurran, Evans, & Duggan, 2007; McMurran, 2009; McMurran, Blair, & Egan, 2002). Social problem-solving profiles have also been found to vary across personality disorder subtypes (McMurran et al., 2007; McMurran, Oaksford, & Christopher, 2010).

Theories of Psychopathy

Psychopathy is not currently a distinct diagnosis in either *DSM* or *ICD*. *ICD-10* lists dissocial PD, with criteria that are largely those traits originally identified by Cleckley (1941) as defining psychopathy, namely lack of guilt, lack of anxiety, inability to learn from punishment, impoverished emotions, inability to form lasting emotional ties, egocentricity, and superficial charm. *DSM-IV* lists antisocial PD, based upon more behavioral criteria, namely law-breaking, recklessness, and irresponsibility. *ICD-10* dissocial PD may mainly tap primary psychopathy, which is characterized by low fear and callous unemotional traits, and *DSM-IV* antisocial PD may mainly tap secondary psychopathy, which is characterized by high anxiety and impulsiveness. The *DSM-5* revision of antisocial PD draws much more heavily on the construct of primary psychopathy, particularly the callous and unemotional traits that many view as the cornerstone of the disorder.

Callous and unemotional traits in children are associated with especially severe aggression and persistent conduct problems, and there is evidence for high levels of heritability of these traits (Viding, Blair, Moffitt, & Plomin, 2005). These traits in children may interfere with early attachment relationships with caregivers, which may exacerbate the absence of concern for others and may also affect the carer's affection for and attention to the child (Saltaris, 2002). Good parenting may have less impact on children with emotional deficits than on those without, in terms of teaching the child to be attentive to the feelings of others, but there may be scope for influence through modeling acceptable means of attaining goals, such that prosocial role models have the potential to divert the child from antisocial means of goal attainment. Indeed, primary psychopathy should not be conflated with criminality. Skeem and Cooke (2010) indicated that omitting measures of criminality and disapproved behaviors produces a purer personality model of primary psychopathy, with three constituent factors: (1) arrogant and deceitful interpersonal style, (2) deficient affective experience, and (3) impulsive and irresponsible behavioral style. However, others are of the view that excluding antisocial behavior from the construct of psychopathy may be to exclude an important dimension (Hare & Neumann, 2010).

The developmental sequence of secondary psychopathy identifies early hyperactivity, impulsivity, and inattention, which flourishes into childhood conduct problems, and presents a direct risk for adult antisocial personality disorder. This developmental pathway has been researched in a number of high quality longitudinal studies, whose findings are summarized by Farrington (2005). Impulsiveness, particularly in association with low verbal intelligence, may be linked to deficits in the executive functions of the brain, and may indicate an impairment in the abilities necessary for forward planning and goal-directed behavior, including attention, abstract reasoning, and behavioral inhibition. This initial risk for antisocial behavior and violence is inflated where parental management of the child is harsh and inconsistent, such that the child is seldom rewarded for good behavior but often punished for bad behavior. The child's experience is that being good is unrewarded and the child may also become desensitized to punishment. The child's difficult behavior and the caregivers' management practices influence each other in a reciprocal relationship, often creating a vicious cycle of adverse effects. Furthermore, there is evidence that some individuals may be more sensitive to stress, and maltreatment in childhood may have a greater effect on their development, leading to increased odds of conduct disorder, antisocial behavior, and violence later in life (Caspi et al., 2002).

Summation

The theories presented above are arguably the major cognitive and behavioral theories of PD that have currency today. Although each of the theories presented here is in accord with a developmental understanding of PD in which adult problems are a product of the individual in reciprocal interaction with his or her social context from infancy onward, each has a different focus. Together, these theories contribute to a broad understanding of the individual. However, they are by no means the only theories. Other theories that are not covered here have an important contribution to make, notably theories from the biological, neuroscience, and evolutionary psychology disciplines. The truth is that there is no single explanation for any one PD, or for the complex picture presented by those with multiple co-occurring disorders. As we shall see later, many therapies adopt a multidimensional approach and the result is complex, multifaceted interventions that may have roots in several of the aforementioned theories.

Treatment Components

Theories that explain different aspects of PD present therapists with the question of what it is they should treat. Should they target basic traits (e.g., negative emotionality; impulsiveness), psychosocially developed core areas of dysfunction (e.g., emotional dysregulation, core beliefs, schemas, identity) or symptoms (e.g., self-harm, aggression, substance use)? Livesley (2005) has proposed a systematic framework for treating personality disorder. This is an eclectic approach, coordinating and integrating both general principles of therapy and specific interventions. The principles acknowledge that PD is multidimensional and that a comprehensive range of interventions will be required, and that these interventions should be coordinated. In general, interventions should address the core issues of PD psychopathology, namely interpersonal dysfunction and a poorly developed sense of self. Therapists should maximize the nonspecific effects of therapy by providing a supportive and validating experience, building a good therapy alliance, and offering the client new learning opportunities. Therapy should be a collaborative endeavor, and interventions should be appropriate to the individual's stage of change. Treatments should target aspects that are amenable to change, namely symptoms, maladaptive thinking styles, attitudes about

the self, and interpersonal patterns. Traits, such as emotional reactivity and impulsiveness, are less amenable to change.

Livesley (2005) proposes a phased approach to treatment with different interventions appropriate within each phase. Phase 1 is *developing safety and managing crises* through defining risk signatures, putting support systems in place, and, if necessary, admitting to hospital for a brief period. Phase 2 is *containment of emotional and behavioral instability* through acknowledging distress, clarifying feelings, and, in some cases, offering medication. Phase 3 is *improving self-management of emotions and impulses* using therapies that teach self-regulation skills, desensitize the individual to the power of triggers for emotional responses, and reframe how triggers are perceived. Phase 4 is *exploration and change* through changing maladaptive beliefs and schemas, interpersonal styles, and self-defeating behaviors. Phase 5 is *integration and synthesis*, where a more coherent sense of self is gradually built up through developing satisfying lifestyles and working toward valued longer-term goals. With this in mind, we turn now to the identification of what specific cognitive and behavioral treatments are empirically supported.

Empirically Supported Cognitive and Behavioral Treatments

Empirically supported cognitive and behavioral treatments do not map exactly onto the major theories of PD just presented. There are two main reasons for this. First, we have presented only those treatments that have the most robust empirical research evidence. According to Chambless and Hollon (1998), for a treatment to be considered empirically supported, at least two independent, well-conducted randomized controlled trials (RCTs) or single-case experiments with a sample size of 3 or more should support the treatment; if only one RCT or single-case experiment supports the treatment, then it is considered promising. Other treatments may be supported by less robust research designs, but these are not reported here. Second, some of the treatments reported here draw on other theories to complement or augment cognitive and behavioral approaches. We have included these if there is research evidence for them, but we have not expounded upon the full range of noncognitive and nonbehavioral approaches.

The most comprehensive and unbiased way of identifying and evaluating the research on any topic is through systematic reviewing. The methodology for conducting a systematic review is rigorous, including precise specification of the research question, explicitly stating the criteria for including and excluding studies, and comprehensively searching the research literature. It seems wise to base this section on existing systematic reviews and meta-analyses of PD treatment outcome studies. Two systematic reviews will form the basis of our overview. Duggan, Huband, Smailagic, Ferriter, and Adams (2007) examined evaluations of psychological treatments for people with personality disorder published up to the end of 2006. Although this meta-analysis included evaluations of dialectical behavior therapy (DBT), it has been superseded by a more recent meta-analysis of this therapy (Kliem, Kröger, & Kosfelder, 2010). Therefore, we will report findings for DBT separately based on the Kliem et al. report. Furthermore, Duggan et al. report on psychodynamic therapies, which are not relevant in this text on cognitive and behavioral therapies, hence will be excluded from our review. However, we have updated Duggan et al.'s (2007) review by searching for RCTs published in English from 2007 to mid-2012.

Cognitive and Behavioral Therapy (CBT)

The core components of CBT are identifying maladaptive core beliefs, negative automatic thoughts, and maladaptive coping strategies through discussion, formal assessment, and self-monitoring. The function of these core beliefs is analyzed, the veracity and utility of core beliefs is challenged, and core beliefs are changed through restructuring, reinterpretation, and behavioral experiments (Beck & Freeman, 1990). Emmelkamp et al. (2006) treated people with avoidant PD, comparing those receiving 20 weekly sessions of CBT (n=21) focusing on anxiety and avoidance as related to individuals' maladaptive beliefs and related thought processes, with those receiving 20 weekly sessions of brief psychodynamic therapy (n=23) and a waitlist control (n=18). At 6-month follow-up, the CBT group showed significantly greater improvements on the Personality Disorder Belief Questionnaire (Arntz, Dreessen, Schouten, & Weertmann, 2004) obsessive and avoidant scales (weighted mean difference [WMD] -18.50; 95% confidence interval [CI] = -33.77, -3.23 and -0.90, 95%CI=-1.68, -0.12, respectively).

Davidson et al. (2006) evaluated the effectiveness of CBT for borderline PD, comparing those who received on average 16 weekly sessions (n=54) with those who received treatment as usual (n=52). Over 24 months postrandomization, those receiving CBT showed significantly fewer suicidal acts (mean difference -0.91; 95%CI=-1.67, -0.15), but no differences in hospitalization episodes, or emergency department contacts. A 6-year follow-up of the same sample, with data available for 82%, showed that this significant difference in suicidal acts was maintained at 2 years (mean difference adjusted for baseline differences in social difficulties = 1.18; 95%CI=-0.31, 2.06), and at 6 years just failed to reach statistical significance (adjusted mean difference = 1.26; 95%CI=-0.06, 2.58) (Davidson, Tyrer, Norrie, Palmer, & Tyrer, 2010).

A comparison of six sessions of manual assisted CBT (MACT) (n=18), that is CBT augmented by self-help booklets, with treatment as usual (n=16) targeting self-harm in people with cluster B PDs, showed that the CBT group had significantly greater improvement on the Social Functioning Questionnaire (Tyrer et al., 2005) at 6 months (WMD=-3.30; 95%CI= -6.38, -0.22), although there were no significant differences in self-harm (Evans et al., 1999). In a further study of MACT for deliberate self-harm, a subsample of persons with any PD who received MACT (n=91) compared those who received treatment as usual (n=90) were not significantly different in incidence of self-harm at 6 or 12-month follow-up, although MACT was cheaper than treatment as usual (Tyrer et al., 2004).

Davidson and Tyrer (1996) delivered cognitive therapy to five men with antisocial PD, who were asked to keep a daily diary of their main problem experiences. After a baseline phase of 16 days, there was a treatment phase of between 2 and 18 sessions (median = 9 sessions). Time series analyses were conducted on 3 patients with a significant improvement on only one rating in one man's case—an improvement in his relationship with his wife. An exploratory RCT with violent men with antisocial PD compared 15 sessions of CBT over 6 months (n=12), 30 sessions of CBT over 12 months (n=13), and treatment as usual (n=27). At 12-month follow-up, both CBT groups together and the treatment as usual group had reduced self-reported verbal and physical aggression, but there were no differences between groups (Davidson et al., 2009). Scores on measures of alcohol consumption, anxiety and depression, and social functioning did not differ between groups at follow-up. However, the authors emphasize that this was a small-scale feasibility study that was not adequately powered to detect a treatment effect.

Svartberg, Stiles, and Selzer (2004) compared cognitive therapy for cluster C PD (*n*=25) versus short-term psychodynamic psychotherapy (*n*=25), each lasting 40 weeks. Over a two-year follow-up, the whole sample of patients made large and significant improvements on measures of distress, interpersonal problems, and psychopathology, although no differences between groups were apparent. This indicates that both treatments worked, but neither was superior.

Schema Therapy

Schema therapy or schema-focused therapy was developed by Jeffrey Young to address the observations that persons with characterological problems find it hard to access core beliefs and associated emotions, they have difficulties building a therapeutic alliance, they are often unclear about what they want to change, and they are frequently pessimistic about change. Its aims are to identify and change maladaptive schemas and ineffective coping strategies. First, maladaptive schemas are identified and their origins are explored. Clients are then helped to become aware of when and how these schemas operate in their everyday lives, to challenge the validity of their maladaptive schemas, and to develop more adaptive beliefs. Emotion regulation strategies are developed and the client is supported in breaking old self-defeating behavior patterns. Throughout, the therapist models a healthy adult mode of operating so that clients can gradually internalize this.

Giesen-Bloo et al. (2006) compared schema-focused therapy (*n*=44) with transference-focused therapy (*n*=42) with borderline PD patients. Treatment sessions were twice weekly over a 3-year period. Significant improvements were found for both treatments on all measures after 1-, 2-, and 3-year treatment periods. After 3 years of treatment, survival analyses demonstrated that significantly more schema-focused therapy patients recovered (relative risk (RR) = 2.18) or showed reliable clinical improvement (RR = 2.33) on the primary outcome measure, the Borderline Personality Disorder Severity Index, fourth version (BPDSI-IV) (Arntz et al., 2003). This group also improved more in general psychopathology and quality of life than the transference-focused therapy group.

Ball (2007) compared Dual Focus Schema Therapy (DFST) (*n*=15), a combination of schema therapy and relapse prevention designed for personality-disordered substance misusers, with 12-step therapy (*n*=15) with opioid-dependent personality-disordered outpatients over a 6-month treatment period. Both groups received methadone maintenance over this period. The DFST group reduced their substance use frequency more rapidly over the treatment period than did the 12-step group (hierarchical linear model estimate -.06, standard error [SE]=.09, *z*=2.25, p<.005), although 12 step therapy produced greater decreases in negative affect. Ball, Maccarelli, LaPaglia, and Ostrowski (2011) conducted a trial of DFST (*n*=54) versus individual drug counselling (*n*=51) for personality-disordered substance misusers in residential treatment with results favoring counseling in reducing psychiatric symptoms measured by the Brief Symptom Inventory (BSI; Derogatis, 1992).

Farrell, Shaw, and Webber (2009) evaluated an 8-month, 30-session schema-focused therapy group (*n*=16) versus usual individual therapy (*n*=16) with women diagnosed with borderline PD. The schema-focused therapy group showed significantly greater improvements both after treatment and at 6-month follow-up on the Borderline Syndrome Index (BSI; Conte, Plutchik, Karasu, & Jerrett, 1980) (Cohen's *d* = 1.97 and 2.81, respectively), the Diagnostic Interview for Borderline Personality Disorder-Revised (DIB-R; Zanarini, Gunderson, Frankenberg, & Chauncey, 1990) (Cohen's *d* = 2.22 and 2.42), the Symptom Checklist-90 (SCL-90; Derogatis, 1994) (Cohen's *d* = 1.35 and 2.20), and the Global Assessment of Functioning (GAF; Endicott, Spitzer, Fleiss, & Coen, 1976) (Cohen's *d* = 1.39 and 3.13).

Using a crossover design, in which the individual serves as his or her own control, Weertman and Arntz (2007) compared the effectiveness of schema-focused therapy with therapy aimed at re-scripting childhood memories with people with personality disorders other than borderline, schizotypal, schizoid, or antisocial. After an alliance-building and assessment phase (12 sessions), there were two 24-session phases—one focused on present schemas and one on childhood memories. The order of these phases was counterbalanced. Analyses of data from 17 patients, using a composite measure of symptoms and schemas, showed that both components of treatment were effective with the focus on current schemas more effective than the focus on childhood memories (Cohen's *d* = 0.70 and 0.54, respectively).

Dialectical Behavior Therapy (DBT)

DBT is a comprehensive treatment program developed by Marsha Linehan for people with borderline PD (see Robins et al., 2001 for an overview). DBT is underpinned by the dialectic that acceptance and change are both necessary; that is, the client needs to accept reality and at the same time strive to change what can be changed. Validation strategies and problem-solving skills are both important components of DBT. Before treatment proper starts, the therapist introduces DBT, agrees on treatment goals with the client, and promotes commitment to the treatment program. The overall aims are to reduce self-harming behaviors, improve emotional stability, develop a more complete sense of self, and expand the capacity for enjoyment of life. DBT does this over the course of a year or more of individual and group sessions teaching and supporting the implementation of behavior chain analysis, mindfulness, distress tolerance techniques, emotion regulation skills, and interpersonal effectiveness skills.

Kliem et al. (2010) conducted a meta-analytic review of both RCTs and non-RCT evaluations of DBT with persons formally diagnosed with borderline PD. They identified 26 studies of 16 separate samples, of which eight were randomized. The sample sizes of these RCTs ranged from 23 to 180 (median = 43). Since studies measure different outcomes, an overall global effect was calculated. The first set of calculations looked at pre-to postintervention differences. The eight RCTs produced positive outcomes of a moderate magnitude (Hedges g = 0.39; 95%CI= 0.10, 0.68). Adding six non-RCTs, which the authors claim are more indicative of how interventions work in actual practice, produced a slightly larger positive effect (Hedges g = 0.44; 95% CI= 0.27, 0.61). Effect sizes were also calculated for specific effects on suicidal and self-injurious behaviors, with six RCTs showing a small effect size (Hedges g = 0.23; 95% CI= 0.00, 0.46) and the addition of five non-RCTs increasing the effect somewhat (Hedges g = 0.37; 95% CI= 0.17, 0.57). The second set of calculations looked at differences between postintervention and longer-term follow-up. Five RCTs produced negative global outcomes of a moderate magnitude (Hedges g = -0.25; 95% CI= -0.25, -0.15). Adding two non-RCTs produced a smaller but still negative effect (Hedges g = -0.05; 95% CI= -0.22, 0.12). Kliem et al. (2010) concluded that DBT has a moderate positive effect compared with treatment as usual, but that these positive effects appear to decay over time, suggesting that more attention needs to be paid to the transfer of DBT skills to daily life.

Acceptance Based Emotion Regulation

Gratz and Gunderson (2006) developed a 14-week emotion-regulation intervention based on Acceptance and Commitment Therapy (Hayes, Strosahl, & Wilson, 1999), DBT (Linehan, 1993), emotion-focused psychotherapy (Greenberg, 2002), and traditional behavior therapy. An RCT with women with borderline PD comparing the emotion regulation intervention (n=12) with treatment as usual (n=10) showed superior improvements posttreatment on the Difficulties in Emotion Regulation Scale (DERS; Gratz & Roemer, 2004) subscales (WMD range = -5.85 to -36.05), the Acceptance and Action Questionnaire (Hayes et al., 2004) emotional-avoidance subscale (WMD=-12.82), and the Depression and Anxiety Stress Scales (Antony et al., 1998) stress scale (WMD=-7.33).

Mentalization-Based Therapy

Although mentalization-based therapy (MBT) is a psychodynamically oriented treatment, it is included here because some of its principles and techniques may be understood within a cognitive and behavioral framework. MBT is used mainly with borderline PD and aims to stabilize the person's sense of self and help the person maintain an optimal level of arousal in interpersonal interactions (Bateman & Fonagy, 2010). Underpinning MBT is the notion that people with BPD have problems "mentalizing," which is the process of making sense of the actions of oneself and others on the basis of mental states such as desires, feelings, and beliefs. This is similar to the concept of theory of mind, in which consideration of the possible thoughts, feelings, and intentions of others enables one to predict or explain their actions. In MBT, therapists "mentalize the transference," which is "encouraging patients to think about the relationship they are in at the current moment (the therapist relationship) with the aim to focus their attention on another mind, the mind of a therapist, and to assist them in the task of contrasting their own perception of themselves with how they are perceived by another, by the therapist or indeed by members of a therapeutic group" (Bateman & Fonagy, 2010, p. 14).

Bateman and Fonagy (1999, 2001) randomized people with borderline PD to receive up to 18 months MBT in a partial hospitalization program (n=19) or general psychiatric services (n=19). The MBT treatment participants attended hospital for a weekly individual psychotherapy session, thrice-weekly group-therapy sessions lasting one hour, and a weekly community meeting for one hour, with other expressive therapies also available. Over the course of treatment, there were significant differences between groups favoring MBT in reducing self-mutilation, suicide attempts, hospital admissions, and medication. There were also greater levels of improvement for the MBT group in self-reported anxiety, depression, social adjustment, and interpersonal functioning (Bateman & Fonagy, 1999). These differential improvements were maintained at follow-up 18 months after the end of therapy (Bateman & Fonagy, 2001) and even at 5 years after the end of therapy (Bateman & Fonagy, 2008). At the 5 year follow-up, the MBT group had fewer suicide attempts (Cohen's d=1.40), borderline symptomatology measured by the Zanarini Rating Scale for Borderline Personality Disorder (ZAN-BPD) (Zanarini et al., 2003) (Cohen's d=1.40), days in hospital (Cohen's d=1.50), emergency department visits (Cohen's d=1.40), years of further outpatient treatment (Cohen's d=0.93), and years of various medications (Cohen's d range = 1.10-2.04). In a different RCT of 18 months of MBT (n=71) versus structured clinical management (n=63), with outpatients with borderline PD, both groups showed reduced self-harm, suicide attempts, and hospital admissions, and improved symptoms, social adjustment, and interpersonal functioning by the end of treatment. Improvements were both quicker and greater in the MBT group for self-harm (Cohen's d=0.62), suicide attempts (Cohen's d=0.65), hospital admissions (RR=0.14), social adjustment (Cohen's d=0.72), and interpersonal functioning (Cohen's d=0.95).

Psychoeducation and Problem-Solving-Based Therapies

Psychoeducation in the management of bipolar disorder for patients with comorbid personality disorder has shown that those who received 20 weeks of psychoeducation (n=15) compared with those who received a nonstructured intervention (n=22) were significantly less likely to relapse at 24-month follow-up (RR=0.67, 95%CI=0.47, 0.95) (Colom et al., 2004).

Focusing on personality disorder *per se*, psychoeducation and problem solving (PEPS) therapy consists of up to four individual sessions of psychoeducation and 12 sessions of group problem-solving skills training. Psychoeducation (Banerjee, Duggan, Huband, & Watson, 2006; D'Silva & Duggan, 2002) is based the International Personality Disorder Examination (IPDE; Loranger, 1999), a structured clinical interview. After conducting

the IPDE, the difficulties identified are discussed with the client, with the aim that the individual should be able to identify his or her difficulties and understand how they relate to his or her individual interpersonal style. Participants are then encouraged to define personal goals for change to be addressed in the problem-solving therapy that follows. Problem-solving therapy teaches the skills required for effective social problem solving (D'Zurilla & Nezu, 2007). These are the ability to recognize problems when they arise, define the problem clearly and accurately, set realistic goals for change, produce a range of possible solutions, think about possible outcomes, devise effective actions plans, and then carry out those action plans to solve problems effectively. In therapy, a great deal of attention is paid to developing the client's optimism about finding solutions to problems and improving the client's confidence for working towards these solutions. Huband et al. (2007) conducted a randomized controlled trial comparing community outpatients with any personality disorder treated with, on average, 12 weekly sessions of psychoeducation and problem-solving therapy (n = 87) with those on a waiting list (n = 89). At follow-up 24 weeks after recruitment, the treated group showed a significantly greater improvement on the Social Functioning Questionnaire (Tyrer et al., 2005) and on the State-Trait Anger Expression Inventory's (Spielberger, 1999) anger control scale (Cohen's d = -.25 and - .37, respectively), as well as improvements on the Social Problem Solving Inventory (D'Zurilla et al., 2002) (Cohen's d = .0.56). A larger-scale trial of PEPS therapy is currently underway (McMurran et al., 2011).

Systems training for emotional predictability and problem solving (STEPPS) is designed for people with borderline PD, whose main difficulty is regulation of emotional intensity (Blum, Pfohl, St. John, Monahan, & Black, 2002). STEPPS is a 20-week group treatment program in three stages. The first is psychoeducation, which involves making patients more aware of their disorder, referred to as "owning the illness." The second is emotion management training, which includes recognizing and being prepared for stressful situations. The third is behavior management training, including teaching skills for communication, coping with challenging thoughts, avoiding self-harming behaviors, and improving interpersonal relationships. Other people within the patient's system can be included, such as family members, partners, friends, and health-care professionals. An RCT comparing STEPPS (n=65) with treatment as usual (*n*=59) for people with borderline PD showed significantly greater improvement for the STEPPS group posttreatment on the ZAN-BPD (Zanarini et al., 2003) (Cohen's *d*=0.84), however this difference was no longer apparent at 1-year follow-up (Blum et al, 2008). Improvements on secondary outcomes, including global assessment of functioning, negative affectivity, depression, impulsiveness, and symptoms, were also significantly greater for the STEPPS group posttreatment but not at 1-year follow-up. STEPPS has also been evaluated in an RCT with borderline PD patients in the Netherlands (Bos, van Wel, Appelo, & Verbraak, 2010). Of those allocated to STEPPS (*n*=42) or treatment as usual (*n*=37), only analyses for those who completed treatment were presented- STEPPS (*n*=33) and treatment as usual (*n*=33). Groups were compared on the Symptom Checklist-90 (SCL-90; Derogatis, 1994) and the Borderline Personality Disorder Checklist (BPD-40; Arntz & Dreessen, 1992), with improvement posttreatment and at 6-month follow-up evident for the whole sample but with no significant group differences. The STEPPS group showed a significantly greater improvement in overall quality of life, particularly in the psychological domain, of the World Health Organization Quality of Life Assessment—BREF (WHOQOL-BREF; Skevington, Lotfy, & O'Connel, 2004).

Cognitive Analytic Therapy (CAT)

Cognitive analytic therapy (CAT) is a brief therapy that draws on both cognitive and psychodynamic approaches. Developed by Anthony Ryle, its aims are to reformulate the patient's difficulties in terms of a procedural model of aim-directed action (Ryle, 2001). The procedural sequence is: appraisal of the context, consideration of the possibility of action and the likely outcomes, selection of a plan, evaluation of the aim and the means in light of the consequences. This has correspondence with a social-problem-solving approach. However, Ryle (2001) goes beyond this to state that the sequence is influenced by the individual's learned repertoire of reciprocal role procedures, that is, the ways by which an individual attempts to elicit an appropriate response from others. Clearly, this resonates with interpersonal theory. Different reciprocal role procedures are located in different "self states," which, in nondisordered people, are appropriate to the current context but, in disordered people, may switch abruptly and inappropriately. Therapy identifies self-states through observation and monitoring,

and these self-states are reformulated by the therapist in a letter summarizing his or her understanding of the client's past experiences, learned coping strategies, and current patterns of coping. From this point, the aim is to enhance the client's capacity for self-reflection and change damaging coping strategies through mapping problematic experiences in a procedural sequence incorporating information about self-states and reciprocal role procedures.

Chanen et al. (2008) compared 24 sessions of CAT (*n*=41) with manualized good clinical care (*n*=37) with young people aged 15 to 18 who met the criteria for borderline PD. Follow-up from baseline was at 6, 12, and 24 months. Both groups improved in psychopathology, measured by the Structured Clinical Interview for Axis II disorders (SCID-II; First, Gibbon, Spitzer, Williams, & Benjamin, 1997) borderline dimension score, internalizing and externalizing problems measured by the Youth Self-Report (Achenbach, 1991) and Young Adult Self-Report (Achenbach, 1997) questionnaires, parasuicidal behavior, assessed by semistructured interview, and global functioning, assessed using the Social and Occupational Functioning Assessment Scale (Goldman, Skodol, & Lave, 1992). Both groups improved on all measures over the 2-year follow-up period, but the rate of improvement was slightly faster for the CAT group. This is the only RCT of CAT with a PD sample, although CAT has been evaluated with other disorders (e.g., anorexia nervosa). There are also a number of published case studies, but with one or two individuals, hence falling short of Chambless and Hollon's (1998) criterion that the sample size should be a minimum of three.

Contingency Management (CM)

Treatments for antisocial PD have focused on reducing substance misuse, which is a common co-occurring problem (Bowden-Jones et al., 2004). CM is a well-evidenced successful approach in substance misuse treatment. The individual receives tangible rewards for behavior change, for example receiving vouchers exchangeable for approved goods and services, when they test negative for alcohol or drugs (Petry, 2006). Duggan et al. (2007) reported two trials of CM in their systematic review, both with persons with antisocial PD. In one study, CM (*n*=20) was compared with methadone substitution for opioid dependence (*n*=23), with CM more successful in getting people transferred to routine care within three months (relative risk [RR] = 0.50; 95% CI= 0.26, 0.97) (Brooner, Kidorf, King, & Stoller, 1998). In another study with cocaine dependent individuals, CM plus methadone maintenance was compared to CM plus methadone maintenance with CBT added (Messina, Farabee, & Rawson, 2003). Both groups reduced cocaine use, as evidenced by urine samples at 16-week follow-up, but there was no difference between groups. The authors concluded that CM is an effective treatment for substance use with this group of antisocial PD individuals. In a more recent study, Neufeld et al. (2008) randomized 100 opioid-dependent outpatients with antisocial PD to CM plus methadone maintenance plus counseling or methadone maintenance plus counseling only. The CM group attended more treatment sessions but, although more of the CM group's urinalysis tests were negative for drugs over 6 months, this difference was not statistically significant.

Summation

Drawing conclusions from the range of outcome evaluations on PD treatments is not straightforward. Recall that, according to Chambless and Hollon (1998), for a treatment to be considered effective, there should be at least two independent, well-conducted RCTs or single-case experiments with a sample size of 3 or more; if there is only one RCT or single-case experiment, then it is considered possibly efficacious. The first issue relates to the quality of the studies. There are several types of threat to the validity of RCTs, one of which is that they are not adequately powered to reliably detect an effect (Nezu & Nezu, 2008). Many of the RCTs of PD treatments have small sample sizes, making them susceptible to erroneous conclusions. A second issue relates to the wide range of outcomes used by researchers, with different degrees of clinical importance (e.g., self-reported changes in personality beliefs versus days in hospital). This variation makes it difficult to draw firm conclusions about any one treatment.

With these issues in mind, the preceding results show that:

• Cognitive and behavioral interventions are probably more effective for reducing personality-disorder beliefs in avoidant PD than usual treatment or brief psychodynamic therapy.

• Cognitive and behavioral interventions are probably more effective for reducing suicidal acts in borderline PD than usual treatment.

• Cognitive and behavioral interventions are probably more effective for improving social functioning in cluster B PDs than usual treatment.

• Cognitive and behavioral interventions are probably just as effective as brief psychodynamic therapy for reducing psychopathology in cluster C PDs.

• Cognitive and behavioral interventions may not be more effective for men with antisocial PD than usual treatment.

• Schema-focused therapy is probably more effective in reducing borderline symptomatology than transference-focused therapy for borderline PD.

• Schema-focused therapy is probably more effective in reducing borderline symptomatology than usual individual therapy for borderline PD.

• Dual focus schema therapy is probably better than 12-step therapy but is probably not better than drug counseling for reducing substance use in dependent PD patients.

• Dialectical behavior therapy (DBT) is more effective than usual treatment for reducing suicide attempts, service use, and borderline symptomatology in borderline PD.

• Acceptance based emotion regulation is probably more effective for improving emotion regulation than usual treatment in borderline PD.

• Mentalization-based therapy (MBT) is probably more effective than usual treatment or structured clinical management for reducing suicide attempts, service use, and borderline symptomatology in borderline PD.

• Psychoeducation and problem-solving therapy (PEPS) is probably more effective than usual treatment for improving social functioning in mixed PD.

• Systems training for emotional predictability and problem solving (STEPPS) is probably more effective in reducing borderline symptomatology than usual individual therapy for borderline PD.

• Cognitive analytic therapy (CAT) is probably more effective than structured clinical management in reducing borderline symptomatology in borderline PD.

• Contingency management shows promise compared to methadone maintenance in moving substance dependent PD patients into routine care.

To establish effectiveness, most of the evaluations need to be replicated by independent groups.

Clinical Guidelines

In contrast to psychosis, depression, and other severe mental health problems, clinical guidelines and treatment recommendations for people with

PD are rare. Those that have been produced have focused almost exclusively on the treatment of people with borderline PD (American Psychiatric Association, 2001; National Institute for Health and Clinical Excellence, 2009a). This probably reflects the high levels of suicidal behavior and service utilization among people with this disorder (Bender et al., 2006). Treatment guidelines for people with borderline PD place a considerable emphasis on general management and the context in which psychological treatments are offered and delivered. These include actively involving people in treatment decisions, the need for contingency and crisis plans, and the importance of explaining boundaries prior to the start of treatment. The positive impact of good clinical management may also help explain why clinical trials of psychological treatments show little or no additional benefit when compared with structured clinical care, which is delivered in a consistent and supportive manner (Bateman & Fonagy, 2009; McMain et al., 2009).

Guidelines also stress the value of being explicit about what patients can expect from treatment. In recognition of the fear that many people with borderline personality disorder have about being neglected or abandoned, treatment guidelines emphasize the need to provide advance information about treatment endings and avoiding sudden breaks or termination of treatment. Guidelines on the treatment of borderline PD by the American Psychiatric Association (2001) describe psychological treatments as the "core" intervention for people with this condition and recommend the use of either psychoanalytic/psychodynamic therapy or DBT. Although these guidelines have not been formally updated, a "Guideline Watch" published in 2005 (Oldham, 2005) recognized the value of other psychological treatments that may be of value, including cognitive therapy and CAT.

National guidelines produced in Britain are more circumspect (National Institute for Health and Clinical Excellence, 2009a). They recommend that women with a history of suicidal behavior are offered DBT, but they fall short of recommending that all people with borderline PD are offered such treatment. Instead, this report suggests that *if* psychological treatments are offered consideration should be given to those that are delivered as part of a package of treatment that involves interventions delivered two or more times a week. The National Institute for Health and Clinical Excellence also recommends that short-term treatments of less than three months duration are avoided.

The National Institute for Health Clinical Excellence has also produced guidelines on the treatment of people with antisocial PD (2009b). These include the recommendation that children aged eight years or older who have conduct problems are offered family-based interventions, and that if it is not possible to deliver these, consideration is given to offering the child cognitive behavioral therapy. For adults with antisocial PD, the recommendation is that if people have a history of offending behavior they should be offered group-based cognitive and behavioral interventions that focus on reducing offending behavior.

Although guidelines on the treatment of people with other forms of PD have not been produced, researchers and those involved in delivering services to people with PD also emphasize the importance of the organizational context in which psychological treatments are offered (Crawford et al., 2007; Crawford et al., 2008). These include support and supervision for those delivering therapy, the value of setting short- as well as long-term goals for therapy, and the benefits, where possible, of involving family members and friends in treatment.

Treatment Engagement

Treatment noncompletion by people in PD treatment programs is a significant problem with, on average, 37% of those recruited to treatment finishing prematurely (McMurran, Huband, & Overton, 2010). In psychotherapies generally, around 20% of people with a PD diagnosis drop out (Swift & Greenberg, 2012). Treatment noncompletion is a matter of concern in that it compromises service efficiency and cost-effectiveness: there are monetary costs to services of carrying an empty place and opportunity costs to wait-list patients who could have had a place in treatment; therapy groups can dwindle in number to the point of necessary dissolution, to the disadvantage of patients who may be engaged in treatment; and noncompletion can lower staff morale and impact adversely the organization's professional reputation. Furthermore, there are societal costs of untreated PD to other people, such as the patient's family members, and other agencies, for example, social services and criminal-justice services. Importantly, treatment noncompleters show poorer treatment outcomes than do treatment completers in having significantly higher hospitalization rates (Karterud et al., 2003; Webb & McMurran, 2009). Offender patients with PD who did not complete treatment have been found to commit more offenses than completers

(McCarthy & Duggan, 2010). Although it may be that those who do not complete treatment are the high-risk and complex cases who would likely have poor outcomes even if they did complete treatment, it is nonetheless possible that creating the conditions that drive people out of treatment rather than maintain their engagement may contribute to treatment failure. It is, therefore, important to attend to issues of engagement.

A study of the barriers to and facilitators of engagement in PD treatments (Tetley, Jinks, Huband, Howells, & McMurran, 2012) has provided direction for improving treatment engagement for people with PD. As with other client groups, people diagnosed with PD who are offered treatment want to receive appropriate treatment when they actually need it, in a convenient location, in a pleasant environment, and from adequately skilled, supported, and motivated staff. Barriers to engagement include practical problems, as well as physical and mental health problems. Engagement is impeded if there is lack of clarity about the treatment being offered, no negotiation of treatment options, and poor treatment contracting. These matters ought to be attended to in therapies with any client group, yet failure to give them due recognition may produce particularly disruptive outcomes with people with PD.

In their review, McMurran, Huband, and Overton (2010) identified a number of risk factors for PD treatment noncompletion that have relevance to the competencies required for therapy engagement: younger age; lower education level; poorer problem-solving abilities; poorer social competence; and less experience with therapy. Some of these risks may be ameliorated in preparatory work that addresses deficits that arise from lack of knowledge and experience of therapy (Ogrodniczuk et al., 2008; Swift, Greenberg, Whipple, & Kominiak, 2012). A variety of strategies can be used prior to entry into treatment proper, including: *role induction*, including education about the rationale of the therapy, the nature of the treatment process, expectations for improvement, and the patient and therapist responsibilities; *vicarious therapy pretraining*, where recorded examples of therapy are discussed; *experiential pretraining*, where the individual is engaged in a simulation of therapy; and *psychoeducational interventions* to develop skills, beliefs, and working relationships that will help the person make best use of therapy (Ogrodniczuk, Joyce, & Piper, 2005; Swift et al., 2012). Despite the potential value of pretreatment preparation in reducing treatment noncompletion, there are few evaluations of these specifically in PD treatments.

Prior to entry into residential therapeutic communities, preparatory work such as pre-admission visits and experiential group work reduced early dropout (Birtle et al., 2007; Chiesa, Wright, & Neeld, 2003). McMurran and colleagues have tested a motivational interview based on the identification of the client's valued goals, obstacles to goal attainment, and clarification of how therapy might help overcome obstacles and thereby improve goal attainment (McMurran, Cox, et al., 2010; McMurran, Cox, Whitham, & Hedges, 2012). Indications are that those who received an interview of about 90 minutes duration showed greater clarity in their therapy goals, better attendance at later therapy sessions, and better treatment engagement as rated by staff (McMurran et al., 2012). Education about PD, instilling beliefs about capability for change, has been found to improve pretreatment knowledge and working alliance with detained PD offenders (Banerjee, Duggan, Huband, & Watson, 2006). A pretreatment intervention piloted by McMurran and Jinks (2012) aimed to teach people how emotions can be useful in solving problems and how emotions are identified; to help people to begin recognizing their own and other people's emotions through guided experiential components and mindfulness techniques; and to practice the skills of discussing emotions in preparation for therapy. Detained personality disordered offenders showed improved interest in emotions as a source of useful information after the intervention.

People with PD may have difficulty trusting and relating to others, and there is evidence that a poor therapeutic alliance is associated with noncompletion of PD treatments (Barnicot, Katsakou, Marougka, & Priebe, 2011). Pretreatment preparation may work not only by helping people develop the skills and confidence that they need for therapy, but also by providing them with the opportunity to gradually build up effective working relationships.

Future Directions

Research over the last 15 years has demonstrated that a number of psychological treatments benefit adults with borderline PD. These studies have successfully challenged the erroneous belief that people with PD cannot be helped. However, only a minority of people with PD have borderline PD and there is a pressing need for better evidence about if and how psychological treatment can help people with other forms of PD. Most people with PD in resource-rich countries do not receive psychological treatments, and in other parts of the world access to psychological treatments for people with PD is either very limited or nonexistent. New approaches, therefore, need to be found to increase access to psychological treatments for people with PD and to deliver them in ways that make the most effective use of limited resources.

Extending the Evidence Base

Although cognitive and behavioral therapies have been shown to help reduce recidivism among offenders (many of whom will have a PD), very few studies have examined the acceptability and effectiveness of psychological treatments for people with antisocial PD in clinical settings. Studies that have been conducted have highlighted problems of engaging people in therapy (Davidson et al., 2009). Providers of mental health services may also be reluctant to provide the structured clinical management that may be needed to help support people during treatment (Crawford, Sahib, Bratton, Tyrer, & Davidson, 2009). If future studies demonstrate that psychological treatments for people with antisocial PD are effective, expanding services for people with these problems has the potential to directly benefit people with this condition and to prevent the harm that they do to others.

Further research is also needed to into psychological treatments for people with other forms of PD. Research by Emmelkamp and colleagues (2006) showing that cognitive and behavioral therapies may improve the mental health of people with anxious and avoidant PDs is encouraging. However, work also needs to be undertaken to establish how best to help people with other forms of Cluster C PD. People with dependent PD experience high levels of emotional distress and poor social functioning and are as likely or even more likely to seek help from mental health services and be prescribed psychotropic mediation (Coid et al., 2009; Crawford et al., 2011). Despite this, studies examining the clinical- and cost-effectiveness of psychological treatment for people with dependent PD have not been conducted to date.

Most services and research studies have focused on delivering and evaluating psychological treatments for working-age adults. However, there is increasing recognition of the impact that PD can have on functioning among the elderly. It is also clear that emerging PD in young people can harm their mental health and educational attainment. The role of cognitive and other psychological treatments in young people and older adults needs to be examined.

Making the Most of Available Resources

PD is not confined to Europe and North America and appears to be as least as prevalent in Asia, Africa and other parts of the world (Huang et al., 2009). Evidence about the effectiveness of psychological treatments in resource-poor nations is limited, but psychological treatments for depression and other common mental health problems appear to be effective (Patel et al., 2007). However, limited funding for health care in many countries means that the great majority of people who may benefit from psychological treatments do not receive them. This is also true in resource-rich nations, where most people with PD and other common mental health problems do not receive evidence-based psychological treatments.

Some of the first approaches that were developed specifically for people with PD were based on inpatient treatment. Although residential treatments appear to be effective in helping people with PD achieve better mental health (Dolan, Warren, & Norton, 1997; Messina, Wish, & Nemes, 1999), the duration and intensity of these programs mean that they do not provide a sound basis for trying to help the large numbers of people who have PD. Similarly, most studies examining outpatient treatment for people with PD have tested interventions that are of greater intensity and duration than those used for the treatment of other mental disorders. Positive findings from studies of relatively short-term psychological treatments (Blum et al., 2002; Huband et al., 2007), challenge the belief that psychological treatments for people with PD need to be long-term. Further work may need to be undertaken to test the clinical- and cost-effectiveness of shorter interventions if more people with PD are to be treated.

In recent years it has also become apparent that people who have used mental health services can play an important part in helping to deliver psychosocial interventions to people with mental disorders (Simpson & House, 2002). People who have used treatment programs for PD highlight the value they get from meeting other people with similar problems and a sense of hope that can come from speaking to people who have overcome personality-related problems (Crawford et al.,

2007). Greater involvement of people with direct experience of PD who have been trained to deliver psychosocial interventions may also provide a means to expand delivery of services to people with PD in the future. Such an approach will require careful evaluation and proper consideration of processes for supporting and supervising those involved.

Conclusion

Our knowledge about the effectiveness of treatments for people with PD has advanced considerably in recent years. Despite this, there is considerable work yet to be done to develop our understanding of PD as a basis for both prevention and treatment, to evaluate treatments more rigorously, and to devise ways of making effective treatments more widely available to the many who might benefit from them.

References

Achenbach, T. M. (1991). *Manual for the youth self-report and 1991 profiles.* Burlington, VT: University of Vermont.

Achenbach, T. M. (1997). *Manual for the young adult self-report and young adult behavior checklist.* Burlington, VT: University of Vermont.

Acton, G. S., & Revelle, W. (2002). Interpersonal personality measures show circumplex structure based on new psychometric criteria. *Journal of Personality Assessment, 79,* 446–471.

American Psychiatric Association (1980). *Diagnostic and statistical manual of mental disorders, 3rd edition.* Washington, DC: Author.

American Psychiatric Association (2000). *Diagnostic and statistical manual of mental disorders, 4th edition, text revision.* Washington, DC: Author.

American Psychiatric Association (2013). *Diagnostic and statistical manual of mental disorders, 5th edition.* Washington, DC: Author.

American Psychiatric Association (2001). Practice guideline for the treatment of patients with borderline personality disorder: American Psychiatric Association Practice Guidelines. *American Journal of Psychiatry, 158*(Suppl), 1–52.

Antony, M. M., Bieling, P. J., Cox, B. J., Enns, M. W., & Swinson, R. P. (1998). Psychometric properties of the 42- item and 21-item versions of the Depression Anxiety Stress Scales in clinical groups and a community sample. *Psycho-logical Assessment, 10,* 176–181.

Arntz, A., & Dreessen, L. (1992). *Borderline personality disorder checklist.* Unpublished document, Maastricht University.

Arntz, A., Dreessen, L., Schouten, E., & Weertmann, A. (2004). Beliefs in personality disorders: A test with the Personality Disorder Belief Questionnaire. *Behaviour, Research and Therapy, 42,* 1215–1225.

Arntz, A., van den Hoorn, M., Cornelius, J., Verheul, R., van den Bosch, W., & de Bie, A. (2003). Reliability and validity of the Borderline Personality Disorder Severity Index. *Journal of Personality Disorders, 17,* 45–59.

Ball, S. A. (2007). Comparing individual therapies for personality disordered opioid dependent patients. *Journal of Personality Disorders, 21,* 305–321.

Ball, S. A., Maccarelli, L. M., LaPaglia, D. M., & Ostrowski, M. J. (2011). Randomized trial of dual-focused vs. single focused individual therapy for personality disorders and substance dependence. *Journal of Nervous and Mental Disease, 199,* 319–328.

Banerjee, P., Duggan, C., Huband, N., & Watson, N. (2006). Brief psychoeducation for people with personality disorder: A pilot study. *Psychology and Psychotherapy: Theory, Research and Practice, 79,* 385–394.

Barnicot, K., Katsakou, C., Marougka, S., & Priebe, S. (2011). Treatment completion in psychotherapy for borderline personality disorder: A systematic review and meta-analysis. *Acta Psychiatrica Scandinavica, 123,* 327–338.

Bartholomew, K., & Horowitz, L. M. (1991). Attachment styles among young adults: A test of a model. *Journal of Personality and Social Psychology, 61,* 226–244.

Bateman, A., & Fonagy, P. (1999). Effectiveness of partial hospitalization in the treatment of borderline personality disorder: A randomized controlled trial. *American Journal of Psychiatry, 156,* 1563–1569.

Bateman, A., & Fonagy, P. (2001). Treatment of borderline personality disorder with psychoanalytically oriented partial hospitalization: An 18-month follow-up. *American Journal of Psychiatry, 158,* 36–42.

Bateman, A., & Fonagy, P. (2008). 8-year follow-up of patients treated for borderline personality disorder: Mentalization-based treatment versus treatment as usual. *American Journal of Psychiatry, 165,* 631–638.

Bateman, A., & Fonagy, P. (2009). Randomized controlled trial of outpatient mentalization-based treatment versus structured clinical management for borderline personality disorder. *American Journal of Psychiatry, 166,* 1355–1364.

Bateman, A., & Fonagy, P. (2010). Mentalization based treatment for borderline personality disorder. *World Psychiatry, 9,* 11–15.

Beck, A. T., & Beck, J. S. (1991). *The personality belief questionnaire.* Bala Cynwyd, PA: Beck Institute for Cognitive Therapy and Research.

Beck, A. T., Butler, A. C., Brown, G. K., Dahlsgaard, K. K., Newman, C. F., & Beck, J. S. (2001). Dysfunctional beliefs discriminate personality disorders. *Behaviour Research and Therapy, 39,* 1213–1225.

Beck, A. T., & Freeman, A. (1990). *Cognitive therapy of personality disorders.* New York, NY: Guilford Press.

Bender, D. S., Skodol, A. E., Pagano, M. E., Dyck, I. R., Grilo, C. M., Shea, M. T., . . . Gunderson, J. G. (2006). Prospective assessment of treatment use by patients with personality disorders. *Psychiatric Services, 57,* 254–257.

Benjamin, L. S. (1974). Structural analysis of social behavior. *Psychological Review, 81,* 392–425.

Bhar, S. S., Brown, G. K., & Beck, A. T. (2008). Dysfunctional beliefs and psychopathology in borderline personality disorder. *Journal of Personality Disorders, 22,* 165–177.

Birtchnell, J., & Shine, J. (2000). Personality disorders and the interpersonal octagon. *British Journal of Medical Psychology, 73,* 433–448.

Birtle, J., Calthorpe, B., McGruer, F., Adie, L., McCullagh, G., & Kearney, S. (2007). Preparing to go to Main House: This week, maybe next week! *Therapeutic Communities, 28,* 127–136.

Blackburn, R. (1998). Psychopathy and personality disorder: Implications of interpersonal theory. In D. J. Cooke, A. E. Forth, & R. D. Hare (Eds.), *Psychopathy: Theory, research and implications for society.* (pp. 269–301). Dordrecht, The Netherlands: Kluwer Academic.

Blackburn, R. (2009). Primary and secondary psychopathy. In M. McMurran & R. Howard (Eds.), *Personality, personality disorder and risk of violence* (pp. 113–132). Chichester, England: Wiley.

Blum, N., Pfohl, B., St. John, D., Monahan, P., & Black, D. W. (2002). STEPPS: A cognitive-behavioral systems-based group treatment for outpatients with borderline personality disorder: A preliminary report. *Comprehensive Psychiatry, 43,* 301–330.

Blum, N., St. John, D., Pfohl, B., Stuart, S., McCormick, B., Allen, J., . . . Black, D. W. (2008). Systems training for emotional predictability and problem solving (STEPPS) for outpatients with borderline personality disorder: A randomized controlled trial and 1-year follow-up. *American Journal of Psychiatry, 165,* 468–478.

Bos, E. H., van Wel, E. B., Appelo, M. T., & Verbraak, M. J. P. M. (2010). A randomized controlled trial of a Dutch version of systems training for emotional predictability and problem solving (STEPPS) for borderline personality disorder. *Journal of Nervous and Mental Disease, 198,* 299–304.

Bowden-Jones, O., Iqbal, M. Z., Tyrer, P., Seivewright, N., Cooper, S., Judd, A., & Weaver, T. (2004). Prevalence of personality disorder in alcohol and drug services and associated comorbidity. *Addiction, 99,* 1306–1314.

Bowlby, J. (1969). *Attachment and loss: Attachment.* New York, NY: Basic Books.

Brooner, R. K., Kidorf, M., King, V. L., & Stoller, K. (1998). Preliminary evidence of good treatment response in antisocial drug abusers. *Drug and Alcohol Dependence, 49,* 249–260.

Butler, A. C., Brown, G. K., Beck, A. T., & Grisham, J. R. (2002). Assessment of dysfunctional beliefs in borderline personality disorder. *Behaviour Research and Therapy, 40,* 1231–1240.

Caspi, A., McClay, J., Moffitt, T. E., Mill, J., Martin, J., Craig, I. W., . . . Poulton, R. (2002). Role of genotype in the cycle of violence in maltreated children. *Science, 297,* 851–854.

Chambless, D. L., & Hollon, S. D. (1998). Defining empirically supported theories. *Journal of Consulting and Clinical Psychology, 66,* 7–18.

Chanen, A. M. Jackson, H. J., McCutcheon, L. K., Jovev, M., Dudgeon, P., Yuen, H. P., Germano, D., . . . McGorry, P. D. (2008). Early intervention for adolescents with borderline personality disorder using cognitive analytic therapy: Randomised controlled trial. *British Journal of Psychiatry, 193,* 477–484.

Cheavens, J. S., Strunk, D. R., & Chriki, L. (2012). A comparison of three theoretically important constructs: What accounts for symptoms of borderline personality disorder? *Journal of Clinical Psychology, 68,* 477–486.

Chiesa, M., Wright, M., & Neeld, R. (2003). A description of an audit cycle of early dropouts from an inpatient psychotherapy unit. *Psychoanalytic Psychotherapy, 17,* 138–149.

Cleckley, H. (1941) *The mask of sanity.* St Louis, MO: Mosby.

Coid, J., Yang, M., Tyrer, P., Roberts, A., & Ullrich, S. (2006). Prevalence and correlates of personality disorder in Great Britain. *British Journal of Psychiatry, 188,* 423–431.

Colom, F., Vieta, E., Sánchez-Moreno, J., Matinez-Arán, A., Torrent, C., Reinares, M., . . . Comes M. (2004). Psychoeducation in bipolar patients with comorbid personality disorders. *Bipolar Disorders, 6,* 294–298.

Coid, J., Yang, M., Moran, P., Brugha, T., Jenkins, R., Farrell, M., . . . Ullrich, S. (2009). Borderline personality disorder: health service use and social functioning among a national household population. *Psychological Medicine, 39,* 1721–1731.

Coid, J., Yang, M., Tyrer, P., Roberts, A., & Ullrich, S. (2006). Prevalence and correlates of personality disorder in Great Britain. *British Journal of Psychiatry, 188,* 423–431.

Conte, H. R., Plutchik, R., Karasu, T. B., & Jerrett, I. (1980). A self-report borderline scale: Discriminative validity and preliminary norms. *Journal of Nervous and Mental Disease, 100,* 428–435.

Crawford, M., Price, K., Rutter, D., Moran, P., Tyrer, P., Bateman, A., . . . Weaver, T. (2008). Dedicated community-based services for adults with personality disorder: Delphi study. *British Journal of Psychiatry, 193,* 342–343.

Crawford, M. J., Kakad, S., Rendel, C., Mansour, N. A., Crugel, M., Liu, K. W., . . . Barnes, T. R. E. (2011). Medication prescribed to people with personality disorder: The influence of patient factors and treatment setting. *Acta Psychiatrica Scandinavica, 124,* 396–402.

Crawford, M., Rutter, D., Price, K., Weaver, T., Josson, M., Tyrer, P., . . . Moran, P. (2007). *Learning the lessons: A multi-method evaluation of dedicated community-based services for people with personality disorder.* London, England: National Co-ordinating Centre for NHS Service Delivery and Organisation.

Crawford, M. J., Sahib, L., Bratton, H., Tyrer, P., & Davidson, K. (2009) Service provision for men with antisocial personality disorder who make contact with mental health services. *Personality and Mental Health, 3,* 165–171.

Davidson, K. M., Norrie, J., Tyrer, P., Gumley, A., Tata, P., Murray, H., & Palmer, S. (2006). The effectiveness of cognitive behaviour therapy for borderline personality disorder: Results from the borderline personality disorder study of cognitive therapy (BOSCOT) trial. *Journal of Personality Disorders, 20,* 450–465.

Davidson, K. M., & Tyrer, P. (1996). Cognitive therapy for antisocial and borderline personality disorders: Single case study series. *British Journal of Clinical Psychology, 35,* 413–429.

Davidson, K. M., Tyrer, P., Norrie, J., Palmer, S. J., & Tyrer, H. (2010). Cognitive therapy v. usual treatment for borderline personality disorder: Prospective 6-year follow-up. *British Journal of Psychiatry, 197,* 456–462.

Davidson, K. M., Tyrer, P., Tata, P., Cooke, D., Gumley, A., Ford, I., . . . Crawford, M. J. (2009). Cognitive behaviour therapy for violent men with antisocial personality disorder in the community: An exploratory randomized controlled trial. *Psychological Medicine, 39,* 569–577.

Derogatis, L. (1992). *Brief Symptom Inventory: Administration, procedures, and scoring manual-II.* Baltimore, MD: Clinical Psychometric Research, Inc.

Derogatis, L. R. (1994). *The SCL-90-R: Administration, scoring and procedures manual (3rd ed.).* Minneapolis, MN: National Computer Systems.

Dolan, B. M., Warren, F., & Norton, K. (1997). Change in borderline symptoms one year after therapeutic community treatment for severe personality disorders. *British Journal of Psychiatry, 171,* 274–279.

D'Silva, K., & Duggan, C. (2002). The development of a psycho-educational programme for personality disordered patients. *Psychiatric Bulletin, 26,* 268–271.

Duggan, C., Huband, N., Smailagic, N., Ferriter, M., & Adams, C. (2007). The use of psychological treatments for people with personality disorder: A systematic review of randomized controlled trials. *Personality and Mental Health, 1,* 95–125.

D'Zurilla, T. J., & Nezu, A. M. (2007). *Problem-solving therapy: A positive approach to clinical intervention* (3rd ed.). New York, NY: Springer Publishing Co.

D'Zurilla, T. J., Nezu, A. M., & Maydeu-Olivares, A. (2002). *Manual for the Social Problem-Solving Inventory—Revised*. North Tonawanda, NY: Multi-Health Systems.

Emmelkamp, P. M. G., Benner, A., Kuipers, A., Feiertag, G. A., Koster, H. C., & van Apeldoorn, F. J. (2006). Comparison of brief dynamic and cognitive-behavioural therapies in avoidant personality disorder. *British Journal of Psychiatry, 189*, 60–64.

Endicott, J. Spitzer, R. L., Fleiss, J. L., & Coen, J. (1976). The Global Assessment Scale: A procedure for measuring overall severity of psychiatric disturbance. *Archives of General Psychiatry, 33*, 766–777.

Evans, K., Tyrer, P., Catalan, J., Schmidt, U., Davidson, K., Dent, J., . . . Thompson, S. (1999). Manual-assisted cognitive-behaviour therapy (MACT): A randomized controlled trial of a brief intervention with bibliotherapy in the treatment of recurrent deliberate self-harm. *Psychological Medicine, 29*, 19–25.

Farrell, J. M., Shaw, I. A., & Webber, M. A. (2009). A schema-focused approach to group psychotherapy for outpatients with borderline personality disorder: A randomized controlled trial. *Journal of Behavior Therapy and Experimental Psychiatry, 40*, 317–328.

Farrington, D. P. (2005). Childhood origins of antisocial behaviour. *Clinical Psychology and Psychotherapy, 12*, 177–190.

First, M. B., Gibbon, M., Spitzer, R. L., Williams, J. B. W., & Benjamin, L. S. (1997). *Structured Clinical Interview for DSM-IV Axis II Personality Disorders*. Arlington, VA: American Psychiatric Publishing, Inc.

Fok, M., Hayes, R., Chang, C-K., Stewart, R., Callard, F., & Moran, P. (2012). Life expectancy at birth and all-cause mortality among people with personality disorder. *Journal of Psychosomatic Research, 73*, 104–107.

Fossati, A., Feeney, J. A., Donati, D., Donini, M., Novella, L., Bagnato, M., . . . Maffei, C. (2003). Personality disorders and adult attachment dimensions in a mixed psychiatric sample: A multivariate study. *Journal of Nervous and Mental Disease, 191*, 30–37.

Frances, A. (2012). DSM-5 in distress: The DSM's impact on mental health practice and research. *Psychology Today*. Retrieved August 14, 2012 from http://www.psychologytoday.com/blog/dsm5-in-distress/201207/two-who-resigned-dsm-5-explain-why.

Frodi, A., Dernevik, M., Sepa, A., Philipson, J., & Bragesjö, M. (2001). Current attachment representations of offenders varying in degree of psychopathy. *Attachment and Human Development, 3*, 269–283.

Giesen-Bloo, J., van Dyck, R., Spinhoven, P., van Tilburg, W., Dirksen, C., van Asselt, T., . . . Arntz, A. (2006). Outpatient psychotherapy for borderline personality disorder: Randomized trial of schema-focussed therapy vs transference-focussed therapy. *Archives of General Psychiatry, 63*, 649–659.

Glenn, C. R., & Klonsky, D. E. (2009). Emotion dysregulation as a core feature of borderline personality disorder. *Journal of Personality Disorders, 23*, 20–28.

Goldman, H., Skodol, A., & Lave, T. (1992). Revising Axis V for DSM–IV: A review of measures of social functioning. *American Journal of Psychiatry, 149*, 1148–1156.

Gratz, K. L., & Gunderson, J. G. (2006). Preliminary data on an acceptance-based emotion regulation group intervention for deliberate self-harm among women with borderline personality disorder. *Behavior Therapy, 37*, 25–35.

Gratz, K. L., & Roemer, L. (2004). Multidimensional assessment of emotion regulation and dysregulation: Development, factor structure, and initial validation of the Difficulties in Emotion Regulation Scale. *Journal of Psychopathology and Behavioral Assessment, 26*, 41–54.

Gratz, K. L., Rosenthal, M. Z., Tull, M. T., Lejeuz, C. W., & Gunderson, J. G. (2006). Experimental investigation of emotion dysregulation in borderline personality disorder. *Journal of Abnormal Psychology, 115*, 850–855.

Greenberg, L. S. (2002). *Emotion-focused therapy: Coaching clients to work through their feelings*. Washington, DC: American Psychiatric Press.

Gunderson, J. G., Stout, R. L., McGlashan, T. J., Shea, T., Morey, L. C., Grilo, C. M., . . . Skodol, A. E. (2011). Ten-year course of borderline personality disorder psychopathology and function from the collaborative longitudinal personality disorders study. *Archives of General Psychiatry, 68*, 827–837.

Gunderson, J. G. & Zanarini, M. C. (2011). Commentary—Deceptively simple or radical shift? *Personality and Mental Health, 5*, 260–262.

Hare, R. D., & Neumann, C. S. (2010). The role of antisociality in the psychopathy construct: Comment on Skeem and Cooke (2010). *Psychological Assessment, 22*, 446–454.

Hayes, S. C., Strosahl, K. D., & Wilson, K. G. (1999). *Acceptance and commitment therapy: An Experiential approach to behavior change*. New York, NY: Guilford Press.

Hayes, S. C., Strosahl, K., Wilson, K. G., Bissett, R. T., Pistorello, J., Toarmino, D., . . . McCurry, S. M. (2004). Measuring experiential avoidance: A preliminary test of a working model. *The Psychological Record, 54*, 553–578.

Hayward, J., McMurran, M., & Sellen, J. (2008). Social problem solving in vulnerable adult prisoners: Profile and intervention. *Journal of Forensic Psychiatry and Psychology, 19*, 243–248.

Hoffart, A., Sexton, H, Hedley, L. M., Wang, C. E., Holthe, H., Haugum, J. A., . . . Holte, A. (2005). The structure of maladaptive schemas: A confirmatory factor analysis and a psychometric evaluation of factor-derived scales. *Cognitive Therapy and Research, 29*, 627–644.

Huang, Y., Kotov, R., de Girolamo, G. Preti, A., Angermeyer, M., Benjet, C., . . . Kessler, R. C. (2009). DSM-IV personality disorders in the WHO World Mental Health Surveys. *British Journal of Psychiatry, 195*, 46–53.

Huband, N., McMurran, M., Evans, C., & Duggan, C. (2007). Social problem solving plus psychoeducation for adults with personality disorder: A pragmatic randomised controlled trial. *British Journal of Psychiatry, 190*, 307–313.

Johnson, J. G., Cohen, P., Smailes, E., Kasen, S., Oldham, J. M., Skodol, A. E., & Brook, J. S. (2000). Adolescent personality disorders associated with violence and criminal behaviour during adolescence and early adulthood. *American Journal of Psychiatry, 157*, 1406–1412.

Jovev, M., & Jackson, H. J. (2004). Early maladaptive schemas in personality disordered individuals. *Journal of Personality Disorders, 18*, 467–478.

Karterud, S., Pederson, G., Bjordal, E., Brabrand, J., Friis, S., Haaseth, Ø., . . . Urnes, Ø. (2003). Day treatment of people with personality disorders: Experiences from a Norwegian treatment research network. *Journal of Personality Disorders, 17*, 243–262.

Kiesler, D. J. (1983). The 1982 interpersonal circle: A taxonomy for complementarity in human transactions. *Psychological Review, 90*, 185–214.

Kliem, S., Kröger, C., & Kosfelder, J. (2010). Dialectical behaviour therapy for borderline personality disorder: A meta-analysis using mixed-effects modelling. *Journal of Consulting and Clinical Psychology, 78*, 936–951.

Kuo, J. R., & Linehan, M. M. (2009). Disentangling emotion processes in borderline personality disorder: Physiological and self-reported assessment of biological vulnerability, baseline intensity, and reactivity to emotionally evocative stimuli. *Journal of Abnormal Psychology, 118*, 531–544.

Leary, T. (1957). *Interpersonal diagnosis of personality*. New York, NY: Ronald Press.

Lenzenweger, M. F., & Clarkin, J. F. (2005). The personality disorders: History, classification, and research issues. In M. F. Lenzenweger & J. F. Clarkin (Eds.), *Major theories of personality disorder* (pp. 1–39). New York, NY: Guilford Press.

Lenzenweger, M. F., Lane, M. C., Loranger, A. W., & Kessler, R. C. (2007). DSM-IV personality disorders in the National Comorbidity Survey Replication. *Biological Psychiatry, 62*, 533–564.

Linehan, M. M. (1993). *Cognitive-behavioral treatment of borderline personality disorder*. New York, NY: Guilford Press.

Livesley, J. (2013). The DSM-5 personality disorder proposal and future directions in the diagnostic classification of personality disorder. *Psychopathology, 46*, 207–216.

Livesley, W. J. (2005). Principles and strategies for treating personality disorder. *Canadian Journal of Psychiatry, 50*, 442–450.

Livesley, W. J., & Lang, K. L. (2005). Differentiating normal, abnormal, and disordered personality. *European Journal of Personality, 19*, 257–268.

Loranger, A. W. (1999). *The International Personality Disorder Examination*. Odessa, FL: Psychological Assessment Resources.

McCarthy, L., & Duggan, C. (2010). Engagement in a medium secure personality disorder service: A comparative study of psychological functioning and offending outcomes. *Criminal Behaviour and Mental Health, 20*, 112–128.

McGlashan, T. H., Grilo, C. M., Skodol, A. E., Gunderson, J. G., Shea, M. T., Morey, L. C., ... Stout, R. L. (2000). The Collaborative Longitudinal Personality Disorders Study: Baseline Axis I/II and II/II diagnostic co-occurrence. *Acta Psychiatrica Scandinavica, 102*, 256–264.

McMain, S. F., Links, P. S., Gnam, W. H., Guimond, T., Cardish, R. J., Korman, L., & Streiner, D. L. (2009). A randomized trial of dialectical behavior therapy versus general psychiatric management for borderline personality disorder. *American Journal of Psychiatry, 166*, 1365–1374.

McMurran, M. (2009). Social problem solving, personality, and violence. In M. McMurran & R. C. Howard (Eds.), *Personality, personality disorder and violence* (pp. 265–279). Chichester: Wiley.

McMurran, M., Blair, M., & Egan, V. (2002). An investigation of the correlations between aggressiveness, impulsiveness, social problem-solving, and alcohol use. *Aggressive Behavior, 28*, 439–445.

McMurran, M., & Christopher, G. (2008). Dysfunctional beliefs and antisocial personality disorder. *Journal of Forensic Psychiatry and Psychology, 19*, 533–542.

McMurran, M., Cox, W. M., Coupe, S., Whitham, D., & Hedges, L. (2010). The addition of a goal-based motivational interview to standardised treatment as usual to reduce drop-outs in a service for patients with personality disorder: A feasibility study. *Trials. 11*, 98. doi: 10.1186/1745-6215-11-98

McMurran, M., Cox, W. M., Whitham, D., & Hedges, L. (2012). The addition of a goal-based motivational interview to treatment as usual to reduce dropouts in a personality disorder treatment service: Results of a feasibility study for a randomized controlled trial. Paper under review.

McMurran, M., Crawford, M. J., Reilly, J. G., McCrone, P. Moran, P. Williams, H., ... Day, F. (2011). Psycho-education with problem solving (PEPS) therapy for adults with personality disorder: A pragmatic multi-site community-based randomized clinical trial. *Trials, 12*, 198.

McMurran, M., Duggan, C., Christopher, G., & Huband, N. (2007). The relationships between personality disorders and social problem solving in adults. *Personality and Individual Differences, 42*, 145–155.

McMurran, M., Egan, V., & Duggan, C. (2005). Stop & Think! Social problem-solving therapy with personality disordered offenders. In M. McMurran & J. McGuire (Eds.), *Social problem solving and offending: Evidence, evaluation, and evolution* (pp. 207–220). Chichester, England: Wiley.

McMurran, M., Huband, N., & Overton, E. (2010). Non-completion of personality disorder treatments: A systematic review of correlates, consequences, and interventions. *Clinical Psychology Review, 30*, 277–287.

McMurran, M., & Jinks, M. (2012). Making your emotions work for you: A pilot brief intervention for alexithymia with personality disordered offenders. *Personality and Mental Health, 6*, 45–49.

McMurran, M., Oaksford, M., & Christopher, G. (2010). Does social problem solving mediate the relationship between personality traits and personality disorders? An exploratory study with a sample of male prisoners. *Personality and Mental Health, 4*, 180–192.

Mennin, D. S., & Heimberg, R. G. (2000). The impact of comorbid mood and personality disorders in the cognitive-behavioral treatment of panic disorder. *Clinical Psychology Review, 20*, 339–357.

Messina, N., Farabee, D., & Rawson, R. (2003). Treatment responsivity of cocaine-dependent patients with antisocial personality disorder to cognitive-behavioral and contingency management interventions. *Journal of Consulting and Clinical Psychology, 71*, 320–329.

Messina, N. P., Wish, E. D., & Nemes, S. (1999). Therapeutic community treatment for substance abusers with antisocial personality disorder. *Journal of Substance Abuse Treatment, 17*, 121–128.

Millon, T., Meagher, S. E., & Grossman, S. D. (2001). Theoretical perspectives. In J. Livesley (Ed.), *Handbook of personality disorders: Theory, research and treatment* (pp. 39–59). New York, NY: Guilford Press.

Monsen, J. T., von der Lippe, A. L., Havik, O. E., Halvorsen, M. S., & Eilersten, D. E. (2007). Validation of the SASB introject surface in a Norwegian clinical and nonclinical. *Journal of Personality Assessment, 88*, 235–245.

National Institute for Health and Clinical Excellence (2009a). *Borderline personality disorder: Treatment and management*. London, England: Author. Retrieved September 25, 2012 from http://www.nice.org.uk/nicemedia/live/12125/43045/43045.pdf.

National Institute for Health and Clinical Excellence (2009b). *Antisocial personality disorder: Treatment, management and prevention.* London, England: Author. Retrieved September 25, 2012 from www.nice.org.uk/Guidance/CG77.

Neufeld, K. J., Kidorf, M. S., Kolodner, K., King, V. L., Clark, M., & Brooner, R. K. (2008). A behavioral treatment for opioid-dependent patients with antisocial personality disorder. *Journal of Substance Abuse Treatment, 34*, 101–111.

Newton-Howes, G., Tyrer, P., & Johnston, T. (2006). Personality disorder and the outcome of depression: Meta-analysis of published studies. *British Journal of Psychiatry, 188*, 13–20.

Newton-Howes, G., Tyrer, P., & Weaver, T. (2008). Social function of patients with personality disorder in secondary care. *Psychiatric Services, 59*, 1033–1037.

Nezu, A. M., & Nezu, C. M. (2008). The devil is in the details: Recognizing and dealing with threats to validity in randomized controlled trials. In A. M. Nezu & C. M. Nezu (Eds.), *Evidence-based outcome research: A practical guide to conducting randomized controlled trials for psychosocial interventions* (pp. 3–24). New York: Oxford University Press.

Noren, K., Lindgren, A., Haellstom, T., Thormaehlen, B., Vinnars, B., Wennberg, P., . . . Barber, J. P. (2007). Psychological distress and functional impairment in patients with personality disorders. *Nordic Journal of Psychiatry, 61*, 260–270.

Nur, U., Tyrer, P., Merson, S., & Johnson, T. (2004). Relationship between clinical symptoms, personality disturbance, and social function: a statistical enquiry. *Irish Journal of Psychological Medicine, 21*, 19–22.

Ogrodniczuk, J. S., Joyce, A. S., Lynd, L. D., Piper, W. E., Steinberg, P. I., & Richardson, K. (2008). Predictors of premature termination of day treatment for personality disorder. *Psychotherapy and Psychosomatics, 77*, 365–371.

Ogrodniczuk, J. S., Joyce, A. S., & Piper, W. E. (2005). Strategies for reducing patient-initiated premature termination of psychotherapy. *Harvard Review of Psychiatry, 13*, 57–70.

Oldham, J. M. (2005) *Guideline watch: Practice guideline for the treatment of patients with borderline personality disorder.* Arlington, VA: American Psychiatric Association.

Patel, V., Araya, R., Chatterjee, S., Chisholm, D., Cohen, A., De Silva, M., . . . van Ommeren, M. (2007). Treatment and prevention of mental disorders in low-income and middle-income countries. *Lancet, 6736*, 44–58.

Patrick, M., Hobson, R. P., Castle, D., Howard, R., & Maughan, B. (1994). Personality disorder and the mental representation of early social experience. *Development and Psychopathology, 6*, 375–388.

Perälä, J., Suvisaari, J., Saarni, S. I., Kuoppasalmi, K., Isometsä, E., Pirkola, S., . . . Lönnqvist, J. (2007). Lifetime prevalence of psychotic and bipolar I disorders in a general population. *Archives of General Psychiatry, 64*, 19–28.

Petrocelli, J. V., Glaser, B. A., Calhoun, G. B., & Campbell, L. F. (2001). Early maladaptive schemas of personality disorder subtypes. *Journal of Personality Disorders, 15*, 546–559.

Petry, N. M. (2006). Contingency management treatments. *British Journal of Psychiatry, 189*, 97–98.

Pincus, A. L. (2005). The interpersonal nexus of personality disorders. In S. Strack (Ed.), *Handbook of personology and psychopathology* (pp. 120–139). Hoboken, NJ: Wiley.

Powers, A. D., & Oltmanns, T. F. (2012). Personality disorders and physical health: A longitudinal examination of physical functioning, healthcare utilization, and health-related behaviors in middle-aged adults. *Journal of Personality Disorders, 26*, 524–538.

Pretzer, J. L., & Beck, A. T. (2005). A cognitive theory of personality disorders. In M. F. Lenzenweger & J. F. Clarkin (Eds.), *Major theories of personality disorder* (pp. 43–113). New York, NY: Guilford Press.

Pukrop, R., Sass, H., & Steinmeyer, E. M. (2000). Circumplex models for the similarity relationships between higher-order factors of personality and personality disorders: An empirical analysis. *Comprehensive Psychiatry, 41*, 438–445.

Reeves, M., James, L. M., Pizzarello, S. M., & Taylor, J. E. (2010). Support for Linehan's biosocial theory from a nonclinical sample. *Journal of Personality Disorders, 24*, 312–326.

Reich, J. (2003). The effect of Axis II disorders on the outcome of treatment of anxiety and unipolar depressive disorders: A review. *Journal of Personality Disorders, 17*, 387–405.

Rendu, A., Moran, P., Patel, A., Knapp, M., & Mann, A. (2002). Economic impact of personality disorders in UK primary care attenders. *British Journal of Psychiatry, 181*, 62–66.

Robins, C. J., Ivanoff, A. M., & Linehan, M. M. (2001). Dialectical behaviour therapy. In W. J. Livesley (Ed.), *Handbook of personality disorders: Theory, research and treatment* (pp. 437–459). New York, NY: Guilford Press.

Rosenstein, D. S., & Horowitz, H. A. (1996). Adolescent attachment and psychopathology. *Journal of Consulting and Clinical Psychology, 64*, 244–253.

Ryle, A. (2001). Cognitive analytic therapy. In W. J. Livesley (Ed.), *Handbook of personality disorders: Theory, research and treatment* (pp. 400–413). New York, NY: Guilford Press.

Saltaris, C. (2002). Psychopathy in juvenile offenders. Can temperament and attachment be considered as robust developmental precursors? *Clinical Psychology Review, 22*, 729–752.

Samuels, J., Eaton, W. W., Bienvenu, O. J., Brown, C. H., Costa, P. T., & Nestadt, G. (2002). Prevalence and correlates of personality disorders in a community sample. *British Journal of Psychiatry, 180*, 536–542.

Seivewright, H., Tyrer, P., & Johnson, T. (2004). Persistent social dysfunction in anxious and depressed patients with personality disorder. *Acta Psychiatrica Scandinavica, 109*, 104–109.

Simpson, E. L., & House, A. O. (2002) Involving users in the delivery and evaluation of mental health services: systematic review. *British Medical Journal, 325*, 1265.

Skeem, J., & Cooke, D. J. (2010). Is criminal behaviour a central component of psychopathy? Conceptual directions for resolving the debate. *Psychological Assessment, 22*, 433–435.

Skevington, S. M., Lotfy, M., & O'Connel, K. A. (2004). The World Health Organization's WHOQOL-BREF quality of life assessment: Psychometric properties and results of the international field trial. A report from the WHOQOL Group. *Quality of Life Research, 13*, 299–310.

Skodol, A. E. (2011). Scientific issues in the revision of personality disorders for DSM-5. *Personality and Mental Health, 5*, 97–111.

Skodol, A. E., Pagano, M. E., Bender, D. S., Shea, M. T., Gunderson, J. G., Yen, S., . . . McGlashan, T. H. (2005). Stability of functional impairment in patients with schizotypal, borderline, avoidant, or obsessive-compulsive personality disorder over two years. *Psychological Medicine, 35*, 443–451.

Soeteman, D. I., Verheul, R., & Busschbach, J. J. V. (2008). The burden of disease in personality disorders: Diagnosis-specific quality of life. *Journal of Personality Disorders, 22*, 259–268.

South, S. C., Turkheimer, E., & Oltmanns, T. F. (2008). Personality disorder symptoms and marital functioning. *Journal of Consulting and Clinical Psychology, 76,* 769–780.

Spielberger, C. D. (1999) *STAXI-2: State-Trait Anger Expression Inventory-2.* Odessa, FL: Psychological Assessment Resources.

Sullivan, H. S. (1953). *The interpersonal theory of psychiatry.* New York, NY: Norton.

Svartberg, M., Stiles, T. C., & Seltzer, M. H. (2004). Randomized, controlled trial of the effectiveness of short-term dynamic psychotherapy and cognitive therapy for cluster C personality disorders. *American Journal of Psychiatry, 161,* 810–817.

Swift, J. K., & Greenberg, R. P. (2012). Premature discontinuation in adult psychotherapy: A meta-analysis. *Journal of Consulting and Clinical Psychology, 80,* 547–559.

Swift, J. K., Greenberg, R. P., Whipple, J. L., & Kominiak, N. (2012). Practice recommendations for reducing premature termination in therapy. *Professional Psychology: Research and Practice, 43,* 379–387.

Tetley, A., Jinks, M., Huband, N., Howells, K., & McMurran, M. (2012). Barriers to and facilitators of treatment engagement for clients with personality disorder: A Delphi survey. *Personality and Mental Health, 6,* 97–110.

Timmerman, I. G. H., & Emmelkamp, P. M. G. (2006). The relationship between attachment styles and Cluster B personality disorders in prisoners and forensic inpatients. *International Journal of Law and Psychiatry, 29,* 48–56.

Torgerson, S., Kringlen, E., & Kramer, V. (2001). The prevalence of personality disorders in a community sample. *Archives of General Psychiatry, 58,* 590–596.

Tyrer, P., Crawford, M., Mulder, R., Blashfield, R., Farnam, A., Fossati, A., . . . Reed, G. M. (2011). The rationale for the reclassification of personality disorder in the 11th revision of the *International Classification of Diseases (ICD-11). Personality and Mental Health, 5,* 246–259.

Tyrer, P., Nur, U., Crawford, M., Karlsen, S., McLean, C., Rao, B., & Johnson, T. (2005). The social functioning questionnaire: A rapid and robust measure of perceived functioning. *International Journal of Social Psychiatry, 51,* 265–275.

Tyrer, P., Tom, B., Byford, S., Schmidt, U., Jones, V., Davidson, K., . . . Catalan, J. (2004). Differential effects of manual assisted cognitive behavior therapy in the treatment of recurrent deliberate self-harm and personality disturbance: The POPMACT study. *Journal of Personality Disorders, 18,* 102–116.

Verheul, R., van den Brink, W., & Hartgers, C. (1995). Prevalence of personality disorders among alcoholics and drug addicts: An overview. *European Addiction Research, 1,* 166–177.

Viding, E., Blair, R. J. R., Moffitt, T. E., & Plomin, R. (2005). Evidence for substantial genetic risk for psychopathy in 7 year olds. *Journal of Child Psychology and Psychiatry, 46,* 592–597.

Webb, D. J., & McMurran, M. (2009). A comparison of women who continue and discontinue treatment for borderline personality disorder. *Personality and Mental Health, 3,* 142–149.

Weertman, A., & Arntz, A. (2007). Effectiveness of treatment of childhood memories in cognitive therapy for personality disorders: A controlled study contrasting methods focusing on the present and methods focusing on childhood memories. *Behaviour, Research and Therapy, 45,* 2133–2143.

West, M., Rose, S. M., & Sheldon-Keller, A. (1994). Assessment of patterns of insecure attachment in adults and application to dependent and schizoid personality disorders. *Journal of Personality Disorders, 8,* 249–256.

Wiggins, J. S. (1982). Circumplex models of interpersonal behaviour in clinical psychology. In P. C. Kendall & J. N. Butcher (Eds.), *Handbook of research methods in clinical psychology* (pp. 183–221). New York, NY: Wiley.

World Health Organisation (1992). *The ICD-10 classification of mental and behavioural disorders.* Geneva: Author.

Young, J. E. (1990). Cognitive therapy for personality disorders: A schema-focused approach. Sarasota, FL: Professional Resource Exchange.

Young, J. E., Klosko, J. S., & Weishaar, M. E. (2003). *Schema therapy: A practitioner's guide.* New York, NY: Guilford Press.

Zanarini, M. C., & Frankenburg, F. R. (2007). The essential nature of borderline psychopathology. *Journal of Personality Disorders, 21,* 518–535.

Zanarini, M. C., Gunderson, J. G., Frankenburg, F. R., & Chauncey, D. L. (1990). Discriminating borderline personality disorder from other axis II disorders. *American Journal of Psychiatry, 147,* 161–167.

Zanarini, M. C., Vujanovic, A. A., Parachini, E. A., Boulanger, J. L., Frankenberg, F. R., & Hennin, J. (2003). Zanarini Rating Scale for Borderline Personality Disorder (ZAN-BPD): A continuous measure of DSM-IV borderline psychopathology. *Journal of Personality Disorders, 17,* 233–242.

PART 4

Special Topics

Multicultural Issues in Cognitive-Behavioral Therapy: Cultural Adaptations and Goodness of Fit

Gordon C. Nagayama Hall *and* Alicia Yee Ibaraki

Abstract

Standard psychotherapies may be useful for those who fit well in mainstream US culture, but they may need to be culturally adapted for those whose fit is not as good. We review the literature on the generalizability of standard cognitive-behavioral therapy (CBT) as well as the literature on cultural adaptations of CBT. We offer a conceptual model for assessing an individual's goodness of fit with his or her sociocultural and cultural environments and for determining implications for interventions. The model considers an individual's fit in the mainstream culture and in the traditional culture and provides treatment recommendations on the basis of relative cultural match or mismatch. Considering goodness of fit with cultural and sociocultural environments may provide guidance on the relative merits of culturally adapted versus unadapted psychotherapy.

Key Words: cultural adaptation, cultural competence, cultural diversity, discrimination, goodness of fit

The scope and breadth of cognitive-behavioral therapy (CBT) is apparent from the range of topics covered in this book. CBT has been demonstrated to be effective in treating multiple disorders in diverse populations. The assumption by many adherents is that CBT is applicable to multiple cultural groups as well. We offer a goodness-of-fit conceptual model to help determine the applicability of CBT across cultural groups. Standard CBT may be useful for those who fit well in mainstream US culture, but it may need to be culturally adapted for those whose fit in mainstream US culture is not as good. We will first review rationales for applying the principles of CBT to multiple cultural groups, evidence of standard CBT's effectiveness across cultural groups, and evidence of the effectiveness of cultural adaptations of CBT. We then explore the utility of using a goodness-of-fit framework to guide assessment and treatment of people of color based on their cultural and sociocultural environments.

As can be seen in the second section of this book, CBT encompasses multiple approaches. However, a commonality across approaches is that cognitions mediate mood, behavior, and physiological reactions in response to the environment (Beck, 1995). Dysfunctional cognitions and behaviors are viewed as the basis of maladjustment and functional cognitions as the basis of adjustment (Dobson, 2001). The focus is on the individual, and environmental influences, such as culture, tend not to be emphasized in most CBT approaches (Hays & Iwamasa, 2006). In this chapter, we do not focus on specific CBT approaches, which are addressed elsewhere in this book, but we discuss how these approaches may be appropriately applied or modified for use with people of color.

A multicultural approach involves the consideration of the cultural influences on the behavior of multiple groups in a single context (Hall & Barongan, 2002). A cultural group shares attitudes, beliefs, norms, roles, and self definitions (S. Sue,

1991). In the United States, the cultures of multiple groups, including African Americans, American Indians, Asian Americans, Latino/a Americans, and European Americans, influence behavior. Although European American cultures have been dominant in the United States and in CBT approaches, European American cultures are by no means the only cultural influence in the United States. The behavior of non–European American groups is often influenced by their cultures of origin as much as it is by European American cultures. Moreover, as the non–European American population of the United States grows, so does its cultural influence on American culture, including European American cultures. However, goodness of fit with the cultural environment is usually a more salient issue for people of color than for European Americans because none of the cultures of people of color is dominant in the United States.

A basic premise of a multicultural approach is that what applies in one cultural context does not necessarily apply in another (Hall, 2010). This means that rather than assume a treatment approach such as CBT generalizes across groups, it is important to determine how well a person fits within a cultural or sociocultural context and then determine how well a treatment approach addresses the person's needs in that context. A multicultural approach is at odds with common assumptions in psychology that its theories are generalizable (Hall, 2010). Nevertheless, there is a conceptual rationale and some evidence that CBT is generalizable to multiple cultural groups, which we will discuss next.

The Cultural Generalizability of CBT

There is emerging evidence that CBT is effective across cultural groups in the United States. CBT has been found to be effective for African American and Latino/a American adults and youth experiencing a range of disorders (Horrell, 2008; Huey & Polo, 2008; Miranda et al., 2005). This evidence of the generalizability of treatment effects might lead some to conclude that CBT is universally effective and that cultural adaptations are unnecessary. Moreover, some CBT researchers and therapists may believe that a "colorblind" approach is the most objective and fair to all clients (Iwamasa, 1997). Cultural adaptation may be viewed as compromising the fidelity of evidence-based treatments. There are also political motivations to maintain the status quo, such as continued funding for a particular treatment approach (Hall & Yee, 2011). Although we concur that unadapted CBT can be beneficial to

people of color, it may be most useful for people of color who have a good fit with mainstream US culture, such as those who are acculturated or who do not experience discrimination.

Limits to the Cultural Generalizability of CBT

Although CBT has been conceptualized as a value-neutral approach, it is embedded in the values of European American cultures (Hays, 2009). European American cultures embrace an atomistic worldview with less emphasis on social or group contexts than on the individual. Not only does CBT focus on the individual, but it tends to focus on the individual's cognitions and less so on how the individual's cultural context might influence these cognitions. Cultural aspects of clients' environments (e.g., respect for elders, interdependence) and sociocultural aspects of clients' environments (e.g., minority status and discrimination) have been largely neglected in CBT (Hays, 2006). Even when CBT does consider the cultural and sociocultural aspects of clients' environments, the individual focus may not address societal-level influences that negatively impact cultural minority groups, including laws, institutional policies, and societal attitudes toward minorities (Organista, 2006). The therapist is not necessarily responsible for directly dealing with societal issues but does need to be aware of their impact on clients.

Although a strength of CBT is its standardization via treatment manuals, some forms of cultural adaptation are likely to occur when CBT is applied to diverse cultural groups even when unadapted treatment manuals are used. Cultural adaptations are not always reported in clinical trials, but accommodations such as language translation, conducting the intervention in a community context (e.g., church), or other seemingly minor methods of making an intervention relevant to a cultural context (e.g., culturally sensitive recruitment methods, therapist–client ethnic matching, using idioms or examples from the community) may qualify as cultural adaptations necessary for the effectiveness of CBT (Huey & Polo, 2008). Such unreported modifications create the impression that unadapted CBT is effective across groups, but these modifications may often be critical to the treatment's effectiveness.

As straightforward as language translation may appear, it may not be possible to literally translate certain CBT concepts across cultural groups without some modification. For example, in our experience we could not identify a concept in the Chinese language that corresponds with assertiveness. To assert one's own rights is aggressiveness in Chinese. Moreover, there is not a term for asserting one's own rights while respecting the rights of others. Any form of asserting one's own rights is aggressiveness, which is not the Western meaning of assertiveness.

It has been contended that all psychotherapy is culturally adapted (Benish, Quintana, & Wampold, 2011). Skilled therapists often seamlessly make such adaptations without acknowledging them. It is likely that some form of cultural adaptation occurs in research on applications of CBT to diverse cultural groups, even if it is unreported (Huey & Polo, 2008). Thus, it cannot be assumed that unadapted CBT generalizes across cultural contexts. Moreover, incorporating unspecified adaptations in studies is not good science because the possible effects of the adaptations are not examined. However, there is a growing body of evidence that cultural adaptations enhance therapeutic outcomes relative to unadapted therapies.

Cultural Adaptations of CBT

Cultural adaptation of a treatment begins with an existing treatment established for one cultural group and making modifications necessary for it to become a good fit for another cultural group (Hall, 2001). Such cultural adaptations may address language translation, the therapist–client relationship, cultural explanations of behavior and problems, therapeutic goals and methods, and the social, economic, and political contexts in which a client exists (Bernal, Bonilla, & Bellido, 1995). Hall and Yee (2014) recently identified nine models of cultural adaptation, most of which have been developed within the last decade. Commonalities across these models include broadening the scope of traditional etiological models to include cultural and sociocultural (e.g., discrimination) influences and the identification of cultural mediators of psychopathology and mental health (e.g., immigration stress, interdependence).

Four meta-analytic studies of the effectiveness of culturally adapted treatments have been conducted (Benish et al., 2011; Chowdhary et al., 2014; Griner & Smith, 2006; Huey & Polo, 2008). In a meta-analysis of 76 studies, Griner and Smith (2006) found a medium effect size for culturally adapted treatments versus unadapted treatments (these two approaches were compared in 77% of the studies) or versus no treatment. Cultural adaptations

in 84% of the studies involved explicitly incorporating cultural values/concepts in the intervention. Interventions that targeted particular ethnic groups (e.g., Latino/a Americans) were four times more effective than interventions that included multiple ethnic groups, which suggests the importance of group-specific cultural adaptations. Interventions conducted in clients' native language other than English were twice as effective as interventions conducted in English. There were also particularly large effect sizes for Latino/a Americans with relatively low levels of acculturation. Culturally adapted CBT was included in five of the studies, although several other studies included cognitive (e.g., psychoeducation) or behavioral (e.g., social skills training) components.

In a subsequent meta-analysis of 20 studies of psychosocial treatments for ethnic minority youth, Huey and Polo (2008) did not find significant differences between the outcomes of culturally adapted and unadapted treatments. Four of the studies involved CBT and three of these four studies involved cultural adaptations. Culturally adapted treatments were defined as intervention or clinician characteristics that made treatment more appropriate for ethnic minority participants. Other CBT-related approaches in studies analyzed included multisystemic treatment, problem solving, assertiveness training, anger management, and anxiety management. Less acculturated youths were poorly represented in the studies analyzed by Huey and Polo (2008), which may account for the lack of an effect. There was only one study in the Huey and Polo (2008) meta-analysis that included an overlapping data set with the Griner and Smith (2006) meta-analysis.

Some of the studies in the Griner and Smith (2006) meta-analysis did not include a control group or included an unspecified treatment (e.g., treatment as usual), which may have artificially inflated the overall effect size of culturally adapted treatments. In a subsequent meta-analysis of 21 studies that compared culturally adapted treatments to bona fide comparison treatments, Benish et al. (2011) again found culturally adapted treatments to be superior, although the effect size was somewhat smaller than in the Griner and Smith (2006) study. Cultural adaptation in the Benish et al. (2011) study was defined as a goal of providing a more effective therapy than conventional therapy for racial or ethnic minorities. Similar to the Griner and Smith (2006) finding of greater effectiveness of treatments adapted for particular groups, Benish et al. (2011)

found that treatments adapted to be consistent with clients' cultural worldviews regarding issues such as etiology, beliefs about the problem and its effects, and expectations about the length and type of treatment were more effective than treatments that were not adapted to clients' cultural worldviews. Unlike Griner and Smith (2006), Benish et al. (2011) did not find a language effect, but they acknowledged that there were few language-match studies in their meta-analysis. Benish et al. (2011) also did not analyze the possible effects of acculturation as a moderator of treatment outcomes. Only two of the studies analyzed by Benish et al. (2011) included culturally adapted CBT, although cognitive (e.g., psychoeducation) or behavioral (e.g., exposure, skills training) components were included in several studies. Only one study in the Benish et al. (2011) meta-analysis included an overlapping data set with the Griner and Smith (2006) meta-analysis, and there were no overlapping studies between the Benish et al. (2011) and Huey and Polo (2008) meta-analyses. However, 11 of the 21 studies in the Benish et al. (2011) meta-analysis included youths under the age of 18 years and client age was not a moderator of the effects.

Most recently, Chowdhary et al. (2014) examined the efficacy of culturally adapted evidence-based psychological treatments for depression compared to unadapted treatments. Their meta-analysis, which included 20 studies, found support for adapted treatments (standardized mean difference, –0.72; 95% confidence interval, –0.94 to –0.49). Through a combination of reviewing published material and contacting authors directly to ask about process of adaptation, the Chowdhary (2014) review also specified the type(s) of adaptations made in each study. The most common form of adaptation was language, which included direct translation as well as the incorporation of colloquial expressions to replace technical terms, and the inclusions of culturally relevant idioms of distress. The second most common adaptation was therapist-level adaptations, which are not always measured or documented in traditional adaptation studies. These strategies include ethnically matching therapist and client, therapists changing how directive they are with clients, or sharing and emphasizing shared personal experiences. Due to small sample sizes, Chowdhary and colleagues were not able to draw conclusions about the relationship between type of adaptation and level of therapy effectiveness. However, their data did illustrate that therapist-level adaptations are quite common

and contribute to the effect of increased efficacy of culturally adapted evidence-based treatments over nonadapted treatments.

Taken together, the findings of these four meta-analyses (Benish et al., 2011; Chowdhary et al., 2014; Griner & Smith, 2006; Huey & Polo, 2008) suggest that psychological treatments, including CBT, are effective with persons of color and that the effectiveness of these interventions is a function of environmental fit. There was almost no overlap in studies reviewed across the meta-analyses, and it appears that the environmental fit of the participants in each of the meta-analyses differed. Most of the participants in the studies reviewed by Huey and Polo (2008) were relatively acculturated, which suggests that they had a good fit with the mainstream US cultural environment. Therefore, it is not surprising that culturally adapted treatments were not more effective than unadapted treatments in these studies. In contrast, there was a broader range of acculturation in the studies reviewed by Griner and Smith (2006) and presumably many of the participants had a relatively poor fit with mainstream US culture. Griner and Smith (2006) found cultural adaptations to be effective, especially when they were adapted for a particular cultural group, or for participants who did not speak English and for Latino/a Americans who were relatively unacculturated. Benish et al. (2011) did not consider participants' acculturation levels, but their finding of greater effectiveness of culturally adapted treatments versus unadapted treatments and the finding similar to that of Griner and Smith (2006) of the greater effectiveness of group-specific adaptations suggests that there was a range of acculturation and that many of the participants were not experiencing a good fit with mainstream US culture.

Objections to Cultural Adaptations of Treatments

Although meta-analytic evidence suggests that culturally adapted treatments, including culturally adapted CBT, are more effective than nonadapted treatments for many clients of color, there may be resistance to modifying an approach for specific groups that is already evidence based for European Americans. Some may object on a practical basis, such as the complexity and cost of culturally adapting treatments. However, it is not true that all adaptations must include the time and expense of a large-scale randomized controlled trial. Lau,

Chang, and Okazaki (2010) propose multiple, cost-effective, empirically supported study designs to address the need for targeted psychological interventions for relatively small and specific, high-risk populations (e.g., first-generation Latina adolescent females). Others may believe that extensive efforts to culturally adapt treatments and to evaluate the effectiveness of these treatments are unnecessary because relatively simple adaptations (e.g., ethnic matching of therapists and clients, language translation) are adequate. However, such approaches may be superficial and overlook complexities, such as language translation, as discussed earlier. Moreover, the effects on treatment outcome of superficial attempts at cultural adaptation, such as ethnic matching, are likely to be small (Maramba & Hall, 2002). Such superficial attempts to culturally adapt treatments have been compared to pouring teriyaki sauce on a non-Japanese entrée and calling it Japanese food (J. Kaplan, personal communication, August 2006).

There are also scientific objections to culturally adapting treatments. Some may contend that there are not adequate conceptual models. However, multiple cultural adaptation models exist, as discussed earlier. One of the earliest models (Bernal et al., 1995) has existed 20 years and has guided cultural adaptations of CBT for depression, which have been demonstrated to be effective (Rosselló & Bernal, 1999; Rosselló, Bernal, & Rivera-Medina, 2008). Others may contend that there are not adequate data to support cultural adaptations. However, as discussed earlier, the results of two meta-analyses of 97 total studies indicate that the effects of culturally adapted treatments are superior to nonadapted treatments for people of color (Benish et al., 2011; Griner & Smith, 2006).

In addition to objections about cultural adaptations of treatments, some may object to devoting attention to treatment studies in diverse cultural groups because generalizability studies are not scientifically compelling or even unnecessary. The basis of this objection and the other objections mentioned earlier may be the low priority of people of color among many policy makers, researchers, and practitioners. Federal mental health policy for people of color in the United States since the 1980s has been a "trickle-down" approach, analogous to President Reagan's trickle-down economics, in which it is assumed that attention to a powerful group will somehow inherently have ancillary benefits to other less powerful groups. CBT and other treatments have generally been developed by and for European Americans, and it is assumed by some that the benefits of these treatments will trickle down to other ethnic and cultural groups once these culturally unadapted treatments are disseminated. This approach overlooks the unique needs of non–European American cultural groups and is not necessarily interested in developing specific treatments that might be the most effective for these groups.

We contend that careful investigation of the unique cultural and sociocultural influences on behavior and how they may moderate treatment outcome is scientifically compelling. Moreover, the investigation of cultural and sociocultural influences on behavior is compelling from a public policy perspective because of the increasing cultural diversity of American society. A scientific approach to identifying which unique cultural influences contextualize the presentation of a mental health disorder also helps to dispel the notion that every intervention must be specifically adapted for every possible combination of demographic factors (Lau, 2006). Instead of targeting all populations equally, the deliberate selection of populations where there is an empirically demonstrated variability in (a) vulnerability or resilience to a target problem or (b) response to the current evidence-based treatment should maximize the impact of an adaptation (Lau, 2006).

We further contend that a cultural community's mental health needs should be the starting point for investigation, rather than starting with an existing treatment such as CBT and attempting to apply it across cultural groups. Unadapted CBT may be quite useful for people of color who have a good fit with the mainstream US cultural environment, but it may require cultural adaptation for those who do not have such a good fit.

Assessing Cultural Competency

It would be erroneous to assume that clinicians of color are inherently capable of delivering culturally sensitive treatment and are naturally free from bias. All clinicians regardless of race, sexual orientation, or gender have inherent bias (D. Sue & Sue, 2008). As ethnic minority clinicians undergo the same training as their nonminority peers, it is unreasonable to expect that ethnic minority clinicians are naturally more skilled in delivering culturally competent treatment than their nonminority counterparts (Iwamasa, 1997). Instead, all therapists, regardless of their background, must assess their ability to deliver culturally sensitive services.

One of the first and most well-known models for measuring cultural competency, the multicultural counseling competencies model, was developed by Derald Wing Sue in 1982. It has since been updated and adopted by the American Psychological Association (2003). This model consists of three core components: (1) attitudes/beliefs—awareness of one's own assumptions, values, and biases; (2) knowledge—understanding the worldview of culturally diverse clients; and (3) skills—the ability to conduct appropriate interventions strategies and techniques.

The ability to be culturally sensitive starts with a therapist's own self-assessment of his or her cultural values, assumptions, biases, and notions of acceptable behavior (Ford-Paz & Iwamasa, 2012; D. Sue & Sue, 2008; S. Sue, Zane, Hall, & Berger, 2009). Therapists should have a clear understanding of their own identity so they can consider how their personal beliefs differ from their client's. Although it is not necessary that therapists and clients share the same values or cultural worldviews, therapists should be comfortable working with these potential differences in a nonjudgmental manner (S. Sue et al., 2009). If differences in lifestyle choices or cultural beliefs are seen not only as different but also as deviant, a therapist might consider referring that client out to work with someone with similar worldviews (D. Sue & Sue, 2008).

In addition to self-assessment, a therapist should have basic knowledge or the willingness to acquire such knowledge about a client's cultural group. This basic knowledge is both broad, such as the conditions surround that group's immigration to the United States, historic treatment by and experiences with other groups, and basic cultural beliefs, as well as specific to the client such as his or her daily living experience (D. Sue & Sue, 2008). Although this knowledge can be obtained through readings and trainings, spending time in that community is particularly valuable, especially if a therapist is planning to work frequently with a specific population. This cultural knowledge will help the therapist assess fit with different treatment modalities. It will also help the therapist to be more aware of important social and environmental stressors such as discrimination, oppression, or economic challenges that are an everyday reality for these clients and are not divorced from their presenting problem (Ford-Paz & Iwamasa, 2012).

Finally, therapists must possess the skill to select and implement culturally appropriate interventions.

In this chapter, we present a decision framework to aid the process of selecting an intervention.

Goodness of Fit of CBT with Populations of Color

Goodness of fit is a statistical concept in which the relative fit of a statistical model with actual data is determined. Person-environment fit has been addressed in the career development literature with the assumption that better fit leads to better work adjustment (e.g., Dawis & Lofquist, 1984; Holland, 1985). It is also possible to determine the goodness of fit between an individual and his or her cultural and sociocultural environments. The cultural environment encompasses the cultural groups in which the individual is situated. People of color are often faced with fit issues in two or more cultural groups, including their cultural group of origin and the mainstream US cultural group (LaFromboise, Coleman, & Gerton 1993). The sociocultural environment involves one's status as a person of color and often involves minority status and discrimination, which may result in a poor environmental fit.

Goodness of fit can also apply to the relevance of a treatment to a client. The ethnic match literature has addressed issues of client–therapist fit. Ethnic matching of clients and therapists creates a good fit in terms of treatment outcomes that are better than those for ethnically mismatched clients and therapists (S. Sue, Fujino, Hu, Takeuchi, & Zane, 1991). Ethnic matching is often a proxy for other mechanisms, such as language match or worldview match between client and therapist (Zane et al., 2005). CBT may be a good fit for clients of color whose worldviews are consistent with the CBT worldview, but CBT may require adaptations for optimal effectiveness with clients whose worldviews diverge from that of CBT.

Proponents of CBT contend that it is naturally a good fit for people of color because its healing principles are universal and are found in the cultures of diverse groups. The cognitive aspects of CBT may be viewed as analogous to the healing wisdom found in many American cultural traditions. For example, it has been proposed that CBT and American Indian healing concepts, such as harmony and wellness, are similar (McDonald & Gonzalez, 2006). The expertise and authority of CBT therapists who impart education and the short-term, problem-focused nature of CBT have been considered beneficial for Latino/a Americans and Asian Americans whose prototype for a healer may be a medical doctor (Hall & Eap, 2007; Iwamasa, Hsia, & Hinton, 2006;

Organista, 2006). The collaborative nature of treatment, with the therapist as the expert on treatment and clients as experts on themselves and their problems, is seen as consistent with African American cultural and community values with respect to the healing process (Kelly, 2006). From a sociocultural perspective, the emphasis of CBT on empowerment could be an asset to those who are marginalized (Kellogg & Young, 2008; Kelly, 2006).

Mindfulness and acceptance-based approaches in CBT have roots in Asian philosophies, which generally may make these approaches a good fit with Asian American cultural values, although there is much variability within and between Asian American cultural groups (Hall, Hong, Zane, & Meyer, 2011). Mindfulness, involving heightened awareness and full engagement, is compatible with Buddhist practices of mindfulness (Kumar, 2002). Similarly, acceptance of events and coping with one's reaction to events rather than attempting to change the events themselves is consistent with indirect coping strategies in Asian and Asian American cultures (Weisz, Rothbaum, & Blackburn, 1984).

A lack of fit can occur when the mainstream American cultural values reflected in CBT do not align with the values of cultural groups. Mainstream American values include a task orientation, independence, expression of feelings, assertiveness, egalitarianism, and intellectualism (Organista, 2006). Although not all mainstream Americans are characterized by these values, these values tend to be emphasized more in mainstream American culture than in the cultures of people of color. For example, many Native American languages lack the word "I," whereas "I" statements are central to many CBT approaches (McDonald & Gonzalez, 2006). In contrast to mainstream American culture, traditional Latino/a cultures value an interpersonal orientation, interdependence, control of emotions and nonverbal communication, deference to others with a goal of interpersonal harmony, hierarchical roles, and religiosity (Organista, 2006). Spiritual and community values emphasized in Asian American and African American communities are not emphases in CBT (Iwamasa et al., 2006; Kelly, 2006). CBT tends to focus on individual solutions to problems (e.g., cognitive restructuring), but such solutions may be of varying effectiveness in cultures in which interpersonal relationships are emphasized.

Even when CBT implements the concepts of non-Western cultures, such as mindfulness and acceptance, these cultural concepts tend to be adapted for Western audiences. For example, Buddhist methods of mindfulness meditation orient the self toward others, such as loving-kindness meditation (Fredrickson, Cohn, Coffey, Pek, & Finkel, 2008). In contrast, a common purpose of meditation in Western therapeutic implementations is orientation toward self, such as in achieving awareness of experiences related to the self in isolation from the experiences of others (Hall et al., 2011). Acceptance in Asian and Asian American contexts includes what might be considered in the West to be passivity or avoidance of experiences, whereas acceptance in Western therapeutic approaches involves an emphasis on actively experiencing events (Hall et al., 2011). These therapeutic adaptations of Asian cultural concepts for Western audiences are not inherently compatible with Asian and Asian American cultural values.

A Goodness-of-Fit Framework to Guide Assessment and Treatment

Figure 25.1 offers a framework for assessing an individual's goodness of fit with his or her sociocultural and cultural environments and for determining the implications of goodness of fit for interventions, including CBT. The assumption of the framework is that competence for people of color both in mainstream US culture and in their traditional culture is optimal (LaFromboise et al., 1993). Thus, assessment and treatment that focus on both mainstream and traditional cultures are warranted. Key assessments of fit include the environment and culture. Level of ethnic identity and experience with discrimination should also be considered when determining fit with a treatment. Each one of these aspects is discussed in turn.

The first step in CBT typically is cognitive-behavioral assessment. Such assessment typically focuses on the individual. Adequate assessment of cultural and sociocultural influences on behavior involves not only the individual and the individual's dyadic relationships but a consideration of the cultural and sociocultural contexts in which the individual exists (Okazaki & Tanaka-Matsumi, 2006). This assessment of the cultural and sociocultural environments is compatible with the assessment of environmental contingencies in CBT.

A logical starting point is to assess an individual's goodness of fit in mainstream US culture because most people of color in the United States live within this cultural context or are influenced by it. If there is a good fit in mainstream culture, then goodness of fit in traditional culture is assessed. If there is

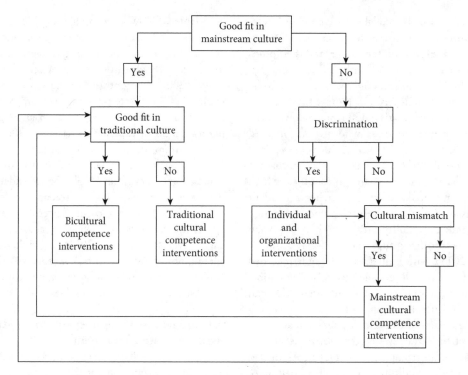

Figure 25.1 Goodness of fit with mainstream and traditional cultural environments: assessment and treatment.

also a good fit in traditional culture, then interventions to enhance bicultural competence are relevant. Existing cultural adaptation models address bicultural competence (Hall & Yee, 2011).

A promising approach to assessing the goodness of fit between the individual and his or her cultural and sociocultural environments is the Scale of Ethnic Experience (SEE), a measure of cognitive ethnicity-related constructs (Malcarne, Chavira, Fernandez, & Liu, 2006). This scale assesses both cultural and sociocultural constructs, as measured by four factors: (a) ethnic identity; (b) perceived discrimination; (c) perceived social affiliation; and (d) mainstream comfort. Ethnic identity, which involves ethnic pride and participation in cultural activities, and perceived social affiliation, which involves preference for and comfort with friendships and romantic relationships in one's own ethnic group, are cultural constructs. Perceived discrimination, which involves perceptions of how one's ethnic group has been mistreated in the United States, and social affiliation, which involves comfort in mainstream US culture, are sociocultural constructs.

The SEE has been demonstrated to have internal and external validity. In a study of four ethnic groups (African Americans, European Americans, Filipino Americans, Mexican Americans), European Americans had higher levels of mainstream comfort

and lower levels of perceived discrimination than the other groups (Malcarne et al., 2006). The opposite pattern was true for African Americans. The groups of color reported greater social affiliation and stronger ethnic identity than did European Americans.

Intercorrelations among the four constructs offer information about person-environment fit (Malcarne et al., 2006). Ethnic identity is positively correlated with social affiliation and perceived discrimination, and negatively correlated with mainstream comfort. Mainstream comfort is negatively correlated with perceived discrimination and social affiliation. Thus, a strong ethnic identity for persons of color may result in fit issues in a mainstream cultural environment, whereas a mainstream identity may result in fit issues for a person of color in an ethnic cultural environment. Persons of color often exist in both ethnic and mainstream environments, facing challenges of adapting to both.

If there is not a good fit in traditional culture, then the intervention focus is on enhancing traditional cultural competence using the methods discussed earlier. However, a poor fit in traditional culture may not appear problematic for some people of color, such as those who do not have access to traditional culture or those who wish to assimilate into mainstream US culture. One option in such cases might be unadapted CBT, which has been demonstrated to be effective with relatively acculturated persons (Huey & Polo, 2008). Nevertheless, even for those for whom traditional cultural fit may not seem to be an issue, it is worth considering enhancing traditional cultural competence because of the mental health benefits it accrues (Hall, 2010; LaFromboise et al., 1993).

If there is not a good fit in mainstream culture, it should be determined whether the lack of fit is because of racially or ethnically based discrimination. Discrimination is considered before other cultural issues because it is a relatively common occurrence for people of color, including those who are not identified with their traditional culture. If discrimination is occurring, the individual and organizational interventions discussed earlier are relevant. When discrimination is not occurring, it may be useful for the CBT therapist to prepare the client to cope with discrimination, as it is relatively likely to happen to people of color. Regardless of whether discrimination is occurring, a cultural mismatch should be considered as the possible basis of psychological distress. A cultural mismatch occurs when one adheres to cultural values, such as interdependence, that are at odds with the mainstream culture. Discrimination or a cultural mismatch or both are common bases for a poor fit for people of color in mainstream US culture. If a cultural mismatch is occurring, interventions to enhance mainstream cultural competence, which are the default mode of CBT, are indicated. After discrimination and cultural mismatch issues are considered, relative fit in one's traditional culture is considered.

Goodness of Fit between Individuals and Their Environments
Discrimination

Dealing with environmental fit in response to discrimination is an issue that many people of color face because they are visible racial or ethnic minorities (Helms, 1994). Because discrimination is a relatively common experience for people of color, it may be productive to address discrimination before other racial/ethnic identity issues are addressed. Moreover, a person's response to discrimination may provide clues to his or her level of racial/ethnic identity. In a clinical or research setting, the SEE could be administered and discrimination could be addressed in a discussion of the client's perceived discrimination score.

Discrimination has been consistently demonstrated to be a risk factor for psychopathology among populations of color (Cook, Alegría, Lin, &

Guo, 2009; Gee, Spencer, Chen, & Takeuchi, 2007; Williams, Neighbors, & Jackson, 2008). Among adults of color, 30%–80% report experiencing race- or ethnicity-based discrimination (Pérez, Fortuna, & Alegría, 2008; Sellers & Shelton, 2003). In contrast, European Americans' experiences of racially/ ethnically based discrimination are quite limited relative to those of persons of color (Romero, Carvajal, Volle, & Orduña 2007; Wei et al., 2010). Thus, it is not surprising that CBT, which has been primarily developed by and for European Americans, does not systematically address discrimination.

CBT tends to focus on the individual and usually not on changing the individual's environment beyond couple and family relationships. We contend that in considering how to cope with discrimination that there should be a strong focus on changing a discriminatory environment rather than a sole focus on changing the individual's cognitions or behavior to adjust to the environment. Such change may involve the client addressing a situation directly (e.g., speaking to a supervisor who is engaging in discrimination) or indirectly (e.g., working with a union steward). Moreover, when efforts to change a discriminatory environment are unsuccessful, moving to a new environment within or outside an organization may be adaptive, given the negative effects of discrimination on mental health (Cook et al., 2009; Gee et al., 2007; Williams et al., 2008).

A challenge in assessing discrimination is that many people of color may minimize the extent to which they experience it (Major et al., 2002). Discrimination may be viewed by some immigrants as an "accepted" aspect of living in the United States (Ayón, Marsiglia, & Bermudez-Parsai, 2010). Persons of color may also minimize their own experiences of discrimination because of the personal/ group discrimination discrepancy (Crosby, 1984). Although a person of color may acknowledge that racially or ethnically based discrimination happens to others, he or she also often has multiple identities and may consider his or her race or ethnicity as one among many. Thus, the person of color may not necessarily attribute mistreatment to membership in a racial or ethnic group but may attribute it to other issues (e.g., inadvertent behavior on the part of the perpetrator, misunderstanding, personality conflict). In addition, individuals may avoid attributing mistreatment to group-based discrimination because it can create a sense of powerlessness. Racial or ethnic biases of others may be perceived as much more difficult to change than interpersonal issues, such as misunderstandings. Thus, minimization of discrimination may represent an attempt to fit into the environment.

Because of tendencies toward not attributing one's personal mistreatment to racial or ethnic discrimination, an observer may be more likely to attribute mistreatment of an actor to discrimination than the actor would (Crosby, 1984). Cognitive-behavioral assessment involves gathering objective evidence of discrimination. For example, are other people of color being mistreated in the same way that the actor is? Does the mistreatment target only people of color? Does the perpetrator of mistreatment have a history or reputation of mistreating people of color? The assessor must be sensitive to actors' tendencies to minimize discrimination, as well as to the powerlessness an actor might experience if he or she did attribute mistreatment to discrimination.

Conversely, people of color with a strong ethnic identity may be particularly sensitive to discrimination (Sellers & Shelton, 2003; Wei et al., 2010). For such persons, the assessor must be careful not to attribute perceptions of discrimination to hypersensitivity but to attempt to objectively assess whether mistreatment constitutes discrimination (Hays, 2009).

How do people of color typically cope with discrimination? Wei and colleagues (2010) identified five common coping methods: (a) education/advocacy; (b) resistance; (c) internalization; (d) detachment; and (d) drug and alcohol use. Education/advocacy involves education or advocacy to deal with discrimination at individual and societal levels. For example, an individual might prepare another individual to cope with the effects of discrimination or might advocate for stronger anti-discrimination policies in an organization or government. Education/advocacy was positively correlated with life satisfaction, self-esteem, and ethnic identity. Resistance involves challenging or confronting individuals for their discriminatory behavior and is consistent with assertiveness in CBT. Resistance is positively associated with self-esteem, but not significantly correlated with life satisfaction or ethnic identity. Although education/advocacy might be viewed as a less direct method of coping with discrimination than resistance, education/advocacy may result in life satisfaction because of its potential societal impact beyond personal incidents. Similarly, individuals who are ethnically identified may be likely to engage in education/advocacy because they view discrimination as a community or societal issue and not simply as an interpersonal issue.

Internalization is the tendency to attribute the cause of a discriminatory incident to oneself. Detachment involves distancing oneself from social support and not knowing how to deal with discrimination. Internalization, detachment, and substance use as methods of coping with discrimination are all maladaptive insofar as they are positively correlated with depression and negatively correlated with life satisfaction, self-esteem, and ethnic identity (Wei et al., 2010). Interestingly, education/advocacy and resistance are not significantly associated with depression. This may imply individual efforts to cope with depression associated with discrimination are not effective and that broader efforts to reduce discrimination, such as policies or interventions with perpetrators of discrimination, are necessary.

A treatment goal for someone experiencing discrimination is to reduce their sense of powerlessness and to develop a plan to address discrimination. Most forms of CBT, including acceptance-based approaches (Hall et al., 2011), encourage active engagement with problems, which may empower a target of discrimination. Such active engagement may include direct confrontation with a perpetrator of discrimination. The research of Wei and colleagues (2010) discussed earlier suggests that confrontation as a method of coping with discrimination is associated with self-esteem.

Direct confrontation, however, is not always possible or effective. Much discrimination is subtle and occurs in the form of microaggressions, which involve denigrating messages to people of color based on their minority group membership (D. Sue et al., 2007). For example, a person of color may observe that people of color are absent from decision-making groups in an organization. This could constitute a microaggression in the form of micro-invalidation insofar as the input of people of color is not valued by the organization. A person could confront the leader of the organization and point out this lack of input from people of color. However, the leader could easily deny that the exclusion of persons of color is systematic and justify the composition of the decision-making group on some grounds, such as that the group is elected by the organization's membership. In this case, effective coping may involve education and advocacy within the organization, which are associated with self-esteem and life satisfaction for targets of discrimination (Wei et al., 2010). In some cases, legal action may be required to change a discriminatory environment. These organizational solutions are typically beyond the scope of CBT interventions, but they may be necessary to augment the individual or interpersonal solutions typically offered by CBT. Solutions beyond the interpersonal level may be particularly important for persons of color who are strongly ethnically identified (Wei et al., 2010).

It might be tempting for a therapist to have the client determine the extent to which he or she is personally responsible for perceived discrimination and to cope with discrimination by modifying the client's cognitions or behaviors. For example, a therapist may want to assess the extent to which the client is misperceiving a situation as discrimination. However, given the tendencies to minimize discrimination as discussed earlier, it is likely that a situation is serious if a person of color is willing to discuss it in therapy. A related example would be a therapist examining the extent to which the client's behavior provokes a discriminatory response. For example, a client could bring attention to his or her ethnicity by discussing family or cultural issues and events or posting culturally related information in the workspace. Nevertheless, discrimination is an inappropriate response to any behavior and the responsibility for discrimination is solely that of the perpetrator. Moreover, attributing responsibility for discrimination to oneself is associated with depression and lower self-esteem and life satisfaction (Wei et al., 2010). Therapists who explore the possibility of the client's responsibility for discrimination may be perceived by the client as racist or naïve (Hays, 2009). Thus, the focus in CBT would be to acknowledge, stop, and prevent discriminatory behavior rather than to focus on the client's personal responsibility (Hays, 2009).

Because ethnic identification is positively correlated with perceived discrimination (Sellers & Shelton, 2003; Wei et al., 2010), another individual therapeutic approach to discrimination might be to help the client assimilate. The assumption is that a lower ethnic identification via assimilation would make a person of color less sensitive to discrimination. Some clients may seek to assimilate, and this may be the reason that they are seeking CBT, which they may perceive as a mainstream cultural approach. However, persons of color having a low ethnic identity may also believe in egalitarianism, which involves an emphasis on individual characteristics (e.g., hard work, self-acceptance) over group membership, such as race or ethnicity (Hughes et al., 2006). Persons of color who believe in egalitarianism may be particularly susceptible to discrimination when it does target them because it violates their assumptions of equality (Brown &

Bigler, 2005). Thus, a person of color having low ethnic identity and seeking to assimilate may still benefit from preparation for bias, which involves becoming aware of discrimination and learning how to cope with it (Hughes et al., 2006). Moreover, not all clients of color are seeking to assimilate. Psychotherapy can often be a coercive acculturative process because of the power differential between the therapist and client (Hall & Malony, 1983). Moreover, reducing ethnic identity via assimilation may concurrently reduce the positive effects of ethnic identity on the mental health of people of color (Hall, 2010).

Although a strong ethnic identity may make a person of color sensitive to discrimination, ethnic identity can also serve as a buffer against it. Ethnic identity has consistently been demonstrated to be associated with mental health among populations of color (Hall, 2010; Wei et al., 2010). Cultural socialization, which helps establish and strengthen ethnic identity, has been found to reduce the psychological impact of discrimination among African American high school and college students (Bynum, Burton, & Best, 2007; Neblett et al., 2008). Cultural socialization involves instilling ethnic and racial pride, teaching about traditions and history, and exposure to and training in cultural practices, such as language, food, and holidays (Hughes et al., 2006). To the extent that it strengthens ethnic identity, which is positively correlated with mental health (Hall, 2010), cultural socialization may be an important component of CBT with clients of color. Despite these potential benefits, ethnic identity and culture are not systematically addressed in CBT. The behavior of people of color is much more strongly influenced by ethnic identity than is the behavior of European Americans (Phinney, Dennis, & Osorio, 2006; Wei et al., 2010); thus, ethnic identity is not viewed as a salient issue for European Americans.

Culture

Acculturation can be conceptualized as an effort to fit into a cultural environment. LaFromboise and colleagues (1993) have described five models of acculturation: assimilation, acculturation, alternation, multicultural, and fusion. Assimilation involves absorption into the dominant or more desirable culture. Acculturation is gaining competence in a second culture but still being identified as a member of the minority culture. Alternation involves competence in two cultures. Multicultural acculturation involves separate and distinct cultural identities that are maintained while cultures coexist within a single multicultural social structure (e.g., national or economic) in which the cultural groups accept one another and work together. Fusion involves cultures fusing together until they are indistinguishable and forming a new culture. Multicultural acculturation and fusion are difficult to achieve in practice because one cultural group tends to be dominant in most societies and it is usually not possible for other cultural groups to achieve equal status with the dominant group. Thus, assimilation, acculturation, and alternation are the primary acculturation options. Alternation is considered an optimal mode of functioning (LaFromboise et al., 1993).

In terms of environmental fit, almost all people of color experience pressure to assimilate, whether it is learning English and mainstream US culture in school or being exposed to individualistic cultural norms in organizational settings. Assimilation may be a good fit for persons of color who desire to assimilate in a mainstream cultural setting. CBT was designed to address mainstream US cultural issues and can be helpful to persons of color in addressing adjustment to mainstream US culture. However, as discussed earlier, a loss of ethnic identity may result in a concurrent loss of the mental health benefits it accrues. Moreover, an assimilation strategy for a person in a traditional cultural context may be a source of conflict. For example, children often assimilate easier and at faster rates than their parents, which may result in acculturative stress (Hwang & Ting, 2008). Conversely, a person who adheres to traditional cultural values may experience conflict in a mainstream cultural context. Pressures to assimilate to an individualist society may result in depression among those whose cultural norms are interdependent (Mak, Law, & Teng, 2011). In these situations, CBT might take a psychoeducational focus on how to alternate effectively between two cultures.

Not all persons of color who wish to assimilate are able to assimilate. In the acculturation model by LaFromboise et al. (1993), gaining competence in a second culture does not inherently result in acceptance in the second culture. Thus, a person may desire to fit with his or her environment but may have difficulties doing so. CBT could focus on helping the person become more competent and accepted in the second culture via increasing social skills or networking relationships. Another strategy would be to recognize that full acceptance into a second culture is not possible and to focus on strengthening one's identity and relationships in the culture of origin. A third strategy would be

to find another context in the second culture in which acceptance is more likely. Yet another strategy would be to create a separatist identity with one's own group. However, a separatist identity may be difficult to achieve in that it would require a critical mass of others similar to oneself (e.g., Chinatown, Little Manila). Some interaction with mainstream culture is usually necessary.

Having both strong ethnic and mainstream identities is considered optimal (LaFromboise et al., 1993). Cultural socialization, which emphasizes the cultural strengths of racial or ethnic groups, may be incorporated into CBT to enhance ethnic identity. CBT's rejection of all-or-nothing thinking can facilitate the concept that one cultural identity need not exist at the expense of another. Because mainstream US culture is the default mode in CBT, the clinician may need to be particularly attuned to cultural strengths that are usually not addressed by CBT, such as interdependence. Analogous to CBT interventions to enhance dyadic relationships, CBT can assist clients in becoming identified with a group and making effective contributions to its functioning, including supporting and assisting others in the group. The group may be one's family, an ethnic or racial group, or some other group, such as one in a school, church, or work setting. Effective groups are essential to the success of most organizations and skills in interdependence are valuable to clients of all racial and ethnic backgrounds. However, many, if not most, organizations in mainstream US culture primarily consist of persons who are individualistic. Thus, an individual's skills in interdependence may not be effective without broader application, such as organizational training in interdependence. Even if broader application of interdependence is not possible or effective, an emphasis in CBT on interdependence for many clients of color may facilitate psychological health, in that interdependence is a component of ethnic identity and a strong ethnic identity is associated with psychological health (Hall, 2010).

The concept of alternation in the LaFromboise et al. (1993) model suggests that traditional and mainstream cultural contexts are nonoverlapping. Optimal fit involves adjusting one's behavior to the cultural setting, whereas introducing cultural behavior from outside the cultural setting would result in a poor fit. Nevertheless, cultural contexts may overlap in that every person is both independent and interdependent to varying degrees (Triandis, 1995), and the growing non–European American population influences mainstream US culture, as discussed at the beginning of this chapter. Moreover, cross-cultural input can be beneficial. We have emphasized the value of interdependence in independent cultural group settings, including families, schools, and organizations. Independence may also be useful in some interdependent contexts. For example, a value of interpersonal harmony may prevent the group from confronting an individual who is creating problems for the group because of his abuse of alcohol. An independent approach would involve confrontation and could be integrated into the interdependent cultural context if the goal was to restore the individual's standing as a productive group member.

Despite the potential benefits of interdependence in family, school, and work settings, CBT has typically emphasized independence over interdependence. For example, interdependence has been associated with negative emotional contagion, in which relationships with persons experiencing negative emotions, such as depression or lowered positive affect, can make an individual vulnerable to experiencing these negative emotions (Joiner & Katz, 1999; Paukert, Pettit, & Amacker, 2008). The therapeutic solution to emotional contagion is seen as buffering the client from the effects of negative emotional contagion and focusing on the welfare of the individual client rather than the welfare of those who are in relationships with the client (Joiner & Katz, 1999). This solution essentially is to reduce interdependence and not to be responsible for the welfare of others experiencing negative emotions, with the expectation that others should seek care for themselves.

The concept of emotional contagion construes awareness of the emotions of others as susceptibility for problems. An alternative construal would be that the person is sensitive and responsive to the emotions of others. Rather than extracting oneself from one's group either psychologically or even physically, the treatment goal in an interdependent context would be to maintain and enhance interpersonal relationships. Although a client experiencing negative emotions may not currently have the resources to assist others experiencing negative emotions, a therapeutic goal more compatible with the values of interdependent cultures might be for the client to learn to reduce his or her negative emotions so that he or she can eventually help others learn to do so as well. The goal in an interdependent cultural context would be to improve personal functioning to be an effective group member and to help other group members improve their personal

functioning with the ultimate goal of enhancing group functioning. Even in individualist cultures, prioritizing the individual over his or her relationships can be maladaptive in any context in which healthy relationships are vital to success.

It is important to recognize that the culture of CBT is not necessarily compatible with clients' cultures. CBT may not be particularly useful for the functioning of clients of any ethnic background in cultural contexts that are not similar to the mainstream US cultural context. For example, CBT typically would address individual adjustment issues for a European American facing conflicts in a school or work setting in which European Americans are part of a small minority. European American clients themselves might view individual adjustment as the solution to any discomfort or conflict that they might experience as a result of minority status. Yet optimal functioning may not involve individual adjustment but finding ways to value the group over the self and to make effective contributions to the group's functioning.

Although many clients of color identify with their ethnic group, some may not be aware of cultural influences on their behavior. They may recognize family or community influences but may not necessarily attribute these influences to ethnicity or culture. It is not necessary for clients to acknowledge that family and community influences are cultural. However, it is useful for clients of color to understand how family and community norms affect their behavior, as well as how these norms might differ from the mainstream culture. It is also important for CBT therapists to understand that culture may be influential even when clients of color do not explicitly acknowledge culture as an influence.

Sociopolitical History

In assessing fit, another important consideration is the importance of tailoring CBT so that it is delivered in the context of an individual's environment and past experiences. This can be at an individual level, as discussed earlier, considering experiences with discrimination and level of assimilation. There may also be past experiences that exist across a specific population that on a group level, such as a shared sociopolitical history, that therapists should be aware of as well. An example of this could be treating a Cambodian refugee, who lived under the Khmer Rouge, for posttraumatic stress disorder (PTSD). Devon Hinton and his colleagues have done extensive work adapting CBT for this population and other South East Asian refugees (e.g., Hinton et al., 2004, 2005; Otto et al., 2003). Cambodian survivors of the Khmer Rouge often display culture-specific panic attacks that are neck focused and orthostatically triggered. These somatic symptoms are tied to cultural beliefs about the catastrophic meaning of dizziness and increased heart rate. They are also related to memories of the physical onset of these symptoms during forced labor, carrying heavy loads on their heads, and starvation under Khmer Rouge rule. Both types of attacks produce high arousal levels and distress and are closely associated with psychopathology.

Flashbacks, a common symptom of PTSD, also carry specific cultural meaning in the Cambodian culture. Specifically, flashbacks indicate mental weakness and are a precursor to insanity and death. They can also indicate that the soul has left its body and returned to the scene of the trauma (Hinton et al, 2005). The culturally ascribed meaning of this PTSD symptom keeps it relevant and prevents extinction over time. As a result, flashbacks continue to occur in this population more than 30 years after the original trauma occurred (Otto et al., 2003). Although the PTSD symptoms of an Iraq veteran and a South East Asian refugee may appear similar on the surface (e.g., panic attacks, flashbacks), the history and sociopolitical context behind their symptoms are quite different. Failure to tailor treatment to a client's past experience may result in a poor fit between problem and treatment.

Conclusions

Optimal treatments for people of color involve much more than simply disseminating unadapted CBT. Considering goodness of fit with cultural and sociocultural environments may provide guidance on the relative merits of culturally adapted versus unadapted CBT for people of color. Culturally adapted CBT has benefits beyond unadapted CBT for people who are identified with traditional cultures. Cultural and sociocultural issues are typically not considered in CBT, but they merit consideration with people of color.

Optimal psychological functioning for many clients of color involves competence in both mainstream and traditional cultures. To provide culturally competent treatment, a clinician must possess self-knowledge of his or her cultural strengths and limitations, as well as knowledge of the cultural and historical contexts in which clients live. This is a more comprehensive approach than the largely individual focus of CBT. A careful assessment of how well a client fits within the mainstream and traditional cultural environments may elucidate salient clinical issues and relevant interventions. Attention to a client's ethnic identity may strengthen it and provide a buffer against psychopathology. However, a sole focus on the individual overlooks systemic protective factors, such as family influences, and systemic risk factors, such as discrimination. Culturally competent treatment may assist a client in mobilizing systemic protective factors and challenging systemic risk factors.

The issues raised in this chapter may help reduce mental health disparities between people of color and other groups, and provide optimal mental health services for people of color. However, these issues are moot unless they become a priority for researchers, practitioners, and funding agencies (Hall, 2006; Hall & Yee, 2011). Nevertheless, cultural and sociocultural factors influence a rapidly growing segment of the US population, and the longer these factors are minimized or ignored by CBT and by psychology more broadly, the less relevant CBT and psychology become in addressing the mental health needs of society.

Author's Note

Work on this chapter was supported by the Asian American Center on Disparities Research (National Institute of Mental Health grant: 1P50MH073511-01A2). We thank Gayle Iwamasa and Janie Hong for their feedback on a previous version of this chapter.

References

American Psychological Association (2003). Guidelines on multicultural education, training, research, practice, and organizational change for Psychologists. *American Psychologist*, 58, 377–402. doi: http://dx.doi.org/10.1037/0003-066X.58.5.377

Ayón, C., Marsiglia, F. F., & Bermudez-Parsai, M. (2010). Latino family mental health: Exploring the role of discrimination and familismo. *Journal of Community Psychology*, 38, 742–756. doi: 10.1002/jcop.20392

Beck, J. S. (1995). *Cognitive therapy: Basics and beyond.* New York: Guilford Press.

Benish, S. G., Quintana, S., & Wampold, B. E. (2011). Culturally adapted psychotherapy and the legitimacy of myth: A direct-comparison meta-analysis. *Journal of Counseling Psychology*, 58, 279–289. doi: 10.1037/a0023626

Bernal, G., Bonilla, J., & Bellido, C. (1995). Ecological validity and cultural sensitivity for outcome research: Issues for the cultural adaptation and development of psychosocial treatments with Hispanics. *Journal of Abnormal Child Psychology*, 23, 67–82. doi: 10.1007/BF01447045

Brown, C. S., & Bigler, R. S. (2005). Children's perceptions of discrimination: A developmental model. *Child Development*, *76*, 533–553. doi: 10.1111/j.1467-8624.2005.00862.x

Bynum, M. S., Burton, E. T., & Best, C. (2007). Racism experiences and psychological functioning in African American college freshmen: Is racial socialization a buffer? *Cultural Diversity and Ethnic Minority Psychology*, *13*, 64–71. doi: 10.1037/1099-9809.13.1.64

Chowdhary, N., Jotheeswaran, A T., Nadkarni, A, Hollon, S. D., King, M., Jordans, M. J. D.,... Patel, V. (2014). The methods and outcomes of cultural adaptations of psychological treatments for depressive disorders: A systematic review. *Psychological Medicine*, *44*, 1131–1146. doi: 10.1017/S0033291713001785

Cook, B., Alegría, M., Lin, J. Y., & Guo, J. (2009). Pathways and correlates connecting Latinos' mental health with exposure to the United States. *American Journal of Public Health*, *99*, 2247–2254. doi: 10.2105/AJPH.2008.137091

Crosby, F. (1984). The denial of personal discrimination. *American Behavioral Scientist*, *27*, 371–386. doi: 10.1177/000276484027003008

Dawis, R. V., & Lofquist, L. H. (1984). *A psychological theory of work adjustment: An individual differences model and its applications*. Minneapolis: University of Minnesota Press.

Dobson, K. (2001). *Handbook of cognitive-behavioral therapies*. New York: Guilford Press.

Ford-Paz, R., & Iwamasa, G. Y. (2012). Culturally diverse children and adolescents. In E. Szigethy, J. R. Weisz, & R. I. Findling (Eds.), *Cognitive-behavioral therapy for children and adolescents* (pp. 75–115). Arlington, VA: American Psychiatric Publishing.

Fredrickson, B. L., Cohn, M. A., Coffey, K. A., Pek, J., & Finkel, S. M. (2008). Open hearts build lives: Positive emotions, induced through loving-kindness meditation, build consequential personal resources. *Journal of Personality and Social Psychology*, *95*, 1045–1062. doi: 10.1037/a0013262

Gee, G. C., Spencer, M. S., Chen, J., & Takeuchi, D. (2007). A nationwide study of discrimination and chronic health conditions among Asian Americans. *American Journal of Public Health*, *97*, 1275–1282. doi: 10.2105/AJPH.2006.091827

Griner, D., & Smith, T. B. (2006). Culturally adapted mental health interventions: A meta analytic review. *Psychotherapy: Theory, Research, Practice, Training*, *43*, 531–548. doi: 10.1037/0033-3204.43.4.531

Hall, G. C. N. (2001). Psychotherapy research with ethnic minorities: Empirical, ethical, and conceptual issues. *Journal of Consulting and Clinical Psychology*, *69*, 502–510. doi: 10.1037//0022-006X.69.3.502

Hall, G. C. N. (2006). Diversity in clinical psychology. *Clinical Psychology: Science and Practice*, *13*, 258–262. doi: 10.1111/j.1468-2850.2006.00034.x

Hall, G. C. N. (2010). *Multicultural psychology* (2nd ed.). Upper Saddle River, NJ: Prentice-Hall.

Hall, G. C. N., & Barongan, C. (2002). *Multicultural psychology*. Upper Saddle River, NJ: Prentice-Hall.

Hall, G. C. N., & Eap, S. (2007). Empirically-supported therapies for Asian Americans. In F. T. L. Leong, A. Inman, A. Ebreo, L. Yang, L. Kinoshita, & M. Fu (Eds.), *Handbook of Asian American psychology* (2nd ed., pp. 449–467). Thousand Oaks, CA: Sage.

Hall, G. C. N., Hong, J. J., Zane, N. W., & Meyer, O. L. (2011). Culturally-competent treatments for Asian Americans: The relevance of mindfulness and acceptance-based therapies. *Clinical Psychology: Science and Practice*, *18*, 215–231. 10.1111/j.1468-2850.2011.01253.x

Hall, G. C. N. & Malony, H. N. (1983). Cultural control in psychotherapy with minority clients. *Psychotherapy: Theory, Research and Practice*, *20*, 131–142. doi: 10.1037/h0088484

Hall, G. C. N., & Yee, A. (2011, April). *Trickle-down mental health policy: Addressing the neglect of Asian Americans*. Invited paper presented at AAPI State of the Science: Mental Health and Treatment Issues for Asian Americans and Pacific Islanders Conference, Los Angeles.

Hall, G. C. N., & Yee, A. (2014). Evidence-based practice. In F. T. L. Leong, L. Comas-Diaz, G. C. N. Hall, V. McLoyd, & J. Trimble (Eds.), *Handbook of multicultural psychology. Vol. 2: Applications and training* (pp. 59–79). Washington, DC: American Psychological Association.

Hays, P. A. (2006). Cognitive-behavioral therapy with Alaska Native people. Cognitive-behavioral therapy with Asian Americans. In P. A. Hays & G. Y. Iwamasa (Eds.), *Culturally responsive cognitive-behavioral therapy: Assessment, practice, and supervision* (pp. 47–71). Washington, DC: American Psychological Association. doi: 10.1037/11433-002

Hays, P. A. (2009). Integrating evidence-based practice, cognitive–behavior therapy, and multicultural therapy: Ten steps for culturally competent practice. *Professional Psychology: Research and Practice*, *40*, 354–360. doi: 10.1037/a0016250

Hays, P. A., & Iwamasa, G. Y. (2006). *Culturally responsive cognitive-behavioral therapy: Assessment, practice, and supervision*. Washington, DC: American Psychological Association. doi: 10.1037/11433-000

Helms, J. E. (1994). The conceptualization of racial identity and other "racial" constructs. In E. J. Trickett, R. J. Watts, & D. Birman (Eds.), *Human diversity: Perspectives on people in context* (pp. 285–311). San Francisco: Jossey-Bass.

Hinton, D. E., Chhean, D., Pich, V., Safren, S. A., Hofmann, S. G., & Pollack, M. H. (2005). A randomized control trial of cognitive-behavior therapy for Cambodian refugees with treatment-resistant PTSD and panic attacks: a cross-over design. *Journal of Traumatic Stress*, *18*(6), 617–629. doi: 10.1002/jts.20070

Hinton, D. E., Pham, T., Tran, M., Safren, S. A., Otto, M. W., & Pollack, M. H. (2004). CBT for Vietnamese with treatment-resistant PTSD and panic attacks. *Journal of Traumatic Stress*, *17*, 429–433. doi: 10.1023/B:JOTS.0000048956.03529.fa

Holland, J. L. (1985). *Making vocational choices*. Englewood, NJ: Prentice-Hall.

Horrell, S. C. V. (2008). Effectiveness of cognitive-behavioral therapy with adult ethnic minority clients: A review. *Professional Psychology: Research and Practice*, *39*, 160–168. doi: 10.1037/0735-7028.39.2.160

Huey, S. J., & Polo, A. J. (2008). Evidence-based psychosocial treatments for ethnic minority youth. *Journal of Clinical Child and Adolescent Psychology*, *37*, 262–301. doi: 10.1080/15374410701820174

Hughes, D., Rodriguez, J., Smith, E. P., Johnson, D. J., Stevenson, H. C., & Spicer, P. (2006). Parents' ethnic-racial socialization practices: A review of research and directions for future study. *Developmental Psychology*, *42*, 747–770. doi: 10.1037/0012-1649.42.5.747

Hwang, W., & Ting, J. Y. (2008). Disaggregating the effects of acculturation and acculturative stress on the mental health of Asian Americans. *Cultural Diversity and Ethnic Minority Psychology, 14,* 147–154. doi: 10.1037/1099-9809.14.2.147

Iwamasa, G. Y. (1997). Behavior therapy and a culturally diverse society: Forging an alliance. *Behavior Therapy, 28,* 347–358. doi: 10.1016/S0005-7894(97)80080-9

Iwamasa, G. Y., Hsia, C., & Hinton, D. (2006). Cognitive-behavioral therapy with Asian Americans. In P. A. Hays & G. Y. Iwamasa (Eds.), *Culturally responsive cognitive-behavioral therapy: Assessment, practice, and supervision* (pp. 117–140). Washington, DC: American Psychological Association.

Joiner, T. E., & Katz, J. (1999). Contagion of depressive symptoms and mood: Meta-analytic review and explanations from cognitive, behavioral, and interpersonal viewpoints. *Clinical Psychology: Science and Practice, 6,* 149–164. doi: 10.1093/clipsy/6.2.149

Kellogg, S. H., & Young, J. E. (2008). Cognitive therapy. In J. L. Lebow (Ed.), *Twenty-first century psychotherapies: Contemporary approaches to theory and practice* (pp. 43–79). Hoboken, NJ: Wiley.

Kelly, S. (2006). Cognitive-behavioral therapy with African Americans. In P. A. Hays & G. Y. Iwamasa (Eds.), *Culturally responsive cognitive-behavioral therapy: Assessment, practice, and supervision* (pp. 97–116). Washington, DC: American Psychological Association.

Kumar, S. M. (2002). An introduction to Buddhism for the cognitive-behavioral therapist. *Cognitive and Behavioral Practice, 9,* 40–43. doi: 10.1016/S1077-7229(02)80038-4

LaFromboise, T. D., Coleman, H. L. K., & Gerton, J. (1993). Psychological impact of biculturalism: Evidence and theory. *Psychological Bulletin, 114,* 395–412. doi: 10.1037/0033-2909.114.3.395

Lau, A. S. (2006). Making the case for selective and directed cultural adaptations of evidence-based treatments: examples from parent training. *Clinical Psychology: Science and Practice, 13,* 295–310. doi: 10.1111/j.1468-2850.2006.00042.x

Lau, A. S., Chang, D. F., & Okazaki, S. (2010). Methodological challenges in treatment outcome research with ethnic minorities. *Cultural Diversity and Ethnic Minority Psychology, 16,* 573–580. doi: 10.1037/a0021371

Major, B., Gramzow, R. H., McCoy, S. K., Levin, S., Schmader, T., & Sidanius, J. (2002). Perceiving personal discrimination: The role of group status and legitimizing ideology. *Journal of Personality and Social Psychology, 82,* 269–282. doi: 10.1037/0022-3514.82.3.269

Mak, W. W. S., Law, R. W., Teng, Y. (2011). Cultural model of vulnerability to distress: The role of self-construal and sociotropy on anxiety and depression among Asian Americans and European Americans. *Journal of Cross-Cultural Psychology, 42,* 75–88. doi: 10.1177/0022022110361713

Malcarne, V. L., Chavira, D. A., Fernandez, S., & Liu, P. (2006). The scale of ethnic experience: Development and psychometric properties. *Journal of Personality Assessment, 86,* 150–161. doi: 10.1207/s15327752jpa8602_04

Maramba, G. G., & Hall, G. C. N. (2002). Meta-analysis of ethnic match as a predictor of drop-out, utilization, and outcome. *Cultural Diversity and Ethnic Minority Psychology, 8,* 290–297. doi: 10.1037/1099-9809.8.3.290

McDonald, J. D., & Gonzalez, J. (2006). Cognitive-behavioral therapy with American Indians. In P. A. Hays & G. Y. Iwamasa (Eds.), *Culturally responsive cognitive-behavioral therapy: Assessment, practice, and supervision* (pp. 23–45). Washington, DC: American Psychological Association.

Miranda, J., Bernal, G., Lau, A., Kohn, L., Hwang, W., & LaFromboise, T. (2005). State of the science on psychosocial interventions for ethnic minorities. *Annual Review of Clinical Psychology, 1,* 113–142. doi: 10.1146/annurev.clinpsy.1.102803.143822

Neblett, E. W., White, R. L., Ford, K. R., Philip, C. L., Nguyên, H. X., & Sellers, R. M. (2008). Patterns of racial socialization and psychological adjustment: Can parental communications about race reduce the impact of racial discrimination? *Journal of Research on Adolescence, 18,* 477–515. doi: 10.1111/j.1532-7795.2008.00568.x

Okazaki, S., & Tanaka-Matsumi, J. (2006). Cultural considerations in cognitive-behavioral assessment. In P. A. Hays & G. Y. Iwamasa (Eds.), *Culturally responsive cognitive-behavioral therapy: Assessment, practice, and supervision* (pp. 247–266). Washington, DC: American Psychological Association.

Organista, K. C. (2006). Cognitive-behavioral therapy with Latinos and Latinas. In P. A. Hays & G. Y. Iwamasa (Eds.), *Culturally responsive cognitive-behavioral therapy: Assessment, practice, and supervision* (pp. 73–96). Washington, DC: American Psychological Association.

Otto, M. W., Hinton, D. E., Korbly, N. B., Chea, A., Ba, P., Gershuny, B. S., & Pollack, M. H. (2003). Treatment of pharmacotherapy-refractory posttraumatic stress disorder among Cambodian refugees: A pilot study of combination treatment with cognitive-behavior therapy vs. sertraline alone. *Behaviour Research and Therapy, 41,* 1271–1276. doi: 10.1016/S0005-7967(03)00032-9

Paukert, A. L., Pettit, J. W., & Amacker, A. (2008). The role of interdependence and perceived similarity in depressed affect contagion. *Behavior Therapy, 39,* 277–285. doi: 10.1016/j.beth.2007.08.001

Pérez, D. J., Fortuna, L., & Alegría, M. (2008). Prevalence and correlates of everyday discrimination among U.S. Latinos. *Journal of Community Psychology, 36,* 421–433. doi: 10.1002/jcop.20221

Phinney, J. S., Dennis, J., & Osorio, S. (2006). Reasons to attend college among ethnically diverse college students. *Cultural Diversity and Ethnic Minority Psychology, 12,* 347–366. doi: 10.1037/1099-9809.12.2.347

Romero, A. J., Carvajal, S. C., Volle, F., & Orduña, M. (2007). Adolescent bicultural stress and its impact on mental well-being among Latinos, Asian Americans, and European Americans. *Journal of Community Psychology, 35,* 519–534. doi: 10.1002/jcop.20162

Rosselló, J., & Bernal, G. (1999). The efficacy of cognitive-behavioral and interpersonal treatments for depression in Puerto Rican adolescents. *Journal of Consulting and Clinical Psychology, 67,* 734–745. doi: 10.1037/0022-006X.67.5.734

Rosselló, J., Bernal, G., & Rivera-Medina, C. (2008). Individual and group CBT and IPT for Puerto Rican adolescents with depressive symptoms. *Cultural Diversity and Ethnic Minority Psychology, 14,* 234–245. doi: 10.1037/1099-9809.14.3.234

Sellers, R. M., & Shelton, J. N. (2003). The role of racial identity in perceived racial discrimination. *Journal of Personality and Social Psychology, 84,* 1079–1092. doi: 10.1037/0022-3514.84.5.1079

Sue, D. W., Bernier, J. B., Duran, M., Feinberg, L., Pedersen, P., Smith, E., & Vasquez-Nuttall, E. (1982). Position paper: Cross-cultural counseling competencies. *Counseling Psychologist, 10,* 45–52. doi: 10.1177/0011000082102008

Sue, D. W., Capodilupo, C. M., Torino, G. C., Bucceri, J. M., Holder, A. M. B., Nadal, K. L., & Esquilin, M. (2007). Racial microaggressions in everyday life: Implications for clinical practice. *American Psychologist, 62*, 271–286. doi: 10.1037/0003-066X.62.4.271

Sue, D. W., & Sue, D. (2008). *Counseling the culturally diverse: Theory and practice* (5th ed.). Hoboken, NJ: Wiley.

Sue, S. (1991). Ethnicity and culture in psychological research and practice. In J. D. Goodchilds (Ed.), *Psychological perspectives on human diversity in America* (pp. 51–85). Washington, DC: American Psychological Association.

Sue, S., Fujino, D. C., Hu, L., Takeuchi, D., & Zane, N. W. S. (1991). Community mental health services for ethnic minority groups: A test of the cultural responsiveness hypothesis. *Journal of Consulting and Clinical Psychology, 59*, 533–540. doi: 10.1037/0022-006X.59.4.533

Sue, S., Zane, N., Hall, G. C. N., & Berger, L. K. (2009). The case for cultural competency in psychotherapeutic interventions. *Annual Review of Psychology, 60*, 525–548. doi: http://dx.doi.org/10.1146/annurev.psych.60.110707.163651

Triandis, H. C. (1995). *Individualism and collectivism.* Boulder, CO: Westview.

Wei, M., Alvarez, A. N., Ku, T., Russell, D. W., & Bonett, D. G. (2010). Development and validation of a Coping with Discrimination Scale: Factor structure, reliability, and validity. *Journal of Counseling Psychology, 57*, 328–344. doi: 10.1037/a0019969

Weisz, J. R., Rothbaum, F. M., & Blackburn, T. C. (1984). Standing out and standing in: The psychology of control in America and Japan. *American Psychologist, 39*, 955–969. doi: 10.1037/0003-066X.39.9.955

Williams, D. R., Neighbors, H. W., & Jackson, J. S. (2008). Racial/ethnic discrimination and health: Findings from community studies. *American Journal of Public Health, 98*, S29–S37.

Zane, N., Sue, S., Chang, J., Huang, L., Huang, J., Lowe, S., . . . Lee, E. (2005). Beyond ethnic match: Effects of client-therapist cognitive match in problem perception, coping orientation, and therapy goals on treatment outcomes. *Journal of Community Psychology, 33*, 569–585. doi: 10.1002/jcop.20067

Combination Treatment for Anxiety and Mood Disorders: Benefits and Issues for the Combination of Cognitive-Behavioral Therapy and Pharmacotherapy

Michael W. Otto *and* Bridget A. Hearon

Abstract

This chapter examines the issues, advantages, and liabilities associated with the combination of pharmacotherapy and cognitive-behavioral therapy (CBT) for the treatment of anxiety and mood disorders. It begins with a brief review of the relative efficacy of CBT and pharmacotherapy in the treatment of depression and anxiety disorders before turning to a discussion of issues that arise from combination treatment for anxiety disorders as well as bipolar disorder, schizophrenia, and adult attention-deficit/hyperactivity disorder. The chapter then considers preference and tolerability with respect to combined treatment modality, along with the availability of each treatment modality. It also asks whether CBT should be added to pharmacotherapy, and vice versa, for mood or anxiety disorders and concludes by outlining new research directions for such combination strategies.

Key Words: combination treatment, cognitive-behavioral therapy, pharmacotherapy, anxiety, depression, affective disorders, relapse, maintenance

Given the strong support for both cognitive-behavioral therapy (CBT) and various forms of pharmacotherapy for the majority of psychiatric disorders, researchers and clinicians alike have hoped that combining these treatment modalities would lead to a particularly powerful intervention. Unfortunately, for many disorders, the expected additive effects for combination treatments have tended to be modest and, in many cases, transient. This chapter provides a review of the issues, advantages, and liabilities of combination treatments for affective disorders. In the current chapter, CBT is defined broadly to encompass any intervention incorporating traditional cognitive techniques such as cognitive restructuring, behavioral techniques such as behavioral scheduling and activation, and other cognitive-behavioral interventions such as exposure and problem solving. Specific treatment elements vary across the studies cited; however, generally speaking, CBT for mood disorders most commonly focuses on cognitive restructuring and behavioral activation components, while treatment for anxiety disorders often relies on exposure and cognitive restructuring techniques.

The greatest attention in this review is placed on anxiety and mood disorders—disorders that have received the most research attention for combination treatments. Nonetheless, later in the chapter, perspectives are given on combination treatments in disorders where pharmacotherapy has been the primary treatment, and hence CBT is delivered typically only in that context. To aid in the evaluation of combination treatment strategies, we will start this chapter with a brief review of the relative efficacy of CBT and pharmacotherapy for anxiety and depressive disorders.

Monotherapy with CBT or Pharmacotherapy

Research in adults has shown strong support for both pharmacological and cognitive-behavioral interventions. For CBT, an abundance of randomized controlled trials and meta-analytic reviews show clear efficacy for the treatment of depression (Cuijpers, Andersson, Donker, & van Straten, 2011; DeRubeis et al., 1999; Jones, 2004) and anxiety disorders (Deacon & Abramowitz, 2004; Hofmann & Smits, 2008). With regard to pharmacotherapy, several classes of pharmacological agent have been shown to reliably decrease mood and anxiety disorder symptom severity, including monoamine oxidase inhibitors (MAO-Is), tricyclic antidepressants, selective-serotonin reuptake inhibitors (SSRIs), and benzodiazepines (Abramowitz, 1997; Gould Buckminster, Pollack, Otto, & Yap, 1997; Hidalgo et al., 2001; Pollack, 2005; Rocha, Fuzikawa, Riera, & Hara, 2012; Vocks et al., 2010).

In a recent meta-analysis, Roshanaei-Moghaddam and colleagues (2011) compared the relative effects of CBT and pharmacotherapy in the treatment of depression and anxiety disorders. Twenty-one studies directly comparing the effects of CBT and pharmacotherapy were examined in each diagnostic category. Results for the anxiety disorders revealed differential effects for each treatment modality depending on the particular disorder examined. A significant advantage, reflecting a medium effect size, was found for CBT over pharmacotherapy for panic disorder, with obsessive-compulsive disorder (OCD) demonstrating a similar effect size that did not reach significance given the reduced number of comparisons. In contrast, there was a nonsignificant trend ($d = .22$) favoring pharmacotherapy over CBT for the treatment of social anxiety disorder. With regard to depression, no advantage was found for either treatment when comparing CBT and pharmacotherapies. These results, based on trials examining both CBT and pharmacotherapy in the same trial, are consistent with the general conclusion of meta-analyses that have compared the controlled effect sizes when CBT and pharmacotherapy are studied independently (Furukawa, Watanabe, & Churchill, 2006; Gould et al., 1997; Otto, Smits, & Reese, 2005).

These data, investigating acute outcomes, have been complemented by trials examining the efficacy of each treatment over the long term. In general, one substantial advantage of CBT is its ability to provide ongoing benefit in the absence of ongoing treatment, whereas relapse is common upon discontinuation of pharmacologic treatment (Keller et al., 2007; Reynolds et al., 2006; Stein, Versiani, Hair, & Kumar, 2002; Walker et al., 2000). Indeed, for the pharmacologic treatment of recurrent major depressive disorder, long-term maintenance therapy using antidepressant medication is recommended to prevent relapse (Anderson, Nutt, & Deakin, 2000), with a trial conducted by Keller and colleagues (2007) indicating continued medication may be required for 2 years or more to adequately prevent relapse. There is evidence that patients who are able to achieve remission from their disorder rather than just symptom reduction may be more successful in avoiding relapse after discontinuing pharmacotherapy (Mavissakalian & Perel, 1999). However, those who achieve remission during the acute phase of treatment represent a minority of individuals who initiate pharmacotherapy, and the remaining majority of patients likely need to continue pharmacotherapy in the long term to maintain treatment gains.

In contrast, short-term CBT interventions have demonstrated much stronger maintenance of treatment gains for both anxiety (Deacon & Abramowitz, 2004; Gould et al., 1997; Otto et al., 2005) and depression (Dobson et al., 2008; Evans et al., 1992; Hollon et al., 2005). Indeed, a recent meta-analytic review of nine studies indicates that patients who receive CBT are significantly less likely to relapse than patients who discontinue their pharmacotherapy on the order of an odds ratio of 2.61. Interestingly, this advantage continued at a trend level (OR = 1.62) even when brief CBT was compared to continued pharmacotherapy.

Also, it is important to note that, due to the need for ongoing pharmacotherapy, the two treatment modalities have different cost efficacy estimates. Studies of anxiety disorders (Heuzenroeder et al., 2004; McHugh et al., 2007; Otto, Pollack, & Maki, 2000) and depression (Haby et al., 2004) indicate that CBT offers a significantly better cost-benefit ratio than pharmacotherapy.

Efficacy of Combination Treatment for Depression

In terms of the effectiveness of combination strategies for depression and anxiety disorders, benefits are again somewhat dependent on the disorder in question. Meta-analysis indicates that the added efficacy of using combination strategies in the treatment of depression offers significant albeit limited ($d = .31$) added effects (Cuijpers et al., 2009). Although the detection of benefits for combination treatments appears to be easier as more treatment-refractory populations are selected (see Lynch et al., 2011; Otto et al., 2005; Spijker et al., 2013), there is recent evidence that combination treatment with CBT does not differentiate itself from alternative augmentation strategies. This evidence comes from the Sequenced Treatment Alternatives to Relieve Depression (STAR*D) trial, the largest trial conducted to date examining the effectiveness of using combination strategies in a medication-nonresponsive population. Treatment of more than 2,800 patients with unipolar depression was examined. Patients who failed to achieve remission through use of clomipramine alone were randomized to one of several augmentation strategies: continued clomipramine, the addition of another pharmacological agent, the addition of CBT, or switching from one treatment modality to another. Results of this trial indicated that no particular augmentation strategy emerged as superior in achieving remission rates for patients who had failed to respond to initial pharmacotherapy (Thase et al., 2007; see also Sinyor, Schaffer, & Levitt, 2010).

Although the addition of CBT is just one of several options for medication-nonresponsive patients with depression, there is clearer evidence for significant benefits for adding CBT for the purpose of maintenance of treatment gains. Specifically, in a meta-analytic review of eight studies (442 patients), Guidi, Fava, Fava, and Papakostas (2011) examined the benefit of adding CBT as well as other psychotherapies to patients who had responded to antidepressant treatment. They found significant reductions in relapse and recurrence of the disorder as well as successful discontinuation of antidepressants. Hence, combination treatment appears to have a modest role as a standard strategy, a useful but not unique role in sequential treatment for patients failing to respond to initial pharmacotherapy, and a useful role in helping patients responding to pharmacotherapy maintain their gains and discontinue their pharmacotherapy.

Efficacy and Issues in Combination Treatment for Anxiety Disorders

For anxiety disorders, several reviews have indicated that combined treatment effects are weaker than initially anticipated (Foa, Franklin, & Moser, 2002; Otto et al., 2005). In the case of OCD, several studies have failed to demonstrate an advantage for combination treatment over CBT alone (Franklin, Abramowitz, Bux, Zoellner, & Feeny, 2002; Hohagen et al., 1998), with a large

multicenter trial conducted by Foa and colleagues (2005) demonstrating no significant differences between CBT-based exposure and response prevention (ERP) used in isolation or in combination with clomipramine. Interestingly, both the combination and CBT treatment alone demonstrated significantly greater effectiveness than clomipramine alone. This result was supported and clarified by another trial finding that the specific components of ERP provided successful augmentation of pharmacotherapy while CBT-based stress management training did not (Simpson et al., 2008). Such findings indicated the importance of disorder-specific treatment tools for influencing outcome. In a meta-analysis examining panic, generalized anxiety, and social anxiety disorders, a significant advantage for combination treatment was only seen reliably for panic disorder and GAD, with each individual therapy showing relatively equal efficacy for each disorder when used in isolation (Bandelow, Seidler-Brandler, Becker, Wedekind, & Ruther, 2007; Hofmann et al., 2009). However, findings examining combination strategies in panic disorder are complex and should be interpreted with caution. Although several studies have demonstrated increased efficacy for combination strategies during the acute and maintenance phases of treatment, discontinuation of medication has led to symptom relapse (Barlow et al., 2000; Marks et al., 1993). This effect has been reflected in meta-analyses of the treatment of panic disorder. Concerning antidepressant treatments, a review of 21 randomized trials indicated that combined therapy outperformed both antidepressant pharmacotherapy and psychotherapy (largely CBT) after the acute phase of treatment (Furukawa, Watanabe, & Churchill, 2007). Yet a different picture on the relative efficacy of combined treatment emerged during follow-up periods following medication discontinuation: combined therapy remained more efficacious than pharmacotherapy but was not more efficacious than psychotherapy alone. Based on a less robust number of studies, meta-analysis has led to similar conclusions for the combination of CBT with benzodiazepine medications for panic disorder (Watanabe, Churchill & Furukawa, 2007), with indications that loss of the advantage of combination treatment over CBT alone over follow-up periods extends to other anxiety disorders as well (Hofmann, Sawyer, Korte, & Smits, 2009).

Also, some of the value of combination treatment appears to be due to expectation (placebo effects) alone. Specifically, a review of three randomized controlled trials indicated that patients receiving CBT plus placebo responded better to treatment than those receiving CBT alone at the end of acute treatment (Furukawa, Watanabe, Omori, & Churchill, 2007). Expectations about pill efficacy and attributions about gains in combination treatment may also detract from CBT efficacy over time. For example, Basoglu and colleagues (1994) reported that attributions of improvement to a study pill significantly predicted relapse in panic disorder patients treated with exposure in combination with medication. Likewise, Biondi and Picardi (2003) reported that making external/medication attributions about the source of treatment efficacy for panic disorder was associated with a 60% relapse rate, whereas making internal attributions was associated with a 0% relapse rate. Finally, in an experimental paradigm with claustrophobic individuals that manipulated expectancy about the effects of placebo, Powers and colleagues (2008) found a relapse rate of 39% among participants who were led to believe that the study pill had a sedating effect, whereas a relapse rate of 0% was observed among participants who were led to believe the pill had a stimulating or no effect. Reduced self-efficacy accounted for the elevated relapse rates associated with the sedating instructional set. Hence, pill taking may account for some of the benefits of combined treatment, but attributions of gains to the pill rather than to learned safety from CBT may leave patients at greater risk of relapse following the cessation of pill use.

Combination Treatment with CBT for Other Disorders

There are also a number of disorders for which combination treatment represents the standard application for CBT. That is, a number of psychiatric disorders have long considered pharmacotherapy to be the core, or only effective, treatment modality. In recent years, studies have shown that CBT can add significantly to the outcomes provided by medication. Reviewed next are treatments for three such disorders: bipolar disorder, schizophrenia, and adult attention-deficit/hyperactivity disorder (ADHD).

Much of the efficacy of CBT for bipolar disorder has emerged over the last two decades, with initial studies of CBT targeting medication adherence (Cochran, 1984), but with later studies targeting relapse prevention more generally as well as treatment of bipolar depression. When applied as a relapse prevention strategy, CBT is introduced during a phase of relative euthymia, typically in patients taking at least a mood stabilizer, and in many cases in patients taking a mood stabilizer plus other antidepressant or anxiolytic agents. In studies of this kind, relatively brief CBT (often in the range of 12 to 18 sessions) has been found to reduce current symptoms as well as the relapse rate over time, particularly for depressive relapse (Lam et al., 2003, 2005; Perry, Tarrier, Morriss, McCarthy, & Limb, 1999; Scott, Garland, & Moorhead, 2001). Recent applications of CBT have included cost-effective group interventions and found significant benefits to bipolar depression and quality of life, as well as the frequency and duration of mood episodes (Costa et al., 2012). Also, CBT that is similar to that used for unipolar depression but includes strategies for relapse prevention as well as early detection and intervention for (hypo)mania have been shown to be efficacious (e.g., Miklowitz et al., 2007; Zaretsky et al., 2008). Indeed, recent findings have shown CBT to be effective in the same cohort of patients taking mood stabilizers for whom antidepressant medication offered no additional efficacy (cf. Miklowitz et al., 2007; Sachs et al., 2007). Also, mindfulness-based CBT has been applied recently to bipolar disorder, in part targeting the cognitive and role dysfunction that accompanies the disorder. Recent open trials have shown promising outcomes, including reductions in depression, increased well-being and psychosocial functioning, and significant improvements in executive functioning, memory, and the ability to initiate and complete tasks (Deckersbach et al., 2012; Stange et al., 2011).

Recent research has also documented an important role for CBT in the management of schizophrenia. Yet, as CBT approaches to schizophrenia have been expanded, there has been some evidence of decreasing effect sizes from the promising initial medium to large effects reported by Gould, Mueser, Bolton, Mays, and Goff (2001). Recent meta-analyses of 34 studies of CBT for the symptoms of schizophrenia indicate effects in the small to medium range for overall and positive symptoms, and in the very small range for negative symptoms (Jauhar et al., 2014). Somewhat larger effect sizes (in the medium range) have been reported when CBT strategies are applied specifically to medication-resistant cases (Burns, Erickson, & Brenner, 2014), perhaps providing a more exact measure of CBT benefit when variability in response to medication is minimized by choosing nonresponsive cases. Regardless of reason, it is promising that CBT can exert beneficial effects to those patients for whom medication offers few benefits.

ADHD is another disorder where medication treatment is the primary intervention. Nonetheless, two trials have shown that CBT interventions can add significant benefit. In an important initial trial, Safren and colleagues (2005) showed that adults with ADHD who were stabilized on medication achieved clinically significant gains, achieving lower severity of ADHD symptoms, as well as lower anxiety and depression. Utilizing a similar design, Emilsson and colleagues (2011) found advantages for CBT compared to usual medication treatment reflecting medium to large effect sizes, with evidence of continued treatment gains over follow-up. Use of a more stringent control group continued to support the efficacy of CBT (Safren et al., 2010). Also, there is tentative evidence that these specialized CBT programs for ADHD are effective for individuals off medication, but the trial was too small to delineate the additive effect of medication to CBT alone (Weiss et al., 2012).

Preference and Tolerability of Combined Treatment Modality

Meta-analytic review makes it clear that psychological treatment for anxiety and mood disorders is preferred to pharmacologic treatment, on the order of a three-fold preference for psychological therapy (McHugh, Whitton, Peckham, Weige, & Otto, 2013). Yet some assume that the time commitment and intensity of work required by CBT during the acute phase of treatment may be less tolerable to patients than simply taking a medication. Research in this area indicates that this is not the case. In a meta-analysis examining treatment discontinuation rates across anxiety disorders treated with CBT and pharmacotherapy either alone or in combination, results revealed that dropout rates in CBT are lower or equivalent to rates for pharmacotherapy alone (Otto et al., 2005). Additionally, this review found that with respect to panic disorder, combined CBT and SSRIs leads to dropout rates that were similar to pharmacotherapy alone, while rates of discontinuation in CBT alone were significantly less. Large-scale studies of OCD (Foa et al., 2005) and social anxiety disorder (Davidson et al., 2004) demonstrated trends toward higher dropout in combined treatment as compared to CBT alone as well. This trend, however, was not observed in a multicenter trial examining panic disorder (Barlow et al., 2000). Nonetheless, evaluation of cost-efficacy for combined treatment for panic disorder indicates that combined treatment has a poorer cost-efficacy profile than CBT alone (McHugh et al., 2007).

Also, in a meta-analysis comparing pharmacological and psychological interventions for depression, Cuijpers and colleagues (2008) found significantly lower dropout rates for psychological interventions as compared to medication. With regard to combination treatment, another review by Cuijpers and colleagues (2009) examining the addition of psychotherapy as an augmentation of pharmacotherapy for depression revealed a significantly lower dropout rate for combined treatment than pharmacotherapy alone, whereas another review examining the differential effects of psychotherapy and pharmacotherapy for depression found that combined treatment yielded similar compliance rates to psychotherapy alone (De Maat et al., 2007). However, there is some evidence that when patients initiate treatment with pharmacotherapy and are given a subsequent choice of additional pharmacotherapy or cognitive therapy, cognitive therapy may be selected by only a minority of patients (Wisniewski et al., 2007), in direct opposition to the near 3:1 preference seen for treatment-seeking samples (McHugh et al., 2013). Hence, initial selection and acculturation to treatment may affect the acceptability of a subsequent switch to an alternative treatment modality. In the STAR*D trial, it was those patients who were better educated and had a family history of a mood disorder who were more likely to accept cognitive therapy as a second-step treatment strategy (Wisniewski et al., 2007).

Taken together, studies indicate that for both anxiety and depression, treatment with psychotherapy is preferred at the outset of treatment and appears equally, if not more, tolerable than pharmacotherapy alone and combined strategies. Given such findings, it is possible to conclude that combination strategies offer no discernible advantage to CBT with regard to retention of patients.

Availability of Each Treatment Modality

Although CBT has proven to be a well-tolerated and efficacious intervention, availability of state-of-the art CBT differs greatly from pharmacotherapy, making the attainment of combination treatment out of reach for many individuals. Whereas both psychiatric specialists and primary care physicians are available to administer pharmacological interventions, the dissemination of CBT to community settings has proceeded slowly. Indeed, despite evidence that CBT can successfully be disseminated to community settings (Addis et al., 2004; Stuart, Treat, & Wade, 2000), studies of patients with anxiety disorders in primary care and specialty care settings indicate that only about one tenth to one third of these patients receive CBT (Goisman, Warshaw, & Keller, 1999; Stein et al., 2004). Despite more recent studies showing some promise for both the implementation and acceptability of computerized CBT (Kaltenthaler et al., 2008), limitations with this method exist and pharmacotherapy still remains the more easily obtained form of treatment.

Should CBT Be Added to Pharmacotherapy for Mood or Anxiety Disorders?

Given the somewhat limited availability of CBT, might it be helpful to add at least some elements of CBT to pharmacotherapy whenever possible? Research in the anxiety disorder literature suggests that using elements of CBT as add-ons to pharmacotherapy can sometimes increase effectiveness. For instance, simply providing instructions in stepwise exposure or short-term CBT protocols administered by non-CBT specialists has been shown to enhance outcomes in individuals already using pharmacotherapy to treat their disorder in both primary care and specialty settings (Craske et al., 2005; Roy-Byrne et al., 2010; Telch, Agras, Taylor, Roth, & Gallen, 1985).

Additionally, improved technology has now made it possible for individuals to access CBT-based treatment through the Internet and by phone, making the augmentation of pharmacotherapy with elements of CBT even more accessible. In a study of a computer-based CBT protocol provided to patients presenting to primary care clinics with anxiety and depression, results indicated that this method of dissemination showed enhanced benefits over treatment as usual for both those assigned to receive the CBT alone or in conjunction with pharmacotherapy (Proudfoot et al., 2003). Such findings have also been extended to CBT-based treatments delivered by phone. For example, in a trial that randomized depressed patients initiating antidepressant medication in the primary care setting to either treatment as usual (e.g., continued medication with the option to independently seek in-person psychotherapy) or the addition of weekly psychotherapy sessions by phone incorporating many elements of CBT, results showed enduring benefits lasting through the 18-month follow-up period for those randomized to the telephone treatment group. The authors also note that these benefits were comparable to the results expected when patients engage in in-person collaborative care models of treatment (Ludman, Simon, Tutty, & Von Korff, 2007). Indeed, several trials have now examined telephone-based CBT treatments as augmentation to pharmacotherapy for depression and found that they lead to higher participation rates and lower overall cost (Hunkeler et al., 2000; Oslin et al., 2003) while at the same time providing near equivalent results to in-person collaborative care models (Ludman et al., 2007; Simon et al., 2004).

Taken together, these results suggest that using elements of CBT as add-ons may enhance the benefits of pharmacotherapy in a cost-effective way when CBT specialists are not available to administer a full program of treatment. However, this is a tentative recommendation at best, as computerized CBT does not utilize the same comprehensive interventions that have demonstrated acceptability, tolerability, and cost-efficacy when used as monotherapies (Deacon & Abramowitz, 2005; Heuzenroeder et al., 2004; Otto, Pollack, & Maki, 2000).

Should Pharmacotherapy Be Added to CBT for Anxiety Disorders?

The decision of whether or not to add pharmacotherapy when full packages of CBT are available is somewhat complex and requires a more in-depth investigation of the proposed mechanisms behind each treatment. Presumably, CBT treats anxiety disorders by helping patients to relearn safety through techniques that alter thoughts, feelings, and behaviors. Foa and Kozak (1986) have hypothesized that higher levels of emotional arousal are important for this learning, positing that new information is added to cognitive fear networks only when these networks are sufficiently activated by exposure to the feared stimuli. Accordingly, they hypothesize that use of anxiolytic medication in the context of CBT interferes with activation of the fear network, making the incorporation of new information more difficult. Therefore, a consequence of the combination treatment strategy may be an initial relief of the anxiety inherent in exposure due to the use of medication but also a reduction in the full benefit of this learning process. Overall, use of medication in the context of exposure may make the task easier to carry out but will be unlikely to provide more than modest enhancement of outcome.

A specific mechanism for interfering effects of pharmacotherapy on safety learning was recently proposed by Otto, McHugh, and Kantar (2010). Rather than focusing on fear activation, they posited a role for glucocorticoid activity in enhancing safety learning, and reviewed evidence for the blockade of acute glucocorticoid activity by antidepressants and benzodiazepine medication. To briefly summarize their accounting: Despite initial evidence suggesting that cortisol inhibits cognition (Heffelfinger & Newcomer, 2001; Newcomer et al., 1999), several more recent studies suggest that this relationship is more complex than initially anticipated (Lupien, Maheu, Tu, Fiocco, & Schramek, 2007). Acute increases in glucocorticoids appear to enhance extinction learning and emotional consolidation. More specifically, research examining the role of cortisol in human populations suggests facilitation of fear extinction (Soravia et al., 2006) as well as enhanced consolidation of verbal and pictorial memory, particularly when emotional stimuli are presented (Abercrombie, Speck, & Monticelli, 2006; Buchanan & Lovallo, 2001; Putnam, Van Honk, Kessels, Mulder, & Koppeschaar, 2004). Indeed, in a recent clinical trial conducted by de Quervain and colleagues (2011), a specific facilitative effect of cortisol on extinction learning was observed. As mentioned earlier, although cortisol may have beneficial effects for CBT-based learning, disruption of this activity is evidenced with both antidepressant and benzodiazepine treatment, making cortisol suppression a possible explanation for the modest gains achieved when medications are added to CBT for anxiety disorders (Otto et al., 2010).

A second theory on interfering effects of pharmacotherapy on extinction learning is that chronic antidepressant treatment can impair amygdala-dependent learning (Burghardt, Sigurdsson, Gorman, McEwen, & LeDoux, 2013). For example, in an animal model, Burghardt and colleagues (2013) showed that 22 days of treatment with the SSRI citalopram reduced the efficacy of extinction. The source of this effect appeared to be downregulation of a subunit of the N-methyl-D-aspartate (NMDA) receptor in the lateral and basal nuclei of the amygdala. Downregulation of this receptor is concerning, given a wealth of evidence that stimulation of the NMDA receptor enhances extinction learning, both in animal models (Davis, 2011) and in clinical trials utilizing the NMDA receptor partial agonist, d-cycloserine (Norberg, Krystal, & Tolin, 2008; see also next section of this chapter). However, the relationship between antidepressant medication and extinction retention is complex, with differences emerging among antidepressants (Yang et al., 2012) and evidence of interactions with genetic factors (Hartley et al., 2012). Accordingly, even though there are a number of current biologic theories for how antidepressants may attenuate the

therapeutic learning from exposure-based (extinction) treatment for anxiety disorders, there is no certainty about these effects or the conditions under which they may be active.

In addition, the context in which therapeutic learning occurs has also been identified as an important factor for determining what is learned during an exposure. In this case, cues can be both internal, such as feeling states and their associated sensations, as well as external, such as time of day, physical environment, or the presence of important objects or people (Bouton, 2002). Animal research has shown that internal states are powerful enough contextual cues to ensure that extinction learning will be contingent upon that state (Bouton, Kenney, & Rosengard; 1990). More simply, patients who undergo CBT in the context of an anxiolytic medication may experience a re-emergence of symptoms when cues are faced following the discontinuation of that medication. Indeed, the effects of internal contextual changes have been directly demonstrated with regard to CBT for anxiety disorders. Mystkowski and colleagues (2003) randomly assigned participants to undergo a single exposure session for spider phobia after having ingested either caffeine or placebo. Although both the caffeine and placebo groups benefited from the exposure session, when participants were asked to confront the spider 1 week later, those who experienced a shift in internal context (i.e., treated on caffeine but assessed on placebo) had a significantly greater return of fear as compared to those who were treated and tested in congruent conditions. In terms of combination treatment of anxiety disorders, as noted earlier, loss of efficacy has been observed when individuals received CBT in the context of medication and then subsequently discontinued the medication (e.g., Barlow et al, 2000; Marks et al. 1993; for further discussion of this effect, see Otto et al., 2005). Engagement in CBT during and after the period of medication discontinuation helps prevent this relapse and can extend treatment gains (e.g., Otto et al., 2010).

With regard to the question of whether pharmacotherapy should automatically be added to CBT protocols, current research suggests that this approach should be used with caution. Combination treatment offers some hope of additional modest treatment benefits acutely, but it appears to offer little benefit over longer term evaluations and may hinder retention of CBT gains for anxiety disorders. As such, we recommend selection of combination treatment on an individualized basis rather than a standard strategy when full protocols of CBT are available.

Combination Strategies for Anxiety Disorders: New Directions

Because combination strategies including traditional pharmacotherapy agents and CBT have proven disappointing, a novel approach that promotes the use of pharmacotherapy to enhance learning during CBT has emerged. Over the past decade, research in this area has focused most closely on one agent in particular, d-cycloserine (DCS). DCS is an N-methyl-D-aspartate (NMDA) partial agonist that has been shown to reliably augment extinction learning in animals (Davis & Myers, 2002; Richardson, Ledgerwood, & Cranney, 2004) and now humans undergoing exposure-based CBT. More simply, the learning of extinction that occurs during exposure-based CBT appears to be better consolidated when patients are administered a single dose of DCS during the memory consolidation window (e.g., administered before or immediately after the therapy session). Indeed, in a recent meta-analysis conducted by Bontemps and colleagues (2012), nine separate trials that utilized DCS augmentation of CBT for the treatment of anxiety disorders found as a whole, those receiving DCS as opposed to placebo close to the time of exposure trials demonstrated significantly greater reductions in anxiety symptoms than those taking placebo. Because DCS is used only at the time of exposure sessions, patients still have the opportunity to practice exposure between sessions while not taking the medication, thereby limiting the concerns of contextual effects. Also, evidence suggests that DCS itself has no direct anxiolytic effects nor does it cause side effects that would change patients' internal context (D'Souza et al., 2000; Hofmann et al., 2006). Although research in this area is still relatively new and further work is needed to clarify the ideal timing and frequency of DCS dosing, in particular in relation to the success of each specific exposure session (Smits et al., 2013a, 2013b), evidence to date suggests that this may be an important new combination strategy for the treatment of anxiety disorders. Moreover, the success of DCS to date has also had a stimulating effect on the search for other novel combination treatment strategies that target the augmentation of CBT effects rather than direct anxiolysis (Hofmann et al., 2011; Nations et al., 2012; Powers et al., 2009); accordingly a number of promising new combination treatment approaches may emerge over the next decade.

Summary and Conclusions

As evidenced in this chapter, the desired additive benefit of traditional combination treatment strategies is observed only selectively across the research literature. For the treatment of anxiety, there is evidence that antidepressants and benzodiazepines offer only modest benefit to standard CBT protocols, perhaps due to the introduction of both hindering and beneficial effects to the therapeutic learning provided by CBT. For the treatment of major depression, adding pharmacotherapy to CBT is more likely to show benefit for more treatment-refractory samples of patients. Adding CBT to pharmacotherapy can help prevent relapse, and, for both anxiety and mood disorders, it can be a strategy for medication discontinuation. In all cases, patients failing to respond to monotherapy with one modality of treatment should be considered for the other modality. Also, when the availability of CBT therapists is limited, use of standard pharmacotherapy augmented by elements of CBT interventions such as telephone sessions or instruction in stepwise exposure may prove beneficial and cost-effective. Additionally, augmentation of CBT with agents that enhance learning, such as DCS, rather than providing direct mood or anxiety reductions appears to be a promising strategy for future use of combination pharmacologic and psychosocial treatment strategies.

References

Abercrombie, H. C., Speck, N. S., & Monticelli, R. M. (2006). Endogenous cortisol elevations are related to memory facilitation only in individuals who are emotionally aroused. *Psychoneuroendocrinology, 31,* 187–196.

Abramowitz, J. S. (1997). Effectiveness of psychological and pharmacological treatments for obsessive-compulsive disorder: A quantitative review. *Journal of Consulting and Clinical Psychology, 65,* 44–52.

Addis, M. E., Haggis, C., Krasnow, A. D., Jacob, K., Bourne, L., & Mansfield, A. (2004). Effectiveness of cognitive-behavioral treatment for panic disorder versus treatment as usual in a managed care setting. *Journal of Consulting and Clinical Psychology, 72,* 625–635.

Anderson, I. M., Nutt, D. J., & Deakin, J. F. (2000). Evidence-based guidelines for treating depressive disorders with antidepressants: A revision of the 1993 British Association for Psychopharmacology guidelines. British Association for Psychopharmacology. *Journal of Psychopharmacology, 12,* 3–20.

Bandelow, B., Seidler-Brandler, U., Becker, A., Wedekind, D., & Ruther, E. (2007). Meta-analysis of randomized controlled comparisons of pharmacological and psychological treatments for anxiety disorders. *World Journal of Biological Psychiatry, 8,* 175–187.

Barlow, D. H., Gorman, J. M., Shear, M. K., & Woods, S. W. (2000). Cognitive-behavioral therapy, imipramine, or their combination for panic disorder: A randomized controlled trial. *Journal of the American Medical Association, 283,* 2529–2536.

Basoglu, M., Marks, I. M., Kilic, C., Brewin C. R., & Swinson, R. P. (1994). Alprazolam and exposure for panic disorder with agoraphobia attribution of improvement to medication predicts subsequent relapse. *British Journal of Psychiatry, 164,* 652–659.

Biondi, M., & Picardi, A. (2003). Attribution of improvement to medication and increased risk of relapse of panic disorder with agoraphobia. *Psychotherapy and Psychosomatics, 72,* 110–111.

Bontempo, A., Panza, K. E., & Bloch, M. H. (2012). D-cycloserine augmentation of behavioral therapy for the treatment of anxiety disorders: A meta-analysis. *Journal of Clinical Psychiatry, 73,* 533–537.

Bouton, M. E. (2002). Context, ambiguity, and unlearning: Sources of relapse after behavioral extinction. *Biological Psychiatry, 52,* 976–986.

Bouton, M. E., Kenney, F. A., & Rosengard, C. (1990). State dependent fear extinction with two benzodiazepine tranquilizers. *Behavioral Neuroscience, 104,* 44–55.

Buchanan, T. W., & Lovallo, W. R. (2001). Enhanced memory for emotional material following stress-level cortisol treatment in humans. *Psychoneuroendocrinology, 26,* 307–317.

Burghardt, N. S., Sigurdsson, T., Gorman, J. M., McEwen, B. S., & LeDoux, J. E. (2013). Chronic antidepressant treatment impairs the acquisition of fear extinction. *Biological Psychiatry, 73*(11), 1078–1086.

Burns, A. M., Erickson, D. H., & Brenner, C. A. (2014). Cognitive-behavioral therapy for medication-resistant psychosis: A meta-analytic review. *Psychiatry Services 1.*

Cochran, S. D. (1984). Preventing medical noncompliance in the outpatient treatment of bipolar affective disorders. *Journal of Consulting and Clinical Psychology, 52,* 873–878.

Costa, R. T., Cheniaux, E., Rangé, B. P., Versiani, M., & Nardi, A. E. (2012). Group cognitive behavior therapy for bipolar disorder can improve the quality of life. *Brazilian Journal of Medical Biological Research, 45,* 862–868.

Craske, M. G., Golinelli, D., Stein, M. B., Roy-Byrne, P., Bystritsky, A., & Sherbourne, C. (2005). Does the addition of cognitive behavioral therapy improve panic disorder treatment outcome relative to medication alone in the primary-care setting? *Psychological Medicine, 35,* 1645–1654.

Cuijpers, P., Andersson, G., Donker, T., & van Straten, A. (2011). Psychological treatment of depression: Results of a series of meta-analyses. *Nordic Journal of Psychiatry, 65,* 354–364.

Cuijpers, P., Dekker, J., Hollon, S. D., & Andersson, G. (2009). Adding psychotherapy to pharmacotherapy in the treatment of depressive disorders in adults: A meta-analysis. *Journal of Clinical Psychiatry, 70,* 1219–1229.

Cuijpers, P., van Straten, A., Andersson, G., & van Oppen, P. (2008). Psychotherapy for depression in adults: A meta-analysis of comparative outcome studies. *Journal of Consulting and Clinical Psychology, 76,* 909–922.

Davidson, J. R. T., Foa, E. B., Huppert, J. D., Keefe, F. J., Franklin, M. E., Compton, J. S., . . . Gadde, K. M. (2004). Fluoxetine, comprehensive cognitive behavioral therapy, and placebo in generalized social phobia. *Archives of General Psychiatry, 61,* 1005–1013.

Davis, M. (2011). NMDA receptors and fear extinction: implications for cognitive behavioral therapy. *Dialogues Clinical Neuroscience, 13*(4), 463–474.

Davis, M., & Myers, K. M. (2002). The role of glutamate and gamma-aminobutyric acid in fear extinction: Clinical implications for exposure therapy. *Biological Psychiatry, 52,* 998–1007.

Deacon, B. J., & Abramowitz, J. S. (2004). Cognitive and behavioral treatments for anxiety disorders: A review of meta-analytic findings. *Journal of Clinical Psychology, 60,* 429–441.

Deacon, B. J., & Abramowitz, J. S. (2005). Patients' perceptions of pharmacological and cognitive-behavioral treatments for anxiety disorders. *Behavior Therapy, 36,* 139–145.

Deckersbach, T., Hölzel, B. K., Eisner, L. R., Stange, J. P., Peckham, A. D., . . . Nierenberg, A. A. (2012). Mindfulness-based cognitive therapy for nonremitted patients with bipolar disorder. *CNS Neuroscience and Therapeutics, 18,* 133–141.

de Maat, S. M., Dekker, J., Schoevers, R. A., & de Jonghe, F. (2007). Relative efficacy of psychotherapy and combined therapy in the treatment of depression: A meta-analysis. *European Psychiatry, 22,* 1–8.

de Quervain, D. J-F., Bentz, D., Michael, T., Bolt, O. C., Wiederhold, B. K., Margraf, J., & Wilhelm, F. H. (2011). Glucocorticoids enhance extinction-based psychotherapy. *Proceedings of the National Academy of Science USA, 108,* 6621–6625.

DeRubeis, R. J., Gelfand, L. A., Tang, T. Z., & Simons, A. D. (1999). Medications versus cognitive behavior therapy for severely depressed outpatients: Mega-analysis of four randomized comparisons. *American Journal of Psychiatry, 156,* 1007–1013.

Dobson, K. S., Hollon, S. D., Dimidjian, S., Schmaling, K. B., Kohlenberg, R. J., Gallop, R. J., . . . Jacobson, N. S. (2008). Randomized trial of behavioral activation, cognitive therapy, and antidepressant medication in the prevention of relapse and recurrence in major depression. *Journal of Consulting and Clinical Psychology, 76,* 468–477.

D'Souza, D. C., Gil, R., Cassello, K., Morrissey, K., Abi-Saab, D., White, J., . . . Krystal, J. H. (2000). IV glycine and oral D-cycloserine effects on plasma and CSF amino acids in healthy humans. *Biological Psychiatry, 47,* 450–462.

Emilsson, B., Gudjonsson, G., Sigurdsson, J. F., Baldursson, G., Einarsson, E., Olafsdottir, H., & Young, S. (2011). Cognitive behaviour therapy in medication-treated adults with ADHD and persistent symptoms: A randomized controlled trial. *BMC Psychiatry, 11,* 116.

Evans, M. D., Hollon, S. D., DeRubeis, R. J., Piasecki, J. M., Grove, W. M., Garvey, M. J., & Tuason, V. B. (1992). Differential relapse following cognitive therapy and pharmacotherapy for depression. *Archives of General Psychiatry, 49,* 802–808.

Foa, E. B, Franklin, M. E., & Moser, J. (2002). Context in the clinic: How well do cognitive-behavioral therapies and medications work in combination? *Biological Psychiatry, 10,* 987–997.

Foa, E. B., & Kozak, M. J. (1986). Emotional processing of fear: Exposure to corrective information. *Psychological Bulletin, 99,* 20–35.

Foa, E. B., Liebowitz, M. R., Kozak, M. J., Davies, S., Campeas, R., Franklin, M. E., . . . Tu, X. (2005). Randomized, placebo-controlled trial of exposure and ritual prevention, clomipramine, and their combination in the treatment of obsessive-compulsive disorder. *American Journal of Psychiatry, 162,* 151–161.

Franklin, M. E., Abramowitz, J. S., Bux, D. A., Zoellner, L. A., & Feeny N. C. (2002). Cognitive-behavioral therapy with and without medication in the treatment of obsessive-compulsive disorder. *Professional Psychology: Research and Practice, 33,* 162–168.

Furukawa, T. A., Watanabe, N., & Churchill, R. (2006). Psychotherapy plus antidepressant for panic disorder with or without agoraphobia: Systematic review. *British Journal of Psychiatry, 188,* 305–312.

Furukawa, T. A., Watanabe, N., & Churchill, R. (2007). Combined psychotherapy plus antidepressants for panic disorder with or without agoraphobia. *Cochrane Database of Systematic Reviews,* CD004364.

Furukawa, T. A., Watanabe, N., Omori, I. M., & Churchill, R. (2007). Can pill placebo augment cognitive-behavior therapy for panic disorder? *BMC Psychiatry, 7,* 73.

Goisman, R. M., Warshaw, M. G., & Keller, M. B. (1999). Psychosocial treatment prescriptions for generalized anxiety disorder, panic disorder, and social phobia, 1991-1996. *American Journal of Psychiatry, 156,* 1819–1821.

Gould, R. A., Buckminster, S., Pollack, M. H., Otto, M. W., & Yap, L. (1997). Cognitive-behavioral and pharmacological treatment for social phobia: A meta-analysis. *Clinical Psychology: Science and Practice, 4,* 291–306.

Gould, R. A., Mueser, K. T., Bolton, E., Mays, V., & Goff, D. (2001). Cognitive therapy for psychosis in schizophrenia: An effect size analysis. *Schizophrenia Research, 48*(2–3), 335–342.

Gould, R. A., Otto, M. W., Pollack, M. P., & Yap, L. (1997). Cognitive-behavioral and pharmacological treatment of generalized anxiety disorder: A preliminary meta-analysis. *Behavior Therapy, 28,* 285–305.

Guidi, J., Fava, G. A., Fava, M., & Papakostas, G. I. (2011). Efficacy of the sequential integration of psychotherapy and pharmacotherapy in major depressive disorder: A preliminary meta-analysis. *Psychological Medicine, 41,* 321–331.

Haby, M. M., Tonge, B., Littlefield, L., Carter, R., & Vos, T. (2004). Cost-effectiveness of cognitive behavioural therapy and selective serotonin reuptake inhibitors for major depression in children and adolescents. *Australia and New Zealand Journal of Psychiatry, 38,* 579–591.

Hartley, C. A., McKenna, M. C., Salman, R., Holmes, A., Casey, B. J., Phelps, E. A., & Glatt, C. E. (2012). Serotonin transporter polyadenylation polymorphism modulates the retention of fear extinction memory. *Proceedings of the National Academy of Sciences USA, 109*(14), 5493–5498.

Heffelfinger, A. K., & Newcomer, J. W. (2001). Glucocorticoid effects on memory function over the human life span. *Developmental Psychopathology, 13,* 491–513.

Heuzenroeder, L., Donnelly, M., Haby, M. M., Mihalopoulos, C., Rossell, R., Carter, R., . . . Vos, T. (2004). Cost-effectiveness of psychological and pharmacological interventions for generalized anxiety disorder and panic disorder. *Australian and New Zealand Journal of Psychiatry, 38,* 602–612.

Hidalgo, R. B., Barnett, S. D., & Davidson, S. D. (2001). Social anxiety disorder: Two decades of progress. *International Journal of Neuropsychopharmacology, 4,* 279–298.

Hofmann, S. G., Pollack, M. H., & Otto, M. W. (2006). Augmentation treatment of psychotherapy for anxiety disorders with D-cycloserine. *CNS Drug Reviews, 12,* 208–217.

Hofmann, S. G., Sawyer, A. T., Korte, K. J., Smits, J. A. (2009). Is it beneficial to add pharmacotherapy to cognitive-behavioral therapy when treating anxiety disorders? A meta-analytic review. *International Journal of Cognitive Therapy, 2,* 160–175.

Hofmann, S. G., & Smits, J. A. (2008). Cognitive-behavioral therapy for adult anxiety disorders: A meta-analysis of randomized placebo-controlled trials. *Journal of Clinical Psychiatry, 69*(4), 621–632.

Hofmann, S. G., Smits, J. A., Asnaani, A., Gutner, C. A., & Otto, M. W. (2011). Cognitive enhancers for anxiety disorders. *Pharmacology, Biochemistry, and Behavior, 99,* 275–284.

Hohagen, F., Winkelmann, G., Rasche-Ruchle, H., Hand, I., Konig, A., Münchau, N., . . . Berger, M. (1998). Combination of behavior therapy with fluvoxamine in comparison with behaviour therapy and placebo. Results of a multicenter study. *British Journal of Psychiatry, 35,* 71–78.

Hollon, S. D., DeRubeis, R. J., Shelton, R. C., Amsterdam, J. D., Salomon, R. M., O'Reardon, J. P., . . . Gallop, R. (2005). Prevention of relapse following cognitive therapy vs medications in moderate to severe depression. *Archives of General Psychiatry, 62,* 417–422.

Hunkeler, E. M., Meresman, J. F., Hagreaves, W. A., Fireman, B., Berman, W. H., Kirsch, A. J., . . . Salzer, M. (2000). Efficacy of nurse telehealth care and peer support in augmenting treatment of depression in primary care. *Archives of Family Medicine, 9,* 700–708.

Jauhar, S., McKenna, P. J., Radua, J., Fung, E., Salvador, R., & Laws, K. R. (2014). Cognitive-behavioural therapy for the symptoms of schizophrenia: Systematic review and meta-analysis with examination of potential bias. *British Journal of Psychiatry, 204*(1), 20–29.

Jones, S. (2004). Psychotherapy of bipolar disorder: a review. *Journal of Affective Disorders, 80,* 101–114.

Kaltenthaler, E., Sutcliffe, P., Perry, G., Beverley, C., Rees, A., & Ferriter, M. (2008). The acceptability to patients of computerized cognitive behavior therapy for depression: A systematic review. *Psychological Medicine, 38,* 1521–1530.

Keller, M. B., Trivedi, M. H., Thase, M. E., Shelton, R. C., Kornstein, S. G., Nemeroff, C. B., . . . Ninan, P. T. (2007). The Prevention of Recurrent Episodes of depression with Venlafaxine for Two Years (PREVENT) Study: Outcomes from the 2-year and combined maintenance phases. *Journal of Clinical Psychiatry, 68,* 1246–1256.

Lam, D. H., Hayward, P., Watkins, E. R., Wright, K., & Sham, P. (2005). Relapse prevention in patients with bipolar disorder: Cognitive therapy outcome after 2 years. *American Journal of Psychiatry, 162,* 324–329.

Lam, D. H., Watkins, E. R., Hayward, P., Bright, J., Wright, K., Kerr, N., . . . Sham, P. (2003). A randomized controlled study of cognitive therapy of relapse prevention for bipolar affective disorder: Outcome of the first year. *Archives of General Psychiatry, 60,* 145–152.

Ludman, E. J., Simon, G. E., Tutty, S., & Von Korff, M. (2007). A randomized trial of telephone psychotherapy and pharmacotherapy for depression: Continuation and durability of effects. *Journal of Consulting and Clinical Psychology, 75,* 257–266.

Lupien, S. J., Maheu, F., Tu, M., Fiocco, A., & Schramek, T. E. (2007). The effects of stress and stress hormones on human cognition: Implications for the field of brain and cognition. *Brain and Cognition, 65*(3), 209–37.

Lynch, F. L., Dickerson, J. F., Clarke, G., Vitiello, B., Porta, G., Wagner, K. D., . . . Brent, D. (2011). Incremental cost-effectiveness of combined therapy vs medication only for youth with selective serotonin reuptake inhibitor-resistant depression: Treatment of SSRI-resistant depression in adolescents trial findings. *Archives of General Psychiatry, 68*(3), 253–262.

Marks, I. M., Swinson, R. P., Basaglu, M., Kuch, K., Nasirvani, H., O'Sullivan, G., ... Sengun, S. (1993). Alprazolam and exposure alone and combined in panic disorder with agoraphobia: A controlled study in London and Toronto. *British Journal of Psychiatry, 162*, 776–787.

Mavissakalian, M., & Perel, J. M. (1999). Long term maintenance and discontinuation of imipramine therapy in panic disorder with agoraphobia. *Archives General Psychiatry, 56*, 821–827.

McHugh, R. K., Otto, M. W., Barlow, D. H., Gorman, J. M., Shear, M. K., & Woods, S. W. (2007). Cost-efficacy of individual and combined treatments for panic disorder. *Journal of Clinical Psychiatry, 68*(7), 1038–1044.

McHugh, R. K., Whitton, S. W., Peckham, A. D., Welge, J. A., & Otto, M. W. (2013). Patient preference for psychological vs pharmacologic treatment of psychiatric disorders: A meta-analytic review. *Journal of Clinical Psychiatry, 74*(6), 595–602.

Miklowitz, D. J., Otto, M. W., Frank, E., Reilly-Harrington, N. A., Kogan, J. N., Sachs, G. S., ... Wisniewski, S. R. (2007). Intensive psychosocial intervention enhances functioning in patients with bipolar depression: Results from a 9-month randomized controlled trial. *American Journal of Psychiatry, 164*, 1340–1347.

Mystkowski, J. L., Mineka, S., Vernon, L. L., & Zinbarg, R. E. (2003). Changes in caffeine states enhance return of fear in spider phobia. *Journal of Consulting and Clinical Psychology, 71*, 243–250.

Nations, K. R., Smits, J. A. J., Tolin, D. F., Rothbaum, B. O., Hofmann, S. G., Tart, C. D., ... Otto, M. W. (2012). Evaluation of the glycine transporter inhibitor ORG 25935 as augmentation to cognitive-behavioral therapy for panic disorder. *Journal of Clinical Psychiatry, 73*, 647–653.

Newcomer, J. W., Selke, G., Melson, A. K., Hershey, T., Craft, S., Richards, K., & Alderson, A. L. (1999). Decreased memory performance in healthy humans induced by stress-levelcortisol treatment. *Archives of General Psychiatry, 56*, 527–533.

Norberg, M. M., Krystal, J. H., & Tolin, D. F. (2008). A meta-analysis of D-cycloserine and the facilitation of fear extinction and exposure therapy. *Biological Psychiatry, 63*(12), 1118–1126.

Oslin, D. W., Sayers, S., Ross, J., Kane, V., Ten Have, T., Conigliaro, J., & Cornelius, J. (2003). Disease management for depression and at-risk drinking telephone in an older population of veterans. *Psychosomatic Medicine, 65*, 931–937.

Otto, M. W., Bruce, S. E., & Deckersbach, T. (2005). Benzodiazepine use, cognitive impairment, and cognitive-behavioral therapy for anxiety disorders: Issues in the treatment of a patient in need. *Journal of Clinical Psychiatry, 66*, 34–38.

Otto, M. W., McHugh, R. K., & Kantak, K. M. (2010). Combined pharmacotherapy and cognitive-behavioral therapy for anxiety disorders: Medication effects, glucocorticoids, and attenuated treatment outcomes. *Clinical Psychology Science and Practice*, 91–103.

Otto, M. W., McHugh, R. K., Simon, N. M., Farach, F. J., Worthington, J. J., & Pollack, M. H. (2010). Efficacy of CBT for benzodiazepine discontinuation in patients with panic disorder: Further evaluation. *Behaviour Research and Therapy, 48*, 720–727.

Otto, M. W., Pollack, M. H., & Maki, K. M. (2000). Empirically-supported treatment for panic disorder: Costs, benefits, and stepped care. *Journal of Consulting and Clinical Psychology, 68*, 556–563.

Otto, M. W., Smits, J. A. J., & Reese, H. E. (2005). Combined psychotherapy and pharmacotherapy for mood and anxiety disorders in adults: Review and analysis. *Clinical Psychology: Science and Practice, 12*, 72–86.

Perry, A., Tarrier, N., Morriss, R., McCarthy, E., & Limb, K. (1999). Randomized controlled trial of efficacy of teaching patients with bipolar disorder to identify early symptoms of relapse and obtain treatment. *British Medical Journal, 16*, 149–153.

Pollack, M. H. (2005). The pharmacotherapy of panic disorder. *Journal of Clinical Psychiatry, 66*(Suppl. 4), 23–27.

Powers, M. B., Smits, J. A. J., Otto, M. W., Sanders, C., & Emmelkamp, P. M. (2009). Facilitation of fear extinction in phobic participants with a novel cognitive enhancer: A randomized placebo controlled trial of yohimbine augmentation. *Journal of Anxiety Disorders, 23*, 350–356.

Powers, M. B., Smits, J. A. J., Whitley, D., Bystritsky, A., & Telch, M. J. (2008). The effect of attributional processes concerning medication taking on return of fear. *Journal of Consulting and Clinical Psychology, 76*, 478–790.

Proudfoot, J., Goldberg, D., Mann, A., Everitt, B., Marks, I., & Gray, J. A. (2003). Computerized, interactive, multimedia cognitive-behavioral program for anxiety and depression in general practice. *Psychological Medicine, 33*, 217–227.

Putnam, P., Van Honk, J., Kessels, R. P., Mulder, M., & Koppeschaar, H. P. (2004). Salivary cortisol and short and long-term memory for emotional faces in healthy young women. *Psychoneuroendocrinology, 29*, 953–960.

Reynolds, C. F., 3rd, Dew, M. A., Pollock, B. G., Mulsant, B. H., Frank, E., Miller, M. D., ... Kupfer, D. J. (2006). Maintenance treatment of major depression in old age. *New England Journal of Medicine, 354*, 1130–1138.

Richardson, R., Ledgerwood, L., & Cranney, J. (2004). Facilitation of fear extinction by D-cycloserine: Theoretical and clinical implications. *Learning and Memory, 11*, 510–516.

Rocha, F. L., Fuzikawa, C., Riera, R., & Hara, C. (2012). Combination of antidepressants in the treatment of major depressive disorder: A systematic review and meta-analysis. *Journal of Clinical Psychopharmacology, 32*, 278–281.

Roshanaei-Moghaddam, B., Pauly, M. C., Atkins, D. C., Baldwin, S. A., Stein, M. B., & Roy-Byrne, P. (2011). Relative effects of CBT and pharmacotherapy in depression versus anxiety: Is medication somewhat better for depression and CBT somewhat better for anxiety? *Depression and Anxiety, 28*, 560–570.

Roy-Byrne, P., Craske, M. G., Sullivan, G., Rose, R. D., Edlund, M. J., Lang, A. J., ... Stein, M. B. (2010). Delivery of evidence-based treatment for multiple anxiety disorders in primary care: A randomized controlled trial. *Journal of the American Medical Association, 303*, 1921–1928.

Sachs, G. S., Nierenberg, A. A., Calabrese, J. R., Marangell, L. B., Wisniewski, S. R., Gyulai, L., ... Thase, M. E. (2007). Effectiveness of adjunctive antidepressant treatment for bipolar depression. *New England Journal of Medicine, 356*, 1711–1722.

Safren, S. A., Otto, M. W., Sprich, S., Perlman, C. L., Wilens, T. E., & Biederman, J. (2005). Cognitive behavioral therapy for

ADHD in medication-treated adults with continued symptoms. *Behaviour Research and Therapy*, *43*, 831–842.

Safren S. A., Sprich, S., Mimiaga, M. J., Surman, C., Knouse, L., Groves, M., & Otto, M. W. (2010). Cognitive behavioral therapy vs. relaxation with educational support for medication-treated adults with ADHD and persistent symptoms: A randomized controlled trial. *JAMA*, *304*, 875–880.

Scott, J., Garland, A., & Moorhead, S. (2001). A pilot study of cognitive therapy in bipolar disorders. *Psychological Medicine*, *31*, 459–467.

Simon, G. E., Ludman, E. J., Tutty, S., Operskalaski, B., & Von Korff, M. (2004). Telephone psychotherapy and telephone care management for primary care patients starting antidepressant treatment: A randomized controlled trial. *Journal of the American Medical Association*, *292*, 935–942.

Simpson, H. B., Foa, E. B., Liebowitz, M. R., Ledley, D. R., Huppert, J. D., Cahill, S., . . . Campeas, R. (2008). A randomized, controlled trial of cognitive-behavioral therapy for augmenting pharmacotherapy in obsessive-compulsive disorder. *American Journal of Psychiatry*, *165*, 621–630.

Sinyor, M., Schaffer, A., & Levitt, A. (2010). The sequenced treatment alternatives to relieve depression (STAR*D) trial: A review. *Canadian Journal of Psychiatry*, *55*, 126–135.

Smits, J. A., Rosenfield, D., Otto, M. W., Powers, M. B., Hofmann, S. G., Telch, M. J., & Tart, C. D. (2013a). D-cycloserine enhancement of fear extinction is specific to successful exposure sessions: Evidence from the treatment of height phobia. *Biological Psychiatry*, *73*, 1054–1058.

Smits, J. A., Rosenfield, D., Otto, M. W., Marques, L., Davis, M. L., Meuret, A. E., . . . Hofmann, S. G. (2013b). D-cycloserine enhancement of exposure therapy for social anxiety disorder depends on the success of exposure sessions. *Journal of Psychiatry Research*, *47*, 1455–1461.

Soravia, L. M., Heinrichs, M., Aerni, A., Maroni, C., Schelling, G., Ehlert, U. . . . de Quervain, D. J. (2006). Glucocorticoids reduce phobic fear in humans. *Proceedings of the National Academy of Sciences USA*, *103*, 5585–5590.

Spijker, J., van Straten, A., Bockting, C. L., Meeuwissen, J. A., & van Balkom, A. J. (2013). Psychotherapy, antidepressants, and their combination for chronic major depressive disorder: A systematic review. *Canadian Journal of Psychiatry*, *58*, 386–392.

Stange, J. P., Eisner, L. R., Hölzel, B. K., Peckham, A. D., Dougherty, D. D., Rauch, S. L., . . . Deckersbach, T. (2011). Mindfulness-based cognitive therapy for bipolar disorder: Effects on cognitive functioning. *Journal of Psychiatric Practice*, *17*, 410–419.

Stein, D. J., Versiani, M., Hair, T., & Kumar, R. (2002). Efficacy of paroxetine for relapse prevention in social anxiety disorder: A 24-week study. *Archives of General Psychiatry*, *59*, 1111–1118.

Stein, M. B., Sherbourne, C. D., Craske, M. G., Means-Christensen, A., Bystritsky, A., . . . Roy-Byrne, P. P. (2004). Quality of care for primary care patients with anxiety disorders. *American Journal of Psychiatry*, *161*, 2230–2237.

Stuart, G. L., Treat, T. A., & Wade, W. A. (2000). Effectiveness of an empirically based treatment for panic disorder delivered in a service clinic setting: 1-year follow-up. *Journal of Consulting and Clinical Psychology*, *68*, 506–512.

Telch, M. J., Agras, W. S., Taylor, C. B., Roth, W. T., & Gallen, C. (1985). Combined pharmacological and behavioral treatment for agoraphobia. *Behaviour Research and Therapy*, *23*, 325–335.

Thase, M. E., Friedman, E. S., Biggs, M. M., Wisniewski, S. R., Trivedi, M. H., Luther, J. F., . . . Rush, A. J. (2007). Cognitive therapy versus medication in augmentation and switch strategies as second-step treatments: A STAR*D report. *American Journal of Psychiatry*, *164*, 739–752.

Vocks, S., Tuschen-Caffier, B., Pietrowsky, R., Rustenbach, S. J., Kersting, A., & Herpertz, S. (2010). Meta-analysis of the effectiveness of psychological and pharmacological treatments for binge eating disorder. *International Journal of Eating Disorders*, *43*, 205–217.

Walker, J. R., Van Ameringen, M. A., Swinson, R., Bowen, R. C., Chokka, P. R., Goldner, E., . . . Lane, R. M. (2000). Prevention of relapse in generalized social phobia: Results of a 24-week study in responders to 20 weeks of sertraline treatment. *Journal of Clinical Psychopharmacology*, *20*, 636–644.

Watanabe, N., Churchill, R., & Furukawa, T. A. (2007). Combination of psychotherapy and benzodiazepine versus either therapy alone for panic disorder: A systematic review. *BMC Psychiatry*, *7*, 70.

Weiss, M., Murray, C., Wasdell, M., Greenfield, B., Giles, L., & Hechtman, L. (2012). A randomized controlled trial of CBT therapy for adults with ADHD with and without medication. *BMC Psychiatry*, *12*, 30.

Wisniewski, S. R., Fava, M., Trivedi, M. H., Thase, M. E., Warden, D., Niederehe, G., . . . Rush, A. J. (2007). Acceptability of second-step treatments to depressed outpatients: A STAR*D report. *American Journal of Psychiatry*, *164*, 753–760.

Yang, C. H., Shi, H. S., Zhu, W. L., Wu, P., Sun, L. L., Si, J. J., & Yang, J. L. (2012). Venlafaxine facilitates between-session extinction and prevents reinstatement of auditory-cue conditioned fear. *Behavioural Brain Research*, *230*, 268–273.

Zaretsky, A., Lancee, W., Miller, C., Harris, A., & Parikh, S. V. (2008). Is cognitive-behavioral therapy more effective than psychoeducation in bipolar disorder? *Canadian Journal of Psychiatry*, *53*, 441–448.

INDEX

Note: Tables, figures, and notes are indicated by *t*, *f*, and *n*.